The Causes of Epilepsy

The Causes of Epilepsy

Common and Uncommon Causes in Adults and Children

Edited by:

Simon D. Shorvon MA MD FRCP
Professor in Clinical Neurology, UCL Institute of Neurology, University College London;

Consultant Neurologist, National Hospital for Neurology and Neurosurgery, London, UK

Frederick Andermann OC MD FRCPC
Professor, Departments of Neurology and Neurosurgery and Pediatrics, McGill University;

Director, Epilepsy Service, Montreal Neurological Institute and Hospital, Montreal, Quebec, Canada

Renzo Guerrini MD
Professor of Child Neurology and Psychiatry, University of Florence;

Director, Pediatric Neurology Unit and Laboratories, Children's Hospital A. Meyer, Florence, Italy

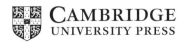

CAMBRIDGE
UNIVERSITY PRESS

CAMBRIDGE UNIVERSITY PRESS
Cambridge, New York, Melbourne, Madrid, Cape Town, Singapore,
São Paulo, Delhi, Dubai, Tokyo, Mexico City

Cambridge University Press
The Edinburgh Building, Cambridge CB2 8RU, UK

Published in the United States of America by
Cambridge University Press, New York

www.cambridge.org
Information on this title: www.cambridge.org/9780521114479

First published 2011

Printed in the United Kingdom at the University Press, Cambridge

*A catalogue record for this publication is available from the British
Library*

Library of Congress Cataloging-in-Publication Data
The causes of epilepsy / edited by Simon D. Shorvon, Frederick
Andermann, Renzo Guerrini.
     p. ; cm.
   Includes bibliographical references.
   ISBN 978-0-521-11447-9 (Hardback)
   1. Epilepsy–Etiology.   I. Shorvon, S. D. (Simon D.)
II. Andermann, Frederick.   III. Guerrini, Renzo.
   [DNLM: 1. Epilepsy–etiology.   2. Epilepsy–diagnosis.
3. Epilepsy–therapy.   WL 385]
   RC372.C38 2011
   616.8′53071–dc22
                                                      2010030379
ISBN 978-0-521-114479 Hardback

Contents

Contributors

Jane E. Adcock
Department of Clinical Neurology,
University of Oxford,
John Radcliffe Hospital,
Oxford, UK

Yahya Aghakhani
Section of Neurology,
Department of Internal Medicine,
University of Manitoba,
Winnipeg, Alberta, Canada

A. Anand
Molecular Biology and Genetics Unit,
Jawaharlal Nehru Center for Advanced Sciences (JNCASR),
Bangalore, India

Eva Andermann
Neurogenetics Unit,
Montreal Neurological Institute and Hospital;
Departments of Neurology and Neurosurgery and Human Genetics,
McGill University,
Montreal, Québec, Canada

Frederick Andermann
Departments of Neurology, Neurosurgery and Pediatrics,
McGill University;
Epilepsy Service,
Montreal Neurological Institute and Hospital,
Montreal, Québec, Canada

Alexis Arzimanoglou
Institute for Children and Adolescents with Epilepsy IDEE,
Department of Epilepsy,
Sleep and Pediatric Neurophysiology,
University Hospitals of Lyon (HCL) and Hôpital
Femme Mère Enfant, Lyon, France

Sandrine Aubert
Service de Neurophysiologie Clinique,
Hôpital de la Timone,
APHM, Marseille, France

Nadia Bahi-Buisson
Department of Pediatric Neurology and Neurophysiology,
Hôpital Necker Enfants Malades,
Université Paris Descartes, Paris, France

Carman Barba
Pediatric Neurology Unit,
Anna Meyer Children's Hospital,
University of Florence, Italy

Agatino Battaglia
Department of Child Neuropsychiatry,
University of Pisa,
Stella Maris Clinical Research Institute, Italy
Division of Medical Genetics,
Department of Pediatrics,
University of Utah School of Medicine,
Salt Lake City, UT, USA

Geneviève Bernard
Pediatric Neurologist and Fellow in Neurogenetics,
CHUM and Saint-Justine's Hospital,
Montreal, Québec, Canada

Nadir E. Bharucha
Departments of Neurology and Neuroepidemiology,
Bombay Hospital Institute of Medical Science,
Mumbai, India

Laurence A. Bindoff
Department of Neurology,
Haukeland University Hospital,
Bergen; Department of Clinical Medicine,
University of Bergen, Norway

William Bingaman
Department of Neurosurgery,
Cleveland Clinic Foundation,
Cleveland, OH, USA

Francesca Bisulli
Department of Neurological Sciences,
University of Bologna, Italy

Thomas P. Bleck
Department of Neurological Sciences,
Neurosurgery, Medicine, and Anesthesiology,
Rush Medical College,
Chicago, IL, USA

Stewart G. Boyd
Department of Clinical Neurophysiology,
Great Ormond Street Hospital for Children,
London, UK

Andreas Brunklaus
Fraser of Allander Neurosciences Unit,
Royal Hospital for Sick Children,
Glasgow, UK

Harry Bulstrode
Division of Clinical Neurosciences,
Faculty of Medicine and Health and Life Sciences,
University of Southampton, UK

Jorge G. Burneo
Department of Neurology,
University of Western Ontario Epilepsy Programme,
London, Ontario, Canada

Laura Canafoglia
Unit of Neurophysiopathology,
Epilepsy Center, IRCCS Foundation C. Besta
Neurological Institute, Milan, Italy

Laura Cantonetti
Bambino Gesu, Santa Marinella, Rome, Italy

Roberto H. Caraballo
Department of Neurology,
Hospital Nacional de Pediatria
"Prof. Dr. Juan P. Garrhan," Buenos Aires,
Argentina

Fernando Cendes
Department of Neurology,
University of Campinas – UNICAMP,
Campinas, SP, Brazil

Kevin E. Chapman
Pediatric Epilepsy, Barrow Neurological Institute,
St. Joseph's Hospital and Medical Center,
Phoenix, AZ, USA

Patrick Chauvel
Laboratoire de Neurophysiologie et Neuropsychologie,
INSERM, Marseille, France

Richard F. M. Chin
Neuroscience Unit,
UCL Institute of Child Health, London;

National Centre for Young People with Epilepsy,
Lingfield, Surrey, UK

H. T. Chong
Division of Neurology,
Faculty of Medicine,
University of Malaya,
Kuala Lumpur, Malaysia

Fahmida A. Chowdhury
King's College Hospital,
London, UK

Catherine J. Chu-Shore
Instructer in Neurology,
Harvard Medical School,
Department of Neurology,
Programs in Pediatric Epilepsy and Neurophysiology,
Massachusetts General Hospital.

Rolando Cimaz Rheumatology Unit,
Department of Pediatrics,
Anna Meyer Children's Hospital,
University of Florence, Italy

Andrew J. Cole
The MGH Epilepsy Service,
Massachusetts General Hospital,
Boston, MA, USA

Bernard Dan
Department of Neurology,
Hôpital Universitaire des Enfants Reine Fabiola,
Brussels, Belgium

The Late Geoffrey Dean
Medical Research Board,
The Health Research Board,
Dublin, Ireland

Alessio De Ciantis
Department of Neuroscience,
Anna Meyer Children's Hospital,
University of Florence, Italy

Fernando De Paolis
Sleep Disorders Center, Department of Neurosciences,
University of Parma, Italy

Rolando F. Del Maestro
Brain Tumor Research Centre,
Department of Neurology and Neurosurgery,
Montreal Neurological Institute and Hospital,
McGill University,
Montreal, Québec, Canada

Irissa M. Devine
Division of Pediatric Neurology,
Department of Neurology,
University of Wisconsin,
Madison, WI, USA

Carlo Di Bonaventura
Epilepsy Unit, Department of Neurological Sciences,
"La Sapienza" University of Rome, Italy

Concezio Di Rocco
Institute of Neurosurgery,
Catholic University Medical School,
Rome, Italy

Henry B. Dinsdale
Queen's University,
Kingston, Ontario, Canada

Maria Alice Donati
Pediatric Neurology and Metabolic and Neuromuscular
Disorders Units, Neuroscience Department,
Anna Meyer Children's Hospital,
University of Florence, Italy

François Dubeau
Department of Neurology and Neurosurgery,
Montreal Neurological Hospital and Institute,
McGill University,
Montreal, Québec, Canada

Michael Duchowny
Comprehensive Epilepsy Program and the Brain Institute,
Miami Children's Hospital,
Miami, FL, USA

Olivier Dulac
Department of Pediatric Neurology and Neurophysiology,
Hôpital Necker Enfants Malades,
Université Paris Descartes, Paris, France

Monika Eisermann
Department of Pediatric Neurology and Neurophysiology,
Hôpital Necker Enfants Malades,
Université Paris Descartes,
Paris, France

Brent Elliott
Department of Neuropsychiatry,
National Hospital for Neurology and Neurosurgery,
London, UK

Bernt A. Engelsen
Department of Neurology,
Haukeland University Hospital,
Bergen; Department of Clinical Medicine,
University of Bergen, Norway

Kevin Farrell
Division of Neurology, Department of Pediatrics,
University of British Columbia and British Columbia's
Children's Hospital,
Vancouver, Canada

Natalio Fejerman
Department of Neurology,
Hospital Nacional de Pediatria
"Prof. Dr. Juan P. Garrhan," Buenos Aires,
Argentina

Rosalie E. Ferner
Guy's and St. Thomas' NHS Foundation Trust,
London, UK

Silvana Franceschetti
Unit of Neurophysiopathology, Epilepsy Center,
IRCCS Foundation C. Besta Neurological Institute,
Milan, Italy

Robert M. Friedlander
Department of Neurosurgery,
Brigham and Women's Hospital,
Boston, MA, USA

Antonio Gambardella
Institute of Neurology, University Magna Graecia,
Catanzaro, Italy

Hector H. Garcia
Cysticercosis Unit, Department of Microbiology,
School of Sciences,
Universidad Peruana Cayetano Heredia,
Lima, Peru

Serena Gasperini
Pediatric Neurology and Metabolic and Neuromuscular
Disorders Units, Neuroscience Department,
Anna Meyer Children's Hospital,
University of Florence, Italy

Lorenzo Genitori
Department of Neurosurgery,
Anna Meyer Children's Hospital,
University of Florence, Italy

Gioia Gioi
Sleep Disorders Center,
Department of Neurology,
Policlinico Monserrato,
Cagliari, Italy

Flavio Giordano
Department of Neurosurgery,
Anna Meyer Children's Hospital,
University of Florence, Italy

Leif Gjerstad
Department of Neurology, Division of Clinical Neuroscience, Rikshospitalet University Hospital, Oslo, Norway

Daniel G. Glaze
Departments of Pediatrics and Neurology, Baylor College of Medicine and Blue Bird Circle Rett Center, Texas Children's Hospital, Houston, TX, USA

Howard P. Goodkin
Department of Neurology, University of Virginia, Charlottesville, VA, USA

Sidney M. Gospe, Jr.
Division of Pediatric Neurology, University of Washington and Seattle Children's Hospital, Seattle, WA, USA

Andrea Grassi
Sleep Disorders Center, Department of Neurosciences, University of Parma, Italy

William P. Gray
Department of Neurosurgery, University of Southampton, UK

Renzo Guerrini
Department of Child Neurology and Psychiatry, University of Florence Pediatric Neurology Unit and Laboratories, Anna Meyer Children's Hospital, University of Florence, Italy

Marie-Christine Guiot
Department of Neuropathology, Montreal Neurological Institute and Hospital, McGill University, Montreal, Québec, Canada

William Harkness
Department of Neurosurgery, Great Ormond Street Hospital, London, UK

Andrew G. Herzog
Department of Neurology, Harvard Medical School, and Neuroendocrine Unit, Beth Israel Deaconess Medical Center, Boston, MA, USA

Linda Huh
Division of Neurology, Department of Pediatrics, University of British Columbia and British Columbia's Children's Hospital, Vancouver, Canada

Margaret J. Jackson
Department of Neurology, Newcastle-upon-Tyne Hospitals Trust, Newcastle-upon-Tyne, UK

Thomas S. Jacques
Neural Development Unit, UCL Institute of Child Health and Department of Histopathology, Great Ormond Street Hospital, London, UK

Anna C. Jansen
Department of Pediatric Neurology, UZ Brussel, Brussels, Belgium

Sigmund Jenssen
Department of Neurology, Hahnemann University Hospital, Philadelphia, PA, USA

Michael R. Johnson
Division of Neuroscience, Imperial College London, UK

Dorothy Jones-Davis
Department of Neurology, University of California, San Francisco, CA, USA

Reetta Kälviäinen
Kuopio Epilepsy Center, Department of Neurology, Kuopio University Hospital, Kuopio, Finland

Peter W. Kaplan
Department of Neurology, Johns Hopkins University School of Medicine, Baltimore, MD, USA

John F. Kerrigan
Department of Clinical Pediatrics and Neurology, University of Arizona College of Medicine, Phoenix; Pediatric Epilepsy Program and Hypothalamic Hamartoma Program, Barrow Neurological Institute, Phoenix, AZ, USA

Autumn Marie Klein
Department of Neurosurgery, Brigham and Women's Hospital, Boston, MA, USA

Matthias Koepp
Department of Clinical and Experimental Epilepsy, UCL Institute of Neurology, London, UK

Edwin H. Kolodny
Department of Neurology, New York University School of Medicine, New York, NY, USA

Kandan Kulandaivel
Department of Neurology,
Hahnemann Hospital,
Drexel University College of Medicine,
Philadelphia, PA, USA

Ruben I. Kuzniecky
NYU Epilepsy Center,
Department of Neurology,
NYU School of Medicine,
New York, NY, USA

Ahmed Lary
Department of Neurosurgery,
Neurosciences Center,
King Fahd Medical City,
Riyadh, Saudi Arabia

Yolanda Lau
Department of Neurology,
University of California,
San Francisco, CA, USA

Anna-Elina Lehesjoki
Folkhälsan Institute of Genetics,
Department of Medical Genetics
and Neuroscience Center,
Biomedicum Helsinki,
University of Helsinki, Finland

Maria K. Lehtinen
Howard Hughes Medical Institute,
Beth Israel Deaconess Medical Center,
Harvard Medical School,
Boston, MA, USA

Holger Lerche
Neurological Clinic and Institute of Applied Physiology,
University of Ulm, Germany

Michael P. T. Lunn
National Hospital for Neurology and Neurosurgery,
London, UK

Snezana Maljevic
Neurological Clinic and Institute of Applied Physiology,
University of Ulm, Germany

Mark R. Manford
Department of Neurology, Addenbrooke's Hospital,
Cambridge, UK

Carla Marini
Pediatric Neurology Unit and Laboratories,
Anna Meyer Children's Hospital,
University of Florence, Italy

Bindu Menon
Department of Neurology,
Narayana Medical College and Superspeciality Hospital,
Nellore, Andhra Pradesh, India

Giulia Milioli
Sleep Disorders Center, Department of Neurosciences,
University of Parma, Italy

Eli M. Mizrahi
Peter Kellaway Section of Neurophysiology,
Department of Neurology and Section of Pediatric Neurology,
Department of Pediatrics, Baylor College of Medicine,
Houston, TX, USA

Manish Modi
Department of Neurology,
Postgraduate Institute of Medical Education and Research,
Chandigarh, India

Márcia Elisabete Morita
Department of Neurology,
University of Campinas – UNICAMP,
Campinas, SP, Brazil

Manuel Murie-Fernandez
Department of Physical Medicine and Rehabilitation,
St. Joseph's Healthcare,
London, Ontario, Canada

Vivek Nambiar
Department of Neurology,
Bombay Hospital Institute of Medical Science,
Mumbai, India

Lina Nashef
King's College Hospital,
London, UK

Vincent Navarro
Epilepsy Unit, Salpêtrière Hospital,
Pierre et Marie Curie University;
Cortex and Epilepsy Unit,
Centre de Recherche de l'Institut du Cerveau
et de la Moelle, Paris, France

Aidan Neligan
UCL Institute of Neurology,
University College London, UK

Ruth E. Nemire
Touro College of Pharmacy,
New York, NY, USA

Charles R. J. C. Newton
The Wellcome Trust,
KEMRI Unit, Kilifi, Kenya

John O'Donavan
Department of Neuropsychiatry,
The National Hospital for Neurology and Neuropsychiatry,
London, UK

Hirokazu Oguni
Department of Pediatrics,
Tokyo Women's Medical University, Tokyo, Japan

Teiichi Onuma
Musasinokokubunnji Clinic, Tokyo, Japan

Andre Palmini
Neurology Service and Faculty of Medicine,
Hospital São Lucas,
Pontifícia Universidade Católica do
Rio Grande do Sul (PUCRS),
Porto Alegre, RS, Brazil

Eleni Panagiotakaki
Institute for Children and Adolescents with Epilepsy (IDEE),
Hôpital Femme Mère Enfant, Lyon, France

Pasquale Parisi
Department of Child Neurology,
II Faculty of Medicine,
"La Sapienza" University of Rome, Italy

Elena Parrini
Pediatric Neurology and Neurogenetics Unit and Laboratories,
Anna Meyer Children's Hospital,
University of Florence, Italy

Liborio Parrino
Sleep Disorders Center, Department of Neurosciences,
University of Parma, Italy

Ignacio Pascual-Castroviejo
University Hospital La Paz, Madrid, Spain

M. Scott Perry
Comprehensive Epilepsy Program and the Brain Institute,
Miami Children's Hospital, Miami, FL, USA

Perrine Plouin
Clinical Neurophysiology Unit,
Hôpital Necker Enfants Malades,
Université Paris Descartes, Paris, France

Charles E. Polkey
Department of Clinical Neurosciences,
Institute of Psychiatry, King's College,
London, UK

Suresh S. Pujar
Neuroscience Unit, UCL Institute of Child Health,
London; National Centre for Young People with Epilepsy,
Lingfield, Surrey, UK

Karthik Rajasekaran
Department of Neurology, University of Virginia,
Charlottesville, VA, USA

R. Eugene Ramsey
International Center for Epilepsy,
University of Miami School of Medicine, Miami, FL, USA

Rahul Rathakrishnan
Department of Neurology and Neurosurgery,
Montreal Neurological Hospital and Institute,
McGill University, Montreal,
Québec, Canada

Roberta H. Raven
Department of Neuroepidemiology,
Bombay Hospital Institute of Medical Science,
Mumbai, India

Guy M. Rémillard
Department of Neurology,
Hôpital du Sacré-Coeur de Montréal,
Montreal, Québec, Canada

David Rosenblatt
Department of Human Genetics and Department
of Pediatrics and Medicine, McGill University,
Montreal, Québec, Canada

M. Elizabeth Ross
Laboratory of Neurogenetics and Development,
Weill Medical College of Cornell University,
New York, NY, USA

Abdulrahman Sabbagh
Department of Neurosurgery,
Neurosciences Center,
King Fahd Medical City, Riyadh, Saudi Arabia

P. Satishchandra
Department of Neurology,
National Institute of Mental Health and Neurosciences
(NIMHANS), Bangalore, India

Swati Sathe
Department of Neurology,
New York University School of Medicine,
New York, NY, USA

Ingrid E. Scheffer
Department of Medicine,
The University of Melbourne,
Victoria;
Department of Pediatrics,
The University of Melbourne,
Royal Children's Hospital,
Melbourne, Victoria, Australia

Philip A. Schwartzkroin
Department of Neurological Surgery,
University of California–Davis,
Davis, CA, USA

Rod C. Scott
UCL Institute of Child Health, London, UK

Frédéric Sedel
Federation of Nervous System Diseases,
Reference Center for Lysosomal Diseases,
Assistance Publique-Hôpitaux de Paris, Paris, France

Michelle J. Shapiro
McMaster University, Hamilton General Hospital,
Hamilton, Ontario, Canada

Elliott H. Sherr
Department of Neurology,
University of California,
San Francisco, CA, USA

Michael Shevell
Departments of Neurology, Neurosurgery and Pediatrics,
McGill University, Montreal, Québec, Canada

Simon D. Shorvon
UCL Institute of Neurology, London; National Hospital for
Neurology and Neurosurgery, London, UK

Adrian M. Siegel
Department of Neurology,
Zuger Kantonsspital, Baar, Switzerland

Gagandeep Singh
Department of Neurology,
Dayanand Medical College and Hospital,
Ludhiana, India

S. Sinha
Department of Neurology,
National Institute of Mental Health and Neurosciences
(NIMHANS), Bangalore, India

Barbara Spacca
Department of Neurosurgery,
Royal Liverpool Children's Hospital NHS Trust,
Liverpool, UK

Waney Squier
Department of Neuropathology,
John Radcliffe Hospital, Oxford, UK

Carl E. Stafstrom
Department of Neurology,
University of Wisconsin, Madison, WI, USA

Bernhard J. Steinhoff
Kork Epilepsy Centre,
Kehl-Kork, Germany

Andrea Taddio
Department of Pediatrics,
IRCCS Burlo Garofolo, Trieste, Italy

Gianpiero Tamburrini
Institute of Neurosurgery,
Catholic University Medical School,
Rome, Italy

C. T. Tan
Division of Neurology, Faculty of Medicine,
University of Malaya,
Kuala Lumpur, Malaysia

Raymond Y. L. Tan
National Hospital for Neurology and Neurosurgery,
London, UK

Erik Taubøll
Department of Neurology,
Division of Clinical Neuroscience,
Rikshospitalet University Hospital,
Oslo, Norway

Robert W. Teasell
Department of Physical Medicine and Rehabilitation,
St. Joseph's Healthcare,
London, Ontario, Canada

Mario Giovanni Terzano
Sleep Disorders Center,
Department of Neurosciences,
University of Parma, Italy

Federica Teutonico
Department of Child Neurology
and Psychiatry, "C. Mondino" Foundation,
University of Pavia, Italy

Suzanne A. Tharin
Department of Neurosurgery,
Brigham and Women's Hospital,
Harvard Medical School,
Boston, MA, USA

Elizabeth A. Thiele
Herscot Center for Tuberous Sclerosis Complex,
Boston, MA, USA

Pierre Thomas
UF EEG-Epileptologie, Service de Neurologie,
University of Nice-Sophia-Antipolis, Nice, France

Paolo Tinuper
Department of Neurological Sciences,
University of Bologna, Italy

Dorothée Kasteleijn-Nolst Trenité
University of Utrecht,
The Netherlands; II Faculty of Medicine,
"La Sapienza" University of Rome, Italy

Sumeet Vadera
Department of Neurosurgery, Cleveland Clinic Foundation,
Cleveland, OH, USA

Pierangelo Veggiotti
Department of Child Neurology and Psychiatry,
"C. Mondino" Foundation,
University of Pavia, Italy

Jean-Pierre Vignal
Service de Neurologie,
Hopital Central CHU de Nancy, Nancy, France

J. M. Walshe
Department of Neurology,
The Middlesex Hospital, London, UK

Elizabeth J. Waterhouse
Department of Neurology,
Medical College of Virginia Commonwealth University,
Richmond, VA, USA

David Watkins
Department of Human Genetics, McGill University,
Montreal, Québec, Canada

Ruth E. Williams
Department of Pediatric Neurology,
Evelina Children's Hospital, London, UK

Yue-Hua Zhang
Department of Pediatrics,
Peking University First Hospital, Beijing, China

Benjamin Zifkin
Epilepsy Clinic, Montreal Neurological Hospital,
Montreal, Québec, Canada

Sameer M. Zuberi
Fraser of Allander Neurosciences Unit,
Royal Hospital for Sick Children,
Glasgow, UK

Foreword

The written history of epilepsy goes back 3000 years with accurate descriptions of epileptic phenomena appearing in the writings of ancient Mesopotamia and the Indian Ayurvedic texts. Although physicians of the Hippocratic school in Greece, about 400 BC, understood that epileptic seizures originated in the brain, as did Galen several hundred years later, epilepsy was generally viewed as a mysterious condition attributed to supernatural causes, at least in the West, until the mid nineteenth century. At that time, the nascent disciplines of basic neuroscience and clinical neurology defined a variety of ictal manifestations, including focal seizures and absences, and recognized them as part of a constellation of disorders referred to as epilepsy. In particular, postmortem clinical pathological correlations not only revealed specific anatomic substrates for different ictal manifestations, but led directly to concepts of localization of function within the human brain, and to surgical treatment for certain types of focal epilepsies. The development of radiology in the twentieth century further improved physicians' abilities to identify "invisible" lesions as responsible for epileptic seizures in some patients, but it was application of the electroencephalogram (EEG), and the subsequent field of both clinical and basic electrophysiology, that provided a means to begin classifying and characterizing different types of epileptic seizures and epilepsy syndromes, and investigating their underlying fundamental pathophysiological neuronal mechanisms.

The careful delineation of different types of ictal phenomena provided the basis for creating experimental animal models for both in vitro and in vivo electrophysiological and microanatomical investigations of epilepsy. EEG localization of the epileptogenic region greatly increased the application of surgical treatment for focal epilepsies, which also provided novel opportunities for parallel invasive in vitro and in vivo electrophysiological and microanatomical investigations in patients. Towards the end of the twentieth century, explosive advances in three-dimensional neuroimaging, first with structural X-ray computerized tomography (CT), then functional positron emission tomography (PET), and finally both structural and functional high-resolution magnetic resonance imaging (MRI) provided intricate insights into the pathophysiologic mechanisms and anatomic substrates of epilepsy disorders in individual patients that could be used to create more informed categorizations and classifications. These efforts were joined by the burgeoning field of neurogenetics, which

not only is identifying an increasing number of "epilepsy genes" responsible for specific types of epilepsy, and further characterizing genetic disorders associated with epilepsy, but also advancing the concept of susceptibility genes, which will explain variable individual predispositions to develop certain forms of acquired epilepsies. Now, in the twenty-first century, we are poised to reap the benefits of these dramatic advances in our understanding of the causes of epilepsy.

Methodology for characterizing different types of epileptic seizures and the disorders associated with them, particularly through electroclinical correlations, that is the association of particular behavioral ictal signs and symptoms with their unique EEG correlates, led the International League Against Epilepsy (ILAE) to propose international classifications for epileptic seizures, and for the epilepsies in 1970. These have undergone several revisions, but the most recent version of the International Classification of Epileptic Seizures was proposed in 1981, and the most recent International Classification of the Epilepsies was proposed in 1989. These were purported to be purely phenomenological, because the authors felt there was, at the time, insufficient mechanistic information on which to base a classification on specific causes of epilepsy. Nevertheless, the inclusion of EEG characteristics permitted categorization of ictal phenomena in a way that implied certain pathophysiologic differences, as well as anatomic substrates. For instance, generalized seizures were distinguished from focal seizures that appeared to originate in a part of one hemisphere. Epilepsies were classified not only based on their characteristic associated seizure types, but also according to broad etiologic categories: idiopathic, meaning epilepsy and nothing else, presumably primary genetic disorders; and symptomatic, meaning secondary to some other disease process. In addition, diseases associated with epilepsy were well described, and some epilepsy diseases were recognized as conditions with a single known cause, but most of the defined epilepsy conditions were syndromes, characterized by specific seizure types, and other clinical features, such as age of onset, response to antiepileptic drugs, and comorbidity. Using this approach, the vast majority of accepted epilepsy syndromes are pediatric idiopathic conditions, while the majority of epilepsies that affect adults, most of which are symptomatic, still defy a reasonable syndromic classification.

For over a decade, the ILAE has attempted to revise the 1981 and 1989 classifications, with multiple reports that have updated the list of epileptic seizure types and epilepsy syndromes. They now recognize certain seizure types as diagnostic entities with associated therapeutic, prognostic, and etiologic implications that can be used when a definitive syndrome or disease diagnosis cannot be made. These deliberations provide a basis for a more scientific classification of epilepsy disorders based on underlying genetic and pathophysiologic mechanisms, as well as anatomic substrates. Ironically, however, as the chapters in this book clearly confirm, with the increasing sophistication of our investigative methodology, the elucidation of distinctive epilepsy conditions as diagnostic entities has become more, rather than less, complicated. The old dichotomies of idiopathic versus symptomatic, and generalized versus focal, are artificial and often impossible to apply. Well-defined classical syndromes, such as childhood absence epilepsy, are not as homogeneous as once believed. Some idiopathic childhood epilepsies, such as Dravet syndrome, are not benign, and there appear to be several distinctly different forms of temporal lobe epilepsy with hippocampal sclerosis. However, the causes of epilepsy discussed in this textbook represent a major effort to put flesh on the bones of what hopefully will ultimately become a biologically based international classification of the epilepsies.

With the hundreds of textbooks that have been published on epilepsy in the past decade or so, it is rather amazing that none have focused specifically on the causes of epilepsy. The editors have undertaken this monumental task and succeeded in documenting the current state of knowledge concerning the genetic and pathological substrates of disorders characterized by epileptic seizures, as well as the situations that provoke ictal events. This comprehensive compendium will not only serve as an important resource for rethinking the organization and classification of epileptic phenomena and epilepsy syndromes and diseases, but will also provide a foundation for basic research attempting to identify the diverse pathophysiological mechanisms at the subcellular, cellular, and systems levels, that are responsible for epileptogenesis and seizure generation. Identification of these fundamental neuronal processes in turn will lead to novel and more effective approaches to treatment, cure, and prevention of epilepsy.

Jerome Engel, Jr.
Los Angeles, California

Medicine is undergoing a remarkable transition as we move from descriptions of disease and a taxonomy based on clinical characteristics to a more detailed and precise understanding of disease pathogenesis. This revolution has been driven by the adoption of a range of molecular tools and, more particularly, by the application of molecular genetics to medicine. These approaches are providing us with insights, often for the first time, of the pathways and precise events associated with disease pathogenesis and this will change forever the foundations on which we base diagnosis and treatment of disease.

The developments in the molecular understanding of disease are nowhere more evident than in neurological disease, particularly the epilepsies. These clinical syndromes, often dramatic in their clinical characteristics, have been associated with a range of taxonomies that have developed over many centuries. The clinical characteristics of seizures and an understanding of the abnormal electrophysiology provided a framework on which taxonomy could be based, but clearly could not address the fundamental issue of the underpinning events in disease pathogenesis. That has had to wait until the past twenty years when the tools available for characterizing both families and individual patients have gradually become available.

Initial progress in this field focused, as with other diseases, on Mendelian forms of epilepsy using family based studies. Although these studies revealed a range of interesting pathophysiological mechanisms, including a number of ion channels, it has been clear that this describes only a portion of the epilepsy syndromes, many of which involve more complex genetics. These now are increasingly tractable with the new tools for genetic association and these are beginning to reveal non-channel molecules and pathways associated with neural excitability. Together, these techniques are providing a crucial framework for redefining the epilepsies based on pathophysiology and, in turn, this will have a profound impact on our ability to predict, diagnose, and, ultimately, treat disease. Anticonvulsive therapy has been remarkably successful, given how little we know about the pathogenic mechanisms of the disease, so it is likely that future therapeutic interventions based on a clearer understanding of the relevant pathways will be even more effective.

Together, these advances have made epilepsy one of the most significant examples in medicine of the importance of genetic tools in clarifying pathophysiology and these disorders demonstrate clearly how powerful the change from pure phenotypic classification of disease to one based on pathophysiology can be. The authors of this important book have been able to bring together a wide range of scientific insight and data on this topic into a single volume that covers the whole range of clinical syndromes. They demonstrate how powerful these new genetic tools have already been in defining pathways in disease and they also clearly demonstrate that, together, their observations are likely to lead to a fundamental new classification of these diseases. Not only is this volume timely, given the recent exciting developments in this field, but it also demonstrates the enormous influence that these key basic insights will have on the way we categorize and, ultimately, treat individuals with disease. Epilepsy and its associated syndromes give us a clear vision of what the future of medicine is likely to look like.

Professor Sir John Bell,
University of Oxford, UK

Preface – an act of supererogation?

An inquiring mind must return again and again to the problem of origin or cause.... physicians have dug away at diverse etiologic theories or facts; physical or psychic; general or individual; genetic or acquired; fundamental or contributory. When a crime is committed, everyone in the vicinity is suspect.
William Lennox, Epilepsy and Related Conditions, 1960

Thus Lennox opened his chapter on "The diverse sources of seizures," and indeed he devoted a great many pages of his famous book to the question of etiology. Yet, 50 years later, causation is an aspect of epilepsy now somewhat neglected in the scientific literature on epilepsy, in the classification of epilepsy, and in the conceptualization of epilepsy at a clinical and experimental level. It was to go some way to remedying this deficiency that this book was conceived.

Kinnier Wilson in 1940 wrote that the listing of all causes of epilepsy would be an *act of supererogation*, but the editors of this book beg to differ. This is the first book ever published, as far as we know, which is devoted to the topic of causation in epilepsy, and we have attempted within its 800 pages to catalog the known causes of epilepsy, and corral these into a single tome.

Such an attempt is only possible because of the great advances made in imaging, molecular biology, and molecular genetics in the last 40 years or so, and we believe that progress has now been sufficient to permit at least a stab at a comprehensive listing of causation. The literature on epilepsy has rapidly increased in recent years. Kinnier Wilson noted that the index catalogue of the US Surgeon-General's office (1925) contained about 3000 titles and the "Gruhle's review for the years 1910–1920 deals with some 1000 articles." In the last 10-year period, a search on PubMed® using the keyword epilepsy produces more than 37 000 references, many of which deal at least tangentially with etiology. It is this literature-base which we have asked our contributors to summarize in the various chapters of this volume.

One striking omission has been the absence of any detailed consideration of etiology in the standard classifications of epilepsy. This is partly because at the time that these schemes were being devised neither modern investigatory imaging methods nor modern molecular biology were available – and the ascertainment of "cause" in life was often simply not possible. Although it was fully recognized that epilepsy was often "a symptom" of neurological disease, the underlying cause of the symptom was completely absent from the current classification schemes, based as they are largely on clinical semiology and electroencephalography, and it is interesting to muse on what form the epilepsy classification might have taken if MRI scanning had preceded EEG as a clinical investigatory tool.

We thus open this book with, in Chapter 2, the presentation of a draft etiological classification which goes some way we hope to filling the nosological void. The main part of the book is organized according to this classificatory scheme. We have divided the etiologies into four categories: idiopathic epilepsies, symptomatic epilepsies, cryptogenic epilepsies, and provoked epilepsies, and these are defined in Chapter 2. In doing so, of course, we recognize, as Lennox, and many before him, frequently reiterated, that epilepsy is in the great majority of cases multifactorial, and frequently has a developmental basis with therefore a temporal dimension. The epilepsy is often the result of both genetic and acquired influences and also influenced by provoking factors, and assignment in such cases to any single etiology is therefore to an extent arbitrary.

The approach to the problem of etiology between 1860 and 1960 forms the subject of the historical introduction (Chapter 1) which ends with Lennox's work, and this is included as we believe it is important to understand the evolution of concepts of causation within its historical context.

In subsequent chapters, we have asked the authors to consider their topic in a consistent fashion, dealing with the phenomenon of epilepsy in each etiology, including its epidemiology, clinical features, and prognosis, and any specific aspects of investigation or treatment.

The purpose of the book is to be a comprehensive reference work, a catalog of all the important causes of epilepsy, and a clinical tool for all clinicians dealing with patients with epilepsy. It is aimed at specialists and the interested generalist and it is hoped provides a distillation of knowledge in a form that is helpful in the clinical setting. We hope too that it will act as a clinical guide to scientists probing the dark interior of the subject.

We have attempted to take a worldwide perspective, and have included chapters on the causes of epilepsy that are rare in the West but common in other parts of the world. To match the worldwide spread of the conditions considered here, we have a distinguished faculty with a similar global reach, and the book has 165 contributors from 21 countries and all continents many of whom are the leaders in their fields.

The editors have exercised a heavy editorial blue pen, have tried to minimize overlap or repetition, and have asked the authors to follow where possible a pre-assigned template. Our contributors have responded magnificently in our opinion, and we extend our grateful thanks for their hard work and for their time and effort. We would like to thank also Professor Jerome (Pete) Engel and Professor Sir John Bell for graciously agreeing to write the foreword to the book. Pete Engel is a famous leader in the field of epilepsy and a prolific author, who has made major contributions to many fields of epilepsy. Sir John Bell is President of the Academy of Medical Sciences and Regius Professor of Medicine at the University of Oxford,

and a renowned medical geneticist. The book is indeed fortunate to have their contributions. We are also enormously grateful to Nicholas Dunton, the Senior Commissioning Editor at Cambridge University Press, who has guided the project since its inception with extraordinary skill and expertise, and without whose assistance the book would not have made it to the shelves. We also thank Assistant Editor Joanna Chamberlin and Production Editor Caroline Brown for their great efforts on behalf of the book. Finally, we would like to thank all our colleagues around the world for their stimulating ideas and knowledge, which have informed and illuminated all the pages of this book.

Simon Shorvon, Renzo Guerrini, and Fred Andermann

Historical introduction: the causes of epilepsy in the pre-molecular era (1860–1960)

– from John Hughlings Jackson to William Lennox

Simon D. Shorvon

The evolution of theories of etiology in epilepsy makes an interesting study at many levels: some theories reflect social and philosophical attitude; some, widely believed and extensively written about at the time, have proved totally erroneous and now even appear ridiculous; and others show scientific insight now lost and worth reappraisal. Much can be learned also from the constructs with which our predecessors conceptualized the process of epilepsy, not least because it puts into perspective our current thought. In this chapter, the theories of etiology for the 100 years since the time of John Hughlings Jackson, whose writing has often been said to announce the dawn of modern epileptology, will be outlined. The chapter ends with William Lennox, a natural break as in many ways Lennox sums up the work of the previous century. After Lennox, the new molecular biology, imaging, and genetic techniques have proved powerful tools in the exploration of etiology and have greatly changed our understanding in the field. Nevertheless, some concepts and ideas of the pre-Lennox period have resonance today and are worth re-evaluation.

In earlier times, epilepsy was almost universally considered to be the result of supernatural or magic forces, or possession by evil spirits or the devil. Leading medical thinkers repeatedly rounded on such superstitious explanations; Hippocrates wrote for instance both that epilepsy was an organic disease of the brain and that "its origin is hereditary, like that of other diseases." Galen divided epilepsy into three etiological groups (remarkably analogous to theories prevalent today): a dyscrasia of the humors of the brain; a stimulation of the brain by an irritating substance brought into the brain from the body (the convulsion being the brain's efforts to repel the irritant); and the invasion of the brain by a pathological humor formed in the extremities. Nevertheless, despite these physical explanations, the majority of physicians and of the public continued to accept supernatural theories right up to the mid nineteenth century and a few continue to do so. In the early nineteenth century, other theories of etiology began to take shape, not least those revolving around heredity. This earlier history is well described by Temkin (1945), whose detailed survey ends in large part in the mid nineteenth century. This chapter starts at this point, when the modern age of epileptology can be said to have been entered.

Theories of the causation of epilepsy 1860–1907

Concepts of etiology in the mid nineteenth century

In the middle of the nineteenth century, there was a recrudescence of interest in epilepsy and its causes, particularly in neurological circles. A number of influential books were written, especially by the English neurologists, which demonstrate a more clinical and physiological view than was previously the case. The first of these books, *Epilepsy and Epileptiform Seizures*, by Edward Sieveking (1861) (Fig. 1.1) provides an interesting starting point for our survey, representing as it does a transition to modern thought. His discussion of etiology starts with a consideration of demonic possession, which he dismisses. The "causes of epilepsy" are divided into "predisposing and exciting components," a common formulation of the period, and Sieveking articulated what was a predominate theory of the time, that the predisposing causes were largely inherited, and formed the *epileptic diathesis*, which he defined using the following rather vivid analogy: "Diathesis may be compared to combustible material of greater or less inflammability, which differs in the facility with which it will take fire, but will infallibly do so if a flame of sufficient intensity is brought into contact with it" (Sieveking 1861). Amongst the predisposing causes, he found "hereditary influences are very palpable" and cites Herpin who "amongst 68 patients with epilepsy found 78 relatives who laboured under some affection of the nervous system" (Table 1.1). The diathesis was embedded in the concept of the "neurological taint," a theory of great influence at the time, and of which more below. However, other mechanisms were also evident to Sieveking who discoursed lengthily on albuminuria, but particularly constipation and other derangement of the bowels. He also emphasized

The Causes of Epilepsy, eds. S. D. Shorvon, F. Andermann, and R. Guerrini. Published by Cambridge University Press. © Cambridge University Press 2011.

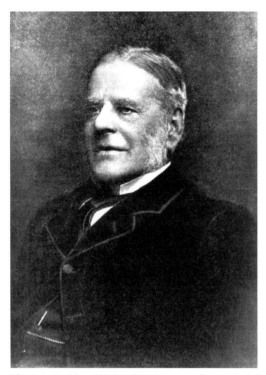

Fig. 1.1. Sir Edward H. Sieveking (1816–1904), appointed physician to the National Hospital Queen Square in 1864.

Table 1.1 Associated neurological conditions in 380 relatives of 68 epileptics

Epilepsy	10
Insanity	24
Suicide	1
Melancholia	2
Hypochondriasis	3
Hysteria	2[a]
Chorea	2
Sleepwalking	2
Nervous excitability	3
Apoplexy	11
Cerebral softening	1
General paralysis	2
Meningitis and chronic hydrocephalus	13
Mortal convulsions	1
Tetanus	1
Total	78

Note:
[a] I cannot but demur to this number, and it is incredible that not more than two relatives of 68 epileptics should have been hysterical.
Source: From Herpin, cited by Sieveking (1861).

the importance of sexual disturbances as a cause of epilepsy, both predisposing and exciting: "Although the unanimous consent of all writers on epilepsy demonstrates the truth of the statement that in this disease, the sexual organs are very frequently at fault … it is by no means determined in how far sexual derangements are to be regarded as a predisposing or exciting cause" and he then cites the ancient proverb attributed to Galen: "*coitus brevis epilepsia est.*" He believed that sexual derangement "enfeebled the system, and by producing excitability gives rise to the epileptic paroxysm." Masturbation was a particular cause, and Sieveking wrote that in nine of 52 of his cases, he found "the sexual system was in a state of great excitement, owing to recent or former masturbation." The theory that sexual practices predisposed to epilepsy was one held by many earlier authors and was again widely but not universally held at this time. Sieveking noted that the influence of the menstrual cycle was most important in females and masturbation in males (evidence of the latter in 31%). Interestingly Sieveking makes no mention of "degeneracy," nor of Morel whose work was published contemporaneously, reflecting the then divergent paths of British and Continental epileptology (see below).

J. Russell Reynolds

In the same year that Sieveking's book appeared, Reynolds (Fig. 1.2), another leading London neurologist, knighted and awarded an FRS, published his book *Epilepsy: Its Symptoms, Treatment and Relation to Other Chronic Convulsive Diseases* (Reynolds 1861) which became extremely influential. Jackson,

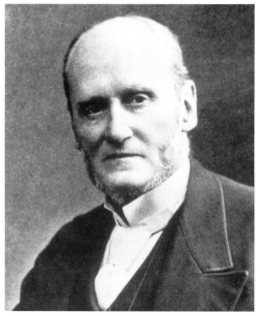

Fig. 1.2. Sir J Russell Reynolds FRS (1828–96) was physician to the royal household and President of the Royal College of Physicians, and physician at the National Hospital Queen Square from 1864.

for instance, extensively cites the book and Gowers dedicated his own book of 1888 to Reynolds ("whose example stimulated and friendship encouraged"). Reynolds considered the "causes

Table 1.2 The classification of epilepsy devised by J. Russell Reynolds (1861)

Category	Comment
1. Idiopathic epilepsy	An internal cause – a *morbus per se*. This may have a basis in heredity or conditions operating after birth.
2. Eccentric epilepsy	Epilepsy due to some systemic disturbance which when cured will result in the cessation of seizures. Reynolds accepted that "eccentric convulsions" can be exacerbated by a predisposing tendency, and he proposed that they had a "reflex" basis.
3. Diathetic epilepsy	Epilepsy in which the convulsions are primarily due to cachexia or toxemia, and in which the nervous system is "involved in that general nutrition-change which is the essential element of the cachexia itself" and have their basis in a general not specific remote causes. These can include patients with an existing predisposition (or not) and other existing symptomatic causes.
4. Symptomatic epilepsy	Epilepsy in which convulsions are due to "more or less contiguous structural disease of the brain. Thus, an intracranial tumor, a chronic inflammatory condition of the meninges, softening or disintegration of the brain substance, or any other structural change in the nervous centres … may set up that peculiar interstitial or molecular change which is the immediate cause of convulsion."

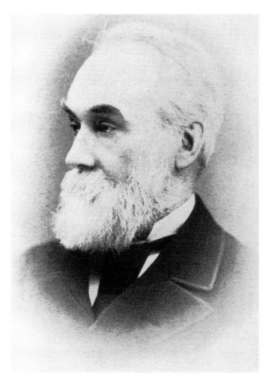

Fig. 1.3. John Hughlings Jackson FRS (1835–1911), the father of modern epileptology, was physician at the National Hospital Queen Square from 1862 to 1906.

of epilepsy" to be divided into proximate and remote categories. The proximate cause is the same in all cases – an abnormal increase in the nutritive changes of the nervous system (a similar concept to the current emphasis on excitatatory changes). He recognized that the remote causes may be very slight in some cases, and in others severe remote disease resulted in very insignificant epilepsy, that there were diverse remote causes but all were mediated though this defect of nutrition, and that the different forms of seizure were due to differing anatomical locations of the abnormal nervous centers – in all this, he anticipated Jackson.

He classified epilepsy into four categories, an excellent scheme worth recording here for its lessons for today's nosologists (Table 1.2). In his category of idiopathic epilepsy, he included other inherited conditions of the neuropathic taint (see below), including mania, idiocy, paralysis, and insanity. He considered an inherited influence was present in 31% of his own cases. The category of "eccentric" epilepsy is very similar to our current concept of "acute symptomatic seizures" and Reynolds listed causes which included teething, worms, and poisons. Diathetic epilepsy seems to be a new category, in which the nutritive change is not confined to the brain but is part of the general systemic disturbance caused by toxemia or cachexia. The causes of cachexia he listed included: tuberculosis,

scrophula, rachitis, syphilis, pyemia, anemia, alcoholism, lead poisoning, typhus, variola, and other exanthemata and diseases which alter nutrition such as pneumonia, carditis, and pericarditis. The term "symptomatic epilepsy" was reserved for epilepsies in which there was a contiguous structural brain disease, a term similar but more narrow than the usage today.

Reynolds viewed the manifestations of epilepsy as the summation of disturbances of structure and function, and considered that the proximate and remote causes cannot be separated from the disease itself.

It is also notable that Reynolds considered that an emphasis on masturbation to be mistaken, and that the ideas of "some mysterious entity taking possession of the body" a theory "long since passed." This then was the state of advanced thinking on etiology at the start of our period, when John Hughlings Jackson began to publish his work on epilepsy.

John Hughlings Jackson

The works of John Hughlings Jackson (Fig. 1.3) are generally agreed to have laid the foundations for much of modern epilepsy studies. An enormous contribution was his observation that "a convulsion is but a symptom, and implies only that there is an occasional, an excessive, and a disorderly discharge of nerve tissue on muscles" (1873). In his Lumlian lectures of 1890, he defined nervous discharge as the liberation of energy by nervous elements and the epileptic discharge as sudden, temporary and excessive in nature, a kind of explosive discharge ... it was "the physiological fulminate" like the gunpowder in a cannon, and just as gunpowder can store energy that is liberated when firing the gun, so the energy stored in nerve cells could be explosively liberated in an epileptic discharge. This definition of epileptic seizures has remained central, ever since, to all thought on the condition and was a quite remarkable insight. The reason for the abnormal levels of stored energy was deranged "nutrition" in Jackson's view. He equated "cause" with "causal mechanism" and was in general not particularly interested in the question of etiology in the sense usual today; his focus was on theories of physiology. The only sustained piece of writing on causation was in his paper, published in 1874, entitled "On the scientific and empirical investigation of epilepsies" (Jackson 1874, pp. 162–273). He wrote that:

> The confusion of two things physiology and pathology under one (pathology) leads to confusion in considering "causes". Thus, for example, we hear it epigrammatically said that chorea is "only a symptom" and may depend on many causes. This is possibly true of pathological causation; in other words it may be granted that various abnormal nutritive processes may lead to that functional change in grey matter which, when established, admits occasional excessive discharge. But physiologically, that is to say, from the point of view of Function, there is but one cause of chorea – viz. instability of nerve tissue. Similarly in any epilepsy, there is but "one cause" physiologically speaking – viz. the instability of the grey matter, but an unknown number of causes if we mean pathological processes leading to that instability.

Jackson defined the term *physiology* in the narrow and specific meaning of:

> the departure of the healthy *function* of nerve tissue. That function is to store up and to expend force ... in epilepsy, the cells store up large quantities and discharge abundantly on very slight provocation: there is what I call instability, or what is otherwise spoken of as increased excitability.

By the term *pathology* he meant "disordered nutrition" and in epilepsy (and excessive discharge) the pathological process was overnutrition which, in Jackson's view, was often caused by congestion of small blood vessels following occlusion of other vessels. He did recognize that there were many possible contributing factors that may result in the vascular disturbance (and thus in overnutrition and thus in the discharge) and those that he mentioned were tubercle, cicatrix, tumor, syphiloma, or hemorrhagic or ischemic stroke. He also realized that there was often no visible cause. His discussion of etiology, though, was not on these conditions but on the nutritional and vascular disturbances itself. He also recognized, *pari passu*, that the position and hierarchical level of the discharging tissue in the nervous system determined the form of the epilepsy.

In summary, Jackson makes the novel and important point that in epileptogenic tissue, the nervous centers are hyperexcitable and that the mechanism by which external or internal factors result in an epileptic seizure is similar and mediated via vascular congestion resulting in metabolic changes in the cells

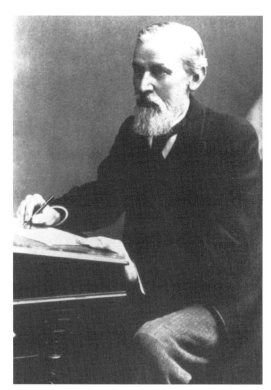

Fig. 1.4. Sir William Gowers FRS (1845–1915) was appointed physician to the National Hospital Queen Square in 1872.

(he defines this mechanism as "the cause of epilepsy"). Many different disease entities can result in this vascular imbalance, but this was not his focus. Furthermore, he held that predisposing factors such as heredity "set" the level of hyperexcitability in individual cases and determine the response of tissue to the stimulus of overnutrition. Like Reynolds and others before him, Jackson really only considered "idiopathic" epilepsy to be true epilepsy, and other forms (symptomatic or organic epilepsies) from the point of view of causation to be worthy of little specific study.

William Gowers

The next important published work on epilepsy was Sir William Gowers' famous book, *Epilepsy and Other Chronic Convulsive Diseases* (Gowers 1881), the first edition of which was published in 1881 with a second edition in 1901, and his views were summarized in this and in his famous and gigantic textbook of neurology of 1888 (*A Manual of Diseases of the Nervous System*; Gowers 1888). Gowers (Fig. 1.4) took a much more empirical approach to causation than Jackson. He classified epilepsy into idiopathic epilepsy and organic epilepsy, and considered only idiopathic epilepsy to be "true epilepsy."

The first chapter of his book was devoted to the causes of idiopathic epilepsy. He divided these into two types, *predisposing* causes and *exciting* causes, the former being "remote" and the latter "immediate" (interestingly a different usage than that of Reynolds for instance). The analogy of gunpowder was used by Gowers (following Sieveking and Jackson) – the gunpowder being the predisposing cause and the spark the exciting cause. It is interesting to note that the terms "eccentric" and "diathetic," used by Reynolds, do not appear in Gowers' book, and his use of the term "reflex" has also changed.

Of the predisposing causes, by far the most important was "heredity." As Gowers put it, "there are few diseases in the production of which inheritance has more manifest influence." The concept of the "neuropathic trait" (the neuropathic tendency; see below) had taken a strong hold by then, and heredity was widely defined. As Gowers wrote:

> It is well known that the "neuropathic tendency" does not always manifest itself in the same form, but is not easy to discern the relation of its varieties ... The chief morbid states (besides epilepsy itself) by which the same neuropathic tendency is manifested is insanity, and, to a much smaller degree, chorea, chronic hysteria, migraine, and some chronic forms of disease of the brain and of the spinal cord. Intemperance is probably also due, in many cases, to a neuropathic disposition.

Of 2400 cases investigated by Gowers, 40% had an inherited tendency in his view, and his later series had even higher rates. Gowers went on to say that, because of the neuropathic trait, epilepsy and insanity were almost interchangeable terms, with three-quarters of those with inherited insanity also having epilepsy. Other predisposing causes were age (74% of epilepsy developed in Gowers' series before the age of 20 years), sex (female cases are greater in number; 52% of 2000 cases in Gowers' series), and inherited syphilis but not other (indirect) inherited conditions such as rheumatism, phthisis, and gout (a common theory at the time). Consanguinity was considered to intensify existing tendencies and only to play a significant part in epilepsy when "neurotic heredity exists in both parents."

The exciting causes in idiopathic epilepsy were, in Gowers' opinion, secondary in importance to inherited causes:

> It may be again pointed out, to prevent misconception, that these exciting causes cannot be regarded as the essential causes of the disease except in a very small number of cases ... The real cause of the disease is the morbid state of the nervous system.

Of 1665 cases, Gowers considered that a reasonable exciting cause could be found in 42% (696 cases). These exciting causes included: difficulty with labor, birth trauma, febrile convulsions (teething fits), rickets, organic lesions of the brain, mental emotion (fright, excitement, anxiety), acute diseases (measles, scarlet fever, typhus, typhoid, rheumatic fever, influenza, diarrhea), reflex seizures, asphyxia, lead poisoning, renal disease, anesthetics, disturbed menstruation, pregnancy, and syphilis. Gowers was doubtful about the relevance of masturbation. Fright, excitement, and anxiety were the most potent of the exciting causes in Gowers' view, of which fright took first place. Emotion was felt to be most important in young adult females. Trauma was included as an exciting cause of idiopathic epilepsy, second only to psychic causes in frequency, and not "organic epilepsy" in most cases where it results in no

lesion. Of the acute infections, Gowers singled out scarlet fever, which he considered especially neurotoxic. Gowers also pointed to "reflex causes" by which he meant causes mediated by irritation of peripheral nerves, visceral or external, and these can excite convulsions which may continue as persistent epilepsy: pain, digestive derangement, or an "anomalous or indigestible meal ... In many cases of tubercular meningitis, the first symptom is a convulsion apparently induced by an indigestible meal."

The "organic epilepsies" (as opposed to "idiopathic epilepsies") were defined as the epilepsies associated with the "many organic diseases of the brain," which Gowers does not go on to list. These are today what would be called the symptomatic epilepsies, and did not attract much interest in Gowers' time.

Finally, Gowers made a unique contribution to "cause" in epilepsy with his theory that

> the malady is self-perpetuating; when one attack has occurred, whether as the result of an immediate excitant or not, others follow either without any immediate cause, or after some very trifling disturbance ... The search for the causes of epilepsy must thus be chiefly an investigation into the conditions with precede the occurrence of the first fit.

This concept ("seizures beget seizures") continues to stimulate debate.

Heredity as a cause of epilepsy 1857–1907: degeneration, and the neurological taint

As was made clear by Gowers, heredity was considered a leading etiological influence of the time. To understand what was meant by "heredity" in this period, the central importance of two related concepts, "degeneration" and the "neurological taint," must be appreciated.

In the early and mid nineteenth century, particularly amongst French writers, the concept of degeneration (*dégénérescence*) replaced the supernatural as the main focus of interest in the causation of epilepsy. Theories of degeneration can be traced back to Ancient Greece, but formal scientific study developed in relation to the concept of speciation. Buffon the French naturalist suggested that living forms could be subject to degeneration (Buffon 1780), and the theme was taken up in relation to art, social science, and politics in the Romantic Movement. In the clinical field, the French psychiatrists, with their practice rooted in institutions, began to develop theories relating to mental and physical degeneration in mental disorders. In 1857 and 1860, Bénédict Morel published his two classic books on the degenerations of the human species and degenerations in mental disorders (Morel 1857, 1860) and these books became standard texts and were widely influential in medicine and beyond. Medical conjectures of degeneration were really part of much wider public concerns about social disintegration and the collapsing state of European cultural identity. There were fears that the rapid urbanization and population growth amongst the peasant and lower classes would sap national intelligence and morality. This was also reflected in the artistic movements of the time, and in studies of criminality and social science, Linked to ideas of *dégénérescence* was the concept that there existed a *neuropathic taint* (also known by various other terms including neurological taint, neuropathic trait, neuropathic predisposition). According to this theory, a wide range of conditions including epilepsy were inherited together. These conditions were not well defined, and different authorities incorporated different categories, but at their core these included, in addition to epilepsy: insanity, psychiatric disorders of various types, mental retardation, general paralysis of the insane, and locomotor ataxy; also moral degeneration such as was found in alcoholics or the criminal; and sexual degeneration evinced by masturbation, perversion, and sexual excess. This belief was widely accepted amongst neurologists, but Jackson earlier had opposed the idea of mixing up conditions with "no evident pathological connection." According to Morel, this inherited tendency resulted in a *progressive* deterioration (degeneration) physically, mentally, and morally, over generations, and this tendency becomes progressively more severe, eventually resulting in the extinction of the line. At about the same time Jacques Joseph Moreau, a student of Esquirol, published his influential text *La Psychologie morbide* (1859) in which he introduced the category of the "neuropathic family," in which hereditary mental disorders were passed down the ancestral line. Epilepsy was central to both Morel and Moreau's writings, and was at the core of the "degenerative endowment." According to these theories, the endowment might for instance cause mild hysteria in one generation, then a more serious epilepsy in the next, and dementia or idiocy in the next. The topic was further developed by Valentine Magnan, a pupil of Morel, and Jules Falret (1864), and ultimately by Charles Féré who divided the "neuropathic family" into a psychopathological arm which included epilepsy and the major psychiatric disorders, and a neuropathological arm which included chorea, migraine, and Parkinson's disease (Féré 1884).

Interestingly, Moreau also included "genius" as a neuropathic feature, and believed that there was a "community of origin" for genius and madness. This was a concept which had its origins at least since Robert Burton's *Anatomy of Melancholy* published in 1621, and was to presage the work of Lombroso who wrote "The creative power of genius may be in the form of degenerative psychosis belonging to the family of epileptic affections" (Lombroso 1889), and later similar pronouncements by Spratling and other stalwarts of the epilepsy establishment.

In parallel to the studies of mental degeneration were investigations of physical stigmata, and particularly physiognomy (Fig. 1.5). The study of physiognomy had a long tradition dating from Ancient Greece, and was considered so subversive that it was banned from university study in England in 1551 by Henry VIII. As a topic of social and medical interest, it had a resurgence in the 1770s following the work of Casper Lavater and Sir Thomas Browne. In psychiatry, an important landmark was the publication of *Mental Maladies* by Jean-Étienne Dominique Esquirol (1838) who found that the insane and the retarded had specific physical appearances which reflected their degenerative taint. Moreau, Falret, and Magnan developed these concepts further.

The notion of degeneration was also linked in this period to the concept of atavism, which had biological plausibility given the theory of recapitulation popularized by Haeckel in 1866 ("Ontogeny recapitulates phylogeny," a theory actually first proposed by Serres in 1824). Degeneration was thought to bring out atavistic characteristics (physical, behavioral, and mental) which were therefore the signs of the degenerative tendency. Epilepsy was seen as one symptom of degeneration, atavistic in nature, in the progressive downward degenerative spiral.

By the end of the nineteenth century almost all writings on the inheritance of epilepsy (of which there were a great number) accepted this concept. Amongst the major writers of the time, Echeverria (1873) reported a heritability rate of epilepsy in 25%, Déjerine (1886) of 66.8% when including other conditions of the neurological taint, Binswanger of 36.3% (1899), and Spratling (1904) of 56.0%. Turner (1907; see below) whose thinking on the topic was a great deal clearer than others, wrote: "in order to ascertain how far definitely neuropathic maladies play a part in the causation of epilepsy, the following table has been constructed to show the percentage frequency of the three main hereditary factors in the ancestral history of epileptics, viz. epilepsy, insanity, and parental alcoholism" (Table 1.3).

Cesare Lombroso

The theories of the neurological taint and degeneration evolved furthest with the writings of Cesare Lombroso on criminality. Lombroso was a physician and psychiatrist by training, and is credited with the first scientific writings on criminality. His scientific method was "measurement" of both physical and mental features. His most enduring work was *L'uomo delinquente* (*Criminal Man*; published in five editions between 1876 and 1896/7) and *Criminal Woman* (*La donna delinquente e la prostituta e la donna normale* (Lombroso and Ferraro, 1893) which are packed with statistical tables of numerous measurements (this cult of anthropomorphic measurement was pioneered by Galton and Pearson, became a fundamental tool of the eugenics movement, and culminated in the anthropometry of the Nazi physicians). In these works, epilepsy was linked to criminality (an idea explored most fully in the fourth edition of *L'uomo delinquente* in 1889), a concept already widely written about in the previous decades (for instance by Echeverria and Maudsley). Lombroso's theory of criminality was based on the demonstration that two-thirds of dangerous criminal individuals were "born criminals" who inherited a criminal trait and possessed "anomalies" (physical and psychological) resembling the traits of primitive man and animals (and even plants).

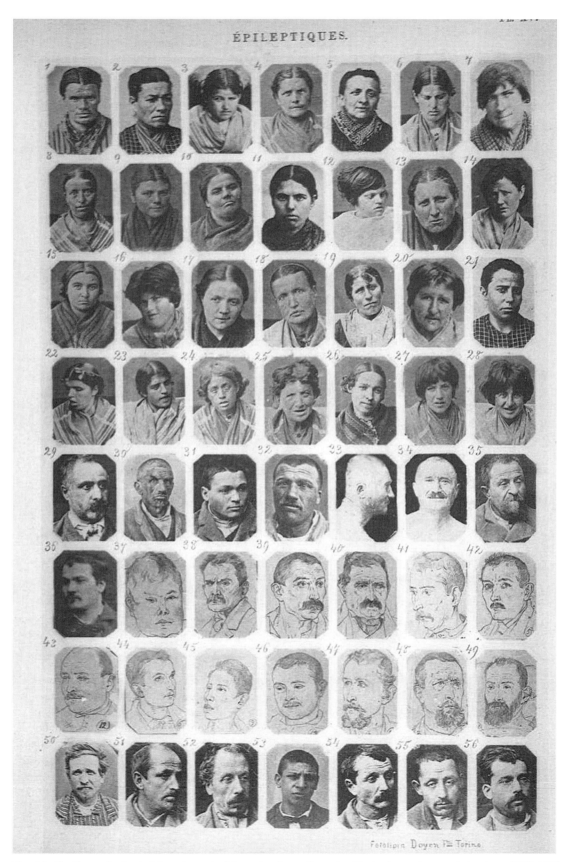

Fig. 1.5. The "faces of epileptics" from the work of Cesare Lombroso, illustrating his physiognomic research. Lombroso (1835–1909) was professor of forensic medicine and hygiene and later professor of psychiatry and criminal anthropology in Turin.

Table 1.3 The table constructed by Turner (1907) showing "The percentage frequency of epilepsy, insanity and alcoholism as hereditary factors in the causation of epilepsy"

	Déjerine (1886)	Binswanger (1899)	Spratling (1904)	Doran (1903)
Epilepsy	21.2%	11%	16%	19.3%
Insanity	16.8%	29.6%	7%	7.9%
Parental alcoholism	51.6%	22%	14%	21.6%

Table 1.4 Lombroso's list of anomalies shared by epileptics and criminals

Skull	Abnormally large, microcephaly, asymmetric (12–37%), sclerosis, med. occ. fossetta, abnormal indices, large orbital arches, low sloping forehead, wormian bones, simple cranial sutures the following characteristics shared by criminals and the morally insane
Face	Overdeveloped jaw, jutting cheekbones, large jug ears, facial asymmetry, strabismus, virility (in women), anomalous teeth
Brain	Anomalous convolutions, low weight, hypertrophied cerebellum, symptoms of meningitis
Body	Asymmetrical torso, prehensile feet, hernia
Skin	Wrinkles, beardlessness, olive skin, tattoos, delayed gray hair/balding, dark and curly hair
Motor anomalies	Left-handedness (10%), abnormal reflexes, heightened agility (16%)
Sensory anomalies	Tactile insensitivity (81%), insensitivity to pain, overly acute eyesight, dullness of hearing, taste, and smell
Psychological anomalies (% in epileptics)	Limited intelligence (30–69%), weak memory (14–91%), hallucinations (20–41%), superstitious, blunted emotions, love of animals, absence of remorse, impulsivity (2–50%), cannibalism and ferocity, pederasty (2–39%), masturbation (21–67%), perversity (15–57%), vanity, sloth, passion for gaming, mania/paranoia, delirium, dizziness, delusions of grandeur (1–3%), irascibility (30–100%), lying (7–100%), theft (4–75%), religious delusions (14–100%)
Causes	Heredity (of alcoholism, insanity, epilepsy, old parents), alcoholism

Note:
List is from editions 4 and 5, with percentages quoted by Lombroso from his own work or that of Cividalli, Tonnini, and Bianchi.

Thus criminals were *atavistic throwbacks* to a primitive stage in human evolution. In his earlier work, he linked criminals with the insane and later with alcoholics, but in the fourth edition of his book turned his attention to epilepsy. He expressed the view that epilepsy was an atavistic characteristic and a fundamental component of the criminal type. He supported this by showing that criminals and epileptics shared the same physiognomy, physical and psychological features, and moral deficiency (Lombroso's list from the fourth and fifth editions of *L'uomo delinquente* is shown in Table 1.4). Lombroso held the same view about epilepsy in females (although the prevalence of crime was less, due to the fact that the female cortex "although as irritable as men's in its motor centre, is much less so in the psychological centres, precisely because there are fewer of these"). Moral insanity, criminality, and epilepsy were closely linked in women, as in men, and as Lombroso wrote about female criminals "I have always been able to find the signs of epilepsy, as in male born criminals." Overall, he wrote that 26.9% of all epileptic men and 25% of all epileptic women have a "full criminal type" from the physiognomic point of view.

Lombroso went further, and suggested that some criminals exhibited "hidden epilepsy" (*epilessia larvata*) manifest by "sharp, sudden outbursts ... the psychological equivalents of physical seizures, marked by unpredictability and ferocity"; and that this hidden epilepsy was responsible for criminal acts, especially acts of physical or sexual violence (this notion became widely accepted, and a classic example of hidden epilepsy is in the character and crimes of Roubaud and Lantier in Zola's *La Bête humaine*, which was greatly influenced by Lombroso's work). In addition to this association with criminality, Lombroso also associated epilepsy with genius (at one point he wrote that all geniuses were epileptic). The association with criminality and genius, two extremes of behavior, was an attempt to explain deviation from the norm in biological terms. Lombroso was a liberal and respected thinker, the leading Italian intellectual of his time, and this view of epilepsy reflected the mountain of stigma which epilepsy carried at the time. His work was widely discussed by the general public. It formed the basis of famous novels (not least by Huysmans and Zola, whom Lombroso even argued was epileptic himself). Lombroso's theories of criminality had a profound influence on social theory for at least the next half century, and his lasting legacies are the medicalization of aberrant behaviors and the demonstration that social behavior had a biological basis. These themes have been the focus of research ever since; perhaps no more so than now.

Reflex theories of causation

The term *reflex epilepsy* also has its roots buried deeply in the historical thought on epilepsy. Galen referred to "sympathetic" epilepsy in which the cause was outside the nervous system and similar concepts have been long prevalent. Marshall Hall and Brown-Sequard preceded Jackson in exploring reflex mechanisms, and Reynolds and Jackson widely discussed the "reflex" theories of causation of epilepsy. The interest in "reflex seizures" in those days was a general interest in the possibility of reflexes underlying epilepsy, rather than in the narrow meaning of reflex seizures today. According to Jackson, "irritation" (of various types) could trigger seizures by draining the cerebral centers of their energy. The irritation could arise in the periphery, ears, eyes, teeth, digestive tract, or sexual organs. These conditions were sometimes classified as "sympathetic epilepsies" – in the sense that they were due not to a primary disorder of the brain but rather to a systemic irritation that triggered a seizure.

In the latter part of the century, a particular and common reflex cause was considered to be eyestrain, particularly in the American literature. Treatment was with eyeglasses and tenotomies (this is well discussed by Friedlander 2001). Other reflexes were induced by pain in a limb, by genital stimulation, and by pathologies in the ear or nose. Gowers in 1881 and 1901 includes pain and gastrointestinal disturbance within his category of reflex epilepsy, but nothing else. Turner (1907) recommended surgical excision of traumatic lesions of the peripheral nerves, removal of a tight prepuce in boys, treatment of coexistent diseases of the ears or nasopharynx and removal of foreign bodies, adenoid growths, and polypi to remove the reflex stimuli. He also mentioned that errors of refraction could be corrected and glasses worn, in view of the dramatic results of such treatment by Dodds, Gould, and Féré, but one senses a lack of enthusiasm about this senseless therapy.

Perhaps because of these obvious absurdities, the reflex theories fell out of fashion in the early twentieth century. However, Pavlov's demonstration of conditioned reflexes reignited interest in the possibility of epilepsy being a reflex phenomenon and Pavlov's theories were favored as the pathogenic mechanism, for instance, in the influential paper on musicogenic epilepsy by MacDonald Critchley (President of the International League Against Epilepsy [ILAE], 1949–53) in 1937. As time passed, the term reflex epilepsy began to refer to very specific sensory precipitants and acquired a meaning not dissimilar to that of today, referring largely to rare and curious cases.

Auto-intoxication

By 1900, a second widely held explanatory model of causation was gaining momentum – the theory of "auto-intoxication." According to this theory, epileptic seizures were caused by toxins produced within the person's own body (not dissimilar to Galen's theory of humors). Most believed that these toxins arose in the bowel, either through fermentation or from bacteria. This was backed up by reports for instance of sigmoidoscopy showing "acute angulation of the sigmoid colon" and "impaction of the sigmoid of an inordinate character" (Axtell 1910), and by radiological examination with bismuth showing "coloptosis" (Clark and Busby 1913; cited by Friedlander 2001). Experiments, which included the injections of blood from epileptic patients into rabbits, or intraperitoneally in guinea pigs, producing "violent convulsions," gave further credence to the auto-intoxication theories. Amongst the toxins actually responsible, much was written about uric acid. As a response to these theories, it was a short step to colectomy as a treatment of epilepsy, discussed further below.

Organic brain disease

During this period, the focus on theories of causation of epilepsy was not on organic brain diseases as such, but on predisposing and exciting factors, on Jackson's emphasis on mechanisms (vascular and nutritive), and on theories of inheritance, degeneration, reflex epilepsy, and auto-intoxication. Indeed, the epilepsies due to organic diseases of the brain (organic epilepsy; symptomatic epilepsy as it is known today) were often considered not "true" epilepsy. All however recognized that cerebral disease could cause epilepsy, and indeed following Jackson that its location determined the nature of the epilepsy. This lack of interest partly reflected the lack of investigatory tools (only postmortem and surgical neuropathology provided any help here) and also the lack of a systematic classification of the degenerative and particularly pediatric conditions. Neuropathology had identified, however, a number of organic disorders that were shown to have some sort of causal relationship with epilepsy. Of these, widely accepted were the developmental disorders (including porencephaly, heterotopy, microcephaly, and brain hypertrophy), asphyxia at birth, infantile hemiplegia and cerebral palsy, brain tumors, cerebral trauma causing a cicatrix, cerebral infection such as abscess, and degenerative conditions resulting in softening of the brain or other pathological findings.

William Aldren Turner 1907

Turner published his classic text on epilepsy in 1907 (Turner 1907) and devoted two chapters to the topic of etiology. These represented the advanced opinion of the day.

First discussed was heredity. Turner (Fig. 1.6) pointed out the difficulties in ascertaining this, citing problems in obtaining family histories and the inclusion of conditions which "do not stand in any causal relation to epilepsy, but are merely thrown in occasional connection with it, such as, tuberculosis, gout, and rheumatism." Turner differentiates these latter conditions from those of the "neuropathic disposition." However, Turner found that the most common feature of the neuropathic trait in an ancestral line of epileptics was epilepsy itself. Amongst his 676 epileptic patients, he found that 37.2% had a family history of epilepsy, and only 3.1% a family history of alcoholism, 5.4% of insanity, and 5.3% a family history of other neurological disorders of relevance ("nervousness," migraine, deaf-mutism, etc.); 49.0% had no known heredity factor. As Turner wrote:

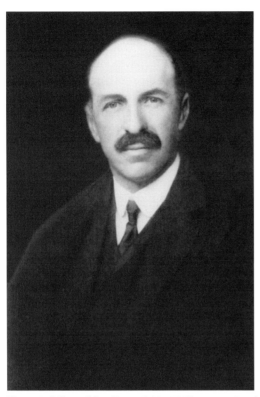

Fig. 1.6. William Aldren Turner (1864–1945) was appointed as full physician to the National Hospital Queen Square in 1900 and visiting physician to the Chalfont Colony in 1902.

Although epilepsy and insanity are the two main elements of the psychopathic hereditary degeneration, the existence in the family history of hysteria, chorea, the drug habit, migraine and paroxysmal headache, are important not so much from any direct bearing which they may have upon the development of epilepsy, but as indications, to some extent, of the neuropathic tendencies of a family. We find such disorders not uncommon in the family and personal histories of epileptics but it is difficult to prove that their occurrence is specially frequent.

The *signs* or *"stigmata" of degeneration* detected by Turner in his epileptic patients included: facial deformities (inequalities of the two sides of the face, irregularities of the nose, prognathism or arrested development of the lower jaw), deformities of the hard palate, dental abnormalities, deformities of the ears, deformities of the iris, abnormal arms, mental aberrations, stammering, and astigmatism. Amongst his own patients, the frequency of such stigmata was 66.5%, and Turner believed these signs were evidence of the "neuropathic disposition."

As he wrote in conclusion:

it is therefore obvious that in the majority of cases of epilepsy, no external exciting cause of the disease is necessary. Many conjectural explanations are given by the patient or his friends ... [e.g. trivial head injury, sunstroke] ... the real explanation is to be found in the rapid brain growth during the first few years of life, the onset of puberty and the full development of the reproductive organs, in

persons anatomically predisposed by heredity to nervous instability and convulsions ... It has also been shown that structural stigmata of degeneration, more particularly of the face, teeth, palate and ears, are frequent phenomena in the subjects of epilepsy, and that their presence is of great importance in determining, not only the degree of inherited predisposition, but also the severity of the disease.

Turner considered that the majority of cases were due to this "predisposition" (usually hereditary) and that an "exciting cause" was present in a minority of cases. The common "determining causes of epilepsy" (the exciting causes) were in his experience:

(1) Physiological causes – puberty, menses, pregnancy, puerperium, lack of sleep, ingestion of certain foods.
(2) Psychical causes – shock, emotional excitement, fear, anxiety, overwork.
(3) Pathological causes – exanthemata and acute infective diseases, organic diseases of the brain and trauma to the head, reflex epilepsies due to morbid conditions of various other organs, auto-infection from the alimentary canal, disorders of bodily metabolism and cerebral palsy.

In Turner's personal case series, psychical causes accounted for 4.1%, head trauma for 7.2%, acute infective causes for 5.6%, syphilis for 0.4%, and "cerebral birth palsy" for 5.9%.

Another important thread within Turner's conception of cause was the fact that once a fit had occurred, an "epileptic habit" is in danger of developing and thereafter fits occur even in the absence of any exciting cause – and here he is following Gowers. Because of this, early and immediate therapy was mandatory, and as Turner showed, many cases of early epilepsy if treated promptly do not go on to develop a chronic condition.

Theories of the causation of epilepsy 1907–1960

In the early part of this period, there were few lasting contributions to the study of etiology in epilepsy. The world wars possibly represented greater challenges to the ingenuity of humankind. In the world of epilepsy, therapeutic advances greatly outstripped interest in causation – and this was a period of major discovery in the fields of antiepileptic drugs and also neurosurgical therapy.

Auto-intoxication

In the early part of this period, interest in the auto-intoxication theory of causation gained momentum and in particular the view that epilepsy (and other conditions such as psychosis) was the symptom of low-grade infection, somewhere in the body. The gastrointestinal tract was the favored site and surgical resection of various parts of the gastrointestinal tract began to flourish. One illustrative, if extreme, enthusiast was the psychiatrist Dr. Henry Cotton who became superintendent of Trenton State Hospital in 1907, a residential institution for mentally handicapped, epileptic, or psychotic patients. He decided to eradicate these pockets of infection by surgical means and after 1916, a program of surgical therapy of extraordinary proportions began, largely for psychotic but also for epileptic patients. In one 12-month period, 6472 dental extractions were performed, as well as 542 tonsillectomies and 79 colon resections. Between 1918 and 1925, 2186 major operations were carried out. By 1921, Dr. Cotton was a national figure, lauded publicly for his remarkable cure rates (85% claimed for psychosis, for instance), interviewed by the national press and in 1921, the President of the American Medical Association declared that Trenton State was one of the country's "great institutions ... a monument to the most advanced civilization" (these details are taken from Nevins 2009).

Epilepsy as a result of lesional cerebral disease

This also was the period when neurosurgical pathology was being systematized and when imaging was beginning to visualize the brain in vivo. X-ray imaging was applied to epilepsy in the first decade of the twentieth century and in 1919 air encephalography followed and then in 1925 contrast ventriculography. In parallel, neurosurgery began to expand, based now not only on clinical semiology but also the results of these investigations.

An emphasis began to be placed on organic theories of causation, and neuropathology and neurosurgery began to reclaim epilepsy as a lesional disease of the brain, at least in Anglo-Saxon practice (it is interesting to note how the pendulum was swinging away from heredity in Britain and the USA, and in the opposite direction in Germany, France and Italy). A landmark in this surgical perspective was Walter Dandy's work, *The Brain*, published in Dean Lewis' *Practice of Surgery* in 1932 (Dandy 1932). Dandy took a very surgical viewpoint:

> Epilepsy is always regarded as an idiopathic disease. The theories of its causation are indeed so numerous as to reflect seriously upon any exclusive stand concerning its etiology or pathology. However, the writer is confident that there is now assembled from experimental, pathologic, clinical and surgical studies a sufficient number of unquestioned facts to place epilepsy unequivocally upon a pathologic instead of idiopathic basis ... the fundamental conception that in every case of epilepsy there is a lesion of the brain can no longer admit of doubt ... The lesions causing epilepsy are most varied. Although superficially of such dissimilar character, fundamentally they act in the same way, i.e., each represents a defect in the nervous paths of the cerebral hemisphere.

He recognized 17 categories of "lesions causing epilepsy" (Table 1.5) which seem by today's standards a rather curious mélange, but no doubt reflected advanced neurosurgical opinion of his time.

The emphasis on the organic basis of epilepsy was systematized in the classic neurological text of the mid 1930s, the three-volume textbook of neurology by SA Kinnier Wilson, published posthumously in 1940 (Wilson 1940) (Fig. 1.7). Seventy-five pages are devoted to *The Epilepsies*, and these

Table 1.5 Dandy's 17 categories of brain lesions causing epilepsy

Congenital malformation and maldevelopment, either general or focal

Tumors

Abscesses

Tubercles

Gummata

Aneurysms

Syphilis with or without demonstrable gummata or vascular occlusions

Areas of cerebral degeneration and calcification

Depressed fractures

Hamartomata

Foreign bodies

Injuries from trauma at birth or subsequently (focal or general)

Connective tissue formation after trauma

Atrophy of the brain after trauma

Thrombosis and embolism

Cerebral arteriosclerosis

Sequelae of obscure inflammatory processes including encephalitis

provide a glimpse of the contemporary Anglo-Saxon thought on the topic, and show the same organic tendencies as Dandy: "Current opinion is ... veering round to the view that all epilepsies are symptomatic, inclusive of the variety [idiopathic epilepsy] whose basis still elude search ... the cause will eventually be revealed." Wilson makes the first reference I can find to the term "cryptogenic" which he feels is preferable to refer to epilepsies of unknown cause.

Regarding etiology, Wilson averred from listing all the known causes – as he put it, this "would be an act of supererogation" – but singled out a few for discussion. On the question of heredity, he is interesting, for this was the time that eugenics was having a major impact on social policy in many parts of the world, and about to reach its ghastly climax in Germany. Wilson thought that inherited epilepsy was uncommon. Myerson (1932) had published an influential survey of the heredity of mental disorders, and Wilson cites his findings that there was a family history of epilepsy amongst 1500 inmates of a hospital for epileptics in only four families (11 persons), and at the same institution 138 marriages of epileptics resulted in 553 offspring among whom a history of fits was got in only 10 or 1.8%. As Wilson put it: "The influence of the factor [heredity] is persistently overvalued; in only about one-fifth of my material has it seemed to be operative." Head trauma is extensively discussed, and Wilson cited a 1920s survey of the UK Ministry of Pension of 18 000 persons with gunshot wounds of the head, finding an incidence of

NEUROLOGY

BY

S. A. KINNIER WILSON

M.A., M.D., D.Sc.(Edin.), F.R.C.P.

FORMERLY PHYSICIAN, NATIONAL HOSPITAL, QUEEN SQUARE ; SENIOR NEUROLOGIST, KING'S
COLLEGE HOSPITAL ; CONSULTING NEUROLOGIST, METROPOLITAN ASYLUMS BOARD (L.C.C.) ;
OFFICER DE L'INSTRUCTION PUBLIQUE, R.F. ; HONORARY FELLOW, ROYAL ACADEMY OF MEDICINE,
TURIN ; HONORARY MEMBER, ROYAL ACADEMY OF MEDICINE, BELGIUM, NATIONAL ACADEMY OF
MEDICINE, RIO DE JANEIRO, NEUROLOGICAL SOCIETIES OF ITALY, POLAND, DENMARK, HOLLAND,
BRAZIL, PARIS, VIENNA, NEW YORK AND PHILADELPHIA, THE JAPANESE ASSOCIATION OF PSY-
CHIATRY AND NEUROLOGY, THE SOCIETY OF GERMAN NEUROLOGISTS, THE MEDICAL SOCIETY OF
COPENHAGEN AND THE AMERICAN NEUROLOGICAL ASSOCIATION ; CORRESPONDING MEMBER,
NEUROLOGICAL SOCIETY OF WARSAW.

EDITED BY

A. NINIAN BRUCE

F.R.C.P.(Edin.), D.Sc.(Edin.), M.D., F.R.S.(Edin.)
Lt.-Col. R.A.M.C.

CONSULTING PHYSICIAN BANGOUR MENTAL HOSPITAL AND ST. ANDREW'S HOSPITAL, STIRCHES ;
LECTURER IN PHYSIOLOGY, NEUROLOGY AND PSYCHIATRY, THE UNIVERSITY, EDINBURGH ;
HONORARY MEMBER AMERICAN PSYCHIATRIC ASSOCIATION ; MEMBRE CORRESPONDANT ÉTRANGER,
SOCIÉTÉ DE NEUROLOGIE DE PARIS ; MEMBRE ASSOCIÉ ÉTRANGER, SOCIÉTÉ MÉDICO-PSYCHO-
LOGIQUE, PARIS.

VOLUME I

LONDON
EDWARD ARNOLD & CO.

Fig. 1.7. Samuel A. Kinnier Wilson (1878–1937) was physician at the National Hospital Queen Square from 1912 until his death. His book was published posthumously in 1940.

post-traumatic epilepsy of only 4.5%. In civilian cases, he cites figures of between 3% and 21%. He dismisses the importance of "bad teeth, septic tonsils, nasal polypi, refractive errors, phimosis, intestinal worm, and what not," but mentions seizures during anesthesia ("ether convulsions"), pleural epilepsy (now we would consider this vasovagal) and cysticercosis (an imperial disease, as he noted that "although infestation may occur in England, the majority contracted the disease in Egypt, India or the Malay states"). He discusses precipitating factors such as cosmic influences (dismissed), sleep, menstrual epilepsy and pregnancy (including eclampsia) and psychical states. Wilson's chapter on epilepsy is a masterpiece, with a detailed elaboration of symptoms, pathogenesis, classification, and treatment. On etiology we see a truly modern view emerging for the first time.

Wilson's influence was evident in all subsequent textbooks, at least until 1960. By 1949, for instance, another standard work, *Neurology* by F. M. R. Walshe (also neurologist to the National Hospital Queen Square and who was appointed editor of *Epilepsia* in 1959/60) could state:

> it is better to speak of "the epilepsies" according to the various known exciting factors than to keep the category of idiopathic epilepsy. Nevertheless, from the practical point of view of diagnosis and treatment the two categories of "idiopathic" and "symptomatic" epilepsy remain useful ... It has always been regarded as a heritable condition, though it obeys no known laws of inheritance, and it is probably that what is inherited – if anything be   is an instability of function in the cells of the cerebral cortex.

As Walshe put it, "nothing is known of the 'exciting' causes of idiopathic epilepsy," and "certainly the heritable causes of epilepsy have been greatly exaggerated in the past, and in consequence severe restrictions upon the liberty of conduct of the epileptic have been imposed in the guise of medical advice" (Walshe 1949). Symptomatic epilepsy "may occur as a symptom of a wide range of diseases of the brain." Walshe singles out head injury, cysticercosis, and cortical venous angioma.

This was a period too when the causes of inherited metabolic diseases of the nervous system began to yield their secrets, as a result of advances in clinical chemistry. The earliest to do so was *phenylketonuria*. The discovery of the metabolic cause of this hereditary condition was the result of painstaking research by the Norwegian physician Ivar Asbjørn Følling in 1934. He found abnormal acid substances in the blood and urine of two affected siblings, screened others in children near Oslo and found eight other patients. After extensive tests, he discovered that the substance was phenylpyruvic acid, and in 1947 the metabolic defect was unraveled (Christ 2003). This superb research work stimulated similar researches in other disorders and the new discipline of inherited metabolic disease arose.

Eugenics

In parallel with the rational and organic views of causation of epilepsy, theories of heredity and degeneration continued to be influential, and out of these came the eugenics movement which played a major role in epileptology in the early twentieth century. Eugenics of course had the advantage of the discovery of Mendelian genetics which was not available to the earlier writers (although Mendel's work was published first in 1866, it was only in the first years of the twentieth century that it became widely appreciated). Many of the early ILAE leaders were active eugenicists, such as Weeks, Munson, Schou, and Lennox. Eugenics permeated not only medical but also social thought and became the "scientific" basis for the Nazi atrocities of the Second World War. Persons with epilepsy were of course extremely vulnerable to eugenic practice, given the theories of degeneration, atavism, and criminality associated with the disease and the stigma of the disease in the public mind, and the undeniable genetic basis in many cases. Eugenic thought permeated many scientific disciplines of the period and influenced social policy. Eugenic solutions were proposed to all the social evils thought to reflect the degeneration of populations, the decline in the civilized social order, the tendencies to atavism, and the downward spiral of morality. Epilepsy became a focus for the eugenics movement, as did insanity, mental deficiency, alcoholism, and racial differences.

According to eugenic theory, epilepsy was inherited by Mendelian mechanisms, and thus by either positive or negative eugenic practices could potentially be removed (or at least minimized) from a population (the evidence of simple Mendelian inheritance is slight now and was slight then, but was glossed over, and the eugenic concepts of heredity were staggeringly simplistic). Enforced sterilization of epileptics was first enacted in the USA (a famous case was that of *Buck* v. *Bell*, in which Judge Wendell Holmes confirmed the legality of sterilization with the words: "It is better for all the world, if instead of waiting to execute degenerate offspring for crime or to let them starve for their imbecility, society can prevent those who are manifestly unfit from continuing their kind ... Three generations of imbeciles are enough"), and followed in several continental countries. In Nazi Germany, eugenic theory was taken further, and mass murder of the unfit (including epileptics) was sanctioned. In the early 1940s, *Action T4*, a program of killings ("euthanasia") of the handicapped was inaugurated. Physicians provided the names, and the victims were gassed or poisoned. It has been estimated that between 200 000 and 250 000 mentally and physically handicapped persons were murdered from 1939 to 1945 under the *Action T4* and other "euthanasia" programs. How many persons with epilepsy perished is not known. When the war was over, eugenicists tried to distance the scientific study of eugenics from these events, but the clear link shamed the topic into scientific obscurity, at least for the next 50 years.

Electroencephalography, hippocampal sclerosis, and temporal lobe epilepsy

As is self-evident, the discovery of "etiology" in epilepsy is heavily dependent on new technology. In the early post-war years, the major methodological advance in the field of epilepsy was of course the electroencephalograph (EEG). The first human EEG recording was published in 1929 by Hans Berger, a German psychiatrist in Jena, but Berger was considered an outcast by his German colleagues and in 1941 committed suicide when the Nazi government removed him from his university post. Berger had coined the term *Elektenkephalogram*, defined the alpha rhythm (the "Berger rhythm"), and in 1933 recorded a partial seizure. His discovery passed initially unnoticed until Adrian and Matthews (1934) confirmed his observations in a celebrated paper in *Brain*. Then the potential of EEG in epilepsy became apparent and rapid advances were made. Fischer and Lowenbach (1934) demonstrated

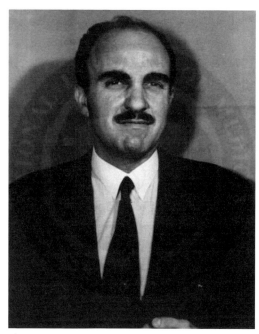

Fig. 1.8. Henri Gastaut (1915–95), President of the ILAE 1969–1973, and founder and physician to the Centre St Paul in Marseilles.

epileptiform spikes, Gibbs, Davis, and Lennox (1935) described interictal spike waves and the three cycles per second pattern of clinical absence seizures, and in 1936 Gibbs and co-workers reported the interictal spike as the signature of focal epilepsy. Electroencephalography, it appeared in these exciting times, was a method of visualizing physiology and it was enthusiastically applied to the discovery of the hidden causes of epilepsy. An immediate discovery was the EEG signature of absence seizures, which from the point of view of discovery of structural causes was in a way unfortunate, as absence seizures are of course a paradigmatic example of idiopathic epilepsy (although, later genetic studies were greatly assisted by the EEG signature of 3 Hz spike and wave as a biomarker of etiology). The EEG changes in brain tumors and other structural lesions were also recognized, but these proved disappointingly non-specific and the diagnostic utility of EEG was soon largely obliterated by the discovery of computed tomography (CT) scanning.

However, EEG proved invaluable in defining temporal lobe epilepsy and in this way led to the recognition of the etiological importance in epilepsy of hippocampal sclerosis. A key player in this regard was Henri Gastaut (Fig. 1.8), who held a landmark conference on the topic of temporal lobe epilepsy in 1953 (Gastaut 1953; Shorvon 2006). The (ictal and interictal) features of temporal lobe epilepsy had been unraveled in the 1940s, and the findings were summarized in Gastaut's papers for the 1956 meeting. Fifty years later, there is really very little to add, and what knowledge has been accrued in this interval is incremental at best. He reported the EEG findings from scalp recordings, electrocorticography, and depth recordings. In regards to underlying pathology, Gastaut clearly recognized that hippocampal sclerosis was often the causal lesion, contrary to the classic opinion of Spielmeyer, still widely held at that time. However, he did not recognize the association with febrile seizures. He believed that trauma was the commonest cause of temporal lobe epilepsy, resulting in contusional damage to the brain as it was compressed against the sphenoid bone or the free edge of the tentorium. He viewed encephalitis as the second most frequent cause (20–25% of cases). The third cause (5% of cases) was obstetrical injury, which in Gastaut's view resulted in herniation of the temporal lobe over the tentorial edge, causing vascular compression of the anterior choroidal (and other) arteries. The consequential ischemia was thought to be responsible for incisural sclerosis.

Not everyone accepted at that time that the mesial temporal structures were the site of temporal lobe seizures, and surprisingly (given his prominence in the field of EEG) Gibbs believed the seizures originated in temporal neocortex and this was the subject of fierce debate. By 1953, Jasper could write that, from the physiological point of view, "the periamygdaloid and rhinencephalic portions of the temporal lobe, including the extent of the hippocampal gyri and often the pes hippocampi, are nearly always severely affected in patients with temporal lobe seizures." The surgical treatment of temporal lobe epilepsy initially was confined to resection to the temporal neocortex, but within a few years, it was fully recognized that the mesial structures needed to be resected to effect a cure (see de Almeida *et al.* 2008; Moran and Shorvon 2009) and the work of Penfield and Murray Falconer reported at the 1953 congress showed how far knowledge had advanced. Perhaps from the clinical point of view, the only really fundamental subsequent clinical advance was the simple visualization of hippocampal atrophy by volumetric magnetic resonance imaging (MRI) (Jack *et al.* 1990; Cook *et al.* 1992; Shorvon *et al.* 1992). The experimental elucidation of the neurochemical and neurophysiological mechanisms of excitotoxic brain damage had to wait a further decade until the seminal work of Meldrum and colleagues in the 1970s (Meldrum and Brierley 1973; Meldrum and Horton 1973; Meldrum *et al.* 1973).

William Lennox

This brings this survey to 1960, and the publication by Lennox of his two-volume book – *Epilepsy and Related Disorders* (Lennox 1960) (Fig. 1.9). Lennox wrote extensively about the then current theories of etiology and his book is a good source of information on this topic. Lennox of course was a committed eugenicist and deeply interested in the genetic predisposition to seizures. His book provides a relatively clear explanation of his views on "causation" which can be summarized as follows:

(1) Epilepsy is due to a combination of: (i) genetic (essential) causes; (ii) acquired causes; and (iii) precipitating causes.

(2) Of these the genetic causes are the most important. As Lennox put it, "we personally believe that nature outnumbers nurture. The relative importance of the latter

is decreasing because of better control of preventable conditions."

He followed his nineteenth-century predecessors in proposing that in many cases (50% in Lennox's view) there were "predisposing" (genetic) and "precipitating" (acquired) causes, and indeed draws an analogy with fire in exactly the same way as Sieveking (Lennox 1960, vol. 1, p. 528). However, it is his "analogy of the reservoir or river" (Fig. 1.10) which encapsulates his thought best, and it is worth quoting directly from Lennox:

> Causes may be represented as the sources of a reservoir. At the bottom is the already present volume of water, which represents the person's predisposition, a fundamental cause. But the reservoir is supplied also by streams which represent the contributory conditions, such as lesions of the brain acquired since conception, certain disorders of bodily function and emotional disturbances. Periodic overflow of the bank represents a seizure.

Another graphic description is the portrayal of the sources of the river (Fig. 1.11).

> The genetic watershed is represented . . . as three generations: parents, grandparents and great-grandparents [e.g. at A, a paternal grandmother has epilepsy]. A confluence of transmitted traits follows into (and through) the patient . . . In addition to these branching streams, there is an independent stream which rises in a lake (the uterus). The outlet is the birth canal and below that are contributing streams: infections [e.g. at B, a viral encephalitis], brain trauma from diverse sources, brain tumor, and circulatory disorders. This side stream enters the main stream at the patient level and combines with the genetic influences which had travelled through three generations to make him epileptic. There is then a third stream which enters below the confluence of the two main streams. This represents transient conditions which may precipitate certain seizures in a person already epileptic, or "all set" to be. This evoking circumstance may be physiologic (say at C, hypoglycaemia) or emotional (say at D, a broken wedding-engagement).

According to Lennox, about 20% of epilepsies are purely genetic, 20% are purely acquired, and about 50% are a mixture of both (leaving 10% in which the cause is quite unknown). The genetic epilepsies were predominant, and in his words "Evidence for this [genetic causation] is relatively simple and convincing: namely, some blood relative who has been subject to seizures which were not the consequence of some acquired brain injury." From a modern perspective, it is a pity that the heredity is not as simple as that. Lennox carried out research based on family trees, much as his eugenic predecessors had done, and particularly on twins.

The acquired causes, less important in Lennox's view than the genetic ones, included a variety of conditions, listed in Table 1.6.

In the category of acquired epilepsy (organic epilepsy), Lennox included developmental defects, but realized that there were strong genetic links ("it would be the channel that joins the genetic river system to the uterine lake"). Lennox used the

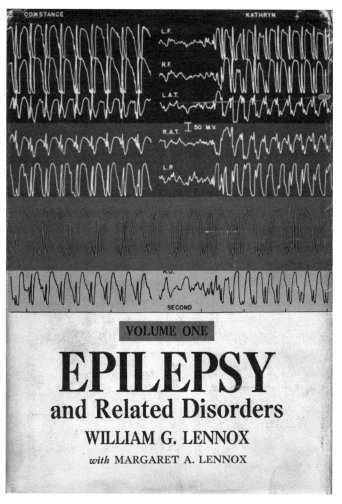 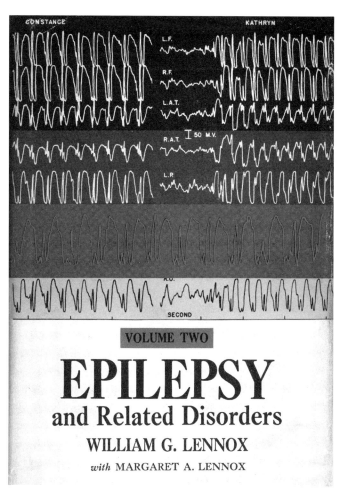

Fig. 1.9. The two volumes of *Epilepsy and Related Disorders* by William Lennox (1884–1960). Lennox was appointed to the Harvard Medical School in 1922 and founded the Seizure Unit in the Children's Hospital in Boston in 1944.

term "hereditary organic epilepsy" to describe inherited genetic conditions that result in structural disorders of the brain. Included here were: mongolism, tuberose sclerosis (epiloia), and various malformations of development.

Lennox also realized that there were other considerations. He cites the use of the term "parahereditary" by continental authors to indicate conditions that are not strictly speaking genetic, but which can alter the sperm or the ovum – and here includes alcohol, syphilis, infections, and intoxications. These were essentially Lamarckian theories which were important in understanding some of the mechanisms of degeneration with which Lennox had considerable residual sympathy despite the by then growing evidence of the Nazi misuse of eugenic and genetic theories.

Finally, Lennox was also interested in the causes and features of mental handicap. He cited Yannet (1950) who categorized mental handicap in his institution as:

(A) Familial defect – 30% of all cases ("probably dependent on multiple dominant genes")
(B) Phenylpyruvic oligophrenia

(C) Congenital ectodermosis ("these include tuberose sclerosis, neurofibromatosis, cerebal angiomatosis")
(D) Hereditary idiocy ("fortunately rare")
(E) Heredodegenerative cerebral diseases, which are of two groups: (i) the ganglion cells are principally affected (e.g. infantile Tay–Sachs disease) and (ii) white matter is principally affected (e.g., Scholz, Krabe, and Schilder disease); 45% of all cases.

Lennox also mentions that "Then there is mongolism, the etiology of which is in question. 10% of cerebral palsy might be of congenital origin. There are also cretinism and cranial anomalies to consider." He also cites Penrose (1949), reporting on the English institutional population of 558 patients (Table 1.7).

In Lennox's own series of 927 patients with acquired epilepsy (out of 1648 persons, 69% office and 31% clinic patients) the distribution of cases is shown in Table 1.8. Where it was possible to assess, 46% of cases developed within 1 year of the causative event, 19% in the subsequent 2 years, and 12% after 10 or more years.

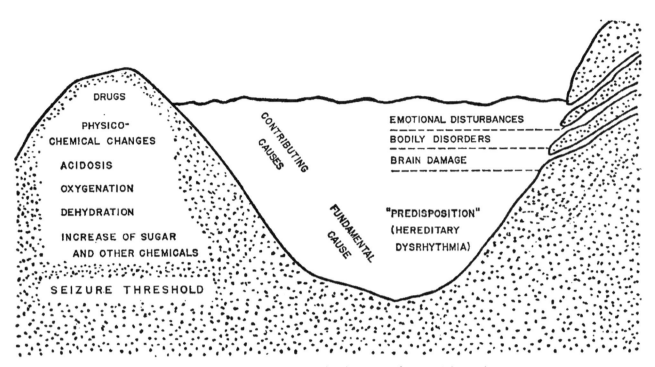

Fig. 1.10. Lennox's pictorial concept of the causes of epilepsy, represented as the sources of a reservoir (see text).

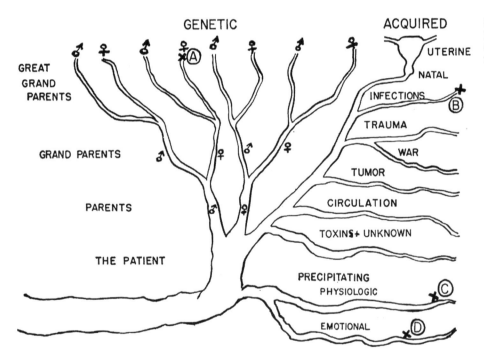

Fig. 1.11. Lennox's pictorial concept of the interaction of the genetic and environmental causes of epilepsy, here represented as tributaries of a river (see text).

Lennox carried out considerable research himself into the genetic basis of epilepsy, and managed to reconcile his eugenic sympathies with his clinical work. His writings mark the end of an era. In the next few decades the scientific advances in imaging, clinical and molecular biochemistry, and molecular genetics would stimulate research in a variety of new directions. Lennox was extremely influential not least in also establishing American epileptology at the forefront of the discipline, and his influence can be still felt today in his picturesque and rather folksy theories of causation and his views on the "epileptic threshold" and on the multifactorial nature of causation. His genetics though now seems thoroughly outdated, and his eugenic writing is rejected.

Table 1.6 Lennox's list of acquired causes of epilepsy

Congenital abnormalities – developmental defects

    Hereditary organic epilepsy

    Mongolism (fetalism)

    Hereditary (Huntington's) chorea

    Tuberose sclerosis

    Amaurotic familial idiocy

    Various other pathologic states

Intrauterine misfortunes

    Embryonic versus fetal timing of insult

    Placental transmission (rubella, toxoplasmosis, erythroblastosis fetalis)

    Intracranial hemangioma

    The cerebral palsies

    Paranatal epilepsy

    Difficulties of parturition

    Postnatal epilepsy

    Infection-derived epilepsy (viral, bacterial, bacillary, spirochetal, protozoan, metazoan)

    Post-traumatic epilepsy (including lobotomy, the wounds of war)

    Brain tumors

    Defects of cerebral circulation

    Toxins and intoxications (alohol, ergot, chemical, lead, radiation)

Table 1.8 The causes of epilepsy in Lennox's series of 927 patients with acquired epilepsy

Cause	Percentage
Paranatal	38.0
Postnatal trauma	25.2
Infections	19.5
Brain tumors	6.7
Circulatory	5.3
Other causes	5.3

Afterthoughts

The purpose of any historical survey should be primarily to put current thought into a proper perspective and to provide a lineage for contemporary ideas. In relation to causation in epilepsy, some general points stand out.

The first is the obvious emphasis on "idiopathic" epilepsy, at the expense of symptomatic epilepsy, at least

Table 1.7 Distribution of causes of mental defect amongst 558 patients in an English Institution, and proportion with epilepsy

	Percent of total	Percent epileptic
Mongolism	11.3	1.6
Endocrine disorder	15.8	14.8
Congenital syphilis	9.0	28.0
Neurologic lesion	22.9	46.1
Cranial malformations	25.4	23.9
Miscellaneous	15.6	25.3
	Total = 100%	25.2%

Source: Penrose (1949).

until the 1930s. This was a period when the assignment of any organic etiology relied on the history and on the pathological findings at operation or postmortem. There were few investigatory methods available, and the lack of emphasis on symptomatic causes was thus in part due to a lack of tools to investigate etiology at a clinical level. It was only with the wider use of neurosurgery that organic etiologies began to take on prominence, and the major early work was that of Walter Dandy, a pioneer neurosurgeon, but his list of etiologies looks peculiar to the modern eye – although his early emphasis on congenital lesions is prescient. Some early studies of "etiology" of such cases (in particular those of Jackson) were focused on the final common pathways of epilepsy in all these cases. Today we make the distinction between the "mechanisms" of epileptogenesis (increased excitation, defects in ion channels, etc.) and the causes of epilepsy, whereas in Jackson's time this was not the case. There is much to commend in Jackson's approach, and exactly how causal lesions translate into epilepsy is still largely unknown – the work discussed in Chapter 63 on epilepsy due to gliomas for instance is a model of how we should proceed. However, the focus on how such a wide range of causes results in the same clinical forms of epilepsy (a focus on "mechanisms" rather than "causes") may be profitable in terms of therapy and certainly it is striking how little we know about any differences in effect of antiepileptic drug therapy in different etiologies.

Linked to the lack of investigatory methods to uncover organic lesions was the emphasis on heredity, using family trees and physiognomic measurements as investigatory tools. There was in this early period a universal agreement that epilepsy had strong hereditary influences. The estimates of the contribution of heredity varied considerably, no doubt partly due to the inclusion of epilepsy within the category of inherited degeneration and the neurological trait. In clinical and family-history studies, the higher rates of an inherited tendency were due to the inclusion of insanity, moral degeneration, and alcoholism for instance. It is interesting to note that the theories of a neurological taint mirror in a striking way the current interest in "comorbidities." Exactly the same types of mental disorder, alcoholism, and dementia are found in contemporary statistical surveys of patients with epilepsy. The fashion for "comorbidity" lacks the unifying theory of a taint or degeneration but in other ways follows the statistically based methods of the early-nineteenth-century physicians closely. Comorbidity is now seldom considered to be genetically based, but it seems to me possible that there are mechanistic links between cryptogenic epilepsy and other neurological diseases (in effect a modern inquiry into the neurological trait), or links between epilepsy and cerebral degenerative mechanisms. Further studies in this area might be well worth conducting, in the hope of uncovering common mechanisms (the Jacksonian meaning of "etiology") that may give a clue to the genetic basis of epilepsy and these other conditions. Recent work on genetic copy-number variants is of great interest in this regard, and deletions or duplications might provide a mechanism for inheritance of comorbidities. Certainly, the current genetic inquiry into the causes of epilepsy has had only limited success, focusing as it has done on the artificially determined phenotypes, syndromes, and seizure classifications. A warning from history, though; in the period under study here, the link of epilepsy to degeneration and to mental disorder resulted in enormous stigma culminating in eugenic measures to restrict reproduction and ultimately in the murder of handicapped persons. Whether similar inquiries would now be ethical or wise, given the societal consequences of previous genetic inquiries into epilepsy (stigma, sterilization, extermination), is questionable. Such considerations are never far from the surface.

It is interesting to note too the impact of social influences on theories of etiology. The anxiety in many areas of social theory about degeneration found a reflection in the degenerative theories of the etiology of epilepsy. Similarly, theories of criminality were incorporated into etiological studies of epilepsy. Eugenic research in epilepsy was driven by political and social forces. Science has a social responsibility and is never neutral or objective, a fact often forgotten in the laboratory, and to ignore these can be disastrous, as was the case in the 1930s.

One delusion of neuroscience (and probably other branches of medicine too) is that its contemporary position inevitably is the most scientifically advanced. The awkward reality is that the march of neuroscience has had an erratic course, veering up many culs de sac. Examples are numerous, and include psychoanalysis, theories of hysteria, eugenics and *dégénérescence* (and more recently some of the work on functional imaging). It has been a trajectory influenced by dominant personalities whose theories are simply wrong, by hubris, by social forces and public fashion – today as much as ever. The evolution of etiological theories of epilepsy illustrates this clearly.

Another rather remarkable feature of "epilepsy" is that the widely used classification schemes do not incorporate etiology. It is often taught, and is a fundamental neurological canon, that epilepsy is a "symptom" not a "condition" but this is not reflected in our classification schemes. This deficiency was recognized too in the period under study, but it was thought, generally, that a comprehensive scheme was not possible. In 1897, Peterson, a leading American epileptologist, wrote: "A classification based strictly on etiology is not possible ... in the light of present knowledge, but such a classification would be more scientific and valuable [than other types of classification]" (cited by Friedlander 2001). However, with the modern neuroimaging, molecular biology, and genetics perhaps for the first time in the modern history of epilepsy, today such a classification could be useful, and might make far more sense than our current semiological or EEG classification schemes. One can muse upon what the classification of epilepsy today might look like if EEG had not been invented before neuroimaging – I suspect, a more useful and valid scheme would have been devised. What can be learnt from the older classification schemes? In my view, Reynolds' was the most interesting, and his concept of eccentric and diathetic epilepsies is superior generally to ours of acute symptomatic epilepsy. In Reynolds' time, there was little distinction made between "causes" and "precipitating factors" – and much more focus on precipitants than currently. This too is a topic worth reappraisal, not least the genetic mechanisms of precipitants (such as stress, menstrual disturbance). Linked to the issues of precipitation are the theories of reflex causation, which were accepted by Jackson and Gowers, and which too warrant modern assessment.

Clinical neurology is essentially an applied science, and the discovery of etiology is to a large extent methodology-driven. The introduction of clinical chemistry, EEG, neuroimaging, and neurogenetics each has changed our perceptions of etiology. Clinical chemistry and molecular genetics unraveled the causes of most of the Mendelian inherited metabolic epilepsies, EEG led in defining the idiopathic generalized epilepsies and epilepsy syndromes, and neuroimaging technologies diverted attention to the structural cerebral changes, leading to the appreciation of the importance of hippocampal sclerosis and disorders of cortical development for instance. I suspect we are now reaching the limits of detection of visible structural change, and whether further inquiry in this direction will yield useful etiological information is doubtful. The most recent focus is on the genetic basis of epilepsy, and the recognition of the role of ion channel defects (see Chapter 3) is the result of the experimental work. However, whilst genetic research has discovered etiologies in rare families, it has not so far illuminated causation in the majority of cases. However, it remains true that there is almost certainly a significant genetic contribution to the causation of many (perhaps most) cases of epilepsy, even if this is currently undefined. It should not be forgotten that epilepsy is essentially a functional disorder (as Jackson pointed out) and future research into the neuronal networks, system changes, and neuronal properties in epilepsy seem to hold most promise for future inquiry into epilepsy. This will require new tools and methodologies, which are likely to be in the fields of molecular genetics, chemistry, and physiology. Today, between 30% and 50% of all cases remain "cryptogenic" to use Kinnier Wilson's term, and the challenge for the next phase of etiological research in epilepsy is surely to understand these functional and molecular mechanisms, and to revert to a concept of etiology, as mechanism, akin to that of Jackson.

References

Adrian ED, Matthews BHC (1934) The Berger rhythm: potential changes from the occipital lobes in man. *Brain* **57**:355–85.

de Almeida AN, Teixeira MJ, Feindel WH (2008) From lateral to mesial: the quest for a surgical cure for temporal lobe epilepsy. *Epilepsia* **49**:98–107.

Axtell W (1910) Acute angulation and flexure of the sigmoid a causative factor in epilepsy: preliminary report of thirty-one cases. *Am J Surg* **24**:385–7.

Binswanger O (1899) *Die Epilepsie*. Vienna: Alfred Hölder.

Buffon G-LL (1780) Treatise on the degeneration of animals. In: *Natural History General and Particular of the Count de Buffon*, vol. **vii**, pp. 392–453. Edinburgh: William Creech.

Christ SE (2003) Asbjørn Følling and the discovery of phenylketonuria. *J Hist Neurosci* **12**:44–54.

Clark L, Busby A (1913) Value of roentgen analysis of gastrointestinal tract in some types of so-called functional nervous disorders: a preliminary report. *Trans Am Neurol Ass* **39**:125–41.

Cook MJ, Fish DR, Shorvon SD, Straughan K, Stevens JM (1992) Hippocampal volumetric and morphometric studies in frontal and temporal lobe epilepsy. *Brain* **115**:1001–15.

Dandy WE (1932) *The Brain*. In: Lewis D (ed.) *The Practice of Surgery*, vol. **XII**. Hagerstown, MD: WF Prior.

Déjerine JJ (1886) *L'Hérédité dans les maladies du système nerveux*. Paris: Asselin and Houzeau.

Doran RE (1903) A consideration of the hereditary factors in epilepsy. *Am J Insanity* **60**:61–73.

Echeverria MG (1873) On epileptic insanity. *Am J Insanity* **30**:1–51.

Esquirol J-ED (1838) *Des maladies mentales considerées sous les rapports médical, hygiénique et médico-légal*. Paris: JB Baillière.

Falret JP (1864) *Maladies mentales et des asiles d'aliénés*. Paris: JB Baillière.

Féré C (1884) La famille névropathique. *Archives de Neurologie* **19**:9–25.

Fischer MH, Lowenbach H (1934) Aktionsstrome des Zentralnervensystems unter des Einwirkung von Krampfgiften 1. Mitteilung. Strychnin und pikrotoxin. *Arch Exper Path Pharmak* **174**:357–82.

Friedlander WJ (2001) *The History of Modern Epilepsy: The Beginning, 1865–1914*. Westport, CT: Greenwood Press.

Gastaut H (1953) International League Against Epilepsy Report of the Quadrennial Meeting: So-called "psychomotor" and "temporal" epilepsy: a critical study. With discussion papers by Falconer M, Fulton J, Fuster B, Gibbs FA, Guillaume J, Mazar G, Mazar Y, Jasper HH, Kaada B, Lennox M, Lennox WG, MacLean PD, Magnus O, Masland R, Paine KWE, Pampiglione G, Penfield W, Schwab RS, Subirana A, with closing remarks by Merlis JK. *Epilepsia* **2**:56–100.

Gibbs FA, Davis H, Lennox WG (1935) The electro-encephalogram in epilepsy and in conditions of impaired consciousness. *Arch Neurol Psychiatry* **34**:1133–48.

Gibbs FA, Lennox WG, Gibbs EL (1936) The electroencephalogram in diagnosis and localization of epileptic seizures. *Arch Neurol Psychiatry* **1936**:1225–35.

Gowers W (1881) *Epilepsy and Other Chronic Convulsive Disorders*. London: Churchill.

Gowers W (1888) *A Manual of Diseases of the Nervous System*. London: Churchill.

Jack CR Jr., Sharbrough FW, Twomey CK, et al. (1990) Temporal lobe seizures: lateralization with MR volume measurements of the hippocampal formation. *Radiology* **175**:423–9.

Jackson JH (1873) On the anatomical, physiological and pathological investigation of epilepsies. *West Riding Lunatic Asylum Medical Reports* **iii**:315.

Jackson JH (1874) On the scientific and empirical investigation of epilepsies. *Med Press Circular* 1874 **18**:325–7, 347–52, 389–92, 409–12, 475–8, 497–9, 519–21.

Lombroso C (1876–1897) *L'uomo delinquente*. Milan: Hoepli.

Lombroso C, Ferrero W (1893) *La donna delinquente, la prostituta e la donna normale*. Turin: Roux.

Meldrum BS, Brierley JB (1973) Prolonged epileptic seizures in primates: ischemic cell change and its relation to ictal physiological events. *Arch Neurol* **28**:10–17.

Meldrum BS, Horton RW (1973) Physiology of status epilepticus in primates. *Arch Neurol* **28**:1–9.

Meldrum BS, Vigouroux RA, Brierley JB (1973) Systemic factors and epileptic brain damage: prolonged seizures in paralyzed, artificially ventilated baboons. *Arch Neurol* **29**:82–7.

Moran D, Shorvon SD (2009) The surgery of temporal lobe epilepsy. I. Historical development, patient selection, and seizure outcome. In: Shorvon SD, Pedley T (eds.) *Blue Book of Neurology*, vol. 3, *The Epilepsies*. Philadelphia, PA: WB Saunders, pp. 294–306.

Moreau LL (1859) *La Psychologie morbide dans ses rapports avec la philosophie de l'histoire*. Paris: Masson.

Morel BA (1857) *Traité des dégénérescences physiques, intellectuelles, et morales des l'espèce humaine*. Paris: JB Baillière.

Morel BA (1860) *Traité des maladies mentales*. Paris: Masson.

Myerson A (1932) *The Inheritance of Mental Diseases*. Baltimore, MD: Williams and Wilkins.

Nevins M (2009) *A Tale of Two "Villages": Vineland and Skillman, NJ*. New York: Universe.

Penrose LS (1949) *The Biology of Mental Defect*. London: Grune and Stratton.

Reynolds JR (1861) *Epilepsy: Its Symptoms, Treatment and Relation to Other Chronic Convulsive Diseases*. London: Churchill.

Shorvon S (2006) An episode in the history of temporal lobe epilepsy: the quadrennial meeting of the ILAE in 1953. *Epilepsia* **47**:1288–91.

Shorvon SD, Fish DR, Andermann F, Bydder GM, Stefan H (1992) *Magnetic Resonance Scanning and Epilepsy*. New York: Plenum Press.

Sieveking E (1861) *Epilepsy and Epileptiform Seizures: Their Causes, Pathology and Treatment*. London: Churchill.

Spratling W (1902) Epilepsy in its relation to crime. *J Nerve Ment Dis* **29**:481–96.

Spratling W (1904) *Epilepsy and Its Treatment*. Philadelphia, PA: WB Saunders.

Temkin O (1945) *The Falling Sickness*. Baltimore, MD: Johns Hopkins University Press.

Turner WA (1907) *Epilepsy: A Study of the Idiopathic Disease*. London: Macmillan.

Walshe FMR (1949) *Diseases of the Nervous System*, 6th edn. Edinburgh: Livingstone.

Wilson SAK (1940) *Neurology*. London: Edward Arnold.

Yannet H (1950) Mental deficiency due to perinatally determined factors. *Pediatrics* **5**:328.

Chapter

2

The etiological classification of epilepsy

Simon D. Shorvon

Introduction

The historical development of concepts of etiology is outlined in the historical introduction (Chapter 1), and as will be clear there are complex issues involved with the assignment of cause, not least the multifactorial nature of epilepsy, the role of genetics and provoking factors, the influence of age and development, and the differentiation between "cause" and "mechanism." Perhaps because of this, remarkably, etiology has been largely ignored in the official classifications of epilepsy in the past 30 years, which were focused more on seizure semiology and electroencephalography, and on syndromic categorization. Etiology was mentioned only in passing in the 1969, 1981, and 1989 ILAE classifications of seizures and syndromes and in other schemes proposed (Gastaut 1969; Commission on Classification and Terminology of the International League Against Epilepsy 1981, 1989; Luders et al. 1993; Engel 2001, 2006). The most recent ILAE Commission report does consider etiology (Berg et al. 2010) but a catalog of causes such as is attempted in this book has never been comprehensively published.

In the opinion of the editors, there is a place for an etiological database or at the very least, a classification which considers etiology as one axis or domain, and this was the impetus for the publication of this book. In this chapter, a classification of the etiology of epilepsy is proposed, and this forms the basis of the sectional divisions in the rest of the book (Table 2.1).

In constructing such a classification, it is furthermore necessary to take cognisance of five particular points:

(a) Definitions – terms must be clearly defined, The usage of the terms *idiopathic* and *symptomatic* for instance has widely differed in the past 150 years. These terms nevertheless are retained in this book, as they are widely understood and widely used. The definitions used in this classification are given below.

(b) Multifactorial cause of epilepsy – as Lennox and many before him frequently reiterated, epilepsy is in the great majority of cases multifactorial. This means that in any individual, the epilepsy is often the result of both genetic and acquired influences and also influenced by provoking factors. Assignment in such cases to any single etiology is therefore to an extent arbitrary. In this scheme, causation is divided into specific etiological categories but it is recognized that epileptogenesis in individual cases will often involve multiple categories, often to a highly significant degree.

(c) Cause versus mechanism – it is also worth recording here that even the meaning of "etiology" has indeed changed over the years. In Jackson's time, it referred largely to the mechanisms of epileptogenesis, the final common pathway in Jackson's view, rather than the causative lesions (this is further discussed in the historical introduction). In this book, we have categorized the epilepsies according to their causal lesions, but recognize that a mechanistic classification is also possible, and further that the mechanisms may often be similar or identical in different etiologies – this is a largely under-researched area. Certainly, though, the mechanisms underpinning idiopathic and symptomatic epilepsy are quite distinct and these are outlined in Chapters 3 and 4.

(d) Focal versus generalized epilepsy – it should be emphasized that an etiological categorization often does not divide the epilepsies into clear-cut focal or generalized subdivisions, and the distinction (problematic as it is) does not map uniformly across the idiopathic versus symptomatic categorization. This, some symptomatic epilepsies are generalized and some idiopathic epilepsies are focal. Furthermore, both generalized and focal seizures may be "provoked," and provoked seizures can be either genetic or acquired.

(e) Flexibility – it is important to recognize that classification may change over time as knowledge of etiology accrues. No classification should be considered to be set in stone. Furthermore, in all classifications there are cases in which the inclusion into any particular category is difficult. In the epilepsies, this particularly applies to some childhood syndromes.

The Causes of Epilepsy, eds. S. D. Shorvon, F. Andermann, and R. Guerrini. Published by Cambridge University Press. © Cambridge University Press 2011.

Table 2.1 An etiological classification of epilepsy

Main category	Subcategory	Subcategory	Examples[a]
Idiopathic epilepsy	Pure epilepsies due to single-gene disorders		Benign familial neonatal convulsions; autosomal dominant nocturnal frontal lobe epilepsy; genetic epilepsy with febrile seizures plus; severe myoclonic epilepsy of childhood; benign adult familial myoclonic epilepsy
	Pure epilepsies with complex inheritance		Idiopathic generalized epilepsy (and its subtypes); benign partial epilepsies of childhood
Symptomatic epilepsy	Predominately genetic or developmental causation	Childhood epilepsy syndromes	West syndrome; Lennox–Gastaut syndrome
		Progressive myoclonic epilepsies	Unverricht–Lundborg disease; dentato-rubro-pallido-luysian atrophy; Lafora body disease; mitochondrial cytopathy; neuronal ceroid lipofuscinoses; Sialidosis and Gaucher disease; myoclonus renal failure syndrome
		Neurocutaneous syndromes	Tuberous sclerosis complex; neurofibromatoses; Sturge–Weber syndrome
		Other neurological single-gene disorders	Angelman syndrome; lysosomal disorders; neuroacanthocytosis; organic acidurias; porphyria; pyridoxine-dependent epilepsy; Rett syndrome; urea cycle disorders; Wilson disease; disorders of cobalamin and folate metabolism
		Disorders of chromosome structure	Down syndrome; fragile X syndrome; 4p syndrome; inverted duplicated chromosome 15; ring chromosome 20
		Developmental anomalies of cerebral structure	Hemimegalencephaly; focal cortical dysplasia; agyria–pachygyria band spectrum; agenesis of the corpus callosum; polymicrogyria and schizencephaly; periventricular nodular heterotopia; microcephaly; arachnoid cysts; malformations of human cerebral cortex
	Predominately acquired causation	Hippocampal sclerosis and perinatal and infantile causes	Hippocampal sclerosis; neonatal seizures and postneonatal epilepsy; cerebral palsy; vaccination and immunization
		Cerebral trauma	Open head injury; closed head injury; neurosurgery; epilepsy after epilepsy surgery; non-accidental head injury in infants
		Cerebral tumor	Glioma; ganglioglioma and dysembryoplastic neuroepithelial tumor; hypothalamic hamartoma; meningioma; metastatic disease
		Cerebral infection	Viral encephalitis; bacterial meningitis and abscess; malaria; neurocysticercosis; other parasitic diseases; tuberculosis; HIV
		Cerebrovascular disorders	Cerebral hemorrhage; cerebral infarction; arteriovenous malformation; cavernous hemangioma
		Cerebral immunological disorders	Rasmussen encephalitis; systemic lupus erythematosus and collagen vascular disorders; inflammatory disorders
		Other cerebral conditions	Psychiatric disorders; Alzheimer disease and other dementing disorders; multiple sclerosis and demyelinating disorders; hydrocephalus; porencephaly
Provoked epilepsy		Provoking factors	Fever; menstrual cycle and catamenial epilepsy; sleep; startle; metabolic and endocrine-induced seizures; electrolyte and sugar disturbances; drug-induced seizures; alcohol- and toxin-induced seizures
		Reflex epilepsies	Photosensitive epilepsies; startle-induced epilepsies; reading epilepsy; auditory-induced epilepsy; eating epilepsy; hot-water epilepsy
Cryptogenic epilepsies[b]			

Notes:
[a]These examples are not comprehensive, and in every category there are other causes.
[b]By definition, the causes of the cryptogenic epilepsies are "unknown." However, these are an important category, accounting for at least 40% of epilepsies encountered in adult practice and a lesser proportion in pediatric practice.

Definitions

In this book, the etiology of the epilepsies is divided into four main categories:

(1) Idiopathic epilepsy – defined here as *an epilepsy of predominately genetic origin and in which there is no gross neuroanatomical or neuropathological abnormality*. The recent advances in genetics have been fruitful in the area of epilepsy etiology, and in the past 10 years a number of new Mendelian idiopathic epilepsy syndromes have been delineated. However, the epilepsies with presumed polygenic or complex inheritance have proved more difficult to elucidate, and their genetic basis has largely eluded explanation, but this is an area in which development is predicted in the next 5–10 years. The question of genetic "susceptibility" is discussed further in Chapters 5 and 6. We have included in this category the conditions which have a presumed polygenic basis, even where this has not been yet identified – and it could be reasonably argued that they would be better moved to a cryptogenic category. However, their general clinical features and age specificity point strongly to a presumed genetic etiology and it is for this reason that these conditions are included here.

(2) Symptomatic epilepsy – defined here as *an epilepsy, of an acquired or genetic cause, associated with neuroanatomical or neuropathological abnormalities indicative of underlying disease or condition*. We thus include in this category developmental and congenital disorders where these are associated with cerebral pathological changes, whether genetic or acquired (or indeed cryptogenic) in origin. Magnetic resonance imaging (MRI) has been of great importance in clarifying the cortical developmental disorders, which are now often classified on imaging grounds, and modern molecular biology and genetics have uncovered the mechanism or genetic causes of many of these conditions. The genetic bases of almost all the single-gene diseases with epilepsy as part of the phenotype have also been identified in the past 20 years. The acquired causes are dealt with in this book within 14 subdivisions, within which we have tried to cover all the important causative types.

(3) Provoked epilepsy – defined here as *an epilepsy in which a specific systemic or environmental factor is the predominant cause of the seizures and in which there are no gross causative neuroanatomical or neuropathological changes*. Some "provoked epilepsies" will have a genetic basis and some an acquired basis. The reflex epilepsies are included in this category (which are usually genetic) as well as the epilepsies with a marked seizure precipitant.

(4) Cryptogenic epilepsy – defined here as *an epilepsy of presumed symptomatic nature in which the cause has not been identified*. The number of such cases is diminishing, but currently this is still an important category, accounting for at least 40% of adult-onset cases of epilepsy.

(nb. 'gross *anatomical* or *pathological abnormality*', is defined as any *identifiable* pathological or anatomical abnormality which can be detected in normal clinical investigation, including clinical microscopy, histology and neurochemistry).

A classification of the etiologies of epilepsy

Bearing the above issues in mind, and adhering to the above definitions, a classification scheme based on etiology is proposed in Table 2.1. This categorization report (Berg *et al.* 2010) in significant ways, including: the retention of the terms 'idiopathic', 'symptomatic', and 'cryptogenic', the inclusion of a category of 'provoked epilepsy' and in the definition of some terms. For a more detailed discussion of these and other issues, see Shorvon (2011). The commission also recommended that a classification should be a database forming the basis of a diagnostic manual; the etological schema in this chapter should be viewed as such for instance in relation to the benign focal epilepsies or even the idiopathic generalized epilepsies; (b) the categorization of some of the childhood syndromes, some of which are included under the "idiopathic" grouping but evidence of a genetic basis is not very strong – for instance, the Panayiotopoulos syndrome – and others are included in the symptomatic epilepsy category, in spite of the fact that there is a presumption of a genetic cause in at least a proportion of cases – for instance in the West or Lennox–Gastaut syndromes.

It is clear that in the future, as further knowledge accrues, some of these epilepsies will be reclassified and the scheme itself will need revision. With these provisos, however, this etiological classification scheme is adopted in this book, and the book is structured according to this scheme.

References

Berg A, Berkovic S, Brodie M, *et al.* (2010) Revised terminology and concepts for organization of seizures and epilepsies: Report of the ILAE Commission on Classification and Terminology, 2005–2009. *Epilepsia* **51**:676–85.

Commission on Classification and Terminology of the International League Against Epilepsy (1981) Proposal for revised clinical and electrographic classification of epileptic seizures. *Epilepsia* **22**:489–501.

Commission on Classification and Terminology of the International League Against Epilepsy (1989) Proposal for revised classification of epilepsies and epileptic syndromes. *Epilepsia* **30**:389–99.

Engel J (2001) A proposed diagnostic scheme for people with epileptic seizures and with epilepsy: Report of the ILAE Task Force on Classification and Terminology. *Epilepsia* **42**:796–803.

Engel J (2006) Report of the ILAE Classification Core Group. *Epilepsia* **47**:1558–68.

Gastaut H (1969) Clinical and electroencephalographical classification of epileptic seizures. *Epilepsia* **10**(Suppl):2–13.

Luders HO, Burgess R, Noachtar S (1993) Expanding the international classification of seizures to provide localization information. *Neurology* **43**:1650–5.

Shorvon S (2011) The etiological classification of epilepsy. *Epilepsia* **52** *in press.*

Chapter

3

Epileptogenesis in idiopathic epilepsy

Snezana Maljevic and Holger Lerche

Introduction

Epilepsy is a disease of the brain characterized by recurring unprovoked epileptic seizures, caused by a transient abnormality of neuronal activity which results in synchronized electrical discharges of neurons within the central nervous system (CNS). Approximately 3% of people are affected by epileptic seizures throughout their lifetime, more frequently during childhood (Hauser et al. 1996). Numerous causes of sporadic or recurrent seizures include trauma, tumors, stroke, altered metabolic states, or inborn brain malformations. However, an estimated 40% of all epilepsy patients have recurrent unprovoked seizures without any other neurological abnormalities. Due to the obscurity of their genesis these seizures are designated as "idiopathic epilepsies," and presumed to be genetic in origin. Various studies within the last 15 years have reported genetic alterations associated with idiopathic epilepsy syndromes (Steinlein 2004; Lerche et al. 2005; Reid et al. 2009), and the number of such reports is likely to increase further with the advance of mutation-detecting technologies. Strikingly, almost all of thus far identified epilepsy genes encode ion channels.

The first inherited ion-channel defects have been found in rare monogenic idiopathic epilepsy syndromes, such as autosomal dominant nocturnal frontal lobe epilepsy (ADN-FLE) or benign familial neonatal seizures (BFNS), but mutations were also identified in a few families with the most common idiopathic generalized epilepsies (IGE), comprising childhood and juvenile absence epilepsy (CAE, JAE), juvenile myoclonic epilepsy (JME), and epilepsy with grand mal seizures on awakening (EGMA). Among the few non-ion-channel genes that have been identified in idiopathic epilepsies so far, are the leucine-rich, glioma-inactivated 1 gene (LGI1), mutations of which cause autosomal dominant lateral temporal lobe epilepsy, or the EFHC1 gene encoding myoclonin, a protein with an EF-hand motif, associated with juvenile myoclonic epilepsy. The pathophysiological mechanisms through which these proteins influence epileptogenesis is still unclear, though an impact on ion-channel function has been proposed, for instance an interaction of

LGI-1 with glutamate (AMPA) receptors or K^+ channels, or of myoclonin with presynaptic Ca^{2+} channels (reviewed in Reid et al. 2009). Recent findings also indicate that metabolic changes can predispose to idiopathic epilepsies, as found for mutations in the glucose transporter GLUT1 which is responsible for transporting glucose, the most important energy carrier of the brain, across the blood–brain barrier. Beside the classical GLUT1 deficiency syndrome, a severe epileptic encephalopathy (De Vivo et al. 1991), GLUT1 mutations have also been found to be associated with milder phenotypes including idiopathic generalized – mainly absence – epilepsy (Roulet-Perez et al. 2008; Suls et al. 2008, 2009; Weber et al. 2008).

This chapter is focused on the most important characteristics of voltage- and ligand-gated ion channels, their role in determining neuronal excitability, and the impact of some reported mutations on epileptogenesis in idiopathic epilepsies. A section describing the importance of the thalamocortical loop and thalamic ion channels for the generation of generalized seizures is also included. The clinical phenotypes of the mentioned syndromes are described in other chapters.

Basic structure and function of ion channels and their relation to neuronal excitability

Ion channels are pore-forming proteins residing in the cell membrane which confer the electrical excitability to a neuron. They are specialized to selectively conduct different ions and have gates, which regulate their opening and closing under well-defined conditions. Two major classes of ion channels most relevant for epileptogenesis are (i) the voltage-gated channels, opening in response to changes in transmembrane voltage, and (ii) the ligand-gated channels controlled by specific ligands, such as neurotransmitters. Whereas voltage-gated channels are responsible for the generation and conduction of action potentials transmitting signals along the axon, ligand-gated channels mediate synaptic transmission and signal transduction from cell to cell.

The Causes of Epilepsy, eds. S. D. Shorvon, F. Andermann, and R. Guerrini. Published by Cambridge University Press. © Cambridge University Press 2011.

Voltage-gated channels

Voltage-gated cation channels have pores selective for Na^+, K^+, or Ca^{2+} ions. These channels consist of a main, pore forming α-subunit responsible for gating and permeation, and accessory subunits (β, γ, or δ) which have modifying effects. The α-subunits of voltage-gated Na^+ and Ca^{2+} channels have a tetrameric structure comprising four homologous domains (I–IV) each with six transmembrane segments (S1–S6) which are all encoded by a single gene (Fig. 3.1A). In contrast, genes of voltage-gated K^+ channels only encode one domain, but nevertheless the channels have a similar structure to the Na^+ channel as four α-subunits assemble into homo- or heterotetramers to give one functional channel (Fig. 3.1B). The three major conformational states of voltage-gated channels are a closed resting state (C), an open conducting state (O), and a closed inactivated state (I) (Fig. 3.1C). At the resting membrane potential, the channels are closed and can be activated by membrane depolarization, causing an outward move of the voltage sensors relative to the rest of the channel which then opens its "activation gate" on a timescale of milliseconds. With sustained depolarization a different, the so-called "inactivation gate" will close spontaneously. The inactivated channels will remain refractory to opening and can only recover from this state after a certain period of membrane repolarization. Some types of K^+ channels do not have an inactivated state and are constitutively open upon membrane depolarization.

The steep depolarizing phase of an action potential is mediated by activation of the Na^+ inward current, and both fast inactivation of Na^+ channels and activation of K^+ channels, carrying an outward K^+ current, account for the membrane repolarization. Thus, both a disruption of the fast Na^+ channel inactivation (resulting in a gain of function with increased Na^+ inward current) and a decrease in outward K^+ conductance (loss of function) can lead to slowed or incomplete repolarization of the cell membrane and result in spontaneous series of action potentials and neuronal hyperexcitability. In contrast, a loss of Na^+ channel function, for example caused by nonsense mutations predicting truncated proteins or by use-dependent Na^+ channel blockers such as phenytoin, carbamazepine and lamotrigine, and a gain of function of a K^+ channel, as the one caused by the new antiepileptic drug retigabine, would both be expected to reduce the excitability of the neurons expressing the affected channels.

One of the main roles of neuronal voltage-gated Ca^{2+} channels is the regulation of transmitter release in presynaptic nerve terminals, but they are also important for other processes such as dendritic and somatic signaling, and burst firing in thalamic and other neurons.

Ligand-gated channels

Ligand-gated channels are activated by neurotransmitters such as acetylcholine (ACh), glutamate, glycine, or γ-amino butyric acid (GABA), or by nucleotides. These channels are found clustered in the postsynaptic membrane of fast chemical synapses and open rapidly after binding of the agonist. They are constituted by tetrameric or pentameric associations of subunits of similar structure (Fig. 3.1D) comprising two to four transmembrane segments (M1–4). The central pore, formed by the M2 segments, is not as selective as in the voltage-gated channels and conducts either cations in excitatory ACh or glutamate receptors, or anions in inhibitory $GABA_A$ or glycine receptors. The binding of transmitters and the coupling to channel opening are complex processes which can consequently be influenced by amino acid changes in many different regions of these channels.

Like the voltage-gated channels, ligand-gated channels have three main conformational states: resting, open, and desensitized (Fig. 3.1E). Binding of the transmitter opens the channel from the resting closed state. However, during constant presence of the transmitter the channel will be transferred to another closed conformational state, the "desensitized" state. Only after removal of the transmitter can the channel recover from desensitization and subsequently will be available for another opening. In channels that have not yet reached the desensitized state, removal of the agonist, as caused by chemical modification for example by acetylcholine esterase or by presynaptic reuptake of the transmitter, induces a faster closing called deactivation. Both processes, deactivation and desensitization, contribute to the termination of the postsynaptic signal. Their disturbance can prolong excitatory or reduce inhibitory signals which both result in a hyperexcitability of the postsynaptic membrane which can promote the generation of epileptic seizures.

Subunit composition, neuronal expression, (sub)cellular localization, and related functional aspects of ion channels

There is considerable molecular diversity of pore-forming subunits of both voltage- and ligand-gated ion channels. This diversity is increased further by the modulating effects of the auxiliary subunits or, as in case of voltage-gated K^+ or ligand-gated channels, by the ability of the channels to form heteromers bearing distinctive gating characteristics. Their physiological role will therefore depend on their spatial and temporal expression pattern. Although some ion-channel proteins have ubiquitous expression, most of the pore-forming subunits are expressed in a tissue-specific manner. This is the reason, for instance, why mutations in different types of Na^+ or K^+ channel genes can either cause myotonia (mutations in the skeletal muscle sodium channel gene *SCN4A*), cardiac arrhythmia with long QT syndrome (mutations in the heart muscle Na^+ channel gene *SCN5A* or the cardiac K^+ channel gene *KCNQ1*), deafness (mutations in the inner ear K^+ channel genes *KCNQ1* and *KCNQ4*), or different forms of epilepsy (mutations in the neuronal Na^+ channel genes *SCN1A*, *SCN2A*, and *SCN1B*, or the neuronal K^+ channel genes *KCNQ2* and

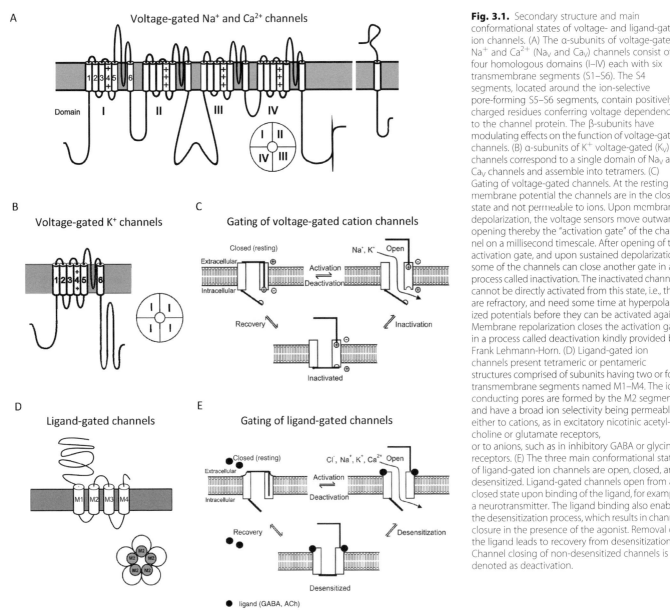

A

Voltage-gated Na$^+$ and Ca^{2+} channels

Domain   I   II   III   IV

B

Voltage-gated K$^+$ channels

C

Gating of voltage-gated cation channels

Closed (resting)   Na$^+$, K$^+$ Open
Extracellular
                          Activation
                          Deactivation
Intracellular

Recovery   Inactivation

                    Inactivated

D

Ligand-gated channels

M1 M2 M3 M4

E

Gating of ligand-gated channels

Closed (resting)   Cl$^-$, Na$^+$, K$^+$, Ca^{2+} Open
Extracellular
                          Activation
                          Deactivation
Intracellular

Recovery   Desensitization

                    Desensitized

● ligand (GABA, ACh)

Fig. 3.1. Secondary structure and main conformational states of voltage- and ligand-gated ion channels. (A) The α-subunits of voltage-gated Na$^+$ and Ca^{2+} (Na$_V$ and Ca$_V$) channels consist of four homologous domains (I–IV) each with six transmembrane segments (S1–S6). The S4 segments, located around the ion-selective pore-forming S5–S6 segments, contain positively charged residues conferring voltage dependence to the channel protein. The β-subunits have modulating effects on the function of voltage-gated channels. (B) α-subunits of K$^+$ voltage-gated (K$_V$) channels correspond to a single domain of Na$_V$ and Ca$_V$ channels and assemble into tetramers. (C) Gating of voltage-gated channels. At the resting membrane potential the channels are in the closed state and not permeable to ions. Upon membrane depolarization, the voltage sensors move outward opening thereby the "activation gate" of the channel on a millisecond timescale. After opening of the activation gate, and upon sustained depolarization, some of the channels can close another gate in a process called inactivation. The inactivated channels cannot be directly activated from this state, i.e., they are refractory, and need some time at hyperpolarized potentials before they can be activated again. Membrane repolarization closes the activation gate in a process called deactivation kindly provided by Frank Lehmann-Horn. (D) Ligand-gated ion channels present tetrameric or pentameric structures comprised of subunits having two or four transmembrane segments named M1–M4. The ion-conducting pores are formed by the M2 segments and have a broad ion selectivity being permeable either to cations, as in excitatory nicotinic acetyl-choline or glutamate receptors, or to anions, such as in inhibitory GABA or glycine receptors. (E) The three main conformational states of ligand-gated ion channels are open, closed, and desensitized. Ligand-gated channels open from a closed state upon binding of the ligand, for example a neurotransmitter. The ligand binding also enables the desensitization process, which results in channel closure in the presence of the agonist. Removal of the ligand leads to recovery from desensitization. Channel closing of non-desensitized channels is denoted as deactivation.

KCNQ3) (Jentsch 2000; George 2005). Furthermore, the localization of ion channels in different brain structures, distinctive neuronal or glial populations, or within different intracellular (neuronal) compartments is decisive for their physiological tasks. Figure 3.2 illustrates the localization of a few selected ion-channel proteins in different types and subcellular compartments of neurons. A nice example is provided by the differential expression of Na$^+$ channels in different types of neurons described in the following paragraph.

Nine different genes encode voltage gated sodium channel α-subunits, and four of them, *SCN1A*, *SCN2A*, *SCN3A*, and *SCN8A*, encoding Na$_V$1.1, Na$_V$1.2, Na$_V$1.3, and Na$_V$1.6 proteins, respectively, are highly expressed in neurons of the CNS. Each sodium channel α-subunit associates with one or more β-subunits, β1–β4, which code for transmembrane proteins with a single extracellular loop (Fig. 3.1A) and influence

α-subunit trafficking, stability, and channel gating. Na$_V$1 subtypes are found in different neuronal subtypes and concentrated in axon initial segments (AISs), the site of action potential generation (Fig. 3.2). Na$_V$1.3 are predominantly expressed in embryonic and neonatal but not adult brain in rodents. In the AISs of the optic nerve and principal neurons, Na$_V$1.2 channels are highly expressed early in development and their expression is diminished towards adult ages, whereas Na$_V$1.6 channel expression increases with maturation largely replacing Na$_V$1.2. In adult brain, Na$_V$1.2 is also highly expressed in unmyelinated axons and Na$_V$1.6 is found at nodes of Ranvier (Liao *et al.* 2010a, 2010b; Vacher *et al.* 2008). In contrast, it has been shown that the Na$_V$1.1 channels reside at the AIS of inhibitory neurons (Ogiwara *et al.* 2007) (Fig. 3.2A), thereby explaining how loss-of-function mutations found in this channel may cause hyperexcitability and seizures (see below).

A

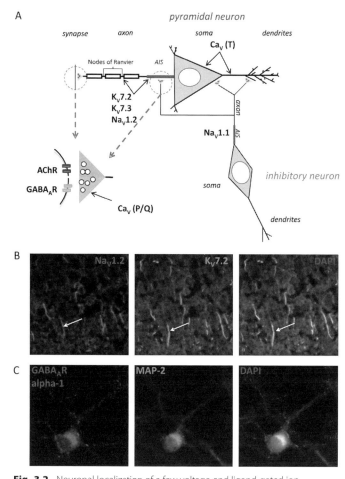

Fig. 3.2. Neuronal localization of a few voltage-and ligand-gated ion channels. (A) Schematic presentation of an excitatory pyramidal (lila) and an inhibitory (green) neuron and their synaptic connections. Distinctive intracellular compartments are targeted by different populations of ion channels. Marked is the localization of several ion channels associated with idiopathic epilepsies: in the somatodendritic compartment–Ca_V T-type channels; at axon initial segments (AIS) and nodes of Ranvier in pyramidal neurons–Na_V1.2, K_V7.2, K_V7.3; at AIS of inhibitory neurons–Na_V1.1; presynaptic terminals–Ca_V P/Q type; postsynaptic compartment–$GABA_A$ and acetylcholine (ACh) receptors. (B) Colocalization of K_V7.2 and Na_V1.2 channels at axon initial segments of cortical neurons in the adult mouse brain shown by immunofluorescent staining using an anti-K_V7.2 (green) and an anti-Na_V1.2 (red) antibody of sections obtained from an unfixed brain. (C) Distribution of $GABA_A$ receptors in a primary cultured hippocampal neuron shown by immunofluorescent staining using an anti-$GABA_A$R α-1 subunit antibody (red). An anti-MAP2 antibody (green) was used as a somatodendritic and DAPI (blue) as a nucleic marker (Maljevic and Lerche, unpublished data). See color plate section.

Voltage-gated K^+ channels are the most diverse ion-channel family with more than 70 genes encoding for the different subunits and most promiscuous oligomerizing potential to generate channels with distinctive electrophysiological properties (Vacher *et al.* 2008). For example there are inactivating (e.g., K_V1) and non-inactivating (e.g., K_V7.1–5) K^+ channels with large differences in the kinetics of activation and inactivation which have a timescale ranging from milliseconds to hundreds of milliseconds. The expression pattern of K_V channels will be illustrated here with a few examples showing their distinctive localization in neurons. For instance, different K_V1 isoforms are expressed along the axons and in presynaptic terminals, playing a role in

action potential generation and propagation. In contrast, K_V4.2 channels show a dendritic localization (Vacher *et al.* 2008). A reduced availability of these channels in dendrites of CA1 pyramidal hippocampal neurons, due to a decrease in the translation process and increased phosphorylation, has been found in an animal model of temporal lobe epilepsy (Bernard *et al.* 2004). Neuronal K_V7 channels (K_V7.2 and K_V7.3), mutated in a neonatal epilepsy, are found at AIS along with Na^+ channels (Vacher *et al.* 2008) (Fig. 3.2A) and modulate the firing frequency of many central neurons.

Voltage-gated Ca^{2+} (Ca_V) channels can have a high or low threshold depending on the membrane potential at which they are activated. High-threshold Ca_V channels are associated with a β-, $α_2$δ-, and sometimes also with a γ-subunit. They comprise L-, N-, P/Q-, and R-types, the latter three mainly located in presynaptic nerve terminals controlling neurotransmitter release. Low-threshold T-type Ca_V channels mediate a burst mode of neuronal firing and are highly expressed in thalamocortical relay and thalamic reticular neurons where they are believed to be involved in the generation of rhythmic spike-and-wave discharges characteristic for generalized absence seizures (see below).

The HCN ("hyperpolarization-activated cyclic nucleotide-gated") channel family comprises four members, expressed in brain and heart. HCN2 and HCN4 are highly expressed in the sinus node and thalamus and act as pacemaker channels to generate spontaneous rhythmic discharges by conducting a cation current activated with increasing membrane hyperpolarization thereby inducing slow, rhythmic depolarizations. HCN1 and HCN2 are found in dendrites regulating the integration of synaptic input (Biel *et al.* 2009).

Neuronal nicotinic ACh receptors (nAChR) have a pentameric structure of two α- and three β-subunits (Fig. 3.1D). Eight α- ($α_{2–9}$) and three β- ($β_{2–4}$) subunit isoforms are known to be expressed differentially in the brain in postsynaptic membranes of neurons under cholinergic control (Fig. 3.2A). Most abundantly found in all brain areas are the $α_4$- and $β_2$-subunits encoded by the genes *CHRNA4* and *CHRNB2*, which are both affected in autosomal dominant nocturnal frontal lobe epilepsy (Hogg *et al.* 2003).

$GABA_A$ receptors belong to the same family of ligand-gated channels, having the same pentameric structure. There are several different subunit classes of $GABA_A$ receptors ($α_{1–6}$, $β_{1–3}$, $γ_{1–3}$, δ, ε, π, $ρ_{1–3}$). The subunit composition most abundantly found in brain is probably $2α_12β_21γ_2$ (Mehta and Ticku 1999; Sieghart *et al.* 1999) (Fig. 3.1D). An example of the subcellular localization of $GABA_A$ receptors is shown in Fig. 3.2A, B.

Idiopathic epilepsy as channelopathy
Sodium channel defects

The first epilepsy syndrome identified as a sodium channel disorder was generalized/genetic epilepsy with febrile seizures plus (GEFS+), in which a variety of febrile and afebrile seizure

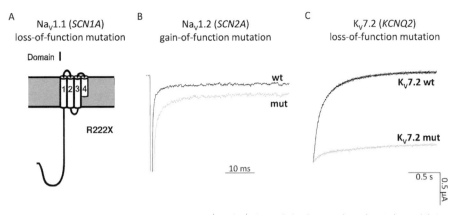

Fig. 3.3. Molecular defects in voltage-gated Na$^+$ and K$^+$ channels leading to idiopathic epilepsy. (A) A truncation R222X in the Na$_V$1.1 channel encoded by the *SCN1A* gene associated with severe myoclonic epilepsy of infancy (SMEI) (Claes *et al.* 2001), indicating a loss-of-function pathophysiological mechanism due to a severely affected, non-functional channel protein (compare Fig. 3.1A for the full length protein). (B) Normalized current traces recorded at 0 mV from cells expressing Na$_V$1.2 wild-type (wt, black) or a BFNIS-associated mutant (muts, gray) channels (Liao and Lerche, unpublished data). The increased persistent current for the mutation designates a gain of function as a pathophysiological mechanism in BFNIS. (C) A BFNS-associated mutation affecting the K$_V$7.2 channel shows reduced potassium currents compared to the WT when expressed in *Xenopus laevis* oocytes. Presented are raw current traces from the WT (black) and mutant (gray) recorded at +40 mV (Maljevic and Lerche, unpublished data).

types can occur in a dominant fashion in one pedigree. Wallace *et al.* (1998) described a mutation in *SCN1B*, encoding the β$_1$-subunit, in a large Australian family, which disrupts a disulfide bridge (C121W) and thereby probably affects the secondary structure of the extracellular loop causing a loss of β$_1$-subunit function, which was subsequently also found in other mutations in this gene (reviewed by Reid *et al.* 2009). However, exactly how these mutations lead to epilepsy is still unclear.

Mutations in *SCN1A*, encoding the α-subunit Na$_V$1.1, cause a wide spectrum of phenotypes. Besides GEFS+ (Escayg *et al.* 2000a), most of the mutations have been described in Dravet syndrome (severe myoclonic epilepsy of infancy, SMEI) (Claes *et al.* 2001), an epileptic encephalopathy with severe refractory seizures and mental decline. Most of the SMEI-associated mutations occur de novo and are nonsense mutations predicting truncated proteins (Fig. 3.3A) or altered splicing. Mutations without function when expressed in heterologous systems have also been described (reviewed by George 2005; Lerche *et al.* 2005; Reid *et al.* 2009).

In two independently generated mouse models, the *SCN1A* gene has been knocked out by introduction of a SMEI-associated premature stop codon or a similar mutation (Yu *et al.* 2006; Ogiwara *et al.* 2007), so that the heterozygous animals represent the genetic mouse homolog of the human disease. Both models show very similar phenotypes with interictal epileptic discharges, decreased thermal seizure threshold, spontaneous seizures, reduced weight, and premature death with much more severe symptoms in the homozygous than in the heterozygous mice. Immunohistochemical studies using Na$_V$1.1-specific antibodies revealed that Na$_V$1.1 channels are specifically localized to AISs of parvalbumine-positive interneurons while they are not detected in excitatory pyramidal cells (Ogiwara *et al.* 2007). Electrophysiological recordings from interneurons revealed a significant reduction of firing with longer and increasing current injections in mutant mice compared to wild-type, which can be explained

by the reduced number of Na$^+$ channels (Yu *et al.* 2006; Ogiwara *et al.* 2007). These studies thus revealed Na$_V$1.1 as the predominant Na$^+$ channel in interneurons and suggest that a loss of interneuron firing is the pathophysiological correlate of seizure generation in SMEI.

One SMEI-associated mutation in the voltage sensor (R1648C) revealed a gain of function with a large persistent Na$^+$ current due to impaired fast channel inactivation when expressed in mammalian cells, which was also described in a less pronounced form for some mutations found in GEFS+ patients. However, most of the other functional alterations found in heterologous expression systems for mutations associated with GEFS+ or simple febrile seizures have resulted in a loss-of-function mechanism, for instance enhanced fast or slow inactivation or an increased threshold for channel activation by a positive shift of the steady-state activation curve, or a complete loss of functional channels (reviewed by George 2005; Lerche *et al.* 2005; Reid *et al.* 2009). It is possible that the mutations associated with milder phenotypes are also due to a loss of Na$^+$ function in inhibitory neurons. The mutations showing a persistent Na$^+$ current might in fact induce a depolarization block, thus depolarizing interneurons beyond the action potential threshold inhibiting their ability to fire. Further studies, in particular in animal models, are needed to test such hypotheses.

A smaller number of mutations have been identified in the *SCN2A* gene, encoding the Na$_V$1.2 channel α-subunit. They have been detected in patients with benign familial neonatal–infantile seizures (BFNIS), a mild syndrome presenting with clusters of partial and generalized tonic–clonic seizures occurring between the neonatal period and the first months of life (Heron *et al.* 2002; reviewed by Reid *et al.* 2009). Studies investigating the functional consequences of a few *SCN2A* mutations using the rat or human isoforms of the channel predicted subtle gain-of-function mechanisms, such as a depolarizing shift of the inactivation curve, a hyperpolarizing shift of the activation curve, a slightly increased persistent current (Fig. 3.3B), or an accelerated recovery from fast inactivation, all of which would result in an increase in neuronal excitability. Only one study suggested a loss-of-function by decreased surface expression for some mutations. A single truncating mutation of *SCN2A* was found to be associated with a severe epilepsy syndrome similar to SMEI, but distinct because of partial seizures, delayed onset, and absence of febrile seizures (reviewed by Reid *et al.* 2009). Immunohistochemical studies in developing mouse brains revealed that Na$_V$1.2 channels are early upregulated in axon initial segments of principal excitatory neurons in cortex and hippocampus and then diminished during further maturation, whereas Na$_V$1.6 channels are not expressed in early development and largely replace Na$_V$1.2 channels later on (Liao *et al.* 2010a). These observations can nicely explain why seizures in BFNIS occur only transiently early in life and disappear spontaneously with further maturation.

Potassium channel defects

Mutations in *KCNQ2* and *KCNQ3*, encoding the voltage-gated neuronal K$^+$ channels K$_V$7.2 and K$_V$7.3, cause benign familial neonatal seizures (BFNS) (Biervert *et al.* 1998; Charlier *et al.* 1998; Singh *et al.* 1998; reviewed by Maljevic *et al.* 2008). This is a dominant epilepsy syndrome, very similar to BFNIS mentioned above, starting within the first days of life with frequent partial and generalized seizures that disappear spontaneously after a few weeks. K$_V$7 (*KCNQ*) channels give rise to the M-current, a slowly activating, non-inactivating K$^+$ current (Fig. 3.3C) which can be suppressed by the activation of muscarinic acetylcholine receptors (Delmas and Brown 2005). These channels control the membrane potential in the subthreshold range of an action potential serving as a brake for neuronal firing. Functional expression of the known mutations has revealed a consistent reduction of the resulting K$^+$ current (Fig. 3.3C) by different molecular mechanisms outlined below, which can lead to a membrane depolarization and increased neuronal firing.

K$_V$7.2 and K$_V$7.3 subunits form heteromers with largely increased current amplitudes compared to homomers. Coexpression of wild-type and mutant K$_V$7.2 with wild-type K$_V$7.3 subunits in a 1 : 1 : 2 ratio, mimicking the in vivo situation in a heterozygous patient, only revealed a 20–25% reduction in current amplitude compared to coexpression of both wild-type subunits, and this suggests that relatively small changes of the M-current could be sufficient to cause epileptic seizures in the neonatal period (Schroeder *et al.* 1998). The pore region, the S4 segment constituting the voltage sensor, and the specifically long C-terminus, which has many regulatory functions and contains the assembly domain for interaction and tetramerization of the channels, are mainly affected by the disease-causing mutations. While some of the C-terminal mutations have been shown to impair surface expression, by different mechanisms, S4 mutations slow and increase the threshold for channel activation. Recently, we described two mutations in the S1–S2 extracellular loop which restrict such changes of

voltage-dependent activation to the subthreshold range of an action potential, thus demonstrating, in human disease, the crucial role of this voltage range for the physiological function of K$_V$7 channels (reviewed by Maljevic *et al.* 2008). Two knock-in models have been generated that carry either a *KCNQ2* or a *KCNQ3* mutation both of which had been identified in BFNS families. Homozygous mice revealed reduced M-currents and showed spontaneous seizures throughout life, not pronounced in an early period of development, whereas the heterozygotes only exhibited a reduced seizure threshold upon the application of convulsant drugs (Singh *et al.* 2008).

A possible explanation for the transient epileptic phenotype during the neonatal period could be the fact that the expression of K$_V$7.2 and K$_V$7.3 channels increases during maturation. In this sense, a small reduction of the M-current by mutations may be sufficient to cause seizures in the neonatal period, when the amount of available K$_V$7 channels needed for control of the subthreshold membrane potential is still critically low, whereas the relatively small reduction of the M-current in adulthood, when channels are abundantly available, is less problematic. Alternatively or complementarily, it has been proposed that the developmental switch of the GABAergic system from excitatory to inhibitory is important for the transient generation of seizures, since the M-current might be particularly important as the main available inhibitory channel in the neonatal period (reviewed by Maljevic *et al.* 2008).

T-type Ca^{2+} and HCN channel defects and thalamocortical loops

Childhood absence epilepsy is characterized by frequent absence seizures with typical 3-Hz generalized spike-and-wave discharges (GSW) starting at 3–8 years of age. There are two rat models that mimic human absence seizures with GSW, although with a different frequency (9–10 Hz): the genetic absence epilepsy rats from Strasbourg (GAERS) and the Wistar Albino Glaxo rats bred in Rijswijk (WAG/Rij). Extensive studies in these two models have revealed that the three main structural elements necessary to generate GSWs within the thalamocortical network are the nucleus reticularis thalami (NRT), thalamocortical relay neurons, and the cortex (Danober *et al.* 1998; Meeren *et al.* 2005) (Fig. 3.4). Furthermore, many alterations in these animals have been described on the molecular level, and have been supported, furthermore, by other studies in mouse models and humans. A selective upregulation of T-type Ca^{2+} currents in neurons of the NRT (Tsakiridou *et al.* 1995), and an upregulation of HCN1 channels and the HCN1/HCN2 ratio together with a reduced cAMP responsiveness of the resulting hyperpolarization-activated cation current (I$_h$) have been described (Budde *et al.* 2005). Since both classes of channels play an important role in burst firing, pacemaker function, and rhythmic activity, these changes can explain enhanced synchronized discharges in the thalamocortical network. Likewise, knock-out mice lacking the T-type Ca^{2+} channel gene *CACNA1G* are resistant to

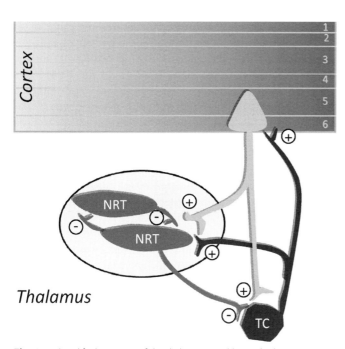

Fig. 3.4. Simplified structure of the thalamocortical loop. The basic thalamocortical loop comprises excitatory (+) projections from glutamatergic pyramidal cortical (light gray) and thalamocortical (TC, dark gray) neurons, and inhibitory (−) projections of GABAergic neurons from the nucleus reticularis thalami (NRT).

GSW induction (Kim *et al.* 2001) and overexpression of the same gene induces absence-like seizures with GSW (Ernst *et al.* 2009). *HCN2* knock-out mice, in which the HCN1/HCN2 ratio is reduced as in WAG/Rij, show spontaneous behavioral arrest with GSWs (Ludwig *et al.* 2003).

In humans, the gene *CACNA1H* encoding another T-type Ca^{2+} channel is mutated in absence and other forms of idiopathic generalized epilepsy. Functional studies of variants found in CAE patients indicated different gating alterations leading to a gain-of-function mechanism which fits well with the data obtained from different rodent models (Chen *et al.* 2003; Vitko *et al.* 2005; Heron *et al.* 2007).

In good agreement with these studies is the fact that some of the most efficient drugs in the treatment of absence seizures, ethusuximide, valproate, and zonisamide, block T-type Ca^{2+} channels. All these studies together indicate that a gain-of-function of T-type Ca_V channels could be one important pathophysiogical mechanism in CAE and other IGE subtypes with generalized spike and wave activity.

Other Ca^{2+} channel defects

Absence-like seizures combined with ataxia in mice can be also caused by mutations in different subunits of P/Q-type Ca^{2+} channels causing a loss of function (Burgess and Noebels 2000). In humans, mutations in *CACNA1A*, encoding the α-subunit of this channel, can cause familial hemiplegic migraine, episodic ataxia type 2, and spinocerebellar ataxia type 6. Direct candidate gene approaches then led to the discovery of a few Ca^{2+} channel variants associated with epilepsy. One variant was discovered in

a patient with juvenile myoclonic epilepsy (JME) in the gene *CACNB4*, encoding the β4-subunit, predicting a premature stop codon (R482X), and another one within the same gene in a father and son affected with juvenile absence epilepsy (JAE) (C104F). The latter mutation was also detected in another family with episodic ataxia type II (EA-2). Functional studies revealed small differences in channel gating for R482X and both mutations lead to a small but significant reduction in current size (Escayg *et al.* 2000b). Furthermore, two mutations were found in *CACNA1A*, predicting (i) a R1820X truncation of the α1-subunit of the same channel complex, in a patient suffering from absence epilepsy, episodic and progressive ataxia, and cognitive impairment, and (ii) a point mutation E147K in a three-generation family with five affected individuals with a similar but more variable combined phenotype of absence epilepsy and episodic/slightly progressive ataxia. Functional studies also showed impaired channel function for both mutations (Jouvenceau *et al.* 2001; Imbrici *et al.* 2004).

The epileptogenic mechanism of these mutations found in mice and humans is not entirely clear. It has been proposed that a compensatory upregulation of T-type Ca^{2+} channels might be responsible for inducing absence seizures with GSW (Song *et al.* 2004).

GABA$_A$ receptors and related genes

Alterations in the genes encoding the γ2-, α1-, and δ-subunits of GABA$_A$ receptors, the major inhibitory ion channels in the mammalian brain, have been found in patients with a wide spectrum of epilepsy phenotypes including simple febrile seizures, GEFS+, absence seizures, and juvenile myoclonic epilepsy. All mutations have in common a reduction in the activity of the pentameric GABA$_A$ receptor when expressed in mammalian cells, in cultured neurons, or in a knock-in mouse model (Fig. 3.5). The molecular mechanisms by which GABA$_A$ receptor function is impaired comprise gating defects such as an acceleration of channel deactivation, a reduced GABA affinity, or reduced surface expression due to protein degradation or trafficking defects (Fig. 3.5A, B) (Baulac *et al.* 2001; Wallace *et al.* 2001; Cossette *et al.* 2002; Dibbens *et al.* 2004; reviewed by Lerche *et al.* 2005; Reid *et al.* 2009). Heterozygous knock-in mice carrying one of the human mutations exhibited frequent episodes of behavioral arrest with spike-and-wave discharges mimicking the human phenotype of absence seizures were observed in patients carrying the same mutation R43Q in the γ2-subunit (Wallace *et al.* 2001; Tan *et al.* 2007). Mutant receptors showed reduced surface expression in neurons and electrophysiological analysis of inhibitory signals in thalamus and cortex suggested that a small reduction in cortical inhibition is the relevant mechanism in the causation of absence-like seizures in these animals (Fig. 3.5C–E).

Genetic variations in a Cl^- channel found in patients with IGE indicate also that a secondary or indirect effect on GABAergic inhibition could predispose to idiopathic epilepsy. ClC-2 is a voltage-gated Cl^- channel which was reported to be

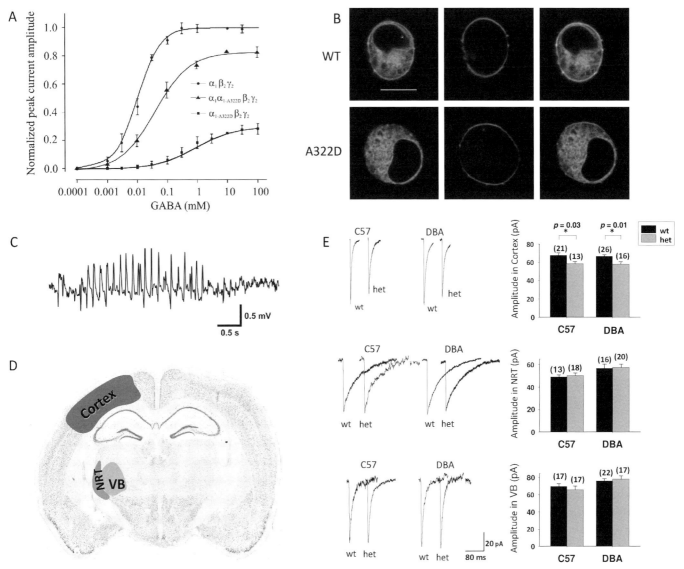

Fig. 3.5. Molecular, cellular, and systemic defects due to mutations in GABA$_A$ receptor subunits leading to idiopathic epilepsy. (A) The A322D mutation of the α$_1$-subunit of GABA$_A$ receptors, detected in a large JME family (Cossette *et al.* 2002), causes reduced GABA sensitivity as shown by a lowered maximal response and a rightward shift in the dose–response curve of the heterologously expressed GABA$_A$ receptors comprising one mutant and one wild-type, or two mutant α$_1$-subunits. (B) A reduced surface expression of the A322D mutation was observed in HEK cells transfected with EGFP-tagged α$_1$ wild-type or mutant together with β$_2$- and γ$_2$-subunits. A membrane marker FM4–64 was used to prove the membrane localization of the mutant channel, which was however reduced compared to the wild-type (modified from Krampfl *et al.* 2005, with permission). (C) EEG from a heterozygous mouse strain harboring the R43Q mutation of the γ$_2$-subunit of GABA$_A$ receptors recorded during a spontaneous absence-like seizure showing rhythmic epileptic discharges. (D) The thalamocortical circuit comprises cortex (here somatosensory), the thalamic reticular nucleus (NRT), and ventrobasal thalamus (VB) containing thalamocortical neurons (compare to Fig. 3.4). Recordings shown in (E) refer to these regions. (E) GABA$_A$ receptor-mediated miniature inhibitory postsynaptic currents (mIPSC) recorded from cortical pyramidal neurons in layer 2/3 of the somatosensory cortex of R43Q heterozygous mouse in two different genetic backgrounds (C57 and DBA are two strains of mice) revealed significantly reduced mIPSC amplitudes for the carriers of the R43Q mutation, indicating that an impaired synaptic inhibition in this layer might play a role in seizure generation, whereas recordings in thalamus did not reveal differences between wild-type and mutant mice (modified from Tan *et al.* 2007, with permission). See color plate section.

expressed in brain, mainly in astrocytes and GABA-inhibited neurons (Sik *et al.* 2000). It has been proposed that this channel plays an important role in neuronal Cl⁻ homeostasis, which is crucial for GABAergic inhibition (Staley *et al.* 1996). Different functional alterations for a few ClC-2 variants have been described, such as truncated proteins, slowing of activation or acceleration of deactivation time courses, and altered cAMP or Cl⁻ sensitivity. These may reduce ClC-2 activity thereby leading to intracellular Cl⁻ accumulation reducing

the effectiveness of GABA$_A$ receptor-mediated inhibition (summarized in Reid *et al.* 2009; Saint-Martin *et al.* 2009).

In summary, GABA$_A$ receptor mutations directly reduce the main mechanism for neuronal inhibition in the brain and this "inhibited inhibition" (disinhibition) could explain the occurrence of epileptic seizures. Hence, there is a broad spectrum of epilepsy syndromes which could be caused by direct or indirect GABAergic disinhibition, ranging from febrile seizures to the classical IGE phenotypes and the epileptic encephalopathies, when *SCN1A* loss-of-function mutations are also considered in this context, as they lead to a loss of firing of inhibitory neurons (see above).

Nicotinic acetylcholine receptors

The first ion-channel mutation detected in an inherited form of epilepsy was identified in the gene *CHRNA4* encoding the α_4-subunit of a neuronal nicotinic acetylcholine receptor (nAChR) in a family with autosomal dominant nocturnal frontal lobe epilepsy (ADNFLE), a disorder characterized by frequent brief seizures originating from the frontal lobe occurring typically in clusters at night (Steinlein *et al.* 1995). To date, several mutations have been identified in *CHRNA4*, and in *CHRNB2* which encodes the β_2-subunit of neuronal nAChRs. One mutation in *CHRNA2*, encoding the α_2-subunit, causing a slightly different phenotype with nocturnal wandering and ictal fear, has recently been reported (De Fusco *et al.* 2000; Phillips *et al.* 2001; Steinlein 2004; Lerche *et al.* 2005; Aridon *et al.* 2006; Reid *et al.* 2009). All these mutations reside in or near to the pore-forming M2 transmembrane segments. Following functional expression of most of the known mutations in *Xenopus* oocytes or mammalian cells, many different effects on gating of heteromeric $\alpha_4\beta_2$ or $\alpha_2\beta_2$ receptors have been reported leading either to a gain or a loss of function (reviewed by Steinlein 2004; Lerche *et al.* 2005; Reid *et al.* 2009). However, a common mechanism evolving from many of the functional studies performed up to now seems to be a relative increase of the response to ACh application (De Fusco *et al.* 2000; Phillips *et al.* 2001; Bertrand *et al.* 2002; Steinlein 2004; Aridon *et al.* 2006). This finding is supported by knock-in mice expressing a hypersensitive α_4-subunit mutation which showed a decreased threshold for ACh-induced seizures (Fonck *et al.* 2003). Thus, a gain of function of the nAChR by increased ACh sensitivity might be the relevant pathophysiological mechanism for ADNFLE. How exactly these changes can induce nocturnal frontal lobe seizures remains to be elucidated. Thalamic neurons under cholinergic control, which are part of thalamocortical loops playing a crucial role for rhythmic activities during sleep and which also occur predominantly in the frontal lobe, could be responsible for the pathophysiology of this disease (Hogg *et al.* 2003).

Concluding remarks and perspectives

The genetic and pathophysiological findings described in this chapter have tremendously advanced our current knowledge of epileptogenesis in idiopathic epilepsies. However, most of the mutations detected so far concern rare monogenic forms of epilepsy and only few have been identified in the common classical forms of IGE. A major task for the near future is therefore to unravel the complex genetics of the common epilepsies. The available results indicate that multiple rare variants may provide the predominant genetic background of the idiopathic epilepsies, but the "common variant – common disease" hypothesis has not been systematically studied to date. Whole genome association studies which can reveal common variants, and large-scale sequencing programs, are expected to detect many more rare variants. These are under way and will hopefully provide this information within the next few years. In this context, the most common genetic alteration predisposing to IGE so far has been recently identified in 1% of a large cohort of IGE patients and is a microdeletion spanning 1.5 Mb on chromosome 15q13.3. The deleted region contains *CHRNA7* encoding the nAChR α_7-subunit as a possible candidate gene (Helbig *et al.* 2009).

Another important question is whether these genetic studies will serve to improve therapy. Most anticonvulsant drugs that are in clinical use today act by modulating the function of ion channels, and we described here how ion channel function can be altered by genetic defects associated with idiopathic epilepsies. This knowledge potentially enables us to develop new therapeutic strategies to counteract the epilepsy-causing mechanisms. Specifically, the defective proteins can be used as new pharmacological targets. For instance, studying the genetic defect of BFNS helped to understand a newly developed strategy in anticonvulsive treatment, as retigabine was identified as an activator of M-currents conducted by neuronal K_V7 channels. By binding within the pore region (Wuttke *et al.* 2005; Schenzer *et al.* 2005), retigabine stabilizes the open state of K_V7 channels and enhances their activity by shifting the voltage dependence of activation of these channels in the hyperpolarizing direction (Rundfeldt and Netzer 2000). The drug thus has an opposing effect to that caused by the mutations described above that induce neonatal seizures, which is a highly potent anticonvulsive mechanism leading to a reduced rate of neuronal firing. None of the other antiepileptic drugs that are in current clinical use displays a similar mechanism of action. Retigabine has been trialed in the treatment of pharmacoresistant partial epilepsies, showing its general anticonvulsant profile, and will be probably licensed soon for this indication. We very much hope that other such genetic and pathophysiological studies will help to improve epilepsy care in the long term.

References

Aridon P, Marini C, Di Resta C, *et al.* (2006) Increased sensitivity of the neuronal nicotinic receptor alpha 2 subunit causes familial epilepsy with nocturnal wandering and ictal fear. *Am J Hum Genet* **79**:342–50.

Baulac S, Huberfeld G, Gourfinkel-An I, *et al.* (2001) First genetic evidence of GABA(A) receptor dysfunction in epilepsy: a mutation in the gamma2-subunit gene. *Nat Genet* **28**:46–8.

Bernard C, Anderson A, Becker A, *et al.* (2004) Acquired dendritic channelopathy in temporal lobe epilepsy. *Science* **305**:532–5.

Bertrand D, Picard F, Le Hellard S, *et al.* (2002) How mutations in the nAChRs can cause ADNFLE epilepsy. *Epilepsia* **43**:112–22.

Biel M, Wahl-Schott C, Michalakis S, Zong X (2009) Hyperpolarization-activated cation channels: from genes to function. *Physiol Rev* **89**:847–85.

Biervert C, Schroeder BC, Kubisch C, *et al.* (1998) A potassium channel mutation in neonatal human epilepsy. *Science* **279**:403–6.

Budde T, Caputi L, Kanyshkova T, *et al.* (2005) Impaired regulation of thalamic pacemaker channels through an imbalance of subunit expression in absence epilepsy. *J Neurosci* **25**:9871–82.

Burgess DL, Noebels JL (2000) Calcium channel defects in models of inherited generalized epilepsy. *Epilepsia* **41**:1074–5.

Charlier C, Singh NA, Ryan SG, *et al.* (1998) A pore mutation in a novel KQT-like potassium channel gene in an idiopathic epilepsy family. *Nat Genet* **18**:53–5.

Chen Y, Lu J, Pan H, *et al.* (2003) Association between genetic variation of CACNA1H and childhood absence epilepsy. *Ann Neurol* **54**:239–43.

Claes L, Del-Favero J, Ceulemans B, *et al.* (2001) De novo mutations in the sodium-channel gene *SCN1A* cause severe myoclonic epilepsy of infancy. *Am J Hum Genet* **68**:1327–32.

Cossette P, Liu L, Brisebois K, *et al.* (2002) Mutation of GABRA1 in an autosomal dominant form of juvenile myoclonic epilepsy. *Nat Genet* **31**:184–9.

Danober L, Deransart C, Depaulis A, Vergnes M, Marescaux C (1998) Pathophysiological mechanisms of genetic absence epilepsy in the rat. *Progr Neurobiol* **55**:27–57.

De Fusco M, Becchetti A, Patrignani A, *et al.* (2000) The nicotinic receptor beta 2 subunit is mutant in nocturnal frontal lobe epilepsy. *Nat Genet* **26**:275–6.

De Vivo DC, Trifiletti RR, Jacobson RI, *et al.* (1991) Defective glucose transport across the blood–brain barrier as a cause of persistent hypoglycorrhachia, seizures, and developmental delay. *N Engl J Med* **325**:703–9.

Delmas P, Brown DA (2005) Pathways modulating neural KCNQ/M (Kv7) potassium channels. *Nat Rev Neurosci* **6**:850–62.

Dibbens LM, Feng HJ, Richards MC, *et al.* (2004) GABRD encoding a protein for extra- or peri-synaptic GABAA receptors is a susceptibility locus for generalized epilepsies. *Hum Mol Genet* **13**:1315–19.

Ernst WL, Zhang Y, Yoo JW, Ernst SJ, Noebels JL (2009) Genetic enhancement of thalamocortical network activity by elevating alpha 1g-mediated low-voltage-activated calcium current induces pure absence epilepsy. *J Neurosci* **29**:1615–25.

Escayg A, MacDonald BT, Meisler MH, *et al.* (2000a) Mutations of *SCN1A*, encoding a neuronal sodium channel, in two families with GEFS+2. *Nat Genet* **24**:343–5.

Escayg AP, De Waard M, Lee DD, *et al.* (2000b) Coding and noncoding variation of the human calcium-channel β4-subunit gene CACNB4 in patients with idiopathic generalized epilepsy and episodic ataxia. *Am J Hum Genet* **66**:1531–9.

Fonck C, Nashmi R, Deshpande P, *et al.* (2003) Increased sensitivity to agonist-induced seizures, straub tail, and hippocampal theta rhythm in knock-in mice carrying hypersensitive alpha 4 nicotinic receptors. *J Neurosci* **23**:2582–90.

George AL Jr. (2005) Inherited disorders of voltage-gated sodium channels. *J Clin Invest* **115**:1990–9.

Hauser WA, Annegers JF, Rocca WA (1996) Descriptive epidemiology of epilepsy: contributions of population-based studies from Rochester, Minnesota. *Mayo Clin Proc* **71**: 576–86.

Helbig I, Mefford HC, Sharp AJ, *et al.* (2009) 15q13.3 microdeletions increase risk of idiopathic generalized epilepsy. *Nat Genet* **41**:160–2.

Heron SE, Crossland KM, Andermann E, *et al.* (2002) Sodium-channel defects in benign familial neonatal-infantile seizures. *Lancet* **360**:851–2.

Heron SE, Khosravani H, Varela D, *et al.* (2007) Extended spectrum of idiopathic generalized epilepsies associated with CACNA1H functional variants. *Ann Neurol* **62**:560–8.

Hogg RC, Raggenbass M, Bertrand D (2003) Nicotinic acetylcholine receptors: from structure to brain function. *Rev Physiol Biochem Pharmacol* **147**:1–46.

Imbrici P, Jaffe SL, Eunson LH, *et al.* (2004) Dysfunction of the brain calcium channel Cav2.1 in absence epilepsy and episodic ataxia. *Brain* **127**:2682–92.

Jentsch TJ (2000) Neuronal KCNQ potassium channels: physiology and role in disease. *Nat Rev Neurosci* **1**:21–30.

Jouvenceau A, Eunson LH, Spauschus A, *et al.* (2001) Human epilepsy associated with dysfunction of the brain P/Q-type calcium channel. *Lancet* **358**:801–7.

Kim D, Song I, Keum S, *et al.* (2001) Lack of the burst firing of thalamocortical relay neurons and resistance to absence seizures in mice lacking alpha1G T-type Ca(2+)channels. *Neuron* **31**:35–45.

Krampfl K, Maljevic S, Cossette P, *et al.* (2005) Molecular analysis of the A322D mutation in the GABA receptor alpha-subunit causing juvenile myoclonic epilepsy. *Eur J Neurosci* **22**:10–20.

Lerche H, Weber YG, Jurkat-Rott K, Lehmann-Horn F (2005) Ion channel defects in idiopathic epilepsies. *Curr Pharm Des* **11**(21):2737–52.

Liao Y, Deprez L, Maljevic S, *et al.* (2010a) Molecular correlates of age-dependent seizures in an inherited neonatal–infantile epilepsy. *Brain* **133**:1403–14.

Liao Y, Anttonen AK, Liukkonen E, *et al.* (2010b) SCN2A mutation associated with neonatal epilepsy, late-onset episodic ataxia myoclonus, and pain. *Neurology* **75**:1454–8.

Ludwig A, Budde T, Stieber J, *et al.* (2003) Absence epilepsy and sinus dysrhythmia in mice lacking the pacemaker channel HCN2. *EMBO J* **22**:216–24.

Maljevic S, Wuttke TV, Lerche H (2008) Nervous system Kv7 disorders: breakdown of a subthreshold brake. *J Physiol* **586**:1791–801.

Meeren H, van Luijtelaar G, Lopes da Silva F, Coenen A (2005) Evolving concepts on the pathophysiology of absence seizures: the cortical focus theory. *Arch Neurol* **62**:371–6.

Mehta AK, Ticku MK (1999) An update on GABAA receptors. *Brain Res Brain Res Rev* **29**:196–217.

Ogiwara I, Miyamoto H, Morita N, *et al.* (2007) Nav1.1 localizes to axons of parvalbumin-positive inhibitory interneurons: a circuit basis for epileptic seizures in mice carrying an *SCN1A* gene mutation. *J Neurosci* **27**:5903–14.

Phillips HA, Favre I, Kirkpatrick M, *et al.* (2001) CHRNB2 is the second acetylcholine receptor subunit associated with autosomal dominant nocturnal frontal lobe epilepsy. *Am J Hum Genet* **68**:225–31.

Reid CA, Berkovic SF, Petrou S (2009) Mechanisms of human inherited

epilepsies. *Progr Neurobiol*
87:41–57.

Roulet-Perez E, Ballhausen D, Bonafé L, Cronel-Ohayon S, Maeder-Ingvar M (2008) Glut-1 deficiency syndrome masquerading as idiopathic generalized epilepsy. *Epilepsia* **49**:1955–8.

Rundfeldt C, Netzer R (2000) The novel anticonvulsant retigabine activates M-currents in Chinese hamster ovary cells tranfected with human KCNQ2/3 subunits. *Neurosci Lett* **282**:73–6.

Saint-Martin C, Gauvain G, Teodorescu G, *et al.* (2009). Two novel CLCN2 mutations accelerating chloride channel deactivation are associated with idiopathic generalized epilepsy. *Hum Mutat* **30**:397–405.

Schenzer A, Friedrich T, Pusch M, *et al.* (2005) Molecular determinants of KCNQ (Kv7) K$^+$ channel sensitivity to the anticonvulsant retigabine. *J Neurosci* **25**:5051–60.

Schroeder BC, Kubisch C, Stein V, Jentsch TJ (1998) Moderate loss of function of cyclic-AMP-modulated KCNQ2/KCNQ3 K$^+$ channels causes epilepsy. *Nature* **396**:687–90.

Sieghart W, Fuchs K, Tretter V, *et al.* (1999) Structure and subunit composition of GABA(A) receptors. *Neurochem Int* **34**:379–85.

Sík A, Smith RL, Freund TF (2000) Distribution of chloride channel-2-immunoreactive neuronal and astrocytic processes in the hippocampus. *Neuroscience* **101**:51–65.

Singh NA, Charlier C, Stauffer D, *et al.* (1998) A novel potassium channel gene, *KCNQ2*, is mutated in an inherited epilepsy of newborns. *Nat Genet* **18**:25–9.

Singh NA, Otto JF, Dahle EJ, *et al.* (2008) Mouse models of human *KCNQ2* and *KCNQ3* mutations for benign familial neonatal convulsions show seizures and neuronal plasticity without synaptic reorganization. *J Physiol* **586**:3405–23.

Song I, Kim D, Choi S, *et al.* (2004) Role of the alpha1G T-type calcium channel in spontaneous absence seizures in mutant mice. *J Neurosci* **24**:5249–57.

Staley KJ, Smith R, Schaack J, Wilcox C, Jentsch TJ (1996) Alteration of GABAA receptor function following gene transfer of the ClC-2 chloride channel. *Neuron* **17**:543–51.

Steinlein OK (2004) Genetic mechanisms that underlie epilepsy. *Nat Rev Neurosci* **5**:400–8.

Steinlein OK, Mulley JC, Propping P, *et al.* (1995) A missense mutation in the neuronal nicotinic acetylcholine receptor alpha 4 subunit is associated with autosomal dominant nocturnal frontal lobe epilepsy. *Nat Genet* **11**:201–3.

Suls A, Dedeken P, Goffin K, *et al.* (2008) Paroxysmal exercise-induced dyskinesia and epilepsy is due to mutations in *SLC2A1*, encoding the glucose transporter GLUT1. *Brain* **131**:1831–44.

Suls A, Mullen SA, Weber YG, *et al.* (2009) Early onset absence epilepsy due to mutations in the glucose transporter GLUT1. *Ann Neurol* **66**:415–19.

Tan HO, Reid CA, Single FN, *et al.* (2007) Reduced cortical inhibition in a mouse model of familial childhood absence epilepsy. *Proc Natl Acad Sci USA* **104**:17 536–41.

Tsakiridou E, Bertollini L, de Curtis M, Avanzini G, Pape HC (1995) Selective increase in T-type calcium conductance of reticular thalamic neurons in a rat model of absence epilepsy. *J Neurosci* **15**:3110–17.

Vacher H, Mohapatra DP, Trimmer JS (2008) Localization and targeting of voltage-dependent ion channels in mammalian central neurons. *Physiol Rev* **88**:1407–47.

Vitko I, Chen Y, Arias JM, *et al.* (2005) Functional characterization and neuronal modeling of the effects of childhood absence epilepsy variants of CACNA1H, a T-type calcium channel. *J Neurosci* **25**:4844–55.

Wallace RH, Wang DW, Singh R, *et al.* (1998) Febrile seizures and generalized epilepsy associated with a mutation in the Na$^+$-channel beta1 subunit gene *SCN1B*. *Nat Genet* **19**:366–70.

Wallace RH, Marini C, Petrou S, *et al.* (2001) Mutant GABA(A) receptor gamma2-subunit in childhood absence epilepsy and febrile seizures. *Nat Genet* **28**:49–52.

Weber YG, Storch A, Wuttke TV, *et al.* (2008) GLUT1 mutations are a cause of paroxysmal exertion-induced dyskinesias and induce hemolytic anemia by a cation leak. *J Clin Invest* **118**:2157–68.

Wuttke TV, Seebohm G, Bail S, Maljevic S, Lerche H (2005) The new anticonvulsant retigabine favors voltage-dependent opening of the Kv7.2 (*KCNQ2*) channel by binding to its activation gate. *Mol Pharmacol* **67**:1009–17.

Yu FH, Mantegazza M, Westenbroek RE, *et al.* (2006) Reduced sodium current in GABAergic interneurons in a mouse model of severe myoclonic epilepsy in infancy. *Nat Neurosci* **9**:1142–9.

Mechanisms of epileptogenesis in symptomatic epilepsy

Philip A. Schwartzkroin

Introduction

A major difficulty in a discussion of epileptogenic mechanisms involved in symptomatic epilepsy is the fact that there is often disagreement about what constitutes "epileptogenesis" and what we mean by "symptomatic epilepsy." It is therefore helpful to consider some components of these concepts – not so much to express any consensus definitions, but rather to provide a working starting point for the discussion.

Epileptogenesis

There is a current belief that "epileptogenic" mechanisms are different from the mechanisms that have been studied/identified underlying seizure genesis and initiation (or, indeed, those processes involved in maintaining the epileptic state). In that sense, the term, "epileptogenesis" certainly implies the existence of an epileptic state (chronic spontaneous seizure discharge? reduced seizure threshold?) – a state that follows, in a *causal* manner, from a previously occurring initiating "insult" or condition. Further, the term "epileptogenesis" suggests a time interval between the physical insult (or the onset of an epileptogenic state) and the resultant epileptic condition. This temporal delay is an important aspect of the epileptogenic concept, since we generally use the term "epileptogenesis" to describe a *process* that requires time. Further, reference to such an epileptogenic process assumes that in some earlier time in the life of the individual, the brain abnormality underlying seizure activity was *not* present, and that the structural changes (molecular or more grossly morphologic) leading to the epileptic state appeared gradually; that is, there is a time at which the epilepsy-inducing abnormalities begin to appear but the epilepsy is not yet present. These assumptions underlie our attempts to identify epileptogenic mechanisms as distinct (and in isolation) from mechanisms that maintain the epileptic state. Thus, when we begin to explore the underlying bases of *epileptogenesis*, we are asking a question that is fundamentally different from asking simply about underlying mechanisms of epilepsy. Given that this separation is very likely to

be an unrealistic oversimplification (see discussion below), I've approached the issue of mechanisms of "epileptogenesis" with a relatively broad perspective.

Symptomatic epilepsy

Descriptions of "symptomatic" epilepsy normally refer to a condition in which there is a physical, morphologically observable brain abnormality ("lesion") that is thought to be causally related to the epilepsy. That is, there is a structural – usually focal – abnormality (as seen histologically or in imaging) associated with seizure activity. When we begin to search for mechanisms of epileptogenesis, we are generally asking about that abnormal structure – how it occurred or developed (as a result of the initiating insult), and how it gives rise to the seizure phenotype (i.e., how the structural abnormality is related to the functional abnormality). Typically, "symptomatic" epilepsies are considered to be "acquired" epilepsies, in which the structural abnormality is a result of a known external insult – an infection, a prolonged bout of high fever, a head injury, etc.

However, it may also be the case that symptomatic structural abnormalities, including focal "lesions," result from aberrant brain development (lissencephalies, tuberous sclerosis, heterotopias) or tumors – i.e., lesions that do not arise from an obvious discrete initiating insult, and that indeed may result from specific genetic mutations. Especially given our modern tools of analysis, "structural symptoms" can even be argued in cases of genetic (i.e., "idiopathic") epilepsies where the structural abnormality is molecular in nature – that is, the "damage" is structural but microscopic.

Major (and not so major) theories explored in experimental studies

We still have relatively limited insight into the cellular/molecular process that might participate in epileptogenesis. In considering various mechanistic hypotheses, investigators have often divided potential participants into two categories (Fig. 4.1):

The Causes of Epilepsy, eds. S. D. Shorvon, F. Andermann, and R. Guerrini. Published by Cambridge University Press. © Cambridge University Press 2011.

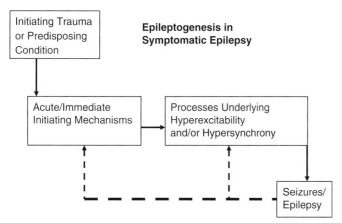

Epileptogenesis in Symptomatic Epilepsy

Fig. 4.1. Flow diagram showing progression of epileptogenesis (including possible feedback pathways).

Table 4.1 Acute/initiating mechanisms

Cell death/injury

Inflammation/blood–brain barrier breakdown

Denervation

Loss of developmental guidance factors

Metabolic changes

Altered gene expression

Table 4.2 Seizure-generating/-sustaining mechanisms

Altered neuronal properties

Loss of inhibitory constraints

Circuitry reorganization

Changes in glial properties and in extracellular environment

Immature regression

Subclinical electrical activity

(1) changes that are a direct result of the insult and which serve to initiate the epileptogenic process (Table 4.1); and (2) processes that give rise to an altered brain condition that is capable of generating/supporting aberrant (hyperexcitable, hypersynchronous) neuronal discharge (Table 4.2). These two sets of mechanisms may overlap (or turn out to be functionally inseparable). However, given the assumed temporal distinction (immediate vs. delayed) between these two categories of processes, it makes some sense to discuss them separately.

Immediate (initiating) processes
Cell death

The prototypical example symptomatic of epilepsy is post-traumatic epilepsy – that is, the epilepsy that develops after physical injury to the brain due to some incident that causes cell injury and/or cell death. Motor vehicle accidents, falls, gunshot and stab wounds, and injuries associated with bomb blasts are all lumped together in this category. Epidemiological data suggest that "penetrating" injuries – the most severe of the traumatic brain injuries – are most likely to have epileptogenic consequences (Herman 2002; Lowenstein 2009). What these insults most obviously have in common is the damage to – and often death of – significant numbers of neurons, often within a focal region of the brain. The "net" injury – including the magnitude of acute cell death – undoubtedly reflects many contributing factors, including the parameters of the physical insult, the brain "state" at the time of injury (e.g., concentration of various circulating hormonal modulators), and underlying genetic predisposition/sensitivity.

Why should cell death, per se, be epileptogenic? The answer to that question is not so obvious as it might seem. At first glance, one might even view neuronal loss as a mechanism of *reduced* brain excitability – since there are fewer cells to contribute to the discharge of the injured brain region. Certainly, if the cell loss is massive and relatively sudden, there may in fact be reduced activity arising from the affected brain region, especially acutely. But the situation is often much more complex. Hyperexcitability (not yet "epilepsy") may arise acutely from brain injury if:

(a) Cell damage is associated with release of molecules from injured cells that have excitatory effects on the remaining neuronal population. For example, investigations have shown that there is a large and prolonged rise in extracellular potassium associated with brain insult in many patients (Reinert *et al.* 2001); this elevated K^+ level may be responsible for acute seizure-like activity (Gorji and Spreckmann 2004) – although such acute and brief K^+ elevations may also lead to a depolarization-induced inactivation of neurons (spreading depression). Further, cell injury is often accompanied by release of neurotransmitter substances, particularly of glutamate which is the excitatory transmitter of choice for many cortical neurons; brain trauma may be associated with a surge of extracellular glutamate (Benardo 2003) that leads to significant excitotoxic damage.

(b) Cells most sensitive to the brain insult are primarily inhibitory. If that were the case – and there are data suggesting that at least some subpopulations of inhibitory interneurons are particularly vulnerable to damage (Buckmaster *et al.* 1999; Sun *et al.* 2007) – then the remaining circuitry would tend toward hyperexcitability because of an acute loss of inhibitory tone.

The proximal cause of cell injury/cell death associated with traumatic brain injury can be quite varied, and many of the mechanisms have been explored experimentally. The physical disruption of cell membranes and/or the rise in intracellular calcium (e.g., associated with glutamate receptor opening and/or calcium release from intracellular stores) can cause mitochondrial dysfunction/degradation, with the subsequent release of cytochrome *c* (Mattson 2003; Niizuma *et al.* 2009). Excitotoxicity may result from the production of reactive oxygen species (Mori *et al.* 2004), and cell injury may follow from DNA injury (or inadequacy of DNA repair mechanisms). Dissecting out the details of the relevant cell death pathway may be helpful in designing treatments that protect at least some cell populations, and/or reduce the epileptogenic consequences of the cell death phenomenon.

Inflammation/blood–brain barrier breakdown

Traumatic brain insults are also typically associated with breaches of the blood–brain barrier (BBB) and with rapid immune reactions that are manifest as inflammation (Vezzani and Granata 2005; Choi and Koh 2008). Physical trauma may cause openings of the BBB, which allow the infiltration of macrophages and the subsequent release of cytokines and related molecules that appear to cause neuronal cell death (Oby and Janigro 2006). Further, trauma leads to the release of these molecules from endogenous brain glia and microglia, contributing to the effects of infiltrating elements from the periphery. The complex effects of these molecules on brain cells are the focus of intense current study; it appears that cytokines not only induce neuronal pathology, but also exert direct excitatory effects on neurons and may be involved in neuronal plasticity (Vezzani *et al.* 2008). Clearly, these direct inflammatory reactions acutely alter the integrity of central nervous system (CNS) structures.

A related potential effect of brain trauma, particularly of brain infections, is the generation of antibodies that target normal brain proteins. Previous studies in an animal model of Rasmussen encephalitis suggested the involvement of autoantibodies that "attacked" elements of the glutamate receptor, leading directly to hyperexcitability and seizures (McNamara *et al.* 1999). Subsequent tests of that hypothesis have yielded unclear results – but the possibility of autoantibody generation in response to an immune challenge remains an interesting possibility, especially as one considers some encephalopathies of early childhood (Pleasure 2008).

Denervation

Physical injury may also have severe consequences for axonal integrity. Shearing forces are known to cause axonal injury (Gaetz 2004), and so various types of head injury (including closed-head trauma) may have significant consequences for cell-to-cell communication, particularly involving long-axon cells. Axonal injury could, at least in theory, result in rapid loss of synaptic activity. Since most long-axon neurons are excitatory projection cells, one might expect to see an acute decrease in excitation following this type of injury. However, given that inhibitory interneurons are also driven by inputs from these projection cells, the net consequences of "denervation" are rather difficult to predict. It should be noted, too, that

denervation has traditionally been associated with reorganization of synaptic inputs and receptors (e.g., "denervation supersensitivity"). These changes, however, are slower and perhaps more appropriately considered as later-stage (delayed) consequences of the injury.

Loss of developmental guidance factors

If one expands the concept of "symptomatic epilepsy" to include those conditions that are due to developmental abnormalities (resulting in structural brain lesions), then it is certainly appropriate to consider how those abnormalities are generated. Gene mutations have been implicated in many such cases – with the gene product culprit generally described as a factor that "guides" normal brain development. This type of abnormality is exemplified in type 1 lissencephaly, where mutations of *LIS1* or *DCX* (which encode microtubule-associated proteins) disrupt neuronal migration in the developing brain (Guerrini and Marini 2006). A similar disruption of cortical organization is seen in lissencephaly with cerebellar hypoplasia, where the mutation in the *RELN* gene leads to loss of reelin (an extracellular matrix-associated protein), a molecule that provides guidance for cell migration (Hong *et al.* 2000). These genetically based developmental syndromes are all highly associated with early-onset epilepsies.

Metabolic changes

For some types of traumatic insult, the challenge may be at the metabolic level. For example, hypoxia (or hypoxic ischemia) or fever may target metabolic pathways, interfere with mitochondrial function, or disrupt normal patterns of phosphorylation/dephosphorylation – all of which are known to affect neuronal function and/or viability. For example, pH changes can directly alter discharge levels, perhaps via the pH sensitivity of N-methyl-D-aspartate (NMDA) receptors.

Changes in gene expression

It is now quite clear that traumatic insult leads directly to altered gene expression (Pitkanen *et al.* 2007). The precise pattern of the change undoubtedly depends on the type of insult and on the intracellular pathways that mediate these changes. For example, expression of various immediate early genes (e.g., various heat shock proteins) is directly inducible by brain insult; these genes can "turn on" other genes to modulate excitability. In many cases, the salient cellular change associated with gene expression is a rise in intracellular calcium – an event common to virtually all brain insults. Increased intracellular calcium not only affects neurons but also glia; in astrocytes, these effects include the release of glutamate (mediated by calcium "waves" that spread across the glial syncytium) (Ding *et al.* 2007; Santello and Volterra 2009). In both neurons and glia, calcium rise has been shown to trigger cell death pathways, including the expression of various apoptotic genes (Raza *et al.* 2004; Fujikawa 2005).

Subsequent (delayed) changes that support epileptiform activities

Altered cell properties

There are, in addition to the immediate changes outlined above, also delayed altered neuronal properties that lead to hyperexcitable discharge properties. Many of the initial changes induced in neurons and glia can also result in delayed alterations of cell properties that affect excitability. For example, these early effects of "trauma" can lead to significant changes in voltage-gated channels (channel loss, movement of channels between intracellular sites and the neuronal membrane, altered channel kinetics due to changes in subunit composition, etc.) (Beck 2007). Similarly, insults – whether physical, metabolic, or genetic – may result in altered receptor distribution and/or properties, changes in uptake/transporter properties, and even affect basic energy-dependent processes such as ionic pump mechanisms (Lima *et al.* 2008).

These changes can be mediated "directly" (e.g., by changes in intracellular ion concentrations, changes in pH, etc.) or result from altered gene expression. A growing number of studies confirm insult-related changes in the pattern of gene expression – often region- (and cell-) specific. Many of the affected genes appear to be associated with immune/inflammatory agents, the consequences of which are still to be determined (Israelsson *et al.* 2008). Some of the gene expression changes also lead directly to altered subunit composition of key channel and receptor proteins (Pitkanen *et al.* 2007; Brooks-Kayal *et al.* 2009). Such changes appear to return the neuron to a relatively immature state – as though the cell were again developing within the still-maturing CNS. For example, following some types of insult, non-NMDA glutamate channels missing the GluR2 subunit reappear, allowing calcium entry and rises in intracellular calcium.

The long-term consequences of trauma appear to be related to direct/acute changes in the level of neuronal activity. For example, seizure activity itself – even acutely – may induce long-term changes in gene expression, channel composition, etc. Such activity-dependent plasticity (Jung *et al.* 2007; Blumenfeld *et al.* 2009) may occur in the absence of dramatic, clinically observable seizure discharge. Interestingly, activity-dependent alterations in cell properties have been proposed as one potential mechanism through which repeated seizure activity becomes progressively more drug-refractory (Beck 2007).

Changes in neuronal properties can be viewed as "homeostatic" – reflecting the neuron's effort to maintain a proper balance between excitation and inhibition. For example, with loss of inhibitory interneurons and/or with increases in discharge level, some cells in some brain regions appear to upregulate inhibitory mechanisms. In contrast, experimental models have shown that loss of excitatory synaptic activity (e.g., via functional deafferentation) leads to an upregulation of excitatory mechanisms that eventually can become "epileptic" (Galvan *et al.* 2000; Echegoyen *et al.* 2007).

Loss of inhibitory constraints

As indicated above, it is quite clear that some neurons are more sensitive to insult than others – and that a subpopulation of inhibitory interneurons (γ-amino butyric acid [GABA] cells) are among the more sensitive. Indeed, irrespective of the type of insult (head trauma, ischemia, status epilepticus), it appears that the same sensitive groups of neurons are lost (and in about the same temporal order). For example, loss of the GABA cells that colocalize somatostatin not only results in loss of GABA-mediated inhibition, but also the loss of inhibitory controls exerted by somatostatin at the level of afferent terminal synapses on pyramidal cell dendrites (Buckmaster *et al.* 1999). Insult-related stimuli can also affect other types of inhibitory mechanisms, such as: (a) alterations in chloride transporters can change inhibitory synapses into depolarizing synapses (although still "controlled" by GABA), thus enhancing excitability (Kahle *et al.* 2008); (b) injury- (or gene-) induced alterations in glial cell properties may not only affect the ability of astrocytes to regulate extracellular potassium and/or glutamate, but may also interfere with the glutamine–glutamate cycle, thereby depriving neurons of a critical raw material (glutamate) for manufacturing GABA (Liang *et al.* 2006). Depending on the nature of the insult, other inhibitory molecules may be affected – e.g., such endogenous antiepileptic molecules as adenosine or endocannabanoids (Chen *et al.* 2007; Boison 2008). Because of the complexity of these molecular systems, it is difficult to predict the net molecular consequences of insults associated with structural brain lesions (i.e., the "symptom" of symptomatic epilepsies).

Altered synaptic and network organization

The hypothesis that tends to dominate discussions about insult-associated epileptogenesis is that of reorganization of brain circuitry. Changes in "intracellular" circuitry do occur (e.g., changes in cell properties) but there are often more "gross" alterations – e.g., morphological changes in the neuron's dendritic tree or axon collateralization – that are easier to identify. Indeed, an early observation of human epileptic tissue gave rise to the idea that dendritic retraction (and spine changes) were a feature of epileptic tissue. More recent descriptions of temporal lobe epilepsy tissue have focused on such phenomena as mossy fiber sprouting and heterotopic neurons (Houser 1990; Nadler 2003; Scharfman *et al.* 2007). These current concepts of epileptogenic morphological changes emphasize the growth, rather than the retraction, of cellular elements. Neurite growth and synaptogenesis have been described (Xu *et al.* 2002), and there is now considerable interest in the possibility that neurogenesis (at least in the dentate region of hippocampus) may contribute to epileptogenic reorganization (Parent and Murphy 2008). Seizure activity does appear to be associated with an increased genesis of granule cell-like neurons; these new cells must be integrated into a functionally appropriate circuit – but are sometimes found in heterotopic positions involved in aberrant synaptic networks (Scharfman *et al.* 2007). These immature cells may contribute not only to epileptogenesis, but also to the restoration of normal neuronal function following trauma-induced cell loss.

Despite all the evidence for trauma-related morphologic plasticity, the question remains if/how these changes give rise to (or support) epileptic activities. Are these changes simply a *result* of seizure activity or really a *cause*? There are, unquestionably, changes in synaptic number, localization, and type associated with events that lead to seizure activity. This type of "plastic" connectivity is most dramatically illustrated by mossy fiber sprouting – involving collaterals of dentate granule cell axons to "replace" the synapses lost when hilar mossy cells die in response to traumatic insult. How are these new axons coaxed into the aberrant circuitry? Investigations suggest that the very molecular machinery that normally provides the signals for brain repair – e.g., neurotrophic factors like brain-derived neurotrophic factor (BDNF) – may also provide signals for aberrant axonal growth into vacated synaptic space or for potentiation of remaining synapses (Gall and Lynch 2004; He *et al.* 2004). If that were the case, then treatments that interfered with such signaling might prevent the formation of abnormal circuits that subsequently support epileptic discharge.

Altered glial function and changes in features of the extracellular space

As indicated above, changes in the properties of glia or of the glial network can have significant consequences for brain excitability. Because glia play such a critical role in maintaining the extracellular ionic environment (pH, K^+ concentration, extracellular glutamate and GABA levels [through glutamine–glutamate metabolism], and a host of other functions), altered astrocyte properties can be devastating. A hint of how astrocyte function may impact excitability can be seen in an animal model of tuberous sclerosis – an example of a "symptomatic" epilepsy syndrome, with a structural brain "lesion" and epileptic phenotype. In conditional knock-out mice in which deletion of one of the tuberous sclerosis complex (TSC) genes is targeted to astrocytes, animals show an epileptic condition associated with aberrant glial properties (Jansen *et al.* 2005). Altered astrocyte function has also been hypothesized for cells in gliomas, and in the reactive glia seen in traumatic brain injury (D'Ambrosio *et al.* 1999; Bordey and Spencer 2004). Changes in gap junction proteins – critical to the formation of the glial syncytium – have also been reported in epileptic tissue (Nemani and Binder 2005).

Another feature typically associated with epileptogenic brain lesions is a change in the nature of the extracellular space (ECS). Decreased ECS may reflect cell swelling (acutely) in response to injury, or may be a function of reactive gliotic growth (more chronically) within the ECS of injured tissue. Changes in ECS are carefully modulated during normal brain function, and studies have shown that decreased ECS can increase brain excitability, presumably through ephaptic influences (Dudek *et al.* 1998).

Reversion of cellular/synaptic properties to an "immature" state

One of the interesting features of epileptic tissue is the presence of many immature-like neuronal features. Trauma appears to trigger "regression" to such immature features (Ben-Ari 2006) as calcium-mediating non-NMDA glutamate receptors, altered chloride co-transporter expression (leading to high intracellular chloride concentration and resultant depolarizing GABA-mediated synaptic potentials), and aberrant dendritic trees. Similarly, one sees in developmental lesions (tuberous sclerosis, lissencephalies, etc.) aspects of the immature brain, including cells that have not differentiated into a mature recognizable phenotype. Even in temporal lobe epilepsy, the prototypical "symptomatic" epilepsy syndrome, one often finds "immature" neurons that appear to have been recently generated (neurogenesis of granule cell-like neurons) but have not migrated properly. These immature cell features not only may contribute to excitability due to their endogenous properties, but also because their connectivity within the already-formed brain may involve inappropriate synaptic contacts. Regression to an immature state may reflect the brain's attempt to reaccess some of the plastic potential of immaturity that might assist with repair of injured elements. Indeed, one might view these features of epileptic tissue as "hyperplastic" processes, distortions of precisely those mechanisms that are essential to normal brain function.

Subclinical electrical activity/oscillatory activity

To a significant extent, much of our attention on epileptogenic mechanisms has been at the molecular level. This focus is in contrast to our preoccupation with the aberrant electrical activity that defines the epileptic state. This change in focus – from electrical to molecular – is almost certainly a consequence of those studies that have shown that antiepileptic drugs, which block seizure activity, have little effect on epileptogenesis (or at least on the development of post-traumatic epilepsy) (Temkin 2009). While it is certainly the case that trauma-induced molecular changes must occur in order to generate new (abnormal) electrical discharge patterns in the brain, it is important to consider the resultant electrical phenomena as potentially epileptogenic. Subclinical seizure discharge, "interictal" discharge patterns (including high-frequency oscillations) (Engel *et al.* 2009), and unique neuronal synchronized output remain potential contributors to the epileptogenic process.

Comments on our current state of understanding

Our need to identify mechanisms of epileptogenesis in symptomatic epilepsies arises from a conviction that a better understanding of these processes will lead to effective *antiepileptogenic* therapies. Toward that end, it would be particularly helpful if we could provide a reasonably precise definition with respect to the targets of our studies. However, as indicated in the introduction to this article, what is meant by "symptomatic" and by "epileptogenesis" is not so clear.

What epilepsies are "symptomatic"?

The focus in this chapter on "symptomatic" epilepsies is intended to contrast with the treatment of "idiopathic" epilepsies taken up in an accompanying chapter. The latter term has traditionally been used to refer to epilepsies of genetic origin, and particularly to those conditions in which there is no apparent pathology. This distinction breaks down, however, as our technical capabilities increase and as our conceptual understanding becomes more sophisticated. Among the issues that confuse this distinction are the following considerations.

There is likely to be a genetic predisposition for "symptomatic" epilepsy. Not everyone who suffers a head injury develops post-traumatic epilepsy. While it is likely that this observation can be "explained" in part by the different details of the insult, it has become increasingly clear that there are genetic factors that predispose some individuals toward post-traumatic epileptogenesis. Such genetic determinants may not be manifest in an overt epileptic condition under normal conditions, but may facilitate the epileptogenic process once it is initiated by a potentially epileptogenic insult. Genetic predisposition has been clearly identified in animal models – for example in different strains of inbred mice (McKhann *et al.* 2003). How should this genetic contribution be factored into a discussion of mechanisms of "symptomatic" epilepsies?

Similarly, genetic abnormalities may have dramatic effects on brain development, with some developmental aberrations reflected in gross brain lesions ("symptoms") that are highly associated with the epileptic condition. In such cases, there is no obvious precipitating event to initiate epileptogenesis – but there is a development time window during which maturational processes give rise to an epileptic (or epileptogenic) state. Such developmental conditions are difficult to categorize as "acquired" epilepsies – but should they be included within the category of "symptomatic" epilepsies? Should the developmental processes that give rise to these brain abnormalities be considered "epileptogenic"?

Finally, the term "idiopathic" has been generally used to describe epilepsies that have no identifiable underlying neuropathology – i.e., no structural basis. However, genetic mutations – even single-gene mutations that affect a single channel or receptor – do have structural underpinnings. Although those structural abnormalities are at the molecular level, modern analysis techniques allow us to "see" many of these microscopic lesions. Thus, the term "idiopathic" has become less and less helpful in describing a category of epilepsy.

What mechanisms are "epileptic" and what mechanisms are "epileptogenic"?

Epileptogenesis is often described as a process that can be initiated in a normal brain, and which reaches fruition when the individual begins to exhibit spontaneous, recurrent seizures. Given this view, what do we make of the concept of seizure propensity? If an individual has a genetic complement that endows him with an innate sensitivity to epileptic insults, when/where does "epileptogenesis" begin (i.e., what is the precipitating "event")? If an individual is born with a genetically determined development brain lesion, is it the gene or the lesion that determines the seizure propensity?

Further, our view of the "latent" period – that time interval between the precipitating event and emergence of an epileptic state – may require modification. We tend to think of this period as a time for processes that lead to seizures, but within which seizures do not yet occur. Some experimental studies now suggest that seizure activity may exist at a very low frequency as an acute consequence of the epileptogenic insult (Williams *et al.* 2009) – that is, the brain is already in an *epileptic* state. Thus, what we call "epileptogenesis" may consist of those processes that increase seizure frequency and/or allow that activity to spread. A correlated issue is the possibility that epileptogenesis does not really "stop" once spontaneous seizure activity has begun. Certainly, the concept of seizures as epileptogenic stimuli remains widespread – and if seizures do "beget" seizures, then the mechanisms underlying epileptic discharge may well be also "epileptogenic."

Finally, how does one separate electrical/behavioral consequences of epileptogenesis – i.e., those criteria that we traditionally use to identify and categorize seizure activity – from other aspects of epileptic syndromes. For example, does post-insult cognitive decline or psychiatric abnormality constitute an "epileptic state" if no gross clinical or electrical signs are readily observable? Might such changes reflect subclinical epileptic processes? Does "epileptogenesis" occur in those cases?

The point of these questions is to emphasize the complexity of the concept of "epileptogenesis." Especially given our current ignorance about epileptogenic mechanisms, it would be unwise to discard potential processes as irrelevant, even if they don't seem to fit our standard definition of epileptogenesis. Further, given the likelihood that epileptogenic mechanisms derive from (are exaggerations of?) normal brain processes, we face the same therapeutic problem in antiepileptogenesis as we've encountered in developing antiepileptic (or anticonvulsant) treatments – the danger of blocking key, normal brain functions as we target the aberrant processes of seizure discharge or development of the epileptic state.

References

Beck H (2007) Plasticity of antiepileptic drug targets. *Epilepsia* 48(Suppl.1): 14–18.

Benardo LS (2003) Prevention of epilepsy after head trauma: do we need new drugs or a new approach? *Epilepsia* 44(Suppl.10):27–33.

Ben-Ari Y (2006) Seizures beget seizures: the quest for GABA as a key player. *Crit Rev Neurobiol* 18:135–44.

Blumenfeld H, Lampert A, Klein JP, et al. (2009) Role of hippocampal sodium channel Na$_v$ 1.6 in kindling epileptogenesis. *Epilepsia* 50:44–55.

Boison D (2008) The adenosine kinase hypothesis of epileptogenesis. *Progr Neurobiol* 84:249–62.

Bordey A, Spencer DD (2004) Distinct electrophysiological alterations in dentate gyrus versus CA1 glial cells from epileptic humans with temporal lobe sclerosis. *Epilepsy Res* 59:107–22.

Brooks-Kayal AR, Raol YH, Russek SJ (2009) Alterations of epleptogenesis genes. *Neurotherapeutics* 6:312–16.

Buckmaster PS, Jongen-Rêlo AL (1999) Highly specific neuron loss preserves lateral inhibitory ciucuits in the dentate gyrus of kainate-induced epileptic rats. *J Neurosci* 19:9519–29.

Chen K, Neu A, Howard AL, et al. (2007) Prevention of plasticity of endocannabinoid signaling inhibits persistent limbic hyperexcitability caused by developmental seizures. *J Neurosci* 27:46–58.

Choi J, Koh S (2008) Role of brain inflammation in epileptogenesis. *Yonsei Med J* 49:1–18.

D'Ambrosio R, Maris DO, Grady MS, Winn HR, Janigro D (1999) Impaired K$^+$ homeostasis and altered electrophysiological properties of post-traumatic hippocampal glia. *J Neurosci* 19:8152–62.

Ding S, Fellin T, Zhu Y, et al. (2007) Enhanced astrocytic Ca^{2+} signals contribute to neuronal excitotoxicity after status epilepticus. *J Neurosci* 27:10 674–84.

Dudek FE, Yasumura T, Rash JE (1998) 'Non-synaptic' mechanisms in seizures and epileptogenesis. *Cell Biol Int* 22:793–805.

Echegoyen J, Neu A, Graber KD, Soltesz I (2007) Homeostatic plasticity studied using in vivo hippocampal activity-blockade: synaptic scaling, intrinsic plasticity and age-dependence. *PLoS One* 2:**e700**.

Engel J Jr., Brain A, Staba R, Mody I (2009) High-frequency oscillations: what is normal and what is not? *Epilepsia* 50:598–604.

Fujikawa DG (2005) Prolonged seizures and cellular injury: understanding the connection. *Epilepsy Behav* 7(Suppl.3):S3–S11.

Gaetz M (2004) The neurophysiology of brain injury. *Clin Neurophysiol* 115:4–18.

Gall CM, Lynch G (2004) Integrins, synaptic plasticity and epileptogenesis. *Adv Exp Med Biol* 548:12–33.

Galvan CD, Hrachovy RA, Smith KL, Swann JW (2000) Blockade of neuronal activity during hippocampal development produces a chronic focal epilepsy in the rat. *J Neurosci* 20:2904–16.

Gorji A, Speckmann EJ (2004) Spreading depression enhances the spontaneous epileptiform activity in human neocortical tissues. *Eur J Neurosci* 19:3371–4.

Guerrini R, Marini C (2006) Genetic malformations of cortical development. *Exp Brain Res* 173:322–33.

He XP, Kotloski R, Nef S, et al. (2004) Conditional deletion of TrkB but not BDNF prevents epileptogenesis in the kindling model. *Neuron* 43:31–42.

Herman ST (2002) Epilepsy after brain insult: targeting epileptogenesis. *Neurology* 59(Suppl.5):S21–S26.

Hong SE, Shugart YY, Huang DT, et al. (2000) Autosomal recessive lissencephaly with cerebellar hypoplasia is associated with human *RELN* mutations. *Nat Genet* 26:93–6.

Houser CR (1990) Granule cell dispersion in the dentate gyrus of human with temporal lobe epilepsy. *Brain Res* 535:195–204.

Israelsson C, Bengtsson H, Kylberg A, et al. (2008) Distinct cellular patterns of upregulated chemokine expression supporting a prominent inflammatory role in traumatic brain injury. *J Neurotrauma* 25:959–74.

Jansen LA, Uhlmann EF, Crino PB, Gutmann DH, Wong M (2005) Epileptogenesis and reduced inward rectifier potassium current in tuberous sclerosis complex-1-deficient astrocytes. *Epilepsia* 46:1871–80.

Jung S, Jones TD, Lugo JN Jr., et al. (2007) Progressive dendritic HCN channelopathy during epileptogenesis in the rat pilocarpine model of epilepsy. *J Neurosci* 27:13 012–21.

Kahle KT, Staley KJ, Nahed BV, et al. (2008) Roles of the cation-chloride cotransporters in neurological disease. *Nat Clin Pract Neurol* 4:490–503.

Liang SL, Carlson GC, Coulter DA (2006) Dynamic regulation of synaptic GABA release by the glutmate-glutamine cycle in hippocampal area CA1. *J Neurosci* 26:8537–48.

Lima FD, Souza MA, Furian AF, et al. (2008) Na$^+$, K$^+$-ATPase activity after experimental traumatic brain injury: relationship to spatial learning deficits and oxidative stress. *Behav Brain Res* 193:306–10.

Lowenstein DH (2009) Epilepsy after head injury: an overview. *Epilepsia* 50(Suppl.2):4–9.

Mattson MP (2003) Excitotoxic and excitoprotective mechanisms: abundant targets for the prevention and treatment of neurodegenerative disorders. *Neuromol Med* 3:65–94.

McKhann GM 2nd, Wenzel HJ, Robbins CA, Sosunov AA, Schwartzkroin PA (2003) Mouse strain differences in kainic acid sensitivity, seizure behavior, mortality, and hippocampal pathology. *Neuroscience* 122:551–61.

McNamara JO, Whitney KD, Andrews PI, et al. (1999) Evidence for glutamate receptor autoimmunity in the pathogenesis of Rasmussen encephalitis. *Adv Neurol* 79:543–50.

Mori A, Yokoi I, Noda Y, Willmore LJ (2004) Natural antioxidants may prevent posttraumatic epilepsy: a proposal based on experimental studies. *Acta Med Okayama* 58:111–18.

Nadler JV (2003) The recurrent mossy fiber pathway of the epilepsy brain. *Neurochem Res* 28:1649–58.

Nemani VM, Binder DK (2005) Emerging role of gap junctions in epilepsy. *Histol Histopathol* 20:253–9.

Niizuma K, Endo H, Chan PH (2009) Oxidative stress and mitochondrial dysfunction as determinants of ischemic neuronal death and survival. *J Neurochem* 109(Suppl.1): 133–8.

Oby E, Janigro D (2006) The blood–brain barrier and epilepsy. *Epilepsia* 47:1761–74.

Parent JM, Murphy GG (2008) Mechanisms and functional significance of aberrant seizure-induced hippocampal neurogenesis. *Epilepsia* 49(Suppl.5):19–25.

Pitkänen A, Kharatishvili I, Karhunen H, *et al.* (2007) Epileptogenesis in experimental models. *Epilepsia* 48(Suppl.2):13–20.

Pleasure D (2008) Diagnostic and pathogenic significance of glutamate receptor autoantibodies. *Arch Neurol* 65:589–92.

Raza M, Blair RE, Sombati S, *et al.* (2004) Evidence that injury-induced changes in hippocampal neuronal calcium dynamics during epileptogenesis causes acquired epilepsy. *Proc Natl Acad Sci USA* 101:17 522–7.

Reinert M, Khaldi A, Zauner A, *et al.* (2000) High level of extracellular potassium and its correlates after severe head injury: relationship to high intracranial pressure. *J Neurosurg* 93:800–7.

Santello M, Volterra A (2009) Synaptic modulation by astrocytes via Ca^{2+}-dependent glutamate release. *Neuroscience* 158:253–9.

Scharfman HE, Goodman J, McCloskey D (2007) Ectopic granule cells of the rat dentate gyrus. *Dev Neurosci* 29:14–27.

Sun C, Mtchedlishvili Z, Bertram EH, Erisir A, Kapur J (2007) Selective loss of dentate hilar interneurons contributes to reduced synaptic inhibition of granule cells in an electrical stimulation-based animal model of temporal lobe epilepsy. *J Comp Neurol* 500:876–93.

Temkin NR (2009) Preventing and treating posttraumatic seizures: the human experience. *Epilepsia* 50(Suppl.2):10–13.

Vezzani A, Granata T (2005) Brain inflammation in epilepsy: experimental and clinical evidence. *Epilepsia* 46:1724–43.

Vezzani A, Ravizza T, Balosso S, Aronica E (2008) Glia as a source of cytokines: implications for neuronal excitability. *Epilepsia* 49(Suppl.2):24–32.

Xu B, Michalski B, Racine RJ, Fahnestock M (2002) Continuous infusion of neurotrophin-3 triggers sprouting, decreases the levels of TrkA and TrkC, and inhibits epileptogenesis and activity-dependent axonal growth in adult rats. *Neuroscience* 115:1295–308.

Williams PA, White AM, Clark S, *et al.* (2009) Development of spontaneous recurrent seizures after kainate-induced status epilepticus. *J Neurosci* 29:2103–12.

Chapter

5

Introduction to the concept of genetic epilepsy

Renzo Guerrini, Simon D. Shorvon, Frederick Andermann, and Eva Andermann

It has been estimated that genetic factors contribute to at least 40% of all epilepsies (Guerrini *et al.* 2003b). In the last decade more than 13 genes have been linked to "idiopathic" epilepsies (Lowenstein and Messing 2007) and most genes encode for components of ion channels or for related molecules. Mutations of these known genes only account for a small fraction of patients, thus many other genes causing seizures are yet to be identified.

Most of the idiopathic epilepsies do not follow single-gene inheritance and their occurrence in large families is rare. Some rare forms of idiopathic epilepsies have Mendelian inheritance where molecular gene defects have been identified. The discovery of these epilepsy genes has been facilitated by the availability of single large families with many affected members, in which a single mutated gene segregates with most affected individuals. However, even in families with apparently single-gene inheritance there is a degree of complexity. The simple correspondence between genotype and phenotype can break down as the same genotype can result in different phenotypes (phenotypic heterogeneity) or, conversely, identical phenotypes may be due to different genotypes (genetic heterogeneity). The phenotypic variability in such families can be attributed to modifier genes or polymorphisms influencing the phenotypic expression or, alternatively, to environmental factors.

Many symptomatic epilepsies are directly linked to genetic factors. Single-gene disorders and structural chromosomal abnormalities can cause developmental brain abnormalities at the macroscopic or ultrastructural level, or metabolic disorders can lead to intracellular changes that are epileptogenic. The propensity to develop epilepsy as a consequence of an acquired brain lesion is also influenced by the individual's genetic background. Provoking factors such as photosensitivity (Chapter 97) can also have a genetic basis, as can some reflex epilepsies (for instance hot-water epilepsy, Chapter 102).

Problems and approaches to genetic studies of the epilepsies

The chief difficulty of genetic studies lies in the fact that the epilepsies are characterized by marked clinical and genetic

Table 5.1 Data acquisition in genetic studies of the epilepsies

(A) Detailed history	
Mother's pregnancy and delivery	Personal and social history
Developmental milestones	Psychiatric history (if any)
Seizure and neurological history	Obstetric history
General medical history	Medication
Educational background	Family history
(B) Seizure history	
Age of onset	
Precipitating factors	
Type(s) of seizures	
Seizure frequency	
Diurnal variation	
Response to medication	
Epilepsy syndrome	
(C) Detailed family history	
Ethnic origin(s)	Congenital malformations
Consanguinity	Mental retardation
Epilepsy	Other genetic diseases
Febrile seizures	Other diseases or surgical procedures
Isolated seizures	

heterogeneity. Other problems include biases in ascertainment, difficulties in determining which relatives are "affected," decreased penetrance, and variable expressivity of genes (Berkovic *et al.* 2006).

Genetic studies of the epilepsies involve two main aspects: detailed gathering of data and data analysis (Table 5.1). The gathering of data with accurate proband ascertainment and phenotyping of family members, as well as detailed family

---

history and pedigree, is key to the success of genetic studies. Data analysis includes segregation analysis to determine the possible mode of inheritance, linkage analysis (parametric or non-parametric), and, more recently, analysis of candidate genes, genome-wide association studies, and the search for pathogenic copy number variations, which may in turn provide insights about the causative role of single genes.

The detailed medical history in the proband should include the features listed in Table 5.1A. The seizure history for the proband and affected family members should include the features in Table 5.1B and lead if possible to the diagnosis of a specific epilepsy syndrome. A detailed family history should be obtained for the patient's immediate family and on the maternal and paternal sides as far up as possible. Information on all diseases, particularly those listed in Table 5.1C, should be sought for each individual in the pedigree, including spouses. If other individuals in the family have a history of seizures, the details listed in Table 5.1B should be documented, for each individual. The relatives should be examined, if possible, and/or the medical records should be obtained.

Genetic versus acquired

Over the years, there have been conflicting opinions on the importance of genetic factors in epilepsy. Lennox (1951), in a study of 20 000 relatives of 4231 patients with epilepsy, found that, both in the essential or genetic (now termed "idiopathic" or, more recently, again, "genetic") and symptomatic types of epilepsy, there was evidence of increased familial predisposition, in that the prevalence of epilepsy in the near relatives of both groups of patients was significantly increased as compared with the general population. Furthermore, the prevalence of epilepsy in the near relatives of the essential group was higher than that in the near relatives of the symptomatic group. These findings were confirmed by twin studies (Lennox 1951, 1960; Lennox and Jolly, 1954), and by the work of other authors (Metrakos 1961). Based on the family studies, Lennox (1960) concluded that the division between idiopathic and symptomatic epilepsy is not clear-cut, and that both genetic and environmental factors are operative to varying degrees in every patient (see Chapter 1). The assessment is complicated by susceptibility to provoking factors, some of which themselves may have a genetic basis (Chapter 88). Recent estimates of the "heritability" of epilepsy, discussed further in Chapter 6, range from 8% to 88%.

Recent twin studies confirmed the original findings of Lennox, indicating that both genetic and environmental factors contribute in varying degrees to the etiology of different epilepsy syndromes (Vadlamudi *et al.* 2004b; Berkovic *et al.* 2006). Vadlamudi *et al.* (2004a) studied the original files of the Lennox twins, and were able to classify the seizure syndromes of the patients according to the current ILAE classification (Commission on Classification and Terminology of the ILAE 1989), and to compare them with the Australian

twin data, resulting in amazing similarities in these two series collected on different continents about 50 years apart.

Increased awareness about the genetic determinants of the epilepsies

Recent advances in genetics of the epilepsies have resulted from various factors:

(1) Improved phenotyping and classification of epilepsy syndromes, with identification of a number of single-gene or Mendelian syndromes (Table 5.2).

(2) Advances in neuroimaging, leading to diagnosis of malformations of cortical development (Table 5.3, and see Chapters 44–52) as well as many other causes of symptomatic epilepsies.

(3) Advances in molecular biology, leading to mapping (Table 5.4, and see Chapters 3 and 4) of genes for a number of epilepsy syndromes, employing molecular genetic techniques.

(4) Advances in genetic epidemiology, specifically analysis of complex genetic traits and genome-wide association studies. The mathematical aspects of these analyses, as well as of mutation and polymorphism databases, and genotype–phenotype correlations, are now included in the new field of bioinformatics.

Genetics and the classification of the epilepsies

Just as the contemporary opinion about the importance of genetic factors in the causation of epilepsy has varied at different times, so too there has been different emphasis applied to genetics in the classification of the epilepsies. In the older literature, the classification was etiological and divided into two main categories: The terms "idiopathic," "cryptogenic," "essential," or "genetic" were employed when there was no known cause to account for the seizures, as opposed to "symptomatic" or "acquired" when an external cause could be identified. The term "cryptogenic" was later separated to indicate a suspected brain lesion, that could not be identified by current diagnostic methods but this term is now considered confusing and included with the symptomatic epilepsies. Even the terms "idiopathic" and "symptomatic", although useful for clinical and didactic purposes, are not necessarily distinct entities (Engel 2001, 2006a,b). Newer molecular evidence has also shown that specific gene mutations can result in both generalized and focal epilepsy syndromes in the same family (e.g., temporal lobe epilepsy in families with GEFS+: Scheffer *et al.* 2007). The relationships between idiopathic and symptomatic epilepsies, and between generalized and focal epilepsies, as well as the concept of the epileptic diathesis, have very recently been reviewed (Luders *et al.* 2009; Rodin 2009). The terms "genetic," "structural–metabolic," and "unknown" have

Table 5.2 Epilepsy syndromes having a single-gene mode of inheritance

Epilepsy syndrome	Type of seizures	Gene	Protein	Locus	OMIM
Generalized epilepsy with febrile seizures plus (GEFS+)	Febrile and afebrile, complex partial, generalized tonic–clonic, absences, myoclonic	SCN1A	Sodium channel, neuronal type 1, α-subunit	2q24.3	182389
		SCN1B	Sodium channel, neuronal type 1, β-subunit	19q13.1	600235
		GABRG2	Gamma-amino butyric acid receptor, γ-2	5q31.1–q33.1	137164
Severe myoclonic epilepsy of infancy (SMEI) or Dravet syndrome	Febrile, partial, absences, myoclonic, generalized or unilateral clonic, generalized tonic–clonic	SCN1A	Sodium channel, neuronal type 1, α-subunit	2q24.3	182389
Benign familial neonatal seizures (BFNS)	Multifocal neonatal convulsions, generalized tonic–clonic	KCNQ2	Potassium channel, voltage-gated, KQT-like subfamily, member 2	20q13.3	602235
		KCNQ3	Potassium channel, voltage-gated, KQT-like subfamily, member 3	8q24	602232
Benign familial neonatal/infantile seizures (BFNIS)	Multifocal neonatal convulsions, generalized tonic–clonic	SCN2A	Sodium channel, voltage-gated, type 2, α subunit	2q23–q24.3	182390
Benign familial infantile seizures (BFIS) with familial hemiplegic migraine	Multifocal neonatal convulsions, generalized tonic–clonic, hemiplegic migraine	ATP1A2	ATPase, Na$^+$/K$^+$ transporting, α-2 polypeptide	1q21–q23	182340
Autosomal dominant nocturnal frontal lobe epilepsy (ADNLFE)	Partial nocturnal motor seizures with hyperkinetic manifestations	CHRNA4	Cholinergic receptor, neuronal nicotinic, α polypeptide 4	20q13.2–q13.3	118504
		CHRNB2	Cholinergic receptor, neuronal nicotinic, β polypeptide 2	1q21	118507
		CHRNA2	Cholinergic receptor, neuronal nicotinic, α polypeptide 2	8p21	118502
Autosomal dominant temporal lobe epilepsy (ADTLE)	Partial seizures with auditory or visual hallucinations	LGI1	Leucine-rich, glioma-inactivated 1	10q24	604619
Childhood absence epilepsy (CAE)	Absences, tonic–clonic	GABRG2	Gamma-amino butyric acid receptor, γ-2	5q31.1–q33.1	137164
		CLCN2	Chloride channel 2	3q26	600570
Absence epilepsy and paroxysmal dyskinesia	Absences, paroxysmal dyskinesia	KCNMA1	Calcium-sensitive potassium (BK) channel	10q22	609446
Juvenile myoclonic epilepsy (JME)	Myoclonic, tonic–clonic, absence	GABRA1	Gamma-amino butyric acid receptor, α-1	5q34–q35	137160
		EFHC1	Protein with an EF-hand motif	6p12–p11	254770
Infantile spasms, West syndrome	Infantile spasms, hypsarrhythmia	ARX	Gene homeobox Aristaless-related	Xq22.13	300382
Early infantile epileptic encephalopathy, infantile spasms	Myoclonic, infantile spasms	CDKL5	Cyclin-dependent kinase 5	Xp22X	300203
Epilepsy and mental retardation restricted to females	Febrile, partial, absences, myoclonic, generalized tonic–clonic	PCDH19	Protocadherin 19	Xq22	300460
Early epileptic encephalopathy with suppression burst (Ohtahara syndrome)	Tonic, infantile spasms	STXBP1	Syntaxin binding protein 1	9q34.1	602926

Table 5.3 Genes associated with epilepsy relating to cortical malformations

Cortical malformation	Pattern of inheritance	Gene	Locus	OMIM
Lissencephaly				
Miller–Dieker syndrome	Autosomal dominant	*LIS1*	17p13.3	601545
Isolated lissencephaly sequence (ILS) or subcortical band heterotopia (SBH)	Autosomal dominant	*LIS1*	17p13.3	601545
Isolated lissencephaly sequence or SBH	X-linked	*DCX*	Xq22.3–q23	300121
Isolated lissencephaly sequence	Autosomal dominant	*TUBA1A*	12q12–q14	602529
X-linked lissencephaly with abnormal genitalia (XLAG)	X-linked	*ARX*	Xp22.13	300382
Lissencephaly with cerebellar hypoplasia	Autosomal dominant	*RELN*	7q22	600514
Periventricular heterotopia				
Classical bilateral periventricular nodular heterotopia (PNH)	X-linked	*FLNA*	Xq28	300017
Ehlers–Danlos syndrome and PNH	X-linked	*FLNA*	Xq28	300017
Facial dysmorphisms, severe constipation, and PNH	X-linked	*FLNA*	Xq28	300017
Fragile-X syndrome and PNH	X-linked	*FMR1*	Xq27.3	309550
Periventricular nodular heterotopia with limb abnormalities (limb reduction abnormality or syndactyly)	X-linked	—	Xq28	
Williams syndrome and PNH	Autosomal dominant	—	7q11.23	
Periventricular heterotopia (PH)	Autosomal dominant	—	5p15.1	
PH	Autosomal dominant	—	5p15.33	
Agenesis of the corpus callosum, polymicrogyria, and PNH	Autosomal dominant	—	6q26–qter	
PH	Autosomal dominant		4p15	
PH	Autosomal dominant	—	5q14.3–q15	
Agenesis of the corpus callosum and PNH	Autosomal dominant	—	1p36.22–pter	
Microcephaly and PNH	Autosomal recessive	*ARFGEF2*	20q13.13	605371
Donnai–Barrow syndrome and PNH	Autosomal recessive	*LRP2*	2q24–q31	600073
Polymicrogyria (PMG)				
Polymicrogyria and rolandic seizures, oromotor dyspraxia	X-linked	*SRPX2*	Xq21.33–q23	300642
Polymicrogyria and agenesis of the corpus callosum (ACC), microcephaly	Autosomal dominant	*TBR2*	3p21.3–p21.2	604615
Polymicrogyria and aniridia	Autosomal dominant	*PAX6*	11p13	607108
Polymicrogyria	Autosomal dominant	—	1p36.3–pter	
Polymicrogyria	Autosomal dominant	*TUBB2B*	6p25.2	610031
Polymicrogyria and microcephaly	Autosomal dominant	—	1q44–qter	
Polymicrogyria and facial dysmorphisms	Autosomal dominant	—	2p16.1–p23	
Polymicrogyria and microcephaly, hydrocephalus	Autosomal dominant		4q21–q22	
Polymicrogyria	Autosomal dominant	—	21q2	
Polymicrogyria and DiGeorge syndrome	Autosomal dominant	—	22q11.2	
Polymicrogyria and Warburg Micro syndrome	Autosomal recessive	*RAB3GAP1*	2q21.3	602536
Polymicrogyria and Goldberg–Shprintzen syndrome	Autosomal recessive	*KIAA1279*	10q21.3	609367

Table 5.4 Chromosomal loci associated with epilepsy syndromes

Epilepsy syndrome	Locus
Juvenile myoclonic epilepsy	6p21, 15q14
Autosomal dominant cortical myoclonus and epilepsy	2p11.1
Familial adult myoclonic epilepsy	8q23.3
Familial idiopathic myoclonic epilepsy of infancy	16p13
Infantile convulsions and paroxysmal coreoathetosis	16p12–q12
Benign familial infantile convulsions	19q
Benign rolandic epilepsy	15q24
Rolandic epilepsy exercise-induced dystonia writer's cramp	16p12
Autosomal dominant nocturnal frontal lobe epilepsy	15q24
Familial partial epilepsy with variable foci	22q11
Febrile seizures	2q24, 5q14, 6q22, 8q13, 19p13, 3q26
Partial epilepsy with pericentral spikes	4p15
Childhood absence epilepsy	8q24
Idiopathic generalized epilepsy	3q26, 2q36, 15q13
Adolescent-onset idiopathic generalized epilepsy	8p12, 18q12

been recently suggested as modified concepts to replace idiopathic, symptomatic, and cryptogenic (Berg *et al.* 2010). However, some recently characterized genetic disorders challenge the distinction between the "pure" genetic epilepsies, which are ideally epitomized by ion-channel alterations, and the structural–metabolic disorders in which a separate abnormality is interposed between the genetic defect and the epilepsy. For example, epilepsy in non-malformation *ARX* phenotypes (at least in relation to some of the mutations of this gene) or in patients with *STXBP1* or *CDKL5* mutations/deletions is difficult to assign to either the "genetic" or the "structural" category. It seems to be a primary expression of the genetic defect: since all patients have severe seizures but no structural lesion is recognizable as far as the diagnostic dimension can be pushed (Guerrini 2010). Neuropathology and molecular pathology will hopefully provide an answer to these queries in the future. The classification scheme, and definitions, applied in this book is outlined further in Chapter 2.

The contribution of genetics to nosology and classification of the epilepsies should be carefully considered. If genetic criteria were prominent, epilepsy syndromes having

heterogeneous clinical expressions would be classified within the same category and homogeneous syndromes caused by different genetic mechanisms would fall in different subcategories. For example, Dravet syndrome and GEFS+ have different clinical expression and severity but can both be caused by intragenic mutations of the *SCN1A* gene. On the other hand, Dravet syndrome can also be caused by copy-number variations leading to genomic deletions or duplications of contiguous genes including *SCN1A* or part of it at the kilobase or megabase level (Marini *et al.* 2009). Etiologic heterogeneity poses insoluble classification problems in common conditions, such as the infantile spasms syndrome, which are caused by mutations in a variety of genes, including *TSC*, *LIS1*, *DCX*, *ARX*, and *CDKL5*, by various copy-number variations or chromosomal or mitochondrial disorders, but are also caused by a number of acquired factors. It is therefore obvious that a genetic classification of the epilepsies can on the one hand offer an objective marker for etiological diagnosis and enlighten prognostic predictions when genotype–phenotype correlations are available, but, on the other hand, could be confusing when the same conditions are caused by different genetic mechanisms.

Modes of inheritance

The genetic mechanisms leading to epilepsy can act through a number of possible modes of inheritance, including single-gene (monogenic or Mendelian) inheritance; polygenic (many genes each with small additive effects), e.g., those determining height, weight, and IQ, which are normally distributed traits; multifactorial or complex inheritance (one or more major genes and/or polygenes interacting with environmental factors); mitochondrial (maternal, cytoplasmic); chromosomal abnormalities (identified by cytogenetic studies, fluorescent in situ hybridization or array comparative genomic hybridization [CGH] techniques). A large number of mental retardation/epilepsy syndromes are caused by copy-number variations, including some recurrent syndromes and a large number of rare syndromes, in which deletions or duplications of a variable number of genes concur in determining the phenotype, with consequent difficulties in identifying the role of specific genes in causing epilepsy.

The analysis of genetic contributions within families is complicated by phenocopies, a term used to refer to individuals in a family with the same phenotype but who do not carry the family mutation (e.g., some patients with simple febrile seizures in GEFS+ families).

Main features of multifactorial or complex inheritance

This mode of inheritance postulates a normally distributed liability or susceptibility in the general population with a threshold effect above which an individual is "affected"

(Falconer 1965). The curve for first-degree relatives is shifted to the right, so that the prevalence in relatives is greater than that in the general population. The vast majority of epilepsies, both generalized and focal, are inherited in this manner.

The main features of multifactorial or complex inheritance are, as follows: high population frequency (prevalence > 1/1000); familial prevalence is higher than that in the general population; does not fit classical Mendelian ratios; and environmental factors are important. The risk to relatives depends on the degree of relationship, and drops rapidly from first-to third-degree relatives, unlike autosomal dominant inheritance where the drop is only by a factor of two for each degree of relationship. In multifactorial inheritance, parents, siblings, and children may be lumped with respect to risks, similar to autosomal dominant inheritance, but differing from autosomal recessive inheritance. The risk to relatives increases according to the number affected in the family, and this is unlike Mendelian inheritance, where the risk remains constant.

Susceptibility genes in common diseases may represent common gene polymorphisms, each with small phenotypic effects, seen in greater than 1% of the general population (e.g., single-nucleotide polymorphisms, SNPs). This is termed the "common disease – common variant" model. There is also a possibility of multiple rare polymorphisms, with relatively greater phenotypic effects, each occurring in less than 1% of the general population, as well as a combination of both (Mulley *et al.* 2005a). Common gene variants contributing to diseases with complex inheritance can be detected by means of genome-wide association studies, unlike the rare variants (Mullen *et al.* 2009). Association studies are considered to be a better tool to elucidate the genetic basis of diseases that show a high familial recurrence rate but are probably not caused by a single gene (Risch and Merikangas 1996). In the last decade more than 50 association studies have been performed but gene defects for common polygenic epilepsies have not yet been identified, leading to some skepticism about the association study approach (Tan *et al.* 2004). The main types of genetic changes contributing to human disease and their means of detection are listed in Table 5.5. In addition to the various genetic influences, the epileptic phenotype can be influenced by environmental, developmental or maturational, and endogenous or hormonal factors.

The issues relating to false-positive findings in association studies (a problem that has bedeviled the field), and the relative merits of the common disease – common variant and common disease – rare variant hypotheses are discussed further in Chapter 6.

Idiopathic generalized epilepsies: a model for complex inheritance

The idiopathic generalized epilepsies constitute a group of syndromes characterized by absence seizures, myoclonus, and generalized tonic–clonic seizures (see also Chapter 12). There is a partial overlap in age of onset, type and frequency of

Table 5.5 Genetic changes contributing to human disease

Monogenic (Mendelian)	– rare mutations with large effects on phenotype
Rare genetic variants	– <1% of the population
	– relatively large effects on phenotype
	– may be pathogenic
Common genetic variants or polymorphisms with small effects on phenotype (e.g., SNPs)	– interact with other genes and/or environmental factors to produce phenotype
Copy-number variation	– deletions, insertions, amplifications involving one or more exons
	– deletions involving a number of genes
	– detected by multiplex ligation-dependent probe amplification (MLPA) and array CGH
Splice site variations	– isoforms with different number of exons
	– may be pathogenic
Epigenetic factors	
DNA methylation	– histone protein modification

seizures, prognosis, and response to treatment. Based on detailed family histories and electroencephalography (EEG) studies in the relatives of patients with idiopathic generalized epilepsies, Metrakos and Metrakos (1969, 1970) suggested that the spike–wave EEG trait, but not the epilepsy, was inherited as an autosomal dominant trait with age-dependent penetrance. This trait had very low penetrance at birth, which rose rapidly to nearly complete penetrance (i.e., expression in almost 50% of first-degree relatives) around the age of 10 years, and declined rapidly to age 20 and gradually to almost no penetrance after age 40. Matthes and Weber (1968) and Doose *et al.* (1973) obtained similar results in parents and siblings of patients with spike–wave absences, although the frequency of spike–wave abnormalities in relatives was lower.

Relatives of probands who had focal EEG abnormalities with or without seizures were also found to have a significantly higher prevalence of 3/s spike–wave EEG abnormalities than control relatives (Metrakos and Metrakos, 1974), but lower than that found in relatives of probands with centrencephalic epilepsy or febrile convulsions (Metrakos and Metrakos 1969, 1970). This method of employing EEG traits as markers of genetic susceptibility would now be termed endophenotyping (Gottesmann and Gould 2003).

Andermann (1972) and Andermann and Metrakos (1972) demonstrated that the families with idiopathic generalized epilepsy fit the model of multifactorial inheritance. This has been further corroborated by various twin studies (Berkovic et al. 1998; Miller et al. 1998; Kjeldsen et al. 2001; Vadlamudi et al. 2004a). Berkovic et al. (1998) and Vadlamudi et al. (2004a) drew the following conclusions:

(1) The high concordance rate for idiopathic generalized epilepsies in monozygotic (MZ) twin pairs (Lennox 75%; Berkovic et al. 65%) strongly supports the primacy of genetic factors.

(2) The concordance using EEG criteria is even higher (Lennox 84%; Berkovic et al. 82%).

(3) The fidelity of subsyndromes in MZ twin pairs (e.g., juvenile myoclonic epilepsy or childhood absence epilepsy) suggested that the subsyndromes are genetically distinct. In particular, childhood absence epilepsy (CAE) and juvenile absence epilepsy (JAE) tend to segregate in different families as compared to juvenile myoclonic epilepsy (Marini et al. 2004; Winawer et al. 2005).

(4) The low rate of concordance in dizygotic (DZ) twin pairs with MZ/DZ ratios >4 and lack of fidelity of subsyndromes in DZ twins excludes simple dominant or recessive inheritance.

These findings led the authors to conclude that a complex or complexes of multiple genes probably underlie the idiopathic generalized epilepsies (IGE). A typical example of the underlying genetic complexity is provided by the absence epilepsies. Absence epilepsies show a complex pattern of inheritance, which, in keeping with other common genetic disorders, is expected to result from the action of a few or many genes of small to moderate effect. Genome-wide linkage analysis of IGE-multiplex families has demonstrated evidence for susceptibility loci on chromosomes 2q36, 3q26, and 14q23 (Sander et al. 2000). Furthermore, loci for three similar forms of absence epilepsy have been identified on chromosomes 8q24, 5q31.1, 3q26, and 3p23–p14 (Fong et al. 1998; Sugimoto et al. 2000; Wallace et al. 2001; Robinson et al. 2002; Chioza et al. 2009). Linkage and association to chromosome 16p12–p13.1, the region containing the calcium channel gene CACNG3 has been demonstrated (Everett et al. 2007). An association in humans has been documented between polymorphisms in CACNA1A (chromosome 19p13.2–p13.1) and IGE including CAE (Chioza et al. 2001). Twelve missense mutations in CACNA1H (chromosome 16p13.3) have been found in 14 sporadic Chinese Han patients with CAE but not in any of 230 unrelated controls (Chen et al. 2003). Mutations in three γ-amino butyric acid (GABA) receptor genes have been identified in families with CAE (sometimes in conjunction with other seizure types): GABRG2 (Wallace et al. 2001), GABRA1 (Maljevic et al. 2006), and GABRB3 (Feucht et al. 1999; Tanaka et al. 2008).

Photosensitivity (Chapter 97) is another clinically associated factor in idiopathic epilepsy which has a strong genetic basis (as is evident from the large familial clusters) but the genetic trait may segregate independently of epilepsy, and the causal genes have eluded detection despite intensive effort. The problem of age-related expression complicates genetic analysis in photosensitivity as it does in idiopathic epilepsy (de Kovel et al. 2010).

The single-gene epilepsies with no structural or metabolic etiology

A number of epilepsy syndromes, or disorders in which epilepsy is a main manifestation, have been recognized, and are caused by single-gene mutations. These disorders are summarized in Tables 5.2 and 5.3 but are not dealt with in this chapter since they are illustrated in detail in other sections of this book. The discovery of these genes has been facilitated by the availability of single large families with many affected members and clear Mendelian inheritance. For most of the idiopathic epilepsies, however, we still do not know why sporadic patients with similar phenotypes do not carry the mutations identified in the families, although no phenotypic differences seem to exist between familial and sporadic patients with idiopathic generalized epilepsies (Briellmann et al. 2001) or between patients with lateral temporal lobe epilepsy harboring LGI1 gene mutations and those who are mutation negative (Bisulli et al. 2004). Genes causing disorders that co-occur with epilepsy, such as migraine (Vanmolkot et al. 2003) or paroxysmal dyskinesia (Du et al. 2005) do not seem to have any substantial effects on the genetic variance of common syndromes either.

Recent identification of the causative genes for a number of early-onset severe epilepsies has led to the possibility of genetic testing (Deprez et al. 2009). Although the clinical impact of genetic testing is considered to be by itself limited, due to the small percentage of patients in whom a mutation can be identified and the lack of specific treatment options, genetic counseling, though complex, can certainly be improved by recognition of a specific etiology and patients can be diagnosed more specifically, reducing the need for unnecessary investigations. Accordingly, although brain malformations, metabolic encephalopathies, and copy-number variations play a major role as causative factors, monogenic severe epileptic encephalopathies presenting with no structural or metabolic etiology are emerging as an important category of disorders whose genetic causes are starting to be disentangled.

The clinical spectrum of Dravet syndrome, which is rather distinctive and closely related to SCN1A mutations (>70%) or deletions/duplications (3%) (Marini et al. 2007, 2009), is also observed in some girls with mutations of the protocadherin 19 (PCDH19) gene (Depienne et al. 2009). However, PCDH19 mutations have been related to epilepsy and mental retardation limited to females (EFMR), an X-linked disorder surprisingly affecting only females and sparing transmitting males, but also often appearing de novo (Marini et al. 2010). It is characterized by a variable clinical presentation, including slow development from birth, normal early development followed by regression starting around seizure onset, and normal development without regression (Dibbens et al. 2008; Deprez et al. 2009). The epilepsy spectrum associated with PCDH19 mutations is in turn variable and includes mild focal epilepsy starting in infancy or epilepsy with recurrent episodes of focal or generalized status epilepticus triggered by fever (Marini *et al.* 2010).

Ohtahara syndrome or early infantile epileptic encephalopathy syndrome with suppression bursts, and infantile spasms, can both be caused by polyalanine expansions of the *Aristaless*-related homeobox (*ARX*) gene (Kato *et al.* 2007; Guerrini *et al.* 2007) and by mutations of the syntaxin binding protein 1 (*STXBP1*) gene. The STXBP1 protein plays an essential role in synaptic vesicle release and secretion of neurotransmitters (Saitsu *et al.* 2008). Available information suggests a mutation rate of about 6% for *ARX* in boys with isolated or X-linked infantile spasms and no brain lesions (Guerrini *et al.* 2007) and up to 37% for *STPBX* in infants with Ohtahara syndrome (Saitsu *et al.* 2008). However, larger series are needed to fully understand the role of these genes. Mutations of both *ARX* and *STXBP1* have also been causally related to non-syndromic mental retardation and epilepsy (Stromme *et al.* 2002; Hamdan *et al.* 2009). The Ohtahara syndrome–infantile spasms spectrum, as well as other forms of very early-onset epilepsies with prominent tonic spasms and profound cognitive impairment, can also be caused by mutations or genomic deletions of the X-linked cyclin-dependent kinase-like 5 (*CDKL5*) gene (Weaving *et al.* 2004; Archer *et al.* 2006; Mei *et al.* 2009). Mutations in *CDKL5* are mainly found in female patients, suggesting gestational lethality in males (Elia *et al.* 2008). Parental germline mosaicism has been reported (Weaving *et al.* 2004). Frequency of *CDKL5* mutations was 17% in females with early-onset epilepsy associated with severe mental retardation of unknown etiology and 10% in girls with infantile spasms (Archer *et al.* 2006); overall, 16.3% of girls with early-onset intractable epilepsy, with or without infantile spasms, exhibited abnormalities of the *CDKL5* gene, including mutations and genomic deletions. (Mei *et al.* 2009).

Chromosomal imbalances and epilepsy: from etiological diagnosis to research

Chromosomal abnormalities are relatively common genetically determined conditions that increase the risk of epilepsy. However, the likelihood of developing seizures varies greatly among the different chromosomal disorders. Chromosomal abnormalities almost constantly result from rearrangements or deletions/duplications that affect the function of more than one gene. As a consequence, even when techniques with the highest resolution such as microarray–CGH are used, patients with chromosomal abnormalities always have a combination of clinical features and only exceptionally have isolated epilepsy. Virtually all known chromosomal abnormalities lead to anatomofunctional impairment of the central nervous system (CNS) and, especially those involving autosomes, are accompanied by cognitive impairment. Tharapel and Summit (1978) found 6.2% of cases of mental retardation to be associated with chromosomal abnormalities, as contrasted with the 0.7% rate found in controls. The ring chromosome 20 syndrome

(see Chapter 43) represents the most striking example in which a highly specific epilepsy phenotype can be, at least in some patients, the only expression of the chromosomal disorder. Most often cognitive impairment and dysmorphic features, even subtle, co-occur with epilepsy. Among patients with epilepsy and intellectual disability, about 6% have chromosomal abnormalities, but this figure climbs to 50% if multiple congenital abnormalities are also present (Singh *et al.* 2002). The use of such current techniques as high-resolution chromosome banding, fluorescent in situ hybridization (FISH), comparative genomic hybridization (array CGH), and multiplex ligand-dependent probe amplification (MLPA) would certainly increase these detection rates. Recently it was estimated that genome-wide molecular cytogenetic techniques can detect cryptic deletions/duplications in no fewer than 20% of individuals with mental retardation and dysmorphic features but apparently normal karyotype (Shaw-Smith *et al.* 2004).

While some conditions are associated with a risk for epilepsy only slightly greater than that in the general population, others carry a risk close to 100% and the epilepsy is a constant phenotypic feature (Guerrini *et al.* 2008). Some chromosomal abnormalities result in intractable seizures, whereas others have a more favorable epilepsy prognosis. Susceptibility to developing epilepsy does not necessarily correlate with the severity of structural abnormalities of the brain or with the extent of the chromosomal derangement. Depending on the specific genes involved, seizure susceptibility is more likely to be related to factors that alter cortical excitability, such as gene-dosage effect in genes involved in ion channel and neurotransmitter function or neural development. Awareness of the associations between syndromes due to chromosomal abnormalities and epilepsy, together with knowledge of their response to treatment and the expected outcome, should help plan rational treatment and counseling for families.

Most chromosomal abnormalities are duplication syndromes (with duplication of a segment of a chromosome), deletion syndromes (absence of a segment), and breakpoint disruption syndromes (only one or a few genes are disrupted). The risk of epilepsy is greater in individuals with chromosomal abnormalities than in the general population (Holmes 1987). However, chromosomal abnormalities do not represent a frequent cause of epilepsy (Jennings and Bird 1981). Epilepsy as a complication of a chromosomal imbalance should be considered in a twofold perspective. First, symptomatic epilepsies have a high probability of causing intractable seizures, leading to further disability. Severe epilepsy may significantly reduce a low-IQ patient's potential for autonomy in everyday life (Guerrini *et al.* 2008). Therefore, early recognition and appropriate treatment of characteristic electroclinical patterns known to be closely associated with chromosomal imbalances will improve a patient's prognosis. For example patients with Angelman syndrome, ring chromosome 20 syndrome, 4p- syndrome, or inverted duplicated chromosome 15 (see Chapters 28, 41–3) are now diagnosed early and treated better because their clinical presentations are widely recognized. Second, when seizures are the main manifestation of a chromosomal disorder or present with peculiar electroclinical patterns, it is important to establish whether these associations result from structural CNS abnormalities caused by the chromosomal changes or from the effect of loci that specifically affect seizure susceptibility. Careful attention to chromosomal abnormalities associated with seizures, together with detailed analysis of electroclinical patterns, may help detect specific genes affecting seizure susceptibility (Singh *et al.* 2002). Epilepsy has been associated with over 400 different chromosomal imbalances (Singh *et al.* 2002; Guerrini *et al.* 2008). Most pathogenic copy-number variations detected by CGH array are rare or unique, making it difficult to collect a sufficient number of patients to identify characteristic features of epilepsy for each chromosomal syndrome. However, at the research level on the causes of epilepsy, the association between cryptic deletions/duplications and epilepsy is improving our ability to clone new critical genes, translating in turn in improved diagnosis. For example, heterozygous missense mutations in the gene encoding syntaxin binding protein 1 (*STXBP1*) in patients with infantile epileptic encephalopathy with suppression bursts (Ohtahara syndrome), were found after a de novo 2.0-Mb microdeletion at 9q33.3–q34.11 in an affected girl prompted analysis of candidate genes mapped to the deleted region in patients with overlapping phenotypes. The diagnostic yield and genotype–phenotype correlations in Dravet syndrome have been improved after the description of microchromosomal rearrangements involving *SCN1A* and contiguous genes in some patients with severe expression of the syndrome (Marini *et al.* 2009).

In clinical practice, a large number of children are brought to medical attention because of seizures and cognitive impairment, variably associated with dysmorphic features and birth defects. Although alterations involving contiguous genes are expected in these patients conventional methods for identifying chromosomal imbalances yield positive results in only a minority. In the last several years, array CGH has greatly improved the diagnostic yield, allowing the identification of new syndromes caused by genomic imbalances as small as a few dozen kilobases. It is estimated that small chromosomal aberrations escaping routine chromosome banding are present in 5–20% of patients with mental retardation/developmental delay and dysmorphisms (Ledbetter 2008). However, little information is available on genome-wide cytogenetic array screening in patients specifically selected for epilepsy. Engels *et al.* (2007) analyzed 60 patients with mental retardation combined with congenital anomalies, 25% of whom also had epilepsy. Novel imbalances were found in six patients (10%), two of whom had epilepsy (Engels *et al.* 2007). Kim *et al.* (2007) reported various copy-number variations in patients with idiopathic generalized or partial epilepsies and febrile seizures. However, absence of genomic data related to the parents and the low resolution of the platform used limited the relevance of these associations (Yamamoto *et al.* 2008). A significant excess of recurrent microdeletions at 1q21.1, 15q11.2, 15q13.3, 16p11.2, 16p13.11, and 22q11.2 has been observed in various neuropsychiatric disorders including autism, intellectual disability, and schizophrenia. A study investigating the impact of these five microdeletions on the genetic risk for common IGE syndromes, using high-density single nucleotide polymorphism arrays, in a large cohort, found significant associations with microdeletions at 15q11.2 and 16p13.11. Familial segregation suggested that these microdeletions, although not in themselves sufficient to cause epilepsy, might be involved in epileptogenesis (de Kovel *et al.* 2010).

How do genetic defects cause epilepsy?

Some genetically determined disorders affecting the CNS are associated with a risk of developing epilepsy equal to, or only slightly exceeding, that of the general population, others with a risk close to 100%. Susceptibility to developing seizures is not necessarily correlated with the severity of structural impairment of the brain, nor with the extent of the chromosome derangement or the type of mutation. It may rather be heavily influenced by imbalance in neurotransmitter activity, abnormal cortical connectivity, or underrepresentation of inhibitory cell types. This is clearly demonstrated by the finding that certain disorders are consistently associated with some epilepsy types or syndromes so that they become part of the phenotype.

Most of the progress in the identification of epilepsy genes has originated from analysis of rare families with Mendelian inheritance. Almost all the identified genes encode for voltage-gated or ligand-gated ion channels (Table 5.2, and see Chapter 3). Genes have been identified also for several Mendelian diseases in which epilepsy is a prominent feature, including several of the progressive myoclonic epilepsies (Table 5.6). As a

Table 5.6 Clinical classification of the progressive myoclonic epilepsies (PMEs)

PME type	Age of onset
Unverricht–Lundborg disease (ULD)	7–16 yrs
Lafora disease (LD)	6–19 yrs
Neuronal ceroid lipofuscinoses (NCLs)	
Infantile (Haltia–Santavuori)	6 months–2 yrs
Late infantile (Jansky–Bielschowsky)	1–4 yrs
Intermediate (Lake or Cavanagh)	5–8 yrs
Juvenile (Spielmeyer–Vogt)	4–14 yrs
Adult (Kufs)	15–50 yrs
Myoclonic epilepsy with ragged red fibers (MERRF)	3–65 yrs
Sialidosis	8–15 yrs
Type 1	
Galactosialidosis (type 2)	
Dentato-rubro-pallido-luysian atrophy (DRPLA)	Childhood
Gaucher disease (type 3)	Variable

Table 5.7 Molecular genetics of progressive myoclonic epilepsies (PMEs)

PME type	Mode of inheritance	Locus	Gene
Unverricht–Lundborg disease (ULD)	Autosomal recessive	21q22.3	EPM1
Lafora disease (LD)	Autosomal recessive	6q 24	EPMA
Neuronal ceroid lipofuscinoses (NCLs)	Autosomal recessive	6p22.3	EPM2B
Infantile		1p32	CLN1
Late infantile		11p15.5	CLN2
Finnish variant		13q21	CLN5
Gipsy variant		15q21–q23	CLN6
Turkish variant		?	CLN7
Juvenile		16p12.1	CLN3
Juvenile variant		8p22	CLN8
Adult	Autosomal recessive and autosomal dominant	?	CLN4
Myoclonic epilepsy with ragged red fibers (MERFF)	Mitochondrial	Mt DNA	tRNA^{Lys}
Sialidosis	Autosomal recessive	6p21.3	NEU
Galactosialidosis		20q13	PPCA
Gaucher disease type 3	Autosomal recessive	1q21	GBA
Dentato-rubro-pallido-luysian atrophy (DRPLA)	Autosomal dominant	12p13.31	CAG repeats

Table 5.8 Diagnostic tools for progressive myoclonic epilepsies (PMEs)

PME type	Methods	Marker
Unverricht–Lundborg disease (ULD)	Molecular biology	EPM1
Lafora disease (LD)	Axillar biopsy	Lafora bodies
	Molecular biology	EPM2A and EPM2B
Neuronal ceroid lipofuscinoses (NCLs)	Biopsy	Storage lipopigment in lysosomes
	Molecular biology	CLN1, 2, 3, 5, 6, 8
Myoclonic epilepsy with ragged red fibers (MERRF)	Muscle biopsy	Ragged red fibers
	Molecular biology	A8344G substitution (90%)
Sialidosis	Urine	↑ Urinary oligosaccharides
	Lymphocytes, fibroblasts	Deficit of α-N-acetyl neuroaminidase
	Molecular biology	NEU
Galactosialidosis	Urine, leukocytes, and fibroblasts	β-galactosidase deficit
	Molecular biology	PPCA
Gaucher disease	Lymphocytes, fibroblasts	Deficit of β-glucocerebrosidase
	Molecular biology	GBA
Deutato-rubro-pallido-luysian atrophy (DRPLA)	Molecular biology	GAC expansion

consequence the diagnostic strategy is now combining genetic testing, and analysis of biopsy tissue or lymphocytes in different ways (Tables 5.7, 5.8). A large number of inherited metabolic disorders have been linked to epilepsy, which is often one clinical manifestation within a complex neurological syndrome but which can sometimes be the prominent, or presenting, symptom (see Chapter 6), and be in some conditions curable. Pyridoxine-dependent seizures (see Chapter 33), a recessive disorder due to mutations of the antiquitin (*ALDH7A1*) gene, respond dramatically to the intravenous injection of pyridoxine and recur within a few days if maintenance therapy is discontinued. Atypical presentations with seizure onset in infancy rather than in the neonatal period and with infantile spasms have been repeatedly reported (Bennett *et al.* 2009). The disorder is caused by a defect of α-amino adipic semialdehyde (α-AASA) dehydrogenase (antiquitin) in the cerebral lysine degradation pathway (Plecko *et al.* 2007). The possibility of determination of specific metabolites such as (α-AASA) (Sadilkova *et al.* 2009) and of mutation analysis has meant that pyridoxine withdrawal is no longer needed to establish the diagnosis.

Epilepsy related to glucose transporter type 1 deficiency syndrome (GLUT1-DS) provides a paradigmatic example of how once the core phenotypic spectrum of a genetically determined inherited neurometabolic disorder has been defined, availability of biological and molecular markers allows progressive delineation of the syndrome spectrum. The cause of GLUT1-DS is heterozygous mutations of the *SLC2A1* gene encoding GLUT1, the molecule that transports glucose across the blood–brain barrier (Seidner *et al.* 1998). Hypoglycorrachia is a key diagnostic laboratory feature. Clinical features classically comprise a combination of infantile-onset seizures, complex movement disorders, ataxia, cognitive impairment, and, in some children, microcephaly (De Vivo *et al.* 1991). Generalized spike-and-wave discharges and a combination of absence, myoclonic, and tonic–clonic seizures have been reported (Leary *et al.* 2003). A syndrome of paroxysmal exercise-induced dyskinesia and epilepsy (Suls *et al.* 2008) and recently an IGE phenotype (Roulet-Perez *et al.* 2008) and more specifically early-onset absence epilepsy (Suls *et al.* 2009) have been associated to *SLC2A1* mutations. A screening in a series of children with early-onset absence epilepsy identified 12% who carried de novo or familial mutations of *SLC2A1* (Suls *et al.* 2009). These observations, although concerning a limited subset of patients, are of great importance since treatment with a ketogenic diet is effective for seizure control (Klepper *et al.* 2007) and, likely, in reducing possible associated clinical manifestations.

Numerous mental retardation syndromes with epilepsy (Table 5.9), and several epileptogenic malformations of cortical development (Barkovich *et al.* 2005; Guerrini *et al.* 2008) have now been characterized and their causative genes identified or mapped.

Large family studies of epilepsy demonstrate that the number of patients with one or more first-degree relatives with epilepsy is 15% in those with IGE and 12% with presumed symptomatic focal epilepsy (12%) (Ottman and Winawer 2008). Most of those with a family history had just one affected relative and only a small minority of families exhibited a pattern of distribution consistent with Mendelian inheritance. It is therefore hypothesized that in non-Mendelian forms of epilepsy genetic influences are determined by a number of genes, each responsible for a small effect, which additively raise the risk, possibly in combination with environmental factors (Ottman 2005). Since most of the genes identified so far in families with Mendelian inheritance encode for voltage-gated or ligand-gated ion channels, it has been assumed that mutations in ion-channel genes may also influence the risk of developing complex epilepsies. However, in spite of large ongoing research projects progress has been slow and no substantial role for genes involved in the Mendelian epilepsies has been demonstrated in the common non-Mendelian forms.

There is increasing evidence about the role of de novo mutations in causing "sporadic" epilepsies. De novo mutations of the *SCN1A* gene are particularly frequent in severe myoclonic epilepsy of infancy (or Dravet syndrome) (Marini *et al.* 2007) or in the early epileptic encephalopathies caused by *CDKL5* or *STPBX* gene variations. Severe disability, as determined by intractable epilepsy and cognitive impairment, will cause reproductive disadvantage, which will in turn heavily contribute to confining the mutation to the affected individual. Genes whose protein product has varied functional domains will, however, also harbor mutations having milder functional consequences and limited reproductive disadvantage, so that members in successive generations can be affected (e.g., some *SCN1A* mutations have familial distributions in GEFS+).

Mosaic mutations affecting a low percentage of ectodermal derivative cells represent an additional, though apparently rare, mechanism that may account for some seemingly de novo germline mutations or for an attenuated phenotype in relatives of affected sibs (Marini *et al.* 2006; Morimoto *et al.* 2006). Mosaic mutations are also responsible for an attenuated phenotype in individuals with malformations of cortical development who are brought to medical attention after onset of seizures. Mosaic mutations of the *FLNA* gene have been described in mildly affected individuals of both sexes having epilepsy and even isolated subependymal nodules (Guerrini *et al.* 2004); mosaic mutations of the *LIS1* gene have been described in individuals with occipital epilepsy and mild posterior subcortical band heterotopia (Sicca *et al.* 2003). Some epilepsies might be caused by somatic mutations that affect limited brain regions and cannot therefore be demonstrated by studies on peripheral blood. Although this mechanism has not yet been demonstrated, there are interesting indications. In one study, mutation analysis in patients with focal cortical dysplasia showed a high frequency of mild and not clearly pathogenic sequence changes in the *TSC1* (but not *TSC2*) gene in cortical dysplasia compared to controls, as well as loss of heterozygosity of markers surrounding the *TSC1* gene in dysplastic tissue surgically removed in patients with intractable seizures compared to control tissue (Becker *et al.* 2002). These results, however, have not been replicated.

Other factors that may influence the expression of genes causing epileptogenic structural abnormalities include the type of mutation and X-inactivation. An interesting example is provided by *DCX* mutations causing subcortical band heterotopia in females. While most carrier mothers are affected, some only have epilepsy without any detectable brain abnormality or are healthy, due either to favorable skewing of X-inactivation or to the mild consequences of missense mutations affecting protein regions with limited functional relevance (Guerrini *et al.* 2003).

Mitochondrial genetic defects have been associated with disorders in which epilepsy is a main phenotypic manifestation. Mutations of the recessive gene polymerase-γ (*POLG*) cause clinically heterogeneous mitochondrial diseases, associated with mitochondrial DNA (mtDNA) depletion or multiple deletions. A characteristic presentation is with syndromic epilepsy with occipital lobe predilection and severe episodes of, often fatal, status epilepticus and should always be considered in teenagers and young adults with sudden onset of intractable seizures or status epilepticus, and acute liver failure (Engelsen *et al.* 2008; Uusimaa *et al.* 2008).

Some of the genetic influences on epilepsy may involve genomic imprinting, in which expression of the genotype is influenced by the sex of parental origin (Ottman and Winawer 2008). There are well-known examples of the influence of imprinting on the expression of epilepsy. Angelman syndrome is caused in about 70% of patients by a deletion involving the maternally inherited chromosome 15q11–q13, encompassing three GABA receptor subunit genes (*GABRB3, GABRA5,* and

Table 5.9 Genetic conditions and rare defects in other genes that have been reported to cause epilepsy

OMIM	Gene or condition	Gene	Locus
606176	Developmental delay, epilepsy, and neonatal diabetes	KCNJ1	11q24
301900	Borjeson–Forssman–Lehmann syndrome (mental deficiency, epilepsy, endocrine disorders)	PHF6	Xq26.3
300607	Hyperekplexia and epilepsy	ARHGEF9	Xq22.1
300491	Epilepsy, X-linked, with variable learning disabilities and behavior disorders	SYN1	Xp11.4–p11.2
300423	Mental retardation, X-linked, with epilepsy	ARX	Xp11.4
235730	Mowat–Wilson syndrome		2q22
610954	Pitt–Hopkins-like syndrome 1 (cortical dysplasia–focal epilepsy syndrome)	CNTNAP2	7q35–q36
604218	Encephalopathy, familial, with neuroserpin inclusion bodies	PI12	3q26
256600	Neurodegeneration with brain iron accumulation 2a (infantile neuroaxonal dystrophy)	PLA2G6	22q13.1
103050	Adenylosuccinase deficiency	ADSL	22q13.1
300032	Alpha-thalassemia/ mental retardation syndrome	ATRX	Xq13
603896	Leukoencephalopathy with vanishing white matter	EIF2B1, EIF2B2, EIF2B3, EIF2B4, EIF2B5	14q24, Chr.12, 1p34.1, 3q27, 2p23.3
300419	X-linked mental retardation, with or without seizures	ARX	Xp22.13
122470	Cornelia de Lange syndrome 1	NIPBL	5p13.1
300590	Cornelia de Lange syndrome 2	SMC1L1	Xp11.22–p11.21
141500	Migraine, familial hemiplegic, 1	CACNA1A	19p13
602481	Migraine, familial hemiplegic, 2	ATP1A2	1q21–q23
609634	Migraine, familial hemiplegic, 3	SCN1A	2q24
607596	Pontocerebellar hypoplasia type 1	VRK1	14q32
277470	Pontocerebellar hypoplasia type 2A	TSEN54	17q25.1
612389	Pontocerebellar hypoplasia type 2B	TSEN2	3p25.1
612390	Pontocerebellar hypoplasia type 2C	TSEN34	19q13.4
313440	Familial epilepsy (with learning disabilities and behavior disorders)	SYN1	Xp11.4–p11.2
245180	Kifafa seizure disorder	—	
160120	Episodic ataxia type 1	KCNA1	12p13
108500	Episodic ataxia type 2	CACNA1A	19p13
117550	Sotos syndrome	NSD1	5q35
606155	Fryns–Aftimos syndrome	—	
609056	Amish infantile epilepsy syndrome	SIAT9	2p11.2
203450	Alexander disease	GFAP	17q21
164180	Oculocerebrocutaneous syndrome	—	
163200	Linear sebaceous nevus syndrome (Schimmelpenning–Feuerstein–Mims syndrome)	—	
200150	Choreoacanthocytosis	CHAC	9q21
300624	Fragile X mental retardation syndrome	FMR1	Xq27.3
300558	Mental retardation, X-linked 30	PAK3	Xq21.3–q24
266100	Epilepsy, pyridoxine-dependent	ALDH7A1	5q31
138140	Epilepsy, exertion-induced dyskinesia, hemolytic anemia	GLUT1 (SLC2A1)	1p35–p31.3
239500	Hyperprolinemia Type I	PRODH	22q11.2
188400	DiGeorge (chromosome 22q11.2 deletion) syndrome	TBX1 del	22q11.2
602066	Convulsions, familial infantile, with paroxysmal choreoathetosis		16p12–q12

Table 5.9 (cont.)

OMIM	Gene or condition	Gene	Locus
609446	Epilepsy, generalized, with paroxysmal dyskinesia	KCNMA1	10q22.3
608500	Epilepsy, progressive myoclonic 1B	PRICKLE1	12q12
271245	Spinocerebellar ataxia, infantile, with sensory neuropathy, epileptic encephalopathy	C10ORF2	10q24
00937	Diabetes mellitus, permanent neonatal, with neurologic features	KCNJ11	11p15.1
602851	Febrile convulsions, familial, 4	MASS1	5q14
158900	Facioscapulohumeral muscular dystrophy 1A	D4Z4 macrosatellite repeat contraction	4q35
600721	D-2-hydroxyglutaric aciduria	D2HGDH	2q37.3
607136	Spinocerebellar ataxia 17	TBP	6q27
602926	Epileptic encephalopathy, early infantile	STXBP1	9q34.1
300203	Epileptic encephalopathy, early infantile	CDKL5 (STK9)	Xp22
608750	Congenital disorder of glycosylation type Id	ALG3	3q27
165240	Pallister–Hall syndrome, hypothalamic hamartoma	GLI3	7p13
606463	Gaucher disease	GBA	1q21
610090	Neonatal epileptic encephalopathy pyridoxamine 5′-phosphate oxidase deficiency	PNPO	17q21.32
609186	D-2-α-hydroxyglutarate aciduria with early infantile-onset epileptic encephalopathy	D2HGDH	2q37.3
609010	3-α Methylcrotonyl-coa carboxylase 1 deficiency	MCCC1	3q25–q27
604369	Sialuria, finnish type	SLC17A5	6q14–q15
601815	Phosphoglycerate dehydrogenase deficiency	PHGDH	1q12
300438	17-β-Hydroxysteroid dehydrogenase X deficiency	HSD17B10	Xp11.2
300105	Mental retardation, X-linked, Snyder–Robinson type	SMS	Xp22.1
300005	Mental retardation, X-linked, syndromic 13	MECP2	Xq28
274270	Dihydropyrimidine dehydrogenase deficiency	DPYD	1p22
236792	L-2-hydroxyglutaric aciduria	L2HGDH	14q22.1
180430	Ribose 5-phosphate isomerase a	RPIA	2p11.2
136430	Neurodegeneration due to cerebral folate transport deficiency	FOLR1	q13.3–q13.5
117000	Central core disease of muscle	RYR1	19q13.1
604149	Myoclonus–dystonia syndrome	SGCE	7q21

Note:
The purpose of this list is to document the extremely wide variety of possible genetic causes of epilepsy, and those genes and conditions which are not featured in other chapters in this book (and so are usually extremely rare). This list is derived from the OMOM database, and included are the OMIM identifying numbers. The list does not include the more common genetic causes of epilepsy, as these are described elsewhere in the book, for instance: the idiopathic epilepsies, the "pure genetic epilepsies," the progressive myoclonic epilepsies, the epilepsies in mitochondrial disease, the epilepsies due to cortical dysplasias, other metabolic conditions featured elsewhere in the book, nor the common genes involved in epilepsy also discussed elsewhere (for instance SCN1A, SCN1B, GABRA1, GABRG2, KCNQ2, KCNQ3. ATP1A2, CHRNA4, CHRNA2, CHRNB2, CLCN2, LIS1, DCX, FLNA, TSC1/2, UBE3A, CRIT1, CRIT2, XH2, FMR1, NF1, LRP2, SRPX2, TBR2, PAX6, TUBA1A and TUBB2B, PCDH19, STXBP1, ARX, and EFHC1). The list is not comprehensive and also excludes conditions in which epilepsy is either a rare accompaniment or may be due to a secondary feature (such as renal failure). Frequencies of epilepsy are not given as some of these conditions are extremely rare, having been reported in few families.

GABRG3). About 3–5% of patients show chromosome 15 uniparental disomy, with both homologs being paternal in origin. This finding has led to the hypothesis that the lack of maternal contribution for the 15q11–q13 region is the main mechanism responsible for Angelman syndrome and that one or more paternally imprinted genes lie within the 15q11–q13 region. About 5% of patients show a mutation in the imprinting center, a large transcriptional regulatory element lying about 1.5 megabases proximal to the GABA receptor cluster. The integrity of the imprinting center ensures the switch from the paternal to the maternal epigenotype at 15q11–q13 in oogenesis, so that imprinting center mutations hamper the expression of paternally imprinted genes from the maternal homolog. A small subset of patients with Angelman syndrome have been shown to harbor intragenic mutations in the UBE3A gene, mapping to 15q12–q13, the expression of which appears to be paternally imprinted in the brain. About 90% of patients with Angelman syndrome have epilepsy, which is often severe and has highly characteristic electroclinical features (Guerrini *et al.* 2003). Prader–Willi syndrome, a contiguous gene syndrome caused by deletion or disruption of one or several genes in the Angelman/Prader–Willi syndrome region at 15q11–q13 or by maternal uniparental disomy 15, is accompanied by epilepsy in fewer than 20% of patients, and exhibits no characteristic electroclinical features (Fan *et al.* 2009). Parental imprinting of the Angelman/Prader–Willi syndrome region therefore influences all aspects of the phenotype, including incidence and type of seizures.

An additional mechanism of genetic influence in the expression of epilepsy is represented by trinucleotide repeat expansions, involving the amplification of tandem repeats rather than a change in the DNA sequence. For example, phenotypes associated with mutations of the *ARX* gene demonstrate remarkable pleiotropy: malformation phenotypes are associated with protein truncation mutations and missense mutations in the homeobox; non-malformation phenotypes, including X-linked infantile spasms (ISS), are associated with missense mutations outside of the homeobox and expansion of the PolyA tracts (Guerrini *et al.* 2007; Friocourt and Parnavels 2010).

Gene–environment interactions should also be considered as an additional element of complexity intervening in the causal pathway leading to the epilepsy phenotype and might explain some of the reduced penetrance observed in the monogenic epilepsies (Ottman and Winawer 2008). Some genotypes might not cause epileptogenesis per se but act by increasing the susceptibility to environmental factors. A risk-raising genotype would not cause seizures unless the carrier individual were exposed to the precipitant environmental factor. Schaumann *et al.* (1994) observed that seizure risk was increased in the relatives of individuals having experienced seizures in relation to either chronic or acute heavy alcohol consumption, possibly indicating that alcohol exposure raises the risk of seizures in individuals with certain genotypes.

While mutations in single genes explain some rare epilepsy syndromes, or sporadic and familial disorders that in turn cause symptomatic epilepsy, the neuronal functions that alter seizure threshold and predispose to symptomatic epilepsy often seem to be influenced by multiple genes (Engel and Pedley 2008). The relative contribution of genetic and acquired factors, and the functional effects of the genetic determinant, will affect whether the epilepsy is manifested as an isolated "idiopathic" disorder or a symptomatic one.

The number of "epilepsy genes" uncovered by family linkage studies has increased slowly over recent years. Their protein products are being characterized using animal models of single-gene mutations and are providing important information about the molecular pathology underlying abnormally regulated control of excitability (Noebels 2003; Engel and Pedley 2008). However, the population of genes encoding for proteins that directly or indirectly contribute to the regulation of cortical excitability at the synaptic or membrane level, as well as signal transduction, is very large. The pathway towards understanding how genetic defects cause human epilepsy is further complicated by the finding, arising from both animal and human data, that some "epilepsy genes" and their protein products had not previously been associated with epileptogenesis; neither is their association with it easy to understand (e.g., *LIG1* mutations in autosomal dominant temporal lobe epilepsy, Cystatin B in Unverricht–Lundborg disease, or *CDKL5* in early epileptic encephalopathy).

Genetic counseling in the epilepsies

Genetic testing can be offered for single-gene or Mendelian epilepsy syndromes, or epilepsy-associated disorders, if the gene has been identified. If not, empirical counseling can be offered, based on the type of epilepsy, mode of inheritance, and penetrance.

Although we can now carry out preclinical and prenatal diagnosis in many cases, the severity and prognosis of the epilepsy in specific individuals, particularly in those with idiopathic epilepsies, is difficult to predict. However, in symptomatic monogenic epilepsies, such as the progressive myoclonus epilepsies, phakomatoses, and malformations of cortical development, carrier detection, prenatal diagnosis, and presymptomatic testing may lead to prevention.

Unfortunately, no curative treatment has emerged from any genetic finding in epilepsy to date (with the possible exception of the ketogenic diet in GLUT1 deficiency syndrome), nor have the many pharmacogenomic studies in epilepsy (which are beyond the scope of this book) yielded any widely applicable treatment advances. This is a disappointing lack of progress, reflecting as it does on the complex nature of epilepsy and its treatment. Counseling needs to consider these issues.

Pathways to the future

The next steps include identifying additional genes both in monogenic epilepsies and epilepsies with complex inheritance, genotype–phenotype correlations, and functional studies of the abnormal proteins. These studies may have practical applications for diagnosis, genetic counseling, and possible treatment, as well as increasing our knowledge of normal brain function and mechanisms of epileptogenesis. Ethical and societal considerations are important in establishing guidelines for both genetic counseling and genetic research in the epilepsies.

Most of the epilepsy syndromes listed above are characterized by marked clinical and genetic heterogeneity. This may be explained by pleiotropic expression of a single-gene mutation, modifying genes, or by several genes producing a similar phenotype, at times because they affect the same developmental or metabolic pathway.

We can now list epilepsy syndromes in which a locus or loci have been mapped, and those in which one or more gene mutations or polymorphisms have been identified. These lists are constantly changing as new loci and genes are identified.

It is hoped that a constantly updated database will be established for all the known gene mutations and polymorphisms and their clinical correlates, so that genotype–phenotype correlations can be determined. This is the objective of the Human Variome project (Cotton *et al.* 2008). For example, over 200 mutations in *SCN1A* associated with Dravet syndrome have now been identified (Nabbout *et al.* 2003; Mulley *et al.* 2005b; Harkin *et al.* 2007; Marini *et al.* 2009), and the severity of the related phenotype can be predicted early, with reasonable accuracy for those recurrent mutations in which sufficient numbers of clinical observations are available.

Appendix: Standard cytogenetic and molecular techniques for diagnosis

Standard karyotype and high-resolution chromosome analysis

The karyotype of an individual (i.e., the number and structure of chromosomes) can be ascertained from readily accessible somatic cells, such as peripheral blood lymphocytes or skin fibroblasts. Cells are grown in tissue culture media until active proliferation occurs, and then single-metaphase chromosomes from cells are prepared for examination by microscopy. Each chromosome can be identified by special staining techniques, using fluorescent dyes or Giemsa staining after treatment with a proteolytic enzyme (trypsin). These techniques produce banding patterns that are specific for each chromosome. A typical standard karyotype from metaphase cells contains 400–550 bands per haploid genome. In general, 15–20 cells should be counted, and three to five analyzed and karyotyped. The "high-resolution" chromosome analysis takes advantage of the synchronization of cells in prometaphase through methotrexate. This makes it possible to visualize up to 2000 bands, although a high-resolution chromosome analysis of standard quality allows the detection of about 850 bands. Given the greatly increased amount of work, the difficulty of the analysis and cost, high-resolution chromosome analysis should not be considered as a routine cytogenetic assay. It is therefore recommended in the case of a precise clinical clue that focuses the search for subtle rearrangements in a particular cytogenetic band.

Fluorescent in situ hybridization (FISH)

The hybridization of a labeled DNA probe to spread metaphase chromosomes allows the detection of small deletions, duplications, or cryptic translocations involving the chromosomal segment complementary to the probe. Briefly, the probe labeled with biotin-modified nucleotides is denatured and then hybridized to denatured metaphase chromosomes, to find its specific counterpart. Fluorochrome-coupled avidin, which has a strong affinity for biotin, is added to the chromosomal slide; the probe signal can then be visualized by fluorescence microscopy. Double or multiple hybridizations can be carried out at the same time using different fluorochromes, and the probe

signals can be amplified by special procedures. Specific centromeric probes or control probes are employed for unequivocal chromosome identification. Although this is a sensitive technique it allows investigation of only a few loci in one experiment. Thus it can be requested when the clinician has a specific clinical suspicion of an abnormality known to be associated with the deletion/duplication of that gene/region (e.g., Angelman syndrome and 15q11–q13 deletion).

Molecular karyotyping with array comparative genomic hybridization

Several techniques defined as molecular cytogenetics have improved in the last 10 years the resolution capability of chromosome banding. The latest technology is the array comparative genomic hybridization (CGH) representing a powerful modification of the classical CGH based on metaphases. With the CGH the DNA of a patient (to be tested) and the DNA of a control are labeled with green and red fluorochromes, respectively, and hybridized on metaphase spreads. The images of both fluorescence signals are captured and the ratio of DNAs intensities quantified by using a dedicated software along each chromosome. The chromosome regions represented in the same amount in both DNAs (patient and control) appear yellow, the deleted regions appear red, and the duplicated regions appear green. The difficulty obtaining sufficiently long metaphases limits the resolution power of this technique to a maximum of 3 Mb. The array CGH technology replaces the use of chromosome spreads with clones or oligomers (targets) that cover the entire genome and its resolution power depends only on the number of targets and their distribution. Recently, microarray having bacterial artificial chromosome (BAC) clones separated by 100 kb have been used. Other platforms, using oligomers as targets, have a higher resolution that theoretically can reach up to a few hundred base pairs. The use of these arrays might allow detecting deletions and duplications below the size of 1 Mb and to precisely define the breakpoints. It has been estimated that among patients with mental retardation and dysmorphic features no fewer than 20% have a cryptic chromosome deletion or duplication causing their condition. This technology has also revealed that the human genome may harbor deletions and duplications devoid of phenotypic effects, having an average size of 2 Mb, which might have a role in multifactorial diseases. It seems obvious that microarray CGH will have a crucial role in pre- and postnatal cytogenetics as well as in oncology; its potential in the etiological diagnosis of epilepsy associated with mental disability and dysmorphic features is extremely high.

Multiplex ligation probe amplification

Multiple ligation-probe amplification (MLPA) is a multiplex polymernse chain reaction (PCR) method with the potential of detecting copy-number variations of up to 50 different genomic DNA sequences in a single assay (Schouten *et al.* 2002). The

MLPA technique is easy to use and can be performed in many laboratories, as it only requires standard laboratory equipment. The results are available within 24 hours. Although MLPA is not suitable for genome-wide research screening, it is a good alternative to array-based techniques for many routine applications. In MLPA assay, MLPA probes that hybridize to the target sequence are amplified but not the target sequences themselves. In contrast to a standard multiplex PCR, a single PCR primer pair is used for amplification. The resulting amplification products of the MLPA reactions range between 130 and 480 nucleotides in length and can be analyzed by capillary electrophoresis. Comparing the peak pattern obtained to that of reference samples indicates which sequences show aberrant copy numbers.

Single-nucleotide polymorphism arrays

Single-nucleotide polymorphisms (SNPs) have received considerable attention as a source of human variation and are particularly amenable to high-throughput genotyping and disease association studies. For this reason, high-density SNP genotyping arrays have become more popular for copy-number detection and analysis. In high-density SNP genotyping platforms, a signal intensity measure is summarized for each allele of a given SNP marker. Hybridizations are not performed using cohybridization of two DNA as in array CGH, but by hybridization of a single DNA. The analysis of signal intensities across the genome can then be used to identify regions with multiple SNPs that support deletions or duplications (Komura *et al.* 2006; Pfeiffer *et al.* 2006). However, there are limitations to the use of SNP genotyping arrays for copy-number variation detection: SNPs in these arrays are not uniformly distributed across the genome and are sparse in regions with segmental duplications or complex variations in copy-number (Carter 2007). To overcome these limitations, the new generations of SNP genotyping arrays have now incorporated additional non-polymorphic markers to provide more comprehensive coverage of the human genome.

References

Andermann E, (1972) Ph.D. thesis, Montreal, Canada McGill University, Genetics of focal epilepsy and related disorders.

Andermann E, and Metrakos JD (1972) A multifactorial analysis of focal and generalized cortico-reticular (centrencephalic) epilepsy. *Epilepsia* **13**:348–9.

Archer HL, Evans J, Edwards S, *et al.* (2006) *CDKL5* mutations cause infantile spasms, early onset seizures, and severe mental retardation in female patients. *J Med Genet* **43**:729–34.

Barkovich AJ, Kuzniecky RI, Jackson GD, Guerrini R, Dobyns WB (2005) A developmental and genetic classification for malformations of cortical development. *Neurology* **65**:1873–87.

Becker AJ, Urbach H, Scheffler B, *et al.* (2002) Focal cortical dysplasia of Taylor's balloon cell type: mutational analysis of the *TSC1* gene indicates a pathogenic relationship to tuberous sclerosis. *Ann Neurol* **52**:29–37.

Bennett CL, Chen Y, Hahn S, Glass IA, Gospe SM Jr. (2009) Prevalence of *ALDH7A1* mutations in 18 North American pyridoxine-dependent seizure (PDS) patients. *Epilepsia* **50**:1167–75.

Berg AT, Berkovic SF, Brodie MJ, *et al.* (2010) Revised terminology and concepts for organization of seizures and epilepsies: Report of the ILAE Commission on Classification and Terminology, 2005–2009. *Epilepsia* **51**:676–85.

Berkovic SF, Howell RA, Hay DA, Hopper JL (1998) Epilepsies in twins: genetics of the major epilepsy syndromes. *Ann Neurol* **43**:435–45.

Berkovic SF, Mulley JC, Scheffer IE, Petrou S (2006) Human epilepsies: interaction of genetic and acquired factors. *Trends Neurosci* **29**:391–7.

Bisulli F, Tinuper P, Avoni P, *et al.* (2004) Idiopathic partial epilepsy with auditory features (IPEAF): a clinical and genetic study of 53 sporadic cases. *Brain* **127**:1343–52.

Briellmann RS, Torn-Broers Y, Berkovic SF (2001) Idiopathic generalized epilepsies: do sporadic and familial cases differ? *Epilepsia* **42**:1399–402.

Carter NP (2007) Methods and strategies for analyzing copy number variation using DNA microarrays. *Nat Genet* **39**(7 Suppl):S16–21.

Chen Y, Lu J, Pan H, *et al.* (2003) Association between genetic variation of *CACNA1H* and childhood absence epilepsy. *Ann Neurol* **54**:239–43.

Chioza BA, Aicardi J, Aschauer H, *et al.* (2009) Genome-wide high density SNP-based linkage analysis of childhood absence epilepsy identifies a susceptibility locus on chromosome 3p23–p14. *Epilepsy Res* **87**:247–55.

Chioza B, Wilkie H, Nashef L, *et al.* (2001) Association between the alpha(1a) calcium channel gene *CACNA1A* and idiopathic generalized epilepsy. *Neurology* **56**:1245–6.

Commission on Classification and Terminology of the International League Against Epilepsy (1989) Proposal for revised classification of epilepsies and epileptic syndromes. *Epilepsia* **30**:389–99.

Cotton RG, Auerbach AD, Axton M, *et al.* (2008) GENETICS: the Human Variome Project. *Science* **322**:861–2.

de Kovel CG, Pinto D, Tauer U, *et al.* (2010a) Whole-genome linkage scan for epilepsy-related photosensitivity: a mega-analysis. *Epilepsy Res* **89**:286–94.

de Kovel CG, Trucks H, Helbig I, *et al.* (2010b) Recurrent microdeletions at 15q11.2 and 16p13.11 predispose to idiopathic generalized epilepsies. *Brain* **133**:23–32.

De Vivo DC, Trifiletti RR, Jacobson RI, *et al.* (1991) Defective glucose transport across the blood–brain barrier as a cause of persistent hypoglycorrhachia, seizures, and developmental delay. *N Engl J Med* **325**:703–9.

Depienne C, Bouteiller D, Keren B, *et al.* (2009) Sporadic infantile epileptic encephalopathy caused by mutations in *PCDH19* resembles Dravet syndrome but mainly affects females. *PLoS Genet* **5**:e1000381.

Deprez L, Jansen A, De Jonghe P (2009) Genetics of epilepsy syndromes starting in the first year of life. *Neurology* **72**:273–81.

Dibbens LM, Tarpey PS, Hynes K, *et al.* (2008) X-linked protocadherin 19 mutations cause female-limited epilepsy and cognitive impairment. *Nat Genet* **40**:776–81.

Doose H, Gerken H, Horstmann T, Völzke E (1973) Genetic factors in spike–wave absences. *Epilepsia* **14**:57–75.

Du W, Bautista JF, Yang H, *et al.* (2005) Calcium-sensitive potassium channelopathy in human epilepsy and paroxysmal movement disorder. *Nat Genet* **37**:733–8.

Durner M, Gorroochurn P, Marini C, Guerrini R (2006) Can we increase the likelihood of success for future association studies in epilepsy? *Epilepsia* **47**:1617–21.

Elia M, Falco M, Ferri R, *et al.* (2008) *CDKL5* mutations in boys with severe encephalopathy and early-onset intractable epilepsy. *Neurology* **71**:997–9.

Engel J (2001) A proposed diagnostic scheme for people with epileptic seizures and with epilepsy: report of ILAE task force on classification and terminology. *Epilepsia* **42**:796–803.

Engel J Jr. (2006a) Report of the ILAE classification core group. *Epilepsia* **47**:1558–68.

Engel J Jr. (2006b) ILAE classification of epilepsy syndromes. *Epilepsy Res* **70**(Suppl 1):S5–10.

Engel J Jr., Pedley TA (2008) Introduction: What is epilepsy? In: Engel J Jr., Peddey TA (eds.) *Epilepsy: A Comprehensive Textbook*, 2nd edn, vol. **3**. Philadelphia, PA: Lippincott Williams and Wilkins, pp. 1–6.

Engels H, Brockschmidt A, Hoischen A, *et al.* (2007) DNA microarray analysis identifies candidate regions and genes in unexplained mental retardation. *Neurology* **68**:721–2.

Engelsen BA, Tzoulis C, Karlsen B, *et al.* (2008) *POLG1* mutations cause a syndromic epilepsy with occipital lobe predilection. *Brain* **131**:818–28.

Everett KV, Chioza B, Aicardi J, *et al.* (2007) Linkage and association analysis of *CACNG3* in childhood absence epilepsy. *Eur J Hum Genet* **15**:463–72.

Falconer DS (1965) The inheritance of liability to certain diseases, estimated from the incidence among relatives. *Ann Hum Genet* **29**:51–76.

Fan Z, Greenwood R, Fisher A, Pendyal S, Powell CM (2009) Characteristics and frequency of seizure disorder in 56 patients with Prader–Willi syndrome. (Letter.) *Am J Med Genet* **149A**:1581–4.

Feucht M, Fuchs K, Pichlbauer E, *et al.* (1999) Possible association between childhood absence epilepsy and the gene encoding GABRB3. *Biol Psychiatry* **46**:997–1002.

Fong GC, Shah PU, Gee MN, *et al.* (1998) Childhood absence epilepsy with tonic-clonic seizures and electroencephalogram 3–4-Hz spike and multispike-slow wave complexes: linkage to chromosome 8q24. *Am J Hum Genet* **63**:1117–29.

Friocourt G, Parnavelas JG (2010) Mutations in *ARX* result in several defects involving GABAergic neurons. *Front Cell Neurosci* **4**:4.

Gottesman II, Gould TD (2003) The endophenotype concept in psychiatry: etymology and strategic intentions. *Am J Psychiatry* **160**:636–45.

Guerrini R (2010) Classification concepts and terminology: is clinical description assertive and laboratory testing objective? *Epilepsia* **51**:718–20.

Guerrini R, Carrozzo R, Rinaldi R, Bonanni P (2003a) Angelman syndrome: etiology, clinical features, diagnosis, and management of symptoms. *Paediatr Drugs* **5**:647–61.

Guerrini R, Casari G, Marini C (2003b) The genetic and molecular basis of epilepsy. *Trends Mol Med* **9**:300–6.

Guerrini R, Moro F, Andermann E, *et al.* (2003c) Nonsyndromic mental retardation and cryptogenic epilepsy in women with doublecortin gene mutations. *Ann Neurol* **54**:30–7.

Guerrini R, Mei D, Sisodiya S, *et al.* (2004) Germline and mosaic mutations of *FLN1* in men with periventricular heterotopia. *Neurology* **63**:51–6.

Guerrini R, Moro F, Kato M, *et al.* (2007) Expansion of the first PolyA tract of *ARX* causes infantile spasms and status dystonicus. *Neurology* **69**:427–33.

Guerrini R, Battaglia A, Carrozzo R, *et al.* (2008a) Chromosomal abnormalities. In: Engel J Jr., Pedley TA (eds.) *Epilepsy: A Comprehensive Textbook*, 2nd edn, vol. **3**. Philadelphia, PA: Lippincott Williams and Wilkins, pp. 2589–601.

Guerrini R, Dobyns WB, Barkovich AJ (2008b) Abnormal development of the human cerebral cortex: genetics, functional consequences and treatment options. *Trends Neurosci* **31**:154–62.

Hamdan FF, Piton A, Gauthier J, *et al.* (2009) De novo *STXBP1* mutations in mental retardation and nonsyndromic epilepsy. *Ann Neurol* **65**:748–53.

Harkin LA, McMahon JM, Iona X, *et al.* (2007) The spectrum of SCN1A-related infantile epileptic encephalopathies. *Brain* **130**:843–52.

Herman ST (2002) Epilepsy after brain insult: targeting epileptogenesis. *Neurology* **59**:S21–6.

Holmes GL (1987) Genetics of epilepsy. In: Holmes GL (ed.) *Diagnosis and Management of Seizures in Children* Philadelphia, PA: WB Saunders, pp. 56–71.

Jennings MT, Bird TD (1981) Genetic influences in the epilepsies. *Am J Dis Child* **135**:450–7.

Kato M, Saitoh S, Kamei A, *et al.* (2007) A longer polyalanine expansion mutation in the *ARX* gene causes early infantile epileptic encephalopathy with suppression–burst pattern (Ohtahara syndrome). *Am J Hum Genet* **81**:361–6.

Kim HS, Yim SV, Jung KH, *et al.* (2007) Altered DNA copy number in patients with different seizure disorder type: by array-CGH. *Brain Devel* **29**:639–43.

Kjeldsen MJ, Kyvik KO, Christensen K, Friis ML (2001) Genetic and environmental factors in epilepsy: a population-based study of 11900 Danish twin pairs. *Epilepsy Res* **44**:167–78.

Klepper J, Leiendecker B (2007) GLUT1 deficiency syndrome: 2007 update. *Dev Med Child Neurol* **49**:707–16.

Komura D, Shen F, Ishikawa S, *et al.* (2006) Genome-wide detection of human copy number variations using high-density DNA oligonucleotide arrays. *Genome Res* **16**:1575–84.

Leary LD, Wang D, Nordli DR Jr., Engelstad K, De Vivo DC (2003) Seizure characterization and electroencephalographic features in Glut-1 deficiency syndrome. *Epilepsia* **44**:701–7.

Ledbetter DH (2008) Cytogenetic technology: genotype and phenotype. *N Engl J Med* **359**:1728–30.

Lennox WG (1951) The heredity of epilepsy as told by relatives and twins. *J Am Med Ass* **146**:529–36.

Lennox WG (1960) *Epilepsy and Related Disorders*, 2 vols. Boston, MA: Little, Brown and Co.

Lennox WG, Jolly DH (1954) Seizures, brain waves and intelligence tests of epileptic twins. *Res Publ Ass Res Nerv Ment Dis* **33**:325–45.

Lowenstein D, Messing R (2007) Epilepsy genetics: yet more exciting news. *Ann Neurol* **62**:549–50.

Lüders HO, Turnbull J, Kaffashi F (2009) Are the dichotomies generalized versus focal epilepsies and idiopathic versus symptomatic epilepsies still valid in modern epileptology? *Epilepsia* **50**:1336–43.

Maljevic S, Krampfl K, Cobilanschi J, *et al.* (2006) A mutation in the GABA(A) receptor alpha(1)-subunit is associated with absence epilepsy. *Ann Neurol* **59**:983–7.

Marini C, Scheffer IE, Crossland KM, *et al.* (2004) Genetic architecture of idiopathic generalized epilepsy: clinical genetic analysis of 55 multiplex families. *Epilepsia* **45**:467–78.

Marini C, Mei D, Helen Cross J, Guerrini R (2006) Mosaic *SCN1A* mutation in familial severe myoclonic epilepsy of infancy. *Epilepsia* **47**:1737–40.

Marini C, Mei D, Temudo T, *et al.* (2007) Idiopathic epilepsies with seizures precipitated by fever and SCN1A abnormalities. *Epilepsia* **48**:1678–85.

Marini C, Scheffer IE, Nabbout R, *et al.* (2009) *SCN1A* duplications and deletions detected in Dravet syndrome: implications for molecular diagnosis. *Epilepsia* **50**:1670–8.

Marini C, Mei D, Parmeggiani L, *et al.* (2010) Protocadherin 19 mutations in girls with infantile onset epilepsy. *Neurology* **75**:646–53.

Matthes A, Weber H (1968) Klinische und elektroenzephalographische Familienuntersuchungen bei Pyknolepsien. *Dtsch Med Wschr* **93**:429–35.

Mei D, Marini C, Novara F, *et al.* (2009) Xp22.3 genomic deletions involving the *CDKL5* gene in girls with early onset epileptic encephalopathy. *Epilepsia* Sep 22. [Epub ahead of print].

Metrakos JD (1961) Heredity as an etiological factor in convulsive disorders. In: Fields WS, Desmond MM (eds.) *Disorders of The Developing Nervous System*. Springfield, I: Charles C. Thomas, pp. 23–37.

Metrakos JD, Metrakos K (1969) Genetic studies in clinical epilepsy. In: Jasper HH, Ward AA, Pope A (eds.) *Basic Mechanisms of the Epilepsies* Boston, MA: Little, Brown and Co., pp. 700–8.

Metrakos JD, Metrakos K (1970) Genetic factors in epilepsy. In: Niedermyer E (ed.) *Modern Problems in Pharmacopsychiatry*, vol. **4** New York: Karger, pp. 71–86.

Metrakos K, Metrakos JD (1974) Genetics of epilepsy. In: Vinken PJ, Bruyn GW (eds.) *The Epilepsies: Handbook of Clinical Neurology*, vol. **15**. Amsterdam: North-Holland, pp. 429–439.

Miller LL, Pellock JM, DeLorenzo RJ, Meyer JM, Corey LA (1998) Univariate genetic analyses of epilepsy and seizures in a population-based twin study: the Virginia Twin Registry. *Genet Epidemiol* **15**:33–49.

Morimoto M, Mazaki E, Nishimura A, *et al.* (2006) *SCN1A* mutation mosaicism in a family with severe myoclonic epilepsy in infancy. *Epilepsia* **47**:1732–6.

Mullen SA, Crompton DE, Carney PW, Helbig I, Berkovic SF (2009) A neurologist's guide to genome-wide association studies. *Neurology* **72**:558–65.

Mulley JC, Scheffer IE, Harkin LA, Berkovic SF, Dibbens LM (2005a) Susceptibility genes for complex epilepsy. *Hum Mol Genet* **14**:R243–R249

Mulley JC, Scheffer IE, Petrou S, *et al.* (2005b) SCN1A mutations and epilepsy. *Hum Mutat* **25**:535–42.

Nabbout R, Gennaro E, Dalla Bernardina B, *et al.* (2003) Spectrum of *SCN1A* mutations in severe myoclonic epilepsy of infancy. *Neurology* **60**:1961–7.

Noebels JL (2003) The biology of epilepsy genes. *Ann Rev Neurosci* **26**:599–625.

Ottman R (2005) Analysis of genetically complex epilepsies. (2005) *Epilepsia* **46**(Suppl 10):7–14.

Ottman R, Winawer MR (2008) Genetic epidemiology. In: Engel J Jr. Pedley TA (eds.) *Epilepsy: A Comprehensive Textbook*, 2nd edn, vol. **3**. Philadelphia, PA: Lippincott Williams and Wilkins, pp. 161–70.

Pfeiffer DA, Le JM, Steemers FJ, *et al.* (2006) High-resolution genomic profiling of chromosomal aberrations using Infinium whole-genome genotyping. *Genome Res* **16**:1136–48.

Plecko B, Paul K, Paschke E, *et al.* (2007) Biochemical and molecular characterization of 18 patients with pyridoxine-dependent epilepsy and mutations of the antiquitin (*ALDH7A1*) gene. *Hum Mutat* **28**:19–26.

Risch N, Merikangas K (1996) The future of genetic studies of complex human diseases. *Science* **273**:1516–17.

Robinson R, Taske N, Sander T, *et al.* (2002) Linkage analysis between childhood absence epilepsy and genes encoding GABA$_A$ and GABA$_B$ receptors, voltage-dependent calcium channels, and the ECA1 region on chromosome 8q. *Epilepsy Res* **48**:169–79.

Rodin E (2009) The epilepsy diathesis. *Epilepsia* **50**:1649–53.

Roulet-Perez E, Ballhausen D, Bonafé L, Cronel-Ohayon S, Maeder-Ingvar M (2008) Glut-1 deficiency syndrome masquerading as idiopathic generalized epilepsy. *Epilepsia* **49**:1955–8.

Sadilkova K, Gospe SM Jr., Hahn SH (2009) Simultaneous determination of alpha-aminoadipic semialdehyde, piperideine-6-carboxylate and pipecolic acid by LC-MS/MS for pyridoxine-dependent seizures and folinic acid-responsive seizures. *J Neurosci Methods* **184**:136–41.

Saitsu H, Kato M, Mizuguchi T, *et al.* (2008) De novo mutations in the gene encoding STXBP1 (MUNC18–1) cause early infantile epileptic encephalopathy. *Nat Genet* **40**:782–8.

Sander T, Schulz H, Saar K, *et al.* (2000) Genome search for susceptibility loci of common idiopathic generalised epilepsies. *Hum Mol Genet* **9**:1465–72.

Schaumann BA, Annegers JF, Johnson SB, *et al.* (1994) Family history of seizures in posttraumatic and alcohol-associated seizure disorders. *Epilepsia* **35**:48–52.

Scheffer IE, Harkin LA, Grinton BE, *et al.* (2007) Temporal lobe epilepsy and GEFS+ phenotypes associated with *SCN1B* mutations. *Brain* **130**:100–9.

Schouten JP, McElgunn CJ, Waaijer R, *et al.* (2002) Relative quantification of 40 nucleic acid sequences by multiplex ligation-dependent probe amplification. *Nucleic Acids Res* **15**:30:e57.

Seidner G, Alvarez MG, Yeh JI, *et al.* (1998) GLUT-1 deficiency syndrome caused by haploinsufficiency of the blood–brain barrier hexose carrier. *Nat Genet* **18**:188–91.

Shaw-Smith C, Redon R, Rickman L, *et al.* (2004) Microarray based comparative genomic hybridisation (array-CGH) detects submicroscopic chromosomal deletions and duplications in patients with learning disability/mental retardation and dysmorphic features. *J Med Genet* **41**:241–8.

Sicca F, Kelemen A, Genton P, *et al.* (2003) Mosaic mutations of the *LIS1* gene cause subcortical band heterotopia. *Neurology* **28**:1042–6.

Singh R, McKinlay Gardner RJ, Crossland KM, Scheffer IE, Berkovic SF (2002) Chromosomal abnormalities and epilepsy: a review for clinicians and gene hunters. *Epilepsia* **43**:127–40.

Stromme P, Mangelsdorf ME, Shaw MA, *et al.* (2002) Mutations in the human ortholog of Aristaless cause X-linked mental retardation and epilepsy. *Nat Genet* **30**:441–5.

Sugimoto Y, Morita R, Amano K, *et al.* (2000) Childhood absence epilepsy in 8q24: refinement of candidate region and construction of physical map. *Genomics* **68**:264–72.

Suls A, Dedeken P, Goffin K, *et al.* (2008) Paroxysmal exercise-induced dyskinesia and epilepsy is due to mutations in *SLC2A1*, encoding the glucose transporter GLUT1. *Brain* **131**:1831–44.

Suls A, Mullen SA, Weber YG, *et al.* (2009) Early-onset absence epilepsy caused by mutations in the glucose transporter GLUT1. *Ann Neurol* **66**:415–19.

Tan NC, Mulley JC, Berkovic SF (2004) Genetic association studies in epilepsy: "the truth is out there". *Epilepsia* **45**:1429–42.

Tanaka M, Olsen RW, Medina MT, *et al.* (2008) Hyperglycosylation and reduced GABA currents of mutated GABRB3 polypeptide in remitting childhood absence epilepsy. *Am J Hum Genet* **82**:1249–61.

Tharapel AT, Summitt RL (1978) Minor chromosome variation and selected heteromorphisms in 200 unclassifiable mentally retarded patients and 200 normal controls. *Hum Genet* **41**:121–30.

Uusimaa J, Hinttala R, Rantala H, *et al.* (2008) Homozygous W748S mutation in the *POLG1* gene in patients with juvenile-onset alpers syndrome and status epilepticus. *Epilepsia* **49**:1038–45.

Vadlamudi L, Andermann E, Lombroso CT, *et al.* (2004a): Epilepsy in twins: insights from unique historical data of William Lennox. *Neurology* **62**:1127–33.

Vadlamudi L, Harvey AS, Connellan MM, *et al.* (2004b) Is benign rolandic epilepsy genetically determined? *Ann Neurol* **56**:129–32.

Vanmolkot KR, Kors EE, Hottenga JJ, *et al.* (2003) Novel mutations in the Na$^+$, K$^+$-ATPase pump gene *ATP1A2* associated with familial hemiplegic migraine and benign familial infantile convulsions. *Ann Neurol* **54**:360–6.

Wallace RH, Marini C, Petrou S, *et al.* (2001) Mutant GABA(A) receptor gamma2-subunit in childhood absence epilepsy and febrile seizures. *Nat Genet* **28**:49–52.

Weaving LS, Christodoulou J, Williamson SL, *et al.* (2004) Mutations of *CDKL5* cause a severe neurodevelopmental disorder with infantile spasms and mental retardation. *Am J Hum Genet* **75**:1079–93.

Winawer MR, Marini C, Grinton BE, *et al.* (2005) Familial clustering of seizure types within the idiopathic generalized epilepsies. *Neurology* **65**:523–8.

Yamamoto T, Páez MT, Shimojima K (2009) Comment on "Altered DNA copy number in patients with different seizure disorder type: by array-CGH" by Kim HS *et al. Brain Dev*; **29**:639–43. *Brain Dev* **31**:94.

The genetic contribution to epilepsy: the known and missing heritability

Michael R. Johnson

Introduction: how much of epilepsy is genetic?

Broad sense heritability (h^2) refers to the proportion of phenotypic variance of a trait from all possible genetic contributions, including additive, dominance, and epistatic (multigenic) effects. There is no agreed estimate of h^2 for epilepsy, reflecting the different approaches used to measure heritability, such as twin and familial aggregation studies and their various specific designs and statistical analyses, as well as the heterogeneity of epilepsy. Thus, published estimates of heritability for epilepsy from twin studies range from 8–27% (Sillanpää *et al.* 1991) to 69–88% (Miller *et al.* 1998; Kjeldsen *et al.* 2001).

An alternative approach to the question of "how much of epilepsy is genetic," is to estimate the percentage of epilepsy that would be prevented if known environmental risk factors were completely eliminated. The proportion of epilepsy attributable to environmental causes can be estimated from knowledge of the relative risk for epilepsy associated with the known environmental risk factors (such as head injury, stroke, tumors, infections, etc.) and exposure frequencies. On this basis, an estimated 68% of all epilepsy may have no cause other than an inherited predisposition (Herman 2002).

Attempts to describe the overall genetic contributions to epilepsy are also confounded by inadequate and non-uniform terminology. Thus, there is no agreed definition as to what constitutes an "epilepsy gene." For example, where epilepsy results from an inherited anomaly of cerebral structure, should the underlying molecular genetic defect be considered an "epilepsy gene" or simply refer to its causal role in determining the underlying brain malformation? Similarly, Alzheimer disease (AD) may account for as much as 2% of all epilepsy (Annegers *et al.* 1996), but genetic risk factors of AD such as ApoE4 as well as the various Mendelian causes of AD are rarely if ever considered to be "epilepsy genes." A full inventory of all the genetic contributions to epilepsy (i.e., its total heritability) must surely contain a list of all the various genetic contributions including those Mendelian and complex disorders where epilepsy is part of the phenotype, even if not a direct consequence of the genetic defect.

In compiling this book, the editors have attempted to draw a loose distinction between the genetically determined "pure epilepsies," where epilepsy is the dominant or sole clinical feature, and those inherited disorders of cerebral structure or metabolism where epilepsy might be considered a consequence of the metabolic or structural derangement. Inevitably there is overlap, not least because of the continuing evolution of our understanding of the genetic etiology of the various epilepsies.

This chapter attempts to provide an overview of the known and unknown heritability of the "pure epilepsies" as we have defined them above. Most but not all of these epilepsies are idiopathic, as in the conventional terminology, but the term idiopathic sits less well when we consider epilepsies such as Dravet syndrome arising as a result of a de novo mutation in *SCN1A*, or Ohtahara syndrome due to a mutation in *STXBP1* or *ARX*. As used in this chapter therefore, the term "idiopathic" is perhaps more closely aligned with that used by J. Russell Reynolds in 1861 ("An internal cause – a *morbus per se*"; see Chapter 1), than the current 2001 ILAE Commission on Classification and Terminology definition of idiopathic requiring "no underlying structural brain lesion or other neurological signs or symptoms" (Engel 2001). It is clear that as our understanding of the genetic contributions to epilepsy evolves, so our definitions and systems of classification of epilepsy will also have to evolve.

Basic genetic considerations

The research method used to detect a causal gene variant varies according to the relative risk conferred by the risk allele (effect size) and its frequency in the population. Thus, a rare mutation that confers very high risk for developing epilepsy will cause the epilepsy to aggregate within an extended family. In such Mendelian situations, the causative gene can be identified using linkage analysis, which examines for co-segregation of the disease with a genetic marker in an extended pedigree before fine mutation detection methods are applied to a restricted area of a chromosome defined by the linked markers. To date, the major successes of epilepsy genetics have

The Causes of Epilepsy, eds. S. D. Shorvon, F. Andermann, and R. Guerrini. Published by Cambridge University Press. © Cambridge University Press 2011.

Table 6.1 Pure epilepsy genes identified by linkage analysis in extended pedigrees

Class	Gene	Gene product	Epilepsy syndrome	Reference
Voltage-gated ion channel genes	SCN1A	Sodium channel α1-subunit	GEFS+, Dravet	Escayg et al. 2000
	SCN1B	Sodium channel β1-subunit	GEFS+	Wallace et al. 1998
	SCN2A	Sodium channel α2-subunit	BFNIS	Heron et al. 2002
	KCNQ2	Potassium channel subunit	BFNC	Singh et al. 1998
	KCNQ3	Potassium channel subunit	BFNC	Charlier et al. 1998
	KCNA1	Potassium channel subunit	EA1 and epilepsy	Zuberi et al. 1999
Ligand-gated ion channel genes	CHRNA4	Acetylcholine receptor α4-subunit	ADNFLE	Steinlein et al. 1995
	CHRNA2	Acetylcholine receptor α2-subunit	ADNFLE	Aridon et al. 2006
	CHRNB2	Acetylcholine receptor β2-subunit	ADNFLE	De Fusco et al. 2000
	GABRA1	GABA$_A$ receptor α1-subunit	AD JME, CAE	Cossette et al. 2002
	GABRG2	GABA$_A$ receptor γ2-subunit	GEFS+, CAE	Wallace et al. 2001
				Baulac et al. 2001
Others	LGI1	Leucine-rich glioma inactivated	ADLTE	Kalachikov et al. 2002
	EFHC1	Protein with EF-hand motif	IGE, particularly JME	Suzuki et al. 2004
	PCDH19	Protocadherin 19	EFMR	Dibbens et al. 2008
	ATP1A2	Na$^+$/K$^+$ ATPase pump	FHM and epilepsy (including BFNIC)	Vanmolkot et al. 2003
	POLGI	Mitochondrial DNA polymerase	Mixed epilepsy phenotypes	Engelsen et al. 2008

Notes:
AD, autosomal dominant; ADNFLE, autosomal dominant frontal lobe epilepsy; ADLTE, autosomal dominant lateral temporal lobe epilepsy; AE, absence epilepsy; BFNC, benign familial neonatal convulsions; BFNIS, benign familial neonatal–infantile seizures; CAE, childhood absence epilepsy; EA1, episodic ataxia type 1; EFMR, epilepsy and mental retardation limited to females; FHM, familial hemiplegic migraine; GEFS+, generalized epilepsy with febrile seizures plus; GLUT-DS, glucose transporter type 1 deficiency syndrome; JME, juvenile myoclonic epilepsy; IGE, idiopathic generalized epilepsy; PED, paroxysmal exercise-induced dyskinesia.

been in the identification of genes for Mendelian epilepsy using linkage analysis (Helbig *et al.* 2008) (Table 6.1). More recently, advances in genomic technology have led to a broadening of the focus of attention to include sporadic forms of epilepsy that manifest either limited or no familial aggregation. Here, two "competing" theories regarding genetic susceptibility have been proposed. The "common disease – common variant hypothesis" (Chakravati 1999) proposes that common genetic variants (defined as having a minor allele frequency >1%) confer low relative risk for the disease but because the risk variant is common in the population, it accounts for a large number of cases. In contrast, the "multiple rare variant – common disease hypothesis" (Pritchard 2001), proposes that individually rare mutations can arise in many different genes so as to confer an overall high mutation rate to the disease class. In this situation, it has been pointed out that the notion of a common disease becomes a misnomer, since in reality the condition is a collection of many genetically distinct conditions (Sawcer 2008). These two competing hypotheses for

common sporadic forms of epilepsy are not mutually exclusive, but necessarily require different approaches to identify the underlying causal variant. In brief, the detection of common variants is by genetic association methodology, which at its simplest compares the frequency of a risk allele in populations of disease cases and matched controls, whilst the identification of rare variants requires the systematic deep resequencing of candidate genes in large cohorts of multiplex families or populations of cases and controls.

Pure epilepsies due to single gene disorders

Table 6.1 lists the known genes implicated in idiopathic ("pure") Mendelian epilepsy. By definition, each gene was identified using linkage analysis in an extended pedigree. Meticulous clinical characterization of epilepsy within each pedigree was instrumental in the discovery of each gene, and the identification of each has been a significant advance in our understanding of epilepsy as is discussed in greater detail in subsequent chapters.

Common variants and common epilepsy

The considerable progress in identifying genes for Mendelian epilepsy is in sharp contrast to the absence of progress in identifying genetic susceptibility to more common sporadic forms of the disease. At the time of writing, there is no validated common variant associated with epilepsy. That is not to say that such variants are unlikely to exist, but rather that the systematic large-scale collaborative efforts required to identify common variants for epilepsy have yet to be undertaken, with the majority of published work focusing on candidate genes in relatively small cohorts. Undoubtedly, this has led to a large number of false-positive reports, as can be explained.

The probability that a reported positive genetic association reflects a true causal relationship with epilepsy depends on the power of the study, the ratio of true to no relationships (i.e., the prior probability of a true causal relationship) and the reported level of significance (p value) for the association (Ioannidis 2005). Bayes' theorem provides a simple algebraic relationship between these parameters which describes the posterior probability that a reported genetic association has a true causal relationship with the disease and is not a false positive report.

Critical to the calculation of the posterior probability of a true causal relationship is the prior probability that any single common variant chosen at random has a causal relationship to epilepsy. This prior probability has been conceptualized as the "needle in the haystack" problem, where the needle is the causal gene variant and the haystack is the great extent of common genetic variation in the human population. Efforts to curate human structural genetic variation such as the HapMap project (http://snp.cshl.org/) suggest that there may be as many as 10 million common variants in the human population (Kruglyak and Nickerson 2001). This provides us with an estimate of the size of the "haystack." It is possible to make estimates of the number of common variants required to explain a common disease such as epilepsy (i.e., the total number of needles in the haystack) based on the frequency of a risk allele, the relative risk for disease conferred by the allele, disease prevalence, and the genetic model (Yang *et al.* 2005). This epidemiological approach suggests that for most common diseases, as few as 20–100 common variants with modest relative risk (1.2 to 1.5) would be sufficient. Thus, for any single common variant chosen at random, the ratio of true relationship to no relationship to epilepsy can be reasonably estimated to be in the region of 1 in 100 000.

Figure 6.1 shows the posterior probability that a genetic association reflects a true causal relationship with epilepsy for any given p-value, assuming a prior probability of a true causal relationship of 1 : 100 000. It can be seen that even for a study with 80% power, a reported positive association is not highly likely to be actually true until the p-value for the association is 1×10^{-7} or less. And where the power of the study is less, then the probability that an association is true for any given p-value

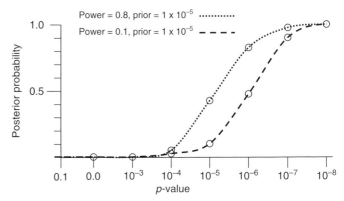

Fig. 6.1. Posterior probability that a reported positive genetic association with epilepsy reflects a true causal relationship.

will also be less, so that for a study with power 10%, an association is not highly likely to be true until the p-value for the association is 5×10^{-8} or less. It is this Bayesian argument that underpins the usual accepted cut-off for "genome-wide significance" in genetic association studies of 5×10^{-8}.

To date, this author is aware of no published association between a common variant and epilepsy that has achieved the accepted cut-off for genome-wide significance. However, better appreciation of the dangers of inadequate power and a stricter adherence to rigorous statistical interpretation of results will ensure that future reported associations between common variants and epilepsy are more likely to be true than false.

Rare variants and common epilepsy

The alternative hypothesis to the common variant explanation of a common disease like epilepsy proposes that instead of a few common variants, a large number of rare variants with large effects underlie genetic susceptibility. Under this model, many hundreds or even thousands of individually rare variants are required to explain epilepsy, even where the risk ratios are large (e.g., relative risk = 10–20) (Yang *et al.* 2005). In recent years, methods for genotyping common genomic variation have advanced more quickly than those for DNA resequencing. As a result, the focus of attention in genomic research has been on the role of common variants in common disease, as opposed to the systematic search for rare variants. This focus on common variants may have obscured the considerable incremental progress that has in fact been made in identifying rare variants for sporadic epilepsy. Here, astute clinical connections made between rare Mendelian forms of epilepsy with known genes and sporadic forms of epilepsy allowed the spectrum of candidate genes that might harbor rare variants to be narrowed to a degree that permitted the detection of rare variants. There is now good evidence for a causal relationship between rare variants in 16 genes and sporadic epilepsy (Table 6.2). As with the identification of genes for Mendelian epilepsy, the identification of each of these is a tribute to the clinical method in epilepsy genetics.

Although the genes listed in Table 6.2 are likely to be only a fraction of the many hundreds of rare variants required to

Table 6.2 De novo arising rare variants associated with sporadic epilepsy

Gene	Gene product	Epilepsy syndrome	Reference
SCN1A	Sodium channel α1-subunit	Dravet syndrome	Claes *et al.* 2001
LGI1	Leucine-rich glioma inactivated	ADLTE	Bisulli *et al.* 2004
GABRA1	GABA$_A$ receptor α1-subunit	IGE	Maljevic *et al.* 2006
CACNA1H	T type calcium channel subunit	IGE	Heron *et al.* 2007
CLCN2	Chloride channel subunit	IGE	Kleefuss-Lie *et al.* 2009
			Saint-Martin *et al.* 2009
GABRD	GABA$_A$ receptor γ2-subunit	GEFS+	Dibbens *et al.* 2004
KCND2	Voltage-gated potassium channel	TLE	Singh *et al.* 2006
SCL2A1	Glucose transporter type 1 (GLUT1)	Early onset AE	Suls *et al.* 2009
KCNJ11	Pore-forming subunit of K(ATP) channel	DEND syndrome	Gloyn *et al.* 2006
ABCC8	ATP binding cassette transporter protein	DEND syndrome	Proks *et al.* 2006
EFHC1	Protein with EF-hand motif	IGE	Stogmann *et al.* 2006
			Medina *et al.* 2008
15q13.3 microdeletion (copy-number variation)		IGE	Helbig *et al.* 2009
			Dibbens *et al.* 2009
POLG1	Mitochondrial DNA polymerase	Mixed epilepsy phenotypes	Uusimaa *et al.* 2008
			Engelsen *et al.* 2008
STXBP1	Syntaxin binding protein	Ohtahara syndrome	Saitsu *et al.* 2008
CDKL5	Cyclin-dependent kinase-like 5	IS and Rett-like syndrome	Bahi-Buisson *et al.* 2008
ARX	Paired type homeobox	West, Ohtahara syndromes	Kato *et al.* 2003, 2007

Notes:
DEND, developmental delay, epilepsy and neonatal diabetes; IS, infantile spasms.

explain heritable epilepsy, they are already sufficient in number to suggest that epilepsy may emerge as predominantly a "rare variant – common disease" condition. Exciting developments in very-high-throughput DNA sequencing technology will soon offer the potential for whole-genome resequencing that will ultimately define all the rare (and common) variant contributions to epilepsy. The challenge will then be how to translate these understandings to better therapies and improved patient care. Subsequent chapters in this book begin to illustrate how this challenge will be met.

References

Annegers JF, Rocca WA, Hauser WA (1996) Causes of epilepsy: contributions of the Rochester epidemiology project. *Mayo Clin Proc* **71**:570–5.

Aridon P, Marini C, Di Resta C, *et al.* (2006) Increased sensitivity of the neuronal nicotinic receptor alpha 2 subunit causes familial epilepsy with nocturnal wandering and ictal fear. *Am J Hum Genet* **79**:342–50.

Bahi-Buisson N, Nectoux J, Rosas-Vargas H, *et al.* (2008) Key clinical features to identify girls with *CDKL5* mutations. *Brain* **131**:2647–61.

Baulac S, Huberfeld G, Gourfinkel-An I, *et al.* (2001) First genetic evidence of

GABA(A) receptor dysfunction in epilepsy: a mutation in the gamma2-subunit gene. *Nat Genet* **28**:46–8

Bisulli F, Tinuper P, Avoni P, *et al.* (2004) Idiopathic partial epilepsy with auditory features (IPEAF): a clinical and genetic study of 53 sporadic cases. *Brain* **127**:1343–52.

Chakravarti A (1999) Population genetics: making sense out of sequence. *Nat Genet* **21**(1 Suppl):56–60.

Charlier C, Singh NA, Ryan SG, *et al.* (1998) A pore mutation in a novel KQT-like potassium channel gene in an idiopathic epilepsy family. *Nat Genet* **18**:53–5.

Claes L, Del-Favero J, Ceulemans B, *et al.* (2001) De novo mutations in the

sodium-channel gene *SCN1A* cause severe myoclonic epilepsy of infancy. *Am J Hum Genet* **68**:1327–32.

Cossette P, Liu L, Brisebois K, *et al.* (2002) Mutation of *GABRA1* in an autosomal dominant form of juvenile myoclonic epilepsy. *Nat Genet* **31**:184–9.

De Fusco M, Becchetti A, Patrignani A, *et al.* (2000) The nicotinic receptor beta 2 subunit is mutant in nocturnal frontal lobe epilepsy. *Nat Genet* **26**:275–6.

Dibbens LM, Feng HJ, Richards MC, *et al.* (2004) *GABRD* encoding a protein for extra- or peri-synaptic GABAA receptors is a susceptibility locus for generalized epilepsies. *Hum Mol Genet* **13**:1315–19.

Dibbens LM, Tarpey PS, Hynes K, et al. (2008) X-linked protocadherin 19 mutations cause female-limited epilepsy and cognitive impairment. *Nat Genet* **40**:776–81.

Dibbens LM, Mullen S, Helbig I, et al. (2009) Familial and sporadic 15q13.3 microdeletions in idiopathic generalized epilepsy: precedent for disorders with complex inheritance. *Hum Mol Genet* **18**:3626–31.

Engel J Jr. (2001) A proposed diagnostic scheme for people with epileptic seizures and with epilepsy: Report of the ILAE Task Force on Classification and Terminology. *Epilepsia* **42**:796–803.

Engelsen BA, Tzoulis C, Karlsen B, et al. (2008) *POLG1* mutations cause a syndromic epilepsy with occipital lobe predilection. *Brain* **131**:818–28.

Escayg A, MacDonald BT, Meisler MH, et al. (2000) Mutations of *SCN1A*, encoding a neuronal sodium channel, in two families with GEFS+2. *Nat Genet* **24**:343–5.

Gloyn AL, Diatloff-Zito C, Edghill EL, et al. (2006) KCNJ11 activating mutations are associated with developmental delay, epilepsy and neonatal diabetes syndrome and other neurological features. *Eur J Hum Genet* **14**:824–30.

Helbig I, Scheffer IE, Mulley JC, Berkovic SF (2008) Navigating the channels and beyond: unravelling the genetics of the epilepsies. *Lancet Neurol* **7**:231–45.

Helbig I, Mefford HC, Sharp AJ, et al. (2009) 15q13.3 microdeletions increase risk of idiopathic generalized epilepsy. *Nat Genet* **41**:160–2.

Herman ST (2002) Epilepsy after brain insult: targeting epileptogenesis. *Neurology* **59**:S21–S26.

Heron SE, Crossland KM, Andermann E, et al. (2002) Sodium-channel defects in benign familial neonatal-infantile seizures. *Lancet* **360**:851–2.

Heron SE, Khosravani H, Varela D, et al. (2007) Extended spectrum of idiopathic generalized epilepsies associated with *CACNA1H* functional variants. *Ann Neurol* **62**:745–9.

Ioannidis JPA (2005) Why most published research findings are false. *PLoS Med* **2**:0696–0701.

Kalachikov S, Evgrafov O, Ross B, et al. (2002) Mutations in *LGI1* cause autosomal-dominant partial epilepsy with auditory features. *Nat Genet* **30**:335–41.

Kato M, Das S, Petras K, Sawaishi Y, Dobyns WB (2003) Polyalanine expansion of *ARX* associated with cryptogenic West syndrome. *Neurology* **61**:267–76.

Kato M, Saitoh S, Kamei A, et al. (2007) A longer polyalanine expansion mutation in the *ARX* gene causes early infantile epileptic encephalopathy with suppression–burst pattern (Ohtahara syndrome). *Am J Hum Genet* **81**:361–6.

Kjeldsen MJ, Kyvik KO, Christensen K, Friis ML (2001) Genetic and environmental factors in epilepsy: a population-based study of 11 900 Danish twin pairs. *Epilepsy Res* **44**:167–78.

Kleefuss-Lie A, Friedl W, Cichon S, et al. (2009) *CLCN2* variants in idiopathic generalized epilepsy. *Nat Genet* **41**:954–5.

Kruglyak L, Nickerson DA (2001) Variation is the spice of life. *Nat Genet* **27**:234–6.

Maljevic S, Krampfl K, Cobilanschi J, et al. (2006) A mutation in the GABA(A) receptor alpha(1)-subunit is associated with absence epilepsy. *Ann Neurol* **59**:983–7.

Medina ST, Suzuki T, Alonso ME, et al. (2008) Novel mutations in Myoclonin1/EFHC1 in sporadic and familial juvenile myoclonic epilepsy. *Neurology* **70**:2137–44.

Miller LL, Pellock JM, DeLorenzo RJ, Meyer JM, Corey LA (1998) Univariate genetic analyses of epilepsy and seizures in a population-based twin study: the Virginia Twin Registry. *Genet Epidemiol* **15**:33–49.

Pritchard JK (2001) Are rare variants responsible for susceptibility to complex disease? *Am J Hum Genet* **69**:124–37.

Proks P, Arnold AL, Bruining J, et al. (2006) A heterozygous activating mutation in the sulphonylurea receptor SUR1 (ABCC8) causes neonatal diabetes. *Hum Mol Genet* **15**:1793–800.

Saint-Martin C, Gauvain G, Teodorescu G, et al. (2009) Two novel *CLCN2* mutations accelerating chloride channel deactivation are associated with idiopathic generalized epilepsy. *Hum Mutat* **30**:397–405.

Saitsu H, Kato M, Mizuguchi T, et al. (2008) De novo mutations in the gene encoding STXBP1 (MUNC18–1) cause early infantile epileptic encephalopathy. *Nat Genet* **40**:782–8.

Sawcer S (2008) The complex genetics of multiple sclerosis: pitfalls and prospects. *Brain* **131**:3118–31.

Sillanpää M, Koskenvuo M, Romanov K, Kaprio J (1991) Genetic factors in epileptic seizures: evidence from a large twin population. *Acta Neurol Scand* **84**:523–6.

Singh B, Ogiwara I, Kaneda M, et al. (2006) A Kv4.2 truncation mutation in a patient with temporal lobe epilepsy. *Neurobiol Dis* **24**:245–53.

Singh NA, Charlier C, Stauffer D, et al. (1998) A novel potassium channel gene, *KCNQ2*, is mutated in an inherited epilepsy of newborns. *Nat Genet* **18**:25–9.

Steinlein OK, Mulley JC, Propping P, et al. (1995) A missense mutation in the neuronal nicotinic acetylcholine receptor alpha 4 subunit is associated with autosomal dominant nocturnal frontal lobe epilepsy. *Nat Genet* **11**:201–3.

Stogmann E, Lichtner P, Baumgartner C, et al. (2006) Idiopathic generalized epilepsy phenotypes associated with different *EFHC1* mutations. *Neurology* **67**:2029–31.

Suls A, Mullen SA, Weber YG, et al. (2009) Early-onset absence epilepsy caused by mutations in the glucose transporter GLUT1. *Ann Neurol* **66**:415–19.

Suzuki T, Delgado-Escueta AV, Aguan K, et al. (2004) Mutations in *EFHC1* cause juvenile myoclonic epilepsy. *Nat Genet* **36**:842–9.

Uusimaa J, Hinttala R, Rantala H, et al. (2008) Homozygous W748S mutation in the *POLG1* gene in patients with juvenile-onset Alpers syndrome and status epilepticus. *Epilepsia* **49**:1038–45.

Vanmolkot KR, Kors EE, Hottenga JJ, et al. (2003) Novel mutations in the Na$^+$, K$^+$-ATPase pump gene *ATP1A2* associated with familial hemiplegic migraine and benign familial infantile convulsions. *Ann Neurol* **54**:360–6.

Wallace RH, Wang DW, Singh R, et al. (1998) Febrile seizures and generalized epilepsy associated with a mutation Na$^+$-channel beta1 subunit gene *SCN1B*. *Nat Genet* **19**:366–70.

Wallace RH, Marini C, Petrou S, et al. (2001) Mutant GABA(A) receptor gamma2-subunit in childhood absence epilepsy and febrile seizures. *Nat Genet* **28**:49–52.

Yang Q, Khoury MJ, Friedman JM, Little J, Flanders WD (2005). How many genes underlie the occurrence of common complex diseases in the population? *Int J Epidemiol* **34**:1129–37.

Zuberi SM, Eunson LH, Spauschus A, et al. (1999) A novel mutation in the human voltage-gated potassium channel gene (Kv1.1) associates with episodic ataxia type 1 and sometimes with partial epilepsy. *Brain* **122**:817–25.

Benign familial neonatal seizures

Perrine Plouin

Recognizing the diagnosis of benign familial neonatal seizures (BFNS) is an important challenge as it allows one to forecast a favorable outcome and a very low risk of subsequent epilepsy. It is then important to know the neurological state of the baby, the description of the seizures, and the personal and familial histories.

Benign familial neonatal seizures is a rare dominantly inherited epileptic syndrome with a penetrance as high as 85%. It was first reported in 1964 by Rett and Teubel. Since then more than 250 cases have been reported. Benign neonatal seizures (BNS) are defined by a favorable outcome, i.e., a normal psychomotor development and the absence of subsequent epilepsy. Benign familial neonatal seizures (BFNS) are of course concerned with a familial history of BNS. The diagnosis of BFNS can be considered as a diagnosis by exclusion if every other etiology has been excluded and if there is a family history of neonatal seizures without any severe epilepsy in family members. The best estimate thus far of the population rate for BFNS comes from a recent prospective, population-based study that involved all obstetric and neonatal units across the province of Newfoundland, Canada (Ronen et al. 1999). Five cases of BFNS were observed among 34 615 live births from January 1, 1990 to December 31, 1994. Thus the incidence of BFNS was 14.4 per 100 000 live births.

By definition, an idiopathic syndrome does not have a specific underlying etiology. This is the case for BFNS (Commission on Classification and Terminology of the ILAE 1989).

Genetics

Basic mechanisms in this syndrome are probably close to those involved in other types of neonatal convulsions. The immature brain is more likely to respond to any kind of injury with epileptic seizures. In this syndrome, genetic susceptibility during the first week of life in full-term neonates is responsible for the appearance of seizures; it is a deficit of a specific channelopathy which is the cause of this epileptic syndrome but the precise mechanism still remains unknown (Kullmann 2008). The fact that seizures occur in premature newborns

when they reach 39 to 41 weeks of gestational age means that a step in maturation has to be reached for the channelopathy to be expressed. Leppert et al. (1989) studied 48 individuals in four generations of a family (Quattelbaum's family), 19 of them having the characteristics of BFNS. They localized the gene to the long arm of chromosome 20, possibly to 20q13.2. These results established the linkage of the gene for BFNS to the long arm of chromosome 20, the first linkage to be reported for an epilepsy syndrome. The BFNS syndrome that maps to chromosome 20q has been designated as EBN1. Linkage to D20S19 and D20S20 was excluded, however, in a three-generation Mexican–American family (Ryan et al. 1991), suggesting locus heterogeneity. Further study of that family (Lewis et al. 1993) demonstrated tight linkage to a locus on 8q, thus indicating heterogeneity (the BFNS syndrome on 8q is designated as EBN2). Suggestive evidence for this second locus was also reported in a northern European pedigree (Steinlein et al. 1995). The sequencing of the genes that are mutated in EBN1 and EBN2 was reported in three papers early in 1998: KCNQ2 located on 20q13.3 and KCNQ3 on 8q24. New families have recently been reported with variations in seizure history and in the type of mutations (de Haan et al. 2006; Heron et al. 2007; Yalçin et al. 2007; Li et al. 2008). The present question is the relationship between BFNS and the developmental changes in KCNQ2 and KNCQ3 expression in the developing brain (Kanaumi et al. 2007; Kullmann 2008).

Clinical presentation

In documented cases, birth was always at full term (except for three cases of Ronen et al. 1993), with normal birth weight and an Apgar score above 7 at the first minute of life. None of these neonates was admitted to an intensive care unit. There was always a seizure-free interval between birth and occurrence of seizures. The sex ratio shows an equal distribution between boys and girls. In 80% of cases, seizures start on the second or third day of life, except in very premature babies who need to reach full-term neurologic state; this point is important, given the strict age-dependence of the syndrome. The neurologic

The Causes of Epilepsy, eds. S. D. Shorvon, F. Andermann, and R. Guerrini. Published by Cambridge University Press. © Cambridge University Press 2011.

state of the babies remains normal in most cases, and they can nurse or drink from a bottle between seizures; mild transitory hypotonia can be noticed in some cases (Plouin and Anderson 2005). None of these babies was transferred to neonatal intensive care units. From different video recordings it appears that in most cases seizures start with a diffuse tonic component, followed by various autonomic and motor changes, which can be unilateral or bilateral, symmetric or not (Hirsch *et al.* 1993; Bye 1994). We had the opportunity to record seizures in five cases with video-electroencephalograph (EEG) monitoring: seizures were stereotyped, starting with diffuse hypotonia and a short apnea, followed by autonomic or oculofacial features and symmetrical or asymmetrical clonic limb movements. No other type of seizure was recorded such as myoclonic jerks or epileptic spasms.

The EEG is normal or mildly abnormal. If recordings are made, the electroclinical presentation of seizures is relatively stereotyped. Nevertheless it seems necessary to exclude any other etiology, metabolic or infectious, and for that purpose a clinical work-up and a lumbar puncture should be performed. Computed tomography (CT) or magnetic resonance imaging (MRI) are not indicated as long as the neurological state of the baby remains normal.

Treatment

No guideline has been proposed concerning the treatment of BFNS. In the past, probably no treatment was given. In some families, mostly coming from around the Mediterranean Sea, the best reported treatment was to put a cold key on the neck of the baby.

Different authors give their own experience in the treatment of these babies. The drug used depends on country, continent, and year of publication.

Most babies were given phenobarbital for 2 to 6 months, rarely for longer periods. In our experience, sodium valproate was effective, leading to rapid cessation of seizures. Some authors have also used diphenylhydantoin. The question remains open about the usefulness of an antiepileptic drug treatment: grandparents of these babies were not treated and did well. If a treatment is initiated at the time of the seizures, it seems reasonable to interrupt it by the third or sixth month.

Outcome

No longitudinal study has been published of BFNS. When reviewing the literature we found that babies with BFNS have a 5% risk for febrile convulsions, which is not very different from the general population risk. Concerning subsequent epilepsy, the mean risk is around 11% among these babies, which is higher than observed in the general population. However no case of severe epilepsy was noticed in this population. Maihara *et al.* (1999) reported two siblings with BFNS who later developed epilepsy with centrotemporal spikes: both stopped having seizures with carbamazepine, and had normal psychomotor development. Recently Steinlein *et al.* (2007) reviewed 17 BFNS families. For 10 families information about outcome was available: in four families at least one affected individual showed delayed psychomotor development or mental retardation. Three of the four mutations were familial, while the fourth mutation was de novo. Mutations associated with an unfavorable outcome tended to be located within the functionally critical S5/S6 regions of the *KCNQ2* gene. The authors raise the question if BFNS can indeed be described as a benign disorder, and which are the genetic and/or environmental factors that influence the outcome.

Summary and conclusion

Recognizing the phenotype of BFNS is important, first because of the prediction of a favorable neurological outcome, and second for the contribution to genetic studies, which comprise a dynamic area of epilepsy research, not only for the idiopathic epilepsies but also for the development of new antiepileptic drugs (Wickenden *et al.* 2000).

The classic phenotype of BFNS comprises the following features: normal pregnancy and delivery; seizure-free interval before onset of seizures (mostly on days 2 and 3); neurologically normal state between seizures; normal interictal EEG; tonic–clonic seizures, symmetric or not; and a familial history of BFNS or other types of epilepsy (mostly idiopathic epilepsies). The families of such babies should be considered for genetic studies.

References

Bye AME (1994) Neonate with benign familial neonatal convulsions: recorded generalized and focal seizures. *Ped Neurol* **10**:164–5.

Commission on Classification and Terminology of the ILAE (1989) Proposal for revised classification of epilepsies and epileptic syndromes. *Epilepsia* **30**:389–699.

de Haan GJ, Pinto D, Carton D, *et al.* (2006) A novel splicing mutation in *KCNQ2* in a multigenerational family with BFNC followed for 25 years. *Epilepsia* **47**:851–9.

Heron SE, Cox K, Grinton BE, *et al.* (2007) Deletions or duplications in *KCNQ2* can cause benign familial neonatal seizures. *J Med Genet* **44**:791–6.

Hirsch E, Velez A, Sellal F, *et al.* (1993) Electroclinical signs of benign neonatal familial convulsions. *Ann Neurol* **134**:835–41.

Kanaumi T, Takashima S, Iwasaki H, *et al.* (2008) Developmental changes in *KCNQ2* and *KCNQ3* expression in human brain: possible contribution to the age-dependent etiology of benign familial neonatal convulsions. *Brain Dev* **30**:362–9.

Kullmann DM (2008) Benign neonatal convulsions and spontaneous network activity in the developing brain: is there a link? *J Physiol* **15**:52–81.

Leppert M, Anderson VE, Quattlebaum T, *et al.* (1989) Benign familial neonatal convulsions linked to genetic markers on chromosome 20. *Nature* **337**:647–8.

Lewis TB, Leach RJ, Ward K (1993) Genetic heterogeneity in benign familial neonatal convulsions: identification of a new locus on chromosome 8q. *Am J Hum Gen* **53**:670–5.

Li H, Li N, Shen L, *et al.* (2008) A novel mutation of *KCNQ3* gene in a Chinese family with benign familial neonatal convulsions. *Epilepsy Res* **79**:1–5.

Maihara T, Tsuji M, Higuchi Y, Hattori H (1999) Benign familial neonatal convulsions followed by benign epilepsy with centro-temporal spikes in two siblings. *Epilepsia* **40**:110–13.

Plouin P, Anderson VE (2005) Benign familial and non-familial neonatal seizures. In: Roger J, Bureau M, Dravet C, Genton P, Tassinari CA, Wolf P (eds.) *Epileptic Syndromes in Infancy, Childhood and Adolescence.* Montrouge, France: John Libbey Eurotext, pp. 3–15.

Quattelbaum TG (1979) Benign familial convulsions in the neonatal period and early infancy. *J Pediat* **95**:257–9.

Rett AR, Teubel R (1964) Neugeborenenkrämpfe im Rahmen einer epileptisch belasten Familie. *Wien Klin Wschr* **76**:609–13.

Ronen GM, Rosales TO, Connolly ME, Anderson VE, Leppert M (1993) Seizure characteristics in chromosome 20 benign familial neonatal convulsions. *Neurology* **43**:1355–60.

Ronen GM, Penney S, Andrews W (1999) The epidemiology of clinical neonatal seizures in Newfoundland: a population-based study. *J Pediat* **134**:71–5.

Ryan SG, Wiznitzer M, Hollman C, *et al.* (1991) Benign familial neonatal convulsions: evidence for clinical and genetic heterogeneity. *Ann Neurol* **29**:469–73.

Steinlein O, Schuster V, Fischer C, Häussler M (1995) Benign familial neonatal convulsions: confirmation of genetic heterogeneity and further evidence for a second locus on chromosome 8q. *Hum Genet* **95**:411–15.

Steinlein OK, Conrad C, Weidner B (2007) Benign familial neonatal convulsions: always benign? *Epilepsy Res* **73**:245–9.

Wickenden AD, Yu W, Zou A, Jegla T, Wagoner PK (2000) Retigabine, a novel anticonvulsant, enhances activation of *KCNQ2/Q3* potassium channels. *Molec Pharm* **58**:591–600.

Yalçin O, Cağlayan SH, Saltik S, *et al.* (2007) A novel missense mutation (N258S) in the *KCNQ2* gene in a Turkish family afflicted with benign familial neonatal convulsions (BFNC). *Turk J Pediatr* **49**:385–9.

69

Chapter

8

Autosomal dominant nocturnal frontal lobe epilepsy

Paolo Tinuper and Francesca Bisulli

The causal disease

In 1981, Lugaresi and Cirignotta described five patients with frequent episodes characterized by violent limb movements and dystonic–tonic posturing during light sleep. The unusual motor behavior, uniform in all patients with stereotyped dystonic-dyskinetic aspects, the lack of clear-cut ictal and interictal abnormalities on electroencephalogram (EEG) and the response to carbamazepine led the authors to label this condition "hypnogenic paroxysmal dystonia." Some years later, the authors better defined this condition, renaming it "nocturnal paroxysmal dystonia" (NPD) (Lugaresi et al. 1986). Since the first descriptions, the epileptic or non-epileptic origin of short-lasting NPD attacks has been debated. However, the similarity of NPD attacks with complex, often bizarre motor behavior, bipedal and bimanual activity, and violent rocking axial and pelvic movements characteristic of frontal seizures recorded in patients undergoing neurosurgical treatment for drug-resistant epilepsy, together with the demonstration of clear-cut epileptiform discharges in some patients, permitted the Bologna group to demonstrate that short-lasting, stereotyped attacks of NPD were in fact epileptic seizures originating in the mesial surface of the frontal lobes (Tinuper et al. 1990, 2002; Provini et al. 1999). The term "nocturnal frontal lobe epilepsy" (NFLE) was therefore adopted.

Meanwhile, in 1994 Scheffer et al. first described a large Australian family with *nocturnal frontal lobe seizures* (NFLS) inherited in an autosomal dominant manner and named this condition "autosomal dominant nocturnal frontal lobe epilepsy" (ADNFLE). Following the initial recognition, more than a hundred families have been described worldwide (Picard et al. 2006). Further molecular genetic studies established linkage to chromosome 20q13.2–q13.13 (Phillips et al. 1995) in some families and subsequent identification of the causative role of the gene coding for the α4-subunit of the neuronal nicotinic acetylcholine receptor (nAChR) (*CHRNA4*) (Steinlein et al. 1995). Subsequently, mutations in genes coding for the α2 and β2 subunits of the acetylcholine receptor (*CHRNA2* and *CHRNB2*) were also identified (De Fusco et al. 2000; Phillips et al. 2000; Aridon et al. 2006), confirming

genetic heterogeneity. At present only two de novo mutations in these genes have been reported (Phillips et al. 2000; Bertrand et al. 2005). Linkage analysis in ADNFLE families without known mutations revealed three additional loci on chromosomes 15q24 (Phillips et al. 1998), 3p22–24, and 8q11.2–q21.1 (De Marco et al. 2007), but causative mutations have not yet been found.

In vitro analyses of the functional properties of nAChR disclosed gain of function (i.e. an increase in acetylcholine sensitivity) (Bertrand et al. 2002) of mutant receptors associated with ADNFLE that may underlie the neuronal network dysfunction responsible for the epileptic seizures. Positron emission tomography (PET) studies in ADNFLE patients suggest a hyperactivation of the cholinergic pathway ascending from the brainstem (Picard et al. 2006). Cholinergic neurons modulate sleep and arousal at both thalamic and cortical level and their involvement in sleep-related disorders is plausible, although the pathophysiological mechanism remains elusive.

Epilepsy in the disease

In both sporadic and inherited (ADNFLE) forms NFLE is a syndromic entity that includes paroxysmal episodes with variable semiology, intensity, and duration, representing different aspects of the same epileptic condition.

A family history of epilepsy may be present and a clear Mendelian autosomal dominant inheritance has been described in some families with marked variation in severity amongst different members. About a third of cases, both sporadic and familial, had a personal and/or family history of true parasomnias (Provini et al. 1999). As recently documented by a large case-control study, among the different parasomnias arousal disorders (sleepwalking, sleep terror, and confusional arousal) have the strongest relation with NFLE, whereas the role of other sleep disturbances like enuresis or sleep-talking, has been excluded. In both the sporadic and inherited forms NFLE typically has a good prognosis with seizure frequency, which may be high during childhood, often diminishing in adulthood, making it a relatively benign clinical

The Causes of Epilepsy, eds. S. D. Shorvon, F. Andermann, and R. Guerrini. Published by Cambridge University Press. © Cambridge University Press 2011.

Table 8.1 Seizures in nocturnal frontal lobe epilepsy (NFLE)

Hypermotor seizures (HS)

Body movements that can start in the limbs, head, or trunk

Complex, often violent behavior

Often with a dystonic–dyskinetic component

Sometimes with cycling or rocking or repetitive body movements

Prevalent in the trunk or legs

The patient may vocalize, scream, or swear

Fear is a frequent expression

  Asymmetric, bilateral tonic seizures

  Sustained non-customary forced position

Paroxysmal arousals (PA)

Bilateral and axial involvement resembling a sudden arousal

Opening of the eyes

Sitting up in bed

Sometimes frightened expression

Epileptic wanderings (EW)

Same beginning as above

Semi-purposeful ambulatory behavior

Mimicking sleepwalking

entity. This is also because seizures occur during sleep and most cases respond to antiepileptic drugs.

There may be an association with structural lesions, usually within the frontal lobe, but a symptomatic etiology is present only in 13% of patients, most cases remaining cryptogenic even after high-resolution magnetic resonance imaging (MRI). Histopathology, performed in a series of 21 patients undergoing surgery for drug-resistant NFLE, demonstrated a Taylor-type focal cortical dysplasia in 16 patients and an architectural focal cortical dysplasia in four (Nobili *et al.* 2007).

Patients with NFLE are usually of normal intelligence, although two families with ADNFLE and intellectual disability have been reported (Khatami *et al.* 1998; Cho *et al.* 2003) and rare families with unusually severe ADNFLE, with associated psychiatric, behavioral, and cognitive features have recently been described (Derry *et al.* 2008).

The spectrum of clinical semiology of nocturnal seizures is listed in Table 8.1 (Tinuper *et al.*, 2005).

Hypermotor seizures

Hypermotor seizures (HS) involve sudden awakening followed by complex body movements in the limbs, head, or trunk, often with a dystonic–diskinetic component. Motor activity may also consist in rocking of the trunk, or cycling or kicking activity of the four limbs. The patient may vocalize, scream, or

swear, often performing semi-purposeful repetitive movements mimicking "primitive" behavior like grasping, spitting, chewing, or sexual activity, sometimes so violent as to risk injury or falling out of bed. Seizures last several seconds and are not followed by a confusional postictal phase. If questioned, the patients may or may not recall a motor attack.

Asymmetric, bilateral tonic seizures represent a subgroup of HS and are characterized by a sudden asymmetric tonic–dystonic position of the four limbs that are kept in this forced position on both sides for some seconds. The tonic contraction may also involve the face and oral muscles. Some vocalization may occur. Usually the patient maintains contact, but is unable to speak.

Paroxysmal arousals

Paroxysmal arousals (PA) were described by Montagna *et al.* (1990). During these very short (1–3 s) attacks the patients open their eyes, sometimes raising their head from the bed, or sitting up with a frightened expression. Sometimes a slight dystonic posture of the fingers or arms may be observed. A short vocalization may occur. These attacks are very stereotyped in a given patient and may be very frequent during the same night, in some cases coexisting in the same patient with full-blown seizures.

Epileptic wanderings

Epileptic wanderings (EW) (Plazzi *et al.* 1995) are characterized by a prolonged seizure (1–2 min) during which the patient has semi-purposeful ambulatory behavior and complex motor activity mimicking sleepwalking. The patient may jump, scream, and try to leave the bedroom, with an agitated frightened expression. In the morning the patient does not recall the episode. These descriptions contributed to clarifying the epileptic nature of prolonged episodes arising during sleep that had been previously reported (Pedley and Guilleminault 1977). The seizures are very frequent, in some patients occurring every night, several times per night. Most patients have seizures of different intensity, often on the same night: 31% paroxysmal arousals and epileptic nocturnal wanderings, 32% paroxysmal arousals and hypermotor seizures, and 2% hypermotor seizures and nocturnal wanderings. Seven percent of the patients presented with the three types of attacks (Provini *et al.* 1999) (Table 8.1).

In at least some patients, attacks had a quasiperiodic occurrence during some portion of non rapid eye movement (NREM) sleep (Tinuper *et al.* 1990; Sforza *et al.* 1993) occurring every 20–40 s and reflecting the pulsatility of arousal mechanisms.

Diagnostic tests

An accurate description of the phenotypic aspects of the patients, including precise clinical and EEG semiology of seizures, is mandatory for a correct diagnosis. Interictal EEG is usually normal, with clear-cut epileptiform discharges present in only 33% of individuals in wakefulness and in 45% during sleep.

Ictal EEG shows no epileptiform activity in almost 50% of patients; focal attenuation or rhythmic theta or delta is the prominent feature in the majority of those presenting EEG abnormalities; only around 10% will show spike-and-wave activity, and another 10% focal fast activity (Provini *et al.* 1999).

Although the inter-observer reliability of NFLE diagnosis by sleep experts and epileptologists, as based on videotaped observation of sleep phenomena, is not satisfactory (Vignatelli *et al.* 2007), in doubtful cases videorecording of the motor phenomenology is necessary to distinguish NFLE from other non-epileptic paroxysmal motor disorders of sleep.

The most frequent diagnostic dilemma is distinguishing NFLE seizures from parasomnic attacks. This difficulty is hampered by the fact that about a third of the patients with NFLE have a personal history of parasomnias (Provini *et al.* 1999). It is difficult to distinguish seizures from parasomnias by clinical history alone. Seizures in NFLE may have a bizarre semiology, with vocalization, complex automatisms, and ambulation, whereas EEG and MRI investigations often show no abnormality. This results in frequent misdiagnosis, with the events being labeled pseudoseizures or parasomnias. Conversely, some parasomnias may be violent and can be confused with NFLE.

While typical parasomnias are often not a minor clinical problem, individuals with severe or frequent events often seek medical attention. A number of historical features have been described which may distinguish NFLE from parasomnias (Derry *et al.* 2006, Tinuper *et al.* 2007) but the value of these features has not been systematically assessed. As such, most authorities recommend video-EEG or video EEG-polysomnography for the diagnosis of paroxysmal nocturnal events. These investigations are the "gold standard" in this situation; they involve monitoring the patient in sleep through neurophysiological, cardiorespiratory, and video modalities, and recording their nocturnal events.

In particular, videorecording is probably sufficient for a reliable diagnosis of nocturnal seizures characterized by major motor activity (hypermotor or asymmetric dystonic seizures).

In those patients with infrequent episodes, due to the difficulty in capturing a paroxysmal event in the sleep laboratory, videorecording performed at home may represent a useful adjunct for diagnosis.

The diagnosis is more difficult in patients with minor events, such as PA. In these cases the diagnosis can be confirmed only if multiple stereotyped and "typical" (abrupt movements of trunk and upper limbs) episodes can be documented on video-polysomnography.

Probably NFLE is a complex disease caused by genetic and environmental factors (multifactorial polygenic model); indeed molecular genetic testing has revealed mutations in *CHRNA2, CHRNA4, CHRNB2* in about a third of NFLE patients with a positive family history and in fewer than 5% of sporadic cases.

Principles of management

Some patients refuse therapy because their seizures are not disturbing, or because they have had a spontaneous reduction in seizure frequency. Carbamazepine, sometimes at very low dosages given at bedtime, completely abolishes the seizures in ~20% of the cases and leads to at least 50% seizure reduction in another half of the patients (Provini *et al.* 1999). Topiramate has also proven effective. An effect of nicotine on the seizures was elegantly demonstrated in a controlled trial (Willoughby *et al.* 2003) and may be explained by considering that the mutant nAChRs are altered and nicotine acts as an acetylcholine receptor agonist. Other studies have confirmed that transdermal nicotine administration may be a suitable treatment option for ADNFLE patients with severe uncontrollable seizures (Brodtkorb and Picard 2006). However, as nicotine is highly addictive, even if the pure form produces fewer cardiovascular complications than cigarette smoking, the advantage of nicotine therapy must be carefully evaluated considering the possible risks and advantages for each individual patient.

A third of patients are drug resistant with frequent and disabling attacks. Surgery may abolish the seizures in some of these cases after appropriate presurgical investigation, usually requiring studies with depth electrodes (Nobili *et al.* 2007).

References

Aridon P, Marini C, Di Resta C, *et al.* (2006) Increased sensitivity of the neuronal nicotinic receptor alpha 2 subunit causes familial epilepsy with nocturnal wandering and ictal fear. *Am J Hum Genet* **79**:342–50.

Bertrand D, Elmslie F, Hughes E, *et al.* (2005) The *CHRNB2* mutation *I312M* is associated with epilepsy and distinct memory deficits. *Neurobiol Dis* **20**:799–804.

Bertrand D, Picard F, Le Hellard S, *et al.* (2002) How mutations in the nAChRs can cause ADNFLE epilepsy. *Epilepsia* **43**(Suppl 5):112–22.

Brodtkorb E, Picard F (2006) Tobacco habits modulate autosomal dominant nocturnal frontal lobe epilepsy. *Epilepsy Behav* **9**:515–20.

Cho YW, Motamedi GK, Laufenberg I, *et al.* (2003) A Korean kindred with autosomal dominant nocturnal frontal lobe epilepsy and mental retardation. *Arch Neurol* **60**:1625–32.

De Fusco M, Becchetti A, Patrignani A, *et al.* (2000) The nicotinic receptor beta2 subunit is mutant in nocturnal frontal lobe epilepsy. *Nat Genet* **26**:275–6.

De Marco EV, Gambardella A, Annesi F, *et al.* (2007) Further evidence of genetic heterogeneity in families with autosomal dominant nocturnal frontal lobe epilepsy. *Epilepsy Res* **74**:70–3.

Derry CP, Duncan JS, Berkovic SF (2006) Paroxysmal motor disorders of sleep: the clinical spectrum and differentiation from epilepsy. *Epilepsia* **47**:1775–91.

Derry CP, Heron SE, Phillips F, *et al.* (2008) Severe autosomal dominant nocturnal frontal lobe epilepsy associated with psychiatric disorders and intellectual disability. *Epilepsia* **49**:2125–9.

Khatami R, Neumann M, Schulz H, Kolmel HW (1998) A family with autosomal dominant nocturnal frontal lobe epilepsy and mental retardation. *J Neurol* **245**:809–10.

Lugaresi E, Cirignotta F, Montagna P (1986) Nocturnal paroxysmal dystonia. *J Neurol Neurosurg Psychiatry* **49**:375–80.

Montagna P, Sforza E, Tinuper P, Cirignotta F, Lugaresi E (1990) Paroxysmal arousals during sleep. *Neurology* **40**:1063–6.

Nobili L, Francione S, Mai R, *et al.* (2007) Surgical treatment of drug-resistant nocturnal frontal lobe epilepsy. *Brain* **130**:561–73.

Pedley TA, Guilleminault C (1977) Episodic nocturnal wandering responsive to anticonvulsant drug therapy. *Ann Neurol* **2**:30–5.

Phillips HA, Scheffer IE, Berkovic SF, *et al.* (1995) Localization of a gene for autosomal dominant nocturnal frontal lobe epilepsy to chromosome 20q13.2. *Nat Genet* **10**:117–18.

Phillips HA, Scheffer IE, Crossland KM, *et al.* (1998) Autosomal dominant nocturnal frontal-lobe epilepsy: genetic heterogeneity and evidence for a second locus at 15q24. *Am J Hum Genet* **63**:1108–16.

Phillips HA, Marini C, Scheffer IE, *et al.* (2000) A de novo mutation in sporadic nocturnal frontal lobe epilepsy. *Ann Neurol* **48**:264–7.

Phillips HA, Favre I, Kirkpatric M, *et al.* (2001) CHRNB2 is the second acetylcholine receptor subunit associated with autosomal dominant frontal lobe epilepsy. *Am J Hum Genet* **68**:225–31.

Picard F, Bruel D, Servent D, *et al.* (2006) Alteration of the in vivo nicotinic receptor density in ADNFLE patients: a PET study. *Brain* **129**:2047–60.

Picard F, Scheffer IE (2005). Recently defined genetic epilepsy syndromes. In: Roger JBM, Dravet C, Genton P, Tassinari CA, Wolf P (eds.) *Epileptic Syndromes in Infancy, Childhood and Adolescence*, Mountrouge, France: John Libbey Eurotext, pp. 519–35

Plazzi G, Tinuper P, Montagna P, Lugaresi E (1995) Epileptic nocturnal wanderings. *Sleep* **18**:749–56.

Provini F, Plazzi G, Tinuper P, *et al.* (1999) Nocturnal frontal lobe epilepsy: a clinical and polygraphic overview of 100 consecutive cases. *Brain* **122**:1017–31.

Scheffer IE, Bhatia KP, Lopes-Cendes I, *et al.* (1994) Autosomal dominant frontal epilepsy misdiagnosed as sleep disorder. *Lancet* **343**:515–17.

Sforza E, Montagna P, Rinaldi R, *et al.* (1993) Paroxysmal periodic motor attacks during sleep: clinical and polygraphic features. *Electroencephalogr Clin Neurophysiol* **3**:67–73.

Steinlein OK, Mulley JC, Propping P, *et al.* (1995) A missense mutation in the neuronal nicotinic acetylcholine receptor alpha 4 subunit is associated with autosomal dominant nocturnal frontal lobe epilepsy. *Nat Genet* **11**:201–3.

Tinuper P, Cerullo A, Cirignotta F, *et al.* (1990) Nocturnal paroxysmal dystonia with short-lasting attacks: three cases with evidence for an epileptic frontal lobe origin of seizures. *Epilepsia* **31**:549–56.

Tinuper P, Lugaresi E, Vigevano F, Berkovich SF (2002) Nocturnal frontal lobe epilepsy. In: Guerrini R, Aicardi J, Andermann F, Hallett M (eds.) *Epilepsy and Movement Disorders in Children*. Cambridge: Cambridge University Press, pp. 97–110.

Tinuper P, Provini F, Bisulli F, Lugaresi E (2005) Hyperkinetic manifestations in nocturnal frontal lobe epilepsy: semiological features and physiopathological hypothesis. *Neurol Sci* (Suppl)**3**:210–4.

Tinuper P, Provini F, Bisulli F, *et al.* (2007) Movement disorders in sleep: guidelines for differentiating epileptic from non-epileptic motor phenomena arising from sleep. *Sleep Med Rev* **11**:255–67.

Vignatelli L, Bisulli F, Provini F, *et al.* (2007) Interobserver reliability of video recording in the diagnosis of nocturnal frontal lobe seizures. *Epilepsia* **48**:1506–11.

Willoughby JO, Pope KJ, Eaton V (2003) Nicotine as an antiepileptic agent in ADNFLE: an N-of-one study. *Epilepsia* **44**:1238–40.

Chapter

9

Genetic epilepsy with febrile seizures plus

Ingrid E. Scheffer and Yue-Hua Zhang

The causal disease

Definition and epidemiology of genetic epilepsy with febrile seizures plus

Genetic epilepsy with febrile seizures plus (GEFS+) was originally called "generalized epilepsy with febrile seizures plus" when we first recognized this familial epilepsy syndrome through family studies. These studies involved careful phenotyping of large families in which multiple individuals had seizures (Scheffer and Berkovic 1997). The GEFS+ spectrum is characterized by a pattern of specific, yet heterogenous, epilepsy phenotypes in different family members. The pattern was initially observed to include febrile seizures and generalized epilepsies and thus GEFS+ was termed "generalized epilepsy with febrile seizures plus." Further research by many groups has widened the spectrum of GEFS+ phenotypes to include partial epilepsies and hence we have recently suggested changing the name from "generalized" to "genetic epilepsy with febrile seizures plus" (Scheffer *et al.* 2009). The pattern of phenotypes seen within the GEFS+ spectrum is quite distinctive and includes at its mildest end, benign seizure disorders such as classical febrile seizures and febrile seizures plus, and at its most severe end, a range of epileptic encephalopathies including Dravet syndrome and myoclonic–astatic epilepsy as described by Doose (Scheffer and Berkovic 1997; Singh *et al.* 1999a, 2001).

The GEFS+ spectrum is a complex concept to understand and derives from clinical genetic studies. The validity of the concept is underpinned by gene discovery. One issue is the heterogeneity of epilepsy phenotypes within a familial, rather than an individual's, epilepsy syndrome. Many previously described genetic epilepsies, such as autosomal dominant nocturnal frontal lobe epilepsy, have a homogeneous phenotype within families although variable severity is usual among family members. In GEFS+, the clinician needs to understand the presentations that form part of the phenotypic spectrum to consider a familial epilepsy syndrome diagnosis of GEFS+. A critical question is what is the minimal number of affected individuals required within a family to make a diagnosis of the familial epilepsy syndrome GEFS+? The minimum number is two individuals who have phenotypes that fall within the GEFS+ spectrum.

There have been no epidemiological studies to date of the frequency of GEFS+; however, many smaller families with GEFS+ would escape diagnosis as GEFS+ has usually been diagnosed in families with a large number of affected individuals. This has led to the assumption that GEFS+ is autosomal dominant, but it is more likely typically to follow complex inheritance where it is due to a number of genes interacting with or without an environmental component. The phenotypes within the GEFS+ spectrum are described below. It is likely that GEFS+ phenotypes are quite common; however, no formal epidemiological studies have been performed. Given the benign nature of many GEFS+ phenotypes, many cases could escape recognition, which would render epidemiological studies challenging.

Pathology, physiology, and clinical features of GEFS+

It is known that GEFS+ is a genetic disorder. To date, four genes have been confirmed as being of significance in GEFS+ and these genes all encode ion-channel subunits. The two sodium channel subunit genes, *SCN1A* and *SCN1B*, encoding the α1- and β1-subunits respectively, have been associated with mutations in GEFS+ families (Escayg *et al.* 2000; Wallace *et al.* 1998, 2001b). In addition, mutations in two γ-amino butyric acid$_A$ (GABA$_A$) receptor subunit genes, *GABRG2* and *GABRD*, encoding the γ2- and δ-subunits respectively, have also been described (Baulac *et al.* 2001; Wallace *et al.* 2001a; Dibbens *et al.* 2004). Mutations in *SCN1A* have been reported in a larger number of families and *SCN1B* mutations in seven families (Wallace *et al.* 1998; Audenaert *et al.* 2003; Scheffer *et al.* 2007). A handful of families have *GABRG2* mutations (Baulac *et al.* 2001; Wallace *et al.* 2001a; Harkin *et al.* 2002). We have reported *GABRD* mutations in two families; this association requires confirmation by another group (Dibbens *et al.* 2004).

The Causes of Epilepsy, eds. S. D. Shorvon, F. Andermann, and R. Guerrini. Published by Cambridge University Press. © Cambridge University Press 2011.

Overall these ion-channel subunits have only been found in a minority (less than 20%) of GEFS+ families studied. A key issue is what does a GEFS+ mutation mean in terms of understanding the genetic determinants of an individual's epilepsy? Given the phenotypic variability within GEFS+, there must be several factors contributing to the more severe phenotypes. They are likely to follow complex inheritance and be due to multiple genes interacting possibly with an environmental contribution. Furthermore, we know that penetrance in large GEFS+ families is in the order of 60% so there are unaffected carriers of genetic mutations. Thus the finding of a genetic mutation for a GEFS+ family is one piece of the genetic puzzle but we still require a lot more information to unravel the genetic architecture of GEFS+.

In general, physiological studies have shown a loss of function on in vitro studies with GEFS+ mutations for most genes (Wallace *et al.* 1998). Interestingly however, functional effects of mutations cannot be specifically predicted as some *SCN1A* mutations in GEFS+ show gain of function with a persistent inward sodium current, whilst others show complete loss of function (Lossin *et al.* 2002, 2003).

In GEFS+, most family members have a predilection to seizures with fever with onset within the typical age range of febrile seizures from 6 months to 6 years of age. A range of later seizure types may follow, producing the characteristic spectrum of GEFS+ phenotypes (see below). Seizures usually cease by adolescent or adult life, except in the more severe phenotypes. In general, the characteristic electroencephalograph (EEG) signature is of irregular generalized spike–wave activity; however, this is not present in all affected individuals. Particularly those patients at the milder end of the GEFS+ spectrum with febrile seizures or febrile seizures plus are likely to have a normal EEG. Imaging studies are usually normal.

Epilepsy in GEFS+

All individuals with GEFS+ have seizures, although some have simple febrile seizures whilst others have more severe phenotypes. The main risk factor is fever in infancy and early childhood, however, some family members also have afebrile seizures of various types. As with all forms of epilepsy, seizures are more likely if the patient is tired or stressed.

Types of epilepsy

Febrile seizures

Febrile seizures (FS) are classical febrile convulsions and comprise the mildest phenotype within the GEFS+ spectrum. Their onset is between 6 months and 6 years of age and they comprise convulsive seizures associated with a fever of greater than or equal to 38 °C.

Febrile seizures plus

Febrile seizures plus (FS+) is a mild form of generalized epilepsy that may have several different presentations of convulsive seizures. We coined the term FS+ to emphasize that the disorder is only marginally worse than typical FS and to recognize that seizures do not always remain within the defined age ranges of classical FS.

The most straightforward FS+ phenotype is where febrile seizures continue past the age of 6 years, which is the upper limit defined for FS. Seizures often peter out by the early teens, but a few later isolated seizures may occur into adult life.

A second type of presentation of FS+ is with febrile and afebrile convulsions limited to the typical age range of FS between 6 months and 6 years.

A third presentation of FS+ is where afebrile convulsive seizures continue after febrile seizures abate. A fourth presentation is where the febrile seizures settle by 6 years and afebrile seizures commence a few years later with a seizure-free period in between.

Febrile seizures or febrile seizures plus with other seizure types

Either FS or FS+ may be associated with one or more other types of seizures. These include absence, myoclonic, atonic, or partial seizures. These patients may not fall into a classically recognized syndrome but have features of febrile seizures with or without afebrile convulsions and other seizure types. Seizures usually resolve by adult life and are relatively easy to treat.

Myoclonic–astatic epilepsy

About one third of children with myoclonic–astatic epilepsy (MAE), described by Doose, have febrile seizures at the onset of their seizure disorder. MAE is characterized by drop attacks due to myoclonic–atonic seizures; children often experience both independent myoclonic seizures and atonic seizures (Oguni *et al.* 2005). They may also have afebrile convulsions. Their EEG is characterized by fast generalized spike–wave activity at a frequency of greater than 3 Hz (Guerrini *et al.* 2005).

Developmental outcome in this severe epileptic encephalopathy is highly variable with some children being of normal intellect whilst others have significant intellectual disability (Guerrini *et al.* 2005). Family studies show that the family history characteristically found in children with MAE is consistent with the GEFS+ spectrum with many family members having FS or FS+ (Singh *et al.* 1999b).

Dravet syndrome

Dravet syndrome, previously known as severe myoclonic epilepsy of infancy, has a very characteristic electroclinical pattern (see Chapter 10). Despite the important finding that >70% of patients with Dravet syndrome have mutations of *SCN1A*, approximately 50% of cases have a family history of epilepsy or febrile seizures (Dravet *et al.* 2005; Harkin *et al.* 2007). Family studies show that the family history found in children with Dravet syndrome is also consistent with the GEFS+ spectrum (Singh *et al.* 2001). It is hard to explain why there is such a significant family history of seizure disorders given that most of the *SCN1A* mutations arise de novo in the child with Dravet syndrome.

Partial epilepsies

Partial epilepsies, most commonly with preceding febrile seizures, are well recognized to be part of the GEFS+ spectrum (Abou-Khalil *et al.* 2001; Ito *et al.* 2002). Patients with partial epilepsies in the setting of GEFS+ family histories have been found with *SCN1A*, *SCN1B*, and *GABRG2* mutations (Abou-Khalil *et al.* 2001; Baulac *et al.* 2001; Ito *et al.* 2002; Scheffer *et al.* 2007). Temporal lobe epilepsy has been reported most frequently; however, frontal lobe epilepsy has also been described (Abou-Khalil *et al.* 2001; Baulac *et al.* 2001; Scheffer *et al.* 2007).

Interestingly, hippocampal sclerosis is seen with some individuals with preceding FS or FS+, but this is not universal in those with focal epilepsies. In many cases, imaging studies are normal. It is now apparent that partial seizures may exist without preceding febrile seizures but this is not a common finding in families with GEFS+ (Scheffer *et al.* 2007). One interesting observation was that we observed a successful surgical outcome following anterior temporal lobectomy in a man with a *SCN1B* mutation and refractory temporal lobe epilepsy and FS+ in the absence of hippocampal sclerosis (Scheffer *et al.* 2007). Thus it remains unclear whether epilepsy surgery is contraindicated in individuals with a genetic epilepsy syndrome and this should be considered on a case-by-case basis.

Diagnostic tests for GEFS+

The EEG in GEFS+ depends on the individual's epilepsy syndrome. The EEG is usually normal in FS. In FS+, the EEG may be normal or show irregular generalized spike–wave. In the moderate to severe phenotypes within the GEFS+ spectrum, there may be irregular generalized spike–wave activity or focal discharges depending on the seizure semiology and epilepsy syndrome. For example, children with Dravet syndrome have generalized and multifocal epileptiform discharges and may show photosensitivity. In MAE, focal discharges are not seen and the EEG shows fast generalized spike–wave activity.

Imaging is usually normal; however, in the partial epilepsies sometimes hippocampal sclerosis may be seen (Scheffer *et al.* 2007).

Intellect is normal for individuals in the mild end of the GEFS+ spectrum, but intellectual disability is usual in the epileptic encephalopathies at the severe end of the GEFS+ spectrum.

In terms of genetic testing, there are no specific gene tests recommended for GEFS+ at present. Research has revealed that a number of ion-channel genes have a role in GEFS+ as noted above; however, these currently remain useful only at a research level. These findings will be key in deciphering the genetic architecture of GEFS+ as more genetic variants or mutations are discovered.

The principal exception to this is Dravet syndrome (Chapter 10) where 70–80% of patients have mutations of the sodium channel α1-subunit gene, *SCN1A*. Around 70% of these mutations are conventional mutations found on sequencing. About 10% of those cases who are negative on conventional mutational analysis have copy-number variants with exonic deletion or duplication causing their Dravet syndrome (Mullen and Scheffer 2009).

Principles of management

Management of the epilepsy in GEFS+ depends upon the exact phenotype. If a patient has FS, reassurance is all that is required and education regarding seizure management.

If they have FS+ often observation and reassurance will be all that is required. Where frequent seizures occur, then the clinician may consider use of an antiepileptic agent such as valproate. The choice of antiepileptic medication in individuals with FS/FS+ and other seizure types will be determined by the specific seizure type. For example, if they have absence seizures, then valproate, ethosuximide, lamotrigine, or topiramate may be considered.

In the more severe phenotypes, multiple antiepileptic agents may be necessary. Often valproate and lamotrigine are useful for MAE. For Dravet syndrome, topiramate and stiripentol are particularly effective whereas lamotrigine may exacerbate seizures (Guerrini *et al.* 1998).

In the partial epilepsies, the usual management for partial epilepsy should be considered. As mentioned above, epilepsy surgery may still be considered (Scheffer *et al.* 2007).

In general, patients with GEFS+ do very well with excellent outcome. This is apart from the severe end of the GEFS+ spectrum where patients carry the poor outcome seen with each specific epileptic encephalopathy.

References

Abou-Khalil B, Ge Q, Desai R, *et al.* (2001) Partial and generalized epilepsy with febrile seizures plus and a novel SCN1A mutation. *Neurology* **57**:2265–72.

Audenaert D, Claes L, Ceulemans B, *et al.* (2003) A deletion in *SCN1B* is associated with febrile seizures and early-onset absence epilepsy. *Neurology* **61**:854–6.

Baulac S, Huberfeld G, Gourfinkel-An I, *et al.* (2001) First genetic evidence of GABA(A) receptor dysfunction in epilepsy: a mutation in the gamma2-subunit gene. *Nat Genet* **28**:46–8.

Dibbens LM, Feng HJ, Richards MC, *et al.* (2004) *GABRD* encoding a protein for extra- or peri-synaptic GABAA receptors is a susceptibility locus for generalized epilepsies. *Hum Mol Genet* **13**:1315–19.

Dravet C, Bureau M, Oguni H, Fukuyama Y, Cokar O (2005) Severe myoclonic epilepsy in infancy (Dravet syndrome). In: Roger J, Bureau M, Dravet C, Genton P, Tassinari CA, Wolf P (eds.) *Epileptic Syndromes in Infancy, Childhood and Adolescence*, 4th edn. Montrouge, France: John Libbey Eurotext, pp. 89–113.

Escayg A, MacDonald BT, Meisler MH, *et al.* (2000) Mutations of *SCN1A*, encoding a neuronal sodium channel, in two families with GEFS+2. *Nat Genet* **24**:343–5.

Guerrini R, Dravet C, Genton P, *et al.* (1998) Lamotrigine and seizure aggravation in severe myoclonic epilepsy. *Epilepsia* **39**(Suppl):508–12.

Guerrini R, Parmeggiani L, Bonanni P, Kaminska A, Dulac O (2005) Myoclonic astatic epilepsy. In: Roger J, Bureau M, Dravet C, Genton P, Tassinari CA, Wolf P (eds.) *Epileptic Syndromes in Infancy, Childhood and Adolescence*, 4th edn. Montrouge, France: John Libbey Eurotext, pp. 115–24.

Harkin LA, Bowser DN, Dibbens LM, *et al.* (2002) Truncation of the GABA(A)-receptor gamma2 subunit in a family with generalized epilepsy with febrile seizures plus. *Am J Hum Genet* **70**:530–6.

Harkin LA, McMahon JM, Iona X, *et al.* (2007) The spectrum of *SCN1A*-related infantile epileptic encephalopathies. *Brain* **130**:843–52.

Ito M, Nagafuji H, Okazawa H, *et al.* (2002) Autosomal dominant epilepsy with febrile seizures plus with missense mutations of the (Na$^+$)-channel alpha 1 subunit gene, *SCN1A*. *Epilepsy Res* **48**:15–23.

Lossin C, Wang DW, Rhodes TH, Vanoye CG, George AL Jr. (2002) Molecular basis of an inherited epilepsy. *Neuron* **34**:877–84.

Lossin C, Rhodes TH, Desai RR, *et al.* (2003) Epilepsy-associated dysfunction in the voltage-gated neuronal sodium channel *SCN1A*. *J Neurosci* **23**:11 289–95.

Mullen SA, Scheffer IE (2009) Translational research in epilepsy genetics: sodium channels in man to interneuronopathy in mouse. *Arch Neurol* **66**:21–6.

Oguni H, Hayashi K, Imai K, *et al.* (2005) Idiopathic myoclonic–astatic epilepsy of early childhood: nosology based on electrophysiologic and long-term follow-up study of patients. *Adv Neurol* **95**:157–74.

Scheffer IE, Berkovic SF (1997) Generalized epilepsy with febrile seizures plus: a genetic disorder with heterogeneous clinical phenotypes. *Brain* **120**:479–90.

Scheffer IE, Harkin LA, Grinton BE, *et al.* (2007) Temporal lobe epilepsy and GEFS+ phenotypes associated with *SCN1B* mutations. *Brain* **130**:100–9.

Scheffer IE, Zhang YH, Jansen FE, Dibbens L (2009) Dravet syndrome or genetic (generalized) epilepsy with febrile seizures plus? *Brain Dev* **31**:394–400.

Singh R, Scheffer IE, Crossland K, Berkovic SF (1999a) Generalized epilepsy with febrile seizures plus: a common, childhood onset, genetic epilepsy syndrome. *Ann Neurol* **45**:75–81.

Singh R, Scheffer IE, Whitehouse W, *et al.* (1999b) Severe myoclonic epilepsy of infancy is part of the spectrum of generalized epilepsy with febrile seizures plus (GEFS+). *Epilepsia* **40**:175.

Singh R, Andermann E, Whitehouse WPA, *et al.* (2001) Severe myoclonic epilepsy of infancy: extended spectrum of GEFS+? *Epilepsia* **42**:837–44.

Wallace RH, Wang DW, Singh R, *et al.* (1998) Febrile seizures and generalized epilepsy associated with a mutation in the Na$^+$ channel beta1 subunit gene *SCN1B*. *Nat Genet* **19**:366–70.

Wallace RH, Marini C, Petrou S, *et al.* (2001a) Mutant GABA(A) receptor gamma2-subunit in childhood absence epilepsy and febrile seizures. *Nat Genet* **28**:49–52.

Wallace RH, Scheffer IE, Barnett S, *et al.* (2001b) Neuronal sodium-channel alpha1-subunit mutations in generalized epilepsy with febrile seizures plus. *Am J Hum Genet* **68**:859–65.

Chapter 10

Severe myoclonic epilepsy of infancy or Dravet syndrome

Carla Marini and Renzo Guerrini

Definition

Dravet syndrome (DS), otherwise known as severe myoclonic epilepsy of infancy (SMEI) (MIM 607208), is an intractable form of epilepsy presenting in the first year of life in an otherwise normal infant (Dravet *et al.* 2005). In the newly proposed diagnostic scheme (Engel 2001), DS is classified among the epileptic encephalopathies, i.e., "the conditions in which the epileptiform abnormalities themselves are believed to contribute to the progressive disturbance in cerebral function." However, SMEI includes a spectrum of conditions with variable severity, from the classical phenotype to "borderline SMEI (SMEB)" in which patients share most but not all the characteristic clinical features (Oguni *et al.* 2001).

Epidemiology

Since its first description in 1978 by Dravet, DS has been increasingly recognized worldwide; yet it remains a rare disorder with an incidence probably less than 1 per 40 000 (Hurst 1990). The prevalence of DS in children with seizure onset in the first year of life varies between 3% to 8% (Yakoub *et al.* 1992; Caraballo *et al.* 1998; Dravet *et al.* 2005).

Seizure types and EEG features

Dravet syndrome presents in all cases before 12 months of age, with repeated *generalized or unilateral clonic* (hemiclonic with alternating sides) seizures, typically triggered by fever. Seizures are often prolonged, up to 20–30 min, tend to recur in clusters in the same day, and may evolve into status epilepticus. Factors that increase body temperature elevation, such as hot-water immersion, can precipitate seizures (Fujiwara *et al.* 1990). Afebrile seizures can also occur, usually in the context of a vaccination.

Between 1 and 4 years other seizure types appear, including myoclonic, absences, focal and exceptionally tonic seizures.

- Most, but not all patients, also exhibit *myoclonic seizures* between the ages of 1 and 5 years; jerks can be massive and

involve the whole body leading to falling or be mild and barely visible. Jerks sometimes only involve a few body segments; they can be single or repetitive, spontaneous or evoked by photic stimulation. In some children myoclonic jerks are often observed in the morning or just preceding a seizure. Polygraphic EEG recordings show that generalized jerks are accompanied by high voltage discharges of generalized spike and wave (GSW,) or polyspike and wave (GPSW) discharges (Fig. 10.1). However, not all myoclonic jerks are accompanied by concomitant paroxysmal EEG activity (Fig. 10.2).

- *Absence seizures* are present in 40–90% of patients (Dravet *et al.* 2005) and appear between ages 1 and 3 years. Absences, lasting several seconds, are classified as atypical and can be associated with a prominent myoclonic component. Ictal EEG shows 2.5–3 Hz GSW discharges.

- About 40% of patients experience *non-convulsive status epilepticus or obtundation status* characterized by impairment of consciousness of variable intensity, with erratic, myoclonic jerks, involving the limbs or the face. Ictal EEG shows diffuse slow waves intermingled with focal or diffuse spikes, sharp-waves or SW.

- More than 50% of patients have *focal seizures*, occurring from 4 months to 4 years of age. Focal seizures can have a main motor component – versive or clonic jerking limited to one limb or one hemiface – or be complex partial with prominent autonomic symptoms.

- *Tonic seizures* have been reported in a limited number of patients and are exceptional in this syndrome.

- *Convulsive seizures* tend to be present along the evolution. The Marseille group, through video-polygraphic recordings, has divided them into several forms: generalized clonic or tonic clonic seizures, unilateral seizures, falsely generalized seizures, and unstable seizures (Dravet *et al.* 2005).

Interictal EEG, normal at onset, during the course of the disorder shows generalized or multifocal paroxysmal activity (Fig. 10.3). About 25% of children are photosensitive and may indulge in self-stimulation.

The Causes of Epilepsy, eds. S. D. Shorvon, F. Andermann, and R. Guerrini. Published by Cambridge University Press. © Cambridge University Press 2011.

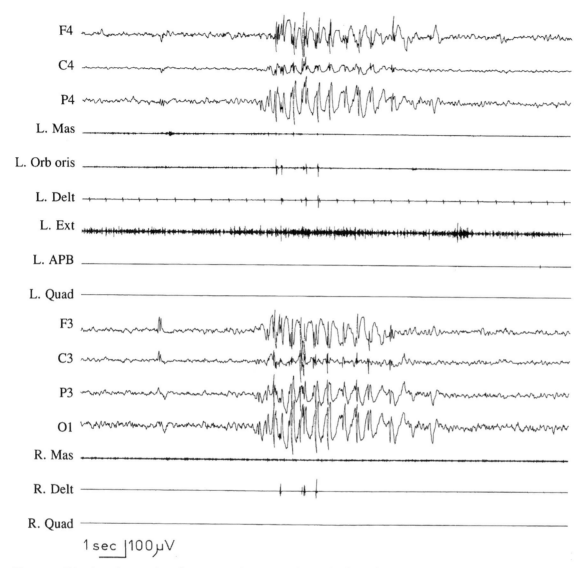

Fig. 10.1. EEG polygraphic recording of a DS patient showing myoclonic jerks of the left orbicular oris and deltoid muscles associated with a bilateral fast spike and polyspike wave discharge.

Cognitive development

Before the onset of the epilepsy, developmental skills and behavior are reported as normal. However, following seizure onset, at around the second year of life, developmental slowing or stagnation becomes evident and moderate to severe mental retardation becomes obvious in most patients before age 6 years (Wolff et al. 2006). Behavioral disturbances with hyperactivity and autistic traits are also frequent. In children with favorable outcome, language skills tend to be better preserved than visuomotor functions. The frequency of convulsive seizures seems to correlate with the severity of developmental delay, suggesting that DS might be considered as a "true" epileptic encephalopathy (Wolff et al. 2006).

Etiology/genetics

A family history of epilepsy is often found in DS patients. Affected relatives have epilepsy phenotypes consistent with the generalized epilepsy with febrile seizure plus (GEFS+) spectrum (Scheffer and Berkovic 1997; Singh et al. 2001) (see Chapter 9). Mutations of the gene coding for the α1-subunit of the sodium channel (SCN1A) were first discovered in GEFS+ (Escayg et al. 2000). This finding prompted the examination of DS patients for SCN1A nucleotide changes, which led to the discovery that an overwhelmingly high number of SCN1A mutations are associated with the DS phenotype (Claes et al. 2001; Mulley et al. 2005).

At present, more than 500 mutations have been associated with DS, including borderline forms. The frequency of

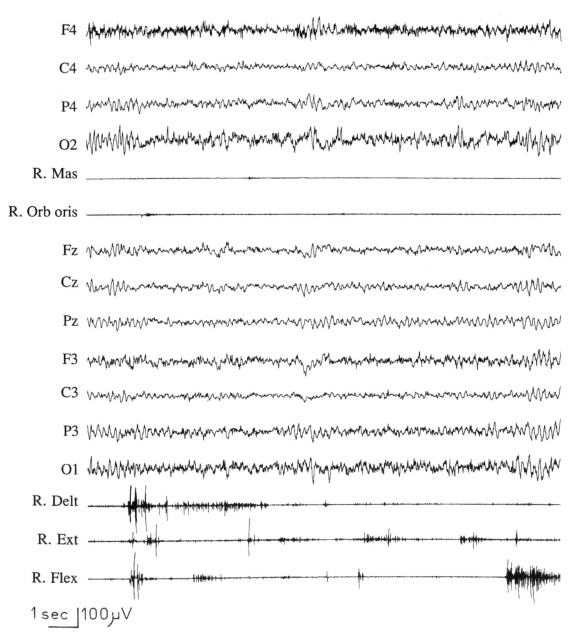

Fig. 10.2. EEG polygraphic recording of a DS patient showing myoclonic jerks of the right deltoid, and wrist flexor and extensor muscles without concomitant, time-locked, paroxysmal EEG activity.

detectable mutations in DS is around 70–80%; truncating mutations account for nearly 50% of the abnormalities with the remaining comprising splice-site and missense mutations. Intragenic deletions and whole gene deletions including only *SCN1A* and/or contiguous genes account for 2–3% of all DS cases and for about 12.5% of DS negative to point mutations (Marini *et al.* 2009). Duplications and amplifications involving *SCN1A* are additional, rare, molecular mechanisms (Marini *et al.* 2009). Most mutations are de novo, but familial *SCN1A* mutations also occur (Claes *et al.* 2001; Sugawara *et al.* 2002; Nabbout *et al.* 2003; Wallace *et al.* 2003). Somatic mosaic mutations have been reported in

some patients, and although rare, demonstration of their existence means they need to be incorporated into recurrence risks in the context of genetic counseling (Depienne *et al.* 2006, 2010; Gennaro *et al.* 2006; Marini *et al.* 2006; Morimoto *et al.* 2006). Mosaic *SCN1A* mutations might explain the phenotypical variability seen in some familial cases.

The clinical data of a significantly higher family history and familial cases of DS are hard to reconcile with the finding that most *SCN1A* mutations in DS are de novo. In such families the model of inheritance is likely to be polygenic and *SCN1A* might be one of the genetic determinants specifically associated with DS but not with the other phenotypes.

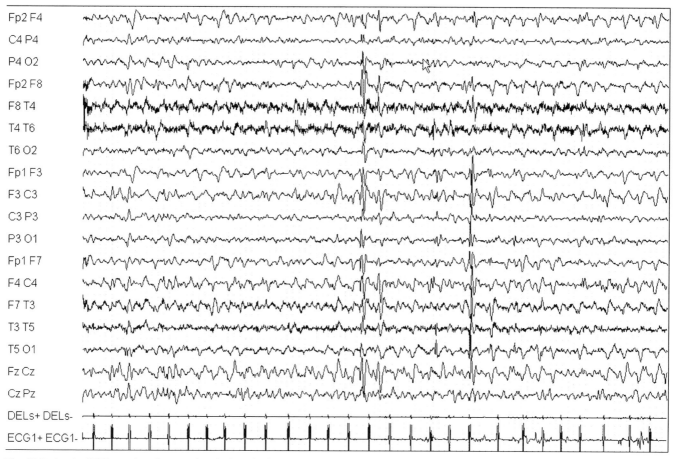

Fig. 10.3. Interictal EEG recording showing: slow rhythmic background activity consisting of predominant theta activity with intermingled spikes over anterior and central regions, and diffuse or left predominant spike–polyspike–wave complexes.

Genotype–phenotype correlations

Mutations in *SCN1A* have been predominantly associated with DS and GEFS+ spectrums but with a phenotypic variability including age of seizure onset, seizure types, and severity. This raises the question: why do mutations in the same gene result in different phenotypes? Some general genotype–phenotype correlations have been suggested: truncating, nonsense, frameshift mutations and partial or whole gene deletions are correlated with a classical DS phenotype and appear to have a significant correlation with an earlier age of seizures onset (Marini *et al.* 2007). The severity of the phenotypes is also correlated with *SCN1A* missense mutations falling into the pore-forming region of the sodium channel while missense changes associated with the GEFS+ spectrum are nearly always localized outside the pore-forming region (Meisler and Kearney 2005). Mutations are randomly distributed across the SCN1A protein both in DS and GEFS+ epilepsies. Mutations in *SCN1A* causing DS in some patients and GEFS+ in others (Escayg *et al.* 2000; Ohmori *et al.* 2002) have been reported suggesting that modifier genes, the genetic background, or environmental factors, within a complex model of inheritance, can also play a role in some patients. The genetic data are summarized in Table 10.1.

Table 10.1 Summary of the genetic findings

Phenotype	Genotype	Gene anomalies/inheritance
Classical DS	*SCN1A*	70–80% pos; point mut, del, dup, amp >90% de novo
Spectrum of phenotypes	*SCN1A*	
SMEB		70% pos; point mut; >90% de novo
ICEGTC		≈30% pos; missense and 1 frameshift mut; > de novo
SIMFE		3/5 patients; 1 truncating + 2 missense mut
Classical DS	*GABRG2*	single case within GEFS+ family
DS-like	*PCDH19*	12/74 (16%) patients (11F); frameshift and missense mut; 1 M with mosaic Del; 4 mut de novo; 5 inherited from asymptomatic fathers

Notes:
amp, amplification; del, deletion; DS, Dravet syndrome; dup, duplication; F, females; GEFS+, generalized epilepsy with febrile seizures plus; IGEGTC, intractable childhood epilepsy with generalized tonic–clonic seizures; M, male; mut, mutations; pos, positive; SMEB, borderline severe myoclonic epilepsy; SIMFE, severe infantile multifocal epilepsy; >, majority.

What causes DS when there is no detectable SCN1A involvement?

A single case with a mutation in the γ2-subunit gene of the γ-amino butyric acid$_A$ (GABA$_A$) receptor, *GABRG2*, has been reported (Harkin *et al.* 2002). Mutations of *PCDH19* have been identified in patients with epilepsy and mental retardation limited to females (EFMR), a disorder with an unusual X-linked inheritance, which is expressed in heterozygous females but not in hemizygous males (Dibbens *et al.* 2008). The *PCDH19* gene encodes a protocadherin 19, a transmembrane protein of the cadherin family of calcium-dependent cell–cell adhesion molecules, which is strongly expressed in the central nervous system. Depienne *et al.* (2009) reported *PCDH19* mutations and one deletion in 12/74 patients (16%) with early-onset epileptic encephalopathy mimicking DS. Patients with *PCDH19* mutations, compared to *SCN1A* mutation positive DS, had a slightly older age of onset, less frequent status epilepticus, rare photosensitivity, seizures were less intractable, mental retardation was less severe, atypical absences and myoclonic jerks were only seen in a few patients. However, clinical similarities between *PCDH19* mutation positive patients and DS, including febrile and afebrile seizures, occurrence of hemiclonic seizures, regression following seizure onset, suggest that *PCDH19* should be tested in those DS patients in whom no *SCN1A* abnormalities can be found; *PCDH19* is a candidate gene for early-onset epileptic encephalopathies within the DS spectrum, at least in females, and accounts for 5% of such patients (Depienne *et al.* 2009). Despite intensive investigation, the etiology of about 20% of patients sharing features with DS remains unknown and more gene mutations are yet to be identified.

Mutations in SCN1A associated with other early onset epileptic encephalopathies: distinct syndromes or DS extended spectrum of phenotypes?

- The term "Borderline severe myoclonic epilepsy of infancy" (SMEB), strictly related to DS, has been coined to describe patients who lack several of the key features of DS such as myoclonic seizures or GSW activity. More than 70% of SMEB patients carry *SCN1A* mutations that are spread throughout the gene with a mixture of mutations including truncating, missense, and splice-site changes (Harkin *et al.* 2007).
- Infants with frequent and intractable generalized tonic–clonic seizures often induced by fever and beginning before 1 year of age have been designated to have "intractable childhood epilepsy with generalized tonic–clonic seizures" (ICEGTC) (Fujiwara *et al.* 2003). The major feature that differentiates DS and ICEGTC is the presence or absence of myoclonic seizures.
- Five patients with early-onset multiple seizure types with the most prominent being focal, developmental delay and abundant multifocal epileptiform activity have been designated as "severe infantile multifocal epilepsy" (SIMFE); three of the five patients carry *SCN1A* mutations (Harkin *et al.* 2007). The clinical keys that distinguish these patients from DS spectrum are the absence or rarity of myoclonic and absence seizures and the lack of GSW on EEG.

Myoclonic seizures, however, are not always present in classical DS. For this reason the term "severe myoclonic epilepsy of infancy" has been considered as misleading and the designation of "severe polymorphic epilepsy of infants" has been proposed (Aicardi 1994). Yet, the question whether myoclonic seizures are an essential component of DS remains controversial. The identification of *SCN1A* mutations in SMEB, ICEGTC, and SIMFE patients (Fujiwara *et al.* 2003; Harkin *et al.* 2007) confirms that these phenotypes share the same genetic determinant in most patients and might be considered as a continuum of the same process, i.e., sodium channel disorder.

Brain imaging

Neuroradiological studies are normal in most patients but structural abnormalities such as cerebral or cerebellar atrophy of various degree and focal arachnoid cysts have been anecdotally reported (Fujiwara *et al.* 2003; Dravet *et al.* 2005). Hippocampal sclerosis (HS) was reported in 10 out of 14 children with clinical diagnosis of DS (Siegler *et al.* 2005). A second study did not support the association between prolonged febrile seizures and HS in DS (Striano *et al.* 2007).

Differential diagnosis

At onset children are often regarded as having febrile convulsions. The repetition of febrile seizures and/or the prolonged convulsions with unilateral clinical features are clues orienting towards a diagnosis of DS. Children may manifest myoclonic seizures at onset and be misdiagnosed as having benign myoclonic epilepsy of infancy. Myoclonic–astatic epilepsy should also be considered in the differential diagnosis because a minority of patients might manifest febrile seizures before the second year of life while the classical myoclonic astatic seizures occur only later on. Exceptionally, patients with DS can be misdiagnosed as having Lennox–Gastaut syndrome in which age at seizure onset – after the second year of life – and the predominant seizure types – tonic, generalized tonic–clonic, and absences – are quite different from DS.

Treatment and outcome

Valproic acid, benzodiazepines, and topiramate have been proven to have some efficacy (Dravet *et al.* 2005). Stiripentol, an inhibitor of the P450 cytochrome, has been demonstrated to be effective in combination with clobazam in a class I trial (Chiron *et al.* (2000). Stiripentol acts by increasing the concentration of norclobazam, an active metabolite of clobazam. Phenytoin, carbamazepine, and lamotrigine can worsen seizures and must be avoided (Guerrini *et al.* 1998; Dravet *et al.* 2005).

Data on long-term evolution are scanty. Seizures persist into adulthood but are less frequent, rarely prolonged, and are usually confined to sleep (Jansen *et al.* 2006). In the course of the disease, cognitive and motor functions might slightly improve but remain at low level. Mortality rates are at around 16% (Dravet *et al.* 2005), mainly as a result of sudden death or seizure-related accidents.

References

Aicardi J (1994) *Epilepsy in Children*. New York: Raven Press.

Caraballo R, Tripoli J, Escobal L, *et al.* (1998) Ketogenic diet: efficacy and tolerability in childhood intractable epilepsy. *Rev Neurol* **26**:61–4.

Chiron C, Marchand MC, Tran A, *et al.* (2000) Stiripentol in severe myoclonic epilepsy in infancy: a randomised placebo-controlled syndrome-dedicated trial. STICLO study group. *Lancet* **356**:1638–42.

Claes L, Del-Favero J, Ceulemans B, *et al.* (2001) De novo mutations in the sodium-channel gene *SCN1A* cause severe myoclonic epilepsy of infancy. *Am J Hum Genet* **68**:1327–32.

Depienne C, Arzimanoglou A, Trouillard O, *et al.* (2006) Parental mosaicism can cause recurrent transmission of *SCN1A* mutations associated with severe myoclonic epilepsy of infancy. *Hum Mutat* **27**:389.

Depienne C, Bouteiller D, Keren B, *et al.* (2009) Sporadic infantile epileptic encephalopathy caused by mutations in *PCDH19* resembles Dravet syndrome but mainly affects females. *PLoS Genet* **5**(2):e1000381.

Depienne C, Trouillard O, Gourfinkel-An I *et al.* (2010) Mechanisms for variable expressivity of inherited *SCNIA* mutations causing Dravet Syndrome. *J Med Genet* **47**:404–10.

Dibbens LM, Tarpey PS, Hynes K, *et al.* (2008) X-linked protocadherin 19 mutations cause female-limited epilepsy and cognitive impairment. *Nat Genet* **40**:776–81.

Dravet C, Bureau M, Oguni H, Fukuyama Y, Cokar O (2005) Severe myoclonic epilepsy in infancy (Dravet syndrome). In: Roger J, Bureau M, Dravet C, Genton P, Tassinari CA, Wolf P (eds.) *Epileptic Syndromes in Infancy, Childhood and Adolescence*, 4th edn. Montronge, France: John Libbey Eurotext, pp. 89–113.

Engel J Jr. (2001) A proposed diagnostic scheme for people with epileptic seizures and with epilepsy: Report of the ILAE Task Force on Classification and Terminology. *Epilepsia* **42**:796–803.

Escayg A, MacDonald BT, Meisler MH, *et al.* (2000) Mutations of *SCN1A*, encoding a neuronal sodium channel, in two families with GEFS+2. *Nat Genet* **24**:343–5.

Fujiwara T, Nakamura H, Watanabe M, *et al.* (1990) Clinicoelectrographic concordance between monozygotic twins with severe myoclonic epilepsy in infancy. *Epilepsia* **31**:281–6.

Fujiwara T, Sugawara T, Mazaki-Miyazaki E, *et al.* (2003) Mutations of sodium channel alpha subunit type 1 (*SCN1A*) in intractable childhood epilepsies with frequent generalized tonic–clonic seizures. *Brain* **126**:531–46.

Gennaro E, Santovelli FM, Bertini E, *et al.* (2006) Somatic and germline mosaicisms in severe myoclonic epilepsy of infancy. *Biochem Biophys Res Commun* **341**: 489–93.

Guerrini R, Dravet C, Genton P, *et al.* (1998) Lamotrigine and seizure aggravation in severe myoclonic epilepsy. *Epilepsia* **39**(Suppl):508–12.

Harkin LA, Bowser DN, Dibbens LM, *et al.* (2002) Truncation of the GABA(A)-receptor gamma2 subunit in a family with generalized epilepsy with febrile seizures plus. *Am J Hum Genet* **70**:530–6.

Harkin L, McMahon JM, Iona X, *et al.* (2007) The spectrum of *SCN1A*-related infantile epileptic encephalopathies. *Brain* **130**:843–52.

Hurst DL (1990) Epidemiology of severe myoclonic epilepsy of infancy. *Epilepsia* **31**:397–400.

Jansen FE, Sadleir LG, Harkin LA, *et al.* (2006) Severe myoclonic epilepsy of infancy (Dravet syndrome): recognition and diagnosis in adults. *Neurology* **67**:2224–6.

Marini C, Mei D, Cross HJ, Guerrini R (2006) Mosaic *SCN1A* mutation in familial severe myoclonic epilepsy of infancy. *Epilepsia* **47**:1737–40.

Marini C, Mei D, Temudo T, *et al.* (2007) Idiopathic epilepsies with seizures precipitated by fever and *SCN1A* abnormalities. *Epilepsia* **48**:1678–85.

Marini C, Scheffer IE, Nabbout R, *et al.* (2009) *SCN1A* duplications and deletions detected in Dravet syndrome: implications for molecular diagnosis. *Epilepsia* [Epub ahead of print].

Meisler MH, Kearney JA (2005) Sodium channel mutations in epilepsy and other neurological disorders. *J Clin Invest* **115**:2010–17.

Morimoto M, Mazaki E, Nishimura A, *et al.* (2006) *SCN1A* mutation mosaicism in a family with severe myoclonic epilepsy in infancy. *Epilepsia* **47**:1732–36.

Mulley JC, Scheffer IE, Petrou S, *et al.* (2005) *SCN1A* mutations and epilepsy. *Hum Mutat* **25**:535–42.

Nabbout R, Gennaro E, Dalla Bernardina B, *et al.* (2003) Spectrum of *SCN1A* mutations in severe myoclonic epilepsy of infancy. *Neurology* **60**:1961–7.

Oguni H, Hayashi K, Awaya Y, Fukuyama Y, Osawa M (2001) Severe myoclonic epilepsy in infants: a review based on the Tokyo Women's Medical University series of 84 cases. *Brain Dev* **23**:736–48.

Ohmori I, Ouchida M, Ohtsuka Y, Oka E, Shimizu K (2002) Significant correlation of the *SCN1A* mutations and severe myoclonic epilepsy in infancy. *Biochem Biophys Res Commun* **295**: 17–23.

Scheffer IE, Berkovic SF (1997) Generalized epilepsy with febrile seizures plus: a genetic disorder with heterogeneous clinical phenotypes. *Brain* **120**: 479–90.

Siegler Z, Barsi P, Neuwirth M, *et al.* (2005) Hippocampal sclerosis in severe myoclonic epilepsy in infancy: a retrospective MRI study. *Epilepsia* **46**:704–8.

Singh R, Andermann F, Whitehouse WP, *et al.* (2001) Severe myoclonic epilepsy of infancy: extended spectrum of (GEFS+). *Epilepsia* **42**:837–44.

Striano P, Mancardi MM, Biancheri R, *et al.* (2007) Brain MRI findings in severe myoclonic epilepsy in infancy and genotype–phenotype correlations. *Epilepsia* **48**:1092–6.

Sugawara T, Mazaki-Miyazaki E, Fukushima K, *et al.* (2002) Frequent mutations of SCN1A in severe myoclonic epilepsy in infancy. *Neurology* **58**:1122–4.

Wallace RH, Hodgson BL, Grinton BE, *et al.* (2003) Sodium channel alpha1-subunit mutations in severe myoclonic epilepsy of infancy and infantile spasms. *Neurology* **61**:765–9.

Wolff M, Cassé-Perrot C, Dravet C (2006) Severe myoclonic epilepsy of infants (Dravet syndrome): natural history and neuropsychological findings. *Epilepsia* **47**(Suppl 2):45–8.

Yakoub M, Dulac O, Jambaqué I, Chiron C, Plouin P (1992) Early diagnosis of severe myoclonic epilepsy in infancy. *Brain Dev* **14**:299–303.

Benign adult familial myoclonic epilepsy

Teiichi Onuma

There were several reports in Japan on cases that had characteristic features of what is now called benign adult familial myoclonic epilepsy (BAFME). They were eight cases of hereditary tremor with epileptic seizure in a family over four generations (Inoue 1975), three families who had grand mal seizures and hereditary tremor (Takahashi *et al.* 1969), 101 cases in a single family over five generations (Wakeno 1975), and 40 cases out of 103 affected members of 12 families giving the term "familial essential myoclonus and epilepsy" (FEME) (Inazuki *et al.* 1990).

Electrophysiological studies on these patients revealed giant somatosensory evoked potential with enhanced long-loop C-reflexes via cortex, and premovement cortical spikes by the jerk-locked averaging method suggesting that involuntary tremor or movements were a form of cortical reflex myoclonus (Ikeda *et al.* 1990; Okino 1997). The term benign adult familial myoclonic epilepsy came from the study on 26 members of two families (Yasuda 1991). Genetic analysis of his patients later gave rise to the discovery of the BAFME gene.

A report of a European family revealed similar symptoms such as cortical tremor, epilepsy, and mental retardation inherited in an autosomal dominant pattern (Elia *et al.* 1998). All four living patients examined were non-progressive. All patients showed diffuse spike–wave complexes on electroencephalogram (EEG), a photoparoxysmal response, giant somatosensory evoked potential, enhanced C-reflex, and premyoclonic spike on jerk-locked averaging methods. However, the two youngest patients had a more severe phenotype, with earlier onset of symptoms (age 5 years) and moderate mental retardation, which were quite unusual as compared with the originally described Japanese cases of BAFME.

Genetic study

Linkage analysis of BAFME on a large Japanese family with 17 affected patients among 27 members over three generations previously reported by Yasuda (1991) revealed that the responsible gene locus was assigned to the distal long arm of chromosome 8q23.3–q24.11 (Mikami *et al.* 1999). Linkage analysis of familial essential myoclonus and epilepsy (FEME) (Araki

2002) also disclosed the responsible gene in the same areas in a 3.37-cM region between D8S1122 and D8S1694 and found that FEME and BAFME were genetically identical disorders.

A genome-wide screen with genetic linkage analysis on what he called familial adult myoclonic epilepsy (FAME) of four previously reported Japanese kindred disclosed the responsible gene on a 4.6-cM region on chromosome 8q24 (Plaster *et al.* 1999). However, Araki stated that the BAFME region had territory widely overlapped on that of FEME, but not of FAME.

European kindred of autosomal dominant cortical myoclonus and epilepsy (ADCME) were reported to have a linkage to chromosome 2p11–q12.2. (Guerrini *et al.* 2001). They described a similar disorder with BAFME in a pedigree in which eight individuals presented a non-progressive disorder with onset between the ages of 12 and 50 years. Most individuals had a normal cognitive level, but three individuals with intractable seizures had mild mental retardation, which was somewhat different from Japanese BAFME. Genome-wide linkage analysis identified new localization of the responsible gene to chromosome 2p11.1–q12.2, with the critical region spanning 12.4 cM between markers D2S2161 and D2S1897 and excluded the locus for BAFME on chromosome 8q23.3–q24.

Linkage analysis of five families with similar disease from southern Italy disclosed significant linkage to chromosome 2p11.1–q12.2. A common 15-Mb haplotype segregated with the disorder was identified in all the families, indicating a founder effect (De Falco *et al.* 2003; Madia *et al.* 2008).

There were two different types of BAFME and the disorder in the Japanese family with chromosome 8q23.3–q24.11 was registered as BAFME1 and those of the European family with chromosome 2p11.1–q12.2 was registered as BAFME2 on OMIM #601068 (Online Mendelian Inheritance in Man, Johns Hopkins University).

Case study

Sixteen members were affected in three generations of this family (Fig. 11.1). There was no sex difference. An autosomal dominant inheritance pattern was clearly seen. Age of onset of

The Causes of Epilepsy, eds. S. D. Shorvon, F. Andermann, and R. Guerrini. Published by Cambridge University Press. © Cambridge University Press 2011.

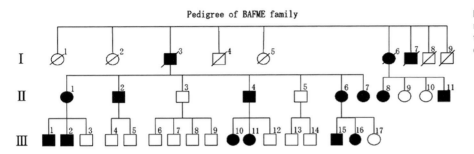

Pedigree of BAFME family

Fig. 11.1. Pedigree of BAFME family. Sixteen members were affected in 37 members over the three generations. Circle, female; square, male; diagonal line, deceased.

Table 11.1 Clinical characteristics of BAFME family

Individual	Age	Sex	Initial symptom	Age of onset	Age of first GTC	Onset of tremor	Slow EEG	Photosensitivity	G-SEP
I–1	73	F	tremor	44	51	44	–	+	+
II–2	71	M	tremor	40	41	40	+	+	+
II–4	65	M	GTC	30	30	40	+	+	+
II–6	62	F	tremor	41	54	41	–	+	+
II–7	55	F	tremor	38	43	38	–	+	+
III–15	34	M	tremor	18	29	18	–	–	+
III–16	31	F	tremor	25	–	25	–	–	–

Notes:
GTC, generalized tonic–clonic seizures; G-SEP, giant somatosensory evoked potential.

tremor, seizure, EEG findings, and somatosensory evoked potential data are shown in Table 11.1.

The initial symptoms in most cases of this family were irregular tremor often accompanied by myoclonic jerks, which started at around the age of 38 to 44 years. Seizures (GTC) were eventually developed in all cases except for the youngest one (III–16) who was too young to have full clinical symptomatology. Seizures were usually infrequent and appeared once in several years. There was slowing in the background EEG in two cases. Excellent driving response to photic stimulation and giant somatosensory evoked potential (G-SEP) were seen in almost all cases except for the youngest ones. The third generation had only partial signs of BAFME; III–15 had tremor, GTC, and G-SEP but not photosensitivity, and III–16 had tremor only. The third generation had slight earlier onset than the second one.

The tremogram (Fig. 11.2) demonstrated the involuntary movements of outstretched arm on all examined affected members of this family. Tremor became larger in amplitude with advancing age, suggesting the possibility of very slow deterioration. However, there was no definite deterioration in the patients' mental and physical condition over a decade of follow-up.

Figure 11.3 shows EEG findings of the second generation of family 1 (II–1, II–2, II–4, II–6, II–7). All showed similar pattern of spikes, and spike–wave complex in occipital areas, particularly on photic stimulation, which often spread to

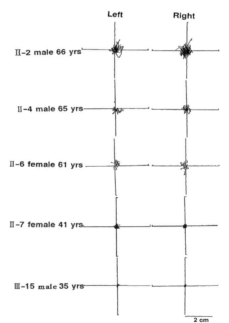

Fig. 11.2. Tremogram. The author's original design showing involuntary tremor and myoclonic jerks of the outstretched arm holding a ballpoint pen.

frontal areas. Light stimulation provoked myoclonic jerks (EOG in individuals II–1 and II–2).

Figure 11.4 shows EEG findings of the third generation (III–15, III–16, III–17) of this family. There were paroxysmal bursts of high-voltage diffuse spike–wave complex in all cases but no photosensitivity. Individual III–17 had EEG

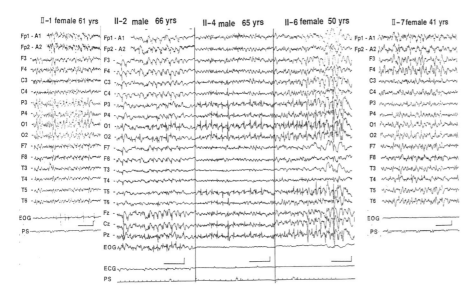

Fig. 11.3. EEG Family 1: tracings. Scale bars show 1 s vs. 50 µV.

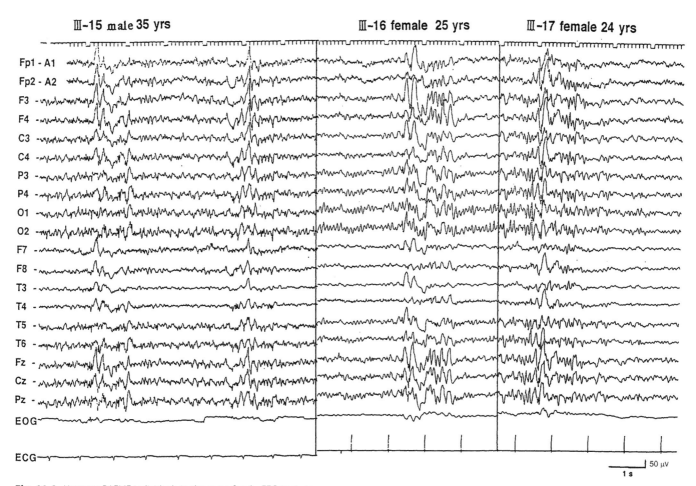

Fig. 11.4. Younger BAFME individuals in the same family: EEG tracings.

abnormality only. They were too young to have full clinical symptomatology.

The somatosensory evoked potential, obtained by right median nerve stimulation at the wrist, produced high-amplitude responses (Fig. 11.5) in all of the second generation and also the oldest individual in the third generation. There was a positive peak at latency of 25 ms and a large negative peak at latency of 29–36 ms. The large negative component became

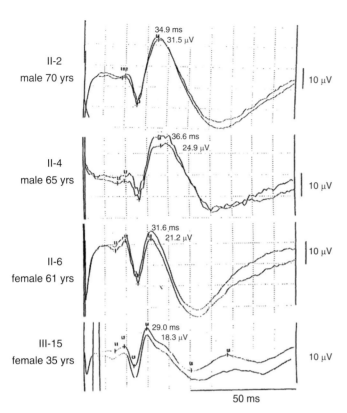

Fig. 11.5. Somatosensory evoked potential (SEP) in the BAFME family.

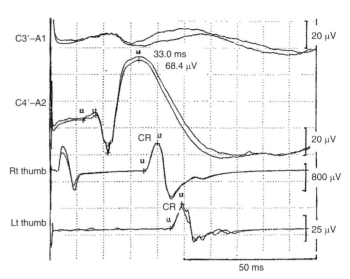

Fig. 11.6. Somatosensory evoked potential and long-loop cortical reflex (CR) in a 35-year-old female. Electrical stimulation was given to the right median nerve at the wrist and it produced G-SEP on the contralateral cortex; CR was recorded on the right thumb as well as on the left thumb.

higher in amplitude and slower in latency as the age of the individuals advanced.

Tremor and myoclonic jerk

Patients with BAFME often had irregular fine dysrhythmic involuntary movement, which became evident on outstretched extended arms. They were a mixture of tremor and myoclonic jerks. The tremor was usually composed of fine irregular rapidly alternative movements from 7 to 9 Hz in frequency with the duration of the electromyogram (EMG) burst over 50 ms which were probably of subcortical origin. Myoclonic jerkes involved several muscle groups or both sides of the extremities having EMG bursts of shorter duration and higher amplitude which were reflex myoclonus of probably cortical origin. This tremor and myoclonic jerks were well demonstrated by the author's original tremogram (Fig. 11.2). The patient was asked to hold a ballpoint pen in his outstretched arms and try to keep in touch with the center of a cross on the paper presented in front of him. The involuntary movement became worse and somatosensory evoked potential became higher as the age advanced. This fact suggested that a considerable time-span would be required for full-blown clinical symptomatology.

Electrophysiology

One of the characteristics of BAFME was G-SEP with enhanced long-loop cortical reflexes and premovement cortical

spikes by the jerk-locked averaging method, suggesting hyperexcitability of cerebral cortex.

Somatosensory evoked potentials were always high in amplitude. Figure 11.6 shows G-SEP and long-loop cortical reflex (CR) in a 36-year-old female BAFME in a family with 12 affected members over four generations. Stimulation given to the right median nerve at the wrist produced high-amplitude SEP of 68.4 μV at a latency of 33.0 ms on the contralateral central areas of the head. In the right thumb after stimulation, there appeared immediate muscle jerks with latency of 5 ms and CR in 40 ms. An interesting finding was the fact that the CR was bilateral. The CR had 40 ms latency in the stimulated right thumb and 49 ms latency in the contralateral left thumb. The left CR probably came from G-SEP transmitted from the left cortex to the right cortex through corpus callosum. Thus a 9-ms delay was considered the time required to cross from the left to the right cortex through the corpus callosum.

Differential diagnosis

Differential diagnosis includs a variety of progressive myoclonus epilepsy, hereditary tremor, and idiopathic epilepsies such as juvenile myoclonic epilepsy (JME) and grand mal on awaking. Most cases of progressive myoclonus epilepsy such as the Unverricht–Lundborg type have a recessive hereditary trait and deteriorate, eventually leading to ataxia and dementia. Dentatorubral-pallidoluysian atrophy (DRPLA) has an autosomal dominant hereditary pattern, similar to BAFME in this respect, but DRPLA is a progressive disorder whereas BAFME is not, so they can be differentiated by follow-up study. DNA analysis can now confirm both DRPLA, Unverricht–Lundborg disease, and mitochondrial disease such as mitochondrial encephalopathy, lactic acidosis, and stroke-like episodes (MELAS) or myoclonic epilepsy with ragged red fibers (MERRF). Idiopathic epilepsy of JME and grand mal on awaking often have a dominant hereditary trait and many cases of BAFME are mistakenly diagnosed as idiopathic generalized epilepsy (IGE). However, careful history-taking reveals that the BAFME family history had a dominant hereditary pattern of almost complete penetrance, which is unusual for IGE. The presence of involuntary hand tremor with seizure strongly suggests the diagnosis of BAFME. The illness usually starts at the age of over 30 and evidence of marked driving response along with spikes to the photic stimulation on the EEG and high amplitude SEP confirms this disorder.

Essential myoclonus has characteristics of myoclonus and/or tremor in a family showing dominant hereditary pattern but who have neither EEG abnormality nor epileptic seizures.

Future perspectives

The clinical symptoms of BAFME may have some variety in each family. For example some individuals had little tremor and others had rather severe tremor. The question arises whether all of the different phenotypes between pedigrees can be included into one single clinical entity. Anticipation and progression are further problems. As seen in the tremogram and G-SEP in the family presented here there is the possibility of deterioration over a long time-span. The onset of illness became earlier in the third generation than in the second one, suggesting possible anticipation. The disorder certainly deserves further genetic study for positional cloning and identification of the specific gene coding BAFME substance.

References

Araki T (2002) Clinical genetic and linkage analysis of familial essential myoclonus and epilepsy (FEME). *Niigata Med J* **116**:535–45.

De Falco FA, Striano P, de Falco A, et al. (2003) Benign adult familial myoclonic epilepsy: genetic heterogeneity and allelism with ADCME. *Neurology* **60**:1381–5.

Elia M, Musumeci SA, Ferri R, et al. (1998) Familial cortical tremor, epilepsy, and mental retardation: a distinct clinical entity? *Arch Neurol* **55**:1569–73.

Guerrini R, Bonanni P, Patrignani A, et al. (2001) Autosomal dominant cortical myoclonus and epilepsy (ADCME) with complex partial and generalized seizures: a newly recognized epilepsy syndrome with linkage to chromosome 2p11.1–q12.2. *Brain* **124**:2459–75.

Ikeda A, Kakigi R, Funai N, et al. (1990) Cortical tremor: a variant of cortical reflex myoclonus. *Neurology* **40**:1561–5.

Inazuki H, Naito A, Ohama E (1990) A clinical study and neuropathological findings of a familial disease with myoclonus and epilepsy. *Seishin Shinkeigaku Zashi* **92**:1–21.

Inoue S (1975) Hereditary epilepsy with epilepsy-like seizure. *Seishin Shinkeigaku Zashi* **77**:1–18.

Madia F, Striano P, Di Bonaventura C, et al. (2008) Benign adult familial myoclonic epilepsy (BAFME): evidence of an extended founder haplotype on chromosome 2p11.1–q12.2 in five Italian families. *Neurogenetics* **9**:139–42.

Mikami M, Yasuda T, Terao A, et al. (1999) Localization of a gene for benign adult familial myoclonic epilepsy to chromosome 8q23.3–q24.1. *Am J Hum Genet* **65**:745–51.

Okino S (1997) Familial benign myoclonus epilepsy of adult onset: a previously unrecognized myoclonic disorder. *J Neurol Sci* **145**:113–18.

Plaster NM, Uyama E, Uchino M, et al. (1999) Genetic localization of the familial adult myoclonic epilepsy (FAME) gene to chromosome 8q24. *Neurology* **53**:1180–3.

Takahashi T, Aoki K, Wada T (1969) Three families of familial tremor with grand mal seizure. *Clin Neurol* **12**:729.

Wakeno M (1975) A family with heredofamilial tremor associated epileptic disorders. *Psychiatr Neurol Jpn* **77**:1–18.

Yasuda T (1991) Benign adult familial myoclonic epilepsy. *Kawasaki Med J* **17**:1–13.

Idiopathic generalized epilepsies

Carla Marini and Renzo Guerrini

Definition of the phenotype

Idiopathic generalized epilepsies (IGEs) are the commonest group of epilepsies in children and adolescents. Based on the main seizure type and their age of onset, the international classification (ILAE 1989) recognizes the following IGE subsyndromes (Table 12.1)

- Benign neonatal convulsions (BNC)
- Benign neonatal familial convulsions (BNFC)
- Benign myoclonic epilepsy of infancy (BMEI)
- Childhood absence epilepsy (CAE)
- Juvenile absence epilepsy (JAE)
- Juvenile myoclonic epilepsy (JME)
- IGE with tonic–clonic seizures alone (IGE–TCS).

Other generalized syndromes typical of childhood such as epilepsy with myoclonic–astatic seizures (EMAS) and epilepsy with myoclonic absences (EMA) were considered at the time to be cryptogenic or symptomatic, due to their less favorable outcome and to the presence of cognitive impairment in some patients. Concepts have evolved and at present both EMAS and EMA are recognized as IGE phenotypes (Table 12.1), at least in some patients, while benign neonatal convulsions and benign familial infantile convulsions are no longer considered to be generalized syndromes.

In general, IGE syndromes are defined by distinct age at onset, seizure types, and characteristic EEG abnormalities, without structural brain lesions and with normal developmental skills.

Epidemiology

The IGEs have a cumulative incidence of approximately 0.7% in the general population; they account for about 40% of all epilepsies up to age 40 and have a general frequency of around 15–20% of all epilepsies (Hauser *et al.* 1993; Forsgren 2004).

Benign myoclonic epilepsy of infancy

Benign myoclonic epilepsy of infancy (BMEI) is the form of IGE with the earliest age at onset. Generalized myoclonic seizures appear at between 4 months and 3–4 years of age in otherwise normal infants. Age of onset as late as 5 years has been reported (Rossi *et al.* 1997). Myoclonic jerks are very brief, isolated, or repetitive, mild and rare at onset but increase gradually in frequency, becoming multiple daily events, and may present in brief clusters. In 30% of children myoclonic seizures are preceded by infrequent simple febrile seizures (Dravet and Bureau 2002). Parents describe head nodding or upward eyes rolling, accompanied by a brisk abduction of the upper limbs. Jerks might vary in intensity; however, jerking with projection of objects or falling are rare and may appear later in the course. When falling occurs, it is followed by immediate recovery, usually without injury. Jerks are typically favored by sleep and, in some patients, can be triggered by a sudden noise or contact (Ricci *et al.* 1995).

Etiology and epidemiology

Benign myoclonic epilepsy of infancy is quite rare, affecting less than 1% of the epilepsy population in specialized centers, and represents around 2% of all IGEs (Dravet and Bureau 2002). It can be diagnosed in 1.3–1.7% of all children with seizure onset in the first year of life and in 2% of those with onset under the age of 3 years (Sarisjulis *et al.* 2000). Boys are affected almost twice as often as girls. There are no familial cases of BMEI, but a family history of epilepsy or febrile seizures is observed in 39% of cases (Dravet and Bureau 2002). These data support the role of genetic factors in the etiology of BMEI.

EEG features

The electroencephalogram (EEG) shows normal background activity; focal interictal EEG abnormalities, occasionally reported, are not a consistent feature of BMEI. Ictal discharges, often observed during sleep, consist of brief bursts (1–3 s) of generalized fast spike-and-waves or polyspike-and-waves and jerks are time-locked with the spike component. A photoparoxysmal response is sometimes observed.

The Causes of Epilepsy, eds. S. D. Shorvon, F. Andermann, and R. Guerrini. Published by Cambridge University Press. © Cambridge University Press 2011.

Table 12.1 Summary of the IGE subtypes included in the ILAE classification (1989) and in the proposed diagnostic scheme (Engel 2001) and their clinical features and of other phenotypes not recognized as discrete IGE entities

IGE subtype	Age of onset	1st seizure type	Other seizure types	EEG	Photosensitivity
Included in ILAE classification					
BMEI	0.4–5 yrs	My	FS	GSW	Rare
CAE	4–10 yrs	Ab	TCS, My	3-Hz GSW	Rare
JAE	10–18 yrs	Ab	TCS, My	3–4-Hz GSW	Rare
JME	12–18 yrs	My	TCS, Ab	4–6-Hz GPSW	Frequent
IGE–TCS	Childhood to early adulthood	TCS	My, Ab	GSW	Rare
EMA	5–10 yrs	MA	TCS	3-Hz GSW	Rare
MAE	2–6 yrs	My–ast	Ab, TCS, non-convulsive SE	GSW	Rare
Not included in ILAE classification and not recognized as discrete IGE entities					
Eyelid myoclonia with absences	3–7 yrs	Ab	TCS	3-Hz GSW	Frequent
Perioral myoclonus with absences	4–6 yrs	Ab	TCS, Ab status	3-Hz GSW	Rare
Absence epilepsy of early childhood	<3 yrs	Ab	TCS	3-Hz GSW	Rare
Intermediate petit mal	<4 yrs	Ab	TCS	2–3-Hz GSW	Rare
Adult onset IGE	19–34 yrs	Ab, My, TCS	—	3–4-Hz GSW	Rare

Notes:
Ab, absences; BMEI, benign myoclonic epilepsy of infancy; CAE, childhood absence epilepsy; EMA, epilepsy with myoclonic absences; FS, febrile seizures; GSW, generalized spike–wave; IGE, idiopathic generalized epilepsy; JAE, juvenile absence epilepsy; JME, juvenile myoclonic epilepsy; MAE, myoclonic absence epilepsy; My, myoclonic; My–ast, myoclonic–astatic; SE, status epilepticus; TCS, tonic–clonic seizures.

Course and outcome

The course of BMEI is said to be benign, an opinion largely based on retrospective studies. One of the proposed criteria for diagnosis was a rapid response to valproate monotherapy, which is clearly also a strong criterion of benignity. However, some children have cognitive or behavioral sequelae indicating that even with these strict criteria a benign outcome cannot be guaranteed, and the difference from the milder cases of myoclonic–astatic epilepsy is not entirely clear.

Absence epilepsies

Absence epilepsies are the prototype of IGEs. Childhood and juvenile forms are recognized in which, by definition, all patients manifest absence seizures associated with an EEG pattern of generalized spike–wave discharges (GSW) (ILAE 1989).

Childhood absence epilepsy

Historical note

Tissot in 1770 first described a 14-year-girl who had suffered from seizures since the age of 7 years, which can now be recognized as typical of childhood absence epilepsy (CAE). Early in the last century CAE was given the Greek name of "pyknolepsy" (Sauer 1916); other synonyms are "petit mal epilepsy," "true petit mal," and "pyknoleptic petit mal."

Epidemiology

Childhood absence epilepsy has an estimated incidence of 6.3–8 per 100 000 in children aged 0 to 15 years (Loiseau 1992) and it accounts for 2–12% of patients with epilepsy (Berg *et al.* 2000).

Clinical characteristics

Childhood absence epilepsy is age related; typical absence seizures are sudden and brief, lasting 5–15 s, periods of loss of awareness with interruption of ongoing activities, followed by immediate and complete recovery. Although absences were initially described as staring spells, only a minority of patients have "simple absences" with unresponsiveness and interruption of ongoing activity (Penry *et al.* 1975). The great majority of children exhibit "complex absences," with additional clinical phenomena such as automatisms, or a tonic, atonic, or autonomic component (Penry *et al.* 1975; Holmes *et al.* 1987).

A mild myoclonic component of the eyelids, often with upward eye deviation, or mild jerking of the perioral region, has traditionally been considered compatible with the diagnosis of CAE. However, Loiseau and Panayiotopoulos (2005) suggested new diagnostic criteria in which eyelid and perioral myoclonias are considered as exclusion criteria. Absences are very frequent, occurring up to 100 times per day. They occur spontaneously but are also influenced by various factors, especially hyperventilation.

The age of onset of CAE is between 4 and 10 years with a peak at 5–7 years, and girls are more frequently affected than boys (Penry et al. 1975; Berkovic 1996). There are no clear-cut boundaries in age of onset, and cases beginning before 3 years or after 10 years have been described (Penry et al. 1975; Cavazzuti 1980).

Most children with CAE exhibit normal developmental skills and normal cognitive functions. However, children with borderline IQ or mild cognitive impairment are not rarely encountered. The lowest scores in neuropsychological tests might be correlated with earlier onset and longer duration of seizures (Sato et al. 1983).

Other seizure types

About 10–15% of patients have febrile convulsions prior to the onset of absences (Penry et al. 1975; Cavazzuti 1980; Rocca et al. 1987). Rare generalized tonic–clonic seizures (TCS) have been reported to develop in a variable percentage of patients with CAE, reaching up to 40%. Indeed, in most cases later TCS appear in adolescence, 5 to 10 years after the onset of absences (Loiseau 1992; Berkovic 1996). Myoclonic seizures can occur in about 8% of cases and mainly in teenagers with persisting CAE (Janz 1985; Camfield and Camfield 2002). It is likely that the number of patients who will experience TCS or myoclonic seizures has been overestimated, due to inclusion of cases of juvenile absence epilepsy or of idiopathic generalized epilepsy with variable phenotypes (Engel 2001). Absence status is exceedingly rare in patients with typical CAE.

Ictal and interictal EEG findings

There is a highly specific EEG pattern consisting of generalized, bilaterally synchronous and symmetrical spike–wave (GSW) discharges. The frequency is around 3.0–3.5 Hz at onset and slows to 2.5–3.0 Hz toward the end of the discharge. More irregular discharges of generalized polyspike–waves (GPSW) changing rhythm inside a discharge can also be observed (Sadleir et al. 2009). Discharges arise suddenly from a normal background and the ending is less abrupt than its onset. Hyperventilation is the most effective activator of the GSW pattern while photic stimulation precipitates absence seizures in only about 15% of cases (Sadleir et al. 2009). Background EEG activity is usually normal although brief GSW may occur. Transient focal epileptiform activity such as centrotemporal spikes may occur (Hedstrom and Olsson 1991).

Prognosis and long-term outcome

The general view is that CAE has a good or excellent prognosis. Absences disappear before adulthood in up to 90% of cases in which no other seizure types are associated (Guiwer et al. 2003). If absences persist, TCS usually appear. Early and late onset (before 4 and after 9 years), initial drug resistance, and photosensitivity have a less favorable prognosis (Guerrini, 2006).

Juvenile absence epilepsy

Historical notes and electroclinical characteristics

Juvenile absence epilepsy (JAE) has only recently been recognized as a syndrome distinct from CAE and brought to general attention (ILAE 1989). Before the ILAE classification introduced the age-related distinction of absence seizure syndromes, the distinction between absence epilepsies in childhood and juvenile forms was used only in German publications (Janz and Christian 1957; Doose et al. 1965). Doose, Janz, and colleagues had clearly recognized that absence epilepsy had a first peak of age of onset at 6–7 years, corresponding to the typical CAE. A second peak was near age 12 years, corresponding to the juvenile form. Thus, JAE typically begins during puberty, between the ages of 10 and 17 years (Wolf 1992; Obeid 1994).

Absence seizures are clinically similar to those seen in CAE; however, loss of awareness appears to be less pronounced and attacks have a much lower frequency, usually occurring a few times per day.

Other seizure types

Tonic–clonic seizures are very common in JAE, occurring in 80% of cases and beginning at the same time or even prior to the onset of absences (Wolf 1992). Sleep deprivation is the main precipitant. About 16% of patients will also have myoclonic seizures, especially early in the morning (Thomas et al. 2002).

Ictal and interictal EEG

On EEG recording absences may have a faster rhythm of GSW at 4–5 Hz, especially at the onset of the attack. Background EEG activity is also normal and interictal GSW are seen. Photosensitivity is rare.

Prognosis and long-term outcome

Absences may persist through adult life, GTCS are common, and episodes of absence status can occur. Only about 60% of patients have a long-term remission (Trinka et al. 2004).

Epilepsy with myoclonic absences

Epilepsy with myoclonic absences (EMA) is the only syndrome with absences, other than CAE and JAE, which is recognized in the international classification amongst the cryptogenic or symptomatic generalized epilepsies (ILAE 1989).

Epilepsy with myoclonic absences is a childhood epilepsy – mean age at onset 7 years – with daily myoclonic absences, and with other infrequent seizure types such as TCS, drop attacks, and atypical absences (Bureau and Tassinari 2005). Myoclonic

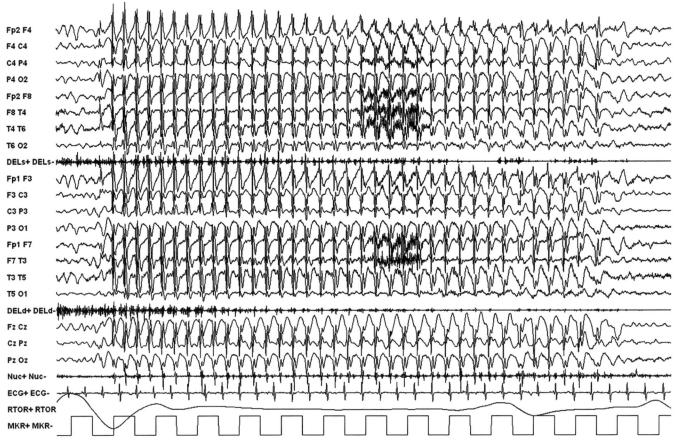

Fig. 12.1. Polygraphic EEG recording of a myoclonic absence seizure showing a high voltage 3-Hz generalized spike–wave discharge associated with myoclonic jerks of the left (DELs) and right (DELd) deltoids and neck muscles (Nuc) (EMG channels). The child was unresponsive, and stopped breathing during the discharge (RTOR, abdominal breath).

absences manifest with rhythmic myoclonic jerks of the head, shoulders, and arms, often associated with a tonic muscle contraction (Fig. 12.1). They usually last from 10 to 60 s, and can be easily precipitated by hyperventilation, or tend to cluster upon awakening. Frequency, calculated in a selected epilepsy population at the Centre Saint Paul, is around 0.5–1% of all epilepsies but the prevalence is probably less among unselected epilepsies (Bureau and Tassinari 2005). Myoclonic absences as a seizure type are by no means limited to a homogeneous syndrome in that they have also been described in association with variable etiologies and in different clinical contexts (Guerrini *et al.* 2005).

There is a male preponderance and mental retardation is present in 45% of patients before the onset of epilepsy (Bureau and Tassinari 2005). Myoclonic absences are associated with 3-Hz GSW similar to those observed in CAE (Fig. 12.1). The prognosis is variable but resistant cases are encountered much more frequently than in CAE and JAE from which this syndrome is clearly distinct in spite of EEG similarities.

Myoclonic–astatic epilepsy

Myoclonic–astatic epilepsy epitomizes a spectrum of IGEs with prominent myoclonic seizures, appearing in previously healthy children. Myoclonic astatic epilepsy represents about 2% of all childhood epilepsies (Guerrini 2006). Onset is between 2 and 6 years of age. Myoclonic seizures and atonic falls might be repeated many times daily and are often associated with episodes of non-convulsive status epilepticus and GTCS. Interictal EEG, often normal at onset, can become very disorganized. Outcome is unpredictable. Remission within a few months or years with normal cognition is possible even after a severe course. About 30% of children experience an epileptic encephalopathy with long-lasting intractability and cognitive impairment (Guerrini 2006).

Other possible syndromes with typical absence seizures

Absences with a mild clonic component, often manifesting as flickering of the eyelids, are well recognized in CAE and JAE. However, no clear-cut boundaries exist in the severity, frequency, and distribution of the jerking component, with the consequence that a confusing nomenclature and several subtypes of absence seizures and epilepsies have been proposed. Whether or not all various syndromes that have been proposed represent distinct clinical and genetic entities is still debated.

Eyelid myoclonia with absences

The hallmark of eyelid myoclonia with absences (Appleton et al. 1993), initially described as a form of photosensitive epilepsy by Jeavons (1977), is eyelid myoclonia somewhat different from the flickering of the eyelids seen in typical absence epilepsies. Age of onset is between 3 and 7 years. Tonic–clonic seizures are infrequent, and usually precipitated by sleep deprivation or photic stimulation. The EEG changes associated with eyelid myoclonia are GPSW discharges at a fluctuating frequency of 3–5 Hz, following eye closure. It has been suggested that eyelid myoclonia would be, at least in some photosensitive patients, a sort of subconscious eye blinking performed in order to self-induce the related absence component (Binnie et al. 1980). The whole population of patients exhibiting such seizure type is extremely heterogeneous, varying from otherwise healthy individuals, who share all the characteristics of an IGE, to patients with severe cognitive impairment and an obvious symptomatic disorder (Guerrini et al. 2005).

Perioral myoclonus with absences

It has been proposed that jaw and lips myoclonus associated with typical absences represents the distinctive feature of a syndrome (Panayiotopoulos et al. 1995) with onset in childhood or adolescence, a high risk for absence status, and possible subsequent GTCS. However, no sufficient evidence has been gathered to consider perioral myoclonus with absence as a recognized distinct epilepsy syndrome; clinical criteria are not sufficient to justify a discrete syndrome, separate from classical CAE or JAE.

Absence epilepsy of early childhood

Doose considered absence epilepsy of early childhood, in which onset is before the age of 5 years (Doose and Baier 1989), as a distinct entity. In his series boys appeared to be more frequently affected than girls, TCS or myoclonic-astatic seizures occurred at onset or later, and, with respect to other forms of absence epilepsy, the EEG exhibited a wider range of abnormalities and the prognosis was often unfavorable. Such a description corresponds to that of children that are now included under the spectrum of myoclonic-astatic epilepsy.

Intermediate petit mal

In 1973, Lugaresi and colleagues described patients with "intermediate" petit mal epilepsy (Lugaresi et al. 1973). The term "intermediate" was meant to suggest that the clinical features of these patients were in between the benign CAE and the more severe symptomatic generalized epilepsy of Lennox–Gastaut. Age of onset was before 4 years in half of the patients; all of them had other seizure types including TCS or tonic seizures, commonly occurring before the onset of absences. Absence seizures were associated with an atypical EEG pattern of slow GSW discharges with a fluctuating

frequency from 3 to 1.5 Hz. More than 50% of patients had some degree of mental retardation. The prognosis was poorer than typical CAE. In clinical practice, similar patients are not frequently observed but pose difficult diagnostic and treatment problems. As with idiopathic generalized epilepsies, no specific etiology can be demonstrated in most.

Typical absence seizures in symptomatic epilepsies

Absence seizures, sometimes typical, may occasionally occur in symptomatic epilepsies, arising as a consequence of a known disorder. Typical absences have been reported following encephalitis, lysosomal storage disorders, and metabolic encephalopathies (Andermann 1967). Hypothalamic hamartomas have also been associated with GSW and with absence attacks (Scherman and Abraham 1963).

Absence epilepsy associated with non-epileptic paroxysmal disorders

Absence epilepsies and more broadly IGEs can sometimes co-occur with paroxysmal movement disorders. Families and sporadic patients in which affected individuals have absence epilepsy or paroxysmal movement disorders or both have been described (Guerrini et al. 2002; Bing et al. 2005; Suls et al. 2008). Age of onset of absences in some of such patients is usually very early, before age 2 years.

Juvenile myoclonic epilepsy
Definition and historical notes

In 1867 Herpin provided the first description of a patient with juvenile myoclonic epilepsy (JME), calling the myoclonic jerks secousses or compulsions that shake the body as does an electric shock (Herpin, 1867). Juvenile myoclonic epilepsy, also known as "impulsive petit mal," is included among the IGEs (ILAE 1989).

Epidemiology

Juvenile myoclonic epilepsy is estimated to account for 3–12% of all epilepsies (Thomas et al. 2002).

Clinical characteristics

The characteristic clinical feature of JME are myoclonic jerks, usually affecting shoulders and arms bilaterally, but not always symmetrically, usually appearing upon awakening in the morning. Jerks can sometimes involve muscles in the face or the legs and very rarely may cause a sudden fall. The patient is usually aware of such symptoms. Myoclonic jerks are single or repetitive and vary in intensity. Subtle jerks are perceived as an internal body electric sensation with no exterior movement; more severe jerks cause objects to be dropped or launched. The age at seizure onset varies between 8 and 26 years, but the great majority of patients exhibit the first manifestations between 12 and 18 years. Males and females are equally affected (Delgado-Escueta et al. 1996).

Ictal and interictal EEG

The characteristic EEG patterns during myoclonic jerks are GPSW complexes or GSW at 3.5–6 Hz. Photosensitivity is found in about 30% of males and 40% of females (Asconape and Penry, 1984; Appleton *et al.* 2000). Background EEG activity is normal.

Other seizure types

Tonic–clonic seizures occur in 90–95% of patients, more frequently in the morning and often preceded by a crescendo of myoclonic jerks (Delgado-Escueta *et al.* 1996) (Fig. 12.2). Myoclonic seizures and TCS may be precipitated by sleep deprivation, awakening, photic stimulation, and excess of alcohol. Absences are reported in 10–33% of cases, and are infrequent, relatively short, and often unnoticed by the patient (Thomas *et al.* 2002). During absence EEG usually shows irregular 3–4-Hz GSW. It has been suggested that 5–15% of patients with CAE will evolve into JME (Janz and Christian 1957; Wirrell *et al.* 1996). We have not observed such a transition in our cohort.

Prognosis and long-term outcome

Juvenile myoclonic epilepsy is described as the prototype of pharmacodependent epilepsies, assuming that treatment will be lifelong (Baruzzi *et al.* 1988), although about 10% appear to have permanent remission in adolescence (Camfield and Camfield 2005).

Idiopathic generalized epilepsy with generalized tonic-clonic seizures

Electroclinical characteristics

Idiopathic generalized epilepsy with generalized tonic–clonic seizures only (IGE–TCS), previously referred to as grand mal epilepsy (Esquirol, Temkin 1971) is a broad and non-specific category including all patients with TCS and an interictal EEG pattern of GSW discharges. The initial defining feature of IGE–TCS was the occurrence of TCS predominantly on awakening or in the evening period of relaxation (ILAE 1989). However, subsequent clinical studies have shown that, in almost half of the patients, seizures do not occur in relation to awakening or relaxation (Reutens and Berkovic 1995). Others have instead proposed the recognition of two separate entities depending upon whether TCSs occur on awakening or not (Unterberger *et al.* 2001). Age of onset ranges from childhood to early adulthood but without clear boundaries; seizures are often infrequent, and provoked by sleep deprivation and excessive alcohol. Some studies have described patients with TCS immediately preceded by 3-Hz GSW or by an absence seizure (Mayville *et al.* 2000). The EEG shows normal background and interictal discharges of GSW or GPSW.

Adult-onset idiopathic generalized epilepsy

Age of onset is one of the main criteria to define the various IGE subsyndromes (ILAE 1989). Most patients have indeed a characteristic childhood or adolescence onset while onset in adulthood is generally considered to be rare. However, in earlier work, Gastaut had reported that 35% of his IGE cases had had seizure onset after adolescence (Gastaut 1981). In 75% of his patients seizures began between the ages of 19 and 34 years and only a minority (5%) were older than 50 years at seizure onset. Infrequent nocturnal TCS, usually provoked by sleep deprivation, appear to be the predominant clinical manifestation, whereas absences and myoclonic jerks accounted for only 1.5% of the epilepsies in this age group. In a more recent study, performed after the international classification was published, 28% of patients seen at a first seizure clinic had adult-onset IGE with predominant TCS but myoclonic and absence epilepsy were also described (Marini *et al.* 2003b).

Adults with TCS and occasional absence status may have unrecognized "phantom" absences beginning in childhood or adolescence (Caraballo *et al.* 2000). Absences in these adult patients may escape recognition, as they are imperceptible to the observer, and described by patients themselves as a momentary lack of concentration and forgetfulness, without practical consequences in their lives. Thus, the diagnosis of phantom absences is possible with appropriate video-EEG recordings.

Patients with adult-onset IGE have normal EEG recordings or show interictal GSW discharges (Yenjun *et al.* 2003); seizures are usually well controlled by medications or by simply removing the provocative factors. A family history of epilepsy is also a common feature in adult-onset cases, suggesting that seizures appear following a provocative factor, commonly sleep deprivation, in subjects with a genetic predisposition (Gilliam *et al.* 2000; Unterberger *et al.* 2001; Marini *et al.* 2003b).

A form of benign familial adult myoclonic epilepsy (BFAME or FAME) has also been described (Okino 1997). Patients have characteristic persistent tremulous fingers, progressively worsening myoclonus, and a familial clustering suggestive of an autosomal dominant mode of inheritance. A locus on chromosome 8q24 has been found in families with FAME but gene defects have not yet been identified (Mikami *et al.* 1999). A similar pattern of myoclonus has also been described in association with familial epilepsy with both focal and generalized seizures (Guerrini *et al.* 2001).

Adult-onset IGE is still a poorly recognized syndrome, yet a real phenomenon that may be encountered in clinical practice. Some patients might experience their first, severe sleep deprivation in relation to their working arrangements only while adults and manifest their initial seizures only after such powerful precipitating circumstances. Because of their age of onset, these patients are often misdiagnosed as having partial epilepsies.

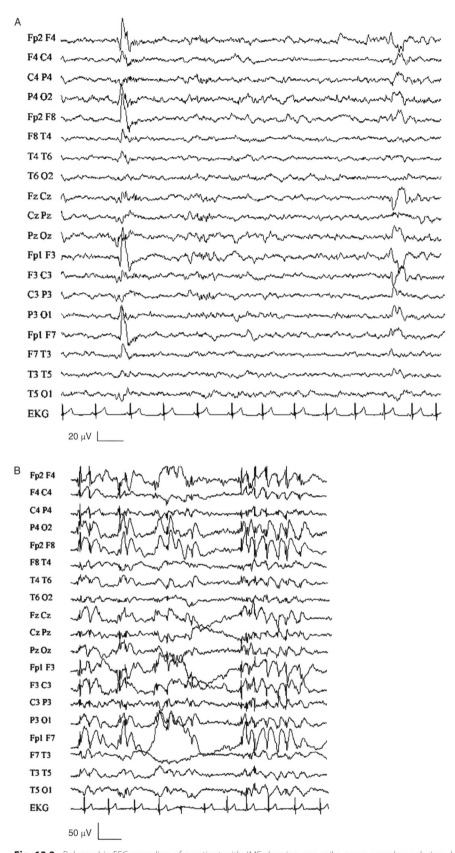

Fig. 12.2. Polygraphic EEG recording of a patient with JME showing rare spike–wave complexes during sleep intermingled with sleep figures (A). A progressive increase of spike–wave discharges is seen upon awakening (B), which translates into a generalized tonic–clonic seizure (C,D).

C

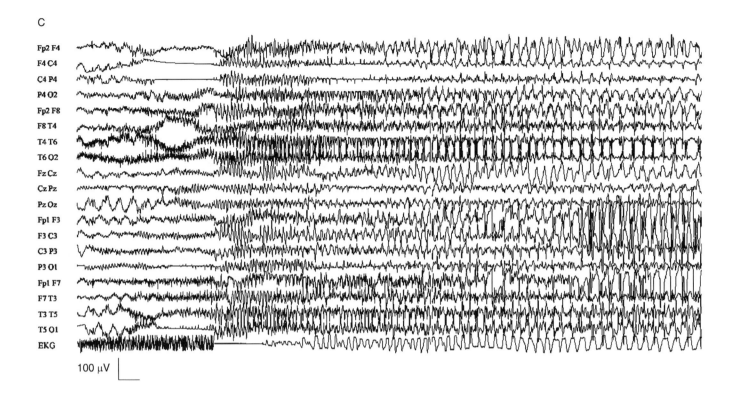

100 μV

D

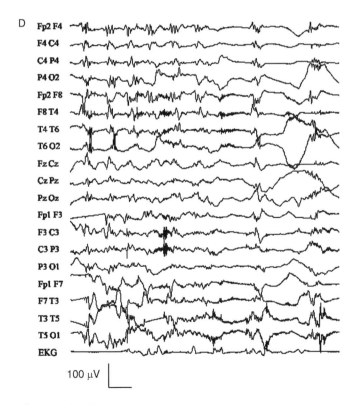

100 μV

Fig. 12.2. (cont.)

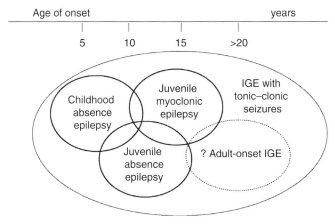

Fig. 12.3. Subsyndromes of IGE: clinical overlap. Each circle represents one of the IGE subsyndromes. The points where the circles cross each other represent the clinical overlap of the IGE subsyndromes (modified from Janz 1992).

Idiopathic generalized epilepsies: discrete or overlapping entities?

In 1960 Lennox formulated the important concept that the division between idiopathic and symptomatic epilepsy does not have a clear-cut boundary, and that in every patient there is a unique combination of genetic and environmental factors interacting to produce the clinical phenotype (Lennox 1960). The semantic distinction of IGE in several subsyndromes based upon age of onset and predominant seizure types offers a nosologic framework within which patients can be placed to facilitate their clinical management. However, patients do not always fit into the widely recognized IGE subsyndromes. Clinical similarities are seen in between subsyndromes and there may be no clear-cut boundaries. Family studies show that relatives of IGE probands often have different IGE subsyndromes (Marini *et al.* 2004). This obvious clinical overlap seen within single individuals and families has led some authors to suggest that generalized epilepsies are different expressions of a continuum (Lennox 1960) (Fig. 12.3). Under the alternative view of the epilepsies as a neurobiological continuum, IGEs might also be regarded as a spectrum with age-dependent expression of particular seizure types and with similar etiology (Janz *et al.* 1992; Berkovic *et al.* 1994). Clinical genetic studies suggest that within the IGE spectrum some subsyndromes have a more similar genetic background. For example, CAE and JAE could be framed within the absence epilepsy syndromes and considered to be rather distinct from JME and IGE–TCS. Within this spectrum one end might be represented by absence epilepsies and the other end by JME and IGT–TCS; halfway along there would be patients with both clinical characteristics, for example CAE evolving into JME, JAE with predominant myoclonic jerks and TCS, or JME with absence seizures. The proposal for recognizing a syndrome category of IGE with variable phenotypes (Engel 2001) seems in keeping with the above concepts and of practical utility, especially for adolescent and adult onset IGEs.

Genetic etiology

The IGEs have a predominant genetic etiology and current data are in favor of a complex model of inheritance with the interaction of two or more genes (Berkovic and Scheffer 2001). Data from twin studies show that monozygous twins concordant for epilepsy have the same IGE subsyndrome and similar EEG patterns (Berkovic *et al.* 1998). Family studies have estimated 4–10% risk of developing epilepsy in close relatives of IGE probands (Annegers *et al.* 1982; Marini *et al.* 2004). The risk is comparable for the subsyndromes of CAE, JAE, and JME (Janz *et al.* 1992). Higher risk is seen in siblings and offspring and is lower in second-degree relatives (Tsuboi 1989). Analysis of epilepsy phenotypes in families with several affected family members shows that, usually, relatives also have an IGE, with about 30% phenotypic concordance (affected relatives have the same IGE subsyndrome as the proband), both for absence epilepsies and JME (Marini *et al.* 2004). In contrast, very few affected relatives of probands with absence epilepsies have JME and vice versa, suggesting that absence epilepsies and JME tend to segregate separately. These findings suggest that, within a polygenic model of inheritance, absence epilepsies are closely related and genetically distinct from JME. Febrile seizures and TCS are equally distributed in affected individuals of all IGEs, perhaps representing the expression of a non-specific susceptibility to seizures.

Rare large IGE families, with a predominant autosomal dominant inheritance, have been reported (Cossette *et al.* 2002; Marini *et al.* 2003a). Other models of inheritance have been suggested for IGEs including two-locus models and autosomal recessive inheritance. The two-locus models would imply two genes, one dominantly and the other recessively inherited or both recessively inherited (Greenberg *et al.* 1989). Possible autosomal recessive inheritance has been observed in consanguineous families (Panayiotopoulos and Obeid 1989).

Thus, despite interest in the genetics of IGEs in the last 50-year period, the extent of the genetic overlap between the IGE subsyndromes is controversial; the mode of inheritance remains uncertain and common genes for IGEs have not yet been identified. Rare families with mutations in genes encoding subunits of voltage- or ligand-gated ion channels have been described (Helbig *et al.* 2008). Genome-wide linkage analyses of large numbers of families with IGEs have shown several loci with putative genes for IGEs (Sander *et al.* 2000; Durner *et al.* 2001; Hempelmann *et al.* 2006). Table 12.2 summarizes current relevant molecular findings.

Sex-related effects

Some authors reported that offspring of mothers with IGEs had a higher risk of developing epilepsy compared to the offspring of affected fathers (Annegers *et al.* 1976; Tsuboi 1989). The cumulative incidence of unprovoked seizures to age 25 years were 8.7% and 2.4% in offspring of affected mothers and fathers, respectively (Ottman *et al.* 1988). Similar

Table 12.2 Summary of the genetic defects identified in some IGE patients or families

Gene	Locus	Protein	Phenotype
GABRG2	5q31–q233	GABA$_A$ receptor γ$_2$-subunit	CAE and FS
GABRA1	5q34–q235	GABA$_A$ receptor α$_1$-subunit	JME, CAE
CLCN2	3q26	ClC-2 voltage-gated Cl$^-$ channel	CAE, JAE, JME, EGMA
EFHC1	6p11–p12	Myoclonin1	JME
CACNA1H	16p13.3	T-type Ca^{2+} channel α$_{1H}$-subunit	CAE
CACNB4	2q22–q23	Ca^{2+} channel β$_4$-subunit	JME, JAE
CACNA1A	19p13	P/Q-type Ca^{2+} channel α$_{1A}$-subunit	CAE with ataxia
—	1p, 2q36, 3q26, 5q12–q14, 5q34, 6p21, 8q24, 8p, 9q32–q33 10q25–q26, 10p11, 11q13, 13q22–q31, 14q23 15q14, 18q21, 19q13	—	IGE, CAE, JME

Notes:
CAE, childhood absence epilepsy; EGMA, epilepsy with grand mal seizures on awakening; FS, febrile seizures; IGE, idiopathic generalized epilepsy; JAE: juvenile absence epilepsy; JME: juvenile myoclonic epilepsy.

findings emerged from other authors where the frequency was also higher in daughters (3.9%) than in sons (3.3%) of epileptic mothers (Tsuboi 1989).

Anatomical changes of brain architecture

Subtle developmental abnormalities of brain architecture (microdysgenesis) have been described in patients with IGE (Meencke and Janz 1984). There were no macroscopic abnormalities, and neurons and glial cells were normal morphologically. However these results were not replicated in a more recent study of five brains of IGE patients (Opeskin *et al.* 2000). Syndrome heterogeneity with different seizure types, the number of convulsive seizures suffered, the small sample sizes, and technical factors could contribute to this discrepancy. In patients with various IGE syndromes quantitative magnetic resonance imaging (MRI) studies have shown volume and structural abnormalities reflecting possible underlying structural abnormalities, supporting the idea that brains of patients with IGE may be morphologically abnormal (Woermann *et al.* 1998). The presence of subtle abnormalities of brain architecture remains an open question yet very interesting as it might represent the morphologic correlate of abnormal synaptic connectivity, due to genetic or acquired intrauterine factors, that underlie diffuse cortical hyperexcitability.

Treatment

Most IGEs are classified amongst the pharmacosensitive epilepsies in which appropriate drug treatment leads to seizure control, followed, after a few years, by spontaneous remission (Guerrini 2006). However, several studies that have evaluated the prognosis of IGEs, especially in the last 20 years, converge in indicating that seizures may persist into adulthood and promptly relapse after drug withdrawal (as typically seen in JME) or even be resistant throughout. This group of "refractory IGEs" includes patients who have more or less typical absences in childhood or adolescence which continue into adulthood, and may be accompanied by other seizure types such as myoclonus, atonic, tonic, or GTCSs. Some IGE patients have a fluctuating evolution; benign forms can manifest transient periods of worsening, whereas some difficult-to-treat patients may later experience spontaneous improvement.

Ethosuximide and valproic acid are the most appropriate drugs and suppress absences in 80% of CAE patients and 60% of JAE (Trinka *et al.* 2004; Grosso *et al.* 2005; Valentin *et al.* 2007). Factors predicting unfavorable prognosis are: TCS in the active stage of absences, myoclonic jerks, eyelid myoclonia or perioral myoclonia, failure of the first appropriate antiepileptic drug, and atypical EEG features (photoparoxysmal response, irregular ictal 3- to 4-Hz spike–wave complexes, excessive slow background activity during the waking record) (Loiseau and Panayiotopoulos 2005).

Juvenile myoclonic epilepsy is regarded as a benign but chronic disorder that may require lifelong treatment. About 80–90% of JME patients are controlled on valproate monotherapy (Thomas *et al.* 2002). Lamotrigine, either in combination with valproate or in monotherapy, can also be effective in a lower number of cases (Wallace 1998). Valproic acid has also been reported as effective in patients with IGE–TCS. However, there is also a significant subgroup of JME patients who pose difficult treatment problems; about 15.5% of JME are resistant to adequate drugs (Gelisse *et al.* 2001).

Aggravation of IGEs by inappropriate antiepileptic drugs is also increasingly recognized as a serious and common problem (Marini *et al.* 2005; Thomas *et al.* 2006). New-generation antiepileptic drugs such as levetiracetam, topiramate, and zonisamide have been proven to be useful in the treatment of pharmacoresistant IGEs (Verrotti *et al.* 2007; Noachtar *et al.* 2008; Marinas *et al.* 2009).

References

Andermann F (1967) Absence attacks and diffuse neuronal disease. *Neurology* 17:205–12.

Annegers JF, Hauser WA, Elveback LR, Anderson VE, Kurland LT (1976) Seizure disorders in offspring of parents with a history of seizures: a maternal–paternal difference? *Epilepsia* 17:1–9.

Annegers JF, Hauser WA, Anderson VE, Kurland LT (1982) The risks of seizure disorders among relatives of patients with childhood onset epilepsy. *Neurology* 32:174–9.

Appleton RE, Panayiotopoulos CP, Acomb BA, Beirne M (1993) Eyelid myoclonia with typical absences: an epilepsy syndrome. *J Neurol Neurosurg Psychiatry* 56:1312–16.

Appleton R, Beirne M, Acomb B (2000) Photosensitivity in juvenile myoclonic epilepsy. *Seizure* 9:108–11.

Asconape J, Penry JK (1984) Some clinical and EEG aspects of benign juvenile myoclonic epilepsy. *Epilepsia* 25:108–14.

Baruzzi A, Procaccianti G, Tinuper P, *et al.* (1988) Antiepileptic drug withdrawal in childhood epilepsies: preliminary results of a prospective study. In: Faienza C, Prati GL. (eds.) *Diagnostic and Therapeutic Problems in Pediatric Epileptology.* Amsterdam: Elsevier Science, pp. 117–23.

Berg AT, Shinnar S, Levy SR, *et al.* (2000) How well can epilepsy syndromes be identified at diagnosis? A reassessment two years after initial diagnosis. *Epilepsia* 41:1267–75.

Berkovic S (1996) Childhood absence epilepsy and juvenile absence epilepsy. In: Wyllie E (ed.) *The Treatment of Epilepsy: Principles and Practice.* Baltimore, MD: Williams and Wilkins, pp. 461–6.

Berkovic SF, Scheffer IE (2001) Genetics of the epilepsies. *Epilepsia* 42(Suppl 5):16–23.

Berkovic SF, Reutens DC, Andermann E, Andermann F (1994) The epilepsies: specific syndromes or a neurobiological continuum? In: Wolf P (ed.) *Epileptic Seizures and Syndromes.* Montrouge, France: John Libbey Eurotext, pp. 25–37.

Berkovic SF, Howell RA, Hay DA, Hopper JL (1998) Epilepsies in twins: genetics of the major epilepsy syndromes. *Ann Neurol* 43:435–45.

Bing F, Dananchet Y, Vercueil L (2005) A family with exercise-induced paroxysmal dystonia and childhood absence epilepsy. *Rev Neurol* 161:817–22.

Binnie CD, Darby CE, De Korte RA, Wilkins AJ (1980) Self-induction of epileptic seizures by eyeclosure: incidence and recognition. *J Neurol Neurosurg Psychiatry* 43:386–9.

Bureau M, Tassinari CA (2005) The syndrome of myoclonic absences. In: Roger J, Bureau M, Dravet C, Genton P, Tassinari CA, Wolf P (eds.) *Epileptic Syndromes in Infancy, Childhood and Adolescence,* 4th edn. Montrouge, France: John Libbey Eurotext, pp. 337–44.

Camfield C, Camfield P (2005) Management guidelines for children with idiopathic generalized epilepsy. *Epilepsia* 46(Suppl 9):112–16.

Camfield P, Camfield C (2002) Epileptic syndromes in childhood: clinical features, outcomes, and treatment. *Epilepsia* 43(Suppl 3):27–32.

Caraballo R, Cersosimo R, Medina C, Fejerman N (2000) Panayiotopoulos-type benign childhood occipital epilepsy: a prospective study. *Neurology* 55:1096–100.

Cavazzuti GB (1980) Epidemiology of different types of epilepsy in school age children of Modena, Italy. *Epilepsia* 21:57–62.

Cossette P, Liu L, Brisebois K, *et al.* (2002) Mutation of *GABRA1* in an autosomal dominant form of juvenile myoclonic epilepsy. *Nat Genet* 31:184–9.

Delgado-Escueta AV, Serratosa JM, Medina MT (1996) Juvenile myoclonic epilepsy. In: Wyllie E (ed.) *The Treatment of Epilepsy: Principles and Practice.* Baltimore, MD: Williams and Wilkins, pp. 484–501.

Doose H, Baier WK (1989) Absences. In: al B-Me (ed.) *Genetics of the Epilepsies.* Berlin: Spinger-Verlag, pp. 34–42.

Doose H, Volzke E, Scheffner D (1965) Verlaufsformen kindlicher epilepsien mit spike-wave-absencen. *Arch Psychiatr Nervenkrh* 207:394–15.

Dravet C, Bureau M (2002) Benign myoclonic epilepsy in infancy. In: Roger J, Bureau M, Dravet C, Genton P, Tassinari CA, Wolf P (eds.) *Epileptic Syndromes in Infancy, Childhood and Adolescence* 3rd edn. Montrouge, France: John Libbey Eurotext, pp. 69–79.

Durner M, Keddache MA, Tomasini L, *et al.* (2001) Genome scan of idiopathic generalized epilepsy: evidence for major susceptibility gene and modifying genes influencing the seizure type. *Ann Neurol* 49:328–35.

Engel J Jr. (2001) A proposed diagnostic scheme for people with epileptic seizures and with epilepsy: report of the ILAE Task Force on classification and terminology. *Epilepsia,* 42:796–803.

Forsgren L (2004) Incidence and prevalence. In: Wallace SJ, Farrel K (eds.) *Epilepsy in Children.* London: Arnold, pp. 21–5.

Gastaut H (1981) Individualisation des epilepsies dites "benignes" ou "fonctionnelles" aux differents ages de la vie. Appreciation des variations correspondantes de la predisposition epileptique a ces ages. *Rev EEG Neurophysiol* 11:346–66.

Gelisse P, Genton P, Thomas P, Rey M, Samuelian JC, Dravet C (2001) Clinical factors of drug resistance in juvenile myoclonic epilepsy. *J Neurol Neurosurg Psychiatry* 70:240–3.

Gilliam F, Steinhoff BJ, Bitterman HJ, *et al.* (2000) Adult myoclonic epilepsy: a distinct syndrome of idiopathic generalized epilepsy. *Neurology* 55:1030–3.

Greenberg DA, Delgado-Escueta AV, Maldonado HM, Widelitz H (1989) Segregation analysis of juvenile myoclonic epilepsy. In: Beck-Mannagetta G, Anderson VE, Doose H, Janz D (eds.) *Genetics of the Epilepsies.* Berlin: Springer-Verlag, pp. 53–61.

Grosso S, Galimberti D, Vezzosi P, *et al.* (2005) Childhood absence epilepsy: evolution and prognostic factors. *Epilepsia* 46:1796–801.

Guerrini R (2006) Epilepsy in children. *Lancet* 367:499–524.

Guerrini R, Bonanni P, Patrignani A, *et al.* (2001) Autosomal dominant cortical myoclonus and epilepsy (ADCME) with complex partial and generalized seizures: a newly recognized epilepsy syndrome with linkage to chromosome 2p11.1–q12.2. *Brain* 124:2459–75.

Guerrini R, Sanchez-Carpintero, Deonna R, *et al.* (2002) Early-onset absence epilepsy and paroxysmal dyskinesia. *Epilepsia* 43:1224–9.

Guerrini R, Bonanni P, Parmeggiani L, Hallett M, Oguni H (2005) Pathophysiology of myoclonic epilepsies. *Adv Neurol* 95:23–46.

Guiwer J, Valenti MP, Bourazza A, *et al.* (2003) Prognosis of idiopathic absence epilepsies. In: Jallon P, Berg A, Dulac O, Hauser A (eds.) *Prognosis of Epilepsies.*

Montrouge, France: John Libbey Eurotext, pp. 249–57.

Hauser WA, Annegers JF, Kurland LT (1993) Incidence of epilepsy and unprovoked seizures in Rochester, Minnesota: 1935–1984. *Epilepsia* **34**:453–68.

Hedstrom A, Olsson I (1991) Epidemiology of absence epilepsy: EEG findings and their predictive value. *Pediatr Neurol* **7**:100–4.

Helbig I, Scheffer IE, Mulley JC, Berkovic SF (2008) Navigating the channels and beyond: unravelling the genetics of the epilepsies. *Lancet Neurol* **7**:231–45.

Hempelmann A, Taylor KP, Heils A, *et al.* (2006) Exploration of the genetic architecture of idiopathic generalized epilepsies. *Epilepsia* **47**:1682–90.

Herpin T (1867) *Des Accès incomplets de l'épilepsies.* Paris, France: J Ballière et Fils.

Holmes GL, McKeever M, Adamson M (1987) Absence seizures in children: clinical and electroencephalographic features. *Ann Neurol* **21**:268–73.

ILAE Commission on Classification and Terminology (1989) Proposal for revised classification of epilepsies and epileptic syndromes. *Epilepsia* **30**:389–99.

Janz D (1985) Epilepsy with impulsive petit mal (juvenile myoclonic epilepsy). *Acta Neurol Scand* **72**:449–59.

Janz D, Christian W (1957) Impulsive-petit mal. *J Neurol* **176**:346–86.

Janz D, Beck-Mannagetta G, Sander T (1992) Do idiopathic generalized epilepsies share a common susceptibility gene? *Neurology* **42**(Suppl 5):48–55.

Jeavons PM (1977) Nosological problems of myoclonic epilepsies in childhood and adolescence. *Dev Med Child Neurol* **19**:3–8.

Lennox WG (1960) *Epilepsy and Related Disorders.* Boston, MA: Little, Brown.

Loiseau P (1992) Childhood absence epilepsy. In: Roger J, Bureau M, Dravet C, Dreifuss FE, Perret A, Wolf P (eds.) *Epileptic Syndromes in Infancy, Childhood and Adolescence* 2nd edn. Montrouge, France: John Libbey Eurotext, pp. 135–50.

Loiseau P, Panayiotopoulos CP (2005) *Childhood Absence Epilepsy.* Available online at www.ilae-epilepsy.org/Visitors/Centre/ctf.

Lugaresi E, Pazzaglia P, Franck L, *et al.* (1973) Evolution and prognosis of primary generalised epilepsy of the petit mal type. In: Lugaresi E, Pazzaglia P, Tassinari CA (eds.) *Evolution and*

Prognosis of Epilepsy. Bologna: Aulo Gaggi, pp. 106–20.

Marinas A, Villanueva V, Giraldez BG, *et al.* (2009) Efficacy and tolerability of zonisamide in idiopathic generalized epilepsy. *Epilept Disord* **11**:61–6.

Marini C, Harkin LA, Wallace RH, *et al.* (2003a) Childhood absence epilepsy and febrile seizures: a family with a GABA(A) receptor mutation. *Brain* **126**:230–40.

Marini C, King MA, Archer JS, *et al.* (2003b) Idiopathic generalised epilepsy of adult onset: clinical syndromes and genetics. *J Neurol Neurosurg Psychiatry* **74**:192–6.

Marini C, Scheffer IE, Crossland KM, *et al.* (2004) Genetic architecture of idiopathic generalized epilepsy: clinical genetic analysis of 55 multiplex families. *Epilepsia* **45**:467–78.

Marini C, Parmeggiani L, Masi G, D'Arcangelo G, Guerrini R (2005) Nonconvulsive status epilepticus precipitated by carbamazepine presenting as dissociative and affective disorders in adolescents. *J Child Neurol* **20**:693–6.

Mayville C, Fakhoury T, Abou-Khalil B (2000) Absence seizures with evolution into generalised tonic–clonic activity: clinical and EEG features. *Epilepsia* **41**:391–4.

Meencke HJ, Janz D (1984) Neuropathological findings in primary generalized epilepsy: a study of eight cases. *Epilepsia* **25**:8–21.

Mikami M, Yasuda T, Terao A, *et al.* (1999) Localization of a gene for benign adult familial myoclonic epilepsy to chromosome 8q23.3–q24.1. *Am J Hum Genet* **65**:745–51.

Noachtar S, Andermann E, Meyvisch P, *et al.* (2008) Levetiracetam for the treatment of idiopathic generalized epilepsy with myoclonic seizures. *Neurology* **70**:607–16.

Obeid T (1994) Clinical and genetic aspects of juvenile absence epilepsy. *J Neurol* **241**:487–91.

Okino S (1997) Familial benign myoclonus epilepsy of adult onset: a previously unrecognized myoclonic disorder. *J Neurol Sci* **145**:113–18.

Opeskin K, Kalnins RM, Halliday G, Cartwright H, Berkovic SF (2000) Idiopathic generalised epilepsy: lack of significant microdysgenesis. *Neurology* **55**:1101–06.

Ottman R, Annegers JF, Hauser WA, Kurland LT (1988) Higher risk of seizures in offspring of mothers than of fathers

with epilepsy. *Am J Hum Genet* **43**:257–64.

Panayiotopoulos CP, Obeid T (1989) Juvenile myoclonic epilepsy: an autosomal recessive disease. *Ann Neurol* **25**:440–3.

Panayiotopoulos CP, Ferrie CD, Giannakodimos S, Robinson RO (1995) Perioral myoclonia with absences. In: Duncan JS, Panayiotopoulos CP (eds.) *Typical Absences and Related Epileptic Syndromes.* London: Churchill Communications, pp. 221–30.

Penry JK, Porter RJ, Dreifuss FE (1975) Simultaneous recording of absence seizures with video tape and electroencephalography: a study of 374 seizures in 48 patients. *Brain* **98**:427–40.

Reutens DC, Berkovic SF (1995) Idiopathic generalized epilepsy of adolescence: are the syndromes clinically distinct? *Neurology* **45**:1469–76.

Ricci S, Cusmai R, Fusco L, Vigevano F (1995) Reflex myoclonic epilepsy in infancy: a new age-dependent idiopathic epileptic syndrome related to startle reaction. *Epilepsia* **36**:342–8.

Rocca WA, Sharbrough FW, Hauser WA, Annegers JF, Schoenberg BS (1987) Risk factors for generalized tonic-clonic seizures: a population-based case-control study in Rochester, Minnesota. *Neurology* **37**:1315–22.

Rossi PG, Parmeggiani A, Posar A, Santi A, Santucci M (1997) Benign myoclonic epilepsy: long-term follow-up of 11 new cases. *Brain Dev* **19**:473–9.

Sadleir LG, Scheffer IE, Smith S, *et al.* (2009) EEG features of absence seizures in idiopathic generalized epilepsy: impact of syndrome, age, and state. *Epilepsia* **50**:1572–8.

Sander T, Schulz H, Saar K, *et al.* (2000) Genome search for susceptibility loci of common idiopathic generalised epilepsies. *Hum Mol Genet* **9**:1465–72.

Sarisjulis N, Gamboni B, Plouin P, Kaminska A, Dulac O (2000) Diagnosing idiopathic/cryptogenic epilepsy syndromes in infancy. *Arch Dis Child* **82**:226–30.

Sato S, Dreifuss FE, Penry JK, Kirby DD, Palesch Y (1983) Long-term follow-up of absence seizures. *Neurology* **33**:1590–5.

Sauer H (1916) Über gehaufte kleine Anfalle hei Kindern (Pyknolepsie). *Mschr Psychiatr Neurol* 1916:40.

Scherman RG, Abraham, K (1963) "Centrencephalic"

electroencephalographic pattern in precocious puberty. *Electroencephalogr Clin Neurophysiol* **15**:559–67.

Suls A, Dedeken P, Goffin K, *et al.* (2008) Paroxysmal exercise-induced dyskinesia and epilepsy is due to mutations in *SLC2A1*, encoding the glucose transporter GLUT1. *Brain* **131**:1831–44.

Temkin O (1971) *The Falling Sickness.* Baltimore, MD: Johns Hopkins University Press.

Thomas P, Genton P, Gelisse P, Wolf P (2002) Juvenile myoclonic epilepsy. In: Roger J, Bureau M, Dravet C, Genton P, Tassinari CA, Wolf P (eds.) *Epileptic Syndromes in Infancy, Childhood and Adolescence*, 3rd edn. Montrouge, France: John Libbey Eurotext, pp. 335–56.

Thomas P, Valton L, Genton P (2006) Absence and myoclonic status epilepticus precipitated by antiepileptic drugs in idiopathic generalized epilepsy. *Brain* **129**:1281–92.

Trinka E, Baumgartner S, Unterberger I, *et al.* (2004) Long-term prognosis for childhood and juvenile absence epilepsy. *J Neurol* **251**:1235–41.

Tsuboi T (1989) Genetic risk in offspring of epileptic patients. In: Beck-Mannagetta G, Anderson VE, Doose H, Janz D (eds.) *Genetics of Epilepsies*. Berlin: Springer-Verlag, pp. 111–18.

Unterberger I, Trinka E, Luef G, Bauer G (2001) Idiopathic generalised epilepsy with pure grand mal: clinical and genetics data. *Epilepsy Res* **44**:19–25.

Valentin A, Hindocha N, Osei-Lah A, *et al.* (2007) Idiopathic generalized epilepsy with absences: syndrome classification. *Epilepsia* **48**:2187–90.

Verrotti A, Greco R, Giannuzzi R, Chiarelli F, Latini G (2007) Old and new antiepileptic drugs for the treatment of idiopathic generalized epilepsies. *Curr Clin Pharmacol* **2**:249–59.

Wallace SJ (1998) Myoclonus and epilepsy in childhood: a review of treatment with valproate, ethosuximide, lamotrigine and zonisamide. *Epilepsy Res* **29**:147–54.

Wirrell EC, Camfield CS, Camfield PR, Gordon KE, Dooley JM (1996) Long-term prognosis of typical childhood absence epilepsy: remission or progression to juvenile myoclonic epilepsy. *Neurology* **47**:912–18.

Woermann FG, Sisodiya SM, Free SL, Duncan JS (1998) Quantitative MRI in patients with idiopathic generalized epilepsy: evidence of widespread cerebral structural changes. *Brain* **121**:1661–7.

Wolf P (1992) Juvenile absence epilepsy. In: Roger J, Dravet C, Bureau M, Dreifuss FE, Wolf P (eds.) *Epileptic Syndromes in Infancy, Childhood and Adolescence*, 2nd edn. Montrouge, France: John Libbey Eurotext, pp. 307–12.

Yenjun S, Harvey AS, Marini C, *et al.* (2003) EEG in adult-onset idiopathic generalized epilepsy. *Epilepsia* **44**:252–6.

Chapter

13

Benign partial epilepsies of childhood

Roberto H. Caraballo and Natalio Fejerman

Introduction

The concept of idiopathic and benign partial epilepsies in childhood is relevant not only from the theoretical point of view, but also as a practical tool because the term implies absence of structural brain lesions and genetic predisposition to present age-dependent seizures. The term "benign" has been questioned for other epilepsy syndromes, because some epileptologists believe that benign implies a natural evolution to remission of seizures and electroencephalographic (EEG) abnormalities even without treatment. In this sense the group of benign partial epilepsies of childhood complies with the mentioned concept even when we must accept that there are exceptions confirming the rule. In agreement with the ILAE´s Commission report, we personally prefer the term "benign focal epilepsies" (Fejerman and Caraballo 2007a).

In 1967, two independent groups reported their series of patients with a peculiar form of epilepsy to be differentiated from other focal epilepsies, mainly from temporal lobe epilepsy. Loiseau et al. (1967) presented 122 cases with the onset of seizures at school age and rolandic paroxysms in the EEG. In 80% of their patients, seizures occurred during sleep and were frequently motor with predominance in the face. Lombroso (1967) made a clear description of the seizures emphasizing somatosensitive symptoms in the tongue, oral mucosa, and gums, along with speech arrest and proposed the term "sylvian seizures" recognizing also the particular focal EEG features. Both Loiseau et al. and Lombroso stressed the benign character of the condition regarding the evolution of the seizures and normalization of the EEG. In 1972 Blom et al. presented a prevalence and follow-up study proposing to name the condition "benign epilepsy of children with centrotemporal EEG foci." Atypical and not-so-benign evolutions have been reported in some patients with this form of epilepsy (Aicardi and Chevrie 1982; Fejerman and Di Blasi 1987; Fejerman et al. 2000, 2007). In the 2001 proposal of the Task Force on classification of the ILAE, "benign childhood epilepsy with centrotemporal spikes" (BCECTS) was included in the group of idiopathic focal epilepsies of childhood (Engel 2001)

and in the report of the Core Group on Classification of ILAE, BCECTS was again clearly identified as a recognized syndrome (Engel 2006). The most common name besides BCECTS appearing in the literature referring to this condition is "benign rolandic epilepsy." We recently reported on benign focal epilepsies in infancy, childhood, and adolescence, and analyzed all focal forms of benign epilepsies in these age groups (Fejerman and Caraballo 2007a).

Gastaut (1982) presented a series of 36 patients with seizures pointing to occipital lobe origin, associated migraine-like symptoms, and occipital paroxysms of spike–waves, and suggested this to be a new epileptic syndrome in childhood. The 1989 ILAE Commission named this syndrome "childhood epilepsy with occipital paroxysms" and included it in the group of localization-related idiopathic epilepsies together with BCECTS (ILAE Commission 1989). In 1989, two cardinal papers of Panayiotopoulos, based on a long follow-up of his patients called attention to the particular cluster of symptoms present in what he called "benign nocturnal childhood occipital epilepsy" (Panayiotopoulos 1989a,b). Vomiting as an ictal symptom and "cerebral insult-like" partial status epilepticus including autonomic symptoms were the main clinical manifestations (Panayiotopoulos 1989a,b). Thereafter, several authors preferred the eponymic nomenclature of "Panayiotopoulos syndrome" (PS) in order to include patients with and without occipital spikes or occipital ictal origin (Caraballo et al. 2000, 2007a; Ferrie et al. 2006; Fejerman and Caraballo 2007b; Fejerman and Panayiotopoulos 2008).

Fejerman and co-workers proposed designating the first syndrome as "Gastaut type of benign childhood occipital epilepsy" in order to distinguish it from the "Panayiotopoulos type of benign childhood occipital epilepsy" or Panayiotopoulos syndrome, which also manifests with occipital EEG paroxysms (Caraballo et al. 1997, 2000, 2007a; Fejerman 2002). These criteria were adopted by the Task Force on Classification and Terminology of the ILAE (Engel 2001).

It is interesting to mention the general and common electroclinical features that are characteristic of all types of benign partial epilepsies of childhood:

The Causes of Epilepsy, eds. S. D. Shorvon, F. Andermann, and R. Guerrini. Published by Cambridge University Press. © Cambridge University Press 2011.

- Normal neuropsychological and neurological exams
- Normal structural neuroimaging
- Significant familial antecedents of epilepsy
- Benign course
- EEG features:

  Normal background activity

  The spikes are broad, diphasic, of high-voltage (100–300 μV), and are often followed by a slow wave

  The spikes may occur isolated or in clusters, be bilateral, unilateral, synchronous, or asynchronous and multifocal

  The discharge rate is increased in drowsiness and in all stages of sleep

  Generalized spike-and-wave discharges may also be found.

In this chapter, we consider the etiologies of the benign partial epilepsies recognized in the Classification and Terminology of ILAE published in 2001 that include BCECTS, early-onset benign childhood occipital epilepsy "Panayiotopoulos type" (PS) and late-onset childhood occipital epilepsy "Gastaut type" (COE of Gastaut).

Benign childhood epilepsy with centrotemporal spikes

Benign childhood epilepsy with centrotemporal spikes accounts for about 15–25% of all epileptic syndromes in children between ages 4 and 12 (Panayiotopoulos 1999; Dalla Bernardina et al. 2005; Fejerman et al. 2007). Its annual incidence has been reported to be between 7.1 and 21 per 100 000 in children under age 15 (Heijbel et al. 1975). It has been recognized all over the world (Panayiotopoulos 1999; Fejerman and Caraballo 2007a). The prevalence of epilepsy is much higher among close relatives of children with BCECTS than in a matched control group (Bray and Wiser 1964). In one study, 15% of siblings had seizures and rolandic spikes, 19% of siblings had rolandic spikes without attacks, and 11% of the parents had had childhood seizures that had disappeared by adulthood (Heijbel et al. 1975).

Clinical features

A high incidence of familial antecedents of epilepsy (18–36%) has been confirmed by all investigators, and we shall see later that there are different genetic interpretations of these findings. About 7–10% of children with BCECTS have a personal history of febrile seizures.

The main clinical features of BCECTS are:

(1) The age of onset is between 4 and 10 years in 90% of the patients and the median age of onset is around 7 years (Dalla Bernardina et al. 2005; Fejerman et al. 2007).

(2) It is seen more frequently in males with a ratio to females of 3 : 2.

(3) Seizures are clearly related to sleep, whether during the night or the day. This is seen in 80–90% of the patients. In about

15% of the cases seizures occur both during sleep and while awake, and in near 10% only in waking states. Typical seizures last from 30–60 s to no more than 2–3 min (Fejerman et al. 2007). Typical clinical manifestation of BCECTS are:

(A) Orofacial motor signs, specially tonic or clonic contractions of one side of the face with predilection of the labial commissure (contralateral to centrotemporal spikes). Involvement of the ipsilateral eyelids is not unusual. More rarely, clonic convulsions may appear simultaneously in the ipsilateral limbs. There are also contractions of the tongue or jaw, guttural sounds, and drooling from hypersalivation and swallowing disturbance.

(B) Speech arrest, constituting anarthric seizures.

(C) Somatosensory symptoms. Unilateral numbness or paresthesia of the tongue, lips, gums, and inner cheek are frequent.

(D) Sialorrhea.

(E) Less frequent ictal manifestations. Although partial seizures are characteristic of this disorder, generalized seizures are not infrequently observed, particularly in younger children. In children aged 2–5 years, hemiclonic seizures last sometimes more than 30 min and may be followed by transient homolateral deficits, generally not including the face (Dalla Bernardina et al. 2005).

Electroencephalographic findings

The characteristic interictal EEG pattern has the following features:

(1) Background EEG activity is normal (Dalla Bernardina et al. 2005).

(2) Interictal epileptic discharges and location of spikes:

(A) Characteristics of spikes: the typical spikes (CTS) are located in centrotemporal or rolandic areas. They are high amplitude, diphasic, high-voltage (100–300 μV) spikes, with a transverse dipole, and they are often followed by a slow wave.

(B) Enhancement of discharges: the centrotemporal spikes are not enhanced by eye opening or closure, by hyperventilation, or photic stimulation. It has been reported that hyperventilation reduces the frequency of rolandic spikes (Fejerman et al. 2007). The discharge rate is increased in drowsiness and in all stages of sleep, and in about one-third of children, the spikes appear only in sleep (Lombroso 1967). Sleep EEG organization is preserved (Dalla Bernardina et al. 2005). In spite of their increasing frequency during sleep, the CTS show the same morphology as in wakefulness. A change in morphology, particularly the appearance of fast spikes or polyspikes, or a marked increase in the slow component, or a brief depression of voltage, evoke an organic etiology even when the ictal features are suggestive of BCECTS (Dalla Bernardina et al. 2005).

Etiology

There is enough evidence regarding the high incidence of a family history for epilepsy and focal EEG abnormalities suggesting the importance of genetic factors in the etiology of BCECTS (Bray and Wiser 1964; Blom et al. 1972; Degen and Degen 1990). Most of the authors suggest an autosomal dominant trait with variable penetrance (Bray and Wiser 1964; Heijbel et al. 1975). This type of inheritance was also suggested by studies of monozygotic twins with rolandic discharges (Kajitani et al. 1980), and human leukocyte antigens and their haplotypes (Eeg-Olofsson 1992). However, in another study of clinical and genetic aspects in children with benign focal sharp waves, including 134 probands with seizures (24% of which had typical rolandic seizures), the findings were in agreement with a multifactorial pathogenesis of epilepsies with "benign" focal epileptiform sharp waves (Doose et al. 1997). Expression of the gene may be influenced by other genetic and environmental factors (Loiseau and Duche 1989; Berkovic and Scheffer 1999). The mentioned series of papers were thoroughly analyzed on account of patient selection and interpretation of the EEGs, and doubts were cast regarding their methodology (Panayiotopoulos 1999). The same criticism is valid for the findings in siblings of patients with BCECTS, especially when they are compared to the known 2–3% of EEG abnormalities in the pediatric population. Nearly 10% of patients have a history of previous febrile seizures and this also suggests a genetic predisposition for febrile seizures expressed at earlier ages in children with BCECTS (Kajitani et al. 1992). However, previous interpretations or speculations regarding genetic influence on BCECTS have recently been questioned. In a study using population-based twin registries of epilepsy from Australia, Denmark, Norway, and the USA, 18 twin pairs were identified (10 monozygous; 8 dizygous) of whom at least one twin was diagnosed with classic BCECTS on the basis of electroclinical criteria with normal neurologic development. Patients with a compatible electroclinical picture but abnormal development were termed non-classic BCECTS. The twin data did not show any concordant twin pair with classic BCECTS, suggesting that non-inherited factors are of major importance in BCECTS. The authors found that genetic factors are probably more important in non-classic BCECTS. The conclusion at present is that the etiology and mode of inheritance are much more complicated than initially thought (Vadlamudi et al. 2006). Linkage to chromosome 15q14 was found in 54 patients from 22 families with BCECTS (Neubauer et al. 1998). However, in a study of 70 families with the same syndrome in Italy, the mentioned linkage could not be found (Pruna et al. 2000). A similar type of seizures and EEG phenotype of BCECTS was found in three children with de novo terminal deletions of the long arm of chromosome 1q and the authors suggested that it could be a potential site for a candidate gene (Vaughn et al. 1996). Recently, Strug et al. (2007) ascertained 38 families with linkage to chromosome 11p12–p13. They assumed a dominant inheritance with incomplete penetrance. More recently, the same

Table 13.1 Diagnosis of BCECTS in children with cerebral pathology

Occasional associations of BCECTS with non-evolutive cerebral lesions
BCECTS "phenotype" and unilateral focal heterotopia
BCECTS in children with cerebral palsy
• As a fortuitous association
• As a peculiar syndrome (not so benign) in children with unilateral polymicrogyria

group hypothesized that a non-coding mutation in elongator protein complex 4 impairs brain-specific elongator-mediated interaction of genes implicated in brain development, resulting in susceptibility to seizures and neurodevelopmental disorders (Strug et al. 2009).

The potassium chloride co-transpoter KCC3 was looked for as a candidate gene in 16 families with rolandic epilepsy, but the results did not support a role of KCC3 in the etiology of BCECTS (Steinlein et al. 2001).

The association of an autosomal recessive rolandic epilepsy with paroxysmal dystonia induced by exercise and writer´s cramp and its gene mapping to chromosome 16p12–p11.2 has been described (Guerrini et al. 1999).

A family with nine affected individuals in three generations was reported showing the features of rolandic epilepsy associated with oral and speech dyspraxia and cognitive impairment (Scheffer et al. 1995; Scheffer 1999). An X-linked French family with a similar phenotype of rolandic seizures with oral and speech dyspraxia and mental retardation has a mutation of SROX2 (Roll et al. 2006). Familial rolandic epilepsy with speech dyspraxia is a rare disorder and the different patterns of inheritance suggest genetic heterogeneity.

Another familial syndrome with rolandic spikes named partial epilepsy with pericentral spikes, linked to chromosome 4p, was described by Kinton et al. (2002); however, no other families have been published.

In Table 13.1 we summarize the alternatives of finding BCECTS phenotypes in children with cerebral pathology. Because of their prevalence, fortuitous associations may be found between BCECTS and non-evolutive brain lesions (Santanelli et al. 1989). Association with neuronal migration disorders has been described by several authors (Ambrosetto 1992; Sheth et al. 1997). The report of five cases of "pseudo-BCECTS" associated with brain tumors raises doubts about how typical their electroclinical phenotype was (Shevell et al. 1996). The last category in Table 13.1 refers to two possibilities: one, that children with cerebral palsy may also have a fortuitous association with CTS and rolandic seizures; the second is constituted by a large series of patients who had congenital hemiparesis associated with unilateral polymicrogyria and behave electroclinically in a quite similar way to our cases of BCECTS who present an atypical evolution with bilateral secondary synchrony in the EEG and transient neuropsychologic deterioration (Caraballo et al. 2007b).

Relations with other idiopathic epileptic syndromes

It is not so difficult to envisage that the non-exceptional findings of two idiopathic benign focal epilepsy syndromes occurring in the same patients might suggest that they constitute phenotypic variants of a single condition. In 1998 we reported 10 neurologically normal children who presented the following features: ictal vomiting in 10 cases, ictal anarthria in 10 cases, oculocephalic deviation in 9 cases, clonic partial seizures in 7 cases, 2 of them with secondary generalization. Seizures were prevalent during sleep. The EEGs showed occipital spikes during sleep in all cases and on wakefulness in 7 patients. The same EEGs showed independent centrotemporal spikes in 9 cases. We disclosed three well-defined groups: five children started with Panayiotopoulos syndrome (PS) and after a certain time presented seizures typical of BCECTS. The second group comprised three patients who featured in the same attack typical seizures of PS and BCECTS. Other two cases presented in different occasions independent seizures of BCECTS and PS (Caraballo *et al.* 1998). The association of BCECTS and childhood absence epilepsy has also been reported (Sarkis *et al.* 2009). Three children had typical BCECTS and 1–4 years after recovering from the electroclinical picture presented typical absences with generalized spike–wave discharges. Their long-term course was excellent (Gambardella *et al.* 1996). Generalized synchronous 3-Hz spike-and-wave complexes, as well as CTS, in the same EEG or in different recordings were also reported in five children. Two of them showed clinically both absences and focal motor seizures. The other two had only absences, and the other patient presented only focal motor seizures (Ramelli *et al.* 1998). Among our 398 cases of BCECTS we observed two patients who later presented typical absences. We have also presented clinical and EEG evidence of cases showing the association of other benign focal epilepsies with absence epilepsy, namely, patients with PS and late-onset occipital epilepsy of the Gastaut type, evolving into typical childhood absence epilepsies (Caraballo *et al.* 2004, 2005). It is also very interesting to quote the report of two siblings with benign familial neonatal convulsions who presented a few years later typical features of BCECTS (Maihara *et al.* 1999). We have mentioned that three of our patients with familial and non-familial benign infantile seizures presented during childhood typical electroclinical features of BCECTS, while another two only showed CTS (Caraballo *et al.* 2007b). It is interesting to note that one of them with benign infantile seizures linked to chromosome 16 (Caraballo *et al.* 2001) had typical electroclinical features compatible with rolandic epilepsy at 5 years of age and clinical manifestations of kinesigenic paroxysmal dyskinesia in the second decade of life. Her father presented with an isolated seizure in adolescence.

Another interesting association to consider is between idiopathic benign focal epilepsies and migraine. The relationship between epilepsies and migraine has been envisaged a long time ago (Andermann and Lugaresi 1987). We know that the prevalence of migraine in children is around 5% (Fejerman *et al.* 2007), while the prevalence of epilepsy is 1%. Therefore chances exist of coincidental co-occurrence of both conditions in the same persons. However, epidemiological data show that the prevalence of migraine in populations with epilepsy is around 10%, and the prevalence of epilepsy in migraineous populations is also significantly higher than in the general population (Andermann and Andermann 1987). Bladin (1987) presented evidence of association between BCECTS and migraine through the 5-to-8-year follow-up of 30 patients with BCECTS. In a more recent report, prevalence of migraine was compared in three cohorts of 53 children each: (a) children with BCECTS; (b) patients with cryptogenic/symptomatic partial epilepsy; (c) children with no history of seizures (Wirrell and Hamiwka 2006). The conclusion was that partial epilepsy, regardless of etiology, is associated with higher rates of migraine in children. In our series of 398 patients with BCECTS we also found an increased history of migraine in first-degree relatives and in the patients. Ion-channel dysfunction may be a common pathophysiological mechanism to explain the association of BCECTS and migraine. However, this intriguing association of two conditions clearly requires further investigations.

Panayiotopoulos syndrome

Panayiotopoulos syndrome (PS) is a clearly recognized syndrome and represents the second most frequent benign focal epilepsy syndrome in childhood, after BCECTS; PS is 4 to 8 times more frequent than the COE of Gastaut.

Three-quarters of patients have their first seizure between the ages of 3 and 6 years. It affects boys and girls almost equally. Seizures occur predominantly during sleep and in two-thirds of patients only during sleep. Onset of seizures occurring while awake may be inconspicuous with pallor, agitation, feeling sick, and vomiting (Fejerman and Caraballo 2007b; Fejerman and Panayiotopoulos 2008).

Seizures are usually of long duration, commonly lasting for more than 5 min, and in around 40% of the cases for longer than 30 min.

Clinical features
Core clinical features

Three groups of symptoms are the most important in PS (Panayiotopoulos 1999; Caraballo *et al.* 2000, 2007a; Ferrie *et al.* 2006, 2007).

(1) Ictal emetic symptoms and other autonomic manifestations: ictal vomiting, which is considered to be exceptional in other epilepsies, occurs in around 80% of the cases with PS. In seizures occurring while awake, other symptoms of the emetic spectrum such as nausea or retching may appear along with or before vomiting (Covanis *et al.* 2003). Pallor is the most frequent autonomic manifestation.

(2) Deviation of the eyes: unilateral deviation of the eyes is as common as vomiting and also occurs in around 80% of

the patients. Eye deviation is frequently accompanied by head deviation.

(3) Impairment of consciousness: consciousness is usually intact at seizure onset but becomes impaired in 80–90% of cases as the attack progresses.

Frequent features of seizures

Unilateral clonic or tonic–clonic seizures: at onset or following vomiting eye deviation is seen in 25–30% of the cases.

Secondarily generalized tonic–clonic seizures: usually follow seizures starting with focal motor manifestations. In one series, this course was seen in near 40% of the cases (Caraballo *et al.* 2000).

Status epilepticus: is usually non-convulsive, lasts longer than 30 min, and occurs in around 30% of cases in all series (Caraballo *et al.* 2000, 2007a; Ferrie *et al.* 2006, 2007).

Less frequent – but not rare – symptoms

Visual symptoms

Migraine-like headaches

Incontinence of urine and feces may occur when consciousness is impaired

Syncope-like manifestations.

Electroencephalographic findings

The most useful laboratory test is the EEG.

Interictal EEG: occipital spikes are bilateral and synchronous, often with voltage asymmetry, or unilateral. While awake, occipital EEG paroxysms of high amplitude with sharp and slow-wave complexes that occur immediately after closing the eyes are often recorded. These paroxysms are eliminated, or markedly attenuated, when the eyes are opened, a phenomenon due to fixation-off sensitivity (Panayiotopoulos 1999).

It has been emphasized that extraoccipital spikes (centrotemporal, frontal, parietal) may also be found in children with PS (Panayiotopoulos 1999; Caraballo *et al.* 2000, 2007a; Covanis *et al.* 2005). Normal EEGs during sleep are exceptional according to a recent consensus report (Ferrie *et al.* 2006).

Etiology

As an idiopathic epilepsy syndrome, PS is by definition not associated with remote symptomatic or acute symptomatic etiology. Most probably, it is genetically determined, although neither a gene nor a chromosomal locus has been found. Affected siblings with PS have been reported (Caraballo *et al.* 2000; Fejerman and Caraballo 2007b). Three siblings were reported in 1987 as having benign occipital epilepsy as described by Gastaut, although reading the paper, those three siblings showed seizures starting at ages 4 and 5 years, and the clinical features were quite compatible with PS (Kuzniecky and Rosenblatt 1987).

There is a high prevalence of febrile seizures in children with PS, ranging from 16% to 45% (Caraballo *et al.* 2000; Covanis *et al.* 2005; Fejerman and Caraballo 2007b). A family history of epilepsy was found in 30.3% of the cases (Caraballo *et al.* 2000).

The finding of several children with PS who had at the same time or later rolandic seizures and centrotemporal spikes typical of BCECTS (Caraballo *et al.* 1998) as well as siblings having either rolandic epilepsy or PS speaks in favor of a genetic linkage of these two syndromes, perhaps expressed as a reversible functional derangement of cortical maturation (Panayiotopoulos 1989b, 1999; Caraballo *et al.* 1998; Caraballo *et al.* 2000; Covanis *et al.* 2003).

Recently, a family with atypical PS has been reported with a *SCN1A* missense mutation in the proband (Grosso *et al.* 2007) and absence of the mutation in the brother with febrile seizures or in the parents. Two siblings with relatively early onset of seizures, prolonged time over which many seizures have occurred and strong association with febrile precipitants even after the age of 5 years (Livingston *et al.* 2009). These data indicate that *SCNIA* mutations when found contribute to a more severe clinical phenotype of PS.

Association of PS with other idiopathic epilepsy syndromes

Occasional findings of isolated cases with electroclinical features of BCECTS in children with idiopathic occipital epilepsies were reported in some series (Panayiotopoulos 1989b, 1999; Fejerman and Caraballo 2007b). In 1998, idiopathic partial epilepsies with rolandic and occipital spikes appearing in the same patients were reported in 10 cases. Five of them first had PS and after 2 or more years presented hemifacial motor seizures with anarthria typical of BCECTS. The other five patients presented anarthria and hemifacial contractions with scialorrhea and ictal vomiting with head deviation as typical seizures of PS and BCECTS in the same epoch and even in the same episodes (Caraballo *et al.* 1998). This finding was later ratified by another group of authors (Covanis *et al.* 2003). This coexistence and/or contiguous expression of PS and BCECTS in the same children is even more clear in our new series of patients presented in this chapter, because 24 out of 192 children with PS had seizures characteristic of BCECTS either concomitantly with typical PS seizures or in the course of the disease. Ten of them had ictal manifestations combining autonomic or occipital and rolandic features, six had both types of seizures independently and eight children developed rolandic seizures after a seizure-free period ranging from 2.5 to 4 years.

Another small series of cases reporting the presence of two idiopathic epilepsy syndromes in the same children showed that absence epilepsy was associated with the Gastaut of COE in five patients and with PS in one child (Caraballo *et al.* 2004).

Childhood occipital epilepsy of Gastaut

Childhood occipital epilepsy (COE) of Gastaut is a rare condition with a probable prevalence of 0.2–0.9% of all epilepsies, and 2–7% of benign childhood focal seizures (Covanis *et al.* 2005). It has been estimated at 0.15% of all focal epilepsies in childhood (Caraballo and Fejerman 2007).

Clinical features

The seizures of COE of Gastaut are always of occipital lobe onset and primarily manifest with visual symptoms, which are the most typical and usually the first ictal symptom, but other types of seizures may be associated. Motor seizures, migraine-like symptoms, and less frequently autonomic manifestations are also seen (Gastaut 1982; Gastaut *et al.* 1992; Caraballo *et al.* 1997, 2008a; Panayiotopoulos 1999; Covanis *et al.* 2005; Caraballo and Fejerman 2007a).

Visual seizures

Visual seizures occurred predominantly during the day at no particular time, but they may appear during sleep causing the patients to awake. They consist of elementary and complex visual hallucinations, visual illusions, blindness or partial visual loss and sensory hallucinations.

(1) The elementary visual hallucinations occur as an initial seizure symptom in the majority of the patients. These hallucinations are brief, seldom exceeding 1–2 min. They are always stereotyped, and usually multicolored and circular, appearing either in the periphery of a hemifield or centrally. They often may be the only ictal manifestation or they may progress to other seizure symptoms.

(2) Complex visual hallucinations are less frequent. The patient may see a face or figures, which often have the same location and movement sequence as that of the elementary visual hallucinations.

(3) Ictal visual illusions such as micropsia, metamorphopsia, palinopsia, and polyopia are probably generated from the non-dominant parietal regions (Covanis *et al.* 2005).

(4) Acute transient blindness is the second most common ictal symptom. It often occurs alone and may be the only ictal symptom in patients who experience visual hallucinations without blindness (Covanis *et al.* 2005; Caraballo *et al.* 2008a).

Motor seizures and other types of seizures

Deviation of the eyes, often associated with ipsilateral turning of the head, is the most common non-visual symptom, occurring in around 70% of patients. Forced eyelid closure and eyelid blinking occur in around 10% of patients.

Elementary visual hallucinations or other ictal symptoms may evolve into hemi or generalized convulsions.

Ictal vomiting is extremely rare in COE of Gastaut and probably represents overlapping between PS and COE of Gastaut (Caraballo *et al.* 1997).

Migraine-like symptoms

Ictal or postictal headache is a common symptom in 30–50% of the patients. As in migraine, the headache occurs immediately or within 5–10 min of the end of the visual hallucinations. The headache is often mild to moderate and diffuse, but may be severe and pulsating, and associated with nausea, vomiting, photophobia, and phonophobia, which may make it indistinguishable from migraine (Andermann and Zifkin 1998).

Electroencephalographic findings

In COE of Gastaut the EEG shows occipital paroxysms, which, in routine recordings, occur when the eyes are closed and disappear or attenuate upon eye opening, reflecting fixation-off sensitivity. EEGs with random occipital spikes, sometimes occurring only during sleep, are frequent.

Only a few patients with COE of Gastaut have occasional occipital spikes and consistently normal EEGs (Caraballo *et al.* 2008a). Centrotemporal, frontal, and giant somatosensory spikes may occur but less often than in PS (Caraballo and Fejerman 2007a).

Etiology

A family history of epilepsy is found in 20–30% of cases and a family history of migraine in 15%, approximately (Gastaut and Zifkin, 1987; Caraballo *et al.* 1997). A personal history of febrile seizures has been reported in 14% of cases with COE of Gastaut (Caraballo *et al.* 1997). Grosso *et al.* (2008) recently described two families with two members having COE of Gastaut.

Taylor *et al.* (2008) in a genetic study using twin and multiplex families in patients with PS and COE of Gastaut, found a single concordant monozygotic and dizygotic twin pair, suggesting that genetic factors play an important role in the etiology. The lack of concordance among monozygotic twins implies that non-conventional genetic influences such as somatic mutations and epigenetic or environmental factors are also likely to play a role (Fraga *et al.* 2005).

In some patients, the overlap between PS and COE of Gastaut has been observed (Caraballo *et al.* 2007a, 2008a; Taylor *et al.* 2008), and these two epileptic syndromes might be on a continuum related to a brain maturation process.

Patients with PS, COE of Gastaut, and BCECTS show EEG features in common with idiopathic generalized epilepsies. For example, generalized spike and wave on EEG has been reported in PS, COE of Gastaut, and BCECTS (Caraballo *et al.* 2007a, 2008a; Fejerman *et al.* 2007). We have also published reports of patients with childhood absence epilepsy and EEG focal abnormalities with or without clinical manifestations (Caraballo *et al.* 2008b). The overlap between idiopathic generalized and idiopathic focal epilepsies occurs at a number of levels, both within individuals and in the relatives. It is probably due to the complex inheritance that underlies the common idiopathic epilepsies where a number of genes contribute to the etiology as well as environmental factors.

Common genetic determinants might explain the finding of patients with idiopathic focal and generalized epilepsies. Further evidence to support this hypothesis has recently been provided by molecular studies. *SCN1A*, the gene encoding the α-subunit of the neuronal type 1 sodium channel, is mutated in generalized epilepsy with febrile seizures plus (Mulley *et al.*

2005). In generalized epilepsy with febrile seizures plus both generalized and focal epilepsies occur (Scheffer *et al.* 2007). On the other hand, a family with atypical PS has been reported with a *SCN1A* missense mutation in the proband (Grosso *et al.* 2007).

Association of COE of Gastaut with other idiopathic epilepsy syndromes

Two girls with typical BCECTS starting at 4 and 5 years of age and easily controlled with AED presented at age 12 years, after several years of freedom from seizures, clinical and EEG features of occipital lobe epilepsy with clear photosensitivity, reinforcing the concept of existence of different idiopathic epilepsy syndromes one after the other in the same children (Guerrini *et al.* 1997). Whether we consider the presence of photosensitivity triggering occipital seizures as part of a different syndrome or as a variant of COE of Gastaut is irrelevant in comparison to the fact that a focal idiopathic epileptic syndrome appeared in these two girls some time after remission of BCECTS. In our series of 33 cases, two girls of 14 and 16 years with photosensitive seizures also had had typical BCETS at ages 7 and 9 respectively. An interval of 3 and 4 years without seizures respectively elapsed between both syndromes (Caraballo *et al.* 2008a).

An association between COE of Gastaut and typical absence seizures in children has been reported by our group. Typical absences appeared at the same time as visual seizures in two patients, and after 1 year in three patients. All patients had occipital EEG paroxysms and 3-Hz generalized spike–wave discharges on the EEG (Caraballo *et al.* 2004). Recently, we published three patients with COE of Gastaut and a particular evolution. The patients had ictal events that were characterized by visual symptoms followed by typical absences. In two of them, the seizures continued despite antiepileptic drug treatment (Caraballo *et al.* 2005). One may interpret that the appearance of typical absences in these three patients might be due to the phenomenon of secondary bilateral synchronies.

We reported a group of patients, predominantly males, with childhood absence epilepsy and EEG focal abnormalities with or without clinical manifestations (Caraballo *et al.*

2008b). Seven had electroclinical features of idiopathic focal epilepsies, three presented seizures characteristic of PS, and the other four had seizures compatible with COE of Gastaut. The association of two different idiopathic focal and generalized epilepsies in the same patient may be merely coincidental, but a close genetic relationship between both epileptic syndromes might be another hypothesis. Another explanation could be that this series of patients represent a subgroup of childhood absence epilepsy.

Conclusions regarding the etiology of benign focal epilepsies in childhood

Despite recent evidence against the genetic etiology of typical cases of BCECTS (Vadlamundi *et al.* 2006), the general impression that there are genetic influences in the etiology of this group of conditions is still valid. Increased incidence of epilepsy in family members, increased incidence of CTS in siblings of children with BCECTS, increased incidence of febrile seizures in patients, occasional cases of siblings with the same syndrome, and association of two of these syndromes or of a focal idiopathic epilepsy with a generalized idiopathic epilepsy in patients constitute strong elements to support the role of genetics in the etiology of the benign focal epilepsies in childhood. Even more, the possibility of a continuum instead of a clear clinico-EEG cut between these syndromes has been repeatedly envisaged (Panayiotopoulos 1999; Fejerman and Caraballo 2007a; Taylor *et al.* 2008).

More information on chromosomal loci associated with these syndromes will help in tracking specific genes. Nevertheless, we have to be aware of coincidental or fortuitous associations with other etiologies. The best examples are the mentioned reported patients with BCECTS and non-evolutive brain lesions, heterotopias or micropolygyria, and brain tumors. Even more, a "malignant rolandic–sylvian epilepsy" was reported in children who ended up having cortical microdysgenesis (Otsubo *et al.* 2001). Of course, one may cast some doubt about the strictness in the recognition of the epileptic phenotypes described in all these apparent "symptomatic" cases of benign focal epilepsies in childhood.

References

Aicardi J, Chevrie JJ (1982) Atypical benign partial epilepsy of childhood. *Dev Med Child Neurol* **24**:281–92.

Ambrosetto G (1992) Unilateral opercular macrogyria and benign childhood epilepsy with centrotemporal (rolandic) spikes. *Epilepsia* **33**:499–503.

Andermann E, Andermann F (1987) Migraine epilepsy relationship: epidemiological and genetic aspects. In: Andermann F, Lugaresi E (eds.) *Migraine and Epilepsy*. Boston, MA: Butterworth, pp. 281–92.

Andermann F, Lugaresi E (eds.) (1987) *Migraine and Epilepsy*. Boston, MA: Butterworth.

Andermann F, Zifkin B (1998) The benign occipital epilepsies of childhood: an overview of the idiopathic syndromes and of the relationship to migraine. *Epilepsia* **39**(suppl 4):59–23.

Berkovic SF, Scheffer IE (1999) Genetics of partial epilepsies: new frontiers. In: Berkovic SF, Genton P, Hirsch E, Picard F (eds.) *Genetics of Focal Epilepsies*. Montrouge, France: John Libbey Eurotext, pp. 7–14.

Bladin PF (1987) The association of benign rolandic epilepsy with migraine. In: Andermann F, Lugaresi E (eds.) *Migraine and Epilepsy*. Boston, MA: Butterworth, pp. 145–52.

Blom S, Heijbel J, Bergfors PG (1972) Benign epilepsy of children with centrotemporal foci: prevalence and follow-up study of 40 patients. *Epilepsia* **13**:609–19.

Bray PF, Wiser WC (1964) Evidence for a genetic etiology of temporal central abnormalities in focal epilepsy. *N Engl J Med* **271**:926–33.

Caraballo R, Fejerman N (2007a) Late-onset childhood occipital epilepsy (Gastaut type). In: Fejerman N, Caraballo R (eds.) *Benign Focal Epilepsies in Infancy, Childhood and Adolescence*. Montrouge, France: John Libbey Eurotext, pp. 145–67.

Caraballo R, Fejerman N (2007b) Benign familial and non-familial infantile seizures. In: Fejerman N, Caraballo R (eds.) *Benign Focal Epilepsies in Infancy, Childhood and Adolescence*. Montrouge, France: John Libbey Eurotext, pp. 31–49.

Caraballo RH, Cersosimo RO, Medina CS, Tenembaum S, Fejerman N (1997) Epilepsias parciales idiopáticas con paroxismos occipitales. *Revista de Neurologia* 25:1052–8.

Caraballo R, Cersosimo R, Fejerman N (1998) Idiopathic partial epilepsies with rolandic and occipital spikes appearing in the same children. *J Epilepsy* 11:261–4.

Caraballo R, Cersosimo R, Medina C, Fejerman N (2000) Panayiotopoulos-type benign childhood occipital epilepsy: a prospective study. *Neurology* 55:1096–100.

Caraballo R, Pavek S, Lemainque A, et al. (2001) Linkage of benign familial infantile convulsions to chromosome 16p12–q12 suggests allelism to the infantile convulsions and choreoathetosis syndrome. *Am J Hum Genet* 68:788–94.

Caraballo RH, Sologuestua A, Granana N, et al. (2004) Idiopathic occipital and absence epilepsies appearing in the same children. *Pediatr Neurol* 30:24–8.

Caraballo RH, Cersosimo RO, Fejerman N (2005) Late-onset, "Gastaut type", childhood occipital epilepsy: an unusual evolution. *Epileptic Disord* 7:341–6.

Caraballo R, Cersósimo R, Fejerman N (2007a) Panayiotopoulos syndrome: a prospective study of 192 patients. *Epilepsia* 48:1054–61.

Caraballo R, Cersósimo R, Fejerman N (2007b) Symptomatic focal epilepsies imitating atypical evolutions of idiopathic focal epilepsies in childhood. In: Fejerman N, Caraballo R (eds.) *Benign Focal Epilepsies in Infancy, Childhood and Adolescence*. Montrouge, France: John Libbey Eurotext, pp. 221–39.

Caraballo R, Cersósimo R, Fejerman R (2008a) Childhood occipital epilepsy of Gastaut: study of 33 patients. *Epilepsia* 49:288–97.

Caraballo R, Fontana E, Darra F, et al. (2008b) Childhood absence epilepsy and electroencephalographic focal abnormalities with or without clinical manifestations. *Seizures* 17:617–24.

Covanis A, Lada C, Skiadas K (2003) Children with rolandic spikes and ictus emeticus: rolandic epilepsy or Panayiotopoulos syndrome? *Epileptic Disorders* 5:139–43.

Covanis A, Ferrie CD, Koutroumanidis M, et al. (2005) Panayiotopoulos syndrome and Gastaut type idiopathic childhood occipital epilepsy. In: Roger J, Bureau M, Dravet C, Genton P, Tassinari CA, Wolf P (eds.) *Epileptic Syndromes in Infancy, Childhood and Adolescence*, 4th edn. Montrouge, France: John Libbey Eurotext, pp. 227–53.

Dalla Bernardina B, Sgro V, Fejerman N (2005) Epilepsy with centrotemporal spikes and related syndromes. In: Roger J, Bureau M, Dravet C, Genton P, Tassinari CA, Wolf P (eds.) *Epileptic Syndromes in Infancy, Childhood and Adolescence*, 4th edn. Montrouge, France: John Libbey Eurotext, pp. 203–25.

Degen R, Degen HE (1990) Some genetic aspects of rolandic epilepsy: waking and sleep EEGs in siblings. *Epilepsia* 31:795–801.

Doose H, Brigger-Heuer B, Neubauer B (1997) Children with focal sharp waves: clinical and genetic aspects. *Epilepsia* 38:788–96.

Eeg-Olofsson O (1992) Further genetic aspects in benign localized epilepsies in early childhood. In: Degen R, Dreifuss FE (eds.) *Benign Localized and Generalized Epilepsies of Early Childhood*. Amsterdam: Elsevier, pp. 117–19.

Engel J Jr. (2001) A proposed diagnostic scheme for people with epileptic seizures and with epilepsy: report of the ILAE Task Force on Classification and Terminology. *Epilepsia* 42:796–803.

Engel J (2006) Report of the ILAE Classification Core Group. *Epilepsia* 47:1558–68.

Fejerman N (2002) Benign focal epilepsies in infancy, childhood and adolescence. *Rev Neurol* 34:7–18.

Fejerman N, Caraballo R (eds.) (2007a) *Benign Focal Epilepsies in Infancy, Childhood and Adolescence*. Montrouge, France: John Libbey Eurotext.

Fejerman N, Caraballo R (2007b) Panayiotopoulos syndrome. In: Fejerman N, Caraballo R (eds.) *Benign Focal Epilepsies in Infancy, Childhood and Adolescence*. Montrouge, France: John Libbey Eurotext, pp. 115–144.

Fejerman N, Panayiotopoulos CP (2008) Early-onset benign childhood occipital epilepsy (Panayiotopoulos type). In: Engel J, Pedley T (eds.) *Epilepsy: A Comprehensive Textbook*, 2nd edn. Philadelphia, PA: Lippincott Williams and Wilkins, pp. 2379–86.

Fejerman N, Di Blasi AM (1987) Status epilepticus of benign partial epilepsies in children: report of two cases. *Epilepsia* 28:351–5.

Fejerman N, Caraballo R, Tenembaum SN (2000) Atypical evolutions of benign localization-related epilepsies in children: are they predictable? *Epilepsia* 41:380–90.

Fejerman N, Caraballo R, Dalla Bernardina B (2007) Benign childhood epilepsy with centrotemporal spikes. In: Fejerman N, Caraballo R (eds.) *Benign Focal Epilepsies in Infancy, Childhood and Adolescence*. Montrouge, France: John Libbey Eurotext, pp. 77–113.

Ferrie CD, Caraballo RH, Covanis A, et al. (2006) Panayiotopoulos syndrome: a consensus view. *Dev Med Child Neurol* 48:236–40.

Ferrie CD, Caraballo R, Covanis A, et al. (2007) Autonomic status epilepticus in Panayiotopoulos syndrome and other childhood and adult epilepsies: a consensus view. *Epilepsia* 48:1165–72.

Fraga MF, Ballestar E, Paz MF, et al. (2005) From the cover epigenetic differences arise during the lifetime of monozygotic twins. *Proc Natl Acad Sci USA* 102:604–9.

Gambardella A, Aguglia U, Guerrini R, et al. (1996) Sequential occurrence of benign partial epilepsy and childhood absence epilepsy in three patients. *Brain Dev* 18:212–15.

Gastaut H (1982) A new type of epilepsy: benign partial epilepsy of childhood with occipital spike-waves. *Clin Electroencephalogr* 13:13–22.

Gastaut H, Zifkin B (1987) Benign epilepsy of childhood with occipital spike and wave complexes. In: Andermann F, Lugaresi E (eds.) *Migraine and Epilepsy*. Boston, MA: Butterworth, pp. 47–81

Gastaut H, Roger J, Bureau M (1992) Benign epilepsy of childhood with occipital paroxysms: update. In: Roger J, Bureau M, Dravet C, Dreifuss FE, Perret A, Wolf P (eds.) *Epileptic Syndromes in Infancy, Childhood and Adolescence*, 2nd edn. Montrouge, France: John Libbey Eurotext, pp. 201–17.

Grosso S, Orrico A, Galli L, et al. (2007) SCN1A mutation associated with atypical Panayiotopoulos syndrome. *Neurology* 69:609–11.

Grosso S, Vivarelli R, Gobbi G, et al. (2008) Late-onset childhood occipital epilepsy (Gastaut type): a family study. Eur J Paediatr Neurol 12:421–6.

Guerrini R, Bonanni P, Parmeggiani L, Belmonte A (1997) Adolescent onset of idiopathic photosensitive occipital epilepsy after remission of benign rolandic epilepsy. Epilepsia 38:777–81.

Guerrini R, Bonanni P, Nardocci N, et al. (1999) Autosomal recessive rolandic epilepsy with paroxysmal exercise-induced dystonia and writer's cramp: delineation of the syndrome and gene mapping to chromosome 16p12–11.2. Ann Neurol 45:344–52.

Heijbel J, Blom S, Rasmuson M (1975) Benign epilepsy of childhood with centrotemporal EEG foci: a genetic study. Epilepsia 16:285–93.

ILAE Commission on Classification and Terminology (1989) Proposal for revised classification of epilepsies and epileptic syndromes. Epilepsia 30:389–99.

Kajitani T, Nakamura M, Ueoka K, Koduchi S (1980) Three pairs of monozygotic twins with rolandic discharges. In: Wada J, Penny J (eds.) Advances in Epileptology: The Tenth International Symposium. New York: Raven Press, pp. 171–5.

Kajitani T, Kimura T, Sumita M, Kaneko M (1992) Relationship between benign epilepsy of children with centrotemporal EEG foci and febrile convulsions. Brain Dev 14:230–4.

Kinton L, Johnson MR, Smith SJ, et al. (2002) Partial epilepsy with pericentral spikes: a new familial epilepsy syndrome with evidence for linkage to chromosome 4p15. Ann Neurol 51:740–9.

Kuzniecky R, Rosenblatt B (1987) Benign occipital epilepsy: a family study. Epilepsia 28:346–50.

Livingston JH, Cross JH, McLellan A, et al. (2009) A novel inherited mutation in the voltage sensor region of SCN1A is associated with Panayiotopoulos syndrome in siblings and generalised epilepsy with febrile seizures plus. J Child Neurol 24:503–8.

Loiseau P, Duche B (1989) Benign childhood epilepsy with centrotemporal spikes. Cleve Clin J Med 56:517–22.

Loiseau P, Cohadon F, Mortureux Y (1967) A propos d'une forme singulière d'épilepsie de l'enfant. Rev Neurol (Paris) 116:244–8.

Loiseau P, Duche B, Cordova S, Dartigues JF, Cohadon S (1988) Prognosis of benign childhood epilepsy with centrotemporal spikes: a follow-up study of 168 patients. Epilepsia 29:229–35.

Lombroso CT (1967) Sylvian seizures and midtemporal spike foci in children. Arch Neurol 17:52–9.

Maihara T, Tsuji M, Higuchi Y, Hattori H (1999) Benign familial neonatal convulsions followed by benign epilepsy with centrotemporal spikes in two siblings. Epilepsia 40:110–13.

Mulley JC, Scheffer IE, Petrou J, et al. (2005). SCN1A mutations and epilepsy. Hum Mutat 25:535–42.

Neubauer BA, Fiedler B, Himmelein B, et al. (1998) Centrotemporal spikes in families with rolandic epilepsy: linkage to chromosome 15q14. Neurology 51:1608–12.

Otsubo H, Chiloku S, Ochi A, et al. (2001) Malignant rolandic–sylvian epilepsy in children: diagnostic, treatment, and outcomes. Neurology 57:590–6.

Panayiotopoulos CP (1989a) Benign childhood epilepsy with occipital paroxysms: a 15-year prospective study. Ann Neurol 26:51–6.

Panayiotopoulos CP (1989b) Benign nocturnal childhood occipital epilepsy: a new syndrome with nocturnal seizures, tonic deviation of the eyes, and vomiting. J Child Neurol 4:43–9.

Panayiotopoulos CP (1999) Benign Childhood Partial Seizures and Related Epileptic Syndromes. Montrouge, France: John Libbey Eurotext.

Panayiotopoulos CP, Igoe DM (1992) Cerebral insult-like partial status epilepticus in the early-onset variant of benign childhood epilepsy with occipital paroxysms. Seizure 1:99–102.

Pruna D, Persico I, Serra D, et al. (2000) Lack of association with the 15q14 candidate region for benign epilepsy of childhood with centro-temporal spikes in a Sardinian population. Epilepsia 41:164.

Ramelli GP, Donati F, Moser H, Vassella F (1998) Concomitance of childhood absence and rolandic epilepsy. Clin Electroencephalogr 29:177–80.

Roll P, Rudolf G, Pereira S, et al. (2006) SRPX2 mutations in disorders of language cortex and cognition. Hum Mol Genet 15:1195–207.

Santanelli P, Bureau M, Magaudda A, et al. (1989) Benign partial epilepsy with centrotemporal (or rolandic) spikes and brain lesion. Epilepsia 30:182–8.

Sarkis R, Loddenkemper T, Burgess RC, et al. (2009) Childhood absence epilepsy in patients with benign focal epileptiform discharges. Pediatr Neurol 41:428–34.

Scheffer IE (1999) Autosomal dominant rolandic epilepsy with speech dyspraxia. In: Berkovic SF, Genton P, Hirsch E, Picard F (eds.) Genetics of Focal Epilepsies. Montrouge, France: John Libbey Eurotext, pp. 109–14.

Scheffer IE, Jones L, Pozzebon M, et al. (1995) Autosomal dominant rolandic epilepsy and speech dyspraxia: a new syndrome with anticipation. Ann Neurol 38:633–42.

Scheffer IE, Harkin LA, Grinton DE, et al. (2007) Temporal lobe epilepsy and GEFS+, phenotypes associated with SCN1B mutations. Brain 130:100–9.

Sheth RD, Gutierrez AR, Riggs JE (1997) Rolandic epilepsy and cortical dysplasia: MRI correlation of epileptiform discharges. Pediatr Neurol 17:177–9.

Shevell MI, Rosenblatt B, Watters GV, et al. (1996) "Pseudo-BECRS": intracranial focal lesions suggestive of a primary partial epilepsy syndrome. Pediatr Neurol 14:31–5.

Steinlein OK, Neubauer BA, Sander T, et al. (2001) Mutation analysis of the potassium chloride cotransporter KCC3 (SLC12A6) in rolandic and idiopathic generalized epilepsy. Epilepsy Res 44:191–5.

Strug LJ, Clarke T, Bali B, et al. (2007) Major locus for centrotemporal sharp waves in rolandic epilepsy families maps to chromosome 11p. Ann Neurol 62:95.

Strug L, Clarke T, Chiang T, et al. (2009) Centrotemporal sharp wave EEG trait in rolandic epilepsy maps to elongator protein complex 4 (ELP4). Eur J Hum Genet 17:1171–81.

Taylor I, Berkovic S, Kivity S, Scheffer I (2008) Benign occipital epilepsies of childhood: clinical features and genetics. Brain 131:2287–94.

Vadlamudi L, Kjeldsen MJ, Corey LA, et al. (2006) Analyzing the etiology of benign rolandic epilepsy: a multicenter twin collaboration. Epilepsia 47:550–5.

Vaughn BV, Greenwood RS, Aylsworth AS, Tennison MB (1996) Similarities of EEG and seizures in del(1q) and benign rolandic epilepsy. Pediatr Neurol 15:261–4.

Wirrell EC, Hamiwka LD (2006) Do children with benign rolandic epilepsy have a higher prevalence of migraine than those with other partial epilepsies or nonepilepsy controls? Epilepsia 47:1674–81.

Introduction to the concept of symptomatic epilepsy

Simon D. Shorvon

The concept of "symptomatic epilepsy" might, at first glance, seem fairly straightforward, but in fact this is not the case. There are conceptual issues, problems with definition, and difficulties in assessing frequency and in differentiating causes. These problems are indeed, given our current level of knowledge, to a large extent insurmountable. The purpose of this chapter is to clarify terminology, to highlight some of the issues surrounding this topic, and to set the clinical context for the chapters that follow. Questions are more easily posed than answered, but what is clear is that more emphasis on etiology in epilepsy would change fundamentally our conceptual approach to the condition.

Definitions

The definition of *symptomatic epilepsy* has changed over time. As discussed in Chapter 1, for most of the nineteenth century symptomatic epilepsy (often previously known as organic epilepsy) was not considered to be a "genuine epilepsy" at all, and was rather ignored. The pendulum swung, and by the middle of the twentieth century, it had become axiomatic that most epilepsies were in fact symptomatic – in the sense that the epilepsy was a symptom of an underlying cause, even if the cause could not be identified (as Wilson [1940] called this, cryptogenic epilepsy). In more recent times, a new meaning has been assigned to the term, largely because the meaning of its opposite, idiopathic epilepsy, has changed. The term *idiopathic epilepsy* was previously used to denote any epilepsy in which there was no demonstrable cause, but is now used for those epilepsies that are primarily genetic in origin and in which there is no gross neuroanatomical or neuropathological abnormality (the change of emphasis in which "idiopathic" was equated with "genetic" was enshrined in the 1989 revision of the classifications of the epilepsies). The current usage of the term excludes the genetic epilepsies in which there are detectable neuropathological changes.

Symptomatic epilepsy was a term originally used to denote any epilepsy in which the cause was identified, but the current definition can usefully be formulated as follows:

Symptomatic epilepsy is an epilepsy, of an acquired or genetic cause, associated with neuro-anatomical or neuropathological abnormalities indicative of an underlying disease or condition.

The term differentiates these epilepsies from the *idiopathic epilepsies* the use of which term is now confined to genetic epilepsies in which there is no gross anatomical or pathological abnormality, and from the *cryptogenic epilepsies* which are those epilepsies in which the cause is not known (but which are often assumed to be covert "symptomatic" cases), and also from the *provoked epilepsies* which are epilepsies precipitated by a systemic non-neurological disturbance in the absence of neuropathological change (see below).

Included in the category of "symptomatic" are thus: (a) all epilepsies due to acquired cerebral causes, whether of known environmental causation or not; and also (b) epilepsies due to genetic causes where these result in either gross anatomical change (for instance the epilepsy due to tuberose sclerosis or neurofibromatosis) or more subtle changes at the molecular pathological level (for example the epilepsies due to Rett syndrome, CDKL5, Angelman syndrome); and also (c) epilepsies due to developmental abnormalities where there are neuropathological changes, despite the fact that these are due to aberrant development rather than to an external acquired cause (some have a genetic basis and others have an external cause producing in utero damage to the developing brain, such as infection, radiation, toxin, etc.). The developmental/congenital disorders are a gray area between core "idiopathic" and core "acquired" epilepsies, and their inclusion under the term symptomatic epilepsy reflects the inevitably artificial nature of all classification schemes.

The term "acquired" is used to refer to "symptomatic" epilepsies excluding the predominately genetic or developmental causes. We do not use the term to mean *due to external or environmental causes*, as some symptomatic epilepsies are due to internal pathological processes which have no known major environmental component (e.g., tumor, neurodegenerative disorders, autoimmune disorders).

The Causes of Epilepsy, eds. S. D. Shorvon, F. Andermann, and R. Guerrini. Published by Cambridge University Press. © Cambridge University Press 2011.

Table 14.1 The classification of epilepsy according to cause[a]

Idiopathic epilepsy	Epilepsy of predominately genetic causation without detectable gross neuropathological abnormality
Symptomatic epilepsy	Epilepsy of predominately acquired causation or genetic causation with gross neuropathological abnormality
Cryptogenic epilepsy	Epilepsy where the cause is unknown
Provoked epilepsy[b]	Epilepsy predominately of non-cerebral causation

Notes:
[a] The causation of epilepsy is often multifactorial.
[b] The inclusion of the category of "provoked epilepsy" is discussed further in the text.

Table 14.2 The categories of symptomatic epilepsy

Symptomatic epilepsy of predominately genetic or developmental causation
Epilepsy syndromes
Progressive myoclonic epilepsies
Neurocutaneous syndromes
Other single-gene disorders
Disorders of chromosomal or genomic structure
Developmental anomalies of cerebral structure
Symptomatic epilepsy of predominately acquired causation
Hippocampal sclerosis
Perinatal and infantile causes
Degenerative and other neurological diseases
Cerebral trauma
Cerebral tumor
Cerebral infection
Cerebral vascular disorders
Cerebral immunological disorders

Also excluded are the epilepsies due to systemic non-neurological diseases (e.g., fever, metabolic change, reflex epilepsy) without neuropathological findings; these are categorized under the term "provoked epilepsy" (see below). This scheme of classification is described in Chapter 2; the main categories are outlined in Table 14.1.

Of course this definition is open to criticisms on a number of fronts:

(1) The *idiopathic epilepsies* might have subtle anatomical abnormalities, or synaptic, membrane, neurotransmitter, or network changes (indeed these are assumed to be present, although none has been identified). The distinction from symptomatic epilepsy, based as it is on the absence of a "gross lesion," is to an extent therefore arbitrary.

(2) Epilepsy etiology is often multifactorial. Many (probably most) epilepsies are caused by a mixture of both genetic and environmental factors (as Lennox [1960] pointed out). In some, one cause may predominate, but it may be difficult to know where to draw the line. The distinction again is to an extent arbitrary.

(3) The assignment of a case to the category of "cyptogenic" versus "symptomatic" epilepsy will depend on the extent of investigation, and the weight put on clinical findings. There are no guidelines on this point, and again the distinction is arbitrary.

(4) Many genetic influences are not "all or none" but confer susceptibility. Where the line is drawn in these cases between a genetic or cryptogenic categorization is arbitrary. Also, some of the provoked epilepsies may occur only in those with an inherited susceptibility, and this point is discussed further in Chapter 88.

(5) Alternative "etiological" classifications can be proposed, of which perhaps the most appealing is the division of the epilepsies into idiopathic/prenatal (developmental and congenital) causes/postnatal causes. This avoids the difficulty of categorizing the developmental/congenital disorders, but poses other nosological problems. What is clear is that the etiological classifications, in common with semiological and electrographic classifications of epilepsy, have gray areas and inconsistencies. Furthermore, although such issues of terminology and definition do not matter much in the clinical care of individual cases (after all, what's in a name?), they are important for communication and in research and for adopting a conceptual approach to the topic of epilepsy.

This section of the book are concerned with symptomatic epilepsy, defined as above. In this book, the category includes the neurocutaneous diseases, progressive myoclonic epilepsies, genetic metabolic disorders, and developmental disorders which have often a strong genetic component, but are included in the symptomatic category because they cause gross cerebral abnormalities. The other symptomatic epilepsies are divided into major categories as shown in Table 14.2. Some of these categories are to an extent artificial and there can be overlap. The provoked seizures are considered separately.

Mechanism versus etiology

As emphasized in Chapter 1, "etiology" in epilepsy, to the nineteenth-century physician, usually referred to "the mechanism of epilepsy" rather than its underlying cause. The mechanistic approach was pioneered by Hughlings Jackson (1874) who considered that all seizures had a final common pathway (an imbalance in excitation due to largely vascular factors) and that this was the "cause" of epilepsy. He was not concerned about the downstream factors contributing to this final common pathway, either genetic or acquired. This is the approach still taken by experimental epileptology, in which the mechanisms of "epileptogenesis" are studied with more or less disregard to the downstream causes (except for a broad distinction often made between the mechanisms of genetic channelopathies and other types of epilepsy – see Chapters 3 and 4).

Frequency of different underlying etiologies

There are difficulties in assessing how commonly different etiologies cause epilepsy, in part due to the facts that:

(1) Epilepsy is multifactorial. Thus, in many cases the assignment of cause is, to some extent, arbitrary. In a patient, for instance, with a history of stroke, alcoholism, and head injury, it is likely that all three contribute to epilepsy, in adition to genetic factors, although their relative contributions can not be assessed, and nor can it be foretold whether the epilepsy would have arisen if only the leading potential cause was present.

(2) Etiology will depend to a very great extent on the population under study. For instance, the range of etiologies is very different in young children compared to adults, in Africa compared to Europe, in hospital practice compared to community practice. Furthermore, the gold standard for minimizing bias is of course the large-scale epidemiologically based case–control study, but in such studies investigatory tools are used (thus, some but not all cases may have had high-quality magnetic resonance imaging [MRI] scanning, full assessment of metabolic status, etc.).

(3) Different investigations have used different investigatory tools. When MRI scanning was introduced, for instance, a causal lesion was found in at least 30% of cases which had been previously undetected. Furthermore, as the technical quality of MRI increases, so too does the yield of more subtle abnormalities. Similarly, in infants and young children, the assessment of etiology may require intensive metabolic or genetic testing not always freely available worldwide.

(4) Definitions are often not standardized (for instance in large-scale registry-based studies). This will affect the assignment of etiology, for instance of alcohol-related epilepsy, epilepsy after head injury (especially where mild), and of epilepsy in vascular disease.

(5) Ideally, case–control studies of comorbidities are needed in order to assign cause. Thus, for instance, in assessing the role of mild vascular disease, it is important to know what the rate of vascular disease is in populations with and without epilepsy. These sorts of calculations have seldom if ever been achieved.

In Table 14.3, very approximate estimates are given for the relative frequency (prevalence) of epilepsy in a typical Western population, where available, based on prevalence rates from community-based studies.

Table 14.3 The approximate relative frequency of different etiological categories

		Approximate frequency[a]
Idiopathic epilepsy	Pure epilepsies due to single-gene disorders	<1%
	Pure epilepsy with complex inheritance and other epilepsy syndromes	15–40%
Symptomatic epilepsy of predominately genetic or developmental causation	Progressive myoclonic epilepsies	<1%
	Neurocutaneous syndromes	<1%
	Other single-gene disorders	<1%
	Disorders of chromosomal/genomic structure	<1%
	Developmental anomalies of cerebral structure	<5%
Symptomatic epilepsy of predominately acquired causation	Hippocampal sclerosis	5–10%
	Perinatal and infantile causes	5%
	Degenerative and other neurological diseases	5%
	Cerebral trauma	5%
	Cerebral tumor	5%
	Cerebral infection	5%
	Cerebral vascular disorders	10–20%
	Cerebral immunological	<5%
Provoked epilepsy[b]		15–40%

Notes:
[a]Rough "best guess" estimates of prevalence based on figures for individual conditions.
[b]Including febrile convulsions. See Chapter 88 for definitions.

Risk factors

The most precise approach to the assignment of etiology is to take a statistical route, and compare the frequency of an etiological factor in the epilepsy population (preferably at the time of diagnosis) with that in a control population (of the same demographic and geographic constitution). This has seldom been attempted, although the reverse study – a case–control study to define the frequency of epilepsy within a defined etiology – has been more commonly performed, for instance in head injury, stroke, and some infections (see for instance Chapters 58, 68, and 77). One exception to this approach can be taken in conditions where epilepsy is almost the rule, the simple epidemiological study of the condition, without case–control methodology, will suffice but such exceptions are rare.

In a case–control study, the following conditions should be met (as noted by Beghi 2004):

(1) A temporal association: exposure to the risk factor should precede epilepsy.
(2) The strength of the association: the greater the difference in incidence between exposed and unexposed populations, the more likely is this to be a true association.
(3) Consistency: the association should be reproducible
(4) Biological gradient: evidence of a "dose–response" effect
(5) Biological plausibility.

In a condition with such variable manifestations and such a multitude of causes, the undertaking of formal case–control studies, complying fully with these conditions, is a formidable task.

Epilepsy as a disease or a symptom – and epilepsy syndromes

One tenacious neurological canon is that epilepsy, like headache or anemia, is a symptom of a neurological condition and not a condition per se. This of course begs the question about the definition of disease in general, a topic beyond the scope of this chapter. The main reason for considering epilepsy a symptom is that there are so many different causes, and it is therefore perhaps ironical to note that the current classifications of epilepsy pay no heed to etiology at all, focused as they are on clinical and electrographic semiology. Nor does etiology have much influence on treatment in most cases, and it is also partly because treatment is largely symptomatic that epilepsy is perceived largely as a symptom.

In spite of this, there is also an increasing tendency to define "syndromes" of epilepsy, and to consider these entities in their own right. Some syndromes are genetic (e.g., severe myoclonic epilepsy of infancy) or presumed genetic (e.g., the idiopathic generalized epilepsies) and others have mixed etiologies (e.g., West syndrome). The definition of "syndrome" is sufficiently vague to allow inclusion of many different groups and subgroups and there is a continuing debate amongst the splitters and lumpers of the epilepsy world about what to include and what not to include. This seems to the author to be largely counterproductive. Furthermore, some conditions are so well defined from the etiological point of view (severe

myoclonic epilepsy of infancy is an example) that it is not really a "syndrome" but an epilepsy etiological type, in the same sense that post-traumatic epilepsy is not considered a syndrome but a specific etiological type of epilepsy.

Thus, whether epilepsy is considered a symptom or a disease, and to what extent epilepsies are grouped into syndromes or not will depend to an extent on the importance placed on etiology; and certainly a classification of epilepsy on etiological grounds has a very different form from that using semiological or electrographic criteria.

Temporal characteristics of acquired epilepsy
Early and late seizures

As mentioned above, one interesting feature of acquired epilepsies is the tendency for the occurrence of early and late seizures which have a different pathophysiological basis and a different clinical and prognostic course. An example is in stroke, where only one-third of those having early seizures will develop later epilepsy and where the risk of ongoing epilepsy is much higher after a first late seizure than after a first early seizure. The physiology of the two conditions is different as is the clinical form, prognosis, and treatment. The distinction between early and late seizures, reflecting as it does a genuine etiological and physiological difference, is valid and probably is the only situation in which the term "acute symptomatic seizure" is appropriate (see p. 626).

The latent period

Linked to the contrast between early and late seizures is the concept of the "latent period." This is the period between the brain insult and the first late seizure. After head injury, for instance, this period can extend for several years although the peak onset of seizures is after about 8 months. Clearly, there is a process of epileptogenesis in these cases which takes a significant time to develop, and current studies focus on changes in neuronal networks or systems, changes in synaptic formation, glial changes, loss of inhibition, cellular and biochemical changes, inflammatory changes, neogenesis, etc. However, there is also some experimental evidence that subclinical seizure activity exists earlier, in other words that the brain is already epileptic, and that the seizures only become apparent clinically as the seizure activity increases in intensity or spread (these aspects are considered further in Chapter 3). Whether there continues to be further development of the epileptic process after the onset of clinical epilepsy is another interesting and largely unanswered point. What is clear, though, is that the distinctive natures of the underlying pathological and physiological processes underlying symptomatic epilepsy after acute brain insults are very different from those underlying idiopathic epilepsy, and so are the clinical, therapeutic, and prognostic features.

Provoked epilepsies

In the classification of etiologies of epilepsy proposed in this book (Chapter 2), the category of provoked epilepsy is differentiated from both idiopathic and symptomatic epilepsy. The importance of distinguishing provoking factors was recognized by Jackson and his successors, who categorized "cause" into (a) predisposing causes (also known as remote, underlying, hereditary, epileptic diathesis, etc.); and (b) exciting causes (also known as determining, proximate, provoking, etc.). In his classification scheme J. Russell Reynolds (1861) also recognized (sensibly in my view) the terms "eccentric" and "diathetic" epilepsy (for definitions see Chapter 1). These terms have been lost over time, but the concept of "provoked epilepsy" remains.

It is sometimes suggested that provoking factors are somehow "different" from real (underlying neurological) causes. However, if one accepts the multifactorial nature of epilepsy causation, it has to be conceded that a "provoking factor" is as much a "cause" as any other factor. It is for this reason that the provoked epilepsies are included here as an etiological category, distinct from the idiopathic or symptomatic epilepsies. Provoked epilepsy is defined as:

An epilepsy in which a systemic or environmental factor is the predominant cause of the seizures and in which there are neuropathological or neuroanatomical changes.

Of course, many patients with provoked seizures have an increased susceptibility to epilepsy (either genetic or acquired) and the term provoked epilepsy should be applied where the overwhelming influence is the provoking factor and not the underlying susceptibility. This is an arbitrary but clinically useful distinction. The provoked epilepsies, and the related topics of reflex epilepsy and acute symptomatic seizures are discussed further in Chapter 88.

References

Beghi E (2004) Etiology of epilepsy. In: Shorvon SD, Fish D, Perucca E, Dodson W (eds.) *The Treatment of Epilepsy,* 2nd edn. Oxford: Blackwell Science, pp. 50–64.

ILAE Commission on Classification and Terminology (1989) Proposal for revised classification of epilepsies and epileptic syndromes. *Epilepsia* **30**:389–99.

Jackson JH (1874) On the scientific and empirical investigation of epilepsies. *Med Press Circular* **18**:325–7, 347–52, 389–92, 409–12, 475–8, 497–9, 519–21.

Lennox WG (1960) *Epilepsy and Related Disorders.* Boston, MA: Little, Brown.

Reynolds JR (1861) *Epilepsy: Its Symptoms, Treatment and Relation to Other Chronic Convulsive Diseases.* London: Churchill.

Wilson SAK (1940) *Neurology.* London: Edward Arnold.

Chapter

15

West syndrome and Lennox–Gastaut syndrome

Renzo Guerrini and Carla Marini

Infantile spasms and West syndrome

Infantile spasms (IS) are a distinctive form of seizure disorder, mainly observed in infants, in the first year of life, and refractory to conventional antiepileptic drugs. Developmental delay or deterioration and a characteristic electroencephalographic (EEG) pattern (*hypsarrhythmia*) are often associated with IS. All these elements occur together in *West syndrome*. The seizure type in itself, irrespective of the age and clinical context, is defined as *epileptic spasm* (Dulac *et al.* 1994) and may rarely occur in childhood or even in adulthood (Egli 1985; Ikeno *et al.* 1985; Bednarek *et al.* 1998; Cerullo *et al.* 1999; de Menezes and Rho 2002). A cumulative incidence of 2.9 per 10 000 live births and an age-specific prevalence of 2.0 per 10 000 in 10-year-old children were observed in the USA (Trevathan *et al.* 1999).

Infantile spasms are manifested as clusters of increasing-plateau–decreasing-intensity brisk (0.5–2.0 s) flexions or extensions of the neck, with abduction or adduction of the upper limbs. Clusters include a few units to several dozens of spasms and are repeated many times per day. After a series, the child is usually exhausted. Other seizure types can coexist. The muscle contraction of IS has distinctive features. It reaches its maximum more slowly than a myoclonic jerk and decreases in an equally slower way (Fusco and Vigevano 1993), though it is faster and less sustained than observed in tonic seizures.

Developmental delay pre-dates the onset of spasms in about 70% of children (Guerrini 2006). Disappearance of social smile, loss of visual attention, or autistic withdrawal is often observed with the onset of spasms.

Electroclinical characteristics

Infantile spasms consist of a sudden, generally bilateral, contraction of muscles of the neck, trunk and extremities. *Flexor spasms* have long been regarded as the hallmark of the syndrome. They consist of a sudden flexion of the head, trunk, and legs, which are usually held in adduction. The arms, also in flexion, can be adducted or abducted. Mixed flexor–extensor spasms are the most common type. They consist of either

flexion of the neck, trunk, and arms with extension of the legs or, less commonly, flexion of the legs and extension of the arms. *Extensor spasms,* involving an abrupt extension of the neck and trunk, with extension and abduction of the arms, are less common (Lombroso 1983). Most affected infants have more than one type of spasm.

The intensity of the contractions and the number of muscle groups involved vary considerably both in different infants and in the same infant with different attacks. The spasms may consist of only slight head nodding, upward eye deviation, or elevation and adduction of the shoulders in a shrugging movement. In some cases, the spasms may be so mild that they can be felt but not seen, or they may be clinically unnoticeable even though they are shown on polygraphic recordings (Kellaway *et al.* 1979). The number of spasms usually is much higher than is reported by parents (Gaily *et al.* 2001). The electromyographic (EMG) tracing in a spasm consists of an abrupt initial contraction lasting less than 2 s, followed by a more sustained contraction lasting 2–10 s (Kellaway *et al.* 1979). The second, or tonic, phase may be absent, the spasm being limited to the initial phasic contraction lasting 0.5 s or less. The contraction may appear diamond-shaped on EMG recordings (Fusco and Vigevano 1993).

In 6–8% of cases, the spasms may be asymmetrical or even unilateral (Kellaway *et al.* 1979; Lombroso 1983). Asymmetrical spasms are associated with a symptomatic etiology, but unilateral lesions can generate symmetrical attacks. Asymmetrical spasms may occur after a partial seizure (Yamamoto *et al.* 1988). Lateralized motor phenomena, including lateral or upward eye deviation and eyebrow contraction, or abduction of one shoulder, may sometimes constitute the entire series of spasms or initiate a series that will eventually develop into bilateral phenomena. Such lateralized manifestations are usually accompanied by unilateral or asymmetric ictal EEG changes.

Spasms are characteristically grouped in series or clusters. The clusters consist of a few units to more than 100 individual jerks, 5–30 s apart. The intensity of the jerks in a series may initially wax and wane, not always regularly. Status of IS has

The Causes of Epilepsy, eds. S. D. Shorvon, F. Andermann, and R. Guerrini. Published by Cambridge University Press. © Cambridge University Press 2011.

been reported (Coulter 1986). The number of series is variable from only 1 to 50 or more daily (Lacy and Penry 1976). Clusters may occur during sleep, usually at the time of awakening or at the transition from slow sleep to rapid eye movement (REM) sleep (Plouin *et al.* 1987). They are frequent in drowsiness. No obvious precipitating stimuli or circumstances are detectable in most infants. However, self-precipitation prompted by complex behaviors is occasionally observed (Guerrini *et al.* 1992). Following a series of spasms, the infant may be left exhausted and lethargic. Spasms may change their characteristics becoming more subtle, spontaneously or as an effect of treatment. Video-EEG monitoring may be necessary to provide firm evidence that spasms have really disappeared in response to medication (Gaily *et al.* 2001).

The hypsarrhythmic EEG is characterized by very high-voltage (up to 500 μV) slow waves, irregularly interspersed with spikes and sharp waves that occur randomly in all cortical areas. The abnormal discharges are not synchronous over both hemispheres, so the general appearance is that of a chaotic disorganization of electrogenesis. Hypsarrhythmia is an interictal pattern observed mainly while the child is awake. During slow sleep, bursts of more synchronous polyspikes and waves often appear. The term "modified hypsarrhythmia" has been used by some investigators to designate EEG patterns with atypical features, such as relatively preserved background activity, generalized synchronous spike–wave discharges, prominent asymmetry, or suppression bursts (Hrachovy *et al.* 1984).

It has been suggested that cognitive and behavioral deterioration, which is typical of the syndrome, might result from persistent hypsarrhythmic EEG activity, possibly representing a variant of non-convulsive status (Dulac 2001). Intravenous diazepam may suppress hypsarrhythmia and unmask focal discharges (Dalla Bernardina and Watanabe 1994).

Hypsarrhythmia tends to disappear in older children, occasionally even when spasms may still be observed (Hrachovy and Frost 1989). The tracings may then become normal or exhibit various abnormalities.

Ictal EEG patterns are variable; the most common is a high-voltage, frontal-dominant, generalized slow-wave transient, with an inverse phase reversal over the vertex, followed by voltage attenuation (Fusco and Vigevano 1993). Bilateral and diffuse fast rhythms in the β-range (occasionally in α-band) coincide with the clinical spasm and with the initial part of the low-voltage record, which lasts 2–5 s. In many cases, only voltage attenuation (decremental discharge) may be observed. Spasms with a more sustained tonic contraction, likewise tonic seizures, are accompanied by a high-amplitude slow wave, followed by fast activity (Vigevano *et al.* 2001). Other ictal patterns include generalized sharp-and-slow wave complexes, generalized slow-wave transients only, or fast rhythms in isolation (Kellaway *et al.* 1983). Asymmetrical and unilateral spasms are usually associated with contralateral EEG activity, suggesting unilateral damage. After the initial spasms of a series, there may be transient suppression of the

hypsarrhythmic pattern, which will not reappear between consecutive spasms. In other cases, hypsarrhythmia resumes between spasms. It has been suggested that disappearance of hypsarrhythmia in the course of a series of spasms might indicate a symptomatic origin, whereas its resumption in between serial spasms would indicate an "idiopathic" condition and carry a favorable prognosis (Dulac 1997). Children with severe structural brain abnormalities, such as tuberous sclerosis, Aicardi syndrome, or lissencephaly, do not usually have typical hypsarrhythmia. It is likely that only children with less severe brain impairment, and higher chances of a better outcome, are able to generate a typical hypsarrhythmic pattern.

Differential diagnosis

A rare condition, termed *benign myoclonus of early infancy,* is characterized by repetitive jerks that closely mimic IS but are not accompanied by EEG abnormalities and have a spontaneously favorable course (Dravet *et al.* 1986; Fejerman and Caraballo 2002) (see Chapter 13). Benign myoclonus, however, although repetitive, never presents with the periodic character of spasms. Another manifestation, called *repetitive sleep starts* (Fusco *et al.* 1999), often observed in children with spasticity, may closely mimic IS. These starts might represent a pathological enhancement of hypnagogic jerks, which are cyclically repeated while the infants are falling asleep. Tonic upgaze deviation, repeated in clusters every few seconds for several minutes, may be seen in *benign tonic upward gaze,* occurring in previously normal children between 6 and 20 months of age (Guerrini *et al.* 1998a). During the attacks, EEG is normal and the child, who is conscious, may maintain visual fixation by bending the head downwards, a maneuver that produces vertical nystagmus. This is an age-related condition that disappears within 1–2 years from onset. *Compulsive self-gratification behavior* (previously termed as *compulsive masturbation*) is a condition that is mainly observed in girls during late infancy or early childhood. Some of the children may present with prolonged episodes of rhythmic contractions of the lower limbs and trunk with eye staring and adducted thighs with an attitude of withdrawal (Guerrini 2006). Early forms of myoclonic epilepsy, especially *benign myoclonic epilepsy,* are mistaken for IS by the inexperienced clinician. The jerks are briefer than spasms and often have a saccadic appearance. Usually, they are not repeated in series, and are accompanied by a short burst of irregular, fast polyspike–wave complexes on a relatively normal background EEG.

Infantile spasms must be differentiated from rarer, earlier-onset conditions with ominous prognosis, such as early infantile epileptic encephalopathy and early myoclonic encephalopathy.

Differentiating IS from the tonic seizures of Lennox–Gastaut syndrome may be difficult (see below), especially when the attacks are in extension and not repeated in clusters. West syndrome may evolve into Lennox–Gastaut syndrome.

Etiological factors

There are multiple causes of IS, and their pathophysiological mechanism is unknown (Table 15.1). Infants with developmental brain abnormalities and those who are small for gestational age are more apt to develop spasms. The age dependency of the disorder is notable. Almost all cases have their onset during the first year of life (Chevrie and Aicardi 1971). Maximum incidence is between 3 and 7 months. Age of onset, however, depends on the proportion of symptomatic versus cryptogenic cases in any particular series. It seems that the location of the cortical lesion(s) may influence age at onset. Koo and Hwang (1996) observed that the earliest onset was seen with occipital lesions; whilst frontal lesions were associated with the latest onset. A family history of IS is only found in about 4% of the cases (Sugai et al. 2001). Familial cases are probably the expression of several genetic disorders, some of which are well characterized, including leukodystrophy (Coleman et al. 1977), tuberous sclerosis (Riikonen 1984), X-linked lissencephaly and band heterotopia (Guerrini and Carrozzo 2001a), X-linked mental retardation and IS due to mutations of the ARX gene (Claes et al. 1997; Stromme et al. 1999, 2002; Guerrini et al. 2007).

Several apparently unrelated phenotypes have been associated with mutations of the ARX gene, including syndromes with and without brain malformations. The former include X-linked lissencephaly with abnormal genitalia (XLAG), severe hydrocephalus and Proud syndrome (agenesis of the corpus callosum with abnormal genitalia), while the latter include X-linked IS (ISS), Partington syndrome, which consists of mental retardation with mild dystonia, and nonspecific X-linked mental retardation (Stromme et al. 2002; Kato et al. 2004). In general, the malformation phenotypes are associated with protein truncation mutations and missense mutations in the homeobox, while the nonmalformation phenotypes are associated with missense mutations outside of the homeobox and expansion of the polyalanine tracts. Boys with X-linked IS due to ARX mutations usually have severe developmental delay and may have microcephaly. Onset of spasms is usually early and hypsarrhythmia is frequent (Stromme et al. 2002; Kato et al. 2003), although not constantly reported. Follow-up data on IS in these patients are not available. A syndrome of early-onset IS, with hypsarrhythmia and severe quadriplegic dyskinesia, in which spasms tend to remit but episodes of status dystonicus complicate the course, has been associated with expansions in the first polyalanine tract of the ARX gene (Guerrini et al. 2007).

A syndrome with microcephaly and early-onset intractable seizures, including spasms with or without hypsarrhythmia, has been associated with mutations or deletions of the X-linked gene CDKL5 (Archer et al. 2006; Elia et al. 2008; Mei et al. 2009). The syndrome is much more frequent in females. No unique EEG pattern seems to be typical for this etiology. The spectrum of clinical manifestations in girls with

Table 15.1 West syndrome and Lennox–Gastaut syndrome: etiologies

Type of etiology	Specific etiology[a]	Syndrome[b]
(1) Malformations of cortical development (30%)	Focal cortical dysplasia	WS
	Tuberous sclerosis TSC1, TSC2 genes	WS–LGS
	Lissencephaly LIS1, DCX, ARX genes	WS–LGS
	Subcortical band heterotopia DCX, LIS1 genes	WS–LGS
	Bilateral perisylvian polymicrogyria	WS
	Bilateral frontoparietal polymicrogyria GPR56 gene mutations	WS
	Diffuse polymicrogyria	WS–LGS
	Hemimegalencephaly	WS
	Neurocutaneous disorders	WS
	Aicardi syndrome	IS
	Schizencephaly	IS
	Periventricular heterotopia/ microcephaly ARFGEF2 gene	IS
	Holoprosencephaly SIX3, SHH, TGIF, ZIC2, PTCH1, GLI2 genes	WS
(2) Pre-, peri-, or post natal damage (20%)	Hypoxic ischemic sequelae	WS
	Hemorrhagic	WS
	Fetal infections	WS–LGS
	Postnatal infection (encephalitis and meningitis)	WS–LGS
	Trauma	WS
	Cardiac surgery with hypothermia	WS
(3) Chromosomal abnormalities and copy-number variations (5%)	15q11.2–q13.1 duplication	LGS
	4p (Wolf–Hirschhorn) syndrome	LGS

Table 15.1 (cont.)

Type of etiology	Specific etiology[a]	Syndrome[b]
	Inverted duplicated chromosome 15	LGS
	Angelman syndrome	WS
	Down syndrome	WS–LGS
	Miller–Dieker syndrome	WS–LGS
	Deletion 1p36	WS
	Deletion 7q11.23–q21.1 (*MAGI2*)	WS
	Pallister–Killian syndrome: mosaic 12p(i[12p])	IS
(4) Inborn errors of metabolism (Rare)	Menkes disease	WS
	Phenylketonuria and TUBP deficiency	WS
	Mitochondrial disease (NARP)	WS
	Complex 1 deficiency	IS
	Hypoglycemia	WS
	Progressive encephalopathy with edema, hypsarrhythmia, and optic atrophy syndrome	WS
	Non-ketotic hyperglycinemia	WS
	Other organic acid disorders	WS
	Pyridoxine dependency	IS
	Biotinidase dependency	WS
	Congenital disorders of glycosylation	WS
(5) Vascular malformations (Rare)	Sturge–Weber syndrome	WS–LGS
(6) Brain tumors (Rare)	All brain tumors	WS
(7) Monogenic: non-malformative – non-metabolic (8%)	*ARX*	WS
	SCN1A	
	CDKL5	
	STPBX1	
(8) No identifiable causes (30%)	50% positive family history of epilepsy	WS–LGS

Notes:
[a]Etiologies are cumulatively intended for West syndrome, the infantile spasms and epileptic spasms, and Lennox–Gastaut syndrome. The column legend indicates the prominent syndrome presentation. For example, girls with Aicardi syndrome most often exhibit infantile spasms, rather than typical West syndrome. However this distinction may not always be feasible.
[b]IS, infantile spasms; WS, West syndrome; LGS, Lennox–Gastaut syndrome.

CDKL5 mutations appears to be broad and includes multiple seizure types with early onset and behavioral features that may, in part, overlap with the most severe forms of Rett syndrome (Weaving *et al.* 2004; Mari *et al.* 2005; Scala *et al.* 2005).

Patients harboring deletions on chromosome 7q11.23 including the *MAGI2* gene, involved in regulation of trafficking, distribution, or function of the glutamate receptors, have IS. This might therefore be considered as a new gene for IS (Marshall *et al.* 2008).

A possibly recessive syndrome of early-onset IS, often preceded and followed by other types of seizures, associated with hypsarrhythmia, facial dysmorphism, optic atrophy, and peripheral edema, has been reported from Finland as PEHO syndrome (progressive encephalopathy with edema, hypsarrhythmia, and optic atrophy) (Riikonen, 2001). Cases exist outside Finland.

Other genetic disorders are more rare and may be of recessive (Fleiszar *et al.* 1977; Caplan *et al.* 1992; Ciardo *et al.* 2001) or of undetermined nature (Reiter *et al.* 2000). West syndrome and IS have also been associated with various mitochondrial disorders, inherited disorders of metabolism, chromosomal abnormalities, and copy-number variations (Table 15.1).

Although IS are traditionally divided into cases of *symptomatic* and *cryptogenic* origin, the meaning of these terms varies among the studies and according to the extent of investigations. The specific nature of the causative lesion also implies a variable prognostic outlook. Most define as symptomatic those cases in which an etiological factor can be clearly identified. Other investigators link symptomaticity to either or both abnormal development prior to the onset of spasms and clinical or imaging evidence of a brain lesion. Cryptogenic spasms are those for which no cause can be identified, or where development was normal before the onset of spasms. In addition, the term cryptogenic does not necessarily mean that a lesion is not present; therefore, a difference in nature between cryptogenic and symptomatic cases is not clearly established.

A few cases that are not included in the symptomatic group, despite increasingly accurate investigations, may belong to an "idiopathic" group (Dulac *et al.* 1986; Vigevano *et al.* 1993). A typical and symmetric hypsarrhythmic pattern, which reappears between individual spasms during a cluster in a previously normal child, would be an electroclinical feature of idiopathic spasms (Plouin *et al.* 1987). However, these features are not fully reliable (Haga *et al.* 1995). In spite of these divergences about definitions the distinction between symptomatic and cryptogenic spasms is of practical significance because a poor prognosis is expected when a structural brain abnormality is present.

Although the IS have multiple causes and it is often stated that this seizure type is but a response of the immature brain to multiple types of insults, some causes are especially likely to result in IS.

Malformations of the cerebral cortex (or of cortical development: Barkovich *et al.* 2005) are a well-established cause of IS and seem to be involved in about 30% of cases.

Tuberous sclerosis is found in 7–25% of the children who present with IS (Curatolo *et al.* 2001). On the other hand about 50% of patients with epilepsy and tuberous sclerosis appear to have or have had IS (Roger *et al.* 1984) and about 85% of infants with tuberous sclerosis who experience seizures in the first year of life have IS (Chevrie and Aicardi 1977). Onset of spasms may be preceded by partial seizures and a combination of partial seizures and spasms is often observed in the same child (Fig. 15.1). Waking EEGs show multifocal or focal spike discharges and irregular slow focal activity (Curatolo 1996; Dulac *et al.* 1996). Abnormalities increase during sleep. Atypical hypsarrhythmia, often asymmetrical, is present in one-third of cases. Video-EEG monitoring and analysis of EEG patterns may suggest a focal origin of the spasms (Curatolo 1996; Dulac 1996). In general, IS in tuberous sclerosis are considered to differ clinically and electroencephalographically from classical IS with typical hypsarrhythmia, the main differences including the frequent association with focal seizures, with asymmetric clinical and EEG features and absence of typical hypsarrhythmia.

Cortical tubers are usually well visualized by MRI scan as enlarged gyri with atypical shape and an abnormal signal intensity, mainly involving the subcortical white matter. In the newborn they are hyperintense with respect to the surrounding white matter on T1-weighted images and hypointense on T2-weighted images. Progressive myelination of the white matter in the older infant gives the tubers a hypointense center on T1 and high signal intensity on T2. The number of tubers is usually multiple. A relationship between location of the tubers and severity of epilepsy has been suggested (Jambaqué *et al.* 1991, 1993). However, some patients with multiple tubers can be asymptomatic, indicating that the relation between the number and location of tubers is a complex one. No obvious phenotypic differences have been found in families linked to the *TSC1* or *TSC2* gene mutations, although it has been suggested that patients with *TSC1*

mutations may have less severe epilepsy and cognitive impairment (Dabora *et al.* 2001).

The association of IS with other neurocutaneous syndromes is less clear. West syndrome has been observed in association with neurofibromatosis, and was said to have a relatively good prognosis (Motte *et al.* 1993) but the association may be coincidental.

Other brain malformations, especially neuronal migration disorders and focal cortical dysplasia have often been associated with IS (Guerrini *et al.* 1996). Some malformations have an elective association with IS. Aicardi syndrome (Chevrie and Aicardi 1986) consists of total or partial agenesis of the corpus callosum, chorioretinal lacunae, and IS that are often asymmetrical and associated with other seizures, especially focal attacks. Neuroimaging demonstrates several brain defects in addition to callosal agenesis or dysgenesis, such as periventricular heterotopia, abnormal gyration, cystic formations around the third ventricle, and gross hemispheric asymmetry (Chevrie and Aicardi 1986). Unlayered polymicrogyria is observed at histopathology (Guerrini *et al.* 1993). The EEG is rarely hypsarrhythmic; typically, the tracings are of the

A

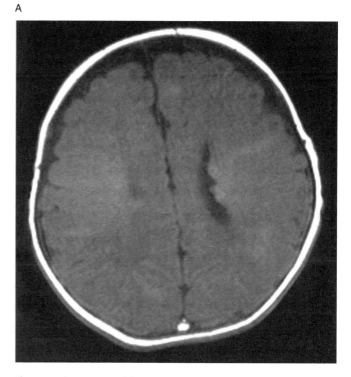

Fig. 15.1. (A) MRI scan of the brain of a 3-month-old boy with tuberous sclerosis. Note the subependymal nodules on both sides and multiple areas of high signal intensity, corresponding to cortical tubers. (B) EEG recording of a focal seizure followed by a series of spasms. (A) and (B) Onset of focal ictal activity is observed on the F3–C3 electrode, with spread over P3 electrode. An initial tonic contraction is recorded in the right wrist extensor and flexor muscles (channels 28–29 and 30–31), followed by activity on the ipsilateral deltoid (A1–A2). Initially arrhythmic and subsequently rhythmic clonic activity is recorded from the same muscles. The whole seizure lasts around 80 s and is followed, around 20 s after its end by a small series of spasms (B).

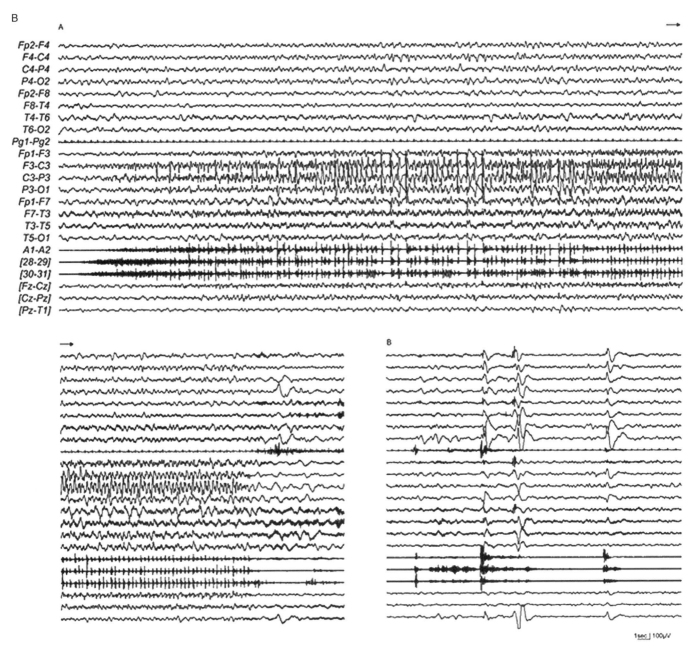

Fig. 15.1. (*cont.*)

so-called split-brain type, with paroxysmal EEG discharges occurring independently over either hemisphere (Fig. 15.2). The onset is often early and may be neonatal. Prognosis is poor; severe developmental delay, neurological abnormalities, and persistence of the spasms are observed in most patients. Aicardi syndrome is not a familial disorder and should be separated from the few cases of familial agenesis of the corpus callosum associated with IS (Cao *et al.* 1977) and from the rare X-linked lissencephaly with callosal agenesis and ambiguous genitalia, which is observed only in boys with *ARX* mutations (see above) (Dobyns *et al.* 1999).

Lissencephaly and pachygyria also have a special relationship with IS (Dulac *et al.* 1983; Gastaut *et al.* 1987; Guerrini and Carrozzo 2001a, b). Although the diagnosis rests on neuroimaging, interictal EEG shows a highly characteristic pattern with high-amplitude fast rhythms, which may alternate with a mixture of high-amplitude theta and delta rhythms that may suggest slow spike–waves or resemble hypsarrhythmia (Gastaut *et al.* 1987; Quirk *et al.* 1993). About 75% of infants with lissencephaly–pachygyria have IS (Guerrini *et al.* 1999). However, since studies defining the electroclinical characteristics of agyria pachygyria were published before the distinction

A

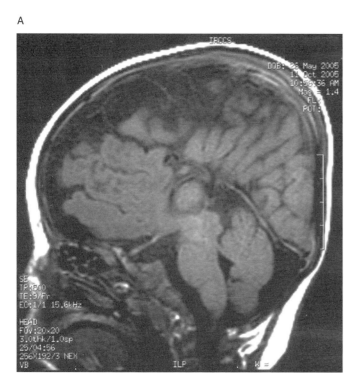

B

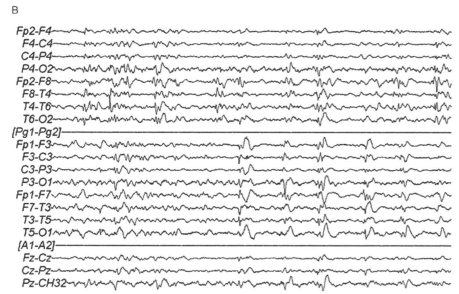

Fig. 15.2. (A) T1-weighted sagittal MRI scan of the brain of a 5-month-old girl with Aicardi syndrome and intractable infantile spasms Note the extremely hypoplastic corpus callosum with an extensive area of polymicrogyria involving the frontal lobe. There is a posterior fossa cyst. (B) Sleep EEG recording of the same girl when aged 9 months. Bilateral asynchronous bursts of repetitive spike-and-wave discharges (Pg1 is the left deltoid EMG and A1–A2 is the right deltoid).

between the different genetic forms was recognized, it is not known whether these have distinctive electroclinical features. Spasms are rarely observed in children with subcortical band heterotopia (Barkovich *et al.* 1994).

Hemimegalencephaly, which is associated with abnormal gyration and dysplasia of one cerebral hemisphere, is a possible cause of IS and may be amenable to hemispherectomy or hemispherotomy. The EEG tracings may include unilateral fast rhythms and suppression bursts, or slow spike–wave patterns (Paladin *et al.* 1989).

Focal cortical *dysplasia* is often detected as abnormal signal on T2-weighted and fluid attenuation inversion recovery (FLAIR) sequences and abnormal folding and thickness of the cortex (Sankar *et al.* 1995). Thin slices and multiplanar reconstruction (Chan *et al.* 1998), as well as additional new MRI techniques (Bastos *et al.* 1999, Eriksson 2001) have enhanced the diagnostic power of neuroimaging. In spite of these increasingly sophisticated techniques, a number of children with IS harbor small areas of dysplasia that escape recognition by MRI. In addition, in children aged less than 2 years even macroscopic dysplasia may be overlooked, as the typical blurring between gray and white matter may not be apparent due to incomplete myelination (Guerrini *et al.* 2008). A repeat MRI scan is therefore advised in children with IS in whom a first early scan was normal, especially if asymmetric EEG or clinical features are present.

It is probable that IS represents the most common seizure type observed in *Down syndrome*. In most children, spasms appear without any evidence of additional brain damage (Stafstrom and Konkol 1994; Silva *et al.* 1996) and remission is obtained on conventional antiepileptic drugs, adrenocorticotrophic hormone (ACTH), steroids or vigabatrin, without relapse of seizures or with later onset of a mild age-related generalized seizure disorders (Silva *et al.* 1996; Nabbout *et al.* 2001).

Metabolic disorders are not a common cause of IS. Phenylketonuria is now unlikely to be a cause of IS in industrialized countries as it is systematically detected by neonatal screening. However, this disorder is electively related to West syndrome (Poley and Dumermuth 1968). A hypsarrhythmic EEG occurs in approximately one-third of untreated phenylketonuric patients. Non-ketotic hyperglycinemia (glycine encephalopathy) is a rare cause of IS. Carbohydrate-deficient glycoprotein disorders and abnormalities of serine metabolism are rare but important causes as they are in part treatable. Pyridoxine dependency can rarely be first manifested by IS (Bankier *et al.* 1983; Krishnamoorthy 1983), and this justifies a systematic trial of intravenous vitamin B_6. The role of pyridoxal phosphate deficiency in causing West syndrome is still unclear.

West syndrome results from acquired brain disorders in 8–14% of cases (Guerrini 2006). Many causes of diffuse brain damage, whether inflammatory (herpes simplex), traumatic (subdural hematomas), anoxic, or ischemic, and, rarely, tumors, have been associated with the syndrome. Some reports have implicated immunization as an etiologic factor, the pertussis component usually being incriminated (Bellman *et al.* 1983). However, the association between IS and immunization is likely coincidental as the onset of spasms is often at an age when infants are normally vaccinated.

Clinical presentation versus etiology

The question as to whether discrete clinical pictures of IS are produced by different etiologic subgroups remains controversial. Some of the causes are associated with relatively specific clinical and EEG patterns, the most obvious examples being Aicardi syndrome, hemimegalencephaly, and, to a lesser extent, the lissencephaly spectrum of malformations and some cases of tuberous sclerosis. Suggestive electroclinical features of idiopathic spasms have been proposed, as summarized above. However, there is no firm evidence suggesting that a subgroup exists with definite characteristics.

It has been suggested that IS might be a peculiar type of age-related secondarily generalized seizures that can be triggered by focal paroxysmal activity arising from limited or more diffuse areas of abnormal cortex (Asano *et al.* 2001). Results of epilepsy

surgery provide unquestionable support to the view that the abnormal cortex plays a key role in the initiation of seizures. Ictal ^{18}F-fluoro-D-glucose positron emission tomography (FDG PET) studies of IS have shown that hypometabolism involves focal cortical areas, as well as the lenticular nuclei and brainstem (Chugani *et al.* 1987; Juhasz *et al.* 2001), which might be in keeping with an interaction between such cortical and subcortical structures during spasms.

Late-onset epileptic spasms

Gobbi *et al.* (1987) described as "periodic spasms" the clinical and EEG features in a series of children with severe encephalopathies. The typical presentation included a frequent onset by a focal seizure or EEG discharge, followed by a series of spasms, often asymmetrical or unilateral, each marked on the EEG by a slow complex with superimposed, low-amplitude, fast rhythms, without resumption of interictal activity between individual spasms. This electroclinical pattern has been repeatedly confirmed (Donat and Wright 1991; Guerrini *et al.* 1992; Pachatz *et al.* 2003), even in adults (Cerullo *et al.* 1999), and appears to be the expression of developmental brain abnormalities. In older children and adults the epileptic spasms are the only manifestation that is reminiscent of the syndrome of IS, the clinical context being very different. Late-onset spasms are almost invariably resistant to treatment. Although the outcome is usually regarded as poor, a number of cases are not associated with mental retardation or neurologic abnormalities. In general, the later the onset of spasms the less the cognitive prognosis is influenced.

Prognosis in relation to etiology, imaging, and EEG

The prognosis of IS is heavily influenced by the pathological process underlying the syndrome. Brain MRI has a high prognostic value, which is closely linked to its diagnostic power. Infants with normal MRI have the best prognosis (Methahonkala *et al.* 2002; Saltik *et al.* 2002). However, MRI may be normal in some metabolic disorders, dysplastic lesions, or genetic non-malformative and non-metabolic conditions, such as *CDKL5* or some *ARX* mutations, which carry a poor prognosis (see also Chapter 4).

Interictal FDG PET in children with IS and normal MRI may show multifocal or diffuse hypometabolic patterns that may correlate with developmental outcome. For example, bilateral hypometabolism in the temporal lobes correlates with an autistic disorder and a poor long-term outcome (Chugani *et al.* 1996).

The prognostic value of the initial EEG characteristics is uncertain. Unilateral and grossly asymmetric tracings predict an unfavorable outcome, whereas a typical hypsarrhythmic pattern may be associated with a more favorable prognosis (Saltik *et al.* 2002). However, there is a limitation in the way studies on the prognostic value of EEG findings have been conducted. Prognosis of spasms and overall developmental prognosis have not been necessarily considered together. Experience with infants with large brain malformations suggests that hypsarrhythmia is often absent and that spasms persist well beyond the typical age range. This observation suggests that the typical hypsarrhythmic pattern requires at least some degree of anatomic and functional integrity of the brain in order to be generated. In addition, it seems that extensive brain malformations determine a sort of archaic or immature functional state whereby only spasms or focal seizure can be generated even at an older age. It is therefore not surprising that prognosis for children exhibiting brain malformations and no typical hypsarrhythmia should be guarded.

Principles of treatment

Vigabatrin and ACTH have proven effective in a few controlled trials, but uncertainties remain regarding the best treatment (Hancock et al. 2002). In three comparative studies, vigabatrin was slightly less effective than, or as effective as ACTH (Vigevano and Cilio 1997; Cossette et al. 1999; Lux et al. 2004), but possibly better tolerated (Vigevano and Cilio 1997). Two randomized trials reported a 78% responder rate (Appleton et al. 1999), and a higher effectiveness of high doses (100–148 mg/kg per day) (Elterman et al. 2001). Particular efficacy has been shown in children with tuberous sclerosis (Jambaqué et al. 2000). Response to 100 mg/kg per day occurs within a few days. Many researchers regard vigabatrin as the first-line drug, despite the risk of visual field constriction (Lewis and Wallace 2001). This side effect appears in 30–50% of patients having received a substantial drug load, but is not ascertainable in small children. According to the Vigabatrin Pediatric Advisory Group (2000) responders should receive vigabatrin for no more than 6 months; non-responders should be switched to ACTH within 3 weeks. The United Kingdom IS Study (UKISS) comparing hormonal treatment against vigabatrin in the management of IS showed that ACTH or prednisolone treatment controlled spasms better than did vigabatrin initially, but not at 12–14 months of age (Lux et al. 2005). In a controlled trial ACTH proved superior to prednisone (Baram et al. 1996); it is used in daily doses from 20 to 40 IU. Non-depot ACTH has a lower risk of causing persistent hypertension. An individualized regimen starting with 3 UI/kg per day progressively increased, by doubling the doses (12 UI/kg per day, daily) every 2 weeks until a response is obtained, can keep dose-related side effects such as hypertension, brain shrinking, adrenal hyporesponsiveness, and cardiac hypertrophy to a minimum (Heiskala et al. 1996). Infections are an ominous complication of ACTH treatment and are responsible for most deaths (Wong and Trevathan 2001). A limit of 4–6 weeks' duration of an ACTH course is advisable. Spasms may respond within days but behavioral improvement needs several weeks. Relapse rate is 30%. A second cycle of ACTH is recommended in cases of relapse after an initial good response. Oral high-dose prednisolone has been suggested as

an alternative to ACTH, providing an equivalent efficacy, with reduced side effects and considerably lower cost (Kossoff et al. 2009). Pulse intravenous methylprednisolone (Mytinger et al. 2010), valproate, topiramate, and benzodiazepines, especially nitrazepam, might represent interesting treatment alternatives. Video-EEG monitoring is necessary to show that the spasms have truly disappeared (Gaily et al. 2001).

Surgical treatment should be considered early when drug resistance is faced and focal epileptogenesis is shown. About 60% of operated children become seizure-free; the best results are obtained when operating on small lesions (Asano et al. 2001). However, most children have large multilobar cortical dysplasia needing extensive resections, with limited cognitive improvement (Pulsifer et al. 2004).

There is some evidence for use of the ketogenic diet in resistant spasms (Kossoff et al. 2002; Kossoff 2010).

Lennox–Gastaut syndrome

Lennox–Gastaut syndrome is characterized by usually intractable brief tonic and atonic seizures, atypical absences, and a generalized interictal EEG pattern of spike and slow wave discharges. It accounts for 2.9% of all childhood epilepsies (Berg et al. 2000). Incidence peaks between 3 and 5 years of age. Cognitive and psychiatric impairment are frequent. About 30% of cases occur in previously healthy children; multiple etiologies are possible but most cases result from neuronal migration disorders and hypoxic brain damage. About 40% of children have previous IS (Guerrini 2006). Persistence of seizures in adulthood is frequent.

The term Lennox syndrome, was proposed by Gastaut et al. (1966) to depict a childhood epileptic encephalopathy with diffuse slow spike–wave complexes, and multiple types of seizures, including tonic seizures, reported by Lennox and Davis (1950). The definition of Lennox–Gastaut syndrome was only adopted years later (Niedermeyer 1969) and accepted by the ILAE in 1989. The term has often been loosely used to designate epilepsy syndromes of childhood featuring multiple types of intractable seizures, including falls. Epilepsy with myoclonic–astatic seizures and Dravet syndrome have likely been designated as Lennox–Gastaut syndrome in the past (Guerrini and Aicardi 2003).

Cognitive impairment is present in most patients and is often associated with behavioral disturbances and psychiatric disorders. Many patients (20–60%) are already developmentally delayed at the onset of the syndrome but the proportion of mentally retarded patients increases to 75–95% at 5 years from onset (Arzimanoglou et al. 2009). In primary cases (30%) the child's development seems normal before the appearance of the first seizures but slowing of mental processing seems to be an almost constant element of the syndrome.

About 80% of patients continue to have seizures later in life, with those of symptomatic origin and early onset having the poorest outcome. Long-term follow-up studies have reported mortality rates of up to 17% (Guerrini 2006).

Electroclinical characteristics

The core seizure types of the syndrome, including tonic, atonic seizures, atypical absences, and episodes of non-convulsive status, are not always present at onset, nor is the interictal EEG pattern of slow spike–wave. Some authors consider the presence of fast (10 Hz) rhythms associated with tonic seizures or occurring with minimal manifestations, especially during non-REM sleep, an essential diagnostic criterion (Beaumanoir 1985; Genton *et al.* 2000).

Tonic seizures, with a "sustained increase in muscle contraction lasting a few seconds to minutes," are the most characteristic type (Blume *et al.* 2001). When the patient is standing, tonic seizures may forcefully throw the patient to the ground, causing sudden drop attacks. During sleep, tonic seizures may have a subtle expression with only opening of the eyes or a short-lasting apnea, or be manifested as full-blown stiffening of the whole body with abduction and elevation of the limbs. Atypical absences can be difficult to identify due to their gradual onset and termination, especially in patients with cognitive impairment. Myoclonic seizures occur in a minority of patients with Lennox–Gastaut syndrome. They are distinctly shorter (<100 ms) than tonic events but may also lead to falls (Blume

et al. 2001) Between 50% and 75% of patients also exhibit episodes of non-convulsive status, manifested as subcontinuous atypical absences with fluctuating responsiveness that may sometimes be interspersed with recurring brief tonic seizures (Arzimanoglou *et al.* 2009). Episodes of non-convulsive status seem definitely to worsen cognitive deterioration (Hoffman-Riem *et al.* 2000). In addition to the main types of attacks, generalized tonic–clonic seizures or focal seizures may be present in a minority of patients.

The classic EEG feature of Lennox–Gastaut syndrome is the slow spike–wave pattern, often repeated in bilaterally synchronous complexes repeated at 1–2 Hz. Although slow spike–wave discharges are often associated with staring, confusion, or at times with an atonic fall, they can be interictal in many cases. Generalized bursts of "polyspikes" or fast rhythms (>10 Hz), also called generalized paroxysmal fast activity, are recorded during slow sleep. Their duration ranges from a few seconds to 15 s, and they tend to recur at relatively brief intervals (Blume *et al.* 1973). They occur as an interictal manifestation or are accompanied by a grading range of clinical manifestations, ranging from opening and upward deviation of the eyes, a brief apnea or a mild EMG axial contraction, to a typical tonic seizure (Fig. 15.3). Sleep EEG recordings may be necessary to elicit their presence.

(a)

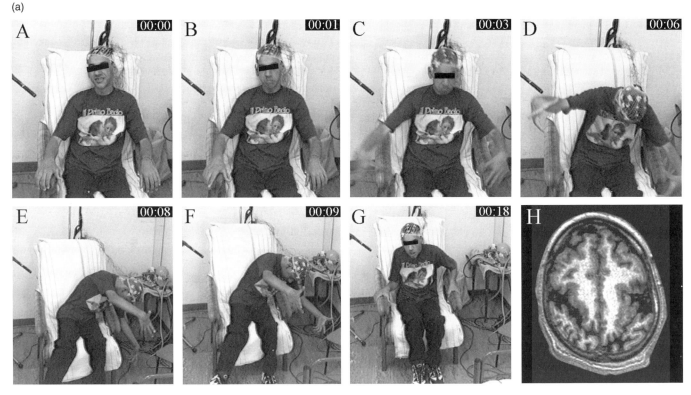

Fig. 15.3. (a) Video recording of a tonic seizure in a patient with symptomatic Lennox–Gastaut syndrome due to bilateral perisylvian polymicrogyria. In (A) the patient is talking with the EEG technician and laughing. Seizure starts in (B) with change of facial expression (pouting). A contraction involves the upper limbs and the axial muscles, producing a relatively slow flexion of the trunk and abduction and extension of both upper limbs (C–F). In (G) the tonic seizure has ended and the patient regains the original posture. Numbers on the top right corner of each picture indicate time from (A) in minutes:seconds format. (H) Axial T1-weighted MRI scan from the same patient. The sylvian fissures appear open and surrounded by a thick cortex. (b) Polygraphic recording of the same seizure shown in Fig. 15.3a. EEG at seizure onset is characterized by a high-amplitude, diffuse slow spike complex, which is followed by a diffuse, high-amplitude, fast, rhythmic activity, which lasts for around 10 s and ends abruptly. EMG from right and left deltoids (R. and L. Delt.) shows an interferential pattern that starts in concomitance with the sharp wave onset and outlasts the fast (recruiting rhythm) polyspike discharge by around 1–2 s. The triangle at lower left indicates when picture (A) was shot.

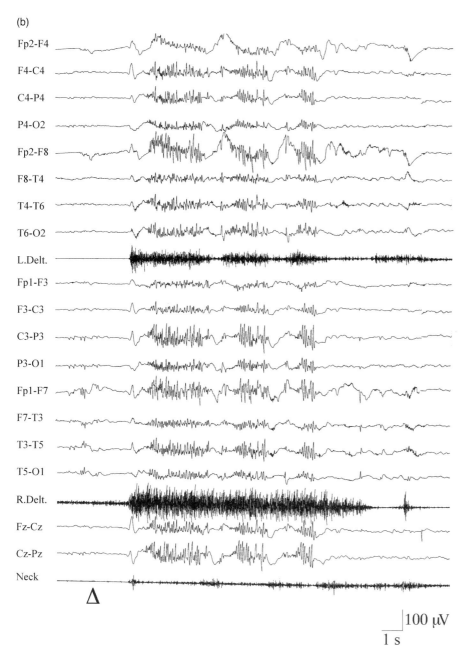

(b)

Fp2-F4
F4-C4
C4-P4
P4-O2
Fp2-F8
F8-T4
T4-T6
T6-O2
L.Delt.
Fp1-F3
F3-C3
C3-P3
P3-O1
Fp1-F7
F7-T3
T3-T5
T5-O1
R.Delt.
Fz-Cz
Cz-Pz
Neck

Δ

100 µV
1 s

Fig. 15.3. *(cont.)*

Differential diagnosis

The typical clinical and EEG manifestations of Lennox–Gastaut syndrome may not be all present at onset, which makes diagnosis difficult especially in cases whose onset is de novo (not resulting as a transition from another syndrome). About 20% of cases of Lennox–Gastaut syndrome gradually evolve after IS and hypsarrhythmia. Distinctions between a prolonged spasm and a short tonic seizure may be arbitrary, although spasms usually appear in clusters while tonic seizures only rarely do so. Drop attacks are also observed in other epilepsy syndromes typical of childhood. In particular, children with myoclonic–astatic epilepsy, aged 2 to 5 years, have prominently myoclonic or myoclonic–astatic seizures, causing drop attacks, and episodes of non-convulsive status epilepticus (also defined as spike-and-wave stupor), interictal spike–wave, and slow spike-and-wave EEG complexes. Some also develop tonic seizures during sleep, which, however, tend to be isolated (Guerrini and Aicardi 2003). Although myoclonic–astatic epilepsy is usually less severe than Lennox–Gastaut syndrome, it fulfills its major diagnostic criteria, making differential diagnosis difficult (Kaminska *et al.* 1999). Difficult problems of differential diagnosis are sometimes posed by epilepsy with continuous spike–waves during sleep (Guerrini *et al.* 1998b) and the so-called atypical benign rolandic epilepsy (Aicardi and Chevrie 1982). Children with this syndrome spectrum present with atypical and atonic absences that may cause repeated falls. Recording of continuous spike–waves during slow sleep and absence of tonic seizures usually permits differential diagnosis.

Etiological factors

Lennox–Gastaut syndrome can appear in the absence of any obvious or suspected etiology (cryptogenic) in otherwise healthy children or be symptomatic. As also observed in West syndrome, the etiology of Lennox–Gastaut syndrome is extremely heterogeneous (Table 15.1). The multiple causes that can be related to the syndrome can play a role for prognosis or sometimes for therapeutic strategies.

A family history of epilepsy is observed in 2.5–28% of cases (Genton and Dravet 2008) but genetic factors, overall, appear to play a minor role. Perinatal hypoxic ischemic brain damage, intrauterine or postnatal infections, malformations of cortical development, chromosomal abnormality syndromes, head trauma, radiotherapy, acute disseminated encephalomyelitis, and brain tumors have been reported (Genton *et al.* 2000). Familial cases of Lennox–Gastaut syndrome have been associated with familial bilateral frontoparietal polymicrogyria due to *GPR56* gene mutations (Parrini *et al.* 2009). In many cases, in spite of normal brain imaging, there is no obvious etiology.

The neurophysiologic bases leading to the interictal and ictal EEG manifestations of Lennox–Gastaut syndrome are poorly understood. Processes related to idiopathic generalized epilepsies seem to play a limited part, if any, since abnormal sleep patterns found in Lennox–Gastaut syndrome seem to originate outside the usual thalamocortical circuit. The cortical process of secondary bilateral synchrony likely plays a major role in the generation of the seemingly generalized discharges. Epileptic myoclonus in Lennox–Gastaut syndrome appears to originate from a stable generator in the frontal cortex, with spread to contralateral and ipsilateral cortical areas, while in myoclonic–astatic epilepsy it appears to be a primary generalized epileptic phenomenon (Bonanni *et al.* 2002). There is no obvious explanation for this abnormal tendency to secondary bilateral synchrony in Lennox–Gastaut syndrome. Blume hypothesized that overwhelming diffuse ictal and interictal discharges at a crucial age play a major role in diverting the brain from physiologic developmental processes towards seizure control mechanisms (Blume 2004).

Principles of treatment

The optimum treatment for Lennox–Gastaut syndrome remains uncertain. Broad-spectrum drugs should be preferred (French *et al.* 2004). Only a few controlled studies are available, usually designed to evaluate efficacy of one drug on one or two types of seizures and no study is available investigating early overall effect of a given drug on the syndrome evolution. Randomized clinical trials in Lennox–Gastaut syndrome have been performed for lamotrigine, topiramate, felbamate, rufinamide, thyrotropin-releasing hormone (TRH) analog, and cinromide (reviewed in Arzimanoglou *et al.* 2009). A recent Cochrane Review (Hancock and Cross 2009) concluded that although the optimum treatment for Lennox–Gastaut syndrome remains uncertain and no study to date has shown any one drug to be highly efficacious, rufinamide, lamotrigine, topiramate, and felbamate may be helpful as add-on therapy. A decrease in the frequency of all seizures was found for lamotrigine (Motte *et al.* 1997), felbamate (Felbamate Study Group 1993), and rufinamide (Glauser *et al.* 2008) whereas for topiramate the decrease in total seizure frequency failed to reach statistical significance (Sachdeo *et al.* 1999). However, there is no guidance on how to combine these drugs and many researchers combine them with valproate, ethosuximide, or benzodiazepines. However, treatment approaches are complicated by the potential of polytherapies for adverse events and seizure aggravation (Guerrini *et al.* 1998).

It has been suggested that vagus nerve stimulation and a ketogenic diet can be useful in some cases (Neal *et al.* 2008). Anterior callosotomy might reduce seizures with drop attacks (Oguni *et al.* 1991).

References

Aicardi J, Chevrie JJ (1982) Atypical benign epilepsy of childhood. *Dev Med Child Neurol* **24**:281–92.

Appleton RE, Peters AC, Mumford JP, Shaw DE (1999) Randomized, placebo-controlled study of vigabatrin as first-line treatment of infantile spasms. *Epilepsia* **40**:1627–33.

Archer HL, Evans J, Edwards S, *et al.* (2006) *CDKL5* mutations cause infantile spasms, early onset seizures, and severe mental retardation in female patients. *J Med Genet* **43**:729–34.

Arzimanoglou A, Guerrini R, Aicardi J (2004) *Aicardi's Epilepsy in Children*, 3rd edn. Philadelphia, PA: Lippincott Williams and Wilkins.

Arzimanoglou A, French J, Blume WT, *et al.* (2009) Lennox–Gastaut syndrome: a consensus approach on diagnosis, assessment, management, and trial methodology. *Lancet Neurol* **8**:82–93.

Asano E, Chugani DC, Juhasz C, Muzik O, Chugani HT (2001) Surgical treatment of West syndrome. *Brain Dev* **23**:668–76.

Bankier A, Turner M, Hopkins IJ (1983) Pyridoxine dependent seizures: a wider clinical spectrum. *Arch Dis Childh* **58**:415–18.

Baram TZ, Mitchell WG, Tournay A, *et al.* (1996) High-dose corticotropin (ACTH) versus prednisone for infantile spasms: a prospective, randomized, blinded study. *Pediatrics* **97**:375–9.

Barkovich AJ, Guerrini R, Battaglia G, *et al.* (1994) Band heterotopia: correlation of outcome with magnetic resonance imaging parameters. *Ann Neurol* **36**:609–17.

Barkovich AJ, Kuzniecky RI, Jackson GD, Guerrini R, Dobyns WB (2005)

A developmental and genetic classification for malformation of cortical development. *Neurology* **65**:1873–87.

Bastos AC, Comeau RM, Andermann F, *et al.* (1999) Diagnosis of subtle focal dysplastic lesions: curvilinear reformatting from three-dimensional magnetic resonance imaging. *Ann Neurol* **46**:88–94.

Beaumanoir A (1985) The Lennox–Gastaut syndrome. In: Roger J, Bureau M, Dravet C, Genton P Tassinari CA, Wolf P (eds.) *Epileptic Syndromes in Infancy, Childhood and Adolescence.* London: Demos, pp. 89–99.

Bednarek N, Motte J, Soufflet C, Plouin P, Dulac O (1998) Evidence of late-onset infantile spasms. *Epilepsia* **39**:55–60.

Bellman MH, Ross EM, Miller DL (1983) Infantile spasms and pertussis immunisation. *Lancet* **1**:1031–4.

Berg AT, Shinnar S, Levy SR, *et al.* (2000) How well can epilepsy syndromes be identified at diagnosis? A reassessment 2 years after initial diagnosis. *Epilepsia* **41**:1269–75.

Blume WT (2004) Lennox–Gastaut syndrome: potential mechanisms of cognitive regression. *Ment Retard Dev Disabil Res Rev* **10**:150–3.

Blume WT, David RB, Gomez MR (1973) Generalized sharp and slow wave complexes: associated clinical features and long-term follow-up. *Brain* **96**:289–306.

Blume WT, Luders HO, Mizrahi E, *et al.* (2001) ILAE Commission Report – Glossary of descriptive terminology for ictal semiology: Report of the ILAE Task Force on Classification and Terminology. *Epilepsia* **42**:1212–18.

Bonanni P, Parmeggiani L, Guerrini R (2002) Different neurophysiologic patterns of myoclonus characterize Lennox–Gastaut syndrome and myoclonic astatic epilepsy. *Epilepsia* **43**:609–15.

Cao A, Cianchetti C, Signorini E, *et al.* (1977) Agenesis of the corpus callosum, infantile spasms, spastic quadriplegia, microcephaly and severe mental retardation in three siblings. *Clin Genet* **12**:290–6.

Caplan C, Guthrie D, Mundy P, *et al.* (1992) Non-verbal communication skills of surgically treated children with infantile spasms. *Dev Med Child Neurol* **34**:499–506.

Cerullo A, Marini C, Carcangiu R, Baruzzi A, Tinuper P (1999) Clinical and video-polygraphic features of epileptic spasms in adults with cortical migration disorder. *Epilept Disord* **1**:27–33.

Chan S, Chin SS, Nordli DR, *et al.* (1998) Prospective magnetic resonance imaging identification of focal cortical dysplasia, including the non-balloon cell subtype. *Ann Neurol* **44**:749–57.

Chevrie JJ, Aicardi J (1971) Le pronostic psychique des spasmes infantiies traités par l'ACTH ou les corticoïdes: analyse statistique de 78 cas suivis plus d'un an. *J Neurol Sci* **12**:351–7.

Chevrie JJ, Aicardi J (1977) Convulsive disorders in the first year of life: etiologic factors. *Epilepsia* **18**:489–98.

Chevrie JJ, Aicardi J (1986) The Aicardi syndrome. In: Pedley TA, Meldrum BS (eds.) *Recent Advances in Epilepsy*, vol. **3**. Edinburgh, UK: Churchill Livingstone, pp. 189–210.

Chugani HT, Mazziota JC, Engel J Jr., Phelps ME (1987) The Lennox–Gastaut syndrome: metabolic subtypes determined by 2-dioxy-2 ^{18}F-fluoro-D-glucose positron emission tomography. *Ann Neurol* **21**:4–13.

Chugani HT, Da Silva E, Chugani DC (1996) Infantile spasms. III. Prognostic implications of bitemporal hypometabolism on positron emission tomography. *Ann Neurol* **39**:643–9.

Ciardo F, Zamponi N, Specchio N, Parmeggiani L, Guerrini R (2001) Autosomal recessive polymicrogyria with infantile spasms and limb deformities. *Neuropediatrics* **32**:325–9.

Claes S, Devriendt K, Lagae L, *et al.* (1997) The X-linked infantile spasms syndrome (MIM 308350) maps to Xp11.4–Xpter in two pedigrees. *Ann Neurol* **42**:360–4.

Coleman M, Hart PN, Randall J, *et al.* (1977) Serotonin levels in the blood and central nervous system of a patient with sudanophilic leukodystrophy. *NeuroPédiatrie* **8**:459–66.

Cossette P, Riviello JJ, Carmant L (1999) ACTH versus vigabatrin therapy in infantile spasms: a retrospective study. *Neurology* **52**:1691–4. Erratum in: *Neurology* (2000) **54**:539.

Curatolo P (1996) Neurological manifestations of tuberous sclerosis complex. *Childs Nerv Syst* **12**:515–21.

Curatolo P, Seri S, Verdecchia M, Bombardieri R (2001) Infantile spasms in tuberous scleroris complex. *Brain Dev* **23**:502–7.

Coulter DL (1986) Continuous infantile spasms as a form of status epilepticus. *J Child Neurol* **1**:215–17.

Dabora SL, Jozwiak S, Franz DN, *et al.* (2001) Mutational analysis in a cohort of 224 tuberous sclerosis patients indicates increased severity of *TSC2*, compared with *TSC1*, disease in multiple organs. *Am J Hum Genet* **68**:64–80.

Dalla Bernardina B, Watanabe K (1994) Interictal EEG: variations and pitfalls. In: Dulac O, Chugani HT, Dalla Bernardina B (eds.) *Infantile Spasms and West Syndrome.* Philadelphia, PA: WB Saunders, pp. 63–81.

de Menezes MA, Rho JM (2002) Clinical and electrographic features of epileptic spasms persisting beyond the second year of life. *Epilepsia* **43**:623–30.

Dobyns WB, Berry-Kravis E, Havernick NJ, Holden KR, Viskochil D (1999) X-linked lissencephaly with absent corpus callosum and ambiguous genitalia. *Am J Med Genet* **86**:331–7.

Donat JF, Wright FS (1991) Simultaneous infantile spasms and partial seizures. *J Child Neurol* **6**:246–50.

Dravet C, Giraud N, Bureau M, *et al.* (1986) Benign myoclonus of early infancy or benign non-epileptic spasms. *Neuropediatrics* **17**:33–8.

Dulac O (1997) Infantile spasms and West syndrome. In: Engel J Jr., Pedley T (eds.) *Epilepsy: A Comprehensive Textbook.* Philadelphia, PA: Lippincott–Raven, pp. 2277–83.

Dulac O (2001) What is West syndrome? *Brain Dev* **23**:447–52.

Dulac O, Plouin P, Perulli L, *et al.* (1983) Aspects électroencéphalographiques de l'agyrie–pachygyrie classique. *Rev EEG Neurophysiol Clin* **13**:232–9.

Dulac O, Plouin P, Jambaqué I, Motte J (1986) Spasmes infantiles épileptiques bénins. *Rev EEG Neurophysiol Clin* **16**:371–82.

Dulac O, Chugani T, Dalla Bernardina B (1994) Overview. In: Dulac O, Chugani T, Dalla Bernardina B (eds.) *Infantile Spasms and West Syndrome.* Philadelphia, PA: WB Saunders, pp. 1–5.

Dulac O, Pinard JM, Plouin P (1996) Infantile spasms associated with cortical dysplasia and tuberous sclerosis. In: Guerrini R, Andermann F, Canapicchi R (eds.) *Dysplasias of Cerebral Cortex and Epilepsy*. Philadelphia, PA: Lippincott–Raven, pp. 217–25.

Egli M, Mothersill I, O'Kane M, O'Kane F (1985) The axial spasm: the predominant type of drop seizure in patients with secondary generalized epilepsy. *Epilepsia* 26:401–15.

Elia M, Falco M, Ferri R, *et al.* (2008) CDKL5 mutations in boys with severe encephalopathy and early-onset intractable epilepsy. *Neurology* 71:997–9.

Elterman RD, Shields WD, Mansfield KA, Nakagawa J (2001) US Infantile Spasms Vigabatrin Study Group: randomized trial of vigabatrin in patients with infantile spasms. *Neurology* 57:1416–21.

Eriksson SH, Rugg-Gunn FJ, Symms MR, Barker GJ, Duncan JS (2001) Diffusion tensor imaging in patients with epilepsy and malformation of cortical development. *Brain* 124:617–26.

Fejerman N, Caraballo R (2002) Appendix to Shuddering and benign myoclonus of early infancy. In: Guerrini R, Aicardi J, Andermann F, Hallett M (eds.) *Epilepsy and Movement Disorders*. Cambridge: Cambridge University Press, pp. 349–51.

Felbamate Study Group in Lennox–Gastaut Syndrome (1993) Efficacy of felbamate in childhood epileptic encephalopathy (Lennox–Gastaut syndrome). *N Engl J Med* 328:29–33.

Fleiszar KA, Daniel WL, Imrey PB (1977) Genetic study of infantile spasms with hypsarrhythmia. *Epilepsia* 18:55–62.

French JA, Kanner AM, Bautista J, *et al.* (2004) Efficacy and tolerability of the new antiepileptic drugs. II. Treatment of refractory epilepsy: report of the Therapeutics and Technology Assessment Subcommittee of the American Academy of Neurology; Quality Standards Subcommittee of the American Academy of Neurology; American Epilepsy Society. *Neurology* 62:1261–73.

Fusco L, Vigevano F (1993) Ictal clinical electroencephalographic findings of spasms in West syndrome. *Epilepsia* 34:671–8.

Fusco L, Pachatz C, Cusmai R, Vigevano F (1999) Repetitive sleep starts in neurologically impaired children: an unusual non-epileptic manifestation in otherwise epileptic subjects. *Epilept Disord* 1:63–7.

Gaily E, Liukkonen E, Paetau R, Rekola R, Granstrom ML (2001) Infantile spasms: diagnosis and assessment of treatment response by video-EEG. *Dev Med Child Neurol* 43:658–67.

Gastaut H, Roger J, Soulayrol R, *et al.* (1966) Childhood epileptic encephalopathy with diffuse slow spike-waves (otherwise known as "petit mal variant") or Lennox Syndrome. *Epilepsia* 7:139–79.

Gastaut H, Pinsard N, Raybaud C, Aicardi J, Zifkin B (1987) Lissencephaly (agyria–pachygyria): clinical findings and serial EEG studies. *Dev Med Child Neurol* 29:167–80.

Genton P, Dravet C (2008) Lennox–Gastaut syndrome. In: Engel J Jr., Pedley TA (eds.) *Epilepsy: A Comprehensive Textbook*, 2nd edn. Philadelphia, PA: Lippincott Williams and Wilkins, pp. 2417–27.

Genton P, Guerrini R, Dravet C (2000) The Lennox–Gastaut syndrome. In: Meinardi H (ed.) *Handbook of Clinical Neurology*, vol. 73, *The Epilepsies, Part II*. Amsterdam: Elsevier, pp. 211–22.

Glauser T, Kluger G, Sachdeo R, *et al.* (2008) Rufinamide for generalized seizures associated with Lennox–Gastaut syndrome. *Neurology* 70:1950–8.

Gobbi G, Bruno L, Pini A, Rossi PG, Tassinari CA (1987) Periodic spasms: an unclassified type of epileptic seizure in childhood. *Dev Med Child Neurol* 27:766–75.

Guerrini R (2006) Epilepsy in children. *Lancet* 367:499–524.

Guerrini R, Aicardi J (2003) Epileptic encephalopathies with myoclonic seizures in infants and children (severe myoclonic epilepsy and myoclonic-astatic epilepsy). *J Clin Neurophysiol* 20:449–61.

Guerrini R, Carrozzo R (2001a) Epilepsy and genetic malformations of the cerebral cortex. *Am J Med Genet* 106:160–73.

Guerrini R, Carrozzo R (2001b) Epileptogenic brain malformations: clinical presentation, malformative patterns and indications for genetic testing. *Seizure* 10:532–47.

Guerrini R, Genton P, Dravet C, *et al.* (1992) Compulsive somatosensory self stimulation inducing epileptic seizures. *Epilepsia* 33:509–16.

Guerrini R, Robain O, Dravet C, Canapicchi R, Roger J (1993) Clinical, electrographic and pathological findings in the gyral disorders. In: Fejerman N, Chamoles NA (eds.) *New Trends in Pediatric Neurology*. Amsterdam: Elsevier, pp. 101–7.

Guerrini R, Andermann F, Canapicchi R, *et al.* (eds.) (1996) *Dysplasias of Cerebral Cortex and Epilepsy*. Philadephia, PA: Lippincott–Raven.

Guerrini R, Belmonte A, Genton P (1998a) Antiepileptic drug-induced worsening of seizures in children. *Epilepsia* 39(Suppl 3):S2–10.

Guerrini R, Genton P, Bureau M, *et al.* (1998b) Multilobar polymicrogyria, intractable drop attack seizures, and sleep-related electrical status epilepticus. *Neurology* 51:504–12.

Guerrini R, Belmonte A, Carrozzo R (1998c) Paroxysmal tonic upgaze of childhood with ataxia: a benign transient dystonia with autosomal dominant inheritance. *Brain Dev* 20:116–18.

Guerrini R, Andermann E, Avoli M, Dobyns WB (1999) Cortical dysplasias, genetics and epileptogenesis. *Adv Neurol* 79:95–121.

Guerrini R, Moro F, Kato M, *et al.* (2007) Expansion of the first PolyA tract of ARX causes infantile spasms and status dystonicus. *Neurology* 69:427–33.

Guerrini R, Dobyns WB, Barkovich AJ (2008) Abnormal development of the human cerebral cortex: genetics, functional consequences and treatment options. *Trends Neurosci* 31:154–62.

Haga Y, Watanabe K, Negoro T, *et al.* (1995) Do ictal, clinical, and electroencephalographic features predict outcome in West syndrome? *Pediatr Neurol* 13:226–9.

Hancock EC, Cross HH (2009) Treatment of Lennox–Gastaut syndrome. *Cochrane Database Syst Rev*: CD003277.

Hancock EC, Osborne JP, Milner P (2002) Treatment of infantile spasms. *Cochrane Database Syst Rev*: CD001770.

Heiskala H, Riikonen R, Santavuori P, *et al.* (1996) West syndrome: individualized ACTH therapy. *Brain Dev* 18:456–60.

Hoffmann-Riem M, Diener W, Benninger C, *et al.* (2000) Nonconvulsive status epilepticus: a possible cause of mental retardation in patients with Lennox–Gastaut syndrome. *Neuropediatrics* 31:169–74.

Hrachovy RA, Frost JD (1989) Infantile spasms. *Ped Clin N Am* 36:311–30.

Hrachovy RA, Frost JD, Kellaway P (1984) Hypsarrhythmia, variations on the theme. *Epilepsia* 25:317–25.

Ikeno T, Shigematsu H, Miyakushi M, *et al.* (1985) An analytic study of epileptic falls. *Epilepsia* **26**:612–21.

ILAE Commission on Classification and Terminology (1989) Proposal for revised classification of epilepsies and epileptic syndromes. *Epilepsia* **30**:389–99.

Jambaqué I, Cusmai R, Curatolo P, *et al.* (1991) Neuropsychological aspects of Tuberous Sclerosis in relation to epilepsy and MRI findings. *Dev Med Child Neurol* **33**:698–705.

Jambaqué I, Chiron C, Dulac O, Raynaud C, Syrota P (1993) Visual inattention in West syndrome: a neuropsychological and neurofunctional imaging study. *Epilepsia* **34**:692–700.

Jambaqué I, Chiron C, Dumas C, Mumford J, Dulac O (2000) Mental and behavioral outcome of infantile epilepsy treated by vigabatrin in tuberous sclerosis patients. *Epilepsy Res* **38**:151–60.

Juhasz C, Chugani HT, Muzik O, Chugani DC (2001) Neuroradiological assessment of brain structure and function and its implication in the pathogenesis of West syndrome. *Brain Dev* **23**:488–95.

Kaminska A, Ickowicz A, Plouin P, *et al.* (1999) Delineation of cryptogenic Lennox–Gastaut syndrome and myoclonic astatic epilepsy using multiple correspondence analysis. *Epilepsy Res* **36**:15–29.

Kato M, Das S, Petras K, Sawaishi Y, Dobyns WB (2003) Polyalanine expansion of *ARX* associated with cryptogenic West syndrome. *Neurology* **61**:267–76.

Kato M, Das S, Petras K, *et al.* (2004) Mutations of *ARX* are associated with striking pleiotropy and consistent genotype–phenotype correlation. *Hum Mutat* **23**:147–59.

Kellaway P, Frost JD, Hrachovy RA (1983) Infantile spasms. In: Morselli PL, Pippenger CE, Penry JK (eds.) *Antiepileptic Drug Therapy*. New York: Raven Press, pp. 115–36.

Kellaway P, Hrachovy RA, Frost JD, Zion T (1979) Precise characterization and quantification of infantile spasms. *Ann Neurol* **6**:214–18.

King M, Stephenson JBP, Ziervogel M, Doyle D, Galbraith S (1985) Hemimegalencephaly: a case for hemispherectomy. *Neuropediatrics* **16**:46–55.

Koo B, Hwang P (1996) Localization of focal cortical lesions influences age of onset of infantile spasms. *Epilepsia* **37**:1068–71.

Kossoff EH (2010) Infantile spasms. *Neurologist* **16**:69–75.

Kossoff EH, Pyzik PL, McGrogan JR, Vining EP, Freeman JM (2002) Efficacy of the ketogenic diet for infantile spasms. *Pediatrics* **109**:780–3.

Kossoff EH, Hartman AL, Rubenstein JE, Vining EP (2009) High-dose oral prednisolone for infantile spasms: an effective and less expensive alternative to ACTH. *Epilepsy Behav* **14**:674–6.

Krishnamoorthy KS (1983) Pyridoxine-dependency seizure: report of a rare presentation. *Ann Neurol* **13**:103–4.

Lacy JR, Penry JK (1976) *Infantile Spasms.* New York: Raven Press.

Lennox WG, Davis JP (1950) Clinical correlates of the fast and slow spike–wave electroencephalogram. *Pediatrics* **5**:626–44.

Lewis H, Wallace SJ (2001) Vigabatrin. *Dev Med Child Neurol* **43**:833–5.

Livingston JH (1988) The Lennox–Gastaut syndrome. *Dev Med Child Neurol* **30**:536–40.

Lombroso CT (1983) A prospective study of infantile spasms: clinical and therapeutic correlations. *Epilepsia* **24**:135–58.

Lux AL, Edwards SW, Hancock E, *et al.* (2004) The United Kingdom Infantile Spasms Study comparing vigabatrin with prednisolone or tetracosactide at 14 days: a multicentre, randomised controlled trial. *Lancet* **364**:1773–8.

Lux AL, Edwards SW, Hancock E, *et al.* (2005) The United Kingdom Infantile Spasms Study (UKISS) comparing hormone treatment with vigabatrin on developmental and epilepsy outcomes to age 14 months: a multicentre randomised trial. *Lancet Neurol* **4**:712–17.

Mari F, Azimonti S, Bertani I, *et al.* (2005) *CDKL5* belongs to the same molecolar pathway of MeCP2 and it is responsible for the early-onset seizure variant of Rett syndrome. *Hum Mol Genet* **14**:1935–46.

Marshall CR, Young EJ, Pani AM, *et al.* (2008) Infantile spasms is associated with deletion of the MAGI2 gene on chromosome 7q11.23–q21.11. *Am J Hum Genet* **83**:106–11.

Mei D, Marini C, Novara F, *et al.* (2009) Xp22.3 genomic deletions involving the *CDKL5* gene in girls with early onset epileptic encephalopathy. *Epilepsia* **51**:647–54.

Metsähonkala L, Gaily E, Rantala H, *et al.* (2002) Focal and global cortical hypometabolism in patients with newly diagnosed infantile spasms. *Neurology* **58**:1646–51.

Motte J, Billard C, Fejerman N, *et al.* (1993) Neurofibromatosis type one and West syndrome: a relatively benign association. *Epilepsia* **34**:723–6.

Motte J, Trevathan E, Arvidsson JF, *et al.* (1997) Lamotrigine for generalized seizures associated with Lennox–Gastaut syndrome. *N Engl J Med* **337**:1807–12.

Mytinger JR, Quigg M, Taft WC, Buck ML, Rust RS (2010) Outcomes in treatment of infantile spasms with pulse methylprednisolone. *J Child Neurol Feb* 8. [Epub ahead of print].

Nabbout R, Melki I, Gerbaka B, Dulac O, Akatcherian C (2001) Infantile spasms in Down syndrome: good response to a short course of vigabatrin. *Epilepsia* **42**:1580–3.

Neal EG, Chaffe H, Schwartz RH, *et al.* (2008) The ketogenic diet for the treatment of childhood epilepsy: a randomised controlled trial. *Lancet Neurol* **7**:500–6.

Niedermeyer E (1969) The Lennox–Gastaut syndrome: a severe type of childhood epilepsy. *Dtsch Z Nervenheilk* **195**:263–82.

Oguni H, Olivier A, Andermann F, Comair J (1991) Anterior callosotomy in the treatment of medically intractable epilepsies: a study of 43 patients with a mean follow-up of 39 months. *Ann Neurol* **30**:357–64.

Pachatz C, Fusco L, Vigevano F (2003) Epileptic spasms and partial seizures as a single ictal event. *Epilepsia* **44**:693–700.

Paladin F, Chiron C, Dulac O, Plouin P, Ponsot G (1989) Electroencephalographic aspects of hemimegalencephaly. *Dev Med Child Neurol* **31**:377–83.

Parrini E, Ferrari AR, Dorn T, Walsh CA, Guerrini R (2009) Bilateral frontoparietal polymicrogyria, Lennox–Gastaut syndrome, and *GPR56* gene mutations. *Epilepsia* **50**:1344–53.

Plouin P, Jalin C, Dulac O, Chiron C (1987) Enregistrement ambulatoire de l'EEG pendant 24 heures dans les spasmes infantiles épileptiques. *Rev EEG Neurophysiol Clin* **17**:309–18.

Poley JR, Dumermuth G (1968) EEG findings in patients with phenylketonuria before and during treatment with a low phenylalanine diet and in patients with some other inborn errors of metabolism. In: Holt KS,

Coffey VP (eds.) *Some Recent Advances in Inborn Errors of Metabolism*. Edinburgh, UK: Churchill Livingstone, pp. 61–9.

Pulsifer MB, Brandt J, Salorio CF, *et al.* (2004) The cognitive outcome of hemispherectomy in 71 children. *Epilepsia* **45**:243–54.

Quirk JA, Kendall B, Kingsley DP, Boyd SG, Pitt MC (1993) EEG features of cortical dysplasia in children. *Neuropediatrics* **24**:193–9.

Reiter E, Tiefenthaler M, Freillinger M, *et al.* (2000) Familial idiopathic West syndrome. *J Child Neurol* **15**:249–52.

Riikonen R (1983) Infantile spasms: some new theoretical aspects. *Epilepsia* **24**:159–68.

Riikonen R (1984) Infantile spasms: modern practical aspects. *Acta Paediatr Scand* **73**:1–6.

Riikonen R (2001) Epidemiological data of West syndrome in Finland. *Brain Dev* **23**:539–41.

Roger J, Dravet C, Boniver C, *et al.* (1984) L'Epilepsie dans la sclérose tubéreuse de Bourneville. *Boll Lega It Epil* **45/46**:33–8.

Sachdeo RC, Glauser TA, Ritter F, *et al.* (1999) Double-blind, randomized trial of topiramate in Lennox–Gastaut syndrome. *Neurology* **52**:1882–7.

Saltik S, Kocer N, Dervent A (2002) Informative value of magnetic resonance imaging and EEG in the prognosis of infantile spasms. *Epilepsia* **43**:246–52.

Sankar R, Curran JG, Kevill JW, *et al.* (1995) Microscopic cortical dysplasia in infantile spasms: evolution of white matter abnormalities. *Am J Neuroradiol* **16**:1265–72.

Scala E, Ariani F, Mari F, *et al.* (2005) *CDKL5/STK9* is mutated in Rett syndrome variant with infantile spasms. *J Med Genet* **42**:103–7.

Seppäläinen AM, Similä S (1971) Electroencephalographic findings in three patients with nonketotic hyperglycinemia. *Epilepsia* **12**:101–7.

Silva ML, Cieuta C, Guerrini R, *et al.* (1996) Early clinical and EEG features of infantile spasms in Down syndrome. *Epilepsia* **37**:977–82.

Stafstrom CE, Patxot CE, Gilmore HE, Wisniewski KE (1991) Seizures in children with Down syndrome: etiology, characteristics and outcome. *Dev Med Child Neurol* **33**:191–200.

Stafstrom CE, Konkol RJ (1994) Infantile spasms in children with Down syndrome. *Dev Med Child Neurol* **36**:576–85.

Strømme P, Mangelsdorf ME, Shaw MA, *et al.* (2002) Mutations in the human ortholog of *Aristaless* cause X-linked mental retardation and epilepsy. *Nat Genet* **30**:441–5.

Stromme P, Sundet K, Mork C, *et al.* (1999) X-linked mental retardation and infantile spasms in a family: new clinical data and linkage to Xp11.4–Xp22.11. *J Med Genet* **36**:374–8.

Sugai K, Fukuyama Y, Yasuda K, *et al.* (2001) Clinical and pedigree study on familial cases of West syndrome in Japan. *Brain Dev* **123**:558–64.

Trevathan E, Murphy CC, Yeargin-Allsopp M (1999) The descriptive epidemiology of infantile spasms among Atlanta children. *Epilepsia* **40**:748–51.

Vigabatrin Pediatric Advisory Group (2000) Guideline for prescribing vigabatrin in children has been revised. *Br Med J* **320**:1404–5.

Vigevano F, Cilio MR (1997) Vigabatrin versus ACTH as first-line treatment for infantile spasms: a randomized, prospective study. *Epilepsia* **38**:1270–4.

Vigevano F, Fusco L, Cusmai R, *et al.* (1993) The idiopathic form of West syndrome. *Epilepsia* **34**:743–6.

Vigevano F, Fusco L, Pachatz C (2001) Neurophysiology of spasms. *Brain Dev* **23**:467–72.

Watanabe K, Iwase K, Hara K (1973) The evolution of EEG features in infantile spasms: a prospective study. *Dev Med Child Neurol* **15**:584–96.

Weaving LS, Christodoulou J, Williamson SL, *et al.* (2004) Mutations of *CDKL5* cause a severe neurodevelopmental disorder with infantile spasms and mental retardation. *Am J Hum Genet* **75**:1079–93.

Wong M, Trevathan E (2001) Infantile spasms. *Pediatr Neurol* **24**:89–98.

Yamamoto N, Watanabe K, Negoro T (1988) Partial seizures evolving to infantile spasms. *Epilepsia* **29**:34–40.

Chapter

16

Unverricht–Lundborg disease

Maria K. Lehtinen, Anna-Elina Lehesjoki, and Reetta Kälviäinen

The causal disease

Progressive myoclonus epilepsy of the Unverricht–Lundborg type (EPM1) is an autosomal recessive neurodegenerative disorder that has the highest incidence among the progressive myoclonus epilepsies worldwide (Berkovic et al. 1986; Marseille Consensus Group 1990). It is characterized by stimulus-sensitive myoclonus, and tonic–clonic epileptic seizures. As EPM1 progresses, patients develop additional neurological symptoms including ataxia, dysarthria, intentional tremor, and decreased coordination, together reflecting widespread neuronal degeneration in the brain (Koskiniemi et al. 1974a, Norio and Koskiniemi 1979). Some patients become wheelchair-bound. Patients may experience emotional lability, depression, and a mild intellectual decline over time, but overall their cognitive functions are less impaired than their motor functions (Koskiniemi et al. 1974a; Lehesjoki and Kälviäinen 2007; Kälviäinen et al. 2008). Loss-of-function mutations in the gene encoding CYSTATIN B (CSTB) are the primary genetic cause of EPM1 (Lalioti et al. 1997; Pennacchio et al. 1998; Joensuu et al., 2008).

Previously EPM1 has been known by the following names: Baltic myoclonus, Baltic myoclonic epilepsy, and Mediterranean myoclonus. With advances in genetic testing, these disorders are now collectively classified as EPM1 (Kälviäinen et al. 2008).

Epilepsy in the disease

At disease onset (6–16 years), EPM1 patients present primarily with myoclonic jerks and/or generalized tonic–clonic seizures. Involuntary action-activated or stimulus-sensitive myoclonus (i.e., triggered by light, physical activity, noise, cognitive stimulus, and/or stress) is observed in the majority of patients (Koskiniemi et al. 1974a; Norio and Koskiniemi 1979). This asynchronized myoclonus occurs primarily in the proximal muscles of the extremities; it may be focal or multifocal, and it may generalize to myoclonic seizures or status myoclonicus (Koskiniemi et al. 1974a).

The most prevalent type of epileptic seizures that EPM1 patients present with is generalized tonic–clonic seizures, which can combine with simple motor or complex partial seizures (Koskiniemi et al. 1974a; Norio and Koskiniemi 1979). However, tonic–clonic seizures are not necessarily observed in all cases, as they may be obscured in part by myoclonic jerks. In rare cases, tonic–clonic seizures are not observed at all. The seizures can be controlled with antiepileptic drugs, which in many cases eliminate them altogether. In the final stages of the disease, care should be taken to distinguish between generalized tonic–clonic seizures and continuous myoclonic and possibly subcortically generated jerks or status myoclonicus (Lehesjoki and Kälviäinen 2007; Kälviäinen et al. 2008).

Diagnostic tests for the disease

Diagnosis should be considered for any previously healthy child who between the ages of 6 and 16 presents with at least one of the following symptoms: (1) involuntary, stimulus and/or action activated myoclonic jerks, (2) generalized tonic–clonic seizures, (3) mild neurological signs in motor function or coordination, (4) photosensitivity, generalized spike-and-wave and polyspike-and-wave paroxysms, and background slowing in the electroencephalogram (EEG), and (5) worsening of neurological symptoms (myoclonus and ataxia) (Koskiniemi et al. 1974b; Kälviäinen et al. 2008). At disease onset, the magnetic resonance imaging (MRI) scan is typically normal; however, cerebral atrophy and neuronal loss in the pons, medulla, and cerebellum have been observed in some patients at later stages of the disease. The clinical examination should also include an evaluation of walking, coordination, handwriting, school performance, and emotional states. An examination of the myoclonus should entail an evaluation of the myoclonus at rest, with action, and in response to stimuli including light, noise, and/or stress (Lehesjoki and Kälviäinen 2007; Kälviäinen et al. 2008).

An EEG should be obtained prior to therapeutic intervention. Abnormalities in the EEG (spike–wave discharges,

The Causes of Epilepsy, eds. S. D. Shorvon, F. Andermann, and R. Guerrini. Published by Cambridge University Press. © Cambridge University Press 2011.

photosensitivity, polyspike discharges during rapid eye movement [REM] sleep, background slowing) are more pronounced at initial diagnosis, when disease onset may be accompanied by generalized tonic–clonic seizures (Koskiniemi *et al.* 1974b; Franceschetti *et al.* 1993). Any physiological sleep patterns that are initially observed disappear in about one-half of the patients after 16 years of having the disease. Some patients also present with focal epileptiform discharges, primarily in the occipital region. In general, EEG abnormalities diminish as the disease stabilizes (Ferlazzo *et al.* 2007; Kälviäinen *et al.* 2008). Navigated transcranial magnetic stimulation (TMS) has also revealed significant neurophysiological changes in cortical excitability in which the motor thresholds are elevated and the silent periods are prolonged in EPM1 patients (Danner *et al.* 2009).

Clinical diagnosis can be complemented with genetic testing. Classical EPM1 is an autosomal recessive disorder associated with mutations in the *CSTB* gene (Lalioti *et al.* 1997; Pennacchio *et al.* 1998; Joensuu *et al.* 2008). The majority of EPM1 patients harbor an unstable dodecamer repeat expansion (5′-CCC-CGC-CCC-GCG-3′) in at least one allele in the *CSTB* promoter region (Lalioti *et al.* 1997; Joensuu *et al.* 2008). While normal alleles typically contain two or three dodecamer repeats, disease-causing expansions contain at least 30 such repeats. Heterozygosity for the dodecamer repeat expansion can be accompanied by a number of additional mutations in the coding region of *CSTB* (Lehesjoki and Kälviäinen, 2007; Joensuu *et al.* 2008). The dodecamer repeat expansion mutation accounts for approximately 90% of EPM1 cases worldwide (Lalioti *et al.* 1997; Lehesjoki and Kälviäinen 2007; Joensuu *et al.* 2008).

Patients presenting with symptoms closely resembling EPM1 but who do not harbor mutations in *CSTB* should be evaluated for additional progressive myoclonic epilepsies (PMEs) that closely resemble EPM1 including the recently described EPM1B. The latter is a variant of EPM1 that arises due to a missense nucleotide mutation in the *PRICKLE1* gene (Bassuk *et al.* 2008). Patients with EPM1B present with symptoms at a slightly younger age than EPM1 patients, and in addition to the classic progressive myoclonus and ataxia observed in EPM1 patients, EPM1B patients may present with an impaired upgaze (Bassuk *et al.* 2008). Another PME syndrome that may be considered in differential diagnosis is action myoclonus–renal failure syndrome (AMRF), which arises from mutations in the gene encoding SCARB2/Limp2 (Berkovic *et al.* 2008). Patients with AMRF present typically at 15–25 years of age with either neurological symptoms including tremor, action myoclonus, seizures, and ataxia, or with proteinuria that progresses to renal failure (Berkovic *et al.* 2008). The PMEs as a whole share many key features that make it difficult to distinguish between distinct PMEs. Thus, completing the differential diagnosis among PMEs is critical as the principles of disease management differ greatly depending on the final diagnosis (Table 16.1).

Principles of management

The primary therapeutic approaches for EPM1 patients include rehabilitation and symptomatic pharmacologic management. Pharmacologic intervention includes: valproic acid (the first drug of choice) (Norio and Koskiniemi 1979; Iivanainen and Himberg 1982; Somerville and Olanow 1982; Shahwan *et al.*, 2005), clonazepam (the only drug approved by the US Food and Drug Administration for the treatment of myoclonic seizures) (Iivanainen and Himberg 1982; Shahwan *et al.* 2005), high doses of piracetam (for myoclonus) (Remy and Genton 1991; Koskiniemi *et al.* 1998), levetiracetam (for myoclonus and generalized seizures) (Genton and Gelisse 2000; Frucht *et al.* 2001; Crest *et al.* 2004; Magaudda *et al.* 2004), and topiramate and zonisamide (as supplements) (Henry *et al.* 1988; Aykutlu *et al.* 2005). Myoclonus is resistant to known therapies, and during time periods when stimulus-activated myoclonus is particularly sensitive, loud noises and bright lights should be avoided and the patient should remain in a quiet, peaceful space. In practice, patients require lifelong clinical follow-up and psychosocial support. However, provided with the appropriate social infrastructure, mental balance can be maintained and depression can be prevented (Lehesjoki and Kälviäinen 2007; Kälviäinen *et al.* 2008).

Several case reports suggest that treatment of EPM1 patients with the antioxidant *N*-acetylcysteine (NAC) alleviates key features of the disorder including dysarthria, ataxia, and seizures (Edwards *et al.* 2002). Although the role of oxidative stress in EPM1-linked neuronal degeneration is not completely understood, a specific decrease in cerebellar defenses against oxidative stress and a concomitant increase in lipid peroxidation occurs in the mouse model for EPM1 (Lehtinen *et al.* 2009).

Phenytoin and fosphenytoin should be avoided as these medications trigger detrimental neurological side effects, specifically exacerbating cerebellar degeneration (Eldridge *et al.* 1983). In addition, other sodium channel blockers (carbamazepine, oxcarbazepine), GABAergic drugs (tiagabine, vigabatrin), gabapentin, and pregabalin should be excluded as they may negatively contribute to myoclonus and myoclonic seizures (Medina *et al.* 2005).

In emergencies, intravenous benzodiazepines (diazepam, lorazepam, clonazepam, and midazolam), valproate, and levetiracetam may be administered (Kälviäinen *et al.* 2008). Phenytoin should be used only if the patient is experiencing a distinct localization-related status epilepticus, such as that due to head trauma (Kälviäinen *et al.* 2008).

Ultimately, some EPM1 patients suffer from drug-resistant forms of progressive myoclonus. Myoclonic seizures can also be easily misdiagnosed as tonic–clonic seizures or even pseudoepileptic seizures, especially as the majority of the myoclonic movements are not time-locked to EEG discharges (Kälviäinen *et al.* 2008). Thus, extreme care should be taken when choosing the correct therapeutic intervention.

Table 16.1 Differential characteristics of progressive myoclonic epilepsies

Disease	EPM1 (Unverricht–Lundborg disease)	EPM1B	Lafora disease	Mitochondrial encephalopathy with ragged red fibers (MERRF)	Neuronal ceroid lipofuscinosis (NCL)	Sialidoses
Inheritance[a]	AR	AR	AR	Maternal	AR/AD[b]	AR
Gene	CSTB	PRICKLE1	EPM2A, NHLRC1	MTTK	TPP1, CLN3, CLN5, CLN6	NEU1
Age of onset (years)	6–16	5–10	12–17	Variable	Variable	Variable
Prominent seizures[c]	Myoclonus	Myoclonus	Myoclonus, occipital seizures	Myoclonus	Variable	Myoclonus
Cerebellar signs	Mild and late	Unknown	Early	Variable	Variable	Gradual
Dementia/ Cognitive decline	Mild and late or absent	Mild or absent	Early, relentless	Variable	Rapidly progressive	Absent in Type I; learning difficulty in Type II
Fundi	Normal	Unknown	Normal	With or without optic atrophy or retinopathy	Macular degeneration and visual failure, except Kuf disease	Cherry-red spot
Dysmorphism	No	No	No	Variable	No	Type II
Evolution/ prognosis	Typically mild/ chronic, occasionally severe	Typically mild/ chronic, occasionally severe	Very severe, death within 2–10 yrs	Variable from very mild to very severe	Severe	Variable, usually severe; late onset usually less severe

Notes:
[a]AR, autosomal recessive; AD, autosomal dominant.
[b]Only Kuf (adult NCL) can be inherited in either an autosomal recessive or autosomal dominant manner.
[c]Prominent features.
Source: Modified and updated from Kälviäinen et al. (2008).

References

Aykutlu E, Baykan B, Gurses C, et al. (2005) Add-on therapy with topiramate in progressive myoclonic epilepsy. *Epilepsy Behav* 6:260–3.

Bassuk AG, Wallace RH, Buhr A, et al. (2008) A homozygous mutation in human PRICKLE1 causes an autosomal recessive progressive myoclonic epilepsy–ataxia syndrome. *Am J Hum Genet* 83:572–81.

Berkovic SF, Andermann F, Carpenter S, Wolfe LS (1986) Progressive myoclonic epilepsies: specific causes and diagnosis. *N Engl J Med* 315:296–305.

Berkovic SF, Dibbens LM, Oshlack A, (2008) Array-based gene discovery with three unrelated subjects shows SCARB2/LIMP-2 deficiency causes myoclonus epilepsy and glomerulosclerosis. *Am J Hum Genet* 82:673–84.

Crest C, Dupont S, Leguern E, Adam C, Baulac M (2004) Levetiracetam in progressive myoclonic epilepsy: an exploratory study in 9 patients. *Neurology* 62:640–3.

Danner N, Julkunen P, Khyuppenen J, et al. (2009) Altered cortical inhibition in Unverricht–Lundborg type progressive myoclonic epilepsy. *Epilepsy Res* 85:81–8.

Edwards MJ, Hargreaves IP, Heales SJ, et al. (2002) N-Acetylcysteine and Unverricht–Lundborg disease: variable response and possible side effects. *Neurology* 59:1447–9.

Eldridge R, Iivanainen M, Stern R, Koerber T, Wilder BJ (1983) "Baltic" myoclonus epilepsy: hereditary disorder of childhood made worse by phenytoin. *Lancet* 2:838–42.

Ferlazzo E, Magaudda A, Striano P, et al. (2007) Long-term evolution of EEG in Unverricht–Lundborg disease. *Epilepsy Res* 73:219–27.

Franceschetti S, Antozzi C, Binelli S, et al. (1993) Progressive myoclonus epilepsies: an electrical, biochemical, morphological, and molecular genetic study of 17 cases. *Acta Neurol Scand* 87:219–23.

Frucht SJ, Louis ED, Chuang C, Fahn S (2001) A pilot tolerability and efficacy study of levetiracetam in patients with chronic myoclonus. *Neurology* 57:1112–14.

Genton P, Gelisse P (2000) Autimyoclonic effect of levetiracetam. *Epilept Disord* 2:209–12.

Henry TR, Leppik IE, Gumnit RJ, Jacobs M (1988) Progressive myoclonus epilepsy treated with zonisamide. *Neurology* 38:928–31.

Iivanainen M, Himberg JJ (1982) Valproate and clonazepam in the treatment of severe progressive myoclonus epilepsy. *Arch Neurol* **39**:236–8.

Joensuu T, Lehesjoki AE, Kopra O (2008) Molecular background of EPM1 Unverricht–Lundborg disease. *Epilepsia*, **49**:557–63.

Kälviäinen R, Khyuppenen J, Koskenkorva P, *et al.* (2008) Chinical picture of EPM1-Unverricht–Lundborg disease. *Epilepsia* **49**:549–56.

Koskiniemi M, Donner M, Majuri H, Haltia M, Norio R (1974a) Progressive myoclonus epilepsy: a clinical and histopathological study. *Acta Neurol Scand* **50**:307–32.

Koskiniemi M, Toivakka E, Donner M (1974b) Progressive myoclonus epilepsy: electro encephalo-graphic findings. *Acta Neurol Scand* **50**:333–59.

Koskiniemi M, Van Vleymen B, Hakamies L, Lamusuo S, Taalas J (1998) Piracetain relieves symptoms in progressive myoclonus epilepsy: a multicentre randomised, double blind, crossover study comparing the efficacy and safety of three doses of oral piracetam with place 60. *J Neurol Neurosurg Psychiatry* **64**:344–8.

Lalioti MD, Scott HS, Buresi C, *et al.* (1997) Molecular background of progressive myoclonus epilepsy. *Nature* **386**:847–51.

Lehesjoki A-E, Kälviäinen R (2007) Unverricht–Lundborg disease. In: GeneReviews at GeneTests. *Medical Genetics Information Resource.* Available online at www.genetests.org.

Lehtinen MK, Tegelberg S, Schipper H, *et al.* (2009) Cystatin B deficiency sensitizes neurons to oxidative stress in progressive myoclonus epilepsy, EPM1. *J Neurosci* **29**:5910–15.

Marseille Consensus Group (1990) Classification of progressive myoclonus epilepsies and related disorders. *Ann Neurol* **28**:113–16.

Magaudda A, Gelisse P, Genton P (2004) Antimyoclonic effect of levetiracetam in 13 patients with Unverricht–Lundborg disease. *Epilepsia* **45**:678–81.

Medina MT, Martinez-Juarez IE, Duron RM, *et al.* (2005) Treatment of myoclonic epilepsies of childhood, adolescence, and adulthood. *Adv Neurol* **95**:307–23.

Norio R, Koskiniemi M (1979) Progressive myoclonus epilepsy: genetic and nosological aspects with special reference to 107 Finnish patients. *Clin Genet* **15**:382–98.

Pennacchio LA, Bouley DM, Higgins KM, *et al.* (1998) Progressive ataxia, myoclonic epilepsy, and cerebellar apoptosis in cystatin-B deficient mice. *Nat Genet* **20**:251–8.

Remy C, Genton P (1991) Effect of high-dose piracetam on myoclonus in progressive myoclonus epilepsy (Mediterranean myoclonus). *Epilepsia* **32**:6.

Shahwan A, Farrell M, Delanty N (2005) Progressive myoclonic epilepsies: a review of genetic and therapeutic aspects. *Lancet Neurol* **4**:239–48.

Somerville ER, Olanow CW (1982) Valproic acid: treatment of myoclonus in dyssynergia cerebellaris myoclonica. *Arch Neurol* **39**:527–8.

Dentato-rubro-pallido-luysian atrophy

Teiichi Onuma

Historical note

Smith et al. (1958) described an unusual case of progressive degenerative disorder of cerebellar ataxia with choreic and dystonic involuntary movement in a sporadic case. Autopsy showed combined degeneration of the dentato-rubral and pallido-luysian systems. Also considering two aditional similar cases in the literature, he postulated a disease entity: dentato-rubro-pallido-luysian atrophy (DRPLA). However, the vast majority of reports of a similar disorder came from Japan. Naito and Oyanagi (1982) described five families with a syndrome of myoclonus, epilepsy, dementia, ataxia, and choreoathetosis.

Naito (1989) summarized a total of 37 cases, 14 of his own and 23 from the Japanese literature, and stated that the characteristic features of this disease were autosomal dominant inheritance, with complete penetrance, and different clinical pictures depending on age of onset. In late-onset cases the presenting symptom was ataxia with choreoathetosis, in early-onset cases progressive myoclonus epilepsy with epileptic seizures and mental decline prevailed. Oyanagi and Naito (1977) described characteristic neuropathological findings in four autopsied cases. All showed degenerative changes in the dentate nucleus, red nucleus, globus pallidus, particularly the lateral segment, and subthalamic nucleus.

Epoch-making evidence was the finding of the DRPLA gene located on chromosome 12p13.31 resulting in unstable expansion of CAG repeats in hereditary DRPLA (Koide et al. 1994). Different clinical pictures were dependent upon the size of the expansion. A greater number of expansions of trinucleotide CAG repeats was accompanied by an earlier onset of the disorder, with epileptic seizures and dementia. Late onset was associated with cerebellar ataxia and choreoathetosis, without seizures or dementia and was related to a relatively smaller expansion of CAG repeats.

Prevalence and racial preponderance

The DRPLA disorder was predominantly seen in the Japanese population. Inazuki et al. (1990) estimated the prevalence rate

of this disorder to be roughly 0.2 to 0.6 per 100 000. He found 15 patients from seven families in the Niigata prefecture which had a population of 2 358 417, estimating the prevalence rate of 0.62. Similarly there were three patients in the Toyama and Tottori prefectures with an estimated prevalence rate of 0.21. This survey was done on a hospital basis, not on a population-based study, and might not be accurate but provides at least an idea about the prevalence of this disease in Japan.

The condition is not very rare in Japan. Nineteen cases of DRPLA, aged from 10 to 80 years old, 11 males and 8 females, are currently being followed up by the Out-Patient Clinic of the National Center Hospital for Mental, Nervous and Muscular Diseases. Two of these patients whom the author has closely investigated in this institution will be described in this chapter. This disease seems to be extremely rare outside Japan, although there have been a few reports arising from a different ethnic background (Burke et al. 1994).

Clinical symptoms

Clinical symptoms are considerably different depending on the age of onset. Juvenile onset, under the age of 20 years, has a poor prognosis with relatively rapid progression. Generalized tonic–clonic seizures and myoclonic seizures are usually the first sign. They are difficult to control. Cerebellar ataxia and mental decline eventually appear. Patients face clinical worsening to the point of being confined to a wheelchair or bedridden.

Late-onset DRPLA, after the age of 20 to 50 years, is rarely accompanied by epilepsy; cerebellar ataxia and choreoathetosis dominate the clinical picture and progression is slow. Onset over the age of 50 years is usually accompanied by cerebellar ataxia without epileptic seizures and little deterioration.

Genetics

Koide et al. (1994) found the causative gene on chromosome 12p13.31, where the unstable CAG repeat was located. There was prominent anticipation. A younger age of onset is accompanied by more severe symptoms and by a larger size of CAG expansion.

The Causes of Epilepsy, eds. S. D. Shorvon, F. Andermann, and R. Guerrini. Published by Cambridge University Press. © Cambridge University Press 2011.

Ikeuchi *et al.* (1995) reported that the number of CAG repeats was usually between 7 and 23 in normal subjects, whereas expansion to over 54 was observed in DRPLA patients. Relatively smaller expansions, between 54 and 67, caused later onset, over the age of 21 years, and milder symptoms, such as cerebellar ataxia with slower progression. Relatively larger expansions, between 62 and 79, caused an earlier age of onset, before 21 years, and symptoms of progressive myoclonus epilepsy with convulsive seizures, myoclonic jerks, ataxia, and progressive mental decline. Offspring from an affected father had larger expansions than those exhibiting maternal inheritance, suggesting increased abnormality in male gametogenesis.

Neurophysiological findings

The electroencephalogram (EEG) of DRPLA frequently shows epileptiform discharges (Inazuki *et al.* 1989). Atypical diffuse spike–wave complexes or slow wave bursts were most frequently seen in the progressive myoclonic epilepsy (PME) type of DRPLA, with onset in childhood or adolescence and epileptic seizures. There appeared to be no epileptiform discharges in cases of late-onset DRPLA with ataxia and without epileptic seizures.

Similar epileptiform abnormalities were commonly seen in other PMEs such as myoclonic epilepsy with ragged red fibers (MERRF) or mitochondrial encephalopathy, lactic acidosis, and stroke-like episodes (MELAS), Lafora body disease, or Unverricht–Lundborg disease. Thus the EEG in DRPLA is not disease-specific but state or symptom dependent. The EEG may change from generalized bilaterally synchronous discharges to more disorganized, multiple independent epileptic discharges when the disease progresses, as illustrated in the EEGs of case 2 (see below).

Somatosensory evoked potentials exhibit interesting characteristics. Electrical stimulation of the median nerve at the wrist produces giant somatosensory evoked potentials (SEP) in most PMEs, whereas in DRPLA such giant SEPs are not usually found (Kasai *et al.* 1998). This finding is therefore helpful for differential diagnosis from the other PME syndromes, especially when gene testing is unavailable.

Case presentations
Case 1

Case 1, a 42-year-old female, had a first seizure at the age of 12 years. She woke up in the middle of night and fell into a generalized convulsion. A year later she had another seizure and since then she has had two to three seizures per month. Anticonvulsant medications failed to control the seizures. After age 15 years, mental decline became evident. She failed to reach senior high school. At age 27 years, she was referred to our clinic. She appeared to be disoriented, had dysarthria, ataxia, and myoclonic jerks. At age 32 years, she was unable to walk unsupported and confined to a wheelchair.

We examined her father and grandfather who showed mild cerebellar ataxia without seizures or definite mental decline. Her father had three other siblings of whom two were said to be affected.

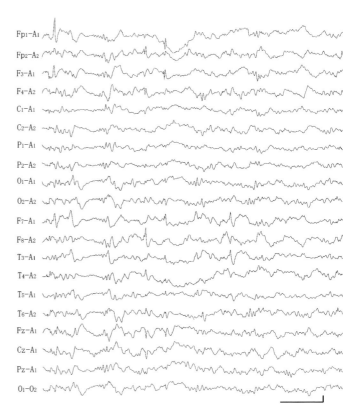

Fig. 17.1. Case 1: EEG at age 31 years. Frequent bilateral asynchronous high-amplitude spikes in the frontotemporal areas and diffuse slow waves. Calibration: 1 s, 50 μV.

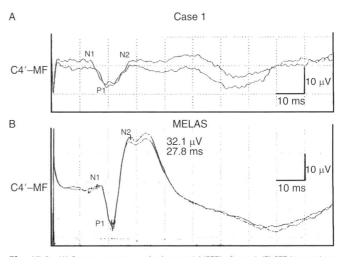

Fig. 17.2. (A) Somatosensory evoked potential (SEP) of case 1. (B) SEP in a patient with progressive myoclonus epilepsy (MELAS) whose clinical symptoms were similar to those of case 1, including seizures and mental deterioration. This case is illustrated for comparison. Case 1 showed the P1 component only whereas the patient with MELAS showed a giant response at the N2 component (27.8 ms, 32.1 μV). There was no giant SEP in DRPLA. Stimulation of the left median nerve at the wrist as recorded at C2′ (2 cm backward from international C) revealed no giant components.

The EEG (Fig. 17.1), taken at age 31 years, showed frequent high-amplitude bilateral asynchronous spikes in frontotemporal areas. Somatosensory evoked potentials (Fig. 17.2) did not show giant responses.

The genetic study (Fig. 17.3) showed a heterozygous change in the DRPLA gene with 15 CAG repeats on one exon and 63 on the twin exon. Exons with 15 repeats were judged to be normal and of maternal origin, 63 repeats were expanded and were of paternal origin. Her father had CAG repeats of 16 and 54 and her grandfather had 19 and 56. Her mother was normal having 15 and 17 repeats. The wife of her grandfather had normal repeats having 16 and 11. Her sister was also normal and had 15 and 16. There was anticipation in which expansion increased from her father's 54 to the patient's 63. However there was no anticipation from her grandfather's 56 to her father's 54. Expansion of 54–56 as seen in her father and grandfather seems to be responsible for late onset and mild progress of their symptoms whereas expansion of her 63 was large enough for an earlier onset and severe symptoms including seizures and mental decline.

Case 2

Case 2 is a 41-year-old female. At age 13 years, the patient became clumsy and was noticed to have myoclonic jerks in her arms activated by action. At age 16 years, she had a first generalized convulsion. Thereafter she has had one or two similar seizures every year. At age 20 years, ataxia became evident and at age 32 she became unable to walk alone. She was disoriented and demented and needed assistance in her daily life.

Her father, aged 67 years, had ataxia from the age of 50 years. He was the fourth child of six siblings, four males and two females. The eldest brother had ataxia from age 53 years and his daughter had ataxia and seizures, and died at age 27 years.

The EEG (Fig. 17.4) taken at age 30 years showed frequent short bursts of high-amplitude diffuse bilaterally synchronous and symmetrical spike–wave complexes. The EEG taken at age 41 years (Fig. 17.5) showed frequent high-amplitude bilateral asynchronous spike discharges in the frontotemporal areas. Somatosensory evoked potentials did not show giant responses.

The genetic study is shown in Fig. 17.6. The patient had 14 and 63 CAG repeats; 14 repeats came from her healthy mother and 63 repeats were expanded and came from her father's 54.

	exon1	twin exon
patient	15	63
sister	15	16
father	16	54
mother	15	17
grandfather	19	56
his wife	16	11

Fig. 17.3. CAG repeats in the family of case 1: numbers of CAG repeats of the patient, her sister, mother, father, grandfather, and his wife. Arrows indicate transmission from parents to children. Short CAG repeats of mother's 15 and father's 16 were stable and transmitted unchanged from parents to children. Larger repeats were unstable and her grandfather's 56 was shortened and transmitted to her father's 54. Expansion was seen in patient's 63 while it was transmitted from her father's 54. It was interesting to note that unstable CAG repeats might not always be expanded but they were at times shortened.

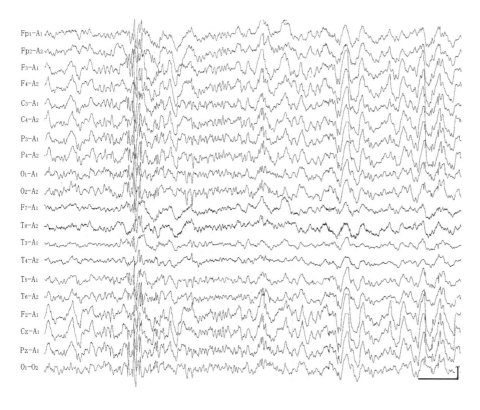

Fig. 17.4. Case 2: EEG at age 30 years. Frequent diffuse bilateral symmetrical and synchronous spike–slow wave complex. Calibration: 1 s, 50 µV.

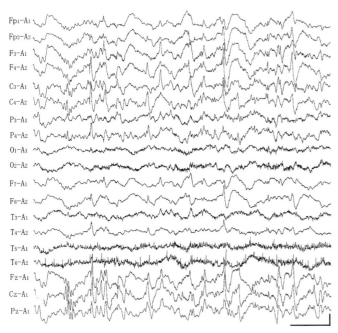

	exon1	twin exon
patient	15	64
father	19	55
mother	15	15

Fig. 17.6. CAG repeats in the family of case 2: normal CAG repeats were stable and transmitted from parents to child without change but larger CAG repeats were unstable and expanded, and were transmitted to child.

Fig. 17.5. Case 2: EEG at age 41 years. Disorganized pattern mixed with frequent high-amplitude spike discharges localized in frontotemporal areas bilaterally and independently, and diffuse high-amplitude slow waves over both sides. Calibration: 1 s, 50 μV.

Summary

Dentato-rubro-pallido-luysian atrophy is an autosomal dominant neurodegenerative disorder caused by abnormal repeat expansions within the DRPLA gene located on chromosome 12p13.31. Ataxia, choreoathetosis, and/or myoclonus and mental decline are the cardinal signs. Epileptic seizures usually occur in patients with an earlier onset. Unstable expanded CAG repeats in one allele in the DRPLA gene are responsible for this disorder and the size of the CAG expansion is well correlated with age of onset and severity of the disease. There are characteristic degeneration of both the dentato-rubral and pallido-luysian systems in the brain. Diffferential diagnosis includes all types of progressive myoclonic epilepsies, hereditary ataxia, and Huntington chorea. An autosomal dominant hereditary pattern and anticipation from the paternal side make the diagnosis more likely. However, a definitive diagnosis is based on genetic testing.

Acknowledgments

DNA analysis was done using triplet repeat primer PCR (TP-PCR) by Dr. Y. Goto and N. Minami in the Section of Molecular Diagnosis and Genetics, Department of Laboratory Medicine, and the outpatient DRPLA survey was done by Dr. M. Watanabe, head of Epilepsy Unit, National Center Hospital of Neurology and Psychiatry, National Center of Neurology and Psychiatry.

References

Burke JR, Wingfield MS, Lewis KE, et al. (1994) The Haw River syndrome: dentatorubural-pallidoluysian atrophy (DRPLA) in an African-American family. Nat Genet 7:521–4.

Ikeuchi T, Koide R, Tanaka H, et al. (1995) Dentatorubral-pallidoluysian atrophy: clinical features are closely related to unstable expansion of trinucleotide (CAG) repeat. Ann Neurol 37:769–75.

Inazuki G, Baba K, Naito H (1989) Electroencephalographic findings of hereditary dentatorubral-pallidoluysian atrophy (DRPLA). Jap J Psychiatry Neurol 43:213–20.

Inazuki H, Kumagai K, Naito A (1990) Geographical distribution of origin of DRPLA in Japan, and prevalence of DRPLA in Niigata prefecture in Japan. Seishinigaku 32:1135–8. (In Japanese).

Kasai K, Onuma T, Kato M, Takeya J, Sekimoto M (1998) Somatosensory evoked potential in DRPLA compared with the other progressive myoclonus epilepsies. J Jap Epilepsy Soc 16:184–92.

Koide R, Ikeuchi T, Onodera O, et al. (1994) Unstable expansion of CAG repeat in hereditary dentatorubral-pallidoluysian atrophy (DRPLA). Nat Genet 6:9–13.

Naito A (1989) DRPLA. In: Progressive Myoclonus Epilepsy. Tokyo: Igakushoin. (In Japanese).

Naito A, Oyanagi S (1982) Familial myoclonus epilepsy and choreoathetosis: hereditary dentatorubral-pallidoluysian atrophy. Neurology 32:798–807.

Oyanagi S, Naito S (1977) Clinicopathological consideration of four cases of autopsy in autosomal dominant myoclonus epilepsy. Seishinshinkeigakuzasshi Zassi 79:113–29. (In Japanese).

Smith JK, Gonda VE, Malamud N (1958) Unusual form of cerebellar ataxia combined dentato-rubral and pallido-luysian degeneration. Neurology 8:205–14.

Chapter

18

Lafora body disease

Anna C. Jansen

Definition and history

Lafora body disease (or Lafora disease) is named after Gonzalo Rodriguez Lafora (1887–1971), a Spanish neuropathologist who reported the presence of spherical inclusions in brains of patients with myoclonus epilepsy, which were called Lafora bodies. These would later prove to be the key feature to distinguish Lafora disease from other myoclonic epilepsies.

The diagnosis is suspected in a previously healthy older child or adolescent with fragmentary, symmetric, or generalized myoclonus, and/or generalized tonic–clonic seizures, visual hallucinations (occipital seizures), and progressive neurological deterioration including cognitive and/or behavioral deterioration, dysarthria, ataxia, and, at later stages, spasticity and dementia. Diagnosis is confirmed by the identification of two mutations in one of the two genes know to be associated with Lafora disease, *EPM2A* or *NHLRC1* (Minassian *et al.* 1998; Chan *et al.* 2003; Ianzano *et al.* 2005).

Epidemiology

Exact prevalence figures for Lafora disease are not available. It occurs worldwide but because of its autosomal recessive inheritance it is more frequent in ethnic isolates and in parts of the world with a high rate of consanguinity. Some mutations occur more frequently in specific populations. Examples include the relatively frequent presence of the p.R241X mutation in *EPM2A* in the Spanish population, the p.C26S mutation in *NHLRC1* in French–Canadian families, and the p.G158fs16 mutation in *NHLRC1* in tribal Oman.

Clinical features and diagnostic criteria

Lafora disease typically starts between ages 12 and 17 years, after a period of apparently normal development. Patients may present with myoclonic jerks, usually precipitated by action or excitement, with a generalized convulsion or with visual hallucinations. They also may be noticed to be depressed and performing poorly at school. Many affected individuals experience isolated febrile or non-febrile convulsions in infancy or earlier in childhood. Intractable seizures rarely begin as early as age 6 years. In families with more than one affected child, clinical signs such as subtle myoclonus, visual hallucinations, or headaches are noted earlier in subsequent affected children than in the proband. Intra- and interfamilial variability in age at onset is considerable.

The course of the disease is characterized by increasing frequency and intractability of seizures. Status epilepticus is common. Cognitive decline becomes apparent at or soon after the onset of seizures. Dysarthria and ataxia appear early while spasticity develops late. Emotional disturbance and confusion are common in the early stages of the disease and are followed by dementia.

By their mid-twenties, most affected individuals are in a vegetative state with continuous myoclonus. Some maintain minimal interactions with the family such as a reflex-like smiling. Affected individuals who are not tube-fed aspirate frequently as a result of seizures; death from aspiration pneumonia is common and death usually occurs in the mid-twenties.

Pathophysiology

The *EPM2A* gene is located on chromosome 6q24 and encodes the dual-specificity phosphatase laforin (Serratosa *et al.* 1999; Tagliabracci *et al.* 2007). By differential splicing of its transcripts, *EPM2A* encodes two laforin isoforms having distinct carboxyl termini (Dubey and Ganesh 2008). The *NHLRC1* gene is located on chromosome 6p22.3 and encodes an E3 ubiquitin ligase called malin (Gentry *et al.* 2005).

Lafora disease-associated mutations are scattered all along the coding regions of the *EPM2A* and *NHLRC1* genes, but also accumulate in discrete spots of high recurrence. For *EPM2A*, these include homozygous deletions of exon 2, followed by the nonsense mutations p.R214X and p.G279S. For *NHLRC1*, recurrent mutations included the frameshift mutation p.G158fs16 and the missense mutation p.P69A.

The mechanisms by which mutations in either *EPM2A* or *NHLRC1* result in Lafora disease and the exact role of the

The Causes of Epilepsy, eds. S. D. Shorvon, F. Andermann, and R. Guerrini. Published by Cambridge University Press. © Cambridge University Press 2011.

Lafora bodies has not been entirely clarified (Ganesh *et al.* 2006). Laforin and malin participate by different mechanisms involved in the regulation of glycogen metabolism (Chan *et al.* 2004; Gentry *et al.* 2007), including the proteasome-dependent degradation of protein targeting to glycogen (PTG) and muscle glycogen synthase (MSG) (Niittyla *et al.* 2006), suppression of excessive glycogen phosphorylation (Worby *et al.* 2008), and degradation of misfolded proteins.

Epilepsy in Lafora disease
Types of epilepsy

The main seizure types in Lafora disease include myoclonic seizures and occipital seizures, although generalized tonic–clonic seizures, atypical absence seizures, and atonic and complex partial seizures may occur.

Myoclonus can be fragmentary, symmetric, or massive (generalized). It occurs at rest and can be exaggerated by action, photic stimulation, or excitement. Both negative (loss of tone) and positive (jerking) myoclonus can occur. Myoclonus usually disappears with sleep. Trains of massive myoclonus with relative preservation of consciousness have been reported. Myoclonus is the primary reason for early wheelchair dependency. In the advanced stages of the disease, affected individuals often have continuous generalized myoclonus.

Occipital seizures present as transient blindness, simple or complex visual hallucinations, photomyoclonic or photoconvulsive seizures, or scintillating scotomata.

Electroencephalography

Early in the course of the disease, electroencephalograms (EEGs) show a normal or slow background. Photosensitivity is common. Alpha-rhythm and sleep features are lost as the disease progresses. At more advanced stages of the disease, EEGs show slow background activity with paroxysms of generalized irregular spike–wave discharges with occipital predominance, as well as focal, especially occipital, abnormalities.

Diagnostic tests
Molecular genetic testing

Diagnosis is confirmed by detection of one of two mutations in *EPM2A* or *NHLRC1* (Lohi *et al.* 2006, 2007). Although some evidence suggests that persons with *NHLRC1*-associated Lafora disease tend to live longer than those with *EPM2A*-associated Lafora disease, the clinical manifestations caused by mutations in either gene are so similar that it is not possible to predict which gene will be mutated in any given individual.

Studies of the combined mutation detection frequency of sequence analysis in *EPM2A* and *NHLRC1* reveal that between 88% and 97% of mutations in these two genes can be detected using sequence analysis alone (Singh and Ganesh 2009). The proportion of mutations in *EPM2A* and *NHLRC1* not detected by sequence analysis that are attributable to deletions is unknown. Deletions should be suspected in affected individuals who have a single heterozygous mutation in one of the genes, and in patients who have an apparently homozygous mutation in one of the genes but when the mutation is carried by only one parent.

Finally, mutations in at least one other gene can cause Lafora disease since two independent studies have provided evidence for the existence of a third locus.

Skin biopsy

Before the advent of molecular genetic testing, diagnosis was confirmed by the presence of Lafora bodies on skin biopsy. Lafora bodies are present in either eccrine duct cells or in apocrine myoepithelial cells. The interpretation of findings on skin biopsy includes a risk of false-negative results, especially in newly symptomatic individuals, and a risk of false-positive results because of the difficulty in distinguishing Lafora bodies from normal periodic acid-Schiff (PAS)-positive polysaccharides in apocrine glands. It is therefore favored to biopsy the skin outside the axilla and genital regions, as eccrine duct cell Lafora bodies are unmistakable.

Results of additional investigations and their evolution over time are summarized in Table 18.1.

Differential diagnosis

Although the occurrence of myoclonus and generalized tonic–clonic seizures in adolescence may raise the possibility of juvenile myoclonic epilepsy, the persistence of EEG background slowing and cognitive deterioration should raise the suspicion of a more severe epilepsy syndrome, such as progressive myoclonus epilepsy.

Later age at onset, more rapid rate of disease progression, and presence of Lafora bodies on skin biopsy differentiates Lafora disease from Unverricht–Lundborg disease.

Careful ophthalmologic examination, including electroretinography, is useful in addressing the possibilities of neuronal ceroid lipofuscinoses and sialidosis.

Other conditions to consider are myoclonic epilepsy with ragged red fibers, subacute sclerosing panencephalitis, or other progressive myoclonus epilepsies.

Management and prognosis
Management

To establish the extent of disease in an individual diagnosed with Lafora disease, a clinical evaluation with special attention to speech, walking, coordination, handwriting, school performance, and emotional status is recommended. Follow-up consists of clinical and psychosocial evaluations at 3- to 6-month intervals throughout the teenage years.

Antiepileptic drugs have a major effect against generalized seizures, sometimes controlling seizures for many months. Valproic acid is the traditional antiepileptic treatment for Lafora disease because it is a broad-spectrum drug that controls

Table 18.1 Clinical evaluation of Lafora disease

Evaluation	At onset	Later in disease course
General physical examination	Normal	Normal
Neurological examination, including fundi and reflexes	Normal	Dysarthria, ataxia, spasticity; fundi remain normal
Mental state examination	Visual hallucinations (epileptic), depressed mood, cognitive deficits	Increased hallucinations, agitation, dementia
EEG	Normal or slow background, loss of α-rhythm and sleep features, photosensitivity is common	Slow background, paroxysms of generalized irregular spike–wave discharges with occipital predominance, and focal, especially occipital, abnormalities
Visual, somatosensory, and auditory brainstem evoked potentials	High-voltage visual and somatosensory evoked potentials	Amplitudes may return to normal size; prolongation of brainstem and central latencies
Nerve conduction studies	Normal	Normal
MRI of the brain	Normal	Normal or atrophy[a]
Proton MR spectroscopy of the brain	Reduced NAA/creatine ratio in frontal and occipital cortex, basal ganglia, and cerebellum[b]	Reduced NAA/creatine ratio in frontal and occipital cortex, basal ganglia, and cerebellum[a]

Notes:
[a]No significant correlation observed with disease evolution.
[b]At least two years after onset of symptoms.
Sources: Minassian 2001; Minassian 2002; Villanueva *et al.* 2006.

both the generalized tonic–clonic seizures and myoclonic jerks. Clonazepam can be used as an adjunctive medication for control of myoclonus. Other possible treatments include zonisamide, piracetam, and levetiracetam.

The use of phenytoin should be avoided. Anecdotal reports describe possible exacerbation of myoclonus with carbamazepine, oxcarbazepine, and lamotrigine.

Myoclonus is often drug-resistant in Lafora disease, and care should be taken not to overmedicate patients for this reason.

Placement by percutaneous endoscopy of a gastrostomy tube for feeding can be helpful in decreasing the risk of aspiration pneumonia in individuals with advanced disease.

Prognosis

Since there is no curative treatment and therapy is mainly supportive and symptomatic, most affected individuals die within 10 years of onset, usually from status epilepticus or from complications related to nervous system degeneration.

References

Chan EM, Young EJ, Ianzano L, *et al.* (2003) Mutations in *NHLRC1* cause progressive myoclonus epilepsy. *Nat Genet* **35**:125–7.

Chan EM, Ackerley CA, Lohi H, *et al.* (2004) Laforin preferentially binds the neurotoxic starch-like polyglucosans, which form in its absence in progressive myoclonus epilepsy. *Hum Mol Genet* **13**:1117–29.

Dubey D, Ganesh S (2008) Modulation of functional properties of laforin phosphatase by alternative splicing reveals a novel mechanism for the *EPM2A* gene in Lafora progressive myoclonus epilepsy. *Hum Mol Genet* **17**:3010–20.

Ganesh S, Puri R, Singh S, Mittal S, Dubey D (2006) Recent advances in the molecular basis of Lafora's progressive myoclonus epilepsy. *J Hum Genet* **51**:1–8.

Gentry MS, Worby CA, Dixon JE (2005) Insights into Lafora disease: malin is an E3 ubiquitin ligase that ubiquitinates and promotes the degradation of laforin. *Proc Natl Acad Sci USA* **102**:8501–6.

Gentry MS, Dowen RH 3rd, Worby CA, *et al.* (2007) The phosphatase laforin crosses evolutionary boundaries and links carbohydrate metabolism to neuronal disease. *J Cell Biol* **178**:477–88.

Ianzano L, Zhang J, Chan EM, *et al.* (2005) Lafora progressive myoclonus epilepsy mutation database: *EPM2A* and *NHLRC1* (*EPM2B*) genes. *Hum Mutat* **26**:397.

Lohi H, Chan EM, Scherer SW, Minassian BA (2006) On the road to tractability: the current biochemical understanding of progressive myoclonus epilepsies. *Adv Neurol* **97**:399–415.

Lohi H, Turnbull J, Zhao XC, *et al.* (2007) Genetic diagnosis in Lafora disease: genotype–phenotype correlations and diagnostic pitfalls. *Neurology* **68**:996–1001.

Minassian BA, Lee JR, Herbrick JA, *et al.* (1998) Mutations in a gene encoding a novel protein tyrosine phosphatase cause progressive myoclonus epilepsy. *Nat Genet* **20**:171–4.

Minassian BA (2001) Lafora's disease: towards a clinical, pathologic, and molecular synthesis. *Pediatr Neurol* **25**:21–9.

Minassian BA (2002) Progressive myoclonus epilepsy with polyglucosan bodies: Lafora disease. *Adv Neurol* **89**:199–210.

Niittyla T, Comparot-Moss S, Lue WL, *et al.* (2006) Similar protein phosphatases control starch metabolism in plants and glycogen metabolism in mammals. *J Biol Chemi* **281**:11 815–18.

Serratosa JM, Gomez-Garre P, Gallardo ME, *et al.* (1999) A novel protein tyrosine phosphatase gene is mutated in progressive myoclonus epilepsy of the Lafora type (EPM2). *Hum Mol Genet* **8**:345–52.

Singh S, Ganesh S (2009) Lafora progressive myoclonus epilepsy: a meta-analysis of reported mutations in the first decade following the discovery of the *EPM2A* and *NHLRC1* genes. *Hum Mutat* **30**:715–23.

Tagliabracci VS, Turnbull J, Wang W, *et al.* (2007) Laforin is a glycogen phosphatase, deficiency of which leads to elevated phosphorylation of glycogen in vivo. *Proc Natl Acad Sci USA* **104**:19 262–6.

Villanueva V, Alvarez-Linera J, Gomez-Garre P, Gutierrez J, Serratosa JM (2006) MRI volumetry and proton MR spectroscopy of the brain in Lafora disease. *Epilepsia* **47**:788–92.

Worby CA, Gentry MS, Dixon JE (2008) Malin decreases glycogen accumulation by promoting the degradation of protein targeting to glycogen (PTG). *J Biol Chemi* **283**:4069–76.

Relevant websites

Online Mendelian Inheritance in Man: Myoclonic Epilepsy of Lafora www.ncbi.nlm.nih.gov/entrez/dispomim. cgi?id=254780

GeneReviews: Progressive myoclonus epilepsy, Lafora type. Jansen AC and Andermann E December 28, 2007 www.ncbi.nlm.nih.gov/bookshelf/br.fcgi? book=gene&part=lafora

The Lafora Progressive Myoclonus Epilepsy Mutation and Polymorphism Database http://projects.tcag.ca/lafora/

Chapter

19

Mitochondrial cytopathies

Laurence A. Bindoff and Bernt A. Engelsen

The causal disease

Mitochondria are subcellular organelles whose major function is the production of adenosine triphosphate (ATP) by the process called oxidative phosphorylation. The energy released by the metabolism of fuels, i.e., glucose and fatty acids, is conserved by the mitochondrial respiratory chain (MRC), an enzyme pathway located in the inner mitochondrial membrane. This enzyme pathway is biologically unique, both because it is the major site of ATP production, but also because it contains subunits encoded by two different genomes. The MRC comprises five large multi-subunit complexes containing >80 proteins (Fig. 19.1). The majority of these proteins are encoded by genes found on chromosomes in the cell nucleus, but 13 are encoded by a genome found inside the mitochondrion (Fig. 19.1). This mitochondrial DNA (mtDNA) also encodes 22 transfer RNA (tRNA) and 2 ribosomal RNA (rRNA) involved in intramitochondrial protein synthesis (Fig. 19.2). Mitochondria, and thus the DNA they contain, are inherited solely from the mother meaning that disease due to mutation in this genome can show strict maternal inheritance. The other respiratory chain proteins encoded on genes located in the nucleus (nuclear DNA [nDNA] defects), show classical patterns of inheritance.

All cells depend on ATP to perform their required functions. Certain cells, such as neurons, skeletal muscle, and retinal ganglion cells appear to have a greater need for readily available energy than others, e.g., skin fibroblasts. This is often cited as one of the reasons why such tissues are more often affected by diseases due to MRC dysfunction. Since all cells contain mitochondria, however, any and indeed all tissues may be involved. The original mitochondrial disease descriptions were of patients with myopathy or encephalopathy and this led to descriptive terms such as mitochondrial encephalomyopathy together with a number of eponymous syndromes. Subsequently, MRC dysfunction has been shown to cause disease including diabetes mellitus, anemia, deafness, and gastric obstruction, as well as epilepsy and other neurological disorders (Zeviani and Carelli 2007; DiMauro and Schon 2008). This has led to problems with nomenclature. For the purposes of this chapter, we will focus only on disorders due to MRC dysfunction and use the collective term *mitochondrial cytopathy*. Disorders arising from disruption of other mitochondrial metabolic pathways such as fatty acid oxidation, urea or citric acid cycle, etc. will not be discussed.

Central nervous system neurons are terminally differentiated cells lacking significant capacity to regenerate, and thereby to select against defective cells. They are also cells with a high energy demand. These factors explain, in large part, their vulnerability to mitochondrial dysfunction and offer a potential explanation for why epileptic seizures occur frequently. Decreased intracellular ATP levels can, moreover, increase neuronal excitability by impairing sodium–potassium ATPase activity and decreasing the membrane potential. Since mitochondria also store intracellular calcium, mitochondrial dysfunction can increase excitability, and thus expose the neuron to damage, by impairing calcium sequestration (Kunz 2002). Other potential factors include lactic acid in high local concentration, which may provoke vasoconstriction sufficient to induce hypoxia. Dysfunction in MRC may also lead to increased free-radical production. It is known that free-radicals are signaling molecules, but they may also initiate damage, for example through apoptosis (Cock 2007). Whatever the initial mechanism, cortical damage can induce further seizures which in turn cause more damage. The resulting vicious circle may constitute an additional factor in the further destruction of surviving neurons.

Mitochondrial diseases are common. Studies in the UK showed that 9.2 in 100 000 people of working age (>16 and <60/65 years for female/male) had a clinically manifest mtDNA disease and a further 16.5 in 100 000 children and adults younger than retirement age were at risk of developing mtDNA disease (Schaefer *et al.* 2008). Studies from Sweden showed that the incidence of mitochondrial encephalomyopathies in preschool children (<6 years) was 1 in 11 000 (Darin *et al.* 2001) and in Australia an estimated minimum birth prevalence of 6.2 per 100 000 was found (Skladal *et al.* 2003). It must be remembered that these figures are based on patients with *known* mtDNA mutations; there is currently no way of

The Causes of Epilepsy, eds. S. D. Shorvon, F. Andermann, and R. Guerrini. Published by Cambridge University Press. © Cambridge University Press 2011.

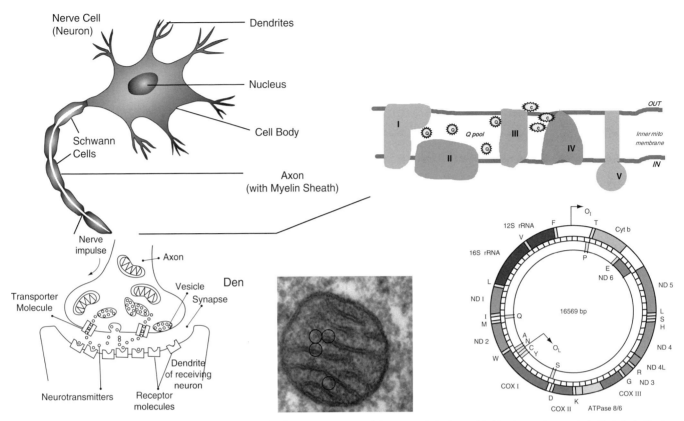

Fig. 19.1. The mitochondrial respiratory chain. Neurons, as all cells, require energy and the vast majority is provided by the respiratory chain that sits in the inner mitochondrial membrane. Reduced co-factors (NADH and flavoproteins) generated by the breakdown of metabolic fuels (e.g., glucose and fatty acids), are reoxidized by respiratory chain complexes and the energy released during this process is conserved and used to drive the phosphorylation of ADP to ATP. This process is called oxidative phosphorylation. The mitochondrial respiratory chain comprises five multi-subunit complexes (depicted by Roman numerals) and four of these contain proteins encoded by the genome found inside mitochondria (mtDNA). MtDNA encodes seven (of a total of 45) proteins in complex I, one (of 11) in complex III, three (of 13) in complex IV, and two (of 14) in complex V. Complex II (succinate dehydrogenase) contains no mtDNA-encoded subunits.

estimating how many more mutations are still to be discovered, but several new mtDNA mutations are published each year. In a major study published in 2008, Chinnery and colleagues determined the frequency of 10 mtDNA mutations in 3168 neonatal-cord-blood samples from sequential live births and found that at least 1 in 200 healthy humans harbors a pathogenic mtDNA mutation that potentially causes disease in the offspring of female carriers (Elliott *et al.* 2008).

Since nuclear genes supply all mitochondrial proteins except for the 13 encoded by mtDNA (Fig. 19.1), defects in nuclear genes can affect the MRC in many ways: by damaging individual components of this pathway or proteins involved in its assembly, by disrupting the transport of proteins/co-factors that must be transferred from the cytosol to the mitochondrion (carriers and chaperone proteins) and by disrupting mtDNA maintenance. Examples of all are now recognized and while many are associated with epilepsy, some are not (DiMauro and Schon 2008).

Epilepsy in the disease

Epilepsy can be a presenting symptom or occur during the course of most forms of MRC disease whether caused by

mtDNA or nDNA defects. Over 150 different mutations in mtDNA (Fig. 19.2) have been described and while many are associated with epilepsy, not all are (Ruiz-Pesini *et al.* 2007). The majority of mutations are also individually rare. In this chapter we will focus on two mtDNA disorders, myoclonus epilepsy with ragged red fibers (MERRF) and mitochondrial myopathy encephalopathy, lactic acidosis, and stroke-like episodes (MELAS). These are typical of the syndromes caused by mtDNA mutation, sufficiently common to permit characterization, and associated with an epileptic semiology representative of mtDNA disease. Both can also be caused by different mtDNA mutations, showing the pleiomorphic nature of mtDNA disease. The reader wishing for detailed descriptions of these and other less common mtDNA diseases, should use the available databases (Ruiz-Pesini *et al.* 2007) and reviews (DiMauro and Schon 2003; Taylor and Turnbull 2005; Zeviani and Carelli 2007) and references contained therein. Nuclear DNA gene defects are increasingly being found, but one group appears common, namely syndromes associated with mutations in the *POLG1* gene (Horvath *et al.* 2006).

No specific type of epilepsy characterizes mitochondrial disease, but interestingly, both mtDNA and nDNA defects demonstrate an occipital lobe predilection, at least initially.

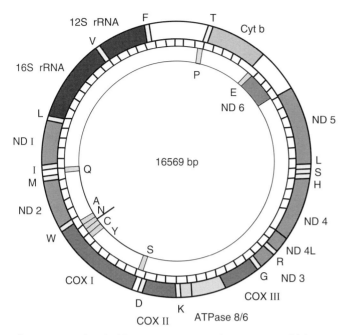

Fig. 19.2. Mitochondrial DNA is a compact circular genome 16.5 kilobases in size with little non-coding sequence. In addition to the 13 proteins, it also encodes 22 transfer RNA (tRNA) and two ribosomal RNA (rRNA) that are involved in intramitochondrial protein synthesis. MtDNA is found in multiple copies inside each mitochondrion. Mutations affecting this genome can therefore affect some or all of the copies. A cellular phenotype arises only when sufficient copies are affected and the level (i.e., the percentage of mutated compared with normal copies) at which this occurs is termed the threshold. The existence of two populations of mtDNA is called heteroplasmy and most mtDNA mutations only produce a phenotype at high levels of heteroplasmy and are thus considered as "functionally" recessive. The common mutations of mtDNA are shown.

Myoclonus occurs in all types of mitochondrial disease, but whether this is purely cortical or brainstem (or both) is unclear and both occur. Most commonly the epilepsy in mitochondrial cytopathy is symptomatic, multifocal, and, thus, secondary generalized epilepsy combining focal and generalized features.

Myoclonus epilepsy with ragged red fibers

Epileptic seizures are one of the defining features of the MERRF syndrome (Fukuhara *et al.* 1980), the other being ragged red fibers, mitochondria accumulation in muscle fibers detected by Gomori-trichrome staining that has become the morphological hallmark of mitochondrial disease (see Fig. 19.5 below). Several different mutations cause this syndrome. The first described was the 8344A>G in the mitochondrial tRNA gene for lysine (Fig. 19.2). Subsequently, two more mutations in this gene were identified and both appeared to cause the same clinical syndrome (8356T>C and 8361G>A). Several other mutations (Ruiz-Pesini *et al.* 2007) have now been described giving clinical syndromes in which myoclonic epilepsy occurs, but which involve other features such as cardiomyopathy or diabetes mellitus. Indeed, overlap syndromes with features of both MERRF and MELAS are described, highlighting the marked phenotypic variability of mitochondrial disorders and the lack of consistent phenotype–

genotype correlation. Nevertheless, the mutations in tRNA lysine cause a syndrome that is now well recognized and, for an mtDNA disorder, relatively frequent.

Patients usually present with progressive myoclonus and most have generalized tonic–clonic (GTC) seizures (9 of 13 cases in Berkovic *et al.* 1989). The myoclonus may be indistinguishable from that seen with other progressive myoclonus epilepsies, e.g., Unverricht–Lundborg or Lafora body disease. Myoclonic jerks may correlate with electroencephalographic (EEG) spike or polyspike activity, and we have seen suppression of epileptic activity following eye opening. The myoclonus can be virtually constant, but may also be intermittent, photosensitive, and intensified by action, such as writing, eating, etc. Focal clonic and atonic seizures have been reported (Berkovic *et al.* 1989; Hirano and DiMauro 1997). Visual or somatosensory symptoms may precede motor symptoms. The GTC seizures are generally easy to control with traditional antiepileptic drugs whereas the myoclonus may be relatively refractory and develop into continuous generalized myoclonus (Berkovic *et al.* 1989). In addition to seizures, patients commonly develop ataxia, deafness, dementia, and a clinical myopathy. Interestingly, there is also an association with multiple symmetrical lipomatosis.

Mitochondrial myopathy encephalopathy, lactic acidosis, and stroke-like episodes

The defining features of MELAS syndrome are the finding of lactic acidosis and the occurrence of stroke-like episodes (SLE) (Pavlakis *et al.* 1984; Montagna *et al.* 1988). Neither, however, is constant and diabetes, deafness, progressive external ophthalmoplegia (PEO), gastroenteropathy and cyclical vomiting, failure to thrive, myopathy, and peripheral neuropathy also occur with variable frequency (DiMauro and Schon 2008). The syndrome can be caused by several different mtDNA mutations (Fig. 19.2), but one, the 3243A>G in the tRNA for leucine(UUR) (Goto *et al.* 1991), is by far the commonest. This mutation can give MELAS, with SLE and epilepsy, or more benign phenotypes such as maternally inherited diabetes, deafness, encephalopathy, or PEO with a proximal myopathy.

Epilepsy occurs primarily in the group of patients that develop stroke-like lesions (SLL) (Fig. 19.3A) and seizures are often preceded by or associated with migraine-like headache. These lesions evolve gradually (Iizuka *et al.* 2003), showing predilection for the occipital and temporal lobes, and seizure semiology often reflects disturbance in these locations. Magnetic resonance imaging (MRI) shows evolving lesions that appear to reflect initial cellular damage followed by vasogenic edema (Tzoulis and Bindoff 2009). Why certain areas of the brain are targeted and what type of pathological process underlies the SLL, i.e., whether the process is primarily vascular or cellular, remain unanswered questions. Thus, whether seizures arise due to ischemic lesions or direct neuronal dysfunction is unknown. Once initiated, however, seizures increase the

149

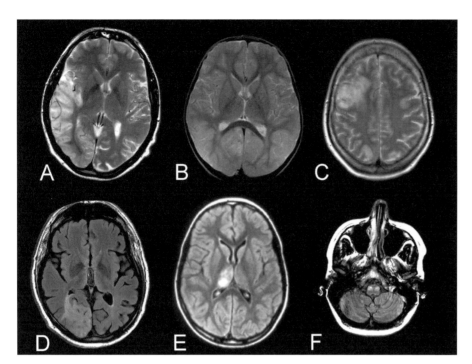

Fig. 19.3. MRI images. (A) T2-weighted image showing a right temporo-occipital high signal lesion (fresh, edematous cortex) in MELAS. This is a typical finding in this disorder and is what can be called a stroke-like lesion. Patient with 3243A > G mtDNA mutation. (B) T2-weighted image showing bilateral temporo-occipital, cortical, high signal lesions in a child with Alpers syndrome and mutation in *POLG1*. (C) T2-weighted image showing right frontal and parieto-occipital and left frontal high signal lesions from a patient with mitochondrial spinocerebellar ataxia and epilepsy (MSCAE) during an episode of status epilepticus and encephalopathy. (D) T2-FLAIR image showing a right occipital high signal lesion developing in a patient with MSCAE and status epilepticus. (E) T2-FLAIR image showing a right thalamic high signal lesion. These are typical for MSCAE and persist in contrast to the lesions depicted in (B), (C), and (D) which are evanescent. (F) T2-FLAIR image showing bilateral inferior olivary high signal lesions. These too are typical for MSCAE, but only one patient had the clinical correlate of palatal myoclonus.

metabolic demand placed on neurons, exposing patients to risk of further damage and therefore further seizures.

In a review of 110 reported cases of MELAS in which SLE was a defining feature, 38% had myoclonus and 96% seizures (Hirano and Pavlakis 1994). In 28% of cases, seizures were the initial clinical manifestation. Both generalized and focal seizures are seen (26/42) and in 10 of 42 patients, generalized epilepsy was defined, including one patient with absence seizures (Hirano and DiMauro 1997). The commonest type of partial seizures they found were motor, followed by visual and temporal lobe seizures. Status epilepticus (SE) occurred in 6/42 in this series (Hirano and DiMauro 1997), but clinical experience shows that SE is frequent in patients with MELAS and similar mitochondrial disorders and can be the initial presentation.

When present, myoclonic seizures appear less severe and less common than in patients with MERRF. Noticeably, there may be overlap syndromes between MELAS and MERFF (Berkovic *et al.* 1989). In a later publication interictal EEG changes in MELAS patients were localized to the parieto-occipital regions or as diffuse sharp wave paroxysms, whereas EEG discharges associated with partial motor seizures had a congruous frontocentral location (Canafoglia *et al.* 2001). Most likely the age of epilepsy debut may influence the seizure semiology in MELAS, absence seizures reflecting young age, whereas complex partial SE with regional epileptic activity in the right posterior quadrant occurred in late onset MELAS (Leff *et al.* 1998).

Syndromes related to *POLG1*

The *POLG1* gene encodes the catalytic subunit of the mitochondrial DNA polymerase, the enzyme that replicates mtDNA. By directly affecting mtDNA, mutations in this nuclear gene can either induce qualitative mtDNA defects (multiple mtDNA deletions or point mutations) or quantitative loss of mtDNA known as depletion. Moreover, mutations in this gene appear to be common and give rise to a variety of disorders ranging from infantile hepatocerebral disease such as Alpers syndrome, ataxia and epilepsy, parkinsonism, and PEO (Hakonen *et al.* 2005; Hudson and Chinnery 2006; Tzoulis *et al.* 2006; Luoma *et al.* 2007).

Alpers–Huttenlocher syndrome

This syndrome comprises refractory seizures, psychomotor retardation, and liver involvement and is caused by a variety of different mutations in the *POLG1* gene (Ferrari *et al.* 2005; Nguyen *et al.* 2005). Initial presentation is most often with SE that can be focal or generalized and from which the child might never recover. Mental retardation can be present before the onset of seizures, or begin thereafter. Liver failure, perhaps the least consistent feature, may be present at onset or only develop during the terminal illness. The majority of children with this disease die within a few months of onset, but some survive several years. Elevated lactate in blood or cerebrospinal fluid is an inconsistent feature. A predilection for involvement of the occipital lobes is seen in MRI (Fig. 19.3B, C); lesions affecting the cortex have features similar to those seen in acute hypoxia. The seizure semiology in this syndrome is very similar if not identical to that we have described for patients with MSCAE and *POLG1* mutation (see below).

Mitochondrial spinocerebellar ataxia and epilepsy

Mitochondrial spinocerebellar ataxia and epilepsy (MSCAE) is a teenage-onset disorder comprising spinocerebellar ataxia, peripheral neuropathy, and epilepsy. Liver failure (cf. Alpers syndrome) occurs spontaneously, but is most often precipitated by exposure to sodium valproate. There is a high prevalence in Scandinavia and Finland, but, similar to Alpers syndrome, MSCAE is also found throughout the world (Winterthun *et al.* 2005; Hakonen *et al.* 2007). Onset of MSCAE can be with ataxia or epilepsy, but all patients will eventually develop ataxia if they survive, while only ~80% appear to develop epilepsy (Engelsen *et al.* 2008). This must be interpreted with caution, however, since patients with MSCAE can develop an explosive and fatal epilepsy >30 years after presenting with ataxia. While several *POLG1* mutations are described giving this later-onset (than Alpers syndrome) disease, two are by far the most common; the c.1399G>A that gives p.A467T and the c.2243G>C giving the p.W748S (Tzoulis *et al.* 2006).

In MSCAE, epilepsy is the presenting symptom in ~65% of patients (Engelsen *et al.* 2008). Occipital lobe epileptic features are the initial symptoms in the majority and seizure phenomena include flickering colored light, that may persist for weeks, months, or even years, ictal visual loss, nystagmus or oculoclonus, dysmorphopsia, micro-/macropsia, and palinopsia often combined with headache and/or emesis. Refractory simple partial seizures (SPS) with visual symptoms in one visual hemifield occurring daily for weeks, months, or even years was seen in over 50% of cases and the epileptic origin of these symptoms could be substantiated by ictal EEG (Fig. 19.4A).

All of the patients with epilepsy develop focal clonic or myoclonic seizures, most often involving an arm, shoulder, neck, and/or head and manifesting as simple partial motor seizures and often continuing to focal motor status. Occasionally, persisting focal or generalized myoclonic jerks can be observed. Palatal myoclonus was seen in one patient who also had involvement of the inferior olivary nuclei. Motor SPS are sometimes accompanied by a clear epileptic EEG correlate, sometimes with rhythmic focal slowing of the contralateral, posterior hemispheric quadrant, or occipital electrodes (Fig. 19.4B). No clear correlation between frequency of focal clonic movements of arm–shoulder–head and frequency of occipital slow waves is seen, but EEG changes can be considered epileptiform in nature (Engelsen *et al.* 2008). Complex partial seizures (CPS) with motor symptoms occur in >50% of patients and may be underreported and GTC seizures, all considered secondary GTC (sGTC), occur in >90% of cases.

All patients who develop epilepsy experience SE and this can begin explosively several decades after disease onset. Status epilepticus can also be the presenting seizure phenomenon, although the median time from onset of epilepsy to the first SE is 2 months.

An EEG showing occipital slow wave and epileptic activity occurs as an early feature in the majority of patients (Engelsen *et al.* 2008) and ictal registrations revealed either severe general slowing, with or without epileptic activity, or, as in the majority of patients, consistent focal occipital, or temporo-occipital, epileptic discharges occurring in T5, T6, O1, and O2 electrodes (Fig. 19.4A–D).

Other mitochondrial cytopathies

There are a large number of reports describing single patients or families with different forms of mitochondrial cytopathy, many of whom have epilepsy. Early work was descriptive and defined mitochondrial disease only in terms of biochemical or morphological abnormalities making it difficult to compare these cases with what we know from genetically defined cytopathies. In our experience, and based on those reviews available, the type of epilepsy seen in these cases does not differ from that seen in the examples we have discussed above. It seems safe to say, therefore, that any and all types of epileptic seizures can occur in mitochondrial cytopathy.

Diagnostic tests for the disease

Diagnosis of mitochondrial diseases is based on the usual algorithm of clinical suspicion and supplementary laboratory investigation (Taylor *et al.* 2004). When faced by a complex systemic disorder, considering the possibility that mitochondrial MRC dysfunction might be the cause is, perhaps, the crucial step. In addition to the clinical findings, the finding of elevated lactate in body fluids is a common, but inconsistent finding in mitochondrial cytopathies. Imaging techniques such as MRI can demonstrate patterns of involvement that suggest mitochondrial etiology, particularly involvement of the occipital lobes (Fig. 19.3), and in MSCAE, involvement of the thalamus and inferior olivary nuclei (Figs. 19.3E, F), but these are not diagnostic. Dystrophic calcification particularly affecting the basal ganglia is seen in MELAS, which has significant epileptic component, but also in Kearns–Sayre syndrome, which does not. Magnetic resonance spectroscopy can demonstrate elevated lactate in regions of the brain, while positron emission tomography (PET) scanning can provide metabolic information suggesting lowered ATP production. Neither of these techniques provides unequivocal evidence of respiratory chain dysfunction, however, and it is usually necessary, therefore, to take a tissue biopsy.

The usual site for tissue sampling is skeletal muscle, which will often show abnormalities even in the absence of clinical myopathy. Proper handling of the muscle sampling is crucial because all investigations are performed on frozen not fixed material. Standard histological and histochemical analysis may demonstrate mitochondrial accumulation (ragged red fibers) or fibers lacking complex IV activity (cytochrome oxidase [COX] negative fibers) (Fig. 19.5). Muscle can also be used for biochemical measurements of respiratory chain complexes and studies of mtDNA. These are techniques that demand a high technical proficiency and it is advisable when faced with the possibility of MRC to contact a specialized laboratory in order to ascertain what is required.

A

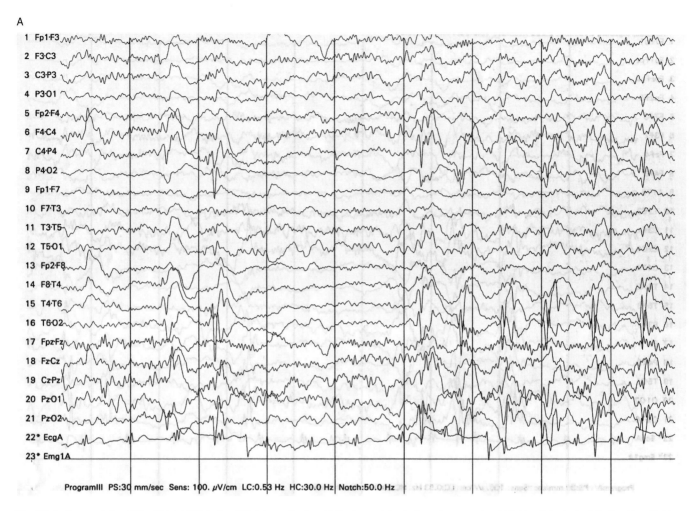

Fig. 19.4. Representative EEGs. (A) Ictal EEG during SPS status epilepticus. Patient complained of continuous colored blinking light in the left visual hemifield. Patient with *POLG1* mutation. (B) Ictal EEG during continuous focal clonic jerking of the left arm, shoulder, and head. Patient with *POLG1* mutation. (C) Diffuse cerebral slowing with epileptiform discharges in the temporal and occipital electrodes, left more than right, during non-convuslive status epilepticus with disorientation, headache, vomiting, and aimless wandering. Patient with *POLG1* mutation. (D) Interictal epileptic discharges in a patient showing transient suppression of epileptic discharges during eye opening. Patient with *POLG1* mutation.

Investigations such as COX/SDH staining provide information concerning where further studies should be directed. A mosaic of COX positive and deficient fibers is a strong indication that the patient has a defect involving mtDNA, but cannot distinguish between primary (i.e., mutation in mtDNA) or secondary (mutation in nuclear gene involved in mtDNA maintenance) defects. A more detailed description of the investigation of mitochondrial cytopathies can be found in the available literature (e.g., Taylor *et al.* 2004).

Since the MRC is controlled by two genomes, establishing the final, genetic diagnosis can be demanding. Unlike the majority of nuclear genes, where we have two copies, mitochondrial DNA is present in multiple copies in every cell. Mutations affecting this genome can affect all or only a proportion of copies (Taylor and Turnbull 2005). In classical genetics we use the concepts of heterozygosity (each gene copy has a different sequence) and homozygosity (both gene copies have identical sequences). Thus, dominant disorders arise when a mutation in one gene copy is sufficient to cause disease and recessive disorders require mutations affecting both copies. In mitochondrial genetics, the situation is complicated by the presence of multiple genomes and an uneven tissue distribution (McFarland *et al.* 2004). Mutations can affect a percentage of mtDNA copies from <1% to >99%. Where all copies in an individual have the same sequence we call this homoplasmy (cf. homozygosity); where there are mtDNAs with two different sequences, e.g. one with a mutation and one normal, this is called heteroplasmy (cf. heterozygosity). In addition, based on factors such as whether the cell retains the capacity to divide and therefore select against cells with impaired energy metabolism, the level of mutation in one tissue can differ dramatically from another. In many mtDNA disorders, particularly those in which the defect is unknown, this will mean that it is not possible to use blood as a source of genetic material since the level will be too low.

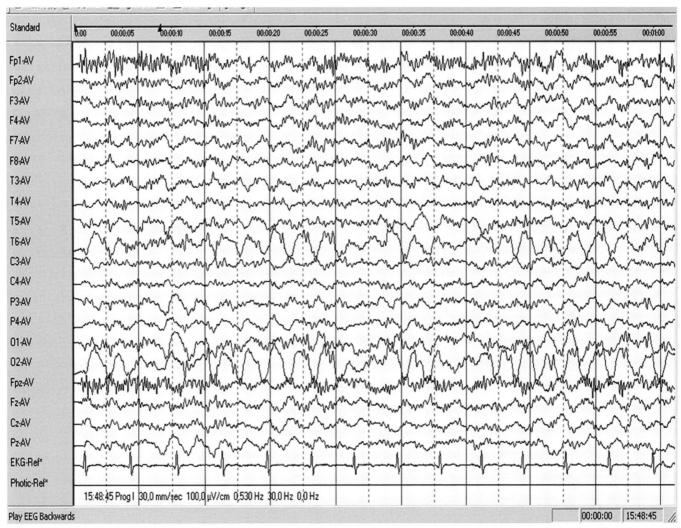

Fig. 19.4. (cont.)

Principles of management

Treatment guidelines

No cures for mitochondrial cytopathies currently exist. Precise diagnosis is vital since this will provide information concerning known potential complications, e.g., development of cardiac involvement or diabetes mellitus. It is important to avoid potential mitochondrial toxins (antibiotics such as tetracyclines, gentamycin, ciprofloxacin), antiviral agents (AZT), and sodium valproate. The latter is absolutely contraindicated in patients with POLG disease. Fasting increases the demand on the MRC, as does fever. This means that care must be taken even when the patient develops a simple viral infection. The use of vitamins, including ubiquinone, has not been shown to have any measurable effect on MRC function, but many still use these, often in combination.

Epilepsy treatment

We advise treating GTC seizures with traditional antiepileptic drugs (AEDs) such as sodium-channel blockers, although we have experienced worsening of myoclonic seizures by lamotrigine and gabapentin (Engelsen *et al.* 2008). Carbamazepine, oxcarbazepine, and phenytoin have proven effective, but in combination with a benzodiazepine, e.g., clobazam or clonazepam, although in some patients it has also been necessary to add a third AED. Levetiracetam or topiramate can also be used against myoclonic seizures. Again, we would stress that patients with known *POLG1* mutations must absolutely avoid sodium valproate and this applies even to patients where the diagnosis is in doubt, so it is best to avoid this drug. The ketogenic diet (Kim and Rho 2008) has been used in the treatment of mitochondrial epilepsy, but we have no experience with this or the modified Atkinson's diet in our patients.

C

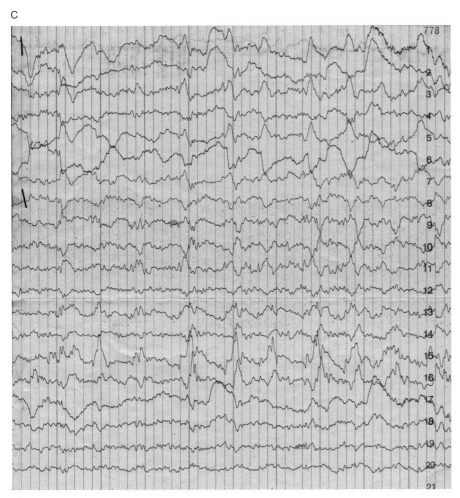

Fig. 19.4. (cont.)

One of our patients tried a modified Atkinson's diet on her own volition, but with no effect on the epilepsy.

Patients with mitochondrial cytopathies such as MELAS and *POLG1* associated disorders have a high risk of SE. Even patients with an apparently benign course can suddenly decompensate and develop focal or generalized SE. While we do not suggest starting AED treatment before the start of any seizure disorders, we do advocate a high index of suspicion and this includes routine and regular EEG monitoring. Due to the potential for generating secondary damage, we strongly advise aggressive treatment once seizures have started. In mtDNA disorders such as MELAS and MERRF, treatment appears to be effective, at least initially. *POLG1*-related disorders, such as Alpers syndrome and MSCAE, can be extremely difficult to treat and we have experience of patients in whom it has been impossible to control focal motor status for long time periods, i.e., weeks, even with combinations of AED in maximal doses.

Convulsive status epilepticus (CSE) is treated aggressively using traditional protocols. Benzodiazepine infusion is evaluated as a first line together with phosphenytoin and occasionally phenobarbital (supervision in intensive care unit).

Subsequently, we use thiopental narcosis where necessary together with cerebral functioning monitoring with the aim of achieving burst suppression for at least 24–48 hr. Daily EEGs are performed including when monitoring protracted recovery periods that may extend to several days. In recent years, we have had some success using propofol as a first-line agent, since the level of narcosis is more easily monitored and can be terminated more rapidly when successful treatment is achieved. Some patients still required thiopental narcosis, however, despite the initial use of propofol. Repeated treatment with thiopental has been successful, but several of our patients, particularly with *POLG1* mutations, have died after a prolonged periods of recurrent CSE and non-convulsive SE with multiple organ failure following the use of every known/ available antiepileptic drug.

Conclusions

Mitochondrial cytopathy due to genetic defects in mtDNA or nDNA may cause epileptic seizures and may even be important in propagating the epileptic process in disorders caused by

D

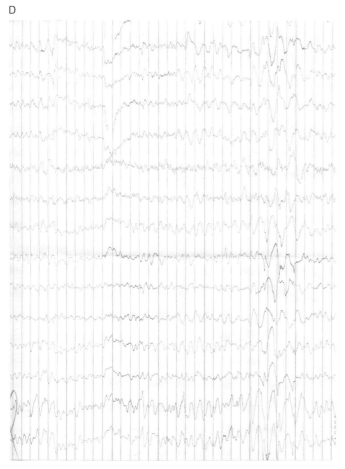

A

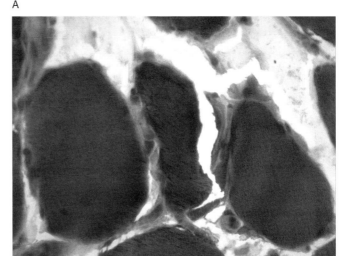

B

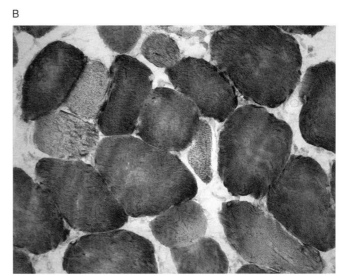

Fig. 19.4. *(cont.)*

Fig. 19.5. Muscle findings. Mitochondrial accumulation, a sign of failing mitochondrial energy production, can be demonstrated using a variety of staining methods. The classical method is the Gomori-trichrome which stains mitochondria red and the background blue. Mitochondrial accumulation distorts the usual regular shape of the muscle fiber giving it an undulated or ragged appearance (A), hence the descriptive name ragged red fiber. As mitochondrial accumulation is an inconsistent feature, it is better to use histochemical investigations that identify specific complex activities. (B) Staining for succinate dehydrogenase (complex II/SDH, no mtDNA-encoded subunits) is combined with staining for complex IV (cytochrome oxidase, three mtDNA-encoded subunits). Where fibers contain both activities, a dark brown color is seen. Fibers lacking COX activity are easily identified since these will only stain with the blue color derived from the succinate dehydrogenase activity. Unfortunately there are currently no available methods for studying complexes I and III. See color plate section.

mechanisms other than MRC defects. Differences in the seizure semiology seen in the different syndromes may reflect age of seizure initiation, e.g., infancy or adulthood, the intracerebral distribution of mtDNA defects, including level of heteroplasmy, or simply phenotypic variation that in itself reflects the different genetic make-up each individual carries. Most seizure types have been reported in mitochondrial cytopathy including generalized ones such as atypical absences, myoclonic seizures, atonic and tonic seizures, GTC, and simple and complex partial seizure types.

The epilepsies in mitochondrial cytopathies often reveal both focal and generalized features. In some cases clearly syndromic epilepsies can be delineated, as for example in *POLG1*-related epilepsy (Engelsen *et al.* 2008), myoclonus epilepsy of MERRF (Berkovic *et al.* 1989), and MELAS (Koo *et al.* 1993). An exceptional feature in mitochondrial cytopathies is the apparent occipital predilection. This can be seen radiologically and in the localization of the epilepsy in *POLG1*-related disorders (Engelsen *et al.* 2008) and MELAS (Koo *et al.* 1993) but not in MERRF (Berkovic *et al.* 1989).

Molecular and biochemical diagnosis of mitochondrial cytopathies are technically demanding areas and best left to

centers that specialize in this area. The major challenge for the general physician is to recognize that mitochondrial dysfunction might be the cause. Thereafter, the decision to investigate or refer to another center will depend on the availability of local genetic and pathological expertise.

Treatment of mitochondrial cytopathies comprises awareness of the potential complications and early and aggressive control of seizures. In the absence of current disease modifying treatments, it is essential to focus on what is achievable. Standard AED treatment appears effective in most of the mtDNA disorders, but *POLG1*-related epilepsy remains a major therapeutic challenge.

Acknowledgments

We would like to thank Charalampos Tzoulis, Department of Neurology, Haukeland, for his help with the manuscript and for Fig. 19.3, and Professor Sigurd Lindal, Neuromuscular Centre of Excellence, Tromsø for the pictures of skeletal muscle.

References

Berkovic SF, Carpenter S, Evans A, *et al.* (1989) Myoclonus epilepsy and ragged-red fibres (MERRF). I. A clinical, pathological, biochemical, magnetic resonance spectrographic and positron emission tomographic study. *Brain* **112**:1231–60.

Canafoglia L, Franceschetti S, Antozzi C, *et al.* (2001) Epileptic phenotypes associated with mitochondrial disorders. *Neurology* **56**:1340–6.

Cock H (2007) The role of mitochondria in status epilepticus. *Epilepsia* **48**:24–7.

Darin N, Oldfors A, Moslemi AR, Holme E, Tulinius M (2001) The incidence of mitochondrial encephalomyopathies in childhood: clinical features and morphological, biochemical, and DNA abnormalities. *Ann Neurol* **49**:377–83.

DiMauro S, Schon EA (2003) Mitochondrial respiratory-chain diseases. *N Engl J Med* **348**:2656–68.

DiMauro S, Schon EA (2008) Mitochondrial disorders in the nervous system. *Ann Rev Neurosci* **31**:91–123.

Elliott HR, Samuels DC, Eden JA, Relton CL, Chinnery PF (2008) Pathogenic mitochondrial DNA mutations are common in the general population. *Am J Hum Genet* **83**:254–60.

Engelsen BA, Tzoulis C, Karlsen B, *et al.* (2008) *POLG1* mutations cause a syndromic epilepsy with occipital lobe predilection. *Brain* **131**:818–28.

Ferrari G, Lamantea E, Donati A, *et al.* (2005) Infantile hepatocerebral syndromes associated with mutations in the mitochondrial DNA polymerase-gamma. *Brain* **128**:723–31.

Fukuhara N, Tokiguchi S, Shirakawa K, Tsubaki T (1980) Myoclonus epilepsy associated with ragged-red fibres (mitochondrial abnormalities): disease entity or a syndrome? Light- and electron-microscopic studies of two cases and review of literature. *J Neurol Sci* **47**:117–33.

Goto Y-I, Nonaka I, Horai S (1991) A new mtDNA mutation associated with mitochondrial myopathy, encephalomyopathy, lactic acidosis and stroke-like episodes (MELAS). *Biocheim Biophys Acta* **1097**:238–40.

Hakonen AH, Heiskanen S, Juvonen V, *et al.* (2005) Mitochondrial DNA polymerase W748S mutation: a common cause of autosomal recessive ataxia with ancient European origin. *Am J Hum Genet* **77**:430–41.

Hakonen AH, Davidzon G, Salemi R, *et al.* (2007) Abundance of the *POLG* disease mutations in Europe, Australia, New Zealand, and the United States explained by single ancient European founders. *Eur J Hum Genet* **15**:779–83.

Hirano M, DiMauro S (1997) Primary mitochondrial diseases. In: Engel J, Pedley TA (eds.) *Epilepsy: A Comprehensive Textbook*. Philadelphia, PA: Lippincott–Raven, pp. 2563–70.

Hirano M, Pavlakis SG (1994) Topical review: Mitochondrial myopathy, encephalopathy, lactic acidosis, and strokelike episodes (MELAS) – current concepts. *J Child Neurol* **9**:4–13.

Horvath R, Hudson G, Ferrari G, *et al.* (2006) Phenotypic spectrum associated with mutations of the mitochondrial polymerase gamma gene. *Brain* **129**:1674–84.

Hudson G, Chinnery PF (2006) Mitochondrial DNA polymerase-gamma and human disease. *Hum Mol Genet* **15**:R244–52.

Iizuka T, Sakai F, Kan S, Suzuki N (2003) Slowly progressive spread of the stroke-like lesions in MELAS. *Neurology* **61**:1238–44.

Kim DY, Rho JM (2008) The ketogenic diet and epilepsy. *Curr Opin Clin Nutr Metab Care* **11**:113–20.

Koo B, Becker LE, Chuang S, *et al.* (1993) Mitochondrial encephalomyopathy, lactic acidosis, stroke-like episodes (MELAS): clinical, radiological, pathological, and genetic observations. *Ann Neurol* **34**:25–32.

Kunz WF (2002) The role of mitochondria in epileptogenesis. *Curr Opin Neurol* **15**:179–84.

Leff AP, McNabb AW, Hanna MG, Clarke CR, Larner AJ (1998) Complex partial status epilepticus in late-onset MELAS. *Epilepsia* **39**:438–41.

Luoma PT, Eerola J, Ahola S, *et al.* (2007) Mitochondrial DNA polymerase gamma variants in idiopathic sporadic Parkinson disease. *Neurology* **69**:1152–9.

McFarland R, Elson JL, Taylor RW, Howell N, Turnbull DM (2004) Assigning pathogenicity to mitochondrial tRNA mutations: when 'definitely maybe' is not good enough. *Trends Genet* **20**:591–6.

Montagna P, Gallassi R, Medori R, *et al.* (1988) MELAS syndrome: characteristic migrainous and epileptic features and maternal transmission. *Neurology* **38**:751–4.

Nguyen KV, Ostergaard E, Ravn SH, *et al.* (2005) *POLG* mutations in Alpers syndrome. *Neurology* **65**:1493–5.

Pavlakis SG, Phillips PC, DiMauro S, De Vivo DC, Rowland LP (1984) Mitochondrial myopathy, encephalopathy, lactic acidosis, and strokelike episodes: a distinctive clinical syndrome. *Ann Neurol* **16**:481–8.

Ruiz-Pesini E, Lott MT, Procaccio V, *et al.* (2007) An enhanced MITOMAP with a global mtDNA mutational phylogeny. *Nucl Acids Res* **35**:D823–8.

Schaefer AM, McFarland R, Blakely EL, *et al.* (2008) Prevalence of mitochondrial DNA disease in adults. *Ann Neurol* **63**:35–9.

Skladal D, Halliday J, Thorburn DR (2003) Minimum birth prevalence of mitochondrial respiratory chain disorders in children. *Brain* **126**:1905–12.

Taylor RW, Turnbull DM (2005) Mitochondrial DNA mutations in human disease. *Nat Rev Genet* **6**:389–402.

Taylor RW, Schaefer AM, Barron MJ, McFarland R, Turnbull DM (2004) The diagnosis of mitochondrial muscle disease. *Neuromusc Disords* **14**:237–45.

Tzoulis C, Bindoff LA (2009) Serial diffusion imaging in a case of mitochondrial encephalomyopathy, lactic acidosis, and stroke-like episodes. *Stroke* **40**:e15–17.

Tzoulis C, Engelsen BA, Telstad W, *et al.* (2006) The spectrum of clinical disease caused by the A467T and W748S *POLG* mutations: a study of 26 cases. *Brain* **129**:1685–92.

Winterthun S, Ferrari G, He L, *et al.* (2005) Autosomal recessive mitochondrial ataxic syndrome due to mitochondrial polymerase-gamma mutations. *Neurology* **64**:1204–8.

Zeviani M, Carelli V (2007) Mitochondrial disorders. *Curr Opin Neurol* **20**:564–71.

Neuronal ceroid lipofuscinoses

Ruth E. Williams

Introduction to the neuronal ceroid lipofuscinoses

The neuronal ceroid lipofuscinoses (NCLs) are a group of inherited neurodegenerative disorders characterized by the accumulation of storage material in lysosomes. They are diagnosed in many different ethnic groups and probably have a worldwide prevalence. In the UK the NCLs are the most commonly diagnosed cause of progressive cognitive and neurological deterioration in children with an incidence of approximately 1.6/100 000 live births. Most have onset in childhood and are autosomal recessive. The key clinical features include a symptomatic generalized (myoclonic) epilepsy syndrome, visual impairment, cognitive and physical regression, and early death. A number of causative genes have now been identified allowing for increased understanding of some of the likely pathological mechanisms involved in this group of disorders, together with enhanced clarity of diagnosis and classification. Table 20.1 summarizes the current classification of NCL disorders and their genetic basis.

In the UK, the most commonly diagnosed NCLs have late infantile (usually caused by mutations in *CLN2*, but also *CLN5*, *CLN6*, and *CLN8*) or juvenile onset (caused by mutations in *CLN3* usually, but also *CLN1* and rarely *CLN2*). Infantile onset NCL (*CLN1*) is also seen in Scotland, Scandinavia, and the USA. Late infantile onset and early juvenile onset variants (*CLN5*, *CLN6*, *CLN7*, and *CLN8*) are seen in Finland, middle and southern Europe, the Middle East, and in families of Indo-Pakistani origin. Congenital (*CTSD*, *CLN10*) and adult onset (putative gene locus *CLN4*) NCLs are rare.

Epilepsy in the NCLs

Juvenile onset NCL (JNCL, usually *CLN3*, occasionally *CLN1* and *CLN2*)

Epilepsy is not an early feature of *CLN3* disease, juvenile. Children lose vision over a 6–18-month period around the age of 5–6 years. They remain essentially well for several years although there may be some learning difficulties.

Epilepsy occurs in all children and is a major feature from the middle school years onwards. In a Finnish series the mean age of onset of seizures was 10 years (Aberg *et al.* 2000). Seizures are often generalized and initially only occasional, becoming more frequent and with the onset of other seizure types (focal onset, atypical absences, and later myoclonic) within 1–2 years. Some seizures are difficult to classify clinically. Epilepsy usually becomes medication resistant. The background electroencephalogram (EEG) may be normal at presentation with focal discharges. Later brief bursts of irregular generalized discharges are seen with slowing of the background. Photic stimulation does not produce an abnormal response.

Around puberty, loss of mobility and communication skills start to become apparent and there is a slow decline in abilities over several years. Teenagers and young adults have a characteristic "parkinsonian-like" gait and stuttering speech. Emotional and psychiatric problems including anxiety, psychosis, and distressing hallucinations are very common. Life expectancy varies greatly from the teenage years to early thirties. The course of the disease varies depending on genotype but also even within the same family. Rating scales have been developed that are helpful in monitoring disease progression (Kohlschütter *et al.* 1988; Marshall *et al.* 2005).

Classic late infantile onset NCL with TPP1 deficiency (*CLN2*)

Most children subsequently found to have tripeptidyl peptidase 1 (TPP1) deficiency and/or mutations in *CLN2* present with seizures between the ages of 2 and 4 years. In a proportion of children concerns about speech and language delay have already been raised before the onset of epilepsy, but seizures quickly become the dominant feature. They may be generalized tonic–clonic, atonic, or focal onset initially. Commonly other seizure types develop and some may be difficult to classify. Seizures may or may not respond initially to medication, but usually become resistant to medication within 12 to 36 months of onset. Myoclonus gradually becomes more

The Causes of Epilepsy, eds. S. D. Shorvon, F. Andermann, and R. Guerrini. Published by Cambridge University Press. © Cambridge University Press 2011.

Table 20.1 Current classification and genetic basis of NCLs

	Gene symbol	Protein/cellular localization	Diseases
Lysosomal enzyme deficiencies	CTSD, CLN10	Cathepsin D	CLN10 disease, congenital
			CLN10 disease, late infantile
			CLN10 disease, juvenile
			CLN10 disease adult
	CLN1	Palmitoyl protein thioesterase 1, PPT1	CLN1 disease, infantile
			CLN1 disease, late infantile variant
			CLN1 disease, juvenile
			CLN1 disease, adult
	CLN2	Tripeptidyl peptidase 1, TPP1	CLN2 disease, classic late infantile
			CLN2 disease, juvenile
			CLN2 disease, adult
Non-enzyme, NCL associated proteins (functions poorly understood at the current time)	CLN3	Transmembrane protein, "battenin" Lysosomal/transport from endoplasmic reticulum to lysosome	CLN3 disease, classic juvenile
	CLN4	Gene not yet identified	Adult
	CLN5	Transmembrane and soluble forms: lysosomal	CLN5 disease, late infantile variant
	CLN6	Endoplasmic reticulum	CLN6 disease, late infantile variant
			CLN6 disease, early juvenile variant
	CLN7		CLN7 disease, late infantile variant
	CLN8	Transmembrane protein: endoplasmic reticulum, endoplasmic reticulum-Golgi	CLN8 disease, EPMR
			CLN8 disease, late infantile variant
	CLN9		CLN9 disease, early juvenile variant
Others – those whose classification is uncertain because of incomplete diagnostic investigations or absence of confirmed gene/mutation designation			Congenital/infantile variants
			Late infantile variants
			Juvenile variants
			Late onset/adult variants
			Chloride transport defect, adult onset

evident as the disease progresses with loss of mobility and communication skills, and often becomes a major symptom in the later stages of disease. Myoclonic status is also seen (Fig. 20.1).

Early EEGs may show a paroxysmal occipital spike response to slow rate photic stimulation (Pampiglione and Harden 1973; Binelli *et al.* 2000), shown in Fig. 20.1. This can alert the physician to the diagnosis and is therefore very

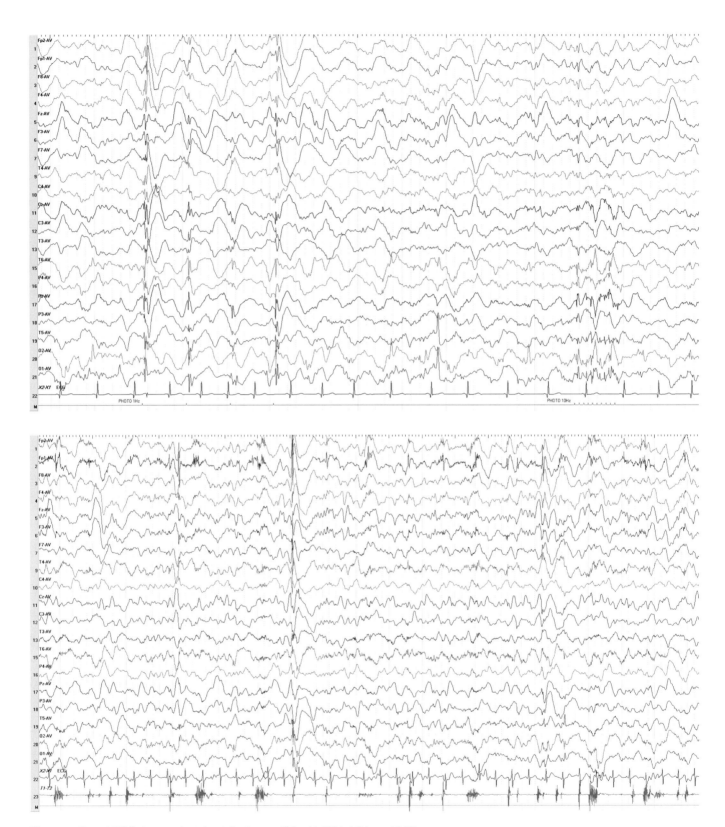

Fig. 20.1. Typical EEG findings in classic late infantile onset NCL with TPP1 deficiency (*CLN2*).

important. The electroretinogram (ERG) may be diminished with an unusually exaggerated visual evoked potential (VEP). As the disease progresses the background EEG slows and epileptiform activity becomes more evident with brief bursts of generalized spike-and-wave discharges.

Variant late infantile and early juvenile NCL (*CLN5, CLN6, CLN7, CLN8* and others)

Children with atypical early features or rate of disease progression often have normal palmitoyl protein thioesterase (PPT) and TPP1 enzyme activities and may then be found to have mutations in one of the other NCL genes (*CLN5, CLN6, CLN7,* and *CLN8*). Children may show learning and behavior difficulties in the early school years and then go on to have seizures later. These are often described as early juvenile variants. As in the other NCLs, seizures become medication resistant, often in association with loss of mobility, play, communication, and feeding skills. Seizure types include atypical absences, focal seizures, atonic and clonic seizures, together with generalized tonic–clonic and myoclonus. Children with mutations in *CLN8* have been described from Turkey and from Italy (Topcu *et al.* 2004; Striano *et al.* 2007). In the majority seizures begin in early childhood and the EEG is characterized by an early occipital spike response to photic stimulation as in *CLN2* disease, classic late infantile.

Classic infantile onset NCL, with PPT1 deficiency (*CLN1*)

This disorder presents within the first 18 months of life with slowing of developmental progress, hypotonia, and irritability. It is most commonly diagnosed in families of Scandinavian heritage. There is a rapid deterioration of skills and onset of seizures with myoclonus. Seizure frequency and severity is highly variable. The EEG is abnormal from presentation with a generalized encephalopathic picture. Myoclonic jerks are associated with irregular generalized spike-and-wave discharges. Later in the course of the disease the sleep and awake organization is lost. The EEG becomes electrically silent after the third year of life. There is no paroxysmal photosensitive response. (Santavuori *et al.* 1974).

Adult NCL

The disease usually starts in young adulthood. Familial cases are well recognized but dominant as well as recessive inheritance patterns are documented. Symptoms include behavioral changes, epilepsy, ataxia, movement disorder, and dementia. Vision is generally preserved. The differential diagnosis includes other progressive myoclonic epilepsies (PMEs): Unverricht–Lundborg, Lafora body disease, mitochondrial disorders, dentatorubral-pallidoluysian atrophy (DRPLA), and new variant Creuzfeldt-Jakob disease (CJD). Some adult onset NCL cases have abnormal storage material in peripheral tissues which leads to the diagnosis. Some are due to mutations in *CLN1* or other known NCL genes but for many an underlying biochemical or genetic defect has not yet been found. Electrophysiology and brain imaging give non-specific results.

Congenital, late infantile, and early juvenile variants due to mutations in *CLN10*

A rare form of NCL has recently been described due to a deficiency of cathepsin D (Siintola *et al.* 2006; Steinfeld *et al.* 2006). Several infants with a very severe disease phenotype characterized by microcephaly, seizures from birth, and early death have been described with cathepsin D deficiency and mutations in *CTSD* (also known as *CLN10*). Furthermore, a child with normal early psychomotor development but presenting with visual symptoms and ataxia in the early school years has also been reported. She went on to show loss of cognitive, communication, and mobility skills and at 17 years of age had severe impairment and was non-ambulant. Thus the clinical spectrum of this disorder may be very wide.

Northern epilepsy, progressive epilepsy with mental retardation (EPMR) (Gene *CLN8*)

This condition is now known to belong to the NCLs and is most frequently diagnosed in Finland (Ranta and Lehesjoki 2000). Children present with generalized seizures at between 5 and 10 years of age. Seizures continue and there is a slow deterioration of cognitive skills. Visual failure is mild and a late symptom. Myoclonus is rare.

Diagnosis of the NCLs

A simplified diagnostic algorithm is given in Fig. 20.2. Children presenting in the early school years with isolated visual failure and electrophysiology suggestive of retinal pathology are most likely to have *CLN3* disease, juvenile onset or *CLN1* disease, juvenile onset. The most helpful diagnostic investigations are therefore peripheral blood sampling for vacuolated lymphocytes, PPT1 activity, and DNA extraction for further genetic studies (*CLN3* and possibly *CLN1*).

Children presenting with refractory seizures and/or developmental regression in early childhood are likely to undergo a number of investigations. Brain imaging is normal initially but as the disease progresses, infratentorial and then generalized atrophy becomes apparent in *CLN1* disease, infantile or late infantile onset and in *CLN2* disease, classical late infantile onset. Early thalamic changes may be suggestive of NCL but there are no features which are diagnostic (Autti *et al.* 1997). Basic biochemistry, liver function, plasma lactate, amino acids, and urine organic acids are normal. The EEG may show characteristic occipital discharges in response to slow photic stimulation in *CLN2*

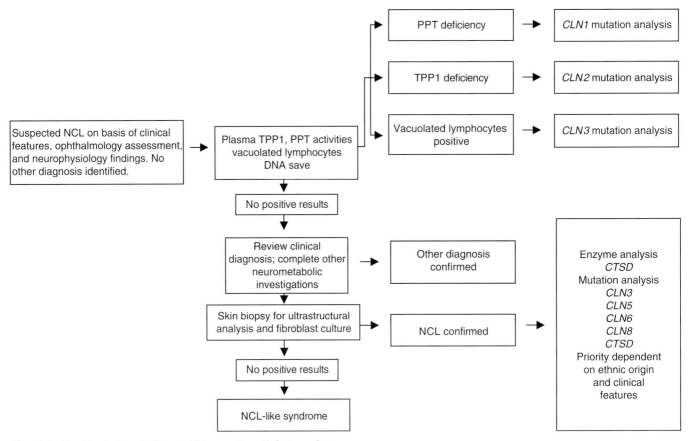

Fig. 20.2. Algorithm for investigation of child presenting with features of NCL.

disease, classic late infantile onset and the other NCLs with onset in the late infantile or early juvenile range (genes: *CLN5, CLN6, CLN7, CLN8*).

When one of the NCLs is being considered as a possible diagnosis, initial samples should be taken for enzyme analysis PPT1, TPP1, and cathepsin D–and DNA saved. If any of the enzymes are deficient, mutation analysis of the relevant gene can then be requested to provide genetic confirmation. If white cell enzyme activities are normal, samples should be sent for ultrastructural analysis. The samples required may depend on local expertise. In the UK, peripheral blood is often sufficient, but in many other countries skin biopsy is preferred. Skin biopsy offers the advantage that fibroblasts can be cultured from the same sample for further enzyme and genetic analysis. Wherever possible a clinical, biochemical, and genetic diagnosis should be established. In unusual cases a description of the ultrastructural findings should be provided to families and professionals.

Principles of management

There is currently no cure for any of the NCLs. Genes *CLN1* and *CLN2* code for lysosomal enzymes and therefore there is much interest in the possibilities that gene therapy, stem cell therapy, enzyme replacement therapy, and/or substrate reduction might offer families some hope in the future.

Antiepileptic drug choices are important once the diagnosis is established. Valproate is probably one of the most effective antiepileptic drugs in the NCLs. Benzodiazepines may be very helpful although tolerance and increased oral secretions are recognized problems.

Lamotrigine may worsen myoclonus in the early stages of *CLN2* disease, late infantile. It has been my personal experience that lamotrigine may hasten apparent progression with worsening of mobility especially in *CLN2* disease. Fortunately mobility usually improves again when lamotrigine is stopped. However for some children lamotrigine works very well! Carbamazepine likewise may work well for a few but for the majority should probably be avoided. Aberg and colleagues reported a favorable response to lamotrigine in a series of 28 children with *CLN3* disease, classical juvenile onset (Aberg *et al.* 1999).

Topiramate has been helpful in many children, as a single agent and as combined therapy with valproate. Topiramate at high doses can of course be associated with word-finding difficulties and changes in mood which can have a profound effect on the abilities of a young adult with *CLN3* disease, juvenile onset. The benzodiazepines (clobazam, clonazepam) and piracetam have been used with good effect for myoclonus. Phenobarbitone has also provided some benefit for prolonged and frequent seizures and for myoclonic status in advanced disease. Phenytoin has recently also been reported to be of benefit for myoclonic status in the advanced stages of NCL (Miyahara *et al.* 2009).

Early anecdotal reports of leviteracetam in both late infantile and juvenile onset NCLs have supported its use (Niezen-de Boer 2005).

Anecdotally, a small number of children with late infantile NCL have been treated using a ketogenic diet with no adverse consequences.

Acknowledgments

I am very grateful to all the children and families I have known and worked with, the Batten Disease Family Association, and professional colleagues of the UK Batten Professional Development Group. I thank Dr. Sushma Goyal, Consultant Pediatric Neurophysiologist, Evelina Children's Hospital, London for providing some of the illustrations and reading and commenting on the script.

References

Aberg L, Kirveskari E, Santavuori P (1999) Lamotrigine therapy in juvenile neuronal ceroid lipofuscinosis. *Epilepsia* **40**:796–9.

Aberg LE, Backman M, Kirveskari E, Santavuori P (2000) Epilepsy and antiepileptic drug therapy in juvenile neuronal ceroid lipofuscinoses. *Epilepsia* **41**:1296–302.

Autti T, Raininko R, Vanhanen S-L, Santavuori P (1997) Magnetic resonance techniques in neuronal ceroid lipofusincosis and some other lysosomal diseases affecting the brain. *Curr Opin Neurol* **10**:519–24.

Binelli S, Canafoglia L, Panzica F, Pozzi A, Franceschetti S (2000) Electrographic features in a series of patients with neuronal ceroid lipofuscinoses. *Neurol Sci* **21**:S83–7.

Kohlschütter A, Laabs R, Albani M (1988) Juvenile neuronal ceroid lipofuscinoses (JNCL): quantitative description of its clinical variability. *Acta Paed Scand* **77**:867–72.

Marshall FJ, de Blieck EA, Mink JW, *et al.* (2005) A clinical rating scale for Batten disease. *Neurology* **65**:275–9.

Miyahara A, Saito Y, Sugai K, *et al.* (2009) Reassessment of phenytoin for treatment of late stage progressive myoclonus epilepsy complicated with status epilepticus. *Epilepsy Res* **84**:201–9.

Niezen-de Boer MC (2005) Levetiracetam therapy in juvenile neuronal ceroid lipofuscinoses. Abstract, 10th International Congress on Neuronal Ceroid Lipofuscinoses, Helsinki.

Pampiglione G, Harden A (1973) Neurophysiological identification of a late infantile form of "neuronal liposis." *J Neurol Neurosurg Psychiatry* **36**:68–74.

Ranta S, Lehesjoki AE (2000) Northern epilepsy, a new member of the NCL family. *Neurol Sci* **21**:S43–7.

Santavuori P, Haltia M, Rapola J (1974) Infantile type of so-called neuronal ceroid lipofuscinoses. *Dev Med Child Neurol* **16**:644–53.

Siintola E, Partanen S, Stromme P, *et al.* (2006) Cathepsin D deficiency underlies human neuronal ceroid lipofuscinoses. *Brain* **129**:1353–6.

Steinfeld R, Reinhardt K, Schreiber K, *et al.* (2006) Cathepsin deficiency is associated with a human neurodegenerative disorder. *Am J Hum Genet* **78**:988–98.

Striano P, Specchio N, Biancheri R, *et al.* (2007) Clinical and electrophysiological features of epilepsy in Italian patients with *CLN8* mutations. *Epilepsy Behav* **10**:187–91.

Topcu M, Tan H, Yalnizoglu D, *et al.* (2004) Evaluation of 36 patients from Turkey with neuronal ceroid lipofuscinoses: clinical, neurophysiological, neuroradiological and histopathologic studies. *Turk J Pediatr* **46**:1–10.

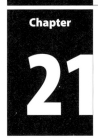

Chapter 21

Sialidosis and Gaucher disease

Silvana Franceschetti and Laura Canafoglia

The epileptic phenotype resulting from sialidoses and from the subtypes of Gaucher disease (GD) presents with myoclonus and generalized seizures and belongs to the category of progressive myoclonus epilepsies (PMEs). Differently from sialidoses, GD also presents a heterogeneous clinical presentation, which may also include seizures with prominent neurological and extraneurological symptoms which do not realize a typical PME picture.

Sialidoses
The causal disease

Sialidoses are classified in two types presenting with different phenotypes. Sialidosis type I presents with the typical features characterizing PMEs (Rapin *et al.* 1978), while the phenotype of sialidosis type II typically includes dysmorphic features. The macular change found in this metabolic disorder led to the definition "cherry-red spot myoclonus" and is caused by intracellular accumulation of metabolic products in the macular area.

Both types of sialidosis are inherited as an autosomal recessive trait leading to α-*N*-acetylneuraminidase (sialidase) deficiency and to sialic acid-rich macromolecular storage and urinary sialyl-oligosaccharide excretion. A subtype of sialidosis type II, called galactosialidosis, results from a deficiency of α-*N*-acetylneuraminidase and β-galactosialidase.

The neuraminidase gene (*NEU1*) has been localized on chromosome 6p21.3 (Bonten *et al.* 1996) and accounts for both sialidoses I and II. Different mutations have been detected and a close correlation between residual activity of the mutant enzymes and clinical severity of the disease has been reported.

The gene responsible for galactosialidosis maps to chromosome 20q13.1 (Rothschild *et al.* 1993) and leads to defective protective protein cathepsin A (PPCA), which, in turn, causes a combined deficiency of β-galactosidase and neuraminidase.

Pathology and pathophysiology

The disease results in lysosomal storage of sialidated glycopeptides and oligosaccharides. Light and electron microscopy reveal cytoplasmic vacuolation involving neurons and perineuronal and interfascicular oligodendroglia, endothelial, and perithelial cells. Vacuolations are associated with diffuse neuronal intracytoplasmic storage of lipofuscin-like pigment detectable in the neocortex, basal ganglia, thalamus, brainstem, and spinal cord, as well in extranervous organs (Allegranza *et al.* 1989). It was found that neuraminidase is a negative regulator of lysosomal exocitosis (Yogalingam *et al.* 2008).

Epilepsy in the disease

Both types of sialidosis are PMEs, because they present with progressively worsening multifocal myoclonus, usually occurring in the second decade of life, variably associated with seizures and ataxia (Lowden and O'Brien 1979).

Sialidosis type II

Sialidosis type II can be suspected early in life because of dysmorphic features (coarse face, short trunk, barrel chest, spinal deformity, and skeletal dysplasia) sometimes associated with corneal clouding, hepatomegaly, and inner-ear hearing loss. Generalized seizures occur in infancy, before the appearance of myoclonic jerks, and are associated with psychomotor delay and ataxia.

Sialidosis type I

Sialidosis type I has a juvenile or adult onset, presenting with rare convulsive seizures (which are often easily controlled by appropriate treatments), severely invalidating action myoclonus, and mild ataxia, in the absence of mental deterioration or dysmorphisms.

In both types of sialidosis, electrophysiological studies performed at onset of seizure or myoclonus show paroxysmal electroencephalographic (EEG) activity, which can either present as polyspike–waves (often associated with spontaneous myoclonus) or as "fast activities" (Fig. 21.1). Jerk-locked back averaging (Franceschetti *et al.* 1980) and coherence analysis (Panzica *et al.* 2003) reveal a consistent temporal relationship

---

The Causes of Epilepsy, eds. S. D. Shorvon, F. Andermann, and R. Guerrini. Published by Cambridge University Press. © Cambridge University Press 2011.

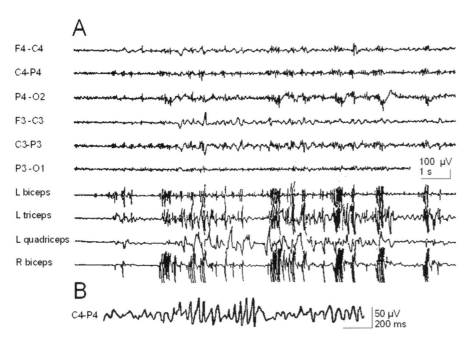

Fig. 21.1. EEG polygraphic recording performed in a 28-year-old patient with sialidosis type 1. Note diffuse discharges of fast activity, prominent on central derivations mixed with polyspikes (A), which are associated with repetitive myoclonic jerks induced by active movements. A fragment of fast activity related to myoclonic jerks is magnified at the bottom (B).

between the EEG spikes and myoclonic jerks, testifying the cortical origin of myoclonus. In some of the reported patients, the presence of high-amplitude somatosensory evoked potentials and of enhanced long-loop reflexes confirms the marked neocortical hyperexcitability, which is responsible for "cortical reflex" and action myoclonus.

Magnetic resonance imaging (MRI) findings in sialidoses are normal in the early stages, while cerebellar, pontine, and cerebral atrophy can appear during the disease progression (Palmeri *et al.* 2000).

This macular change may finally lead to visual failure. However, it can be clinically undetectable for many years and lead to visual failure only late in the course of the disease. Cherry-red spot can disappear in the latest stages, due to loss of the ganglion cells, which results in optic atrophy (Kivlin *et al.* 1985).

Prognosis

Patients with sialidosis type II progressively develop multiple neurological defects and severe mental impairment. Patients with sialidosis type I exhibit progressive visual impairment. All patients, with sialidosis of either type, become wheelchair-bound in a few years, due to severe motor disability, mainly resulting from severe myoclonus.

Diagnostic tests for the disease

A positive diagnosis is based on the detection of high urinary sialyloligosaccharides and upon confirmation of the lysosomal enzyme deficiency in leucocytes or cultured fibroblasts (Lowden and O'Brien 1979).

Gaucher disease
The causal disease

Gaucher disease is an autosomal, recessively inherited lysosomal storage disorder caused by mutations in the gene encoding acid β-gluco(cerebro)sidase (*GBA*), which maps to chromosome 1q21 (Koprivica *et al.* 2000). To date, more than 200 causative mutations have been identified, including recombination events within the *GBA* locus (Horowitz *et al.* 1989).

Traditionally, GD has been divided into three clinical types, based upon the presence and rate of progression of neurologic symptoms. Type 1 GD (MIM 230800) has no associated neurologic symptoms. Type 2 GD (acute neuronopathic form, MIM 230900) presents with a rapidly progressive neurologic deterioration leading to death in utero or within the first 2–3 years of life. Type 3, or chronic neuronopathic GD (MIM 606463), typically includes neurologic symptoms, beginning in childhood or early adulthood. It may be divided into subtypes 3a, 3b, and 3c, based upon the nature of the neurologic manifestations (Patterson *et al.* 1993). Type 3a typically identifies forms presenting with progressive PME (Park *et al.* 2003).

The clinical features are not strictly linked to the type of mutation. Indeed a wide genotypic heterogeneity is described in patients sharing a similar phenotype, while the same genotype is not necessarily associated with the same symptoms (Sidransky *et al.* 1994). Goker-Alpan *et al.* (2003) described a phenotype with intermediate severity between GD type 2 and 3, characterized by a delayed age of onset but a rapidly progressive neurological disease with refractory seizures, suggesting

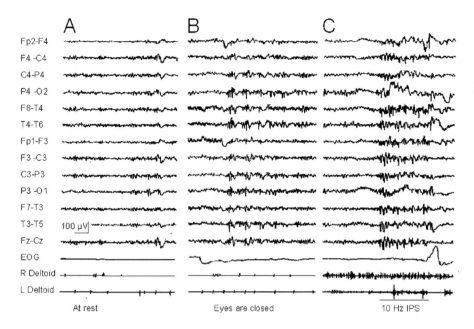

Fig. 21.2. EEG polygraphic recording of an 18-year-old patient with Gaucher disease. Note diffuse polyspikes and waves, diffuse but prominent on posterior regions, which are enhanced at eye closure (B) and during intermittent photic stimulation (IPS), sometimes associated with irregular myoclonic jerks (C).

that neuronopathic GD is likely to be a continuum of phenotypes from the severe perinatal to mildly impaired cases.

A distinctive form of GD is termed the "Norrbottnian type" because of its origin from the province of Norrbotten, in the northern Sweden. Affected patients have short stature with splenomegaly, abnormal eye movements, and sometimes seizures, but no myoclonus. Although all Norrbottnian patients are believed to share the same genotype (L444P/L444P), the course of the disease may vary markedly (Blom and Erikson 1983).

Pathology and pathophysiology

The deficient glucocerebrosidase activity causes accumulation of glucosylceramide (glucocerebroside), a breakdown product of membrane glycosphingolipids, within lysosomes of reticuloendothelial cells, particularly in the liver, bone marrow, spleen, and lung. The so-called Gaucher cells invade various tissues and may result in organ dysfunction. It is hypothesized that pathology is caused by material storage and macrophage activation. Moreover, evidences suggest that glucoylceramide accumulation is correlated with defective calcium homeostasis in neurons (Jmoudiak and Futerman 2005).

The most common mutation found in myoclonic phenotypes is N188S, which is supposed to alter protein structure and processing, leading to neuronal cell death (Kowarz *et al.* 2005). Neuronal loss has been found in the hippocampal regions, calcarine cortex, and brainstem in patients with GD type 2 and type 3 with progressive myoclonic encephalopathy, whereas astrogliosis has been found in GD type 1 (Wong *et al.* 2004). Patients with GD type 3 show cerebellum–dentate degeneration that may play a role in subcortical myoclonus (Verghese *et al.* 2000).

Epilepsy in the disease

According to Park *et al.* (2003), patients presenting with PME exhibit heterogeneity in age at onset and rate of progression. Myoclonus manifests between 16 months and 50 years, combining with variable symptoms including horizontal gaze abnormality, progressive dementia, generalized seizures, ataxia, and spasticity. A few of the adult patients also have parkinsonian-like symptoms. Among PME patients, there are two partially distinct subgroups, the first with onset of myoclonus in early childhood associated with significant cognitive deficits, delayed development, severe visceral involvement, and early death. The second group has a later onset, generally with slower deterioration and less severe systemic involvement. Almost all adult patients have generalized seizures, in addition to myoclonus, and EEG abnormalities.

Most patients have normal MRI findings or mild changes, including T2 hyperintensities in the periventricular white matter, the pons, and the cerebellum, and cerebral atrophy or dural thickening.

The EEG can show slow-waves in the posterior and temporal areas and focal or diffuse paroxysmal epileptiform discharges (Fig. 21.2).

The amplitude of somatosensory evoked potentials is typically enlarged in patients with GD type 3 in comparison to those with GD type 1 (Garvey *et al.* 2001). This finding has been correlated with cognitive impairment. Multimodal evoked potentials were used to obtain information about nervous subclinical damage in GD type 1; transcranial magnetic stimulation is considered to be a good tool to detect an enhanced cortical motor threshold in preclinical stages (Perretti *et al.* 2005).

Prognosis

Due to the heterogeneity of the GD phenotypes, prognosis is also variable among the PME phenotypes.

Diagnostic tests for the disease

The positive diagnosis can be based on the determination of very low blood glucocerebrosidase enzyme activity. This can be confirmed by measuring glucocerebrosidase activity in cultured fibroblasts, obtained from skin biopsy. The identification of mutations in the GBA gene confirms the diagnosis and facilitates genetic counseling since genetic analysis is the only test that can accurately identify heterozygous healthy individuals.

Principles of management

For both sialidoses and Gaucher disease, pharmacological treatment does not differ from that of other PMEs. Valproate can be considered as the first-line drug; however, treatment of severe myoclonus usually needs two or three associated drugs, including benzodiazepines, levetiracetam, or zonisamide.

Sialidoses

In sialidosis, even if enzyme replacement therapy is a possible approach to treatment, there is no supporting evidence in humans. In mice, restored neuraminidase activity can persist for some days and give a significant reduction in lysosomal storage. However, the injected enzyme could not cross the blood–brain barrier. In addition, its use is hampered by the risk of severe anaphylactic responses (Wang *et al.* 2005).

Gaucher disease

A European consensus (Vellodi *et al.* 2001) recommended enzyme replacement therapy (ERT) in all GD subtypes, using chronic intravenous administration of macrophage-targeted recombinant human glucocerebrosidase. Enzyme replacement therapy is aimed at increasing the residual capacity to degrade glucosylceramide, which was found to ameliorate systemic involvement in the majority of patients with GD type 1, but unable to cross the blood–brain barrier and prevent central nervous system complications in patients with GD type 3. Nevertheless, it has been suggested that high-dose ERT might stabilize neurological manifestations in some patients with GD type 3, either by forced penetration of recombinant GBA into the cerebrospinal fluid due to systemic overload or by clearance of perivascular Gaucher cells located outside the blood–brain barrier (Zimran and Elstein 2007). Myoclonus is not reported to improve with ERT (Park *et al.* 2003).

Another proposed treatment is substrate reduction therapy (SRT), which is based on chronic oral administration of an inhibitor of the biosynthesis of glucosylceramide and higher glycosphingolipids (miglustat), This inhibitor can cross the blood–brain barrier and might help reducing central nervous system complications in some GD patients. Data reported for an individual GD patient from Capablo *et al.* (2007) indicated that a combination of miglustat and ERT may improve neurologic clinical deficits and epilepsy and reduce epileptic EEG discharges.

References

Allegranza A, Tredici G, Marmiroli P, *et al.* (1989) Sialidosis type I: pathological study in an adult. *Clin Neuropathol* **8**:266–71.

Blom S, Erikson A (1983) Gaucher disease–Norrbottnian type: neurodevelopmental, neurological, and neurophysiological aspects. *Eur J Pediatr* **140**:316–22.

Bonten E, van der Spoel A, Fornerod M, Grosveld G, d'Azzo A (1996) Characterization of human lysosomal neuraminidase defines the molecular basis of the metabolic storage disorder sialidosis. *Genes Dev* **10**:3156–69.

Capablo JL, Franco R, de Cabezón AS, *et al.* (2007) Neurologic improvement in a type 3 Gaucher disease patient treated with imiglucerase/miglustat combination. *Epilepsia* **48**:1406–8.

Franceschetti S, Uziel G, Di Donato S, Caimi L, Avanzini G (1980) Cherry-red spot myoclonus syndrome and alpha-neuraminidase deficiency: neurophysiological, pharmacological and biochemical study in an adult. *J Neurol Neurosurg Psychiatry* **43**:934–40.

Garvey MA, Toro C, Goldstein S, *et al.* (2001) Somatosensory evoked potentials as a marker of disease burden in type 3 Gaucher disease. *Neurology* **56**:391–4.

Goker-Alpan O, Schiffmann R, Park JK, *et al.* (2003) Phenotypic continuum in neuronopathic Gaucher disease: an intermediate phenotype between type 2 and type 3. *J Pediatr* **143**:273–6.

Horowitz M, Wilder S, Horowitz Z, *et al.* (1989) The human glucocerebrosidase gene and pseudogene: structure and evolution. *Genomics* **4**:87–96.

Jmoudiak M, Futerman AH (2005) Gaucher disease: pathological mechanisms and modern management. *Br J Haematol* **129**:178–88.

Kivlin JD, Sanborn GE, Myers GG (1985) The cherry-red spot in Tay–Sachs and other storage diseases. *Ann Neurol* **17**:356–60.

Koprivica V, Stone DL, Park JK, *et al.* (2000) Analysis and classification of 304 mutant alleles in patients with type 1 and type 3 Gaucher disease. *Am J Hum Genet* **66**:1777–86.

Kowarz L, Goker-Alpan O, Banerjee-Basu S, *et al.* (2005) Gaucher mutation N188S is associated with myoclonic epilepsy. *Hum Mutat* **26**:271–3.

Lowden JA, O'Brien JS (1979) Sialidosis: a review of human neuraminidase deficiency. *Am J Hum Genet* **31**:1–18.

Palmeri S, Villanova M, Malandrini A, *et al.* (2000) Type I sialidosis: a clinical, biochemical and neuroradiological study. *Eur Neurol* **43**:88–94.

Panzica F, Canafoglia L, Franceschetti S, *et al.* (2003) Movement-activated myoclonus in genetically defined progressive myoclonic epilepsies: EEG–EMG relationship estimated using autoregressive models. *Clin Neurophysiol* **114**:1041–52.

Park JK, Orvisky E, Tayebi N, *et al.* (2003) Myoclonic epilepsy in Gaucher disease:

genotype–phenotype insights from a rare patient subgroup. *Pediat Res* **53**:387–95.

Patterson MC, Horowitz M, Abel RB, *et al.* (1993) Isolated horizontal supranuclear gaze palsy as a marker of severe systemic involvement in Gaucher's disease. *Neurology* **43**:1993–7.

Perretti A, Parenti G, Balbi P, *et al.* (2005) Study of multimodal evoked potentials in patients with type 1 Gaucher's disease. *J Child Neurol* **20**:124–8.

Rapin I, Goldfisher S, Katzman R, Engel J Jr., O'Brien JS (1978) The cherry-red spot myoclonus syndrome. *Ann Neurol* **3**:234–42.

Rothschild CB, Akots G, Hayworth R, *et al.* (1993) A genetic map of chromosome 20q12–q13.2. *Am J Hum Genet* **52**:110–23.

Sidransky E, Bottler A, Stubblefield B, Ginns E (1994) DNA mutational analysis of type 1 and type 3 Gaucher patients: how well do mutations predict phenotype? *Hum Mutat* **3**:25–8.

Vellodi A, Bembi B, de Villemeur TB, *et al.* (2001) Neuronopathic Gaucher Disease Task Force of the European Working Group on Gaucher Disease: Management of neuronopathic Gaucher disease–a European consensus. *J Inherit Metab Dis* **24**:319–27.

Verghese J, Goldberg RF, Desnick RJ, *et al.* (2000) Myoclonus from selective dentate nucleus degeneration in type 3 Gaucher disease. *Arch Neurol* **57**:389–95.

Wang D, Bonten EJ, Yogalingam G, Mann L, d'Azzo A (2005) Short-term, high dose enzyme replacement therapy in sialidosis mice. *Mol Genet Metab* **85**:181–9.

Wong K, Sidransky E, Verma A, *et al.* (2004) Neuropathology provides clues to the pathophysiology of Gaucher disease. *Mol Genet Metab* **82**:192–207.

Yogalingam G, Bonten EJ, van de Vlekkert D, *et al.* (2008) Neuraminidase 1 is a negative regulator of lysosomal exocytosis. *Dev Cell* **15**:74–86.

Zimran A, Elstein D (2007) No justification for very high-dose enzyme therapy for patients with type III Gaucher disease. *J Inherit Metab Dis* **30**:843–4.

Action myoclonus–renal failure syndrome

Eva Andermann

The progressive myoclonus epilepsies (PMEs) are a group of genetically determined disorders characterized by myoclonus and generalized tonic–clonic seizures, and are usually associated with neurodegeneration leading to dementia and other neurological involvement, particularly ataxia and dysarthria. Inheritance is usually autosomal recessive, but autosomal dominant and maternally inherited PMEs also occur, the former including the adolescent or adult forms of neuronal ceroid lipofuscinosis (Kufs disease) and dentatorubral-pallidoluysian atrophy (DRPLA). The various forms of PME have previously been reviewed (Berkovic and Andermann 1986; Berkovic et al. 1986, 1991, 1993; Marseille Consensus Conference 1990; Shahwan et al. 2005; Ramachandran et al. 2009).

Action myoclonus–renal failure syndrome (AMRF) is a form of progressive myoclonus epilepsy first described in four French–Canadian patients belonging to three apparently unrelated sibships living in different regions of Quebec (Andermann et al. 1986).

Clinical features

The main clinical features and their ages of onset in the original patients were quite stereotyped: tremor of the fingers and hands and proteinuria with onset at 17–18 years, followed by onset of action myoclonus at 19–23 years, renal failure at 20–22 years, and onset of ataxia and dysarthria as well as infrequent generalized tonic–clonic seizures at 21–23 years. A patient with a very similar phenotype had been described by Horoupian and Ross in Winnipeg in 1977. Her mother was of French origin, but it was unclear whether she also originated from Quebec, and her father was born in the south of England.

No further communications on AMRF appeared in the literature until 2004, when 15 patients in nine sibships were described by the same group (Badhwar et al. 2004), including an update on the four original patients. In addition to four French–Canadian sibships, the families originated from English Canada, USA, Australia, Cuba, and Germany. The disease now had a much wider geographic and ethnic distribution, and was not confined to French–Canadians.

In this larger series, there was a more variable presentation of the symptoms with onset of tremor between 17 and 26 years (mean 19.8 years); progressively disabling action myoclonus between 14 and 29 years (mean 21.7 years); infrequent generalized seizures in 11 out of 15 patients between 20 and 28 years (mean 22.7 years). Proteinuria was detected between 9 and 30 years (mean 20.1 years) in all patients and progressed to renal failure requiring dialysis and/or renal transplantation in 12 of 15 patients within 0–8 years (mean 3.8 years) after detection of proteinuria.

All patients with AMRF develop action myoclonus and seizures. Seizures can be precipitated by movement or startle, as well as the usual factors, such as fatigue, stress, and sleep deprivation. Patients have diurnal variation, and can have "good" or "bad" days. The patients do not show significant cognitive deterioration. Indeed, in most patients, intelligence was remarkably normal and preserved, even in the later stages of the disease. Predominantly axonal peripheral neuropathy was found in at least two patients, although this was not symptomatic.

Most patients died between 25 and 34 years of age, mainly of complications related to dialysis or rejection of the renal transplant, although some died of respiratory effects of the severe myoclonus. Several patients did not receive a compatible renal transplant in time, and died of renal failure.

The first clinical symptoms in this disease can be either renal or neurological. The progression of renal and neurological disorders appears to be separate, suggesting pleiotropic effects of a single molecular lesion, differentially affecting the two organ systems (Andermann et al. 1986; Badhwar et al. 2004). The disease is probably underdiagnosed, since patients presenting with renal symptoms are probably thought to have neurological complications of uemia.

Segregation analysis in these families, using several different models of ascertainment and the a priori method, was compatible with autosomal recessive inheritance (Badhwar et al. 2004).

The Causes of Epilepsy, eds. S. D. Shorvon, F. Andermann, and R. Guerrini. Published by Cambridge University Press. © Cambridge University Press 2011.

Neurophysiology

The main EEG findings are generalized epileptiform abnormalities, often photosensitive, as well as diffuse slow-wave disturbance of background activity, beginning in the early stages of the disease. At times, single spike and slow-wave discharges were recorded, corresponding to the myoclonic jerks (Badhwar *et al.* 2004).

Neuroimaging

Most of the patients showed diffuse cerebral and cerebellar atrophy, although some patients had normal computed tomography (CT) and magnetic resonance imaging (MRI) findings.

Neuropathology

Autopsy of one of the original patients, who died at 25 years due to complications related to rejection of his renal transplant, showed marked atrophy of the patient's kidneys, which each weighed 30 g. The brain was normal in size without convolutional atrophy. However, there was mild but definite dilatation of the lateral ventricles (Andermann *et al.* 1986).

Microscopic examination showed no neuronal loss or significant gliosis. The only abnormality was the presence of pigment granules, which appeared to be in astrocytes and in certain cells in the meninges.

Numerous small pigment granules were seen in the hippocampus in glial cells and in the molecular layer of the dentate gyrus, and were prominent in the layer of the Bergmann glia in the cerebellum (Andermann *et al.* 1986). These findings strongly resembled those of the patient described by Horoupian and Ross (1977), and were confirmed by postmortem examination of an Australian patient (Badhwar *et al.* 2004).

The renal pathology based on renal biopsy specimens showed focal glomerulosclerosis in all patients examined, with features of collapsing glomerulopathy in some (Andermann *et al.* 1986; Badhwar *et al.* 2004).

Molecular findings

In 2008, the causative gene for AMRF was found to be *SCARB2/LIMP-2*, and at least nine additional sibships have been reported in Australia, Quebec, Portugal, and Italy (Balreira *et al.* 2008; Berkovic *et al.* 2008; Dardis *et al.* 2009; Dibbens *et al.* 2009). One of the Australian families was of Turkish–Cypriot origin.

There are presently 12 known mutations of *SCARB2*, including missense, nonsense, and splice-site mutations (Dibbens *et al.* 2009). Ten of these were homozygous and two were compound heterozygotes.

In a study of 41 "Unverricht–Lundborg disease-like" patients with PME beginning at age 5 years or older, in whom the principal clinical manifestations were action myoclonus,

tonic–clonic seizure, and ataxia, without evidence of significant intellectual decline or other neurological features, and in whom mutation in *cystatin B* had not been found, five were found to have mutations in *SCARB2* (Dibbens *et al.* 2009). None of these patients had renal failure, although one was found to have proteinuria.

Pathophysiology

SCARB2/LIMP-2 is a lysosomal membrane protein which has specific functions in maintaining endosomal transport and lysosomal biogenesis (Eskelinen *et al.* 2003). More specifically, LIMP-2 is a receptor for lysosomal mannose-6-phosphate independent targeting of β-glucocerebrosidase (β-GC), the enzyme that is deficient is Gaucher disease.

Patients with AMRF have been reported to have normal or low normal β-GC in leukocytes, but very low levels in cultured fibroblasts, and elevated levels in serum (Balreira *et al.* 2008; Dardis *et al.* 2009), suggesting missorting of β-GC (Reczek *et al.* 2007). Interestingly, one of two siblings with type 3 neuronopathic Gaucher disease who had a more severe phenotype than his sibling was also found to be heterozygous for a mutation in *SCARB2/LIMP-2* (De Paolo *et al.* 2009), suggesting that this additional mutation may result in a more severe phenotype.

Blanz *et al.* (2010) recently performed functional studies on the first six *SCARB2* mutations described (Balreira *et al.* 2008; Berkovic *et al.* 2008) and found that all six mutations led to a retention of LIMP-2 in the endoplasmic reticulum, but affected the binding to β-GC differentially. Of three nonsense mutations, only the Q288X mutation was still able to bind to β-GC as efficiently as wild-type LIMP-2, whereas the other two nonsense mutations lost their β-GC-binding capacity almost completely (Blanz *et al.* 2010).

The animal model of LIMP-2/LGP85 deficiency in mice has a somewhat different phenotype to AMRF, with ureteric pelvic junction obstruction, deafness and peripheral neuropathy.

Diagnostic testing

A high level of suspicion should be present if a patient has onset of PME in the late teens or early twenties, preceded by tremor and associated with proteinuria and renal failure. Low levels of β-GC in fibroblasts without other evidence of Gaucher disease is also suggestive. Even without evidence of renal failure, the diagnosis should still be suspected.

A molecular diagnosis with mutation detection in the *SCARB2/LIMP-2* gene has been possible since 2008, although this test is not yet commercially available. Identification of the causative mutation is important for genetic counseling, including carrier detection, presymptomatic and prenatal diagnosis, and prevention. In regions where there is high consanguinity and/or a founder effect, resulting in a high prevalence of the disease, such as the province of Quebec, Canada, population screening for heterozygote status may be contemplated.

Principles of management

The main neurological feature of the disease is severe action myoclonus, which can interfere with the patient's daily activities, such as walking, eating, and writing. The patients are often confined to a wheelchair because of the severe myoclonus. The most common treatment is valproic acid and clonazepam. Piracetam is also a very effective antimyoclonic agent. More recently, levetiracetam has been utilized for these patients, and other derivatives are now in clinical trials.

It is important to avoid antiepileptic medications that can aggravate the myoclonus such as phenytoin, carbamazepine, and possibly lamictal.

With respect to the renal pathology, dialysis and/or renal transplantation become necessary when the patient develops renal failure. Despite the correction of renal function, the neurological symptoms continue to progress, and require continuous treatment.

It is hoped that, with the rapid progress in studying the functional aspects of the *SCARB2/LIMP-2* gene, innovative treatments will be discovered to counteract the effects of specific pathological mutations.

References

Andermann E, Andermann F, Carpenter S, *et al.* (1986) Action myoclonus-renal failure syndrome: a previously unrecognized neurological disorder unmasked by advances in nephrology. In Fahn S, Marsden D, van Woert M (eds.) *Myoclonus*. New York: Raven Press, pp. 87–103. (*Adv Neurol* **43**:87–103).

Badhwar A, Berkovic SF, Dowling JP, *et al.* (2004) Action myoclonus–renal failure syndrome: characterization of a unique cerebro-renal disorder. *Brain* **127**:2173–82.

Balreira A, Gaspar P, Caiola D, *et al.* (2008) A nonsense mutation in the *LIMP-2* gene associated with progressive myoclonic epilepsy and nephrotic syndrome. *Hum Mol Genet* **17**:2238–43.

Berkovic SF, Andermann F (1986) The progressive myoclonus epilepsies. In Pedley TA, Meldrum BS (eds.) *Recent Advances in Epilepsy*, vol. **3**, Edinburgh, UK: Churchill Livingstone, pp. 157–87.

Berkovic SF, Andermann F, Carpenter S, Wolfe LS (1986) Progressive myoclonus epilepsies: specific causes and diagnosis. *N Engl J Med* **315**:296–305.

Berkovic SF, Cochius J, Andermann E, Andermann F (1993) Progressive myoclonus epilepsies: clinical and genetic aspects. *Epilepsia* **34**(Suppl 3):S19–30.

Berkovic SF, Dibbens LM, Oshlack A, *et al.* (2008) Array-based gene discovery with three unrelated subjects shows SCARB2/LIMP-2 deficiency causes myoclonus epilepsy and glomerulosclerosis. *Am J Hum Genet* **82**:673–84.

Berkovic SF, So NK, Andermann F (1991) Progressive myoclonus epilepsies: clinical and neurophysiological diagnosis. *Clin Neurophysiol* **8**:261–74.

Blanz J, Groth J, Zachos C, *et al.* (2010) Disease-causing mutations within the lysosomal integral membrane protein type 2 (LIMP-2) reveal the nature of binding to its ligand β-glucocerebrosidase. *Hum Mol Genet* **19**:563–72.

Dardis A, Filocamo M, Grossi S, *et al.* (2009) Biochemical and molecular findings in a patient with myoclonic epilepsy due to a mistarget of the β-glucosidase enzyme. *Mol Genet Metab* **97**:309–11.

DePaolo J, Goker-Aplan O, Tayebi N, *et al.* (2009) A mutation in lysosomal integral membrane protein type 2 (LIMP-2) associated with myoclonic epilepsy in a patient with type 3 Gaucher disease. Abstract #2085, American Society of Human Genetics Annual Meeting, Honolulu, Hawaii, USA.

Dibbens LM, Michelucci R, Gambardella A, *et al.* (2009) *SCARB2* mutations in progressive myoclonus epilepsy (PME) without renal failure. *Ann Neurol* **66**:532–6.

Eskelinen E-L, Tanaka Y, Saftig P (2003) At the acidic edge: emerging functions for lysosomal membrane proteins. *Cell Biol* **13**:137–45.

Gamp A-C, Tanaka Y, Lullmann-Rauch R, *et al.* (2003) LIMP-2/LGP85 deficiency causes ureteric pelvic junction obstruction, deafness and peripheral neuropathy in mice. *Hum Mol Genet* **12**:631–46.

Horoupian DS, Ross RT (1977) Pigment variant neuronal ceroid-lipofusinosis. *Can J Neurol Sci* **4**:67–75.

Marseille Consensus Group (1990) Classification of progressive myoclonus epilepsies and related disorders. *Ann Neurol* **28**:113–16.

Ramachandran N, Girard J-M, Turnbull J, Minassian BA (2009) The autosomal recessively inherited progressive myoclonus epilepsies and their genes. *Epilepsia* **50**(Suppl 5):29–36.

Reczek D, Schwake M, Schröder J, *et al.* (2007) LIMP-2 is a receptor for lysosomal mannose-6-phosphate-independent target of β-glucocerebrosidase. *Cell* **131**: 770–83.

Schroen B, Leenders JJ, van Erk A, *et al.* (2007) Lysosomal integral membrane protein 2 is a novel component of the cardiac intercalated disc and vital for load-induced cardiac myocyte hypertrophy. *Exp Med* **204**: 1227–35.

Shahwan A, Farrell M, Delanty N (2005) Progressive myoclonic epilepsies: a review of genetic and therapeutic aspects. *Lancet Neurol* **4**:239–48.

Chapter 23

Progressive myoclonus epilepsies: other rare causes

Frederick Andermann and Eva Andermann

The progressive myoclonus epilepsies (PMEs) are a rare group of disorders with varied causes manifested by myoclonus, often activated by movement or action, but also occurring at rest. In the majority of patients, there are generalized seizures, often clonic tonic clonic in appearance, followed at times by a period of suppression of the myoclonus only to gradually build up again (Berkovic and Andermann 1986; Berkovic *et al.* 1986a, 1993; Shahwan *et al.* 2005).

There is in some of the progressive myoclonus epilepsies progressive dementia, but in others this is not a feature. There may also be ataxia which is slowly progressive. The limiting factor however is usually the myoclonus which leads to the patients becoming wheelchair-bound. Most of the PMEs start in late childhood or adolescence, although some occur de novo later in life.

Until a generation ago, PME was considered to be the final diagnosis that could be reached. Over the years, progress in neuropathology and particularly in neurogenetics has enabled a specific diagnosis to be made in the majority of patients. In our series of almost 100 patients with PME, a specific diagnosis was possible in all but three patients. New causes of PME have been identified over time. The benefit of a specific diagnosis lies in our ability to provide a clearer explanation to the patient and the family, and in improved genetic counseling. In some instances, prenatal diagnosis is now possible.

The early diagnosis of PME may be difficult and a form of idiopathic generalized epilepsy such as juvenile myoclonic epilepsy may be suspected, with eventual clarification of the diagnosis because of progressive deterioration not attributable to the use of inappropriate medication. The electroencephalogram (EEG) usually shows generalized, sometimes predominantly occipital discharges, associated with the clinical myoclonus. However, with some myoclonic jerks, there is no visible EEG discharge suggesting that some of these discharges originate in subcortical or brainstem structures and fire downstream without cortical involvement. No specific diagnosis can be made reliably by electroencephalography (Berkovic *et al.* 1991).

The best known forms of PME are: Lafora disease (Chapter 18), including the late-onset form; Unverricht–Lundborg disease (Chapter 16); the neuronal ceroid lipofuscinoses (Chapter 20), particularly the ones with later onset; mitochondrial disease (Chapter 19), in particular mitochondrial encephalomyopathy with ragged red fibers (MERRF); and the sialidoses (Chapter 21). There still remain a number of rarer forms of PME and most are difficult or impossible to distinguish from the forms just mentioned on clinical grounds alone.

Juvenile neuroaxonal dystrophy

The onset is with myoclonic jerks between the ages of 9 and 12 years. There is progressive deterioration and absences or generalized seizures supervene. The disorder progresses relentlessly (Dorfman *et al.* 1978). There is a decline in cognitive ability, with dysarthria, ataxia, chorea, and lower motor neuron involvement. The pathological findings consist of neuroaxonal spheroids, cerebellar atrophy, and degeneration of the long fiber tracts of the brain and spinal cord. The disorder should be distinguished from pantothenate-kinase-associated degeneration by the absence of pigmentary changes. In our series of almost 100 patients with PME only one had the juvenile form of this disorder. Juvenile neuroaxonal dystrophy does not seem to have preponderance for any racial group. The patient described by Thibault (1972) had a positive family history which was difficult to interpret, raising the possibility of recurrence in other generations, although this was not conclusively proven.

Pantothenate-kinase-associated neurodegeneration or Hallervorden–Spatz disease

The presence of myoclonic jerking in the adult form of the disease has been suggested, but the literature is not entirely conclusive (Rozdilsky *et al.* 1968). Additional symptoms are dementia, generalized seizures, dysarthria, rigidity, spasticity,

The Causes of Epilepsy, eds. S. D. Shorvon, F. Andermann, and R. Guerrini. Published by Cambridge University Press. © Cambridge University Press 2011.

and athetoid movements. The biochemical basis of the disorder has recently been clarified. Pathologically the changes are those of neuroaxonal dystrophy, but in addition there is extensive pigmentation and iron deposits are present in the globus pallidus and the substantia nigra.

Neuroserpin inclusion body disease

This is a recently identified form of PME with onset late in the second decade, including generalized seizures and dementia (Berkovic et al. 1986b). Collins bodies contain neuroserpin, a neuron-specific protease inhibitor as a predominant component (Davis et al. 2002). There is also a dominant form of the disease with dementia as a prominent symptom and onset later in adult life (Jansen et al. 2008). Patients with the adult form are not described to have myoclonus. Peripheral biopsies are not helpful in the diagnosis, which can only be made by brain biopsy. In our series, a single patient with this disorder was identified. There were additional white-matter changes that were difficult to interpret and which originally were considered to indicate the presence of a mitochondrial disorder. The diagnosis was made at post mortem.

Leukoencephalopathy with vanishing white matter

This disorder is caused by mutations in the genes encoding for one of the five subunits that constitute the eukaryotic initiation factor 2B (eIF2B). It is characterized by a highly suggestive magnetic resonance imaging (MRI) pattern indicating progressive vanishing of the cerebral white matter. The corpus callosum is extremely thin. Seizures are well known to occur in this disorder, but usually do not represent a prominent feature. One of our patients, a 40-year-old man, was diagnosed with PME in his twenties. There was extensive white-matter involvement with very striking thinning of the corpus callosum. In his late thirties, the myoclonus abated (Jansen et al. 2008). Paraparesis and dementia were the most striking features. Mutation analysis of the eIF2B5 gene revealed a homozygous c338G>A (p.Arg 113His) mutation. The frequency or incidence of PME in this condition is unknown. The diagnosis should be suggested by the imaging studies.

Biotin-responsive infantile encephalopathy

Progressive lethargy, scarce scalp hair, autistic-like behavior, myoclonus and drug-resistant generalized seizures have been reported. There is an increased urinary excretion of two keto-glutaric acids and a small peak of 3-hydroxyvaleric acid. Serum biotinidase activity is reduced to a lesser extent in the parents. There are multifocal EEG abnormalities with generalized tonic–clonic attacks, myoclonus, and excessive startle. Dramatic improvement was obtained in a child by treatment with biotin 5 mg twice daily. The frequency of this disorder remains uncertain.

Late-onset GM2 gangliosidosis

This autosomal recessive disorder due to partial hexosaminidase α deficiency is at times associated with myoclonus in the later stages of the illness (Brett et al. 1973). This however is usually overshadowed by other neurological symptoms, primarily quadriparesis and dementia.

Celiac disease

Malabsorption was well documented in two patients with progressive cerebellar dysarthria, ataxia of the arms and legs, spontaneous and action cortical reflex myoclonus, and occasional major seizures. They had mild intellectual impairment with brisk tendon reflexes and extensor plantar responses. They were described by Lu et al. from the University Department of Neurology and Psychiatry at King's College Hospital in London (Lu et al. 1986). The neurological features did not respond to dietary treatment of the malabsorption syndrome. The frequency of the disorder is uncertain, but it is not a clinical feature of the many patients with celiac disease and bioccipital calcifications reported from Italy and Argentina, where the disorder predominates in people of Italian origin.

Early-onset Alzheimer disease, dementia, and myoclonus

This form of PME is particularly striking in many family members affected by autosomal dominant Alzheimer disease linked to chromosome 14. The presenting features are cognitive decline with prominent seizures and myoclonus. In the differential diagnosis, Creutzfeldt-Jakob disease must be considered (Edwards-Lee et al. 2005).

Occasional sporadic patients with progressive myoclonus epilepsy beginning around the age of 30 have been shown to have the pathological changes of Alzheimer disease (Berkovic et al. 1995).

Myoclonus is frequently described as an early feature of patients with amyloid precursor (16) protein gene mutation pedigrees who have limb dyspraxia, brisk reflexes, visual disorientation, and slow gait (see Edwards-Lee et al. 2005) for review).

Familial cortical myoclonic tremor with epilepsy

The terms used to describe affected patients include autosomal dominant cortical myoclonus and epilepsy, benign adult familial myoclonic epilepsy, cortical tremor, familial adult myoclonic epilepsy, familial cortical myoclonic tremor, familial cortical tremor with epilepsy, familial essential myoclonus and epilepsy, familial benign myoclonus epilepsy of adult onset, and hereditary familial tremor and epilepsy (van Rootselaar et al. 2005). There is an obvious overlap between some of these families and the ones reported in this volume as benign adult familial myoclonic epilepsy and probably also with hereditary essential myoclonus.

In a large group of families from Japan and Europe, cortical myoclonic tremor and epilepsy has been reported under various names. Van Rootselaar *et al.* (2005) reviewed the available literature and concluded that adult onset distal action tremor and low amplitude myoclonus, epileptic seizures, autosomal dominant inheritance, a benign course, effectiveness of antiepileptic drugs and possibly cognitive decline are characteristic. Patients have giant somatosensory evoked responses and long latency reflexes, usually a family history suggestive of autosomal dominant inheritance, and no additional symptoms such as ataxia, parkinsonism, or dementia. Clear-cut larger-amplitude myoclonus was present in a minority of families. Linkage to chromosome 2p11.1–p12.2 was identified in a family by Guerrini *et al.* (2001), but there seems to be genetic heterogeneity in this condition. Linkage to chromosome 8q was found in some Japanese families (Mikami *et al.* 1999).

An additional condition in which myoclonus may be present is *dementia with Lewy bodies*, which in most cases consists of sporadic small and infrequent myoclonic jerks, focal and predominating in the distal upper limbs. It is frequently induced by action and posture of the limbs (Caviness 2003).

Creutzfeldt–Jakob disease is characterized by myoclonus and rapidly evolving dementia. The association with focal neurological signs should suggest the diagnosis. Myoclonus is generalized, non-rhythmic or rhythmic, occurring in continuous fashion with a periodicity of 0.6–1.2 Hz. Focal, segmental, or multifocal myoclonus can occur in the course of the disease (Caviness 2003).

Differential diagnosis

At the Marseille Consensus Meeting in 1989 (Aicardi *et al.* 1990) it was agreed that action myoclonus in the setting of slowly progressive ataxia with no recognized etiology would be called progressive myoclonic ataxia, and progressive myoclonus epilepsy, if seizures are the main symptom. Thus the clinical presentation may vary enormously even within the same family. Among the causes of progressive myoclonic ataxia not discussed above are spinocerebellar degenerations such as Friedreich ataxia or ataxia telangiectasia and prion diseases (Caviness 2003). It is generally accepted that there are a number of patients who develop progressive myoclonic ataxia in adult life and remain undiagnosed even after detailed evaluation.

New causes of PME are still being identified. The most recent *Prickle1*, also known as RILP for REST/NRSF, an interacting LIM domain protein, blocks the PRICKLE1 and REST interaction in vitro and disrupts the normal function of *Prickle1* in an in vivo zebrafish overexpression system. *Prickle1* is expressed in brain regions implicated in epilepsy and ataxia in mice and humans and, to our knowledge, is the first molecule in the non-canonical WNT signaling pathway to be directly implicated in human epilepsy (Bassuk *et al.* 2008).

Symptomatic causes of myoclonus include post-anoxic myoclonus, occasionally heat stroke, electric shock, decompression injury, and post-traumatic brain injury. Myoclonus may be focal, multifocal, segmental, or generalized and it may be associated with seizures and/or neurological deficits (Borg 2006).

Toxic causes of myoclonus include the sialysis syndrome characterized by myoclonus, asterixis, speech disorder, seizures, personality changes, and progressive dementia. Aluminum has been inculpated in degenerative acute or chronic encephalopathies due to oral phosphate-binding agents that contain aluminum. Methylbromide intoxication can induce multifocal action myoclonus as can bismuth, toxic cooking oil, chronic toluene abuse, gasoline sniffing, and intake of l-tryptophan-containing products (see Borg 2006 for review).

The use of serotonin reuptake inhibitors commonly used as antidepressants may lead to severe myoclonus described with the use of citalopram and risperidone (Yee and Wijdicks 2010). Cephalosporin toxicity (Grill and Maganti 2008), levetiracetam accumulation in renal failure (Vulliemoz *et al.* 2009), amlodipine (Wallace *et al.* 2009), and verapamil, diltiazem, and nifedipine can induce acute myoclonic jerking without convulsive seizures. Metformin in the presence of endstage renal disease (Jung *et al.* 2009) and pregabalin (Yoo *et al.* 2009) may induce myoclonus in patients receiving hemodialysis, but again, no seizures were reported.

Finally, myoclonus may be found in patients with multiple system atrophy, corticobasal degeneration, progressive supranuclear palsy, frontotemporal dementia, Huntington disease, particularly with early onset, and in some forms of Parkinson disease (Bassuk *et al.* 2008). Many of these disorders are noted for the sake of completeness, and the myoclonus is often not well described. These disorders are beyond the scope of this volume and are not associated with epileptic seizures.

References

Aicardi J, Andermann E, Andermann F, *et al.* (1990) Marseille Consensus Group Consensus Statement: classification of progressive myoclonus epilepsies and related disorders. *Ann Neurol* **28**:113–16.

Bassuk AG, Wallace RH, Buhr A, *et al.* (2008) A homozygous mutation in human *PRICKLE1* causes an autosomal-recessive progressive myoclonus epilepsy–ataxia syndrome. *Am J Hum Genet* **83**:572–81.

Berkovic SF, Andermann F (1986) The progressive myoclonus epilepsies. In: Pedley T A, Meldrum BS (eds.) *Recent Advances in Epilepsy.*

Edinburgh, UK: Churchill Livingstone, pp. 157–87.

Berkovic S, Andermann F, Carpenter S, *et al.* (1986a) Progressive myoclonus epilepsies: specific causes and diagnosis. *N Engl J Med* **315**:296–305.

Berkovic S F, Carpenter S, Andermann F, (1986b) Atypical inclusion body progressive myoclonus epilepsy: a fifth case? (Letter.) *Neurology* **36**:1275–6.

Berkovic S, Cochius J, Andermann E, *et al.* (1993) Progressive myoclonus epilepsies: clinical and genetic aspects. *Epilepsia* **34**:S19–30.

Berkovic SF, So NK, Andermann F, *et al.* (1991) Progressive myoclonus epilepsies: clinical and neurophysiological diagnosis. *J Clin Neurophysiol* **8**:261–74.

Berkovic SF, Melanson M, Andermann F (1995). Dementia and myoclonus: differential diagnosis of early onset Alzheimer's disease. *Ann Neurol.* **37**:412.

Borg M (2006) Symptomatic myoclonus. *Neurophysiol Clinique*, **36**:309–18. (In French).

Brett EM, Ellis RB, Haas L, *et al.* (1973). Late onset G$_{m2}$–gangliosidosis: clinical, pathological and biochemical studies on 8 patients. *Arch Dis Childh* **48**:775–85.

Caviness JN (2003) Myoclonus and neurodegenerative disease: what's in a name? *Parkinsonism Related Dis*, **9**:185–192.

Colamaria V, Burlina AB, Gaburro D, *et al.* (1989) Biotin-responsive infantile encephalopathy: EEG-polygraphic study of a case. *Epilepsia* **30**:573–8.

Davis RL, Holohan PD, Shrimpton AE, *et al.* (1999) Familial encephalopathy with neuroserpin inclusion bodies. *Am J Pathol* **155**:1901–13.

Davis RL, Shrimpton AE, Carrell RW, *et al.* (2002) Association between conformational mutations in neuroserpin and onset and severity of dementia. *Lancet* **359**:2242–7.

Dorfman LJ, Pedley TA, Tharp BR, Scheithauer BW (1978) Juvenile neuroaxonal dystrophy: clinical, electrophysiological, and neuropathological features. *Ann Neurol*, **3**:419–28.

Edwards-Lee T, Ringman JM, Chung J, (2005) An African American family with early-onset Alzheimer disease and an APP (T714I) mutation. *Neurology* **64**:377–9.

Grill MF, Maganti R(2008) Cephalosporin-induced neurotoxicity: clinical manifestations, potential pathogenic mechanisms, and the role of electroencephalographic monitoring. *Ann Pharmacol* **42**:1843–50.

Guerrini R, Bonanni P, Patrignani A, *et al.* (2001) Autosomal dominant cortical myoclonus and epilepsy (ADCME) with complex partial and generalized seizures: a newly recognized epilepsy syndrome with linkage to chromosome 2p11.1–q12.2. *Brain* **124**:2459–75.

Jansen AC, Andermann E, Niel F, *et al.* (2008) Leucoencephalopathy with vanishing white matter may cause progressive myoclonus epilepsy. *Epilepsia* **49**:910–13.

Jung EY, Cho HS, Seo JW, *et al.* (2009) Metformin-induced encephalopathy without lactic acidosis in a patient with contraindication for metformin. *Hemodialysis Int.* **13**:172–5.

Lu CS, Thompson PD, Quin NP, Parkes JD, Marsden CD (1986) Ramsay Hunt syndrome and coeliac disease: a new association? *Movement Disord*, **1**:209–19.

Mikami M, Yasuda T, Terao A, *et al.* (1999) Localization of a gene for benign adult familial myoclonic epilepsy to chromosome 8q23.3q24.1. *Am J Hum Genet* **65**:745–51.

Rozdilsky B, Cumings JN, Huston AF (1968) Hallervorden–Spatz disease: late infantile and adult types, report of two cases. *Acta Neuropathol* **10**:1–16.

Shahwan A, Farrell M, Delanty N (2005) Progressive myoclonic epilepsies: a review of genetic and therapeutic aspects. *Lancet Neurol*, **4**:239–48.

Thibault J (1972) Neuroaxonal dystrophy: a case of non-pigmented type and protracted course. *Acta Neuropath (Berlin)* **21**:232–8.

van Rootselaar AF, van Shaik IN, van den Maagdenberg AM JM, *et al.* (2005) Familial cortical myoclonic tremor with epilepsy: a single syndromic classification for a group of pedigrees bearing common features. *Movement Disord* **20**:665–73.

Vulliemoz S, Iwanowski P, Landis T, Jallon P (2009) Levetiracetam accumulation in renal failure causing myclonic encephalopathy with triphasic waves. *Seizure* **18**:376–8.

Wallace EL, Lingle K, Pierce D, Satko S, (2009) Amlodipine-induced myoclonus. *Am J Med* **10**:36.

Yee AH, Wijdicks EFM (2010) A perfect storm in the Emergency Department. *Neurocrit Care* **12**:258–60.

Yoo L, Matalon D, Hoffman RS, Goldfarb DS (2009) Treatment of Pregabalin toxicity by hemodialysis in a patient with kidney failure. *Am J Kidney Dis* **54**:1127–30.

Chapter

24

Tuberous sclerosis complex

Catherine J. Chu-Shore and Elizabeth A. Thiele

The causal disease

Tuberous sclerosis complex (TSC) is an autosomal dominant, multiorgan disease which is estimated to occur in at least 1 in 6000 live births, although the true prevalence is thought to be higher due to undiagnosed mild variants of the disease (Webb and Osborne 1995; Crino et al. 2006). It is clinically characterized by multisystem involvement and the presence of dysgenic and hamartomatous lesions in multiple organs, although expression is widely variable between individuals.

The brain is frequently affected in TSC. Epilepsy is the most common symptom and often the cause of highest morbidity. Approximately half of patients with TSC are cognitively impaired and up to 40% of patients have autism or autism spectrum disorder with or without mental retardation (Webb et al. 1991; Winterkorn et al. 2007). Other frequent neurological and psychiatric manifestations include symptoms of mood disorder, anxiety, attention-deficit hyperactivity disorder, and aggressive or self-injurious behaviors (Muzykewicz et al. 2007; Staley BA 2008).

Genetics and molecular physiology

Approximately 85% of patients with TSC are found to have a mutation in one of two genes, TSC1 or TSC2. The TSC1 gene encodes hamartin, is located on chromosome 9p34 and, consists of a 3.4-kb coding region with 21 exons. The TSC2 gene encodes tuberin, is located on chromosome 16p13, and consists of a 5.4-kb coding region with 41 exons. Mutations in TSC2 accounted for approximately two-thirds of identified mutations. Approximately one-third of cases are familial and two-thirds are the result of either spontaneous mutations or rare germline mosaicism. The only genotype–phenotype relationship that has been established in TSC is that more severe multiorgan disease is seen in patients with the TSC2 gene mutations (Dabora et al. 2001; Sancak et al. 2005). Patients with TSC2 mutations tend to exhibit a higher frequency of seizures and moderate and severe mental retardation, and to have more severe kidney, brain, skin,

and lung involvement than patients with TSC1 mutations, although there is considerable overlap between genotypes. There is wide variability in phenotype between family members and monozygotic twins suggesting the role for other genetic and environmental modifiers in this disease (Lyczkowski et al. 2007).

Hamartin and tuberin, the protein products of the TSC1 and TSC2 genes, form a heterodimer (TSC1–TSC2 complex) which inhibits the mammalian target of rapamycin (mTOR) signaling cascade. The mTOR pathway is a well-characterized signal transduction pathway which is intimately involved in regulating cellular division and growth in response to growth factors and nutrients (Kwiatkowski and Manning 2005). Many cancer-promoting mutations activate this pathway via dysregulation of the TSC1–TSC2 complex. Loss of p53 tumor suppressors or mutations that lead to neurofibromatosis 1 result in altered mTOR regulation via inhibition of the TSC1–TSC2 complex. In TSC, the abnormal TSC1–TSC2 complex does not appropriately inhibit mTOR complex 1 (mTORC1) kinase activity, leading to increased activity of downstream effectors, including translation regulator eukaryotic translation initiation factor 4E (4EBP1), and ribosomal S6 kinase 1 (S6K1) and subsequent upregulation of many anabolic processes promoting cell growth and protein synthesis (Sabatini 2006). Increased mTORC1 and subsequent S6K1 activity simultaneously suppresses phosphatidylinositol-3-kinase (PI3K)–Akt signaling, thereby providing a feedback loop that may contribute to the benign nature of TSC-related tumors (Manning et al. 2005).

Pathology

In TSC, inadequate suppression of the mTORC1 pathway results in dysgenic lesions and tumor growth in multiple organ systems (Richardson 1991). Cortical tubers are characterized by areas of chaotic disruption of cortical lamination on histological evaluation. Within the disorganized cortex and underlying subcortical white matter, abnormal cell types including dysmorphic neurons, large balloon-type

The Causes of Epilepsy, eds. S. D. Shorvon, F. Andermann, and R. Guerrini. Published by Cambridge University Press. © Cambridge University Press 2011.

cells, and prominent reactive astrocytes are present. The neuropil is composed of increased glial fibers and decreased myelinated fibers. The appearance of the cortex between the cortical defects and tubers is generally normal, but subtle changes in the organizational pattern of the neurons and gliosis can often be demonstrated even in parts of the brain that are grossly normal. Subependymal nodules are found as smooth excrescences of varying sizes projecting into the third and lateral ventricles and histologically are composed of large cells with irregular nuclei and often contain multiple calcifications. The hamartomas found in other organ systems are typically named after the cell types of which they are composed. Facial angiofibromas are fibrous vascular tumors. Shagreen patches are composed of increased collagenous bundles. Cardiac rhabdomyomas are composed of large swollen myocytes called "spider cells" with radial cytoplasmic extensions. Renal angiomyolipomas are hamartomas composed of abnormal fat, smooth muscle, and blood vessels. Lung tissue affected by lymphangioleiomyomatosis (LAM) is composed of abnormally dilated distal air spaces and diffuse infiltration of the pulmonary interstitium, including spaces surrounding airways, vessels, and lymphatics, with atypical smooth muscle cells.

Evaluations of cells from angiomyolipomas, cardiac rhabdomyomas, and subependymal giant cell tumors reveal loss of heterozygosity of the *TSC1* or *TSC2* genes and supports a two-hit tumor suppressor model for pathogenesis of TSC-related tumors. The giant cells classically found in cortical tubers do not exhibit loss of heterozygosity, however nuclear accumulation of hamartin in giant cells may prevent normal hamartin–tuberin heterodimer interactions (Boer *et al.* 2008).

Epilepsy in the disease

Epilepsy is the most common neurological symptom, affecting approximately 85% of TSC patients, and is a significant source of morbidity and mortality (Shepherd *et al.* 1991; Webb *et al.* 1991; Thiele 2004; Holmes *et al.* 2007).

Approximately one-third of patients develop infantile spasms within the first 2 years of life with the median age of onset between 3 and 6 months of age. Classic infantile spasms are characterized by brief, massive clusters of flexor or extensor tonic contractions of the axial musculature; however, subtle spasms may involve brief head nods or clusters of stereotyped eye deviation. These seizure clusters typically occur just before falling asleep or soon after awakening. The presence of infantile spasms is a significant risk factor for the development of mental retardation in TSC patients; approximately two-thirds of patients with a history of infantile spasms have an IQ < 70 on formal testing. Recognition and prompt treatment of infantile spasms is critical as delayed cessation is highly correlated with poor cognitive outcome (Goh *et al.* 2005). Infantile spasms in TSC frequently develop concurrently with partial epilepsy and poor control of seizures types other than spasms is also correlated with poor outcome. The

interictal electroencephalogram (EEG) in infantile spasms can range from normal to modified or classic hypsarrhythmia patterns. The severity of EEG abnormalities at the time of treatment correlates with poor cognitive outcome (Muzykewicz 2009). Current work is evaluating whether treating abnormal EEG features without clinical seizures may be beneficial (Jozwiak *et al.* 2007). Age of onset does not correlate with intellectual outcome and patients with infantile spasms due to TSC may have better cognitive outcome compared with other causes of symptomatic infantile spasms (Goh *et al.* 2005; Chu-Shore *et al.* in press).

More than half of TSC patients with epilepsy will have multiple seizure types. Complex partial seizures are the classic clinical seizure phenotype seen in TSC; however, approximately one-fourth of patients will develop multiple generalized seizure types and EEG features consistent with a diagnosis of Lennox–Gastaut syndrome.

Seizure onset can occur at any time from gestation to adulthood, though in our experience, approximately two-thirds of patients have seizure onset during the first year of life and 80% by age 3. Adults remain at risk, as 12% of adults without a previous epilepsy history will subsequently develop epilepsy. Epilepsy is refractory to multiple anticonvulsant medication trials in nearly two-thirds of patients; however, approximately one-third of epilepsy patients enter remission through medical management, surgical intervention, or the natural course of their disease.

Many features are predictive of epilepsy prognosis. Patients with infantile spasms are more likely to develop subsequent refractory epilepsy and Lennox–Gastaut syndrome. Mutation in *TSC2* is also correlated with more severe epilepsy. History of epilepsy, infantile spasms, seizure onset before 3 years of age, and refractory epilepsy are each correlated with poor cognitive outcome while epilepsy remission correlates with better cognitive outcomes (Chu-Shore *et al.* in press).

Mechanisms of epileptogenicity remain largely unknown in TSC, though due to the known genetic, biochemical, and cortical structural abnormalities seen in this disease, this is an active and exciting area of research. Cortical tubers are areas of disorganized cortex, thought to be the result of abnormal cellular proliferation, differentiation, or migration during fetal corticogenesis. Tubers exhibit abnormal cellular expression of excitatory glutamate receptors (Talos *et al.* 2008) and cortex adjacent to tubers may be the source of epileptiform activity (Major *et al.* 2009). Some cortical tubers are clearly epileptic foci while others are not (Jacobs *et al.* 2008). Cortical tubers that exhibit cyst-like characteristics on neuroimaging are present in approximately half of TSC patients and correlate with more severe epilepsy (Chu-Shore *et al.* 2009). However, epileptic foci can also originate from cortex without apparent tuber and some TSC patients without any cortical tubers evident on neuroimaging have epilepsy.

The role of mTOR dysregulation and epilepsy is an active area of research. The mTORC1 pathway is necessary for regulation of synaptic remodeling as seen in long-term potentiation (Tsokas *et al.* 2007; Ehninger *et al.* 2008) and dysregulation at the molecular level has been implicated in epileptogenesis in TSC in animal models (Meikle *et al.* 2008; Zeng *et al.* 2008).

Diagnostic tests for the disease

Tuberons sclerosis complex remains a clinical diagnosis, as approximately 15% of patients have no mutation identified on genetic testing. According to the diagnostic criteria developed by a consensus conference in 1998, definite diagnosis of TSC requires the presence of two major features or one major and two minor features (Roach *et al.* 1998). Major clinical features of TSC include facial angiofibromas, ungual or periungual fibromas, three or more hypomelanotic macules, shagreen patch, multiple retinal nodular hamartomas, cortical tuber, subependymal nodule (SEN), subependymal giant cell tumor, cardiac rhabdomyoma, pulmonary LAM, and renal angiomyolipoma. Minor clinical features of TSC include multiple pits in dental enamel, hamartomatous rectal polyps, bone cysts, cerebral white-matter radial migration lines, gingival fibromas, non-renal hamartomas, retinal achromic patch, "confetti" skin lesions, and multiple renal cysts. The presence of one major plus one minor feature suggests probable TSC, and the presence of one major feature or two minor features suggests possible TSC.

Initial evaluation of a patient with known or suspected TSC should focus on confirmation of the diagnosis by identifying major and minor diagnostic features. Proper diagnosis allows for appropriate surveillance and preventative health measures in identified patients. Diagnostic evaluation requires skin examination (including Wood's lamp), neurologic examination, dilated ophthalmologic evaluation with slit lamp, electrocardiogram (EKG) or echocardiogram, renal imaging (ultrasound, computed tomography [CT], or magnetic resonance imaging [MRI], and neuroimaging with brain MRI. High-resolution chest CT should be performed in young adults to identify subclinical LAM.

Confident diagnosis of TSC in a young child can be difficult, as different organs are preferentially involved at distinct developmental stages. Cardiac rhabdomyomas are present in utero and typically regress in early childhood. Cortical tubers are present by 19 weeks gestation, though they may become more apparent on neuroimaging after age 2 years when myelination patterns are more mature. Hypopigmented macules (which may be easier to detect with a Wood's lamp) are present at birth but become easier to appreciate as the skin surface area increases. Shagreen patches and facial angiofibromas are typically evident in early childhood. Periungual fibromas, and LAM tend to develop after puberty. Subependymal nodules can develop at any age; however, these growths lose their propensity to develop into subependymal giant cell tumors after approximately age 20 years. Renal lesions can be present at any age but are thought to develop increasingly with age.

Because TSC may be extremely variable within families and because some patients with TSC have very few manifestations, it is often necessary to evaluate the parents and other relatives of a patient with known TSC to determine their status and genetic risks. If a disease-causing TSC mutation is identified, family members can be tested for the known genetic mutation and prenatal testing can also be offered.

After diagnosis is confirmed, surveillance tests are recommended depending on age and findings. Neuroimaging findings include subependymal glial nodules, cortical or subcortical tubers, and radial glial migration lines. New cortical tubers do not form after corticogenesis is complete; however, tubers can develop progressive calcification and cyst-like characteristics over time. Subependymal giant cell tumors develop de novo or from existing subependymal nodules in approximately 20% of all patients with TSC (Adriaensen *et al.* 2009) and because enlarging tumors can block cerebrospinal fluid outflow near the foramen of Monroe, annual imaging is recommended in all patients with clinical TSC until age 21 years. Continued surveillance neuroimaging beyond age 21 may be indicated if there is a known subependymal giant cell tumor. Renal imaging findings include renal cysts and angiomyolipomas. Surveillance renal imaging should be repeated every other year in pediatric and adult patients without known lesions, and annually, or more frequently, in patients with known renal involvement, depending on disease burden. Although LAM was previously thought to affect only women (approximately one-third), several men with LAM have now also been identified and therefore both men and women with TSC should be evaluated with a high resolution chest CT after puberty. Neurodevelopmental testing should be performed on all children to identify developmental delay, school performance problems, or a history of behavioral difficulties at home or in school.

Principles of management

Management of TSC involves attention to multiple organ systems and is best achieved in a multidisciplinary TSC clinic. Follow-up for patients diagnosed with TSC should include anticipatory guidance and genetic counseling for families at all stages of disease. Children with TSC should have annual neurological and developmental assessments. An epileptologist is frequently involved to manage seizures. A mental health specialist should be involved with all patients suffering from mood or anxiety symptoms, which may be significant. Rapidly progressive or symptomatic subependymal giant cell tumors may require surgical resection. Large angiomyolipomas may require treatment with embolization to prevent spontaneous bleeding. Patients with significant or symptomatic dermatological disease may require laser therapy by an experienced dermatologist.

Management of epilepsy in TSC has many unique features. In our experience, the likelihood of developing epilepsy after presenting with a single seizure in patients with TSC is nearly 100% and treatment with anticonvulsant medications after a first seizure should therefore be considered. The vast majority of patients with infantile spasms present with or subsequently develop a different seizure phenotype and more than half of TSC patients with epilepsy develop multiple seizure types. Therefore, frequent surveillance for new paroxysmal events is necessary. Although half of patients are cognitively impaired at baseline, sudden or fluctuating changes in cognitive function could indicate epileptic encephalopathy and EEG should be considered. The EEG features may be misleading in TSC since tubers may obstruct underlying electrographic signals leading to a false-negative surface EEG (Major *et al.* 2009). Although non-epileptic seizures do occur in this population, practitioners should have a high suspicion for epileptic seizures when evaluating recurrent, stereotyped, paroxysmal events in this population.

Infantile spasms in TSC are uniquely sensitive to vigabatrin with spasm cessation reported in 74–100% of patients within 2–4 weeks of treatment, and this therapy should be used as the first-line treatment in any infant with TSC presenting with infantile spasms (Willmore *et al.* 2009). Vigabatrin is a structural analog to γ-aminobutyric acid (GABA) that irreversibly inhibits GABA-transaminase. Spasm cessation is typically seen shortly after onset of treatment and if no response is seen by 12 weeks, vigabatrin should be discontinued and other therapies pursued. Even in spasm-free patients, the EEG should be followed and may warrant treatment if features of hypsarrhythmia persist (Muzykewicz *et al.* 2009). If spasms are controlled, patients should be maintained on vigabatrin, often at doses of 150 mg/kg per day (though higher doses may be needed for complete spasm control), until they are at least 1 year spasm-free and then a slow taper should be initiated. The efficacy and recurrence rate of infantile spasms following shorter treatment courses is being investigated. Up to 15% of children and 25–50% of adults develop a peripheral visual field defect on vigabatrin, though central acuity is almost always preserved. Therefore, it is recommended that infants taking vigabatrin should be evaluated by an experienced pediatric ophthalmologist at baseline and at regular intervals. Hyperintensities on T2-weighted and diffusion-weighted imaging in the basal ganglia and brainstem on brain MRI have also been observed in infants treated with vigabatrin. These changes are reversible with discontinuation of the drug and are of unknown significance (Milh *et al.* 2009). Adrenocorticotropin hormone (ACTH) therapy is a second-line treatment for infantile spasms in TSC; ACTH may cause growth of cardiac rhabdomyomas and serial echocardiograms are recommended in patients with large or obstructive lesions (Hishitani *et al.* 1997; Hiraishi *et al.* 2000). The ketogenic diet has shown some success in the treatment of infantile spasms in TSC and may be appropriate to consider as an alternative second-line treatment, though further studies are needed to establish its efficacy. In our experience, carbamazepine may exacerbate infantile spasms and should be used with caution in patients with active infantile spasms.

In TSC, even classic generalized seizure phenotypes are thought to have a focal onset with rapid secondary generalization and should be treated accordingly with appropriate anticonvulsant agents. For medical management of patients with multiple seizure types, a broad-spectrum anticonvulsant such as levetiracetam, lamotrigine, topiramate, or valproic acid can be useful. Another issue to consider when treating epilepsy in TSC is that hormonal therapies to modulate epilepsy may be contraindicated. The observation that pulmonary LAM is overwhelmingly more common in women than men has led to the hypothesis that hormones, including estrogen and progesterone, may play a role in regulating mTOR signaling. As such, it is generally recommended that women with TSC avoid oral contraceptive therapy and pregnancy, particularly if there is evidence of LAM on chest CT.

Refractory epilepsy develops in approximately two-thirds of patients and non-pharmacologic options may be warranted. Dietary therapy, including low-glycemic index therapy and the ketogenic diet, can be very effective in refractory epilepsy. The ketogenic diet has been shown to reduce seizures by more than 90% in two-thirds of patients and by at least 50% in the vast majority of TSC patients (Kossof *et al.* 2005).

Surgical options should also be evaluated, including the vagal nerve stimulator (VNS) and epilepsy surgery. In our experience, the VNS reduced seizure frequency by at least 50% in half of TSC patients with refractory epilepsy (Major and Thiele 2008). Patients with refractory epilepsy should undergo presurgical evaluation with video-EEG and a high-resolution brain MRI. Additional tests including positron emission tomography (PET), single-photon emission computed tomography (SPECT), and magnetoencephalography may also be helpful in identifying the epileptogenic lesion. Patients in whom a primary epileptogenic tuber can be identified in presurgical evaluation may be good surgical candidates. A recent review of epilepsy surgery outcomes found that seizure frequency was improved by at least 50% in 90% of TSC patients and seizure-freedom was achieved in approximately 60% (Jansen *et al.* 2007). A history of tonic seizures, mental retardation, multifocal abnormalities on SPECT, and epilepsy surgery consisting of corpus callosotomy were each associated with increased risk of seizure recurrence after epilepsy surgery. These features should not be considered exclusion criteria since many of these patients can achieve seizure-freedom and quality of life may be significantly improved by seizure reduction in the absence of complete seizure control. There may be a role for corpus callosotomy for treatment of drop seizures and a possible role of this surgical intervention to help localize a focal onset for seizures with rapid secondary generalization.

Approximately one-third of TSC patients with epilepsy achieve epilepsy remission and approximately one-third of these patients are able to be successfully weaned off anticonvulsant medication. Thus, carefully selected, well-controlled patients may be considered for medication taper even in this high-risk population.

Much work is currently focusing on the role of pharmacologic mTOR inhibitors for treatment of tumors and symptoms seen in TSC, although the role of these therapies for epilepsy remains uncertain. Rapamycin, which is a pharmacologic inhibitor of mTORC1 activity, has shown some success in inducing regression of subependymal giant cell tumor and angiomyolipoma growth in patients with TSC; however, regrowth occurs with medication discontinuation (Franz *et al.* 2006; Bissler *et al.* 2008). Rapamycin has been shown to have antiepileptic activity in animal models. In mice with conditional inactivation in the *TSC1* gene in glia, rapamycin administration prevented the development of epilepsy in animals treated at young ages and suppressed seizures in older animals (Zeng *et al.* 2008). In a mouse model with conditional knockout of the *TSC1* gene in neurons, rapamycin treatment completely abolished spontaneous clinical seizures (Meikle *et al.* 2008).

Few data are available regarding the effects of pharmacologic mTOR inhibition on epileptogenesis or epilepsy treatment in TSC patients; however, this is an exciting and active area of research. Multiple rapamycin analogs designed to specifically target the mTORC1 pathway are undergoing development and evaluation in animal models at this time. Multicenter clinical trials evaluating rapamycin and other structurally similar chemical analogs are currently underway for use in TSC.

Tuberous sclerosis complex is a fascinating and multifaceted genetic epilepsy syndrome that will undoubtedly teach us broader insights into mechanisms of epileptogenesis, treatment, and prevention.

References

Adriaensen ME, Shaefer-Prokop CM, Stignen T, *et al.* (2009) Prevalence of subependymal giant cell tumors in patients with tuberous sclerosis and a review of the literature. *Eur J Neurol* **16**:691–6.

Bissler JJ, McCormack FX, Young LR, *et al.* (2008) Sirolimus for angiomyolipoma in tuberous sclerosis complex or lymphangioleiomyomatosis. *N Engl J Med* **358**:140–51.

Boer K, Troost D, Jansen F, *et al.* (2008) Clinicopathological and immunohistochemical findings in an autopsy case of tuberous sclerosis complex. *Neuropathology* **28**:577–90.

Chu-Shore CJ, Major, P, Montenegro M, Thiele E (2009) Cyst-like tubers are associated with TSC2 and epilepsy in tuberous sclerosis complex. *Neurology* **72**:1165–9.

Chu-Shore CJ, Major P, Camposano S, Muzykewicz D, Thiele EA The natural history of epilepsy in tuberous sclerosis complex. *Epilepsia* (in press).

Crino PB, Nathanson KL, Petri Henske E (2006) The tuberous sclerosis complex. *N Engl J Med* **355**:1345–56.

Dabora SL, Jozwiak S, Franz DN, *et al.* (2001) Mutational analysis in a cohort of 224 tuberous sclerosis patients indicates increased severity of TSC2, compared with TSC1, disease in multiple organs. *Am J Hum Genet* **68**:64–80.

Ehninger D, Han S, Shilyansky C, *et al.* (2008) Reversal of learning deficits in a *Tsc+/−* mouse model for tuberons sclerosis. *Nat Med* **14**:843–8.

Franz DN, Leonard J, Tudor C, *et al.* (2006) Rapamycin causes regression of astrocytomas in tuberous sclerosis complex. *Ann Neurol* **59**:490–8.

Goh S, Kwiatkowski DJ, Dorer DJ, Thiele EA (2005) Infantile spasms and intellectual outcomes in children with tuberous sclerosis complex. *Neurology* **65**:235–8.

Hiraishi S, Iwanami N, Ogawa N (2000) Images in cardiology: enlargement of cardiac rhabdomyoma and myocardial ischaemia during corticotrophin treatment for infantile spasm. *Heart* **84**:170.

Hishitani T, Hoshino K, Ogawa K, *et al.* (1997) Rapid enlargement of cardiac rhabdomyomas during corticotropin therapy for infantile spasms. *Can J Cardiol* **13**:72–4.

Holmes GL, Stafstrom CE, Tuberous Sclerosis Study Group (2007) Tuberous sclerosis complex and epilepsy: recent developments and future challenges. *Epilepsia* **48**:617–30.

Jacobs J, Rohr A, Moeller R, *et al.* (2008) Evaluation of epileptogenic networks in children with tuberous sclerosis complex using EEG-fMRI. *Epilepsia* **49**:816–25.

Jansen FE, van Huffelen AC, Algra A, van Nieuwenhuizen O (2007) Epilepsy surgery in tuberous sclerosis: a systematic review. *Epilepsia* **48**:1477–84.

Jozwiak S, Domanska-Pakiela D, Kotulska K, Kaczorowska M (2007) Treatment before seizures: new indications of antiepileptic therapy in children with tuberous sclerosis complex. *Epilepsia* **48**:1632.

Kossof EH, Thiele EA, Pfeifer HH, McGrogan JR, Freeman JM (2005) Tuberous sclerosis complex and the ketogenic diet. *Epilepsia* **46**:1684–6.

Kwiatkowski DJ, Manning BD (2005) Tuberous sclerosis: a GAP at the crossroads of multiple signaling pathways. *Hum Mol Genet* **14**:R251–8.

Lyczkowski DA, Conant KD, Pulsifer MG, *et al.* (2007) Intrafamilial phenotypic variability in tuberous sclerosis complex. *J Child Neurol* **22**:1348–55.

Major P, Thiele EA (2008) Vagus nerve stimulation for intractable epilepsy in tuberous sclerosis complex. *Epilepsy Behav* **13**:357–60.

Major P, Rakowski S, Simon MV, *et al.* (2009) Are cortical tubers epileptogenic? Evidence from electrocorticography. *Epilepsia* **50**:147–54.

Manning BD, Logsdon MN, Lipovsky AI, *et al.* (2005) Feedback inhibition of Akt signaling limits the growth of tumors lacking TSC2. *Genes Dev* **19**:1773–8.

Meikle L, Pollizzi K, Egnor A, *et al.* (2008) Response of a neuronal model of tuberous sclerosis to mammalian target of rapamycin (mTOR) inhibitors: effects on mTORC1 and Akt signaling lead to improved survival and function. *J Neurosci* **28**:5422–32.

Milh M, Villeneuve N, Chapon F, *et al.* (2009) Transient brain magnetic resonance imaging hyperintensity in basal ganglia and brain stem of epileptic infants treated with vigabatrin. *J Child Neurol* **24**:305–15.

Muzykewicz DA, Newberry P, Danforth N, Halpern EF, Thiele EA (2007) Psychiatric comorbid conditions in a clinic population of 241 patients with tuberous sclerosis complex. *Epilepsy Behav* **11**:506–13.

Muzykewicz DA, Costello DJ, Halpern EF, Thiele EA (2009) Infantile spasms in tuberous sclerosis complex: prognostic utility of EEG. *Epilepsia* **50**:290–6.

Richardson EP (1991) Pathology of tuberous sclerosis: neuropathologic aspects. *Ann N Y Acad Sci* **615**:128–39.

Roach ES, Gomez MR, Northrup H (1998) Tuberous sclerosis complex consensus conference: revised clinical diagnostic criteria. *J Child Neurol* **13**:624–8.

Sabatini DM (2006) mTOR and cancer: insights into a complex relationship. *Nature Rev* **6**:729–34.

Sancak O, Nellist M, Goedbloed M, *et al.* (2005) Mutational analysis of the *TSC1* and *TSC2* genes in a diagnostic setting: genotype–phenotype correlations and comparison of diagnostic DNA techniques in tuberous sclerosis complex. *Eur J Hum Genet* **13**:731–41.

Shepherd CW, Gomez MR, Lie JT, Crowson CS (1991) Causes of death in patients with tuberous sclerosis. *Mayo Clin Proc* **66**:792–6.

Staley BA, Montenegro MA, Muzykewicz DA, *et al.* (2008) Self-injurious behaviors and tuberous sclerosis complex: frequency and possible associations in a population of 257 patients. *Epilepsy Behav* **13**:650–3.

Talos DM, Kwiatkowski DJ, Cordero K, Black PM, Jensen FE (2008) Cell-specific alterations of glutamate receptor expression in tuberous sclerosis complex cortical tubers. *Ann Neurol* **63**:454–65.

Thiele EA (2004) Managing epilepsy in tuberous sclerosis complex. *J Child Neurol* **19**:680–6.

Tsokas P, Ma T, Iyengar R, Landau EM, Blitzer RD (2007) Mitogen-activated protein kinase upregulates the dendritic translation machinery in long-term potentiation by controlling the mammalian target of rapamycin pathway. *J Neurosci* **27**:5885–94.

Webb DW, Osborne JP (1995) Tuberous sclerosis. *Arch Dis Childh* **72**:471–4.

Webb DW, Fryer AE, Osborne JP (1991) On the incidence of fits and mental retardation in tuberous sclerosis. *J Med Genet* **28**:395–7.

Webb DW, Fryer AE, Osborne JP (1996) Morbidity associated with tuberous sclerosis: a population study. *Dev Med Child Neurol* **38**:146–55.

Willmore LJ, Abelson MB, Ben-Menachem E, Pellock JM, Shields WD (2009) Vigabatrin: 2008 update. *Epilepsia* **50**:163–73.

Winterkorn EG, Pulsifer MB, Thiele EA (2007) Cognitive prognosis of patients with tuberous sclerosis complex. *Neurology* **68**:62–4.

Zeng LH, Xu L, Gutmann DH, Wong M (2008) Rapamycin prevents epilepsy in a mouse model of tuberous sclerosis complex. *Ann Neurol* **63**:444–53.

Chapter

25

Neurofibromatoses

Rosalie E. Ferner and Margaret J. Jackson

Neurofibromatosis 1 (NF1) and neurofibromatosis 2 (NF2) are inherited tumor predisposition syndromes that have a major impact on the nervous system but are clinically and genetically distinct disorders. Epilepsy is a recognized association of NF1, but there have been no systematic studies of the frequency, etiology, and type of seizures in NF2. This chapter discusses the clinical characteristics and genetics of the neurofibromatoses and presents the current knowledge about their relationship with epilepsy.

Neurofibromatosis 1

Formerly termed von Recklinghausen disease, neurofibromatosis 1 (NF1) is a complex, neurocutaneous disorder with a birth incidence of 1 in 3000 and a minimum prevalence of 1 in 4–5000. There is an autosomal dominant pattern of inheritance and new mutations occur in approximately 50% of patients (Huson *et al.* 1988). It is a tumor suppressor disorder and loss of *NF1* gene function through mutation predisposes affected individuals to the development of benign and malignant tumor. Two of the principal disease manifestations are required for diagnosis–a family history of NF1, café au lait patches, skinfold freckling, benign peripheral nerve sheath tumors called neurofibromas, iris Lisch nodules, optic pathway glioma, and distinctive bony dysplasia involving the sphenoid wing and the long bones (National Institutes of Health 1988). Although NF1 affects the skin, peripheral nervous system, and skeletal system predominantly, the complications are widespread and vary even within families (Huson *et al.* 1988; Ferner 2007) (Table 25.1).

Distinction should be made between NF1 and other forms of neurofibromatosis (see section on NF2 and schwannomatosis). Individuals with mosaic NF1 have either mild generalized disease or cutaneous features of NF1 restricted to one or more body segments (Ruggieri and Huson 2001). Multiple, symmetrical spinal nerve root neurofibromas and café au lait patches are characteristic of the rare hereditary spinal neurofibromatosis. The recently described Legius syndrome overlaps with NF1 and is characterized by *SPRED1* mutations and a mild phenotype of café au lait patches, axillary freckling, and macrocephaly (Brems *et al.* 2007).

The *NF1* gene was cloned on chromosome 17q11.2, has 60 exons and spans 350 kb of genomic DNA (Viskochil *et al.* 1991). The function of the three embedded genes *EVI2A*, *EVI2B*, and oligodendrocyte myelin glycoprotein (*OMGP*) is uncertain, but *OMGP* has a putative role in central nervous system myelination (Viskochil *et al.* 1991; Johannessen *et al.* 2005). Neurofibromin, the cytoplasmic protein product of *NF1*, acts as a tumor suppressor and is ubiquitously expressed with high levels in the nervous system. Neurofibromin reduces cell growth and proliferation by negative regulation of the cellular proto-oncogene p21RAS and by control of the serine threonine kinase MTOR (mammalian target of rapamycin) in a common biochemical pathway with the *TSC2* gene (Xu *et al.* 1990; Daston *et al.* 1992; Johannessen *et al.* 2005). SPRED1 is a member of the SPROUTY/SPRED family of proteins that control the RAS pathway and mitogen-activated protein kinase signaling (Brems *et al.* 2007).

Epilepsy in NF1

Estimates of seizure frequency in NF1 adults and children have ranged from 4% to 13% partly due to different methods of ascertainment and study design. Overall the studies suggest that having NF1 increases the lifetime risk of having epilepsy about tenfold. A South Wales population study identified 4.4% of 135 individuals with epilepsy without known etiology and a further 2.2% had seizures secondary to NF1 complications (Huson *et al.* 1988). In retrospective hospital-based assessments Korf and colleagues diagnosed epilepsy in 6.1% of 359 patients and a cross-sectional database review identified 4.2% of 499 patients with seizures including all causes (Korf *et al.* 1993; Kulkantrakorn and Geller 1998). Vivarelli *et al.* noted 7% of 198 NF1 patients referred to a specialist center from general practitioners and regional hospitals had unprovoked recurrent seizures (Vivarelli *et al.* 2003). We performed a cross-sectional study of cognitive impairment in 103 NF1 adults and children with age, gender, and socioeconomically matched sibs, close

The Causes of Epilepsy, eds. S. D. Shorvon, F. Andermann, and R. Guerrini. Published by Cambridge University Press. © Cambridge University Press 2011.

Table 25.1 Neurological complications of NF1

Complication	Frequency	Clinical manifestation
Brain and spinal cord glioma	2–3%	Related to site; often indolent; brainstem and cerebellum commonest sites
Optic pathway glioma	15%	Asymptomatic or visual signs/visual loss Symptomatic mainly in children <6 years Progressive visual loss requires chemotherapy
Macrocephaly	45%	Asymptomatic
Aqueduct stenosis	1.5%	Hydrocephalus Subependymal glial cell proliferation around aqueduct
Sphenoid wing dysplasia	1%	Asymptomatic or pulsating exophthalmos Temporal lobe herniates into orbit; occasionally requires surgery
Cognitive impairment IQ < 70	4–8%	Usually IQ in low average range
Learning problems	>70%	Problems with language, reading, maths, coordination, visual spatial ability, executive function, socialization
Attention deficit hyperactivity disorder (ADHD)	38%	(ADHD) responds to methylphenidate Lovostatin (inhibits RAS pathway and corrects learning problems in mice) clinical trial
T2 hyperintensities on brain MRI	80%	Probably abnormal myelination or gliosis; no mass effect, enhancement, or symptoms; disappear in adulthood
Cerebrovascular disease	2.5% (children)	Stenosis/occlusion internal carotid and cerebral arteries; moya moya in children; aneurysm
Multiple sclerosis		Usually primary progressive form although relapsing–remitting also reported; not linked to mutations of OMGP
Spinal neurofibromas causing cord compression	<5%	Frequently high cervical. Decision to operate should be based on progressive neurological deficit and not on MRI appearances alone
Malignant peripheral nerve sheath tumor	Lifetime risk 7–12%	Present with pain, rapid increase in size, neurological deficit, hard texture; symptoms overlap with benign plexiform neurofibromas; diagnose on [18]FDG PET CT; treat with surgery, radiotherapy for high-grade tumor, chemotherapy for metastases
Neurofibromatous neuropathy	1.5%	Mild symmetrical axonal sensorimotor neuropathy with thickened peripheral nerves
Epilepsy	6–7%	All seizure types but mainly complex partial seizures

relatives, or friends as controls (Ferner *et al.* 1996). We recorded epilepsy in 12.6% patients with NF1 but in only one control. Subsequently in an unselected retrospective audit of 450 NF1 individuals attending our NF1 clinic, we identified 6.1% of NF1 adults and children with seizures including 1.78% with an established underlying cause (Ferner and Jan 2001). Szudek *et al.* undertook a database analysis of 4402 NF1 individuals looking for associations between clinical manifestations in NF1. They documented an association between learning problems and epilepsy in probands and this relationship would probably account for the high frequency of seizures in our study on cognitive impairment (Szudek *et al.* 2000). In Northern Ireland, geneticists studying their register of patients with NF1 found epilepsy in 4% of 75 children under 17 years old (McKeever *et al.* 2008). A recent three-center Italian study reported infantile spasms in 0.76% of NF1 children compared with 0.02–0.05% in the general population (Ruggieri *et al.* 2009). Although commoner than in the general population, infantile spasms occur considerably less frequently in NF1 than in tuberous sclerosis.

Evidence exists for an underlying cortical dysgenesis in NF1; neurofibromin plays a role in the formation of the central nervous system and ablation of *Nf1* function in neurons of transgenic mice produces cortical astrogliosis and hippocampal dysplasia (Zhu *et al.* 2001). A neuropathological study in 10 NF1 patients detected disordered cerebral architecture with random orientation of neurons, disarray of normal cortical lamination, and subcortical heteropias (Rosman and Pearce 1967). Neuroimaging of children with NF1 has revealed transient T2 hyperintensities on brain magnetic resonance imaging (MRI) that do not cause overt symptoms or neurological deficit and the postulated etiology is aberrant myelination or gliosis (Ferner *et al.* 1993; Hyman *et al.* 2007). There is no evidence to suggest that these children have an increased propensity to develop seizures, and current research suggests

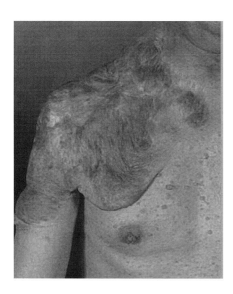

Fig. 25.1. Plexiform neurofibroma and cutaneous neurofibromas in NF1 patient.

that apart from lesions in the thalamus, they are not significantly related to learning disability (Hyman *et al.* 2007).

As neurofibromin acts as a tumor suppressor, NF1 individuals are at increased risk of developing benign and malignant tumors, particularly pilocytic astrocytomas, although pilomyxoid astrocytomas and glioblastoma multiforme can also occur (Ferner 2007) (Fig. 25.1). Anecdotal reports link ganglioglioma and dysembryoblastic neuroepithelial tumor (DNET) in association with NF1 and we have encountered three patients with DNET in our clinic. However, Fedi and colleagues did not demonstrate loss of the *NF1* gene in either type of tumor on molecular analysis, implying that they may not be causally related (Fedi *et al.* 2004). Chiari malformation, cerebrovascular disease, and multiple sclerosis are recognized associations of NF1 and potential causes of epilepsy (Ferner 2007).

The age at onset of seizures in NF1 has been described at any time between infancy and late middle age and we have assessed 30 patients who presented with seizures from age 2 weeks to 52 years (mean 18 years) (Ferner and Jan 2001). The type and etiology of seizures associated with NF1 are protean, the clinical presentation is often mild and the presence of epilepsy is not invariably associated with a more severe underlying NF1 phenotype. We have been referred NF1 patients with generalized epilepsy or focal epilepsies secondary to trauma or infection that are unrelated to the pathology of NF1. Unsurprisingly focal epilepsies predominate in NF1 in accordance with our personal experience. In 13 of 103 NF1 patients diagnosed with epilepsy we identified generalized tonic–clonic seizures (4/13), typical absences (1/13), focal seizures (FS) (7/13), and infantile spasms (1/13) (Ferner *et al.* 1996). In our retrospective assessment of 30 NF1 patients with epilepsy, the seizure types were 22/30 FS, 1 child with infantile spasms, 7/30 generalized seizures, and three individuals had a history of febrile seizures (Ferner and Jan 2001).

Epilepsy syndromes associated with NF1 in childhood include infantile spasms, febrile convulsions, and focal epilepsy. In a proportion of children with infantile spasms, the epilepsy syndrome can evolve into a localization-related type with FS (Ruggieri *et al.* 2009). Psychomotor delay and symmetrical spasms are encountered in about half of individuals with infantile spasms (Ruggieri *et al.* 2009). In adults FS predominate but there is not any particular location for seizure onset (Korf *et al.* 1993). There does not appear to be an increased risk of status epilepticus and only one of our NF1 patients, a 52-year-old male with cerebrovascular disease, required intensive care therapy for non-convulsive status epilepticus.

Few neuroimaging studies have addressed the role of microdysgenesis in NF1 and epilepsy. Korf *et al.* and Kulkantrakorn *et al.* detected no significant cortical dysplasias in their patients (Korf *et al.* 1993; Kulkantrakorn and Geller 1998). Vivarelli *et al.* (2003) performed brain MRI in a subset of three patients with unusually severe seizures and profound learning disability and single-photon emission computed tomography (SPECT) and position emission tomography (PET) in two of these individuals. Magnetic resonance imaging demonstrated transmantle cortical dysplasia, gray matter heterotopia, pachygyria, and polymicrogyria. Furthermore, the areas of abnormality were identified as hypoperfusion on SPECT and hypometabolism on PET. A fourth child with intractable epilepsy had a normal MRI but hypometabolism in the left temporo-occipital region on PET that correlated with electroencephalographic (EEG) findings, supporting the hypothesis of an underlying cortical microdysgenesis (Vivarelli *et al.* 2003). Mesial temporal sclerosis has also been identified in NF1 patients and we have encountered three such individuals with poorly controlled FS (Vivarelli *et al.* 2003).

No features on the EEG are pathognomonic of NF1. Records usually reflect the focal nature of the epilepsy associated with NF1 and may become normal with remission of the epilepsy (Vivarelli *et al.* 2003). Infantile spasms have been reported with "typical" hypsarrhythmia in 8/10 and "modified" hypsarrythmia in 2/10 in the Italian study and described as being usually continuous, rarely fragmented, by Motte and colleagues (Motte *et al.* 1993; Ruggieri *et al.* 2009). Additional focal slow waves found in the latter study were associated with a clinical semiology suggestive of a focal abnormality (head turning). In children who have developed FS subsequent to infantile spasms in NF1, the clinical evolution is reflected in the EEG changes (Vivarelli *et al.* 2003).

Diagnosis of NF1

In most patients the diagnosis can be made according to the National Institutes of Health clinical diagnostic criteria (see above) and the majority of adults will have café au lait patches, axillary freckling, and cutaneous neurofibromas (National Institutes of Health 1988). The *NF1* mutation can be identified in 95% of cases with optimal laboratory techniques. Diagnostic testing should be considered in patients with atypical clinical presentations and for prenatal diagnosis, although patients should be informed that the individual phenotype cannot be predicted (Ferner 2007).

Management of epilepsy in NF1

No specific antiepileptic drugs are recommended for people with epilepsy associated with NF1. Given that the epilepsy seen most frequently with NF1 is focal antiepileptic drugs shown to be most effective for focal seizures such as carbamazepine and lamotrigine are usually the mainstay of therapy (Marson *et al.* 2007). Anecdotal evidence suggests corticosteroids may be more effective in the treatment of NF1-related infantile spasms than vigabatrin (Ruggieri *et al.* 2009). Neurofibromatosis 1 is associated with an increased frequency of mild intellectual impairment with a mean full-scale IQ in the low average range, specific learning problems, and behavioral difficulties (Ferner *et al.* 1996). Some antiepileptic drugs, most notably levetiracetam, can be associated with worsening of behavior in people with intellectual disability and care should be taken to warn relatives of this possibility (Hurtado *et al.* 2006). There is an increased risk of early development of osteoporosis in NF1 due to impaired maintenance of bone structure and a reduction in bone density (Ferner 2007). Patients on long-term anticonvulsants or who have received corticosteroids may require monitoring with hip and spine tone mineral density scans and bone chemistry. Individuals with epilepsy associated with structural lesions such as DNET or mesial temporal sclerosis should undergo appropriate investigation to determine whether surgical resection is feasible as it can be curative.

The treatment of NF1 is based on assiduous monitoring for disease complications and treatment of the specific disease manifestations (Ferner *et al.* 2007). Advances in molecular biology and in mouse models of disease have permitted the development of drugs that block the RAS pathway. Statins reverse p21RAS activity and the learning deficits in a mouse model of NF1 and their efficacy is being assessed in NF1 children with learning problems (Krab *et al.* 2008).

About 60–70% of people with epilepsy should enter a remission with appropriate treatment. There are few data published on remission of epilepsy associated with NF1 but outcomes appear to be better than in other similar disorders. For example, infantile spasms in children with NF1, in contrast to those with other neurocutaneous syndromes, have relatively good rates of remission (14/15 with corticosteroids in one series) and better intellectual outcome (Motte *et al.* 1993) Other series of NF1-associated epilepsy report good seizure control (albeit with few details of the length of remission) in 8/9 patients with CPS, complete remission in 7/12 children available to follow up, and greater than 1 year remission in 11/21 children and young adults (Kulkantrakorn and Geller 1998; Vivarelli *et al.* 2003). These data suggest that people with epilepsy and NF1 have equal or only slightly lower frequency of remission than average and better than with neurocutaneous disorders such as tuberous sclerosis.

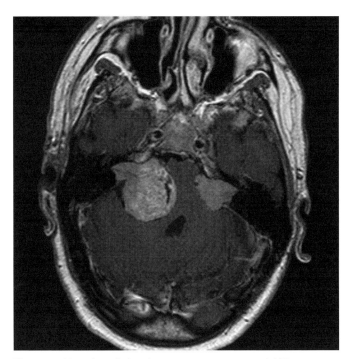

Fig. 25.2. Bilateral vestibular schwannomas in a patient with NF2.

Neurofibromatosis 2

Neurofibromatosis 2 was previously referred to as bilateral acoustic or central neurofibromatosis and is a rare autosomal dominant condition with a birth incidence of 1 in 25 000 and a diagnostic prevalence of 1 in 210 000 (Evans *et al.* 1992). Bilateral vestibular schwannomas are the hallmark of NF2 but schwannomas can form on other cranial, spinal, and peripheral nerves (Baser *et al.* 2002; Ferner 2007) (Fig. 25.2). Additional diagnostic features include meningiomas, ependymomas, and posterior subcapsular lens opacities. Cutaneous manifestations are less conspicuous than in NF1, there are fewer café au lait patches, and skin tumors occur as predominantly schwannomas. Malignancy is uncommon and NF2 disease complications are confined to the eye and nervous system, including retinal hamartomas, neurofibromatous neuropathy, facial mononeuropathy, and focal amyotrophy (Evans *et al.* 1992; Ferner 2007). Mild generalized disease or cranial tumors localized to one area of the brain betokens NF2 mosaicism. Neurofibromatosis 2 should be distinguished from schwannomatosis, a rare condition characterized by the development of painful schwannomas involving the cutaneous, peripheral, and spinal nerves (MacCollin *et al.* 2005). The disease is mostly sporadic, but familial cases have been described and some patients have localized schwannomas, consistent with mosaicism.

Genetics of NF2

The *NF2* tumor suppressor gene was identified on chromosome 22q11.2 and the gene encodes the protein merlin (Trofatter *et al.* 1993). Merlin is related to the moesin–ezrin–radixin proteins which link the actin cytoskeleton to cell surface glycoproteins controlling growth and cellular remodeling. Merlin is widely expressed in Schwann, lens, and leptomeningeal cells and regulates proliferation of these cells. Merlin is involved in the coordination of cellular adhesion and growth factor receptor signaling. The gene for schwannomatosis has been identified on chromosome 22 proximal to the NF2 gene and mutations have been described in *INI1* in 7% of sporadic disease and 30% of familial patients (Boyd *et al.* 2008).

Epilepsy in NF2

Seizures are reported in association with NF2 within the context of large clinical studies, but there has been no systematic assessment of seizure frequency in NF2. In a genetic-based study 8 out of 100 adults with NF2 were reported to have epilepsy (Evans *et al.* 1992). We diagnosed epilepsy in 9.8% of 61 patients with mosaic or classical NF2 in our multidisciplinary NF2 service.

Loss of *NF2* function predisposes to tumor formation, predominantly the development of meningiomas (frequently multiple) and gliomas that are potentially epileptogenic (Evans *et al.* 1992; Trofatter *et al.* 1993; Ferner 2007). Neuropathological studies have demonstrated a microdysgenesis including glial hamartomas that cluster in the gray matter of the cerebral cortex and the thalamus (Wiestler *et al.* 1989). Meningioangiomatosis is rare and usually sporadic but has been associated with NF2 in 16 out of 100 cases in the literature, although only a minority of these patients presented with seizures (Omeis *et al.* 2006). It involves the leptomeninges and underlying cortex with meningiovascular proliferation and leptomeningeal calcification (Wiestler *et al.* 1989; Omeis *et al.* 2006). In NF2 the site is predominantly in the frontal cortex, but lesions can be multiple. Intracranial calcifications unrelated to tumor were described in the choroid plexus, cerebral and cerebellar hemispheres in 7 out of 11 patients imaged with brain computerized tomography (CT) but the frequency in large NF2 populations, etiology, and relationship with epilepsy is uncertain (Mayfrank *et al.* 1990).

There are no published studies on the types of epilepsy in NF2. Our NF2 patients with epilepsy had varying severity of NF2 and a mixture of seizure types but focal becoming generalized was predominant. Seizures were the presenting manifestation of severe NF2 in two of our patients aged 7 years and 19 years, but the age range of first seizure was from 7 to 52 years. The six patients with seizures all had meningiomas, but there was no difference in the site or number of meningiomas between patients with epilepsy and the 22 NF2 individuals without seizures. We have not detected meningioangiomatosis or any other dysgenesis on imaging in any of our patients. We are unable to evaluate the frequency of calcification because CT scanning is not routinely performed in NF2 patients.

Diagnosis of NF2

The diagnosis of NF2 is made according a combination of skin, eye, and central and peripheral nervous system manifestations (Baser *et al.* 2002). Mutations in *NF2* can be identified in 95% of patients with classical disease. Genetic testing is undertaken in all patients as in contradistinction to NF1 there is phenotype–genotype correlation. Missense mutations and large deletions indicate mild disease whilst nonsense and frameshift mutations result in a truncated protein and are associated with severe NF2 (Ferner 2007). Mutation testing is also available for presymptomatic assessment for at risk relatives and for prenatal screening.

Management of NF2

The majority of our patients have received treatment with carbamazepine with good seizure control. One individual required levetiracetam and one had intractable seizures due to a meningioma in the middle cranial fossa, which did not respond to temporal lobectomy or multiple drug therapy.

The management of NF2 is complex as individuals can have multiple symptomatic nervous system tumors. Treatment requires the involvement of a multidisciplinary team of surgeons, clinicians, and hearing therapists (Evans *et al.* 2005).

There is no doubt that epilepsy occurs in association with both NF1 and NF2, but there is a clear need for further well-documented clinical, neuroradiological, and neurophysiological studies in a large cohort for evaluation of seizure type, etiology, and prognosis in these conditions.

Acknowledgments

We are grateful to Dr. Michael Johnson and Dr. Karine Lascelles for their help in managing our NF1 patients with epilepsy.

References

Baser ME, Friedman JM, Wallace AJ, *et al.* (2002) Evaluation of clinical diagnostic criteria for neuro-fibromatosis 2. *Neurology* 59:1759–65.

Boyd C, Smith MJ, Kluwe L, *et al.* (2008) Alterations in the *SMARCB1* (*INI1*) tumor suppressor gene in familial schwannomatosis. *Clin Genet* 74:358–66.

Brems H, Chmara M, Sahbatou M, *et al.* (2007) Germline loss-of-function mutations in *SPRED1* cause a neurofibromatosis 1-like phenotype. *Nat Genet* 39:1120–6.

Daston MM, Scrable H, Nordlund M, *et al.* (1992) The protein product of the neurofibromatosis type 1 gene is expressed at highest abundance in neurons, Schwann cells, and oligodendrocytes. *Neuron* 8:415–28.

Evans DG, Huson SM, Donnai D, *et al.* (1992) A clinical study of type 2 neurofibromatosis. *Q J Med* 84:603–18.

Evans DG, Baser ME, O'Reilly B, *et al.* (2005) Management of the patient and family with neurofibromatosis 2: a consensus conference statement. *Br J Neurosurg* **19**:5–12.

Fedi M, Mitchell A, Kalnins RM, *et al.* (2004) Glioneuronal tumors in neurofibromatosis type 1: MRI–pathological study. *J Clin Neurosci* **11**:745–7.

Ferner RE (2007) Neurofibromatosis 1 and neurofibromatosis 2: a twenty-first century perspective. *Lancet Neurol* **6**:340–51.

Ferner RE, Jan W (2001) Epilepsy in neurofibromatosis. *J Neurol Sci* **819**:S280.

Ferner RE, Chaudhuri R, Bingham J, Cox T, Hughes RA (1993) MRI in neurofibromatosis 1: the nature and evolution of increased intensity T2-weighted lesions and their relationship to intellectual impairment. *J Neurol Neurosurg Psychiatry* **56**:492–5.

Ferner RE, Hughes RA, Weinman J (1996) Intellectual impairment in neurofibromatosis 1. *J Neurol Sci* **138**:125–33.

Ferner RE, Huson SM, Thomas N, *et al.* (2007) Guidelines for the diagnosis and management of individuals with neurofibromatosis 1. *J Med Genet* **44**:81–8.

Hurtado B, Koepp MJ, Sander JW, Thompson PJ (2006) The impact of levetiracetam on challenging behavior. *Epilepsy Behav* **8**:588–92.

Huson SM, Harper PS, Compston DA (1988) Von Recklinghausen neurofibromatosis: A clinical and population study in south-east Wales. *Brain* **111**:1355–81.

Hyman SL, Gill DS, Shores EA, Steinberg A, North KN (2007) T2 hyperintensities in children with neurofibromatosis type 1 and their relationship to cognitive functioning. *J Neurol Neurosurg Psychiatry* **78**:1088–91.

Johannessen CM, Reczek EE, James MF, *et al.* (2005) The NF1 tumor suppressor critically regulates TSC2 and mTOR. *Proc Natl Acad Sci USA* **102**:8573–8.

Korf BR, Carrazana E, Holmes GL (1993) Patterns of seizures observed in association with neurofibromatosis 1. *Epilepsia* **34**:616–20.

Krab LC, De Goede-Bolder A, Aarsen FK, (2008) Effect of simvastatin on cognitive functioning in children with neurofibromatosis type 1: a randomized controlled trial. *J Am Med Ass* **300**:287–94.

Kulkantrakorn K, Geller TJ (1998) Seizures in neurofibromatosis 1. *Pediatr Neurol* **19**:347–50.

Maccollin M, Chiocca EA, Evans DG, *et al.* (2005) Diagnostic criteria for schwannomatosis. *Neurology* **64**:1838–45.

Marson AG, Al-Kharusi AM, Alwaidh M, *et al.* (2007) The SANAD study of effectiveness of carbamazepine, gabapentin, lamotrigine, oxcarbazepine, or topiramate for treatment of partial epilepsy: an unblinded randomised controlled trial. *Lancet* **369**:1000–15.

Mayfrank L, Mohadjer M, Wullich B (1990) Intracranial calcified deposits in neurofibromatosis type 2: a CT study of 11 cases. *Neuroradiology* **32**:33–7.

McKeever K, Shepherd CW, Crawford H, Morrison PJ (2008) An epidemiological, clinical and genetic survey of neurofibromatosis type 1 in children under sixteen years of age. *Ulster Med J* **77**:160–3.

Motte J, Billard C, Fejerman N, *et al.* (1993) Neurofibromatosis type 1 and West syndrome: a relatively benign association. *Epilepsia* **34**:723–6.

National Institutes of Health Consensus Development Conference (1988) Neurofibromatosis: Conference statement. *Arch Neurol* **45**:575–8.

Omeis I, Hillard VH, Braun A, *et al.* (2006) Meningioangiomatosis associated with neurofibromatosis: report of two cases in a single family and review of the literature. *Surg Neurol* **65**:595–603.

Rosman NP, Pearce J (1967) The brain in multiple neurofibromatosis (von Recklinghausen's disease): a suggested neuropathological basis for the associated mental defect. *Brain* **90**:829–38.

Ruggieri M, Huson SM (2001) The clinical and diagnostic implications of mosaicism in the neurofibromatoses. *Neurology* **56**:1433–43.

Ruggieri M, Iannetti P, Clementi M, *et al.* (2009) Neurofibromatosis type 1 and infantile spasms. *Childs Nerv Syst* **25**:211–16.

Szudek J, Birch P, Riccardi VM, Evans DG, Friedman JM (2000) Associations of clinical features in neurofibromatosis 1 (NF1). *Genet Epidemiol* **19**:429–39.

Trofatter JA, MacCollin MM, Rutter JL, *et al.* (1993) A novel moesin-, ezrin-, radixin-like gene is a candidate for the neurofibromatosis 2 tumor suppressor. *Cell* **72**:791–800.

Viskochil D, Cawthon R, O'Connell P, (1991) The gene encoding the oligodendrocyte–myelin glycoprotein is embedded within the neurofibromatosis type 1 gene. *Mol Cell Biol* **11**:906–12.

Vivarelli R, Grosso S, Calabrese F, (2003) Epilepsy in neurofibromatosis 1. *J Child Neurol* **18**:338–42.

Wiestler OD, Von Siebenthal K, Schmitt HP, Feiden W, Kleihues P (1989) Distribution and immunoreactivity of cerebral micro-hamartomas in bilateral acoustic neurofibromatosis (neurofibromatosis 2). *Acta Neuropathol* **79**:137–43.

Xu GF, O'Connell P, Viskochil D, *et al.* (1990) The neurofibromatosis type 1 gene encodes a protein related to GAP. *Cell* **62**:599–608.

Zhu Y, Romero MI, Ghosh P, *et al.* (2001) Ablation of NF1 function in neurons induces abnormal development of cerebral cortex and reactive gliosis in the brain. *Genes Dev* **15**:859–76.

Chapter

26

Sturge–Weber syndrome

Alexis Arzimanoglou and Eleni Panagiotakaki

Sturge–Weber syndrome (SWS) is a rare, sporadic, congenital disorder arising from an early developmental lesion affecting the facial skin (usually a unilateral facial skin malformation, referred to as port-wine stain or PWS), the eye (glaucoma and associated choroidal or episcleral hemangioma), and the central nervous system (leptomeningeal angioma). Associated common neurological symptoms include epileptic seizures, hemiparesis, visual field deficits, and mental retardation. The degree of disability associated with SWS varies significantly between patients and some may remain seizure-free with no neurological deficits while others may present severe intractable epilepsy with profound neurological deficits and developmental delay. The incidence of the syndrome has not been formally assessed but it is estimated to be about 1 in 50 000 live births.

This syndrome was first reported, in 1860, by Schirmer who identified an association between bilateral facial angiomatous nevus and bilateral buphthalmos (eye enlargement). In 1879 Sturge described a relationship between facial and ocular angiomatous lesions and cerebral pathology that led to focal seizures, as well as hemiparesis contralateral to the facial angioma. Later, in 1897 Kalischer provided neuropathological confirmation of the cerebral lesions and in 1922 Weber described radiological evidence of intracranial calcifications that may be associated with the syndrome.

Clinical features

Based on the commonality of both skin and nervous system disorders, SWS belongs to a group referred to as phakomatoses. These are neurocutaneous syndromes and congenital neuroectodermal dysplasias and include neurofibromatosis, tuberous sclerosis, and von Hippel–Lindau syndromes, although unlike other phakomatoses, SWS is not associated with intracranial neoplasms (Di Rocco and Tamburrini 2006).

The classic features of SWS include facial port-wine stain (PWS or nevus flemus; predominantly in trigeminal V1–V3 distribution), congenital glaucoma, and leptomeningeal angiomatosis that leads to neurological sequelae such as epilepsy and progressive mental retardation. Other neurological symptoms include focal deficits, such as chronic hemiparesis, hemianopia, and stroke-like episodes with transient visual field defects or unilateral weakness. Episodes of migraine-like headaches are also reported that may be accompanied by transient hemiparesis. The association of neurological and developmental deterioration and the onset of seizures means that patients with SWS often suffer considerable disability.

The presence of PWS at birth may lead to a suspicion of SWS, although in most cases neurological deficits are absent. The extent of lesions that affect the facial skin, eyes, and central nervous system vary between patients, and in some cases only a single tissue may be affected. Roach (1992) designated different subtypes associated with the extent of angioma. Type 1 (reported in up to one-third of cases): both PWS and leptomeningeal angiomatosis and sometimes glaucoma. Type II (most common): PWS without evidence of leptomeningeal angiomatosis, with or without glaucoma. Type III (least reported): leptomeningeal angiomatosis without PWS and usually without glaucoma. Whereas the presence of PWS may be indicative of leptomeningeal angiomatosis, the advent of available magnetic resonance imaging (MRI) and computed tomography (CT) scanning techniques has identified cases of leptomeningeal angioma without PWS (type III). Types II and III are often referred to as incomplete SWS. In the authors' view the presence of leptomeningeal angiomatosis is a prerequisite for retaining the diagnosis of SWS.

Facial skin malformation

Usually PWS is the first symptom of the syndrome to be observed since it is visible at birth. In the general population, PWS affects 3 in 1000 people, but only about 8% of these individuals develop glaucoma or leptomeningeal angioma. The cutaneous malformation may be initially flat and pale pink, becoming more nodular with a deeper red or dark purple with age, although the extent of the malformation does not increase with age. Port-wine stain results from a vascular, rather than neural, disorder and is is caused by an increase in number and size of dermal capillaries (Parsa 2008).

The Causes of Epilepsy, eds. S. D. Shorvon, F. Andermann, and R. Guerrini. Published by Cambridge University Press. © Cambridge University Press 2011.

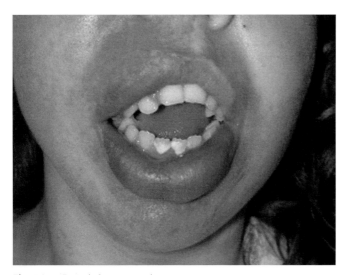

Fig. 26.1. Extended port-wine skin angioma.

Facial and leptomeningeal angiomas in the same patient may be ipsilateral or bilateral. The leptomeningeal angioma may be bilateral and facial angioma unilateral (Bebin and Gomez 1988; Aicardi 1992). In a recent study of 55 patients with leptomeningeal angioma, PWS was bilateral in 31% patients, unilateral in 65.5% patients, and absent in 5.5% patients (Pascual-Castroviejo *et al.* 2008). Extension of the lesion to both sides of the face, as well as other facial areas (Fig. 26.1) such as lips, palate, tongue, and larynx are common with possible involvement of the neck, trunk, and limbs, either ipsilateral or contralateral to the facial nevus. The PWS itself is benign, although the psychological impact of such a feature may lead patients to pursue cosmetic surgery. Patients with no cutaneous involvement appear to be at very low risk of any ocular manifestations.

Ocular manifestations

Ocular manifestations commonly include glaucoma in 28–70% of cases (Boltshauser *et al.* 1976; Cibis *et al.* 1984; Sullivan *et al.* 1992; Sujansky and Conradi 1995a; Mallea *et al.* 1997). Glaucoma may be present at birth but can develop at any age, even in adults. For almost half of bilateral PWS cases, glaucoma is also bilateral. Contralateral glaucoma is relatively rare and the greatest risk of ocular problems is associated with ipsilateral PWS that affects both the ophthalmic and maxillary areas (Uram and Zubillaga 1982; Enjolras *et al.* 1985). In a report by Sullivan *et al.* (1992) of 51 patients, 71% had glaucoma (onset before age 24 months), 69% had conjunctival or episcleral hemangiomas, and 55% had choroidal hemangiomas. Other secondary changes may also develop following choroidal hemangioma: retinal pigment epithelium degeneration, fibrous metaplasia, cystic retinal degeneration, and retinal detachment. Other ocular disorders associated with SWS include buphthalmos, retinal vascular tortuosity, iris heterochromia, optic disk coloboma, and cataracts.

The effect of choroidal or ciliary body hemangioma in SWS interferes with the angle of the eye, causing elevated episcleral venous pressure or hypersecretion of fluid. In children, glaucoma is due to an altered angle of the anterior chamber; in late-onset cases, glaucoma is largely due to an increased episcleral venous pressure. Left untreated, glaucoma leads to decreased vision and even blindness with increased intraocular pressure that damages the optic nerve.

Abnormalities of the central nervous system

The leptomeningeal angioma more frequently involves the parieto-occipital region (Fig. 26.2) but also the entire hemisphere (Fig. 26.3), usually unihemispheric but also bihemispheric. The extent or location of the angioma does not necessarily correlate with severity and whereas bihemispheric angioma is reported to be associated with poor outcome (Pascual-Castroviejo *et al.* 1993), many reports also indicate that global cognitive impairment is present in patients with unihemispheric angioma. The leptomeningeal angioma consists of a complex of distorted blood vessels that involve the pia mater and subarachnoid space. The deep medullar veins and choroid plexus are typically enlarged with blood (Fig. 26.4), whilst the cortical veins are reduced in number. The natural history of the disease is characterized by the development of cortical calcifications, gliosis and cerebral atrophy. The presence of a choroidal angioma leads to the association of glaucoma.

Epilepsy

Epileptic seizures are the predominant symptom of SWS and occur in about 80% of cases presenting PWS and leptomeningeal angioma. The onset of seizures is variable and reported to occur anywhere between birth and 23 years of age. Of those that develop epilepsy, most do so early in life, with 63–75% within the first year (Sujansky and Conradi 1995a; Bourgeois *et al.* 2007). For these patients, epilepsy may be difficult to control and is associated with progressive neurological deterioration, intellectual impairment, hemiparesis and episodes of status epilepticus (Hoffman *et al.* 1979; Oakes 1992; Sujansky and Conradi 1995b). These early seizures may be triggered by fever in about one-third of cases, and are often long-lasting and consist of unilateral status epilepticus. Early seizure onset is also associated with bilateral involvement and a worse developmental prognosis. Most seizure types are reported to be focal with frequent secondary generalization (Hoffman *et al.* 1979; Ogunmekan *et al.* 1989; Erba and Cavazzuti 1990; Arzimanoglou and Aicardi 1992). Status epilepticus, occurring as prolonged clonic seizures, is reported in 50% of cases, and less commonly, infantile spasms and myoclonic seizures (Arzimanoglou and Aicardi 1992).

Unilateral convulsive status, reported in about half of cases that present epilepsy or an episode of serial seizures is often followed by hemiplegia during the first year of life (Arzimanoglou and Aicardi 1992). These acquired hemiplegias closely resemble

A   B

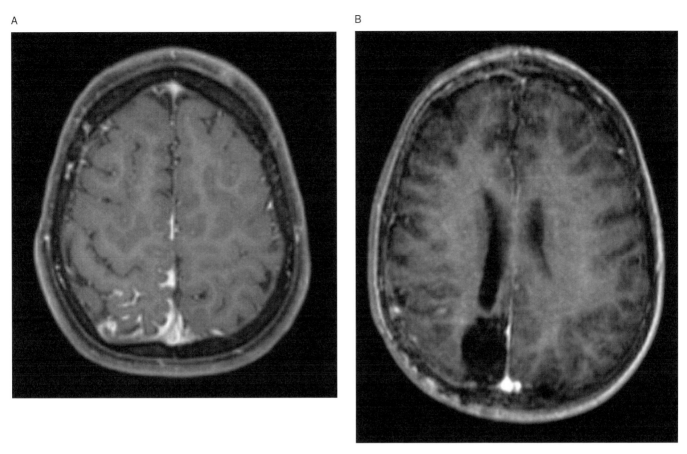

Fig. 26.2. Pial angioma investigated by gadolinium-enhanced MRI: (A) pre-operative; (B) post-operative confirming complete resection following simple lesionectomy; patient seizure-free.

those observed in the hemiconvulsion–hemiplegia–epilepsy (HHE) syndrome. Cases of transient hemiplegia, not preceded by epileptic seizures, also occur. These transitory phenomena often present with headache, vomiting, and other features reminiscent of migraine and may result from a temporary circulatory deficit or subclinical ictal activity.

There is a strong association between the presence of seizures and the occurrence of other neurologic abnormalities; for example, in one large study, mental retardation was only reported in patients with seizures (Bebin and Gomez 1988). Transient neurological sequelae are generally considered to be the result of epileptiform activity, as seizures are the most common symptom of the syndrome. However, such sequelae may result from temporary ischemia of the cortex that underlies the vascular malformation. The occurrence of transient focal deficits therefore presents a diagnostic challenge and adequate differentiation between epileptic and ischemic origins is important with regards to therapy.

Electroencephalograms (EEGs) vary between patients and include focal or generalized discharges as well as non-epileptiform background amplitude asymmetry. The interictal EEG in SWS typically shows focal or unilateral depression of background activity over the area of the leptomeningeal

angiomatosis. A characteristic feature of EEG patterns in patients with SWS is the attenuation and excess of slow activities. Polymorphic delta activity (classically associated with ischemia) colateralizes with angiomatosis when unilateral (Arzimanoglou and Aicardi 1992; Arzimanoglou *et al.* 2000) and was reported to be related to severe mental retardation in one study (Sassower *et al.* 1994). The absence of interictal spiking and the presence of EEG seizure discharges only in the periphery of the lesion may indicate focal ischemia (Sassower *et al.* 1994).

For bilateral lesions, EEG abnormalities may be identified earlier than for unilateral lesions. Bilateral paroxysmal activity may be associated with more frequent seizures and lower IQ and the occurrence of apparently generalized seizures, including occasional infantile spasms (Fukuyama and Tsuchiya 1979; Chevrie *et al.* 1988). Despite the presence of bilateral EEG abnormalities, such cases may respond well to resective surgery (Rosen *et al.* 1984; Chevrie *et al.* 1988).

Etiology

Little is known of the etiology of SWS. The incidence is very low within families and the syndrome is not shared between monozygotic twins. The sporadic, non-hereditary nature of the

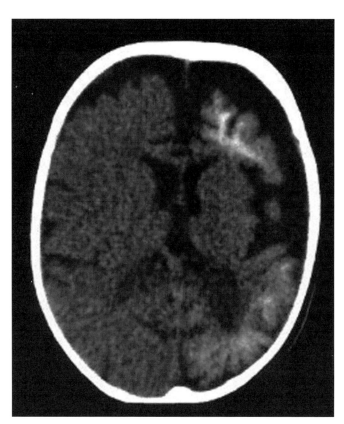

Fig. 26.3. CT scan of hemispheric SWS with atrophy and calcifications.

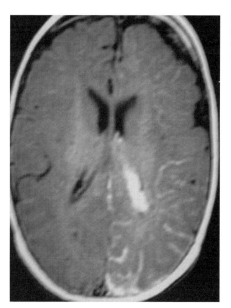

Fig. 26.4. MRI scan showing extended pial angiomatosis and enlarged choroid plexus.

disorder therefore indicates that somatic mutations are responsible. Happle (1987) proposed that SWS is due to a sporadic autosomal dominant mutation that occurs during development but is non-transmissible since it imparts lethality at an earlier stage of development. The resultant somatic mosaicism would likely thus affect development of the neural crest during the first trimester of pregnancy (Di Rocco and Tamburrini 2006). Abnormalities of cerebral vascularization are believed to start between 4 and 8 weeks' gestation. At this early stage, the ectoderm that will become the forehead skin is juxtaposed to the part of the neural tube, destined to become the occipital lobe of the cerebral hemisphere (Etchevers *et al.* 2001). The facial dermis, leptomeninges, and ocular choroid are all mesenchymal derivatives of the neurectodermal germ layer or mesectoderm.

The pathogenesis of SWS is believed to originate from localized primary venous dysplasia, and the severity of symptoms to be dependent on the extent and location of venous dysplasia (Parsa 2008). This may occur in one or both cerebral hemispheres. The resultant leptomeningeal angiomatosis is caused by the lack of cortical bridging veins and persistence of the vascular plexus, leading to engorgement of veins by redirected blood flow. The cortical bridging veins ensure bidirectional cerebral blood flow between the superficial parts of the brain (leptomeningeal and facial that are primarily drained by the superior sagittal sinus) and the deeper structures (choroidal plexus veins and ophthalmic veins that are drained by the cavernous sinus, straight sinus, and other deep veins). Venous engorgement is worsened by an increase in blood flow as a consequence of increased oxygen and glucose demand during normal brain development and seizures (Parsa 2008). Reduced blood flow (Probst 1980; Chiron *et al.* 1989) and glucose utilization (Chugani *et al.* 1989) have been reported in SWS patients. Evidence using position emission tomography (PET) indicates that hypometabolism may be more widespread than the area of hemangioma (Chugani *et al.* 1989).

Treatment

The treatment of SWS is symptomatic. Port-wine stain may be reduced or removed using laser therapy (commonly with a pulsed dye laser) as early as possible. Drug therapy (β-blocker drops) may be used to treat glaucoma and photodynamic therapy for choroidal hemangioma. Stroke-like episodes and hemiparesis may be treated with physical or occupational therapy. Low-dose aspirin is reported to reduce stroke-like episodes by improving blood flow and preventing potential thrombus formation (Maria *et al.* 1998); however, it is controversial whether this is appropriate for young children (Greco *et al.* 2008) and controlled studies are not available. Behavioral problems are treated with relevant therapy and medication (e.g., methylphenidate, clonidine).

Seizures are reported to be benign in as many as one-fourth of patients in one study (Erba and Cavazzuti 1990) and could be controlled with antiepileptic drugs in 40–50% of patients in others (Arzimanoglou and Aicardi 1992; Sujansky and

Table 26.1 Sturge–Weber syndrome: clinical symptoms suggesting progression

Initially focal seizures evolving to frequent episodes with secondary generalization
Increasing frequency and duration of seizures
Increasing duration of postictal deficits
Installation of a hemi-deficit
Evolution of focal or diffuse atrophy in serial CT scans
Progressive enlargement of the calcified lesions
Signs of psychomotor regression

Conradi 1995a). All available antiepileptic drugs for the treatment of focal seizures are indicated.

The potential consequence of seizures on the development of neurological sequelae, which often impose serious disability, necessitates prolonged and aggressive antiepileptic treatment. A particular risk occurs with repeated episodes of status epilepticus or prolonged seizures, which can result in a step-wise progression of focal deficits (Table 26.1). In about 40–60% cases, seizures become progressively refractory to medical treatment and surgery is considered (Erba and Cavazzuti 1990; Arzimanoglou and Aicardi 1992; Di Rocco and Tamburrini 2006).

Surgery

When patients with SWS are not seizure-free with medical treatment they should be considered as candidates for epilepsy surgery early in the course of the disorder. Recently proposed criteria (Kwan et al. 2010) for the definition of drug resistance (i.e., failure of two antiepileptic drugs) particularly apply to SWS and other lesional epilepsies.

For children with hemispheric unilateral leptomenigeal angiomatosis, *hemispherotomy*, in order to maximize developmental progress and reduce the chance of neurologic deterioration (Ogunmekan et al. 1989; Hoffman 1997; Arzimanoglou et al. 2000) is the treatment of choice. Issues to be considered are the presence or absence of hemiplegia. For patients that present with transient postictal hemiplegia and drug-resistant epilepsy (Kwan et al. 2010) early surgery is the option. This is particularly true when the postictal hemiparesis is becoming progressively longer, as this usually rapidly leads to a permanent deficit. Early surgery also prevents psychomotor regression. Late surgery may also control seizures (Kossoff et al. 2002) but psychomotor regression by that time may become irreversible.

More recently, the success of surgery in controlling seizures was shown not to be dependent on patient age at all at the time of surgery, but rather the extent of resection or disconnection of affected tissue (Bourgeois et al. 2007). Consequently, criteria for surgery in patients with SWS are similar to those applied to other lesional epilepsy cases, i.e., is it possible to completely remove the epileptogenic zone (in that case the region related to the leptomeningeal angioma) without creating additional irreversible neurological sequelae (Arzimanoglou and Aicardi 1992; Arzimanoglou et al. 2000;)

As a prerequisite to surgery, the full extent of the pial angioma is investigated firstly by gadolinium-enhanced MRI. This technique is preferred over CT since it is more sensitive to identify and determine the extent of leptomeningeal enhancement and parenchymal atrophy (Benedikt et al. 1993) and is also useful for the identification of pial angioma in pre-symptomatic patients (Griffiths 1996). Magnetic resonance imaging should be performed at a distance of a seizure event to avoid false interpretation of gadolinium enhancement, due to contrast leakage because of alteration of the blood–brain barrier. Short echo and long repetition time and/or echo time studies should be conducted. Gyriform calcifications are best identified using gradient-echo MRI sequences or particularly CT, which in this case, is more sensitive than MRI (Fig. 26.3). An enhanced CT scan does not outline the superficial angiomatosis, but it does demonstrate cortical enhancement due to post-epileptic increases in the blood–brain barrier permeability. Single photon emission computed tomography (SPECT) or position emission tomography (PET) scanning may provide additional information (Chiron et al. 1989; Chugani et al. 1989).

The outcome of resective surgery (lesionectomy, lobectomy, or circumscribed cortical resection) is reported to be satisfactory in a number of reports (Hoffman et al. 1979; Rosen et al. 1984; Erba and Cavazzuti 1990; Ito et al. 1990; Aicardi 1992; Arzimanoglou and Aicardi 1992; Arzimanoglou 1997; Arzimanoglou et al. 2000). In cases with more extensive lesions and in children with pre-existing hemiplegia, hemispherectomy is advocated. In a study of 20 patients surgically treated using different approaches, including callosotomy (1 patient), hemispherectomy (5 patients), and cortical resection (14 patients), 13 became seizure-free and almost all benefited from the surgery irrespective of age at seizure onset and type of operation (Arzimanoglou et al. 2000).

In cases with a unilateral leptomeningeal angioma and bilateral EEG abnormalities or generalized seizures, surgery is not contraindicated. Decision-making for cases with bilateral angiomatosis is much more difficult and no controlled studies are available.

The early onset of seizures is strongly associated with progression of neurological sequelae and development of intellectual deficits. The decision to undertake surgery is thus complex and a multidisciplinary approach (between the epilepsy team, patient, and family) is required for each individual case early in the course of the disorder (Comi 2007).

References

Aicardi J (1992) *Diseases of the Nervous System in Childhood.* London: McKeith Press.

Arzimanoglou A (1997) The surgical treatment of Sturge–Weber syndrome with respect to its clinical spectrum. In: Tuxhorn I, Holthausen H, Boenigk H (eds.) *Pediatric Epilepsy Syndromes and Their Surgical Treatment.* London: John Libbey, pp. 353–63.

Arzimanoglou A, Aicardi J (1992) The epilepsy of Sturge–Weber syndrome: clinical features and treatment in 23 patients. *Acta Neurol Scand* (Suppl.) **140**:18–22.

Arzimanoglou AA, Andermann F, Aicardi J, *et al.* (2000) Sturge–Weber syndrome: indications and results of surgery in 20 patients. *Neurology* **55**:1472–9.

Bebin EM, Gomez RM (1988) Sturge–Weber syndrome. In: Gomez RM (ed.) *Neurocutaneous Diseases: A Practical Approach.* London: Butterworth-Heinemann, pp. 356–67.

Benedikt RA, Brown DC, Walker R, *et al.* (1993) Sturge–Weber syndrome: cranial MR imaging with Gd-DTPA. *AJNR Am J Neuroradiol* **14**:409–15

Bioxeda P, de Misa RF, Arrazola JM, *et al.* (1993) Facial angioma and the Sturge–Weber syndrome: a study of 121 cases. *Med Clin (Barc)* **101**:1–4.

Boltshauser E, Wilson J, Hoare RD (1976) Sturge–Weber syndrome with bilateral intracranial calcification. *J Neurol Neurosurg Psychiatry* **39**:429–35.

Bourgeois M, Crimmins DW, de Oliveira RS, *et al.* (2007) Surgical treatment of epilepsy in Sturge–Weber syndrome in children. *J Neurosurg* **106**(1 Suppl):20–8.

Chevrie JJ, Specola N, Aicardi J (1988) Secondary bilateral synchrony in unilateral pial angiomatosis: successful surgical treatment. *J Neurol Neurosurg Psychiatry* **51**:663–70.

Chiron C, Raynaud C, Tzourio N, *et al.* (1989) Regional cerebral blood flow by SPECT imaging in Sturge–Weber disease: an aid for diagnosis. *J Neurol Neurosurg Psychiatry* **52**:1402–9.

Chugani HT, Mazziotta JC, Phelps ME (1989) Sturge–Weber syndrome: a study of cerebral glucose utilization with positron emission tomography. *J Pediatr* **2**:244–53.

Cibis GW, Tripathi RC, Tripathi BJ (1984) Glaucoma in Sturge–Weber syndrome. *Ophthalmology* **91**:1061–71.

Comi AM (2007) Sturge–Weber syndrome and epilepsy: an argument for aggressive seizure management in these patients. *Expert Rev Neurother* **7**:951–6.

Di Rocco C, Tamburrini G (2006) Sturge–Weber syndrome. *Childs Nerv Syst* **22**:909–21.

Enjolras O, Riche MC, Merland JJ (1985) Facial port-wine stains and Sturge–Weber syndrome. *Pediatrics* **76**:48–51.

Erba G, Cavazzuti V (1990) Sturge–Weber syndrome: natural history and indications for surgery. *J Epilepsy* **3**(Suppl.):287–91.

Etchevers HC, Vincent C, Le Douarin NM, Couly GF (2001) The cephalic neural crest provides pericytes and smooth muscle cells to all blood vessels of the face and forebrain. *Development* **128**:1059–68.

Fukuyama Y, Tsuchiya S (1979) A study on Sturge–Weber syndrome: report of a case associated with infantile spasms and electroencephalographic evolution in five cases. *Eur Neurol* **18**:194–209.

Greco F, Fiumara A, Sorge G, Pavone L (2008) Subgaleal hematoma in a child with Sturge–Weber syndrome: to prevent stroke-like episodes, is treatment with aspirin advisable? *Childs Nerv Syst* **24**:1479–81.

Griffiths PD (1996) Sturge–Weber syndrome revisited: the role of neuroradiology. *Neuropediatrics* **27**:284–94.

Happle R (1987) Lethal genes surviving by mosaicism: a possible explanation for sporadic birth defects involving the skin. *J Am Acad Dermatol* **16**:899–906.

Hoffman HJ (1997) Benefits of early surgery in Sturge–Weber syndrome. In: Tuxhorn I, Holthausen H, Boenigk H (eds.) *Pediatric Epilepsy Syndromes and Their Surgical Treatment.* London: John Libbey, pp. 364–70.

Hoffman HJ, Hendrick EB, Dennis M, Armstrong D (1979) Hemispherectomy for Sturge–Weber syndrome. *Childs Brain* **5**:233–48.

Ito M, Sato K, Ohnuki A, Uto A (1990) Sturge–Weber disease: operative indications and surgical results. *Brain Dev* **12**:473–7.

Klapper J (1994) Headache in Sturge–Weber syndrome. *Headache* **34**:521–2.

Kossoff EH, Buck C, Freeman JM (2002) Outcomes of 32 hemispherectomies for Sturge–Weber syndrome worldwide. *Neurology* **59**:1735–8.

Kossoff EH, Hatfield LA, Ball KL, Comi AM (2005) Comorbidity of epilepsy and headache in patients with Sturge–Weber syndrome. *J Child Neurol* **20**:678–82.

Kwan P, Arzimanoglou A, Berg AT, *et al.* (2010). Definition of drug resistant epilepsy: consensus proposal by the ad hoc Task Force of the ILAE Commission on Therapeutic Strategies. *Epilepsia* **51**:1069–77.

Mallea MJ, Heras GI, Aguirre BP, *et al.* (1997) Sturge-Weber syndrome: experience with 14 cases. *An Esp Pediatr.* **46**(2):138–42.

Maria BL, Neufeld JA, Rosainz LC, (1998) Central nervous system structure and function in Sturge–Weber syndrome: evidence of neurologic and radiologic progression. *J Child Neurol* **13**:606–18.

Mazereeuw-Hautier J, Syed S, Harper JI (2006) Bilateral facial capillary malformation associated with eye and brain abnormalities. *Arch Dermatol* **142**:994–8.

Oakes WJ (1992) The natural history of patients with the Sturge–Weber syndrome. *Pediatr Neurosurg* **18**:287–90.

Ogunmekan AO, Hwang PA, Hoffman HJ (1989) Sturge–Weber–Dimitri disease: role of hemispherectomy in prognosis. *Can J Neurol Sci* **16**:78–80.

Parsa CF (2008) Sturge–Weber syndrome: a unified pathophysiologic mechanism. *Curr Treat Options Neurol* **10**:47–54.

Pascual-Castroviejo I, Díaz-Gonzalez C, García-Melian RM, Gonzalez-Casado I, Muñoz-Hiraldo E (1993) Sturge–Weber syndrome: study of 40 patients. *Pediatr Neurol* **9**:283–8.

Pascual-Castroviejo I, Pascual-Pascual SI, Velazquez-Fragua R, Viaño J (2008) Sturge–Weber syndrome: study of 55 patients. *Can J Neurol Sci* **35**:301–7.

Probst FP (1980) Vascular morphology and angiographic flow patterns in Sturge–Weber angiomatosis: facts, thoughts and suggestions. *Neuroradiology* **20**:73–8.

Roach ES (1992) Neurocutaneous syndromes. *Pediatr Clin N Am* **39**:591–620.

Rosen I, Salford L, Starck L (1984) Sturge–Weber disease: neurophysiological evaluation of a case with secondary epileptogenesis, successfully treated with lobe-ectomy. *Neuropediatrics* **15**:95–8.

Sassower K, Duchowny P, Jayakar T, (1994) EEG evaluation of children with Sturge–Weber syndrome and epilepsy. *J Epilepsy* **7**:285–9.

Sujansky E, Conradi S (1995a) Sturge–Weber syndrome: age of onset of seizures and glaucoma and the prognosis for affected children. *J Child Neurol* **10**:49–58.

Sujansky E, Conradi S (1995b) Outcome of Sturge–Weber syndrome in 52 adults. *Am J Med Genet* **57**:35–45.

Sullivan TJ, Clarke MP, Morin JD (1992) The ocular manifestations of the Sturge–Weber syndrome. *J Pediatr Ophthalmol Strabismus* **29**:349–56.

Tallman B, Tan OT, Morelli JG, *et al.* (1991) Location of port-wine stains and the likelihood of ophthalmic and/or central nervous system complications. *Pediatrics* **87**:323–7.

Uram M, Zubillaga C (1982) The cutaneous manifestations of Sturge–Weber syndrome. *J Clin Neuroophthalmol* **2**:245–8.

Other neurocutaneous syndromes

Ignacio Pascual-Castroviejo

Introduction

Tuberous sclerosis complex (TSC) and Sturge–Weber syndrome (SWS) are the neurocutaneous disorders (NCD) that are most frequently associated with epilepsy. Neurofibromatosis type 1 (NF1), on the contrary, is one of the most common NCD, but is associated with a low prevalence (between 3% and 7%) of epilepsy.

Seventy different NCD have been described in a recent publication (Ruggieri *et al*. 2008). Several of these, in addition to TSC, SWS, and NF1, are associated with epilepsy in an important number of cases. These NCD mainly are the following.

Hypomelanosis of Ito and related disorders (pigmentary mosaicism)

The term hypomelanosis of Ito (HI) (OMIM #30033) encompasses a heterogeneous group of cutaneous disorders characterized by hypopigmented whorls and streaks following the lines of Blaschko. Seizures may occur in about 50% of cases (Pascual-Castroviejo *et al*. 1998) commonly appear early, within the first year of life, and are associated with severe electroencephalographic (EEG) changes. Seizures frequently are refractory to anticonvulsant drugs and in 8% of cases manifest as infantile spasms (Pascual-Castroviejo *et al*. 1998). Mental retardation is observed in 50–60% of cases. Seizures and mental retardation are often caused by underlying neuronal migration disorders, and may be accompanied by macrocephaly or microcephaly. The most frequent intracranial structural anomalies are cerebellar hypoplasia or atrophy, generalized or focal cerebral atrophy, cerebral dysplasias, and/or other migration abnormalities, often associated with hemimegalencephaly. Other anomalies include gray matter heterotopia, agyria, polymicrogyria, and porencephaly.

Chromosomal mosaicism is recognized as the pathogenic basis of many cases of HI and related disorders. It can explain the protean clinical manifestations of this condition and their often asymmetrical expression. Several different chromosomal abnormalities have been documented in about 30–60% of the reported cases and in a recent literature review different types of mosaicism have been identified (Taibjee *et al*. 2004).

Incontinentia pigmenti

Also known as Bloch–Sulzberger syndrome (OMIM #308310), incontinentia pigmenti (IP) is a rare ectodermal dysplasia that segregates as an X-linked dominant disorder and is usually lethal to affected males in utero. The gene responsible for IP maps to Xq28, a region known to encode the nuclear factor kB essential modulator (NEMO).

The prominent skin signs occur in four classic cutaneous stages: (1) perinatal inflammation with erythematous and vesicular rash; (2) verrucous patches; (3) a distinctive pattern of hyperpigmentation; and (4) dermal scarring.

Other tissues and organs, such as hair, nails (with subungual painful keratotic tumors which must be radically removed despite their histologic benignity), eyes, teeth, breast, skeletal, and other systems can be also involved. The central nervous system (CNS) is affected in 30–50% of patients, with consequent mental retardation, seizures, spasticity, microcephaly, somatic malformations secondary to unilateral or bilateral cerebral lesions, and cerebellar ataxia. Generalized or mainly focal seizures are present in 25% of patients (Pascual-Castroviejo *et al*. 2006). Bilaterality of the brain lesions and seizures in the first week of life may indicate a poor prognosis and betoken subsequent developmental delay.

Magnetic resonance imaging (MRI) does not reveal abnormalities in IP patients without neurologic disease. Cerebral lesions of IP patients commonly extend radially through cortical and subcortical zones, involving cortex, subcortical and deep white matter, ependymal and subependymal zones of one or both cerebral hemispheres (Fig. 27.1).

Nevus sebaceous syndrome or Schimmelpenning/nevus sebaceous syndrome

This condition has two different entries in the OMIM catalogue (OMIM #163200 and OMIM #165630). Nevus sebaceous (NS) is a relatively common type of cutaneous lesion characterized by epidermal acanthosis and hyperplasia of the sebaceous glands

---

The Causes of Epilepsy, eds. S. D. Shorvon, F. Andermann, and R. Guerrini. Published by Cambridge University Press. © Cambridge University Press 2011.

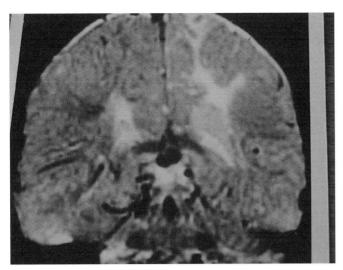

Fig. 27.1. Incontinentia Pigmenti (IP): coronal T2-weighted (2000/100) image shows asymmetric increased signal in the deep white matter of both cerebral hemispheres, more extensively on the left side, which also presents cortical and ependymal involvement.

which, when coupled with extracutaneous manifestations (mostly of the central nervous, ocular or skeletal systems), gives the name to a complex malformation syndrome (NS syndrome or NS of Jadassohn), The prevalence of NS rages from 1 to 3 per 1000 live births. Males and females are equally affected. Histological rather than clinical characteristics of the lesions appear to be more reliable to distinguish the type of epidermal nevus. The clinical and histological appearance of the lesions changes with age. The lesion is typically flat during early infancy, but at puberty often thickens. The cutaneous lesions may take a verrucous appearance at any time during the course of the disease.

The most common associated neurological abnormalities are seizures, mental retardation, and/or developmental delay. The seizure disorders are often of early onset, almost always occurring during the first 8 months of life. Prevalence of seizures in NS syndrome as described in the international literature vary from 38% to 96% and in a review of the British literature a percentage higher than 50% in patients with epidermal naevi of the NS and keratinocytic types (Gurecki *et al.* 1996). Seizures in NS are often resistant to medical therapy and cause severe neurological sequelae. The neurological picture is more severe in the presence of many types of seizures, such as focal, generalized, and infantile spasms, which are often followed by Lennox–Gastaut syndrome. Major hemispheric malformations predispose patients to neonatal seizures, infantile spasms and the Lennox–Gastaut variant.

Linear scleroderma (morphea) "en coup de sabre"

This disorder represents a unique form of localized scleroderma that primarily affects the pediatric population. It is characterized by atrophic, band-like regions of indurations involving the frontoparietal area of the forehead and scalp,

most frequently unilaterally, although bilateral involvement has been described in some patients. The internal area of the eyebrow, eyelid, ala nasi, and lateral zone of the nose may also be involved with progressive involution of the craniofacial bones, resulting in mild to severe hemifacial atrophy similar to that seen in the Parry–Romberg syndrome (Untenberger *et al.* 2003).

The most frequent neurologic manifestations are seizures, most commonly focal, followed in order of frequency by depressive mood, low self-esteem, decreased school performances of variable degree, and hemiparesis. Skull and cerebral atrophy in the tissues subjacent the affected skin may be found some years after the onset of the disorder. The pathogenesis is not completely understood.

Progressive facial hemiatrophy (Parry–Romberg syndrome)

This disease (OMIM #141300) is characterized by progressive and self-limited shrinking and deformation of one side of the face, which involves different tissues, scar-like cutaneous changes, subcutaneous connective and fatty tissue atrophy, circumscribed osteoporosis, bone deformation commonly accompanied by contralateral focal epilepsy, trigeminal neuralgia, and changes in the eyes and hair. Epilepsy usually appears after a variable period of evolution when the subcortical lesions are apparent in the cerebral hemisphere ipsilateral to the facial hemiatrophy (Dupont *et al.* 1997). Cerebral lesions can be demonstrated by standard imaging (computed tomography ([CT] or MRI) techniques (Moon *et al.* 2008).

Pascual-Castroviejo type II syndrome

Pascual-Castroviejo type II syndrome (P-CIIS) is also known as PHACE association (OMIM #606519). The relationship of two main cutaneous vascular anomalies, hemangiomas and vascular malformations, with intracranial and/or extracranial vascular and non-vascular abnormalities and the higher presentation in females were established by Pascual-Castroviejo (1978; Pascual-Castroviejo *et al.* 1995, 1996). The P-CIIS is the most frequent neurocutaneous syndrome (Pascual-Castroviejo *et al.* 1996; Pascual-Castroviejo 2008). Both types of cutaneous lesions, hemangioma (a vascular tumor with rapid endothelial cell proliferation and spontaneous involution) and vascular malformations (composed of dysplastic vessels without cellular proliferation) can be located in any area of the body (Fig. 27.2). They are frequently associated with internal abnormalities, such as absence of cerebral arteries (mainly carotid, vertebral, or anterior cerebral arteries), presence of persistent embryonic arteries (trigeminal or proatlantal arteries), cerebellar malformation, coarctation of the aortic arch, and cardiac malformation, preferentially in patients with facial, neck, and chest cutaneous vascular anomalies (Pascual-Castroviejo 1978, 2008; Pascual-Castroviejo *et al.* 1995, 1996, 2007), and brain migration or cortical organization disorders.

A

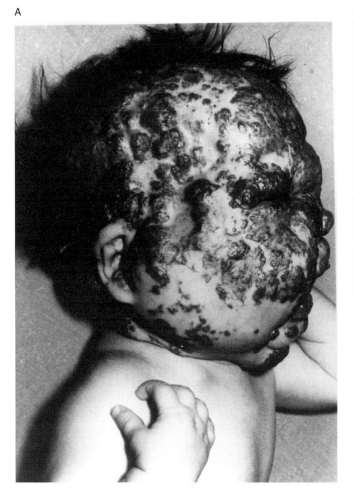

B

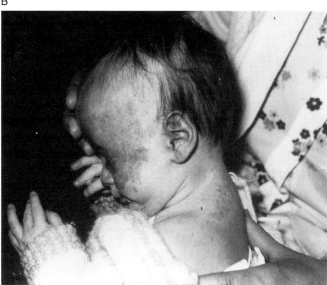

Fig. 27.2. Pascual-Castroviejo type II syndrome. (A) Voluminous right hemifacial hemangioma; (B) left hemifacial vascular malformation.

Seizures, usually of focal type, are present almost exclusively in patients with cortical dysplasia or hemispheric migration disorders (Pascual-Castroviejo *et al.* 1995, 2007). Pharmacological control of the seizures is possible in most of the patients with P-CIIS (Pascual-Castroviejo *et al.* 2007).

Neurocutaneous melanosis

This disease is a rare syndrome that affects males and females with the same frequency. The cutaneous lesions are present at birth as single or numerous giant melanotic nevi with abundant hair. The color of the skin and hair is similar; it may be very dark and light brown, but darker in persons of African descent. Neurological manifestations are caused by leptomeningeal melanosis, occur before the age of 2 years, and most often during the first year of life. The most frequent manifestations are caused by increased intracranial pressure. Increased head circumference, headaches, vomiting, meningeal signs, cranial nerve paralysis, generalized or focal seizures and papilledema are the most frequent features.

Oculocerebrocutaneous syndrome

This is a rare disease (OMIM #164180) characterized by bilateral anophthalmia and orbital cysts, typical skin lesions consisting of skin appendages, focal dermal hypoplasia/aplasia and punch-like defects, complex brain malformations (mostly of the Dandy–Walker type) associated with mental retardation and seizures. It has been suggested that the disorder is due to an autosomal dominant lethal somatic mutation that survives by mosaicism. Corticosubcortical anomalies, mainly polymicrogyria and heterotopia, and defects of corpus callosum may contribute to causing seizures (Pascual-Castroviejo *et al.* 2005).

Unilateral somatic intracranial hypoplasia

This is a rare syndrome that probably affects only females. The main clinical features are: unilateral hypoplasia that involves the upper and lower extremities, breast, and trunk, mental retardation, and partial epilepsy. Unilateral hypoplasia of a polymicrogyric cerebral hemisphere, of the brainstem, cerebellum, and of the intracranial arteries on the same side and a hypoplastic hemibody commonly occur (Pascual-Castroviejo et al. 1997).

The presence of seizures in other neurocutaneous disorders, such as nevus of Ota, Costello syndrome (Pascual-Castroviejo and Pascual-Pascual 2005), Proteus syndrome, Hallermann–Streiff syndrome, and others is possible in some cases, but is only rarely seen.

References

Dupont S, Catala M, Hasdboun D, et al. (1997) Progressive facial hemiatrophy and epilepsy: a common underlying dysgenetic mechanism. *Neurology* **48**:1013–18.

Gurecki PJ, Holden KR, Sahn EE, et al. (1996) Developmental neural abnormalities and seizures in epidermal nevus syndrome. *Dev Med Child Neurol* **38**:716–23.

Moon WJ, Kim HJ, Roh HG, et al. (2008) Diffusion tensor imaging and fiber tractectomy and Parry–Romberg syndrome. *AJNR Am J Neuroradiol* **29**:714–15.

Pascual-Castroviejo I (1978) Vascular and nonvascular intracranial malformations associated with external capillary hemangiomas. *Neuroradiology* **16**:82–4.

Pascual-Castroviejo I, Pascual-Pascual SI (2005) Síndrome de Costello: presentación de un caso con seguimiento durante 35 años. *Neurología* **20**:144–8.

Pascual-Castroviejo I, Viaño J, Pascual-Pascual SI, et al. (1995) Facial hemangioma, agenesis of internal carotid artery and cerebral cortex dysplasia: case report. *Neuroradiology* **37**:693–5.

Pascual-Castroviejo I, Viaño J, Moreno F, et al. (1996) Hemangiomas of the head, neck and chest with associated vascular and brain anomalies: a complex neurocutaneous syndrome. *AJNR Am J Neuroradiol* **17**:461–71.

Pascual-Castroviejo I, Pascual-Pascual SI, Viaño J, Martinez V (1997) Unilateral somatic and intracranial hypoplasia. *Neuropediatrics* **28**:341–4.

Pascual-Castroviejo I, Roche C, Martínez-Bermejo A, et al. (1998) Hypomelanosis of Ito: a study of 76 infantile cases. *Brain Dev* **20**:36–43.

Pascual-Castroviejo I, Pascual-Pascual SI, Velazquez-Fragua R, et al. (2005) Oculocerebrocutaneous (Delleman) syndrome: report of two cases. *Neuropediatrics* **36**:50–4.

Pascual-Castroviejo I, Pascual-Pascual SI, Velazquez-Fragua R, et al. (2006) Incontinentia pigmenti: Hallazgos clínicos y radiológicos en una serie de 12 pacientes. *Neurologia* **21**:239–48.

Pascual-Castroviejo I, Pascual-Pascual SI, López-Gutierrez JC, et al. (2007) Facial hemangioma and hemispheric migration disorder: presentation of five patients. *AJNR Am J Neuroradiol* **28**:1609–12.

Pascual-Castroviejo I (2008) Vascular birthmarks of infancy: PHACE association (Pascual-Castroviejo type II syndrome) and Cobb syndrome. In: Ruggieri M, Pascual-Castroviejo I, Di Rocco C (eds.) *Neurocutaneous Disorders: Phakomatoses and Hamartoneoplastic Syndromes*. New York: Springer-Verlag pp. 19–49.

Ruggieri M, Pascual-Castroviejo I, Di Rocco C (eds). (2008) *Neurocutaneous Disorders: Phakomatoses and Hamartoneoplastic Syndromes*. New York: Springer-Verlag.

Taibjee SM, Bennett DC, Moss C (2004) Abnormal pigmentation in hypomelanosis of Ito and pigmentary mosaicism: the role of pigmentary genes. *Br J Dermatol* **151**:269–82.

Untenberger I, Trinko E, Engelhardt K, et al. (2003) Linear scleroderma "en coup de sabre" coexisting with plaque-morphea: neuroradiological manifestations and response to corticosteroids. *J Neurol Neurosurg Psychiatry* **74**:661–4.

Angelman syndrome

Bernard Dan and Stewart G. Boyd

Angelman syndrome is characterized by developmental delay, absence of speech, motor impairment, epilepsy, and a peculiar behavioral phenotype with happy demeanor (Dan 2008). It is caused by lack of expression of the *UBE3A* gene, which can result from various abnormalities of chromosome 15q11–q13. Similar chromosome 15q11–q13 abnormalities result in either Angelman syndrome if they concern the chromosome inherited from the mother, or Prader–Willi syndrome (a clinically distinct condition with hypotonia, learning difficulties, obesity, and hypogonadism) if they concern the chromosome of paternal origin, illustrating the phenomenon of genomic imprinting. In about 70% of patients, Angelman syndrome is due to a de novo 15q11–q13 microdeletion on the maternally inherited chromosome that can be detected with fluorescence in situ hybridization (FISH). Approximately 2–3% of patients have inherited both copies of chromosome 15 from the father and none from the mother, i.e., paternal uniparental disomy. As a result, no functional copy of *UBE3A* is inherited from the mother. These patients statistically show a less severe phenotype than those with a deletion, with larger head circumference, less severe epilepsy, and more words, although eventual speech remains extremely limited (Lossie *et al.* 2001). Another 3–5% of patients have an imprinting defect resulting in the absence of the typical maternal pattern of DNA methylation. Phenotypically, they are indistinguishable from patients with uniparental disomy (Lossie *et al.* 2001). There is a mutation in the maternal *UBE3A* gene in 5–10% of patients, with high occurrence of private, de novo mutations. Finally, no cytogenetic or molecular abnormality can be found in up to 10% of typical cases.

Patients with Angelman syndrome have a remarkably high risk of epilepsy compared to many other neurodevelopmental disorders. In particular, early-childhood onset of refractory epilepsy with atypical absences and myoclonic seizures with susceptibility to non-convulsive status epilepticus is a common presentation. This may be due to propensity to hypersynchronous neuronal activity, which might be related to abnormal γ-amino-butyric acid

(GABA)-mediated transmission due to lack of *UBE3A* expression, or other factors. In recent years, there has been increasing awareness of the possibility of seizure disorder in adult patients.

Interictal electroencephalographic patterns

Interictal high-amplitude rhythmic electroencephalographic (EEG) patterns are distinctive and should be differentiated from epileptic activity (Boyd *et al.* 1988; Dan and Boyd 2003; Valente *et al.* 2003). They are included in the diagnostic criteria (Williams *et al.* 2006).

Pattern I (Fig. 28.1A) is most commonly identified. It consists of runs of high-amplitude, rhythmic 2–3/s activity seen predominantly over the frontal regions. It often appears continuously in young children, tends to become intermittent in later childhood, and may persist into adulthood, when it can be continuous (Laan *et al.* 1997). Several variants have been described (Valente *et al.* 2003), including a "Pattern IB" (Dan and Boyd 2003) which consists of runs of sharp slow waves (Fig. 28.1B).

Pattern II (Fig. 28.1C) consists of prolonged runs of moderate to high-amplitude rhythmic 4–6/s activity with centro-temporal predominance. It is common in young children but becomes uncommon after puberty.

Pattern III (Fig. 28.1D) consists of bursts or runs of high-amplitude 3–6/s rhythmic activity, sometimes containing small spikes, maximal over the occipital regions. It is often markedly facilitated by eye closure, drowsiness, and sleep (Boyd *et al.* 1988; Viani *et al.* 1995; Rubin *et al.* 1997). It may persist into adulthood.

Seizure disorder

Seizures occur in about 90% of patients (Pelc *et al.* 2008). Epilepsy is often more severe in patients with 15q11–q13 microdeletion (including genes encoding GABA_A receptor subunits) than in other molecular classes. This is consistent with generally milder neurobehavioral features in patients without a deletion (Lossie *et al.* 2001), although seizures tend

The Causes of Epilepsy, eds. S. D. Shorvon, F. Andermann, and R. Guerrini. Published by Cambridge University Press. © Cambridge University Press 2011.

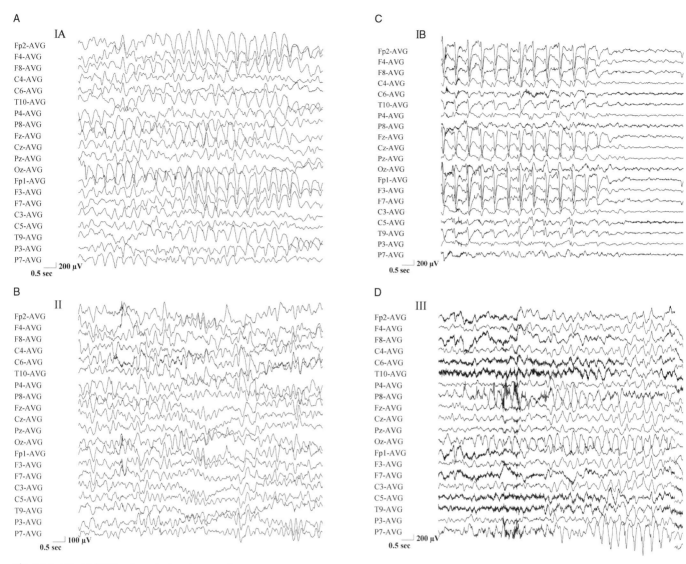

Fig. 28.1. Interictal EEG patterns in Angelman syndrome.

to occur in clusters alternating with seizure-free periods whatever the molecular class. The clusters occur apparently spontaneously or may be precipitated by factors such as infection, excitement, physical effort, intense fatigue, etc.

Epilepsy onset often precedes the diagnosis of Angelman syndrome. Seizure onset is often between 1 and 3 years. Fewer than 25% develop seizures before 12 months of age (Saitoh *et al.* 1994), 30% before 24 months (Buntinx *et al.* 1995). In infants, seizures tend to occur in a febrile context. Seizure types may evolve with age. As in other developmental conditions with epilepsy, the seizure disorder often improves in late childhood, though epilepsy can persist or reappear in adulthood, and be difficult to control.

Many seizure types, both generalized and focal, have been reported, including epileptic spasms, myoclonic absences, myoclonic, atonic, tonic and tonic–clonic seizures (Viani *et al.* 1995; Laan *et al.* 1997; Pelc *et al.* 2008), but absences and myoclonic seizures have been particularly emphasized.

Multiple seizure types occur in about half of the patients with a 15q11–q13 deletion.

Patterns of seizures, including type, age of onset, other clinical features, and EEG features of patients with Angelman syndrome may show some resemblance to defined epileptic syndromes. Correct characterization of their epilepsy is therefore important for both management and prognosis. West syndrome (infantile spasms), for example, has rarely been documented convincingly in Angelman syndrome; EEG patterns seen in Angelman syndrome can usually be differentiated easily from hypsarrhythmia (Dan and Boyd 2003; Valente *et al.* 2003). Similarly, although tonic seizures and complex absences can occur in Angelman syndrome, confusion with Lennox–Gastaut syndrome can be avoided without much difficulty in many cases. In contrast, myoclonic status in non-progressive encephalopathies has been appropriately recognized in a number of patients with Angelman syndrome (Dalla Bernardina *et al.* 1995) (and in other conditions, e.g., Wolf–Hirschhorn syndrome or non-ketotic hyperglycine-mia). Epilepsy with continuous spike–wave discharges during sleep has rarely been documented in Angelman syndrome (Rubin et al. 1997).

Both convulsive and non-convulsive status epilepticus (NCSE) may occur. The latter is particularly common during childhood, but it can occur in infancy (Ogawa et al. 1996) and adulthood (Espay et al. 2005). The EEG shows continuous epileptic discharges which are distinct from the typical rhythmic EEG features of Angelman syndrome (Dan and Boyd 2003). Frequent or prolonged episodes of NCSE may contribute to a poor cognitive outcome, as suggested in other conditions with epilepsy.

In adolescents or adults, particularly, prolonged disabling tremor has been ascribed to cortical myoclonus (Guerrini et al. 1996) or myoclonic status (Ogawa et al. 1996). The underlying mechanism remains unclear. It seems to be non-epileptic in some cases, where response to levodopa (Harbord 2001), reserpine or topiramate (Stecker and Myers 2003) has been documented. Some cases suggestive of cortical myoclonus responded to piracetam (Guerrini et al. 1996).

Pathophysiology

Although epilepsy has been one of the most studied aspects of Angelman syndrome, the underlying pathophysiology is still a matter of speculation. It has been hypothesized to be related to GABA$_A$ receptor dysfunction, primarily because the common 15q11–q13 microdeletion contains genes for three of its subunits (α5, β3, and γ3). These genes are expressed in several regions of the adult brain and are even more abundant in the embryonic and neonatal brain (Laurie et al. 1992). Hemizygosity of these genes has been suggested to underlie deficits in GABA-related neural synchrony mechanisms (Egawa et al. 2008). This could explain the propensity for more severe epilepsy in patients with a 15q11–q13 microdeletion. Knockout mice for Gabrb3, Gabrg3, and Gabra5 (Culiat et al. 1994) or for Gabrb3 alone (DeLorey et al. 1998) have been proposed as animal models for Angelman syndrome. The most relevant of these models appears to be the latter, which shows epilepsy and other abnormalities that show similarities to Angelman syndrome (DeLorey et al. 1998). In double knock-out Gabrb3$^{-/-}$ mice, virtual abolition of GABA-mediated reciprocal inhibition specifically in the thalamic reticular nucleus and dramatically increased oscillatory synchrony were demonstrated in vitro (Huntsman et al. 1999) and correlated with in vivo studies in these mice (Handforth et al. 2005), although no rhythmic EEG activities were observed and only irregular seizure-related discharges were recorded from the cortex in Gabrb3$^{-/-}$ mice (DeLorey et al. 1998). Disruption of GABRB3 does not account for all features of Angelman syndrome. For example, patients with other 15q11–q13 cytogenetic alterations (e.g. Prader–Willi syndrome, inverted duplicated chromosome 15 syndrome) have distinct clinical phenotypes. Furthermore, about 30% of patients with Angelman syndrome do not have a

deletion involving the GABRB3 gene, i.e., those with imprinting defect, uniparental disomy, UBE3A mutation, or no detectable 15q11–q13 abnormality.

In contrast, all patients with a molecular diagnosis of Angelman syndrome have a functional absence of the maternally inherited UBE3A gene. The gene product (UBE3A) acts as an E3 ubiquitin–protein ligase along the ubiquitin pathway. The best-characterized function of ubiquitination is to mark target proteins for specific proteolysis by proteasomes. Ubiquitin-mediated proteolysis may be important in a number of neuronal processes, including synaptogenesis and mechanisms of long-term memory. The ubiquitin pathway may also be involved in regulating abundance of postsynaptic receptors (Burbea et al. 2002). Functional absence of UBE3A may thus impair the regulation of GABA$_A$ receptors (Dan and Boyd 2003). In this hypothesis, altered regulation of β3-subunit-containing GABA$_A$ receptors would lead to "compensation" involving isoforms of the GABA$_A$ receptor that do not contain the β3-subunit, possibly changing the receptors' kinetics and desensitization properties. Although these changes are expected to be subtle, they may have extensive effects during brain maturation as well as through the patient's life.

Another mouse model with inactivated maternally inherited Ube3a gene showed deficits in hippocampal long-term potentiation (Weeber et al. 2003), pointing to a possible role of glutamatergic neurotransmission. In this model, electrocorticography showed almost continuous rhythmic 3/s activity mixed with polyspikes and slow waves (Jiang et al. 1998).

Other less specific mechanisms are likely to play major roles in epilepsy seen in Angelman syndrome and other neurodevelopmental disorders. Synaptic modulation and plasticity probably deserve more attention. In addition, the potential role of non-synaptic mechanisms of neuronal synchrony, such as gap junctions, has not been investigated (except in the cerebellum [Cheron et al. 2005]). The complexity of these interactions throughout brain maturation suggests that late, targeted molecular intervention cannot be expected to restore normal functioning.

Management

Seizures may be difficult to control, particularly in childhood. However, in a study of 68 patients, 91% of whom had epilepsy, 43% were controlled by the initial therapeutic option (Artigas y Pallarés et al. 2005). Surveys of antiepileptic drugs used in patients with Angelman syndrome have suggested that valproic acid is the most commonly used (Thibert et al. 2009). The use of clonazepam has also been reported in a number of cases. These drugs have been recommended on the basis of early reports of retrospective, open studies of limited patients series. The effectiveness of other benzodiazepines, such as nitrazepam and clobazam, seems to be similar to that of clonazepam. However, in the majority of patients, the use of benzodiazepines does not appear to be justified as a first-line treatment. Phenobarbital can be effective and well tolerated in infants. Because of sedative or cognitive side effects, it is less used in children and older patients, but has been suggested as an option in adults (Clayton-Smith and Laan 2003). Levetiracetam, topiramate, ethosuximide, and lamotrigine have been successfully used in many cases, but there is a lack of controlled studies. It is noteworthy that although lamotrigine has no direct effect on GABA$_A$ receptors, chronic treatment increases *GABRB3* gene expression in primary cultured rat hippocampal cells (CA1, CA3, and dentate gyrus) (Wang *et al.* 2002).

Some antiepileptic drugs (including carbamazepine, oxcarbazepine, vigabatrin, tiagabine, and gabapentin) may paradoxically increase in the risk of seizures and precipitate NCSE (Pelc *et al.* 2008). However, these drugs may prove useful in some patients. This aggravation due to antiepileptic drugs is not specific to Angelman syndrome, where it appears to be more marginal than in some epileptic syndrome, notably idiopathic generalised epilepsies.

The response of NCSE to treatment is variable. Oral benzodiazepines, corticosteroids, and ketamine (Mewasingh *et al.* 2003) may be early options, but there has been a marked lack of well-designed studies. Morbidity associated with aggressive treatment may outweigh the risk of therapeutic abstention.

Non-pharmacological management is rarely considered, despite the relatively high prevalence of drug resistance. Ketogenic diet has been effective in a few cases.

References

Artigas y Pallarés J, Brun-Gasca C, Gabau-Vila E, Guitart-Feliubadaló M, Camprubí-Sánchez C (2005) Aspectos médicos y conductuales del síndrome de Angelman. *Rev Neurol (Madrid)* **41**:649–656.

Boyd SG, Harden A, Patton MA (1988) The EEG in early diagnosis of the Angelman (happy puppet) syndrome. *Eur J Pediatr* **147**:508–13.

Buntinx IM, Hennekam RC, Brouwer OF, *et al.* (1995) Clinical profile of Angelman syndrome at different ages. *Am J. Med Genet* **56**:176–83.

Burbea M, Drier L, Dittman JS, Grunwald ME, Kaplan JM (2002) Ubiquitin and AP180 regulate the abundance of GLR-1 glutamate receptors at postsynaptic elements in *C. elegans. Neuron* **33**:107–20.

Cheron G, Servais L, Wagstaff J, Dan B (2005) Fast cerebellar oscillation associated with ataxia in a mouse model of Angelman syndrome. *Neuroscience* **130**:631–7.

Clayton-Smith J, Laan L (2003) Angelman syndrome: a review of the clinical and genetic aspects. *J Med Genet* **40**: 87–95.

Culiat CT, Stubbs LJ, Montgomery CS, Russell LB, Rinchik EM (1994) Phenotypic consequences of deletion of the gamma 3, alpha 5, or beta 3 subunit of the type A gamma-aminobutyric acid receptor in mice. *Proc Natl Acad Sci USA* **91**:2815–18.

Dalla Bernardina B, Fontana E, Zullini E, *et al.* (1995) Angelman syndrome: electroclinical features of 10 personal cases. *Gaslini* **27**(Suppl. 1):75–8.

Dan B (2008) *Angelman Syndrome*. London: Wiley-Blackwell.

Dan B, Boyd SG (2003) Angelman syndrome reviewed from a neurophysiological perspective: The *UBE3A–GABRB3* hypothesis. *Neuropediatrics* **34**:169–76.

DeLorey TM, Handforth A, Anagnostaras SG, *et al.* (1998) Mice lacking the beta3 subunit of the GABA$_A$ receptor have the epilepsy phenotype and many of the behavioral characteristics of Angelman syndrome. *J Neurosci* **18**:8505–14.

Egawa K, Asahina N, Shiraishi H, *et al.* (2008) Aberrant somatosensory-evoked responses imply GABAergic dysfunction in Angelman syndrome. *Neuroimage* **39**:593–9.

Espay AJ, Andrade DM, Wennberg RA, Lang AE (2005) Atypical absences and recurrent absence status in an adult with Angelman syndrome due to the UBE3A mutation. *Epileptic Disord* **7**:227–30.

Guerrini R, De Lorey TM, Bonanni P, *et al.* (1996) Cortical myoclonus in Angelman syndrome. *Ann Neurol* **40**:39–48.

Handforth A, Delorey TM, Homanics GE, Olsen RW (2005) Pharmacologic evidence for abnormal thalamocortical functioning in GABA receptor β3 subunit-deficient mice, a model of Angelman syndrome. *Epilepsia* **46**:1860–70.

Harbord M (2001) Levodopa responsive Parkinsonism in adults with Angelman syndrome. *J Clin Neurosci* **8**:421–2.

Huntsman MM, Porcello DM, Homanics GE, Delorey TM, Huguenard JR (1999) Reciprocal inhibitory connections and network synchrony in the mammalian thalamus. *Science* **283**:541–3.

Jiang YH, Armstrong D, Albrecht U, *et al.* (1998) Mutation of the Angelman ubiquitin ligase in mice causes increased cytoplasmic p53 and deficits of contextual learning and long-term potentiation. *Neuron* **21**:799–811.

Laan LAEM, Renier WO, Arts WFM, *et al.* (1997) Evolution of epilepsy and EEG findings in Angelman syndrome. *Epilepsia* **38**:195–9.

Laurie DJ, Wisden W, Seeburg PH (1992) The distribution of thirteen GABA$_A$ receptor subunit mRNAs in the rat brain. III. Embryonic and postnatal development. *J Neurosci* **12**:4151–72.

Lossie AC, Whitney MM, Amidon D, *et al.* (2001) Distinct phenotypes distinguish the molecular classes of Angelman syndrome. *J Med Genet* **38**:834–45.

Mewasingh LD, Sekhara T, Aeby A, Christiaens FJ, Dan B (2003) Oral ketamine in pediatric non-convulsive status epilepticus. *Seizure* **12**:483–9.

Ogawa K, Ohtsuka Y, Kobayashi K, Asano T, Oka E (1996) The characteristics of epilepsy with Angelman syndrome. *Epilepsia* **37**(Suppl. 3):83–4.

Pelc K, Boyd SG, Cheron G, Dan B (2008) Epilepsy in Angelman syndrome. *Seizure* **17**:211–17.

Rubin DI, Patterson MC, Westmoreland BF, Klass DW (1997) Angelman' syndrome: clinical and electroencephalographic findings. *Electroencephalogr Clin Neurophysiol* **102**:299–302.

Saitoh S, Harada N, Jinno Y, *et al.* (1994) Molecular and clinical study of 61 Angelman syndrome patients. *Am J Hum Genet* **52**:158–63.

Stecker MM, Myers SM (2003) Reserpine responsive myoclonus and hyperpyrexia in a patient with Angelman syndrome. *Clin Neurol Neurosurg* **105**:183–7.

Thibert RL, Conant KD, Braun EK (2009) Epilepsy in Angelman syndrome: a questionnaire based assessment of the natural history and current treatment options. *Epilepsia* **50**:2369–76.

Valente KD, Andrade JQ, Grossmann RM, *et al.* (2003) Angelman syndrome: difficulties in EEG pattern recognition and possible misinterpretations. *Epilepsia* **44**:1051–63.

Viani F, Romeo A, Viri M, *et al.* (1995) Seizure and EEG patterns in Angelman's syndrome. *J Child Neurol* **10**:467–71.

Wang JF, Sun X, Chen B, Young LT (2002) Lamotrigine increases gene expression of GABA$_A$ receptor β3 subunit in primary cultured rat hippocampal cells. *Neuropsychopharmacology* **26**: 415–21.

Weeber EJ, Jiang YH, Elgersma Y, *et al.* (2003) Derangements of hippocampal calcium/calmodulin-dependent protein kinase II in a mouse model for Angelman mental retardation syndrome. *J Neurosci* **23**:2634–44.

Williams CA, Beaudet AL, Clayton-Smith J, *et al.* (2006) Angelman syndrome 2005: updated consensus for diagnostic criteria. *Am J Med Genet* **140**:413–18.

Chapter 29

Lysosomal disorders and Menkes syndrome

Edwin H. Kolodny and Swati Sathe

Seizures are a major manifestation of several lysosomal storage diseases. These have in common the accumulation within neurons of lipids or glycoconjugates which would normally be degraded by hydrolytic enzymes within the lysosome. These include the neuronal ceroid lipofuscinoses, the gangliosidoses, the sialidoses, and two of the mucopolysaccharidoses, Hunter syndrome and Sanfilippo disease. The galactolipidoses, Krabbe disease, and metachromatic leukodystrophy also qualify for inclusion in this chapter because they secondarily affect neurons and clinically present with seizures. Finally, two transport disorders, one lysosomal, Niemann–Pick disease type C, and the other, Menkes disease, a non-lysosomal X-linked disorder, join these other seizure-provoking hereditary metabolic syndromes because of identifiable metabolic abnormalities within neurons. With the exception of Hunter syndrome and Menkes disease all the other diseases described here are inherited as autosomal recessive traits.

Different cellular mechanisms may be involved. In the case of the G_{M2}-gangliosidoses, the neuronal membrane is altered by the formation of new dendritic spines increasing neuronal excitability. Psychosine (galactosphingosine), a toxic metabolite in Krabbe disease, which leads to destruction of oligodendroglial cells, may secondarily interfere with nerve cell viability. In the case of Menkes disease, absence of copper transport into the nerve cell impairs a vital energy-producing pathway within neurons. However much remains to be learned about each of these disorders, their association with seizures confirms the centrality of the neuron in their pathogenesis. For comprehensive reviews of each disorder described in this chapter the reader may wish to consult the textbook of Lyon *et al.* (2006) and the Online Metabolic and Molecular Bases of Inherited Disease (www. ommbid.com).

Gangliosidoses
G_{M1}-Gangliosidosis

Deficiency of lysosomal β-galactosidase is characteristic of G_{M1}-gangliosidosis, galactosialidosis, and Morquio disease type B. The phenotypic spectrum of G_{M1}-gangliosidosis includes patients presenting as newborns with hydrops fetalis and failure to thrive, infants with developmental arrest between 3 and 6 month of age, late infantile/juvenile patients who lose motor and language skills later in the first year, or in their second or third year and individuals with progressive central nervous system (CNS) disease beginning after the third year. In all but the latter variant, there is easy startle and hypotonia. Subsequently, the patients develop spastic quadriparesis, decerebrate rigidity, tonic–clonic seizures, and blindness. Corneal clouding and cherry-red maculae are observed in many of these patients. Extraneural manifestations include a dysmorphic facial appearance, bony deformities, and cardiomyopathy.

G_{M1}-ganglioside, a sphingoglycolipid with a galactose residue at its non-reducing end, accumulates in the brain and to a lesser extent in the liver and spleen. The connective tissue and skeletal abnormalities are due to storage of galactose-containing oligosaccharides and keratin sulfate-like proteoglycans in tissues outside the nervous system. Diagnosis of G_{M1}-gangliosidosis can be made by assay of β-galactosidase activity in plasma or leukocytes, bone X-rays for dysostosis multiplex, a search for vacuoles within lymphocytes, the appearance of foam cells in the bone marrow, and urinary oligosacchariduria. One juvenile onset patient appears to have stabilized neurologically during treatment with an inhibitor of glycosphingolipid synthesis.

G_{M2}-Gangliosidoses

The G_{M2}-gangliosidoses result from the accumulation of G_{M2}-ganglioside within neurons throughout the CNS. Onset may be in the infantile, juvenile, or adult years. In the classical late-infantile variant, Tay–Sachs disease, hexosaminidase A (Hex A) is deficient whereas patients with another variant, Sandhoff disease, lack both hexosaminidases A and B (Hex A and B). Two other forms, a B_1 variant with clinical features similar to early juvenile G_{M2}-gangliosidosis and a very rare variant with deficiency of the G_{M2} activator protein, are also known. G_{M2}-gangliosidosis occurs with an incidence of

The Causes of Epilepsy, eds. S. D. Shorvon, F. Andermann, and R. Guerrini. Published by Cambridge University Press. © Cambridge University Press 2011.

approximately 1 in 120 000 live births. Prior to carrier screening, Tay–Sachs disease was most common among the Ashkenazi Jewish population.

Seizures are most common in the late-infantile forms of Tay–Sachs and Sandhoff disease (Nalini and Christopher 2004). The earliest signs in these patients are poor visual fixation and an exaggerated startle response. Developmental delay is evident by age 4–6 months. Other clinical signs are hypotonia, poor head control, and absence of vocalizations. A cherry-red spot is present in both maculas and by the second year there is megalencephaly, blindness, and spasticity. During this phase, stiffening progressing to myoclonic or generalized tonic–clonic seizures may be elicited by stimuli such as touch or sound. Occasional unmotivated laughing spells resembling gelastic seizures occur spontaneously. The electroencephalogram (EEG) shows paroxysmal slow-wave activity and polyspikes. The cerebrospinal fluid and nerve conduction velocities are normal.

Diagnosis is by enzyme analysis using artificial substrates, 4-MU-N-acetylglucosamine and its sulfated substrate. Patients with Sandhoff disease excrete hexosamine-containing oligosaccharides in their urine and demonstrate foam cells in their bone marrow. Pseudodeficiency is a recognized cause of apparently low Hex A activity in some normal individuals who should be genotyped to distinguish them from presymptomatic adult-onset patients. Neither stem cell transplantation with umbilical cord cells nor substrate synthesis inhibition has been effective in preventing progression of G_{M2}-gangliosidosis. Adult-onset patients are currently being recruited for a study of chemical chaperone therapy designed to enhance the activity of residual Hex A and B.

Gaucher disease

Gaucher disease, which is considered in more detail in Chapter 21, results in storage of glucocerebroside within macrophages of the reticuloendothelial system leading to hepatosplenomegaly, anemia, thrombocytopenia, bone pain, and osteonecrosis. There is a wide phenotypic spectrum including some individuals with seizures (Grabowski et al. 2006). The most common of these are the type 3 patients who present with developmental delay, gaze initiation failure and visceromegaly. A convergent squint due to bilateral 6th cranial nerve palsies is observed in some patients. Myoclonic seizures develop and increase in frequency becoming less and less responsive to anticonvulsant medication. The most common glucocerebrosidase gene mutation in type 3 patients is L444P but other rarer genotypes specific to individual populations may be associated with similar clinical manifestations. Onset is usually early in childhood with variable degrees of progression so that some patients may succumb in childhood or adolescence to intractable myoclonic seizures whereas others live into middle age. Myoclonic seizures are especially common in patients with the N1885 mutation (Kowarz et al. 2005). Death

in these patients typically occurs in early adolescence from congestive heart failure.

Approximately 1 per 1 000 000 individuals have a severe infantile type 2 variant of Gaucher disease with an onset from birth to 4 months of age. Clinical manifestations include bulbar signs with frequent choking episodes resulting in chronic pulmonary infection. Fulminant CNS deterioration including frequent seizures leads to death by age 3 years.

The EEG in type 3 patients can be abnormal even in the absence of overt seizure activity. Characteristic findings include background slowing with generalized epileptiform discharges, marked photosensitivity, and multiple spikes especially over the posterior regions. Brainstem auditory evoked responses and somatosensory evoked potentials are also abnormal. Assay of leukocyte β-glucosidase activity is the gold standard for diagnosis but mutation analysis is a useful adjunct for classification into subtypes. Patients with even one allele for the N370S mutation are generally free of neurologic complications.

Enzyme replacement therapy (ERT) with imiglucerase is effective in treating type 1 non-neuronopathic disease and the extraneural complications in type 2 and 3 patients but even in high doses has not halted the progression of myoclonic epilepsy. Measurement of serum chitotriosidase activity is a useful marker for responsiveness to ERT. Oral substrate reduction therapy is available for patients who are unable to tolerate ERT. The use of chemical chaperones for enhancement of residual enzyme activity is being investigated as an alternative therapy.

Niemann–Pick disease type C

Niemann–Pick disease type C (NP-C) is a devastating pan-ethnic autosomal recessive disorder with a minimum estimated incidence of 1 in 150 000 (Wraith et al. 2009a). Mutations in the NPC1 gene result in approximately 90–95% cases of NP-C while 4% result from mutations in the NPC2 gene and mutations are undetected in the remainder. The NPC1 protein is involved in the transport of glycosphingolipids, sphingosine, and cholesterol. Abnormal lipid transport leads to accumulation of lipids in diverse tissues. The accumulation of gangliosides in the CNS causes functional and structural damage to neurons. Visceral tissues, mostly the liver and spleen, are almost universally affected. Niemann–Pick disease type C develops primarily in children and adolescents and is categorized as early-childhood presentation (younger than 6 years of age), late-childhood presentation (6–11 years), and juvenile or adult presentation (12 years or older). With very early onset of disease, systemic manifestations are prominent but neurological manifestations eventually dominate the clinical picture in all subtypes. Supranuclear gaze palsy with deficit in vertical eye movements is often the earliest presenting feature though it may not be easily recognized in young children. Progressive neuropsychiatric deterioration appears from the late infantile period manifesting as ataxia, dystonia, dysphagia, dysarthria, seizures, cataplexy, and cognitive deterioration.

Gelastic cataplexy, which is sometimes disabling, occurs in 20% of affected individuals but it is considered characteristic of NP-C. Episodes vary from fully developed attacks of atonia to subtle presentation such as head nodding. Cataplexy generally responds well to treatment with tricyclic antidepressants. Epilepsy is reported in 50% of patients with NP-C. Both partial and generalized seizures occur; cortical myoclonus has been described. Standard antiepileptic drugs are effective in controlling seizures although in some cases seizures may be refractory to medical therapy. Neuronal fallout with progressive involvement of CNS leads to better control of seizures.

Brain magnetic resonance imaging (MRI) may be normal initially, but late in the course of the disease shows cerebellar and cortical atrophy, myelin loss, and thinning of the corpus callosum. Electron microscopy of skin, rectal, or conjunctival biopsies shows polymorphous cytoplasmic bodies, which are highly suggestive of NP-C. The definitive diagnosis is obtained by cholesterol esterification studies with filipin staining on fibroblasts grown from a skin biopsy sample (Wraith *et al.* 2009b). Substrate reduction therapy with miglustat, a small iminosugar molecule that acts as a competitive inhibitor of glucosylceramide synthase, blocks glycosphingolipid synthesis, and reduces accumulation of potentially neurotoxic gangliosides G_{M2} and G_{M3}. Miglustat has shown to be effective in stabilizing the course of illness with improvements in eye movements, swallowing, ambulation, and cognition.

Cherry-red spot, myoclonus, epilepsy syndrome (sialidosis I)

This disorder begins in late childhood or early adolescence with ataxia and myoclonus (Shahwan *et al.* 2005). There is gradual visual failure and generalized tonic–clonic seizures. Fundoscopy reveals a macular cherry-red spot and optic atrophy. Intention and action myoclonus become constant and interfere with all motor activities. Intelligence deteriorates and the patient becomes bedbound. There are no dysmorphic features. Patients do not survive past the third decade.

Vacuoles are present in lymphocytes and the bone marrow contains foamy histiocytes. A characteristic pattern of sialyloligosaccharides is present on thin-layer chromatography of urine. Accumulation of this material is due to deficiency of α-neuraminidase resulting from mutations in the *NEU1* gene (Seyrantepe *et al.* 2003; Shahwan *et al.* 2005). Attempts to control the myoclonus with benzodiazepines, 5-hydroxytryptophan, and levetiracetam have been only partially successful.

Sialidosis II

Deficiency of α-neuraminidase is also responsible for a Hurlerlike phenotype which may be present prenatally, in infancy, or in later childhood The congenital onset form manifests as hydrops fetalis with ascites and hepatosplenomegaly. In the early infantile form dysmorphic facial features, skeletal dysplasia, short stature, hepatosplenomegaly, intention myoclonus, seizures, and mental retardation are present. Juvenile sialidosis appears as a mild clinical phenotype.

X-rays disclose dysostosis multiplex, membrane-bound inclusions are found in biopsies of skin, liver, and bone marrow, and sialylated oligosaccharides appear in urine on thin-layer chromatography (Shahwan *et al.* 2005).

Galactosialidosis

The phenotype in galactosialidosis resembles sialidosis type II while the molecular defect is in the gene for the protective protein cathepsin A (PPCA). The consequence is a combined deficiency of α-neuraminidase and β-galactosidase. The EEG shows low-voltage fast activity with slowing present in patients with dementia. Trains of 10–20-Hz myoclonus is associated with small vertex positive spikes.

Neuronal ceroid lipofuscinoses (Batten disease)

The neuronal ceroid lipofuscinoses (NCL) are the most common cause of inherited progressive neurodegenerative disease in childhood (see Chapter 20). Their combined incidence ranges from 1 in 12 500 in the USA and Scandinavian countries to 1 in 100 000 worldwide. Eleven different disorders have been delineated and nine human genes identified yet this genetically heterogeneous group of diseases share many common features (Shahwan *et al.* 2005; Williams *et al.* 2006). Clinically, there is progressive decline in intellectual and motor functions, and retinopathy leading to blindness and seizures in nearly all patients. Autofluorescent ceroid lipopigments accumulate within tissues and nerve cells degenerate. Age of onset varies widely with premature death in affected individuals. The main storage materials are subunit C of mitochondrial ATP synthase (CLN2, CLN3, CLN4, CLN5, CLN6, CLN7, CLN8, CLN9, CLCN7) and sphingolipid activator proteins A and D (CLN1, CLN10). The ultrastructural appearance of the stored material can vary with granular osmiophilic dense material predominating in CLN1, curvilinear bodies in CLN2 and a pattern of fingerprint bodies in CLN3. In each circumstance where the disease protein is known it is either a soluble lysosomal enzyme (CLN1, CLN2, CLN5, CLN10) or a transmembrane protein (CLN3, CLN6, CLN7, CLN8).

Classical infantile-onset NCL is caused by mutations in the *CLN1* gene coding for the enzyme palmitoyl protein thioesterase 1 (PPT1). Seizures and myoclonus are accompanied by visual failure and increasing spasticity. The EEG progresses from decreased reactivity to passive eye opening and closing at age 1 year, to loss of sleep spindles at 2 years, to isoelectric at 3 years along with extinction of somatosensory evoked potentials, then of the electroretinogram (ERG), and finally of the visual evoked potentials.

The classical form of late-infantile NCL results from mutations in the gene for tripeptidyl-peptidase 1 (TPP1). Beginning in the third year, generalized tonic–clonic or partial, frequently myoclonic seizures develop which may become resistant to drug treatment. In the EEG, there are posterior spikes on slow photic stimulation suggestive of retinal deterioration. Evoked potentials are increased and the ERG is reduced or absent. The preference in anticonvulsant therapy for these patients is valproic acid as carbamazepine and lamotrigine may cause worsening of the seizures. A phase 1 trial of an adeno-associated virus expressing *CLN2* in 10 children has shown slower progression of neurological deterioration than was expected (Worgall *et al.* 2008).

Late-infantile NCL has also been described in Finnish patients with mutations in the *CLN5* gene and in Turkish patients with mutations in *CLN2*, *CLN7*, and *CLN8*. On EEG, the Finnish patients demonstrate posterior spikes to low-frequency photic stimulation and generate giant somatosensory evoked potentials. A variant late-infantile NCL caused by mutations in *CLN6* has also been found in Europe and Central and South America.

The first sign of juvenile NCL (JNCL), formerly known as the Spielmeyer–Vogt syndrome, is visual failure due to pigmentary retinopathy occurring at about 5 years of age. Progressive cognitive impairment follows leading up to epileptic seizures beginning at 10 years of age. Generalized tonic–clonic seizures predominate but partial seizures and myoclonic jerks also occur. Cerebellar and/or extrapyramidal signs develop in the early teens and the patient becomes bedridden by age 20. Death occurs a few years later.

The brain MRI is normal until age 14 when cerebral and cerebellar atrophy appear. Vacuolated lymphocytes are found in the peripheral blood and by electron microscopy contain fingerprint profiles. Patients with JNCL have a 1-kb deletion in *CLN3*, which codes for the CLN3 transmembrane protein. The JNCL phenotype may also be seen in some patients deficient in PPT1 due to *CLN1* mutations and in some children with *CLN5* mutations.

Krabbe disease (globoid cell leukodystrophy)

When seizures occur in a lysosomal storage disease, they are usually a late manifestation and infrequent. A notable exception is Krabbe disease in which seizures may be a presenting sign. In approximately 90% of all cases, symptom onset is before 6 months. Presenting symptoms in these early-onset patients include inconsolable crying, marked irritability, poor head control with opisthotonus, fisting, stiffness, and poor feeding. About one-fifth have seizures at the time of diagnosis. Both generalized tonic–clonic and myoclonic seizure activity can occur. Two-thirds of symptomatic infants with early-onset disease have EEG abnormalities. These can include background slowing with synchronous or asynchronous irregular spike–wave complexes and independent multifocal spikes. Later the background becomes nearly flat in between periodic spike–wave complexes. With clinical progression, there is loss of vision, hyperreflexia, quadriparesis, stiffness, polyneuropathy,

and stimulus-provoked myoclonus. Survival beyond 3 to 4 years is rare (Duffner *et al.* 2009).

Initial computed tomography (CT) and MRI scans can appear normal but with progression diffuse cerebral atrophy occurs in association with diffuse symmetrical high-intensity signal in the deep white matter in T2-weighted images and an abnormal low signal in the thalami. Evoked potentials are delayed and abnormal and nerve conduction velocities reduced due to concomitant peripheral nerve demyelination. Cerebrospinal fluid protein concentration is elevated.

A juvenile onset variant is recognized in children 2 to 13 years of age. The earlier the onset the more likely these children are to progress to blindness and rapid deterioration whereas a later onset phenotype presents with gait ataxia and motor regression or delay and longer survival. Some of these patients also experience seizures (Morse and Rosman 2006). Other rarer variants become symptomatic in later adolescence or adult life. Globoid cell leukodystrophy is used to describe all cases not of the classical early infantile Krabbe variant.

Krabbe disease is believed to affect 1–2 per 100 000 newborns but the true incidence may be higher because of undiagnosed later-onset forms. This disease causes degeneration of central and peripheral myelin due to a deficiency in the activity of galactocerebroside β-galactosidase. The enzyme is required for the metabolism of galactocerebroside, an essential myelin glycolipid. Macrophages within the brain white matter engulf the galactocerebroside transforming themselves into multinucleated globoid cells. Bone marrow transplantation has led to prolonged survival and improved quality of life in affected newborns and early symptomatic cases (Escolar *et al.* 2005).

Metachromatic leukodystrophy

Metachromatic leukodystrophy (MLD) is the most common of the inherited dysmyelinating disorders with an estimated frequency of 1 in 40 000. The myelin lipid galactocerebroside sulfate (sulfatide) accumulates in brain white matter and in peripheral nerves due to a deficiency in arylsulfatase A or, in very rare cases, in the non-enzymatic activator protein saposin B. As in globoid cell leukodystrophy, several clinical forms with different ages of onset can be observed. Late-infantile patients usually present in their second year with an unsteady gait and progressive polyneuropathy. Hypotonia evolves to hypertonia, speech deteriorates, and the neuropathy becomes painful. The child becomes bedridden and feeding difficulties ensue because of bulbar palsy. It is at this relatively late stage that epileptic seizures are encountered in about half of the patients (Balslev *et al.* 1997). Optic atrophy, blindness, and loss of contact with their surroundings characterize the final stage of this illness, usually within 5 years of onset.

Early juvenile MLD occurs with an equal incidence to the late juvenile form but the age of onset is later and the illness is accompanied by behavioral changes, loss of walking ability, and spasticity also progressing to quadriparesis and brainstem dysfunction. Seizures in this variant also occur in about one-half of the patients. These include primary generalized tonic–clonic seizures, myoclonic jerks, and partial complex seizures. Startle myoclonus is also encountered (Balslev et al. 1997).

The EEG may be normal in the earliest stages but as the disease progresses, mild slowing of the background activity develops. Epileptiform discharges with simple and multiple focal spikes then begin to appear. One late juvenile patient has been described who had a startle response and an ictal EEG showing rhythmic 6–7-Hz wave bursts at the beginning of the seizures. Whilst in MLD convulsions may occur at any stage of the disease, they are more frequent in the later stages. Late infantile patients more often have generalized seizures while the juvenile onset patients are more likely to experience partial seizures (Wang et al. 2001; Nalini and Christopher 2004).

Seizures are rare in the late juvenile and adult phenotypes. Leukocyte arylsulfatase A is deficient in all patients except for those with the very rare deficiency of saposin B. However, in all patients, the concentration of urinary sulfatides is increased, thus aiding in differentiating cases of MLD from the relatively common occurrence of pseudodeficiency of arylsulfatase A. In infantile and juvenile cases the cerebrospinal fluid protein concentration is elevated and nerve conduction velocities are slowed. Brain computed tomography (CT) and magnetic resonance imaging (MRI) reveal a diffuse symmetrical signal change throughout the periventricular and subcortical white matter involving also the internal capsule and corticospinal tracts. On MR spectroscopy, there is a marked reduction in N-acetylaspartate in both gray and white matter indicative of neuroaxonal degeneration. Nitrazepam has been used to treat seizures in MLD. Bone marrow transplantation has been reported in juvenile and adult MLD and trials of enzyme replacement therapy are currently underway.

Multiple sulfatase deficiency

The clinical features of multiple sulfatase deficiency (MSD) overlap MLD and the mucopolysaccharidoses (MPS). There is early psychomotor retardation such as occurs in late infantile MLD and the dysmorphic facial features and skeletal deformities typical of a mucopolysaccharidosis. Ichthyosis is an important distinguishing feature. The disorder results from mutations in SUMF1 which encodes a formylglycine generating enzyme involved in post-translational modification of at least 12 different sulfatases. As a result, the urine of patients contains increases in heparin and dermatan sulfates as well as sulfatide. The activity of arylsulfatases A, B, C, and other sulfatases involved in the degradation of MPS are deficient.

Generalized and myoclonic seizures occur frequently (Nalini and Christopher 2004) and may be refractory to anticonvulsant therapy. The prevalence of MSD is estimated at 1 per 1.4 million.

Mucopolysaccharidoses

The mucopolysaccharidoses (MPS) are a group of heterogeneous disorders resulting from deficiency of lysosomal glycosidases and sulfatases with a collective incidence estimated at ~1 in 25–50 000. Hunter syndrome (MPS II), the only X-linked recessive MPS subtype caused by deficiency of the lysosomal enzyme iduronate-2-sulfatase (I2S), is characterized by progressive storage of glycosaminoglycans in nearly all cell types, tissues, and organs. Two forms are recognized: severe and attenuated (Schwartz et al. 2007). The age at diagnosis is between 18 and 36 months for the severe forms, by which time developmental delay is usually apparent followed by a developmental plateau between 3 and 5 years of age. By the time of death in their second decade, most patients with CNS involvement are demented. Other clinical manifestations include airway obstruction, skeletal deformities, and cardiomyopathy. Seizures were reported in 13% of cases with MPS II. They are usually tonic–clonic in nature and respond to standard anticonvulsant treatment. Abnormal measurements of urinary glycosaminoglycans indicate presence of an MPS disorder. Definitive diagnosis is established by enzyme assay in leukocytes, fibroblasts, or plasma. Enzyme therapy with recombinant I2S was recently approved. A multidisciplinary approach is essential for management of systemic complications of MPS II (Wraith et al. 2008).

Sanfilippo B syndrome (MPS III) is an autosomal recessive disorder caused by deficiency of one of the four enzymes involved in the degradation of heparan sulfate. Syndromes MPS IIIA, B, C, and D are differentiated based on the deficient enzyme but have similar clinical course characterized by three stages. Stage I, presents between 1 and 4 years of age with developmental delay followed by behavioral problems and progressive mental decline leading to dementia (stage II) at around 3 to 4 years of age. In the third stage, spasticity and swallowing difficulties predominate with progressive loss of function. Death ensues by the end of the second decade. Somatic features such as coarse facies, hepatosplenomegaly, and skeletal changes are absent or only mildly expressed. Seizures can be troublesome especially in older patients, but most respond to appropriate anticonvulsant medication. Occasionally an unusual seizure pattern such as nocturnal bouts of laughing or panting has been reported. Fifty percent of adult patients with Sanfilippo B were reported to have seizures (Valstar et al. 2008). Grand mal seizures were common and half of the patients were well controlled on antiepileptic drugs. A probable diagnosis of MPS III is suspected with increased concentration of heparan sulfate in the urine and confirmed by enzymatic assays in the leukocytes or fibroblasts.

There is no definitive therapy for MPS III but substrate reduction therapies as well as gene therapy are under investigation.

Menkes (kinky hair) disease

This X-linked disease is characterized by a general deficiency in copper within the brain leading to dysfunction of several copper-dependent enzymes. As a result, severe mental retardation, hypothermia, laxity of skin and joints, hypopigmentation, arterial degeneration, and osteoporosis are present by age

2–3 months. Hair growth is sparse, the hair poorly pigmented, and the shafts twisted and broken. The incidence is estimated to range between 1 in 40 000 to 1 in 350 000. Survival beyond 18 months is unusual. Seizures are almost constant and include asymmetric myoclonic jerks that can be stiumulus-provoked. On the EEG, multifocal spike, polyspikes, and slow wave activity predominate.

Serum copper and ceruloplasmin are very low and the content of copper in the brain is reduced due to mutations in the copper transport gene *ATP7A*. Plasma dopamine and dihydroxyphenylacetic acid are elevated due to low dopamine-β-hydroxylase activity. Early treatment with copper histidine administered subcutaneously leads to improved survival and neurological outcome (Kaler *et al.* 2009).

References

Balslev T, Cortez MA, Blaser SI, Haslam RHA (1997) Recurrent seizures in metachromatic leukodystrophy. *Pediatr Neurol* 17:150–4.

Duffner PK, Jalal K, Carter RL (2009) The Hunter's Hope Krabbe family database. *Pediatr Neurol* 40:13–18.

Escolar ML, Poe MD, Provenzale JM, *et al.* (2005) Transplantation of umbilical-cord blood in babies with infantile Krabbe's disease. *N Engl J Med* 352:2069–81.

Grabowski GA, Kolodny EH, Weinreb NJ, *et al.* (2006) *The Online Metabolic and Molecular Bases of Inherited Disease. Chap 146.1 Gaucher disease phenotype and genetic variation.* New York: McGraw-Hill. Available on line at www.ommbid.com.

Kaler SG, Holmes CS, Goldstein DS, *et al.* (2009) Neonatal diagnosis and treatment of Menkes disease. *N Engl J Med* 358:605–14.

Kowarz L, Golker-Alpan O, Banerjee-Basu S, *et al.* (2005) Gaucer mutation N1885 is associated with myoclonic epilepsy. *Hum Mutat* 26:271–3.

Lyon G, Kolodny EH, Pastores GM (2006) *Neurology of Hereditary Metabolic Diseases of Children*, 3rd edn. New York: McGraw-Hill.

Morse LE, Rosman NP (2006) Myoclonic seizures in Krabbe disease: a unique presentation in late-onset type. *Pediatr Neurol* 35:154–7.

Nalini A, Christopher R (2004) Cerebral glycolipidoses clinical characteristics of 41 pediatric patients. *J Child Neurol* 19:447–52.

Schwartz IV, Ribeiro MG, Mota JG, *et al.* (2007) A clinical study of 77 patients with mucopolysaccharidosis type II. *Acta Paediatr* (Suppl.) 96(455):63–70.

Seyrantepe V, Poupetova H, Froissart R, *et al.* (2003) Molecular pathology of *NEU1* gene in sialidosis. *Hum Mutat* 22:343–52.

Shahwan A, Farrell M, Delanty N (2005) Progressive myoclonic epilepsies: a review of genetic and therapeutic aspects. *Lancet Neurol* 4:239–48.

Valstar MJ, Ruijter GJG, van Diggelen OP, *et al.* (2008) Sanfilippo syndrome: a mini-review. *J Inherit Metab Dis* 31:240–52.

Wang P-J, Hwu W-L, Shen Y-Z (2001) Epileptic seizures and electroencephalographic evolution in genetic leukodystrophies. *J Clin Neurophysiol* 18:25–32.

Williams RE, Aberg L, Autti T, *et al.* (2006) Diagnosis of the neuronal ceroid lipofuscinoses: an update. *Biochim Biophys Acta* 1762:865–72.

Worgall S, Sondhi D, Hackett NR, *et al.* (2008) Treatment of late infantile neuronal ceroid lipofuscinosis by CNS administration of a serotype 2 adeno-associated virus expressing *CLN2* cDNA. *Hum Gene Ther* 19:463–74.

Wraith JE, Scarpa M, Beck M, *et al.* (2008) Mucopolysaccharidosis type II (Hunter syndrome): a clinical review and recommendations for treatment in the era of enzyme replacement therapy. *Eur J Pediatr* 167:267–77.

Wraith JE, Guffon N, Rohrbach M, *et al.* (2009a) Natural history of Niemann–Pick disease type C in a multicentre observational retrospective cohort study. *Mol Genet Metab* 98:250–4.

Wraith JE, Baumgartner MR, Bembi B (2009b) Recommendations on the diagnosis and management of Niemann–Pick disease type C. *Mol Genet Metab* 98:152–65.

Chapter 30

Neuroacanthocytosis

Anna C. Jansen

Definition and history

The term acanthocyte derives from the Greek ακανθα meaning "thorn." Acanthocytes or spur cells are spiculated red cells with a few projections of varying size and surface distribution. The cells appear contracted, dense, and irregular. In general, the formation of acanthocytes depends on alteration of the lipid composition and fluidity of the red cell membrane (Stevenson and Hardie 2001). Up to 3% of acanthocytes in the peripheral blood smear may be considered normal; ranges beyond this are often associated with disease.

Neuroacanthocytosis syndromes form a genetically heterogeneous group of disorders characterized by the association of neurological abnormalities with acanthocyte (Andermann *et al.* 2005; Walker *et al.* 2007, 2008). The neuroacanthocytosis syndromes may be divided in three groups: (1) syndromes with basal ganglia degeneration, comprising autosomal recessive chorea-acanthocytosis (ChAc: MIM #200150) due to mutation of the *VPS13A* gene on chromosome 9q21, and X-linked McLeod syndrome (MLS: MIM #314850) due to mutation of the *XK* gene on the X-chromosome; (2) conditions with decreased lipoproteins, including abetalipoproteinemia or Bassen–Kornzweig syndrome (ABL: MIM #200100), and hypobetalipoproteinemia (MIM #107730), which are characterized by peripheral neuropathy and ataxia; and (3) conditions in which acanthocytosis is occasionally seen, such as neurodegeneration with brain iron accumulation (NBIA1: MIM #234200)) or Hallervorden–Spatz disease which is caused by mutations in the *PKAN2* gene on chromosome 20p13–p12.3, and Huntington disease-like-2 (HDL2: MIM #606438) which can be caused by an expanded CAG/CTG repeat in the *JPH3* gene on chromosome 16q24.3.

Seizures are part of the phenotype in chorea-acanthocytosis which was reported by Levine and Critchley in the late 1960s (Critchley *et al.* 1967; Estes *et al.* 1967; Levine *et al.* 1968), and in McLeod syndrome which was first described in 1961 by Allen *et al.* who named the disorder after the propositus, a dental student at Harvard. Both chorea-acanthocytosis and McLeod syndrome will be described in more detail in this chapter.

Chorea-acanthocytosis
Epidemiology and clinical features

Chorea-acanthocytosis (ChAc) is a neurodegenerative disorder which is estimated to affect 500 to 1000 individuals worldwide. Its clinical expression is variable and includes a progressive movement disorder, cognitive and behavioral changes, neuropathy, myopathy, and acanthocytosis. Mean age of onset is 35 years, ranging from the first to seventh decade. The diagnosis should be considered in patients who have both seizures and a movement disorder, have one and later develop the other, or have a family history of both movement disorders and epilepsy.

Most characteristic of ChAc are involuntary movements affecting the face, mouth, tongue, pharynx, and larynx. Involuntary vocalizations, belching, spitting, and bruxism are common. Limb chorea including flinging arm and leg movements, shoulder shrugs, pelvic thrusts, and violent trunk spasms with head banging is the most common movement disorder in individuals with ChAc. Dystonia is often present and affects the oral region and the tongue in particular, causing dysarthria and serious dysphagia with resultant weight loss. Habitual tongue and lip biting are characteristic. Subtle eye movement abnormalities such as impaired upgaze or slowed saccades may be found.

As the hyperkinetic orofacial state progresses to mutism, the choreiform and dystonic syndrome gradually evolves into parkinsonism in about one-third of patients, although in some cases parkinsonism may be the presenting feature.

Changes in personality and behavior affect almost all individuals with ChAc and vary from apathy and depression to hyperactivity and emotional instability. Obsessive–compulsive behavior, paranoia, aggression, self-neglect, and suicidal ideation are part of the disease (Rampoldi *et al.* 2002). The cognitive deterioration is characterized mainly by frontal lobe dysfunction. Nerve and muscle involvement cause ankle areflexia, reduced vibration sense, and raised creatine kinase levels, as well as muscle atrophy and weakness. Seizures occur

---

The Causes of Epilepsy, eds. S. D. Shorvon, F. Andermann, and R. Guerrini. Published by Cambridge University Press. © Cambridge University Press 2011.

in almost half of affected individuals and may be the presenting symptom (Tiftikcioglu *et al.* 2006).

Pathophysiology

In the majority of ChAc families, the disease is inherited as an autosomal recessive trait, and is caused by mutations in the *VPS13A* (vacuolar protein sorting 13A) gene on chromosome 9q21, encoding for chorein.

Based on studies in yeast it is hypothesized that chorein may play a role in protein sorting and trafficking, with dysfunction impairing plasma membrane structure.

McLeod syndrome

Epidemiology and clinical features

McLeod syndrome is a rare X-linked neurodegenerative disorder resulting from heterozygous mutations in the *XK* gene (Danek *et al.* 2001; Jung *et al.* 2007. Approximately 150 cases are known worldwide. Males who inherit the mutation will be affected and will pass the disease-causing mutation to all of their daughters and none of their sons. Females who inherit the mutation will be carriers and will usually not be affected. The chance of transmitting McLeod syndrome is 50% with each pregnancy. McLeod syndrome is characterized hematologically by the absence of Kx red blood cell antigen, weak expression of Kell red blood cell antigens, acanthocytosis, and compensated hemolysis. Neuromuscular manifestations include myopathy, sensorimotor axonal neuropathy, and cardiomyopathy. Central nervous system manifestations consist of a choreatic movement disorder, "subcortical" neurobehavioral deficits, psychiatric abnormalities, and generalized seizures. The age of onset of neurological manifestations is between 18 and 61 years with the majority of individuals becoming symptomatic before age 40 years.

Pathophysiology

McLeod syndrome is caused by mutations of the *XK* gene encoding the XK protein which carries the Kx red blood cell antigen. Although the exact function of the human XK protein is still unknown, it is suggested to play an important role in apoptosis.

Epilepsy in neuroacanthocytosis

Epilepsy in chorea-acanthocytosis

Seizures are one of many neurological manifestations of chorea-acanthocytosis and occur in almost half of the patients. Although they usually occur after the onset of involuntary movements or late in the course of the disease, seizures can be the presenting symptom and may precede the onset of movement disorders by several years (Swartz *et al.* 1992).

The nature of the epileptic syndrome(s) in ChAc is not well characterized in the literature except for a study on the epilepsy phenotype in two French–Canadian families with ChAc

where six patients in three sibships presented with seizures (Al-Asmi *et al.* 2005). Age at seizure onset ranged from 22 to 38 years. The epileptic aura consisted of a sensation of déjà-vu, fear, hallucinations, palpitations, and vertigo. Electroencephalography (EEG) with video-telemetry showed epileptiform discharges originating either from one or both temporal lobes. Epilepsy was generally well controlled, but some patients had periods of increased seizure frequency requiring treatment with multiple antiepileptic drugs.

Although ChAc patients have many symptoms of temporal lobe epilepsy, they do not clearly fit any of the familial temporal lobe epilepsy syndromes previously described. The prognosis in ChAc families is worse than is usually the case in familial temporal lobe epilepsy. Seizures seem to be more difficult to control, and cognitive functioning deteriorates, resulting in loss of autonomy.

It still remains unclear why ChAc patients develop epilepsy, and the anatomical substrate for the epilepsy in ChAc requires further study. Unlike many neurodegenerative disorders with diffuse histopathological changes and generalized seizures, ChAc causes focal epilepsy, most frequently of temporal lobe origin. Autopsy studies in ChAc showed that the abnormal histopathological findings in the central nervous system were mainly confined to the striatum, where the putamen and caudate nuclei showed moderate to severe atrophy, correlating with the involuntary movements. Lesions or focal changes in the temporal lobe structures have never been mentioned in autopsy studies of ChAc patients with epilepsy. It is possible that ChAc represents another example of pseudotemporal epilepsy. Furthermore, a subcortical origin of the epileptic activity cannot be entirely excluded. Further studies of the expression pattern and function of chorein, the *VPS13A* gene product, might shed light on the epileptogenesis of ChAc.

Epilepsy in McLeod syndrome

The epilepsy phenotype in McLeod syndrome has not been studied in detail. Seizures may be the presenting symptom in about 20% of individuals with McLeod syndrome. Up to 40% develop seizures in the course of the disease. Seizures are usually described as generalized.

Diagnostic tests

Chorea-acanthocytosis

When clinical findings suggest the diagnosis of ChAc, peripheral blood smears should be examined for acanthocytosis. The proportion of acanthocytes in ChAc may vary from 5% to 50% and does not correlate with the severity of the disease. In some patients, acanthocytosis may be absent or may occur only late in the course of the disease.

To facilitate genetic testing, chorein detection by Western blot analysis has proven useful but is currently only available on a research basis.

The diagnosis of ChAc is confirmed by the detection of two mutations in the *VPS13A* gene. Mutations are dispersed throughout the gene and comprise missense, frameshift, nonsense, splice-site, and deletion mutations. The mutation detection rate is not known.

McLeod syndrome

When a diagnosis of McLeod syndrome is suspected, it can be confirmed by the immunohematological determination of absent expression of the Kx erythrocyte antigen and reduced expression of the Kell blood group antigens using human anti-Kx and anti-Kell human alloantibodies, respectively.

Acanthocytosis is found in virtually all males with McLeod syndrome, particularly if analyses are repeated. Unfortunately no data are available on the age at which acanthocytosis develops.

The *XK* gene is the only one currently known to be associated with McLeod syndrome. The majority of *XK* mutations include deletions, nonsense mutations, or splice-site mutations predicting absent or truncated XK protein. Large X-chromosomal deletions including the *XK* gene may result in a contiguous gene syndrome, comprising X-linked chronic granulomatous disease, Duchenne muscular dystrophy, and X-linked retinitis pigmentosa.

Differential diagnosis

The differential diagnosis includes a wide range of disorders, such as parkinsonian syndromes, choreiform and other movement disorders, epilepsy, and neuromuscular disorders.

The presence of a neurodegenerative disorder with acanthocytes should evoke other neuroacanthocytosis syndromes including abetalipoproteinemia and hypobetalipoproteinemia, neurodegeneration with brain iron accumulation (formerly Hallervorden–Spatz syndrome), and Huntington-disease-like 2.

Management and prognosis
Management of the epilepsy in chorea-acanthocytosis and McLeod syndrome

The treatment of epilepsy in patients with chorea-acanthocytosis or McLeod syndrome represents a challenge, since seizures may at times be intractable and some antiepileptic drugs may worsen the involuntary movements.

Antiepileptic drugs are known to have a potential influence on involuntary movements in patients with underlying movement disorders. Carbamazepine is known to induce various movement disorders, not necessarily related to toxic levels. This can occur in an idiosyncratic and transient fashion, and does not always necessitate drug discontinuation. Reversible lamotrigine-induced tic disorder has also been reported.

Epilepsy surgery is not an option in these patients, mainly because of the progressive nature of the underlying disease.

Management of chorea-acanthocytosis

When an individual is diagnosed with ChAc, the extent of the disease should be evaluated including a swallowing assessment, cardiac evaluation, electroencephalography, neuropsychological assessment, electromyography, and nerve conduction testing as well as physical therapy evaluation.

Botulinum toxin may be helpful in decreasing the oro-facio-bucco-lingual dystonia that interferes with eating. Tube feeding by gastrostomy may be necessary in later stages of the disease to provide sufficient intake and prevent aspiration. Mechanical protective devices may be needed for complications such as teeth grinding, head banging, and repeated falls. Splints can be tried for foot drop. Psychiatric medications such as antidepressants or antipsychotic medications as well as the management of cardiomyopathy are based on conventional approaches.

Management of McLeod syndrome

At present there is no cure for McLeod syndrome and treatment is focused on symptom relief. Evaluations to be performed at initial diagnosis include neurologic and neuropsychological examination, serum creatine kinase (CK) concentration and liver function tests, cardiac examination including electrocardiogram (ECG), Holter ECG and cardiac ultrasound, cerebral magnetic resonance imaging (MRI) and electroencephalography (EEG). The choreatic movement disorder can be treated with dopamine antagonists such as tiapride, clozapine, or quetiapine, as well as tetrabenazine. Psychiatric problems and cardiac manifestations should be treated based on conventional approaches. Continuous multidisciplinary psychosocial support for affected individuals and their families is mandatory.

Individuals with McLeod syndrome who receive multiple transfusions are at risk for transfusion hazards caused by allogenic antibody production. If possible, Kx-negative blood or banked autologous blood should be used for transfusions. Surveillance consists of Holter ECG and cardiac ultrasound every 2 to 3 years in those without known cardiac complications; monitoring for seizures; monitoring serum CK concentrations for evidence of rhabdomyolysis if excessive movement disorders are present of if neuroleptic medications are being used.

Prognosis

Chorea-acanthocytosis is a neurodegenerative disorder leading to major disability within a few years. Life expectancy is reduced with age of death ranging from the third to sixth decade.

Patients with McLeod syndrome usually show a slow progression of disease with duration varying from 7 to over 50 years. Mean age at death is in the fifth decade, ranging from the third to sixth decade. Cardiovascular events, seizures and aspiration pneumonia are the major causes of death in the older McLeod patients.

References

Al-Asmi A, Jansen AC, Badhwar A, *et al.* (2005) Familial temporal lobe epilepsy as a presenting feature of choreoacanthocytosis. *Epilepsia* **46**:1256–63.

Andermann E, Danek A, Irvine G, *et al.* (2005) Second International Neuroacanthocytosis Symposium: Expanding the spectrum of choreatic syndromes. *Movement Disord* **20**:1673–84.

Critchley EMR, Clark DB, Wikler A (1967) An adult form of acanthocytosis. *Trans Am Neurol Ass* **92**:132–7.

Estes JW, Morley TJ, Levine IM, Emerson CP (1967) A new hereditary acanthocytosis syndrome. *Am J Med* **42**:868–81.

Danek A, Rubio JP, Rampoldi L, (2001) McLeod neuroacanthocytosis: genotype and phenotype. *Ann Neurol* **50**:755–64.

Jung HH, Danek A, Frey BM (2007) McLeod syndrome: a neurohaematological disorder. *Vox Sanguinis* **93**:112–21.

Levine IM, Estes JW, Looney JM (1968) Hereditary neurological disease with acanthocytosis: a new syndrome. *Arch Neurol* **19**:403–9.

Rampoldi L, Danek A, Monaco AP (2002) Clinical features and molecular bases of neuroacanthocytosis. *J Mol Med* **80**:475–91.

Swartz MS, Monro PS, Leigh PN (1992) Epilepsy as the presenting feature of neuroacanthocytosis in siblings. *J Neurol* **239**:261–2.

Stevenson VL, Hardie RJ (2001) Acanthocytosis and neurological disorders. *J Neurol* **248**:87–94.

Tiftikcioglu BI, Dericioglu N, Saygi S (2006) Focal seizures originating from the left temporal lobe in a case with chorea-acanthocytosis. *Clin EEG Neurosci* **37**:46–9.

Walker RH, Danek A, Dobson-Stone C, *et al.* (2006) Developments in neuroacanthocytosis: expanding the spectrum of choreatic syndromes. *Movement Disord* **21**:1794–805.

Walker RH, Jung HH, Dobson-Stone C, (2007) Neurological phenotypes associated with acanthocytosis. *Neurology* **68**:92–8.

Walker RH, Saiki S, Danek A (2008) *Neuroacanthocytosis Syndromes II.* Dordrecht, The Netherlands: Springer-Verlag.

Organic acid, amino acids, and peroxisomal disorders

Maria Alice Donati, Serena Gasperini, and Renzo Guerrini

Definition and epidemiology

Inherited disorders of amino acid, organic acid, and peroxisomal metabolism are individually rare but have a high cumulative frequency. The underlying biochemical defect is heterogeneous. Neurological manifestations are common. Epilepsy can be observed during the course of many disorders, usually as part of a larger clinical spectrum.

Deficiencies of enzymes involved in amino acid catabolism of phenylalanine or glycine frequently result in the accumulation of toxic substances and these "catabolic" aminoacidopathies are known to be responsible for brain damage with mental retardation and seizures. Phenylketonuria was one of the first neurogenetic disorders to be identified (by Folling in 1934) and the first inborn error of metabolism to be treated successfully with diet (Bickel 1953). In the 1960s, neonatal screening was introduced for the diagnosis of phenylketonuria (Guthrie and Susi 1963) and later extended to several other disorders (Scriver *et al.* 2001). At the moment, in many countries, phenylketonuria and hyperphenylalaninemias are recognized by newborn screening with Guthrie test or tandem mass spectroscopy (LC-MS/MS) and therapy can begin in the neonatal period to prevent chronic neurological damage. Neonatal screening by LC-MS/MS, recently introduced in some countries, allows the diagnosis of many disorders of intermediary metabolism (aminoacidopathies, organic acidurias, fatty acid oxidation disorders, and some urea cycle defects).

Non-ketotic hyperglycinemia is the most common amino acid disorder causing epilepsy in countries in which phenylketonuria is detected by newborn screening (Fernandes *et al.* 2000; Scriver *et al.* 2001).

Early-onset seizures have been described in new "anabolic" disorders of amino acids. Such disorders are caused by defects in the biosynthesis of serine or glutamine, resulting in serine deficiency and congenital glutamine deficiency (de Koning *et al.* 2004; Häberle *et al.* 2006).

The classic organic acidurias are disorders of intermediary metabolism with characteristic accumulation of carboxylic acids identified by gas chromatography–mass spectrometry

(GC–MS) analysis in the urine (Fernandes *et al.* 2000; Scriver *et al.* 2001). The most common organic acidurias result from an abnormality of specific enzymes involving the catabolism of branched-chain amino acids (leucine, isoleucine, valine). Maple-syrup urine disease, isovaleric acidemia, propionic aciduria, and methylmalonic acidurias represent the most commonly encountered abnormal organic acidurias. These four organic acidurias often present in neonates, after a free interval from birth. Clinical symptoms are neurologic distress of an intoxication type with either ketosis or ketoacidosis and hyperammonemia. In the comatose state, most patients have characteristic changes in muscle tone with myoclonic jerks or abnormal movements (boxing or pedaling) which are often mistaken for convulsions; true convulsions occur later. Characteristic organic aciduria, cutaneous, and neurologic symptoms with frequent seizures are present in holocarboxylase synthetase and biotinidase deficiencies. Both disorders in biotin metabolism lead to multiple carboxylase deficiency and respond dramatically to biotin therapy (Kalayci *et al.* 1994; Scriver *et al.* 2001).

Several organic acidurias show mainly cerebral symptoms without metabolic or lactic acidosis, hyperammonemia, or hypoglycemia. In these "cerebral" organic acidurias, an epileptic encephalopathy has been frequently reported, in association with variable clinical features. Some examples from this group are D-2-hydroxyglutaric aciduria, succinic semialdehyde dehydrogenase deficiency, malonic aciduria, and Canavan disease; in the latter, onset is in the first months of life with progressive psychomotor retardation, progressive epileptic encephalopathy, macrocephaly, leukodystrophy, and optic atrophy (Fernandes *et al.* 2000; Scriver *et al.* 2001).

In early-onset seizures, particularly if associated with multiple extraneurological abnormalities, peroxisomal disorders should also be considered. The peroxisomal disorders are subdivided into two groups: the peroxisome biogenesis disorders and the single peroxisome enzyme deficiencies. The peroxisome biogenesis disorders group comprises rhizomelic chondrodysplasia punctata type I and the Zellweger spectrum disorders that constitute a triad of overlapping disorders. The

---

The Causes of Epilepsy, eds. S. D. Shorvon, F. Andermann, and R. Guerrini. Published by Cambridge University Press. © Cambridge University Press 2011.

most severe is Zellweger syndrome, followed by neonatal adrenoleukodystrophy and infantile Refsum disease (Steinberg *et al.* 2006).

In all these metabolic defects, epileptic seizures may complicate a metabolic attack or arise from a background of diffuse neurological involvement. However, in some defects, epilepsy can be the presenting or main symptom. When dealing with new-onset epilepsy of unknown origin, it is always helpful to search for clinical keys, e.g., dysmorphic traits, macrocephaly, or skin, liver, skeletal system, and heart involvement that may suggest the cardinal signs and symptoms for differential diagnosis. A set of laboratory studies will effectively reaffirm clinical impressions and confirm the diagnosis. Most of these disorders are autosomal recessive. In some instances an inborn error of metabolism is suspected because of informative family history, e.g., consanguineous parents, neurological diseases, and early death in siblings, which may provide important information.

Pathogenesis of epilepsy and central nervous system involvement

The pathogenesis of seizures is not fully understood. It has been demonstrated for some of these diseases that the accumulation of pathological metabolites is directly involved. Various patho-mechanisms have been reported in different in vitro and in vivo models, including impairment of brain energy metabolism, imbalance of excitatory and inhibitory neurotransmission, altered transport across the blood–brain barrier and between glial cells and neurons, impaired myelination, and neuronal efflux of metabolic water (Kölker *et al.* 2008). In some inborn errors of metabolism (e.g., peroxisomal disorders, glutaric aciduria type II) the defect in brain structure, produced by the inherited metabolic disorder in uterus, results in various types of malformations, such as neuronal migration disorders.

Understanding patho-mechanisms is important for developing therapeutic approaches. In non-ketotic hyperglycinemia the knowledge that glycine, which is inhibitory in the brainstem and spinal chord (explaining apnea, hiccups, and severe hypotonia), is excitatory and epileptogenic in the cortex by activation of *N*-methyl-D-aspartate-(NMDA) receptors, is the basis for treatment using dextromethorphan. This molecule is converted into its active metabolite, dextrorphan, a non-competitive inhibitor of the NMDA-receptor-channel complex (Hamosh *et al.* 1998). Knowledge of these basic mechanisms has prompted further trials with other receptor-channel blockers.

In phenylketonuria the most conclusive explanation for neurological manifestations is the "large neutral amino acid (LNAA) hypothesis": elevation of phenylalanine in plasma impairs transport of LNAA. As a consequence of competition at the blood–brain barrier, LNAA are depleted into the central nervous system (CNS), resulting in decreased protein synthesis

and decreased production of serotonin, catecholamines, histamine and S-adenosylmethionine. Supplementation with LNAA can reduce phenylalanine levels in the brain despite high serum levels. In addition to LNNA depletion, high phenylalanine levels in the CNS have implications in glutamatergic neurotransmission (Kölker *et al.* 2008; van Spronsen *et al.* 2009).

In organic acidurias there is no unifying and generally accepted hypothesis for neuropathogenesis. Recent pathophysiological hypotheses for organic acidurias (toxic metabolite hypothesis) point to the contribution of toxic metabolites to neurological disease involving excitotoxic cell damage and mitochondrial dysfunction (Kolker *et al.* 2004; Sauer *et al.* 2006; Zinnanti *et al.* 2007). In glutaric acidemia type I it has recently been demonstrated that glutaric and 3-hydroxyglutaric acids accumulate in the brain, following de novo intracerebral synthesis with a very limited efflux from brain to blood (trapping hypothesis) (Sauer *et al.* 2006). It has been hypothesized that in certain organic acidurias, secondary to very limited efflux, a pathological accumulation of dicarboxylic acids is present in the brain (Kölker 2006). The blood–brain barrier contributes to the patho-mechanism underlying neurological manifestations (Kölker *et al.* 2008).

Impaired mitochondrial glutamate transport (*SLC25A22* gene) has been reported in an autosomal recessive neonatal myoclonic epilepsy. Expression studies showed that, during human form of development, *SLC25A22* is specifically expressed in the brain, within territories supposed to contribute to genesis and control of myoclonic seizures. This study provides evidence that, despite normal oxidative phosphorylation, impaired mitochondrial glutamate import/metabolism leads to an alteration of neuronal excitability, possibly linking glutamate transport to the pathogenesis of myoclonic seizures (Molinari *et al.* 2005).

Clinical manifestations

Epileptic seizures may be the inaugural or the main symptom in rare inborn errors of intermediary metabolism (e.g., non-ketotic hyperglycinemia and serine deficiency). Most often seizures occur late and inconsistently.

In a neonate with unexplained and refractory epilepsy, besides well-known vitamin-responsive epilepsies (e.g., pyridoxine or pyridoxal phosphate-dependent seizures), disorders of amino acid metabolism such as non-ketotic hyperglycinemia, methylene tetrahydrofolate reductase deficiency, serine deficiency, and congenital glutamine deficiency should be considered.

In many cases of neonatal onset epilepsy the picture can be defined as "early myoclonic encephalopathy."

In neonatal-onset non-ketotic hyperglycinemia, neurological depression with coma, apnea, seizures, and a burst suppression pattern on the electroencephalogram (EEG) are present in the first days of life. Hiccupping is frequent and brain imaging may show defects of the corpus callosum (Fig. 31.1). Affected neonates may need ventilatory support during a short period of respiratory depression. Patients develop moderate to profound mental retardation and often a severe seizure disorder (Fig. 31.2). A few patients have been reported as affected by a transient form, in which the biochemical abnormalities disappear in infancy with a corresponding clinical recovery (Applegarth and Toone 2004). A late-onset non-ketotic hyperglycinemia often starts in infancy or childhood with severe seizures requiring multiple anticonvulsants;

some patients exhibit moderate to mild mental retardation and a mild seizure disorder (Table 31.1). Non-ketotic hyperglycinemia is caused by deficient activity of the glycine cleavage system that consists of four subunits. Mutations have been reported in the genes coding for the P-, T-, and H-protein subunits, most cases show mutation in gene *GLDC* coding for P-protein (Applegarth and Toone 2004). The disorder is biochemically characterized by elevated glycine in urine and cerebrospinal fluid (CSF); glycine is disproportionately high in the CSF and an elevated CSF/plasma glycine ratio is diagnostic; plasma glycine has been reported in the normal range in some patients. Treatment with oral sodium benzoate (250–750 mg/kg per day), or NMDA receptor antagonist as dextrometorphan and folinic acid (5–15 mg per day) can modify the early neonatal course of severe non-ketotic hyperglycinemia but does not prevent a poor long-term outcome (Scriver *et al.* 2001; Korman and Gutman 2002).

Patients with maple-syrup urine disease rarely show seizures without first presenting coma or hypoglycemia. Also in urea cycle defects and in the more frequent organic acidurias (e.g., methylmalonic aciduria, propionic aciduria, isovaleric acidemia), poor feeding, lethargy, and coma in acute metabolic decompensation, with severe hyperammonemia and acidosis generally precede seizures or status epilepticus in the neonatal period.

Early infantile epileptic encephalopathy, progressive psychomotor retardation, severe microcephaly, and lens dislocation are present in sulfite oxidase deficiency and molybdenum co-factor deficiency, disorders of the metabolism of sulfur amino acids. The sulfite test in fresh urine is positive; plasma amino acids analysis shows elevated taurine and sulphocysteine. In molybdenum co-factor deficiency uric acid is very low in serum.

Intractable seizures occur in the first months of life in congenital serine deficiency, a defect of de novo biosynthesis of the

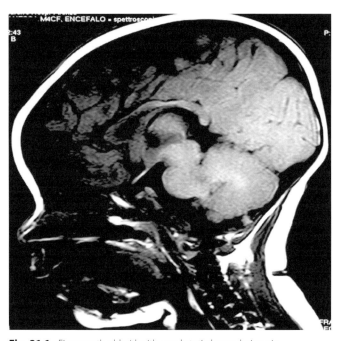

Fig. 31.1. Five-month-old girl with non-ketotic hyperglycinemia. Brain MRI: T1-weighted sagittal section passing through the midline. Note the typical thinning of the corpus callosum, more prominent on its anterior and central part.

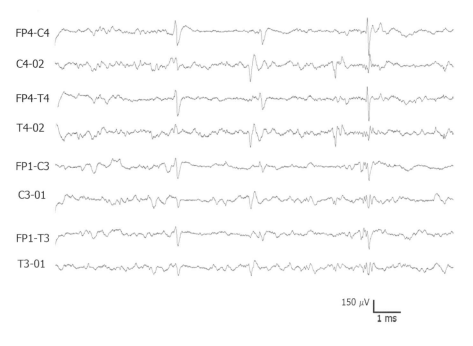

Fig. 31.2. Three-month-old boy with non-ketotic hyperglycinemia. EEG recording. Note the repetitive biphasic or triphasic sharp waves followed by burst suppressions, which are typical of the condition.

Table 31.1 Clinical and biochemical features in non-ketotic hyperglycinemia (NKH)

Disorder	Findings		Clinical presentation	Outcome
Neonatal NKH	Plasma glycine CSF glycine CSF/plasma glycine ratio >0.08 (normal value <0.04)		Neonatal period: hypotonia, lethargy developing into coma, apnea, hiccups, neonatal seizures, and burst-suppression on EEG	**Severe** No developmental progress. Severe seizures requiring multiple anticonvulsants. Brain malformations (corpus callosum dysgenesis) **Moderate** Some developmental progress, moderate to severe mental retardation. Seizures responding to a single anticonvulsant
Mild NKH	Plasma glycine CSF glycine CSF/plasma glycine ratio >0.08	Biochemistry persists	Neonatal coma and seizures	Good outcome
Transient NKH	Plasma glycine CSF glycine CSF/plasma glycine ratio >0.08	Normalization after months	Neonatal coma and seizures, or infantile seizures	Good outcome or mental retardation
Late-onset NKH: severe	Plasma glycine CSF glycine CSF: plasma glycine ratio >0.06		In infancy with increasingly severe seizures. Occasionally, degenerative course in late infancy or early childhood	No developmental progress. Severe seizures requiring multiple anticonvulsants
Late-onset NKH: mild	Plasma glycine CSF glycine CSF/plasma glycine ratio >0.04		Mild seizures starting in infancy or childhood	Moderate to mild cognitive impairment Mild seizures

amino acid L-serine due to 3-phosphoglycerate dehydrogenase deficiency (de Koning and Klomp 2004; de Koning 2006). The serine biosynthetic pathway plays an important role in multiple cellular reactions, particularly in brain tissue: neurons lose the ability to synthesize L-serine after their final differentiation so that only astrocytes can supply this amino acid. Serine is a precursor of nucleotides, phospholipids, and neurotransmitters glycine and D-serine. Some studies have established a fundamental link between the glia/astrocyte serine biosynthesis and the energetic metabolism that leads to the differentiation of neurons and other glia cells in the gray and white matter. The symptoms of this disease are congenital microcephaly, seizures, severe psychomotor retardation, and polyneuropathy (de Koning and Klomp 2004). Biochemical abnormalities are low concentrations of serine (<14 μmol/L, nv 42–86) and glycine with low 5-methyltetrahydrofolate in CSF. Fasting plasma levels of serine and glycine can be low or normal. Molecular and enzymatic assay on fibroblasts confirm this diagnosis (Tabatabaie *et al.* 2009). This disorder is potentially treatable with L-serine and glycine oral supplementation at the dosage respectively of 500 mg/kg and 200 mg/kg per day. Prenatal and postnatal supplementation have been effective (de Koning *et al.* 2004; Pearl 2009).

Glutamine synthetase deficiency has recently been described in two newborns with an early fatal course of disease (Haberle *et al.* 2006). From observation in the first patients,

seizures and hypotonia, in the first day of life, related to severe brain malformation are the leading signs. Brain magnetic resonance imaging (MRI) showed cerebral and cerebellar atrophy associated with delayed gyration, and marked white matter changes with multiple subependymal cysts. One of the patients exhibited severe enteropathy and necrolytic erythema of the skin. The amino acid assay revealed a largely diminished level or absence of glutamine in plasma, urine, and CSF. In both patients fibroblasts failed to grow when cultured; glutamine synthetase activity in immortalized lymphocytes and molecular analysis of the glutamine synthetase gene confirmed the inherited glutamine synthetase deficiency.

An autosomal recessive impaired mitochondrial glutamate transport and homozygosity for a missense mutation in the *SLC25A22* gene have been reported in a family with neonatal epilepsy (Molinari *et al.* 2005). The family history showed four affected children born to consanguineous Arab Muslim parents; all affected children showed, a few hours after birth or in the first days of life, intractable seizures and hypotonia with progressive microcephaly. The EEG showed myoclonic seizures with burst suppression. Brain MRI showed progressive brain atrophy, especially in the frontal regions.

In cases of neonatal onset seizures, peroxisomal disorders should also be considered. Seizures with onset in the first months of life have been frequently reported among the group

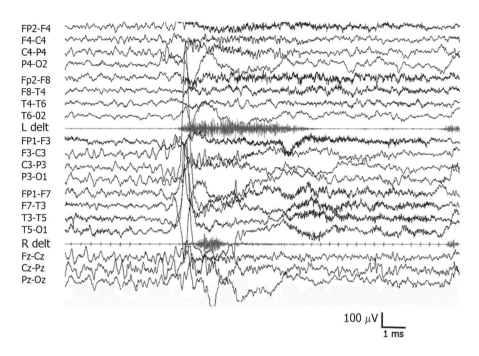

FP2-F4
F4-C4
C4-P4
P4-O2
Fp2-F8
F8-T4
T4-T6
T6-O2
L delt
FP1-F3
F3-C3
C3-P3
P3-O1
FP1-F7
F7-T3
T3-T5
T5-O1
R delt
Fz-Cz
Cz-Pz
Pz-Oz

100 μV
1 ms

Fig. 31.3. Two-month-old girl with Zellweger syndrome. EEG recording. There is slowing of background activity. A focal seizure is recorded with rhythmic theta activity in the frontocentroparietal leads of both hemispheres, much more prominent on the right, lasting for about 9 s, accompanied by a sustained tonic contraction of the left arm and a mild contraction in the contralateral limb.

of Zellweger spectrum disorders but also in single peroxisome enzyme deficiencies such as acyl-CoA oxidase deficiency and D-bifunctional protein deficiency. Common to all three Zellweger spectrum disorders (Zellweger syndrome, neonatal adrenoleukodystrophy, infantile Refsum disease) are liver disease, variable neurodevelopmental delay, retinopathy, and perceptive deafness with onset in the first months of life. Zellweger syndrome (cerebrohepatorenal syndrome) is a multiple congenital syndrome characterized by craniofacial abnormalities: high forehead, large anterior fontanel, shallow orbital ridges, epicanthus, redundant folds of the neck, external ear deformities, low and broad nasal bridge, and midface hypoplasia. In the neonatal period profound hypotonia with the absence of neonatal and deep reflexes, inability to feed, and seizures are present. The ocular abnormalities may include corneal clouding, cataracts, glaucoma, optic atrophy, and retinopathy. Hepatomegaly and renal cysts are present. In approximately 50% of patients there is bony stippling at the patella and in other bones. The main seizure type is focal clonic epileptiform potentials and seizure patterns in EEG are mainly seen at central and centroparietal regions reflecting the underlying cortical abnormalities (Figs. 31.3, 31.4). The brain shows a striking abnormality of neuronal migration; there are areas of polymicrogyria, Purkinje cell heterotopia, and abnormalities of the olivary nucleus. Affected children fail to acquire any developmental skill and usually die in the first year of life (Steinberg *et al.* 2006).

Neonatal adrenoleukodystrophy and infantile Refsum disease exhibit milder presentations and longer lifespans. Most children have the initial symptoms in the neonatal period, others are brought to medical attention later. Seizures may likewise be present in the neonatal period or later. Craniofacial abnormalities are less pronounced; renal cysts and bony stippling are not seen routinely. Sensorineural hearing loss and retinitis pigmentosa are the most common manifestations. Most children show hypotonia but, unlike in Zellweger syndrome, they can achieve developmental milestones such as head control and sitting unsupported, and may even walk independently. In some patients leukodystrophy develops, accompanied by loss of previously acquired skills and spasticity. In neonatal adrenoleukodystrophy patients have hypotonia, seizures, and progressive white matter disease, may have polymicrogyria, and usually die in late infancy (Steinberg *et al.* 2006).

In rhizomelic chondrodysplasia punctata seizures are common. The main clinical features include rhizomelia, coronal clefts of the vertebral bodies, chondrodisplasia punctata, and contractures. Affected infants also have cataracts, craniofacial abnormalities with frontal bossing, depressed nasal bridge, and small nose. Ichthyosis can develop. Milder incomplete phenotypes have been described. Cerebral and cerebellar atrophy, alterated myelination, and neuronal migration defects involving the midbrain have been reported (Steinberg *et al.* 2006).

Seizures have been described in several isolated peroxysomal enzyme deficiencies. D-bifunctional protein deficiency is a relatively frequent peroxisomal β-oxidation deficiency, second to X-adrenoleukodystrophy, but problably understimated. Nearly all patients show neonatal hypotonia (98%) and seizures (93%) within the first months of life; some patients (15%) have shown infantile spasms. Failure to thrive has been observed in nearly half of patients. Like Zellweger syndrome, dysmorphisms (68%) and virtual absence of any developmental skill are observed; patients affected by D-bifunctional protein deficiency die within the first 17 months.

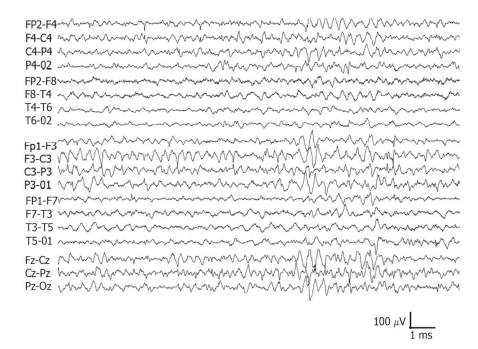

FP2-F4
F4-C4
C4-P4
P4-O2
FP2-F8
F8-T4
T4-T6
T6-O2

Fp1-F3
F3-C3
C3-P3
P3-O1
FP1-F7
F7-T3
T3-T5
T5-O1
Fz-Cz
Cz-Pz
Pz-Oz

100 μV
1 ms

Fig. 31.4. Same patient as in the previous figure. Sleep EEG recording. There is slowing of background activity, with absence of physiological sleep patterns and bursts of high-amplitude, asynchronous, irregular slow and sharp wave activity that is at times organized in quasi-rhythmic sequences.

Patients affected by acyl-CoA oxidase deficiency show moderate neonatal hypotonia, frequent, but less severe, seizures with onset between 2 and 4 months and are more responsive to therapy than those with D-bifunctional protein deficiency. Renal, skeletal, and liver involvements are usually not observed; polydactyly has been reported. Most patients do not show craniofacial dysmorphisms (Wanders and Waterham 2006).

Biochemical analyses in Zellweger spectrum disorders show elevated plasma very long chain fatty acids (VLCFA) and usually deficient erythrocyte membrane plasmalogens. Patients affected by rhizomelic chondrodysplaia punctata have deficient plasmalogens but normal VLCFA. Since 15–20% of patient present clinical phenotypes similar to Zellweger and elevated VLCFA have a single defect in peroxisomal fatty acid metabolism, further biochemical analysis is often vital. If the phenotype is suggestive of mild or variant Zellweger spectrum disorders, it is important, even when VLCFA are normal, to measure erythrocyte plasmalogens and plasma phytanic, pristanic acids, pipecolic acid, and bile acids. If abnormalities have been detected in at least one pathway or there is a strong clinical suspicion, skin biopsy and biochemical studies in cultured fibroblasts should be performed.

In acyl-CoA oxidase deficiency and D-bifunctional protein deficiency the only anomaly observed in plasma is elevated VLCFA. In some patients with D-bifunctional protein deficiency, plasma VLCFA are normal and abnormal VLCFA profiles are detected in fibroblasts.

The Zellweger spectrum disorders are known to be associated with mutations in 12 different *PEX* genes; mutations of the same gene can lead to three phenotypes, whereas mutations in *PEX7* are associated with rhizomelic chondrodysplaia

punctata type I but not with the Zellweger spectrum disorders (Wanders and Waterham 2006). Molecular analysis shows *PEX1* deficiency in 70% of all patients with peroxisome biogenesis disorders; two common alleles *I700fs* (Nt2098insT) and *G843D* (Nt2528G>A) have been reported. In patients with rhizomelic chondrodysplasia punctata, analysis of the *PEX7* gene shows a common allele, L292X (Nt875T>A), with a frequency of 50–52%. Prenatal diagnosis is feasible by biochemical and molecular analysis (Steinberg *et al.* 2006).

No specific therapy is available; current treatment is supportive and targets seizures, hearing, and ophthalmologic manifestations: oral bile acid administration improved hepatobiliary function in several Zellweger syndrome infants.

Seizures and psychomotor retardation are often combined in inborn errors of metabolism but are not specific. In peroxisomal disorders and a number of other metabolic defects, highly specific symptoms can be excellent keys to diagnosis. In multiple carboxylase deficiency (holocarboxylase synthetase deficiency and biotinidase deficiency) characteristic manifestations are cutaneous symptoms, such as skin rash and alopecia, seizures, ataxia, hypotonia, impaired consciousness, and metabolic acidosis (Scriver *et al.* 2001).

Both disorders respond dramatically to oral therapy with pharmacological doses of biotin (10–80 mg per day); restriction of protein intake is not necessary except in very severe cases of holocarboxylase synthetase deficiency. In biotinidase deficiency low doses of biotin stop the seizures and prevent brain damage if started early (Desai *et al.* 2008).

Biotinidase deficiency is a metabolic disorder characterized by the inability to recycle biotin and hence multiple carboxylase deficiency. The age of onset of symptoms varies from

1 week to 2 years, with median and mean ages of 3 and 5.5 months. Neurological manifestations are major features and seizures occur in over 50% of patients and may often be the presenting and only obvious symptom, so testing for biotinidase deficiency is warranted in any patient with unexplained seizures. The most frequent seizure types are generalized convulsive or myoclonic, in some patients they only occur with fever, or intermittently in some periods only; sometimes, infantile spasms may be the presenting feature. Ataxia is another prominent feature and may also be intermittent; hypotonia has been observed in over half of the patients and development may be delayed. Other common initial symptoms include seborrheic or atopic dermatitis, partial or complete alopecia, and conjunctivitis. Without treatment most of these patients show progressive encephalopathy with psychomotor regression or bulbar symptoms; 75% of the patients have ketolactic acidosis at some time with lethargy leading to coma and death. Breathing problems such as hyperventilation, stridor, or apnea, and sensorineural hearing loss and visual loss associated with optic atrophy have been reported (Fernandes et al. 2000; Scriver et al. 2001; Wolf et al. 2009).

Metabolic abnormalities in biotinidase deficiency include lactic acidemia and characteristic organic aciduria that consists of 3-methylcrotonylglycine, 3-hydroxyisovaleric acid, 3-hydroxypropionic acid, and 2-methylcitric acid. Some patients have been reported not to have organic aciduria. The diagnosis is made by the assay of biotinidase in serum. A method of neonatal screening for biotinidase deficiency is a semiquantitative colorimetric assessment of biotinidase activity on blood spotted on filter paper used for phenylketonuria screening. Samples with biotinidase activity show a characteristic purple color upon addition of developing reagents after incubation with biothynil p-aminobenzoate, whereas those with little or no activity remain straw-colored. Positive screening tests can be confirmed by a quantitative assay of enzyme activity using additional samples of serum.

Isolated 3-methylcrotonyl-CoA carboxylase deficiency shows a variable phenotype that ranges from severe neonatal onset with seizures, infantile spasms and hypsarrhythmia and hypotonia to asymptomatic adult forms. Elevated excretion of 3-methylcrotonylglycine and 3-hydroxyisovaleric acid are present. A biotin-responsive form has been described (Scriver et al. 2001; Baumgartner et al. 2004).

In early onset cobalamin C/D deficiencies (vitamin B_{12}-responsive methylmalonic aciduria) partial seizures, both simple and complex, and convulsive status epilepticus may be the first manifestation. The EEG may show multifocal epileptiform abnormalities while awake, which increase during slow sleep, leading to a nearly continuous slow spike-and-wave activity. Diffuse delta rhythms, probably due to metabolic derangement, prevalence with superimposed focal and multifocal EEG abnormalities associated with slow background activity can also be observed. Cobalamin C/D deficiency is an inborn error of intracellular cobalamin metabolism with high levels of methylmalonic acid, homocysteine, and homocystine.

The early onset is characterized by feeding difficulties, failure to thrive, hypotonia, seizures, microcephaly, developmental delay, hematologic abnormalities (macrocytic anemia, thrombocytopenia, leukopenia), and sometimes hemolytic uremic syndrome presenting in the first year of life. There is no typical EEG pattern and thus we suggest that an assay of plasma amino acids and urinary organic acids is performed in infants with seizures associated with failure to thrive and hematologic abnormalities. Neuroradiological findings include a variable degree of supratentorial white matter atrophy with thinning of the corpus callosum (Biancheri et al. 2002).

Cerebellar atrophy, moderate mental retardation, cerebellar ataxia, and seizures have been reported in mevalonic aciduria, an inborn error in the biosynthesis of cholesterol due to mevalonate kinase deficiency (Breton et al. 2007).

L-2-Hydroxyglutaric aciduria, a "cerebral organic aciduria," is a chronic progressive neurodegenerative disorder. Clinical findings include mild psychomotor delay in the first years of life, followed by progressive cerebellar ataxia, dysarthria, mental deterioration, pyramidal and extrapyramidal signs, seizures, and macrocephaly. Brain MRI shows characteristic lesions in the subcortical white matter, cerebellar atrophy, and abnormal signal in the dentate nuclei and putamen. The centripetal extension of the white matter involvement is a distinctive feature with respect to other leukodystrophies. L-2-Hydroxyglutaric acid is increased more than 4–10-fold in plasma, urine, and CSF. Amino acid assays in plasma, urine, and CSF have shown increased levels of L-lysine in some patients. It has been demonstrated that a gene encoding for a putative FAD-dependent L-2-hydroxyglutarate dehydrogenase is mutated in L-2-hydroxyglutaric aciduria (Wajner et al. 2002; Rzem et al. 2004).

A severe early-onset epileptic encephalopathy has been reported in association with D-2-hydroxyglutaric aciduria due to D-2- hydroxyglutarate dehydrogenase. The severe neonatal or early infantile onset form is characterized by severe generalized hypotonia, irritability, developmental delay, generalized, mostly tonic, seizures, lethargy, cardiomyopathy, and dysmorphic features such as a flat face with broad nasal bridge and external ear abnormalities. Patients with a mild phenotype exhibit psychomotor retardation, macrocephaly, and hypotonia (Struys et al. 2005). Typical neuroradiological findings include enlargement of the lateral ventricles, subependymal cysts, and delayed myelination (van der Knaap et al. 1999). The mild phenotype has a more variable clinical presentation and less consistent MRI findings than the severe form. The biochemical marker of this disorder is a persistently elevated urinary excretion of D-2-hydroxyglutaric acid with mildly increased urinary 2-ketoglutarate, succinate, fumarate, lactate, and L-2-hydroxyglutaric acid. There may also be increased levels of γ-aminobutyric acid (GABA) and lactate in the CSF (Wajner et al. 2002; Rzem et al. 2004).

Gamma-aminobutyric acid, the major inhibitory neurotransmitter of the brain, is synthesized primarily from glutamate, the major excitatory neurotransmitter. Up to one-third of the brain's synapses utilize GABA, a four-carbon amino acid which also exists in the form of a dipeptide with histidine, know as homocarnosine. The disorders of GABA metabolism are succinic semialdehyde dehydrogenase deficiency, GABA transaminase deficiency, and homocarnosinosis. The latter are extremely rare and require CSF determination of GABA concentrations for laboratory diagnosis. Succinic semialdehyde dehydrogenase deficiency, also called 4-hydroxybutirric aciduria or γ-hydroxybutirric aciduria, is a rare autosomal recessive disorder of the GABA degradation pathway. In succinic semialdehyde dehydrogenase deficiency transamination of GABA to succinic semialdehyde is followed by reduction to 4-hydroxybutyric acid. The disorder has been described in at least 350 individuals worldwide but is probably underdiagnosed. The most constant clinical features are developmental delay, hypotonia, and mental retardation. Seizures, ataxia, behavior problems, and hyporeflexia are reported in nearly half of patients. Generalized tonic–clonic, absence, and myoclonic seizures and convulsive status epilepticus have all been described. Studies with EEG have shown a variety of abnormalities including background slowing, focal and generalized epileptiform discharges, and, rarely, a photoparoxysmal response. Sleep spindle asynchrony and absence of the rapid eye movement (REM) phase were reported in one study (Pearl et al. 2003). Magnetic resonance imaging typically reveals bilaterally increased T2-weighted signal in the globus pallidus, with variable involvement of the white matter and dentate nucleus in the cerebellum. Magnetic resonance spectroscopy for the standard neuronal markers has been reported to be normal; however, special edited sequences for GABA and GABA metabolites have revealed significant increases in these compounds in the occipital cortex providing the first in vivo evidence of increase GABA concentration in patients with epilepsy. In contrast to other organic acidurias or other metabolic disorders, in this defect, metabolic acute decompensation or intermittent vomiting, ataxia, and altered mental status are not reported. In contrast to the progressive course of inherited metabolic diseases, ataxia is not progressive and has been noted to improve with age. The diagnosis may be suspected in cases of seizures if accompanied by a mental retardation–ataxia syndrome of unknown etiology. The increased signal intensity involving the globus pallidus is an important key. Screening by urine organic acids is essential for laboratory detection of 4-hydroxybutyric acid; careful organic acid analysis is important as measuring 4-hydroxybutyric acid is sometimes difficult because the compound has a high volatility and may be obscured on GC–MS studies by a high urea peak. The inclusion of selective ion monitoring mass spectrometry for 4-hydroxybutyric acid in organic acid analyses increases the number of diagnosis. Dicarboxylic aciduria, with elevations of glutaric, adipic, and suberic acids occurs secondarily to the inhibition of mitochondrial β-oxidation and these elevations may mislead towards suspecting another disorder but the accumulation of 4-hydroxybutyric aciduria is specific to succinic semialdehyde dehydrogenase deficiency. Diagnosis is confirmed by enzymatic assay in isolated cultured lymphoblasts. A retrospective study in the cerebrospinal fluid from 13 patients showed significant increases in 4-hydroxybutyric aciduria, GABA, and homocarnosine, while glutamine levels were low to borderline-low. Decreased glutamine, coupled with elevated GABA, suggests disruption of the "glutamine–glutamate shuttle" essential for the maintenance of neurotransmitter pools of glutamate and GABA. Disruption of the GABA–glutamate axis resulting in a significant imbalance between glutamatergic excitatory activity and GABAergic inhibition and may be responsible for the seizures. Vigabatrin, an irreversible inhibitor of GABA transaminase, should theoretically inhibit the formation of succinic semialdehyde and therefore 4-hydroxybutyric aciduria. This drug has been widely used in succinic semialdehyde dehydrogenase deficiency but its long-term clinical efficacy is marginal (Gibson et al. 1995; Pearl et al. 2003). Other antiepileptic drugs have been used with varying success, including carbamazepine and lamotrigine; valproate is contraindicated as it may inhibit any residual succinic semialdehyde dehydrogenase enzyme activity. In the experimental homozygous-deficient mice with 4-hydroxybutyric aciduria receptor antagonist (NCS-382) enhance survival.

Diagnostic assessment should also consider diseases that are usually tested in newborn screening programs as some cases may have been missed, false negatives are possible, and not all countries have neonatal screening programs. Untreated phenylketonuria subjects constantly exhibit delayed developmental skills and a mousy odor is detectable in the urine; infantile spasms with hypsarrhythmia, often with progressive microcephaly, begin after the first few months of life in one-third of infants. In older phenylketonuria patients mental handicap and disturbed behavior are common; about 25% have generalized seizures at some time (Fig. 31.5). As in classical phenylketonuria, patients with hyperphenylalaninemia due to tetrahydrobiopterin (BH4) defects will develop a progressive epileptic encephalopathy (such patients might not have been included in newborn screenings or have been false negative). However, neurotransmitters are involved in a wide spectrum of neurological diseases (e.g., truncal hypotonia with distal hypertonus, bradykinesia, dystonia with diurnal fluctuations, oculogyric spasms, and autonomic instability). Tetrahydrobiopterin (BH4) plays an essential role in the regulation of tyrosine and tryptophan hydroxylase, the initial and rate-limiting steps in the biosynthesis of dopamine, norepinephrine, epinephrine, and serotonin. Aromatic L-amino acid decarboxylase deficiency and tyrosine hydroxylase deficiency are rare disorders of biogenic amine metabolism, with hyperhenilalaninemia, rare disorders of monoamine metabolism are aromatic L-amino acid decarboxylase deficiency and tyrosine hydroxylase deficiency. The first defect combines serotonin and catecholamine deficiency and the clinical features are hypotonia and paroxysmal movement disorders; neurological symptoms become evident in all patients during the first 6 months and in some generalized and complex partial seizures and paroxysmal EEG abnormalities have been reported,

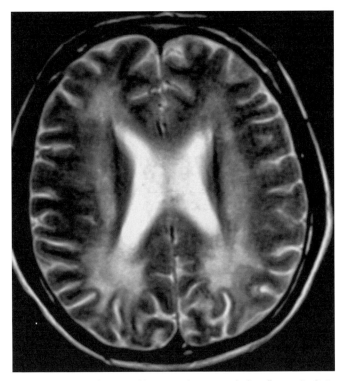

Fig. 31.5. Twenty-five-year-old man with untreated phenylketonuria. Brain MRI: T2-weighted axial section. Note the widespread areas of white matter abnormality, manifested as high signal intensity, lesions.

Table 31.2 Laboratory tests

Initial metabolic work-up

- Basic laboratory tests:
  In blood: glucose, lactate, ammonia, acid–base status, blood counts; liver function tests; creatine kinase levels; uric acid; acetest in urine

Additional tests

- Urine: organic acids, Sulfitest
- Plasma/serum: amino acids, homocysteine
- Acylcarnitine profile
- Biotinidase activity

In specific suspected disease

- CSF: amino acids, neurotransmitters, pterins
- Peroxisomal studies (very long chain fatty acids, phytanic acids, plasmalogens)

Secondary metabolic work-up

- Skin biopsy: cultured fibroblasts
- Enzymatic assays
- Molecular analysis

although none developed severe epilepsy. Seizures may be difficult to differentiate from oculogyric crises and paroxysmal dystonia. Typically the patients initially receive a diagnosis of cerebral palsy, epilepsy, or hyperekplexia. In both defects neuroimaging is generally unremarkable or, in the advanced stages, shows progressive cerebral atrophy (Ito *et al.* 2008; Manegold *et al.* 2009).

Diagnostic tests and therapy

All infants with unexplained seizures should be evaluated for an underlying inborn error of metabolism. It is important to recognize these disorders early, before irreversible consequences occur, since a specific therapy may be effective.

Basic laboratory tests (glycemia, blood counts, liver function, acid–base balance, lactate, ammonia) can be important keys for diagnosis. Metabolic acidosis with ketosis (elevated anion gap, urine pH below 5, and positive acetest) is suggestive of organic acidurias such as methylmalonic aciduria, propionic aciduria, and isovaleric acidemia, and may indicate a large number of rarer and less known organic acidurias. Some organicoacidurias induce thrombocytopenia, anemia, and granulocytopenia (e.g., methylmalonic aciduria CblC). A positive family history (parental consanguinity and other family members having neurological disorders) together with clinical or radiological features can suggest an inborn error of metabolism or even a specific defect. In "cerebral" organic acidurias basic laboratory tests are often not informative.

Unexplained seizures in infants should prompt careful routine metabolic screening in the blood and urine with plasma amino acids and urinary organic acid analysis (Table 31.2). It is obviously important to diagnose treatable disorders, such as phenylketonuria and hyperphenilalaninemias due to BH4 deficiency, biotinidase defect, some organic acidurias, and serine deficiency, as early as possible.

In BH4 defects, diagnosis is based on the measurement of plasma phenylalanine, pterin metabolites in the urine, BH4 loading test, neurotransmitters and pterins in CSF, enzyme activity in red blood cells (such as dihydropteridine reductase), or in fibroblasts and molecular analysis. The outcome is no longer negative if diagnosis is early and therapy with a low phenylalanine diet and/or BH4 and L-dopa, carbidopa, 5-hydroxytryptophan, and folinic acid is introduced.

In neonates, lumbar puncture should be performed immediately to rule out infection, non-ketotic hyperglycinemia, disorders of biogenic amine metabolism, or the folinic acid-responsive seizure disorder. Analysis of CSF should include glucose, lactate, amino acids (mainly serine and glycine), and neurotransmitters. Confirmatory tests include skin biopsy for enzyme assays on fibroblasts and molecular studies of causative genes.

Extraneurologic findings

Extraneurologic findings can be the clue for a specific diagnostic approach in consideration of the relevant associated signs:

(1) Disorder of the respiratory rhythm: hyperpnea and apnea may result from metabolic acidosis (organic aciduria), brainstem lesions, or the direct action of a toxic metabolite

(hyperammonemia in propionic and methylmalonic acidemia and urea cycle disorders) on the respiratory center.

(2) Dysmorphic facial features: in peroxisomal diseases.

(3) Abnormalities of skin and hair: alopecia and skin rash may occur in disorders of biotin metabolism (biotinidase or holocarboxylase synthetase deficiency).

(4) Hepatomegaly: enlargement or dysfunction of the liver is often present in Zellweger syndrome (cerebrohepatorenal syndrome).

(5) Nephropathy: renal cysts and dysplastic changes are a feature of Zellweger syndrome and glutaric aciduria type II. Nephrolithiasis is present in molybdenum co-factor deficiency.

(6) Skeletal changes: patellar calcification is present in Zellweger disease.

(7) Ocular abnormalities: cataract, corneal opacities, glaucoma, and retinal degeneration are characteristic of a number of inborn errors of metabolism but are not specific. Brushfield spots are frequently observed in Zellweger syndrome. A characteristic lens dislocation may be present in the neonatal period but is usually noted after a few weeks of life in molybdenum co-factor deficiency.

(8) Head circumference: the majority of infants affected by inborn errors of metabolism show a normal head circumference at birth but head growth tends to slow down after a few months or weeks. Progressive microcephaly is suggestive of inborn error of metabolism; an early progressive head enlargement is characteristic of a few disorders (glutaric aciduria type I, Canavan disease). In 3-phosphoglycerate dehydrogenase deficiency (serine deficiency) congenital microcephaly and intractable seizures are almost always present.

In suspected Zellweger spectrum disorders, plasma VLCFA assay must be performed and then other biochemical analyses such as erythrocyte membrane plasmalogens, plasma phytanic and pristanic acids, pipecolic acid, and bile acids. If abnormalities have been detected in at least one pathway or there is a strong clinical suspicion skin biopsy and biochemical studies in cultured fibroblasts and then molecular analysis should be performed.

The list of genetically determined metabolic diseases that produce seizures in infancy is quite long (Table 31.3). In the newer group of disorders associated with defects of serine, glutamate and GABA pathways, CSF analysis is necessary for diagnosis.

Table 31.3 Organic acidurias, aminoacidopathies, and peroxisomal disorders that can present with seizures as a prominent manifestation

Inborn error of metabolism	Epilepsy	Other neurological manifestations	Brain MRI	Non-neurological signs	Diagnostic tests
Non-ketotic hyperglycinemia (NKH)	Myoclonic and generalized in the classical neonatal form, infrequent in the late form	Severe hypotonia in classical neonatal NKH. In mild NKH hyperactivity or aggressiveness, though uncommon	Inconsistently white matter involvement, corpus callosum dysgenesis (classical form)	Hiccup–apnea in classical neonatal form	Plasma and CSF aminoacids, CSF/plasma glycine ratio, glycine cleavage system activity, mutation analysis
Maple-syrup urine disease	Intractable seizures during severe decompensation	Coma Stupor Abnormal movements (pedaling–boxing) Opisthotonus	Possible signs of cerebral edema (increased intracranial pressure)	Maple-syrup-like odor Poor feeding and drowsiness Hypoglycemia	Plasma and urine amino acids, organic acids in urine, enzyme activity in fibroblasts, mutation analysis
Sulfite oxidase deficiency/ molybdenum co-factor deficiency	Intractable seizures in the postnatal period	Progressive psychomotor impairment, severe hypotonia	Chronic dysmyelination early cystic white matter damage, with severe cerebral atrophy	Severe microcephaly, lens dislocation	Plasma and urine aminoacids, sulfite test in fresh urine, serum uric acid, urine purines, enzyme studies, mutation analysis
Congenital serine deficiency	Seizures in the first year of life, often West syndrome with hypsarrhythmia	Severe psychomotor delay	Hypomyelination and severe white matter attenuation	Congenital microcephaly	Plasma, urine, and CSF serine levels, enzyme activity in fibroblasts, mutation analysis

Table 31.3 (cont.)

Inborn error of metabolism	Epilepsy	Other neurological manifestations	Brain MRI	Non-neurological signs	Diagnostic tests
Glutamine synthetase deficiency	Seizures in the first days of life	Hypotonia Brain malformations Coma	Cerebral and cerebellar atrophy with delayed gyration, marked white matter changes with subependymal cysts	Severe enteropathy, necrolytic erythema of the skin	Plasma, urine, and CSF aminoacids, enzyme activity in lymphocytes, mutation analysis
Mitochondrial glutamate transport impaired	Neonatal onset myoclonic seizures with burst suppression	Hypotonia, coma	Progressive brain atrophy especially in the frontal regions	Progressive microcephaly	Mutation analysis
Zellweger syndrome (cerebrohepatorenal syndrome)	Neonatal and infantile seizures, partial epilepsy with focal clonic epileptic potentials especially in central and centroparietal regions reflecting cortical abnormalities	Severe developmental delay, loss of acquired skills, absence of deep reflexes in newborn, exitus generally in the first year	Leukodystrophy, neuronal migration abnormalities, Purkinje cell heterotopia, abnormalities of olivary nucleus	Craniofacial abnormalities: high forehead, large anterior fontanel, shallow orbital ridges, epicanthus, redundant folds of neck, broad nasal bridge, midface hypoplasia, external ear deformities, poor feeding, cataracts, corneal clouding, glaucoma, optic atrophy, retinopathy, hepatomegaly, renal cysts bony stippling of patella	Plasma VLCFA, biochemical studies in fibroblasts, mutation analysis
Adrenoleukodystrophy and infantile Refsum disease	Neonatal and infantile seizures	Mild developmental delay, leukodystrophy, loss of acquired skills, hypotonia	White matter disease, polymicrogyria	Craniofacial abnormalities, sensorineural hearing loss, retinitis pigmentosa, renal cysts (rare), bone stippling (rare)	Plasma VLCFA, erythrocytes membrane plasmalogens, plasma phytanic and pristanic acids, pipecolic acid, and bile acids, biochemical studies in fibroblasts, mutation analysis
Rhizomelic chondrodysplasia punctata	Neonatal and infantile seizures	Developmental delay	Cerebral and cerebellar atrophy Hypomyelination, neuronal migration disorders	Failure to thrive, rhizomelia, chondrodysplasia punctata, vertebral abnormalities, craniofacial abnormalities, cataracts, ichthyosis	Plasma VLCFA, erythrocytes, membrane plasmalogens, biochemical studies in fibroblasts, mutation analysis

Table 31.3 (cont.)

Inborn error of metabolism	Epilepsy	Other neurological manifestations	Brain MRI	Non-neurological signs	Diagnostic tests
D-bifunctional protein deficiency	Neonatal seizures, infantile spasms	Neonatal hypotonia, developmental delay	Hypomyelination, neuronal migration disorders	Failure to thrive Dysmorphisms	Plasma VLCFA, biochemical studies in cultured fibroblasts, mutation analysis
Biotinidase deficiency	First months of life: generalized tonic–clonic, myoclonic, infantile spasms, febrile seizures, dramatic response to biotin	Lethargy, ataxia, hypotonia, developmental delay (without treatment)	White matter involvement, cerebral and cerebellar atrophy and widened extracerebral CSF spaces	Skin rash, alopecia, breathing impairment, hearing and visual loss	Organic acids in urine, biotinidase activity in serum, mutation analysis
Holocarboxylase synthetase deficiency	Generalized tonic–clonic, myoclonic, febrile seizures, infantile spasms, response to biotin	Progressive encephalopathy with psychomotor regression (without treatment), ataxia, hypotonia, coma	White matter involvement	Skin rash, alopecia, breathing impairment, hearing and visual loss	Organic acid in urine, carboxylase activity in fibroblasts, mutation analysis
Isolated 3-methylcrotonyl-CoaA carboxylase deficiency	Neonatal seizures, infantile spasms, EEG: hypsarrhythmia, recurrent status epilepticus	Developmental delay, hypotonia	Confluent and multiple foci of leukodystrophy		Organic acids in urine and plasma, enzyme activity in cultured fibroblasts
Methylmalonic aciduria/cobalamin C/D deficiencies	Partial seizures EEG: multifocal abnormalities and delta rhythm, convulsive status epilepticus vitamin B_{12} responsive	Developmental delay, hypotonia	Supratentorial white matter atrophy with thinning corpus callosum	Progressive microcephaly, feeding difficulties Failure to thrive, hematologic abnormalities (megaloblastic anemia, thrombocytopenia, leukopenia), hemolytic uremic syndrome	Organic acids in urine and plasma (methylmalonic acid), plasma homocysteine and homocystine, biochemical studies in fibroblasts (e.g., complementation analysis), mutation analysis
Mevalonic aciduria	Partial seizures, febrile seizures	Moderate developmental delay, cerebellar ataxia	Cerebellar atrophy	Dysmorphic features, cataracts, recurrent febrile crises with vomiting, diarrhea, rash, hematological abnormalities (normocytic hypoplastic anemia, leukocytosis, thrombocytopenia)	Urinary mevalonic acid levels, enzyme activity in fibroblasts, mutation analysis
D-2-Hydroxyglutaric aciduria	Neonatal seizures	Irritability, developmental delay, lethargy, severe hypotonia	Enlarged lateral ventricles, subependymal cysts, delayed myelination	Macrocephaly, cardiomyopathy, dysmorphic features	D-2-hydroxyglutaric acid in plasma, urine, and CSF, amino acids assay in plasma, urine, and CSF, mutation analysis

Table 31.3 (cont.)

Inborn error of metabolism	Epilepsy	Other neurological manifestations	Brain MRI	Non-neurological signs	Diagnostic tests
L-2-Hydroxyglutaric aciduria	Generalized seizures, most cases with good response to conventional therapy	Mild to moderate developmental delay, progressive cerebellar ataxia, behavioral disturbances	Leukodystrophy (particularly U-fibers) combined with progressive cerebellar atrophy and signal changes in basal ganglia and the dentate nuclei	Macrocephaly	2-Hydroxyglutaric acid in urine, FAD-dependent 1–2-enzyme activity in fibroblasts, mutation analysis
4-Hydroxybutyric aciduria or succinic semialdehyde dehydrogenase deficiency	50% of the cases: generalized tonic–clonic, partial seizures, some patients may be resistant to conventional therapy, some others EEG abnormalities without seizures, EEG: background slowing focal and diffused abnormalities	Mild to moderate developmental delay, behavior abnormalities (autistic-like, attention deficit hyperactivity) Hypotonia, hyporeflexia, cerebellar non-progressive ataxia	Increased T2-weighted signal of white matter globus pallidus, dentate nucleus, increase of GABA metabolites in the occipital cortex (MRI spectroscopy) In 40% of the cases cerebellum atrophy		Organic acids in urine, plasma, and CSF, GABA/glutamine levels in CSF, enzyme activity in fibroblasts, mutation analysis
Phenylketonuria	Infantile spasms with hypsarrhythmia, generalized focal seizures, status epilepticus	From preserved intelligence to mild developmental delay	From normal pattern to severe white matter damage	Mousy odor of urine, progressive microcephaly	Amino acids in plasma, mutation analysis
BH4 defects	Generalized focal seizures, status epilepticus	Metabolic encephalopathy, bradykinesia, dystonia and paroxysmal movement disorders, diurnal fluctuation, autonomic instability	Unremarkable in the first years, progressive cerebral atrophy		Amino acids in plasma, prolactin, urinary pterins, dihydropteridine reductase (DHPR) assay on blood spot, neurotransmitter assay in CSF, mutation analysis
Homocystinuria, classical form	Not common	From preserved intelligence to mild developmental delay, depression, obsessive–compulsive and personality disorders, cerebrovascular accidents	Normal or arterial/venous strokes	Marfanoid habitus, lens dislocation, thrombotic vascular disease	Plasma and urine amino acids, total homocystinemia, mutation analysis

Table 31.3 (cont.)

Inborn error of metabolism	Epilepsy	Other neurological manifestations	Brain MRI	Non-neurological signs	Diagnostic tests
Homocystinuria, N(5,10)-methylenetetra hydrofolate reductase deficiency	Generalized focal seizures, infantile spasms	Hypotonia, developmental delay Motor and gait abnormalities, psychosis, cerebrovascular accidents	White matter involvement, arterial/venous strokes, progressive brain atrophy	Thrombotic vascular disease, Marfanoid habitus, progressive microcrania	Plasma and urine amino acids, total homocystinemia, biochemical studies in fibroblasts, mutation analysis
Urea cycle disorders	Neonatal seizures, status epilepticus	Metabolic encephalopathy triggered by high protein intake or catabolism, nausea, vomiting, cephalalgia, confusion, psychiatric symptoms, ataxia, coma, stroke-like episodes, paraplegia	Normal or cerebral edema or high signal intensity in the cortex (T2)		Blood ammonia, amino acids in plasma, orotic acids in urine, mutation analysis

Careful study of patients will continue to identify new inborn errors of metabolism or to clarify biochemically or genetically old defects.

Therapies with specific vitamins, diet, drugs, and neurotransmitters are possible for some inborn errors of metabolism. Diet in phenylketonuria and some aminoacidopathies removes the offending metabolites with the use of special formulas with low specific metabolites (e.g., phenylalanine, protein, isoleucine–valine–leucine). Another approach in correcting the metabolic abnormalities is to stimulate an alternative pathway as for example with betaine in homocystinuria. In some defects it is possible to detoxify the toxic metabolite by binding it to another substance which converts it into a nontoxic and readily eliminated conjugate (e.g., benzoate and phenylbutyrate in hyperammonemias and glycine in isovaleric acidemia). In biotinidase deficiency low doses of biotin have remarkable effects on neurological and cutaneous symptoms.

Biotin can be life-saving in patients with biotinidase or holo-carboxylase synthetase deficiency as well as in hydroxycobalamin and in some forms of methylmalonic aciduria. Therapy with biotin in biotinidase deficiency and with vitamin B_6 in vitamin B_6-dependency represent two of the most successful therapies for inborn errors of metabolism. It is important that clinicians are aware of these disorders because treatment is simple and the results can be very successful.

Some metabolic disorders are not responsive or only partially responsive to treatment. Recently, successful treatment of molybdenum co-factor deficiency type A with intravenous cyclic pyranopterin monophosphate has been reported (Veldman *et al.* 2010). Use of drugs that induce metabolic acidosis (acetazolamide and topiramate) should be avoided in patients with pre-existing metabolic acidosis. Biochemical and molecular analysis are important for a definitive diagnosis and open the way to genetic counseling and prenatal diagnosis.

References

Applegarth DA, Toone JR (2004) Glycine encephalopathy (nonketotic hyperglycinaemia): review and update. *J Inherit Metab Dis* **27**:417–22.

Baumgartner MR, Dantas MF, Suormala T, *et al.* (2004) Isolated 3-methylcrotonyl-CoA carboxylase deficiency: evidence for an allele-specific dominant negative effect and responsiveness to biotin therapy. *Am J Hum Genet* **75**:790–800.

Biancheri R, Cerone R, Rossi A, *et al.* (2002) Early-onset cobalamin C/D deficiency: epilepsy and electroencephalographic features. *Epilepsia* **43**:616–22.

Breton Martinez JR, Canovas Martinez A, Casana Perez S, *et al.* (2007) Mevalonic aciduria: report of two cases. *J Inherit Metab Dis* **30**:829.

de Koning TJ (2006) Treatment with amino acids in serine deficiency disorders. *J Inherit Metab Dis* **29**:347–51.

de Koning TJ, Klomp LW (2004) Serine-deficiency syndromes. *Curr Opin Neurol* **17**:197–204.

de Koning TJ, Klomp LW, van Oppen AC, *et al.* (2004) Prenatal and early postnatal treatment in 3-phosphoglycerate-dehydrogenase deficiency. *Lancet* **364**:2221–2.

Desai S, Ganesan K, Hegde A (2008) Biotinidase deficiency: a reversible metabolic encephalopathy: neuroimaging and MR specroscopic findings in a series of four patients. *Pediatr Radiol* **38**:848–56.

Fernandes J, Saudubray J-M, van den Berghe G (2000) *Inborn Metabolic Diseases: Diagnosis and Treatment*, 3rd edn. Heidelberg: Springer-Verlag.

Friebel D, Von Der Hagen M, Baumgartner ER, *et al.* (2006) The first case of 3-methylcrotonyl-CoA carboxylase (MCC) deficiency responsive to biotin. *Neuropediatrics* **37**:72–8.

Gibson KM, Jacobs C, Ogier H, *et al.* (1995) Vigabatrin therapy in six patients with succinic semialdehyde dehydrogenase deficiency. *J Inherit Metab Dis* **18**:143–6.

Guthrie R, Susi A (1963) A simple phenylalanine method for detecting phenylketonuria in large populations of newborn infants. *Pediatrics* **32**:338–43.

Häberle J, Görg B, Toutain A, *et al.* (2006) Inborn error of amino acid synthesis: human glutamine synthetase deficiency. *J Inherit Metab Dis* **29**:352–8.

Hamosh A, Maher JF, Bellus GA, Rasmussen SA, Johnston MV (1998) Long-term use of high-dose benzoate and dextromethorphan for the treatment of nonketotic hyperglycinemia. *J Pediatr* **132**:709–11.

Ito S, Nakayama T, Ide S, *et al.* (2008) Aromatic L-aminoacid decarboxylase deficiency associated with epilepsy mimicking non-epileptic involuntary movements. *Dev Med Child Neurol* **50**:876–8.

Kalayci O, Coskun T, Tokatli A, *et al.* (1994) Infantile spasms as the initial symptom of biotinidase deficiency. *J Pediatr* **124**:103–4.

Kölker S, Koeller DM, Sauer S, *et al.* (2004) Excitotoxicity and bioenergetics in glutaryl-CoA dehydrogenase deficiency. *J Inherit Metab Dis* **27**:805–12.

Kölker S, Sauer S, Surters RAM, *et al.* (2006) The aetiology of neurological complications of organic acidaemias: a role for the blood–brain barrier. *J Inherit Metab Dis* **29**:701–4.

Kölker S, Sauer S, Hoffmann GF, *et al.* (2008) Pathogenesis of CNS involvement in disorders of amino and organic acid metabolism. *J Inherit Metab Dis* **31**:194–204.

Korman SH, Gutman A (2002) Pitfalls in the diagnosis of glycine encephalopathy (nonketotic hyperglycinemia). *Dev Med Child Neurol* **44**:712–20.

Manegold C, Hoffmann GF, Degen I, *et al.* (2009) Aromatic L-amino acid decarboxylase deficiency: clinical features, drug therapy and follow-up. *J Inherit Metab Dis* **32**:371–80.

Molinari F, Raas-Rothschild A, Rio M, *et al.* (2005) Impaired mitochondrial glutamate transport in autosomal recessive neonatal myoclonic epilepsy. *Am J Hum Genet* **76**:334–9.

Neumaier-Probst E, Harting I, Seitz A, Ding C, Kolker S (2004) Neuroradiological findings in glutaric aciduria type I (glutaryl-CoA dehydrogenase deficiency). *J Inherit Metab Dis* **27**:869–76.

Pearl PL (2009) New treatment paradigms in neonatal metabolic epilepsies. *J Inherit Metab Dis* **32**:204–13.

Pearl PL, Novotny EJ, Acosta MT, Jakobs C, Gibson KM (2003) Succinic semialdehyde dehydrogenase deficiency in children and adults. *Ann Neurol* **54**:S73–80.

Rzem R, Veiga-da-Cunha M, Noël G, *et al.* (2004) A gene encoding a putative FAD-dependent L-2-hydroxyglutarate dehydrogenase is mutated in L-2-hydroxyglutaric aciduria. *Proc Natl Acad Sci USA* **101**:16 849–54.

Sauer SW, Okun JG, Fricker G, *et al.* (2006) Intracerebral accumulation of glutaric and 3-hydroxyglutaric acids secondary to limited flux across the blood–brain barrier constitute a biochemical risk factor for neurodegeneration in glutaryl-CoA dehydrogenase deficiency. *J Neurochem* **97**:899–910.

Scriver CR, Beaudet AL, Valle D, *et al.* (2001) *The Metabolic and Molecular Bases of Inherited Disease,* 8th edn. New York: McGraw-Hill.

Steinberg SJ, Dodt G, Raymond GV, *et al.* (2006) Peroxisome biogenesis disorders. *Biochim Biophys Acta* **1763**:1733–48.

Struys EA, Salomons GS, Achouri Y, *et al.* (2005) Mutations in the D-2-hydroxyglutarate dehydrogenase gene cause D-2-hydroxyglutaric aciduria. *Am J Hum Genet* **76**:358–60.

Tabatabaie L, de Koning TJ, Geboers AJ, *et al.* (2009) Novel mutations in 3-phosphoglycerate dehydrogenase (PHGDH) are distributed throughout the protein and result in altered enzyme kinetics. *Hum Mutat* **30**:749–56.

Van der Knaap MS, Jacobs C, Hoffmann GF, *et al.* (1999) D-2-Hydroxyglutaric aciduria: further clinical delineation. *J Inherit Metab Dis* **22**:404–13.

van Spronsen FJ, Hoeksma M, Reijngoud D-J (2009) Brain dysfunction in phenylketonuria: is phenylalanine toxicity the only possible cause? *J Inherit Metab Dis* **32**:46–51.

Veldman A, Santamaria-Araujo JA, Sollazzo S (2010) Successful treatment of molybdenum cofactor deficiency type A with cPMP. *Pediatrics* **125**:e1249–54.

Wajner M, Vargas CR, Funayama C, *et al.* (2002) D-2-Hydroxyglutaric aciduria in a patient with a severe clinical phenotype and unusual MRI findings. *J Inherit Metab Dis* **25**:28–34.

Wanders RJ, Waterham HR (2006) Peroxisomal disorders: the single peroxisomal enzyme deficiencies. *Biochim Biophys Acta* **1763**:1707–20.

Wolf NI, Garcia-Cazorla A, Hoffmann GF (2009) Epilepsy and inborn errors of metabolism in children. *J Inherit Metab Dis* **32**:609–17.

Zinnanti WJ, Lazovic J, Housman C, *et al.* (2007) Mechanism of age-dependent susceptibility and novel treatment strategy in glutaric acidemia type I. *J Clin Invest* **117**:3258–70.

Chapter

32

Porphyria

Geoffrey Dean and Simon D. Shorvon

... I found
A thing to do, and all her hair
In one long yellow string I wound
Three times her little throat around,
And strangled her.
Robert Browning, *Porphyria's Lover* (1842)

Introductory note

This chapter was commissioned from Dr. Geoffrey Dean, who sadly died on September 7, 2009, before the chapter was completed. We publish here a short autobiographical recollection by Dr. Dean and then a summary of the clinical aspects of the condition as it relates to epilepsy. Dr. Dean was one of the pioneering physicians in South Africa who documented and clarified the many difficult aspects of this group of conditions, a true porphyrinologist as Professor Peter Meissner of the University of Cape Town has written, and this chapter is dedicated to his memory. Dr. Dean's autobiography (Dean 2002) provides more detail of his life and work with porphyria.

Dr. Geoffrey Dean's autobiographical recollections

In 1947 I emigrated from England to South Africa and decided to settle in practice in Port Elizabeth, the main city of the eastern Cape. In February 1951, I was called to see a nurse in a nearby hospital. Following an unhappy love affair, she could not sleep and started taking barbiturate tablets. She was crying and very emotional and complained of abdominal pain and pains in her arms and legs. Her doctor had suspected an intestinal obstruction and the previous day had undertaken an exploratory abdominal operation. Sodium thiopental was used to induce anaesthesia. After the operation her pains became much worse. Her arms and legs became weak and she needed a respirator to aid her breathing. She did not have seizures. Her urine was normal in colour when passed and it became deeply red on standing for two or three hours and I suspected she had acute porphyria. Her urine showed a brilliant fluorescence in ultraviolet light

using a Wood's lamp. In spite of all our care and intravenous drip, oxygen and the use of a respirator, she died two days later. I asked Nurse van Rooyen's father to come and see me and he told me that he had had twelve children and that three others of his daughters had already died from similar symptoms to that of Nurse van Rooyen and that none of them had been diagnosed as having porphyria. Mr. van Rooyen had scars and blisters on the back of his hands and he told me that this was due to the 'van Rooyen skin' and that many men in his very large family had this skin disorder going back at least to his great grandfather. With the help of Nurse van Rooyen's father and a very old aunt, I decided to trace all of his relatives on the side of the family which had a sensitive skin over six generations. Among those who were alive over the age of 18, 60 had inherited porphyria, 24 men and 36 women [Dean 1956]. Professor Jan Waldenström of Lund University, Sweden [who had named acute intermittent porphyria (AIP)] invited me to come to Sweden to see some of his patients, and on returning to South Africa, I continued to see patients with acute porphyria, and by March 1953 I had attended 13 patients with acute attacks of porphyria, two of whom died. Among these 13 family groups, 216 porphyrics were found [Dean 1953]. With the help of a nineteenth-century book about the genealogy of the early South African settlers (Der Oude Kaapsche Familiën) and of the scribe who kept the church records and the central records in Cape Town, all of the first 32 family groups we studied on the porphyria side were traced back to Gerrit Jansz who came from Deventer in Holland in 1685 [Fig. 32.1]. In 1688 he married Ariaantje Adriaansse (Jacobs), one of eight orphans sent to the Cape of Good Hope by the Lord's Seventeen (*Die Heeren 17*) on a 5-year contract, but really to become wives of the first free burghers at the Cape who had been provided with land to produce food for the spice ships that called at the Cape on the way to the East. The first child of Gerrit Jansz to be a forebear of porphyric families was Jacomijntje who married the first van Rooyen to come to South Africa, Cornelius, who came from Gorkum in Holland. Other porphyria families trace back to three of the other children of Gerrit Jansz van Deventer or his wife Adriaantje van Rotterdam [Dean 1963]. In 1996 the Cape Town porphyria research group working in collaboration with colleagues from Wales and

The Causes of Epilepsy, eds. S. D. Shorvon, F. Andermann, and R. Guerrini. Published by Cambridge University Press. © Cambridge University Press 2011.

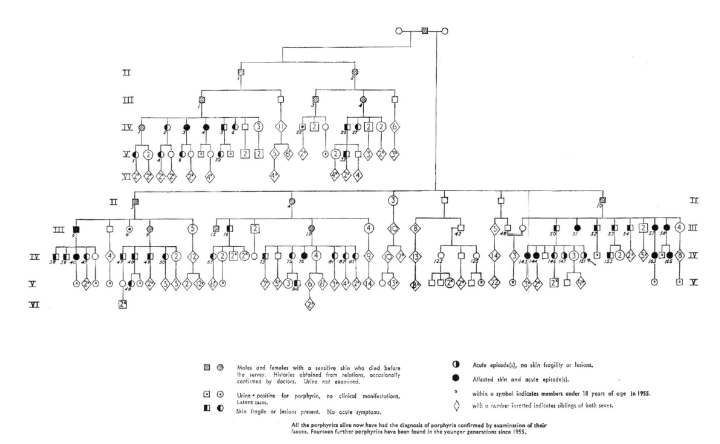

Fig. 32.1. Genealogical tree of G. R. van Rooyen, born 1814.

the United States found that the gene responsible for South African variegate porphyria (VP) was *R59W*. Today 94% of those with VP in South Africa carry this gene and the other 6% are more recent immigrants and carry different genes (Meissner *et al.* 1996).

[Not least due to the work of Dr. Dean and others] the incidence of acute porphyria has fallen rapidly in South Africa since the replacement of barbiturate sedatives by tranquilizers and other sedatives. It has also been greatly reduced by the study of family trees undertaken today so well by the porphyria research group in Cape Town and by the increased awareness among doctors. Before the introduction of modern drugs, those who had inherited VP had as many children on average as the general population, as can be seen in the increase of their numbers.

Porphyria and epilepsy

The porphyrias are a group of conditions in which there are deficiencies in one of the eight enzymes of the heme biosynthetic pathway (the porphyrin pathway): four of the enzymes are located in the mitochondria and the other four in the cytosol. The enzyme deficiency leads to underproduction of heme and the accumulation of porphyrins which are heme precursors. It is this accumulation, rather

than the deficiency of heme, that causes the symptoms in most cases.

The disorders are often inherited but can be secondary to severe liver disease (porphyria cutanea tarda). The inherited conditions are classified into the acute porphyrias (hepatic porphyrias) and cutaneous (erythropoietic) porphyrias, depending on the site of accumulation of porphyrins or precursors.

Neurological disturbance, including epilepsy, is the predominant features of the inherited acute porphyrias (hepatic porphyrias), and the major symptoms including pain are due to acute neurological dysfunction. There are three acute porphyrias which cause epilepsy and other neurological symptoms: acute intermittent porphyria (AIP), variegate porphyria, and hereditary coproporphyria (HCP) (Kadish *et al.* 2006).

Epilepsy may coexist with porphyria by chance, and in these cases, care needs to be exercised in choosing appropriate long-term therapy. Dr. Dean calculated that, in 1951, for instance, there were 8000 persons descended from the van Deventer family in South Africa, possibly now $13\,000 \pm 2000$, and taking a low estimate of epilepsy as 30 per 1000, this would mean that there may be approximately 400 epileptics who also have variegate porphyria in South Africa (Dean 1971).

The only epidemiological study carried out specifically to determine the incidence of epilepsy seizures was a postal

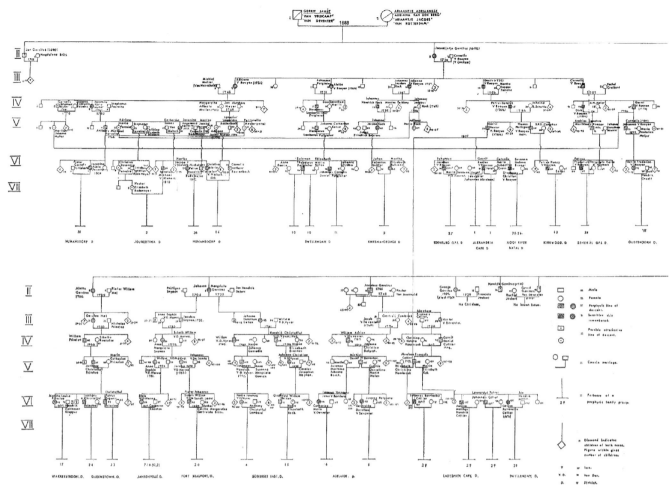

Fig. 32.2. Porphyria Variegate in South Africa.

survey carried out in Sweden amongst all those with known AIP. Seizures were self-reported in only 2.2% of all cases and in 5.1% of all those with manifest AIP (Bylesjo *et al.* 1996).

Clinical features of the acute porphyrias that can cause epilepsy

Acute intermittent porphyria (AIP) is the commonest hepatic porphyria and the most commonly associated with epilepsy. This condition is inherited in an autosomal dominant fashion and is caused by a deficiency of porphobilinogen deaminase (PBGD; synonym – hydroxymethylbilane synthase [HMB synthase] and uroporphyrinogen I-synthase).

The majority of persons with this deficiency are asymptomatic (i.e., are carriers). Furthermore, in symptomatic cases, the deficiency often becomes evident only when the susceptible individual is exposed to provoking factors which include: intercurrent infection, hormonal changes (especially estrogen or progesterone changes), low calorific diet or other dietary changes, or medicinal drugs. The drugs which

can induce or worsen an attack are those that induce amino-levulinic acid synthetase or PBGD in the liver, and these include most enzyme-inducing antiepileptic drugs which therefore should be avoided (Table 32.1). Oral contraceptives, some analgesics, some cardiovascular and antihypertensive drugs, ergotamine derivatives, chloramphenicol, erythromycin, rifampicin, trimethoprin, ketaconizole, nitrofurantoin, and sulfonamide antibiotics are amongst the other drugs which frequently precipitate attacks. (A full list of drugs that can be safely used in porphyria are to be found at www.drugs-porphyria.com/ or www.porphyria-europe.com/03-drugs/selecting-drugs.asp.)

The clinical and biochemical features of the acute attacks of variegate porphyria are identical to AIP, except for cutaneous photosensitivity which occurs in one-third of cases. The condition presents after puberty, particularly in women, due to hormonal changes. The symptoms take the form of attacks that evolve over hours or days. The predominant symptoms are caused by acute neuropathy and include abdominal pain, nausea, vomiting, constipation, acute neuropathy, muscle weakness, severe neuropathic pain, urinary retention,

233

Table 32.1 Safe and unsafe drugs for patients with acute intermittent porphyria or variegate porphyria

Safe drugs	Unsafe drugs
Acetaminophen	Barbiturates
Acetazolamide	Captopril
Acyclovir	Chloramphenicol
Allopurinol	Chlorpropamide
Amiloride	Diazepam
Ampicillin	Diltiazem
Aspirin	Diphenhydramine
Atropine	Doxycycline
Bumetanide	Ergot compounds
Bupivacaine	Erythromycin
Chlorothiazide	Estrogen
Codeine phosphate	Ethanol
Corticosteroids	Furosemide
Deferoxamine	Griseofulvin
Demerol	
Digoxin	Hydralazine
Fentanyl	Hydrochlorothiazide
Follicle-stimulating hormone (FSH)	Impramine
Gabapentin	Lidocaine
Gentamicin	Methyldopa
Glipizide	Metoclopramide
Haloperidol	Metronidazole
Heme arginate	Nifedipine
Heparin	Oral contraceptives
Insulin	Orphenadrine
Iron	Oxycodone
Lithium salts	Pentazocine
Meperidine	Phenobarbital
Mequitazine	Phenytoin
Metformin	Piroxicam
Metoprolol	Pivampicillin
Morphine	Progesterone
Nadolol	Pyrazinamide
Oxytocin	Sodium valproate
Penicillin	Terfenadine
Procaine	Tetracyclines
Propofol	Theophylline
Propylthiouracil	Trimethoprim
Quinine	Verapamil
Ranitidine	
Salbutamol	
Senna	
Temazepam	
Thyroxine	
Warfarin	

Source: American Porphyria Foundation website, at www.porphyriafoundation.com

encephalopathy, delerium, coma, mental confusion, hallucinations, and epileptic seizures. Pain is often severe and the neuropathic picture can predominate mimicking a Guillain–Barré syndrome. The abdominal symptoms may be misdiagnosed as a primarily gastrointestinal disease (Solinas and Vajda 2008).

Seizures are relatively common in the acute attacks although chronic epilepsy is seldom a problem. The epilepsy may occur as a neurologic manifestation of the condition or secondary to metabolic disturbance such as hyponatremia (Birchfield and Cowger 1966). It has been estimated that about one-third of children and one-fifth of adult cases have seizures during the acute attacks. Status epilepticus can occur (Bhatia *et al.* 2008).

Diagnostic tests

The index of suspicion must be high as many cases are overlooked. A family history is an important clue.

Biochemical tests

The diagnosis of acute porphyria depends on demonstrating increased levels of urinary δ-aminolevulinic acid (ALA) and porphobilinogen (PBG) in urine. The diagnosis of AIP is confirmed if there is a deficiency of PBGD in red blood cells, a test which is however not always positive in all cases. In some patients, only hepatic PBGD is deficient, requiring liver biopsy to confirm the diagnosis. Estimations of PBGD in red blood cells is a sensitive way of detecting latent porphyria in asymptomatic family members.

In an acute attack, the measurement of porphobilinogen (PBG) in a random urine sample is a useful screening test, and if positive followed by a 24-hour collection of ALA, PBG, and/or porphyrin. Estimation of fecal porphyrins helps to diagnose VP and HCP (see Table 32.2)

Interpretation of the tests can be complex (Sedel *et al.* 2007). In some patients, porphyrins or precursor levels may be virtually normal in between attacks, and false-positive mild to moderate elevations occur in other conditions. In an attack, ALA and PBG levels are usually increased, but

Table 32.2 The diagnostic tests in the acute porphyrias associated with epilepsy

	Plasma ALA and PBG levels	Urine porphyrin levels	Fecal prophyrin levels	Red cell porphyrin levels
Acute intermittent porphyria	Normal	Increased URO (may be normal if not in an acute attack)	Normal	Decreased
Variegate porphyria	Increased (may be normal if not in an acute attack)	Increased COPRO	Increased COPRO and PROTO	Normal
Hereditary coproporphyria	Normal	Increased COPRO	Increased COPRO	Normal

Notes:
URO, uroporphyrins; COPRO, coproporphyrins; PROTO, protoporphyrins.

ALA levels are less specific. The pattern of elevation is different in each type of porphyria.

Genetic tests

Genetic testing can confirm the disease, but as there are many different mutations in the PBGD gene it is not used widely for screening purposes. Detection is easier if the familial mutation has been identified. Members of a family can be tested to identify asymptomatic cases in order to counsel about avoiding precipitants.

Treatment and prognosis

The patient should be hospitalized in an acute attack and pain, nausea, vomiting, and electrolyte imbalance treated. A high intravenous or oral glucose intake can suppress the attack. Intravenous hematine (Panhematin®) or heme arginate (NormoSang) are effective therapies, given preferably early in an attack or before the attack develops. Heme arginate can be given prophylactically. Provoking drugs should be immediately discontinued.

Prevention is possible with simple measures. Patients at risk of attacks should eat a normal or high-carbohydrate diet. Dieting or weight loss should be avoided or carried out only under medical supervision and a diet with 90% of the normal heme intake is recommended. Drugs that are known precipitants should be avoided and infection and intercurrent illness treated quickly, with special attention to electrolyte balance.

The treatment of epilepsy

All the enzyme-inducing antiepileptic drugs can exacerbate or precipitate attacks and such drugs should be avoided in the treatment of acute seizures (and also in the therapy of chronic epilepsy). Barbiturates have a particularly bad reputation in this regard. Non-enzyme-inducing drugs such as gabapentin, pregabalin, topiramate, or levetiracetam are much safer. For acute therapy, diazepam and clonazepam are relatively safe. Magnesium sulfate has also traditionally been used (Sergay 1979; Kalman and Bonkovsky 1998).

Prognosis

With early recognition of the condition, prevention of provoking factors, and early therapy in an attack, the prognosis is excellent. Long-term effects include chronic pain, peripheral nerve damage, and muscle weakness. Refractory epilepsy can occur but is uncommon.

References

Bhatia R, Vibha D, Srivastava MV, *et al.* (2008) Use of propofol anesthesia and adjunctive treatment with levetiracetam and gabapentin in managing status epilepticus in a patient of acute intermittent porphyria. *Epilepsia* **49**:934–6.

Birchfield RI, Cowger ML (1966) Acute intermittent porphyria with seizures: anticonvulsant medication-induced metabolic changes. *Am J Dis Child* **112**:561–5.

Bylesjo I, Forsgren L, Lithner F, Boman K (1996) Epidemiology and clinical characteristics of seizures in patients with acute intermittent porphyria. *Epilepsia* **37**:230–5.

Dean G (1953) Porphyria. *Bri Med J.* **ii**:1291–301.

Dean G (1956) Porphyria: a familial disease: its diagnosis and treatment. *S A Med J* **30**:377–81.

Dean G (1963) *The Porphyrias: A Story of Inheritance and Environment.* London: Pitman Medical.

Dean G (1971) *The Porphyrias: A Story of Inheritance and Environment,* 2nd edn. London: Pitman Medical.

Dean G (2002) *The Turnstone: A Doctor's Story.* Liverpool, UK: Liverpool University Press.

Kadish K, Smith K, Guilard R (2006) *Medical Aspects of Porphyrins.* Oxford, UK: Elsevier.

Kalman DR, Bonkovsky HL (1998) Management of acute attacks in the porphyrias. *Clin Dermatol* **16**:299–306.

Meissner PN, Dailey TA, Hift RJ, *et al.* (1996) ARS9W mutation in human protoporphyrinogen oxidase results in decreased enzyme activity and is prevalent in South Africans with variegate porphyria. *Nat Genet* **13**:95–7.

Sedel F, Gourfinkel-An I, Lyon-Caen O, *et al.* (2007) Epilepsy and inborn errors of metabolism in adults: a diagnostic approach. *J Inherit Metab Dis* **30**:846–54.

Sergay SM (1979) Management of neurologic exacerbations of hepatic porphyria. *Med Clin N Am* **63**:453–63.

Solinas C, Vajda FJ (2008) Neurological complications of porphyria. *J Clin Neurosci* **15**:263–8.

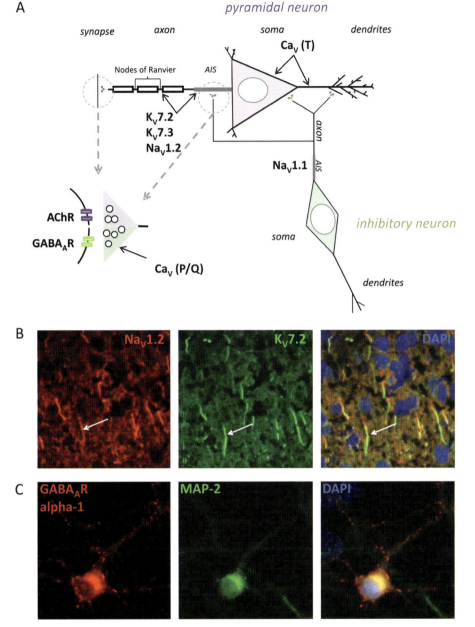

A

pyramidal neuron

synapse   axon   soma   dendrites

Nodes of Ranvier   AIS

Ca$_V$ (T)

K$_V$7.2
K$_V$7.3
Na$_V$1.2

Na$_V$1.1

AChR

GABA$_A$R

Ca$_V$ (P/Q)

inhibitory neuron

soma

axon

AIS

dendrites

B

Na$_V$1.2   K$_V$7.2   DAPI

C

GABA$_A$R
alpha-1   MAP-2   DAPI

Fig. 3.2. Neuronal localization of a few voltage- and ligand-gated ion channels. (A) Schematic presentation of an excitatory pyramidal (lila) and an inhibitory (green) neuron and their synaptic connections. Distinctive intracellular compartments are targeted by different populations of ion channels. Marked is the localization of several ion channels associated with idiopathic epilepsies: in the somatodendritic compartment–Ca$_V$ T-type channels; at axon initial segments (AIS) and nodes of Ranvier in pyramidal neurons–Na$_V$1.2, K$_V$7.2, K$_V$7.3; at AIS of inhibitory neurons–Na$_V$1.1; presynaptic terminals–Ca$_V$ P/Q type; postsynaptic compartment–GABA$_A$ and acetylcholine (ACh) receptors. (B) Colocalization of K$_V$7.2 and Na$_V$1.2 channels at axon initial segments of cortical neurons in the adult mouse brain shown by immunofluorescent staining using an anti-K$_V$7.2 (green) and an anti-Na$_V$1.2 (red) antibody of sections obtained from an unfixed brain. (C) Distribution of GABA$_A$ receptors in a primary cultured hippocampal neuron shown by immunofluorescent staining using an anti-GABA$_A$R α-1 subunit antibody (red). An anti-MAP2 antibody (green) was used as a somatodendritic and DAPI (blue) as a nucleic marker (Maljevic and Lerche, unpublished data).

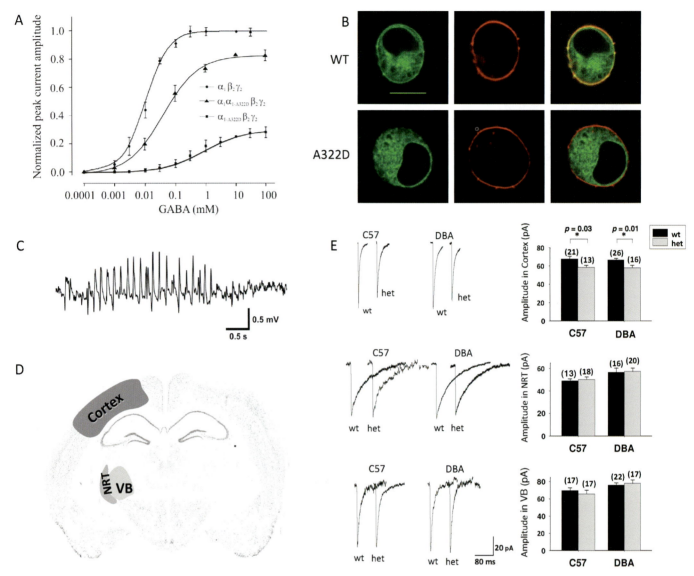

Fig. 3.5. Molecular, cellular, and systemic defects due to mutations in GABA_A receptor subunits leading to idiopathic epilepsy. (A) The A322D mutation of the α_1-subunit of GABA_A receptors, detected in a large JME family (Cossette *et al.* 2002), causes reduced GABA sensitivity as shown by a lowered maximal response and a rightward shift in the dose–response curve of the heterologously expressed GABA_A receptors comprising one mutant and one wild-type, or two mutant α_1-subunits. (B) A reduced surface expression of the A322D mutation was observed in HEK cells transfected with EGFP-tagged α_1 wild-type or mutant together with β_2- and γ_2-subunits. A membrane marker FM4–64 was used to prove the membrane localization of the mutant channel, which was however reduced compared to the wild-type (modified from Krampfl *et al.* 2005, with permission). (C) EEG from a heterozygous mouse strain harboring the R43Q mutation of the γ_2-subunit of GABA_A receptors recorded during a spontaneous absence-like seizure showing rhythmic epileptic discharges. (D) The thalamocortical circuit comprises cortex (here somatosensory), the thalamic reticular nucleus (NRT), and ventrobasal thalamus (VB) containing thalamocortical neurons (compare to Fig. 3.4). Recordings shown in (E) refer to these regions. (E) GABA_A receptor-mediated miniature inhibitory postsynaptic currents (mIPSC) recorded from cortical pyramidal neurons in layer 2/3 of the somatosensory cortex of R43Q heterozygous mouse in two different genetic backgrounds (C57 and DBA are two strains of mice) revealed significantly reduced mIPSC amplitudes for the carriers of the R43Q mutation, indicating that an impaired synaptic inhibition in this layer might play a role in seizure generation, whereas recordings in thalamus did not reveal differences between wild-type and mutant mice (modified from Tan *et al.* 2007, with permission).

A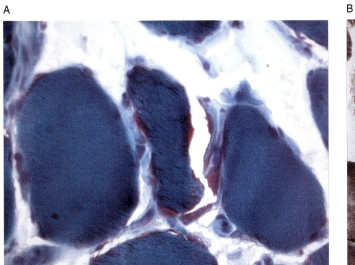

B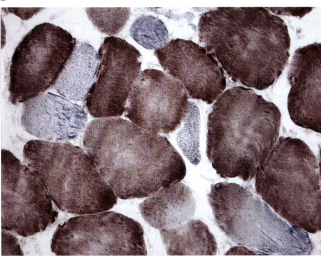

Fig. 19.5. Muscle findings. Mitochondrial accumulation, a sign of failing mitochondrial energy production, can be demonstrated using a variety of staining methods. The classical method is the Gomori-trichrome which stains mitochondria red and the background blue. Mitochondrial accumulation distorts the usual regular shape of the muscle fiber giving it an undulated or ragged appearance (A), hence the descriptive name ragged red fiber. As mitochondrial accumulation is an inconsistent feature, it is better to use histochemical investigations that identify specific complex activities. (B) Staining for succinate dehydrogenase (complex II/SDH, no mtDNA-encoded subunits) is combined with staining for complex IV (cytochrome oxidase, three mtDNA-encoded subunits). Where fibers contain both activities, a dark brown color is seen. Fibers lacking COX activity are easily identified since these will only stain with the blue color derived from the succinate dehydrogenase activity. Unfortunately there are currently no available methods for studying complexes I and III.

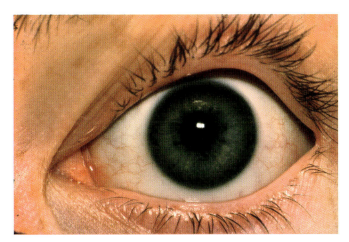

Fig. 36.1. Kayser Fleischer ring. This shows a brown ring as viewed over a blue iris. The pigment is densest in the top crescent where it is always first laid down.

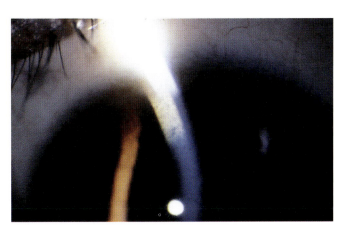

Fig. 36.2. Slit lamp photograph of a Kayser Fleischer ring showing the granular nature of the pigment in the inner layer of Descemet's membrane.

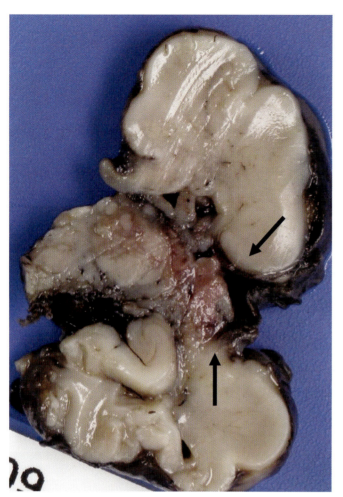

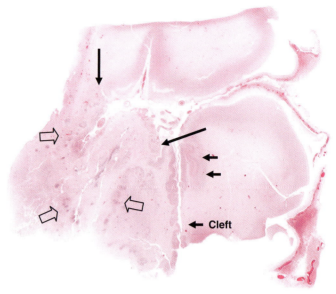

Fig. 52.2. Stained section of mid part of cerebral hemisphere. (Original magnification × 1). The area of infarction is indicated by long arrows. Note an area of polymicrogyria at the junction with normal cortex (short arrows) and a cleft lined by abnormal cortex extending deep into the brain from the surface. Groups of immature unmigrated neurons are seen in the white matter of the damaged area (open arrows).

Fig. 52.1. Fetus 32 weeks gestation: fixed brain slice. Softening and collapse of the tissues in the middle cerebral artery territory are indicated by arrows. A large cystic cavity is covered by thickened and hemorrhagic meninges.

A

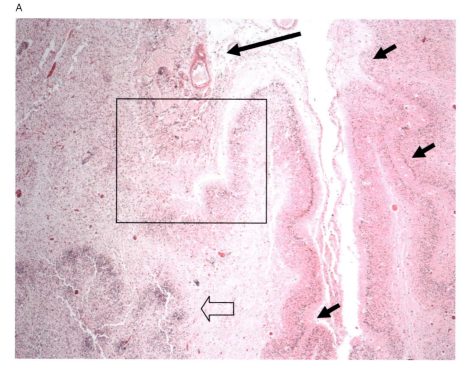

B

C

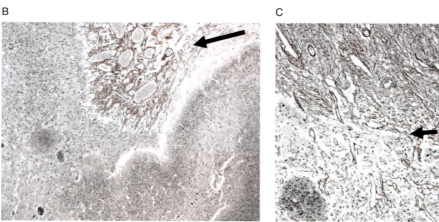

Fig. 52.3. (A) Necrotic cortex (arrow) with loss of nerve cells and proliferation of blood vessels and surface connective tissue; area in box is shown at higher magnification in (B). The open arrow indicates groups of immature cells in the white matter which have failed to migrate to the cortex. Three short arrows mark abnormal areas of cortex bordering the infarcted area; this is developing polymicrogyria (hematoxylin and eosin [H&E] stain original magnification ×2). (B) Extensive proliferation of capillaries (arrow) in the leptomeninges overlying the necrotic cortex (reticulin stain ×4). (C) Higher-power image showing nuclei of cortical neurons which appear as black dots in the cortex and extending between the new capillaries in the leptomeninges. Note many new capillaries in the cortex. An arrow marks the border of cortex and the leptomeninges (reticulin ×10).

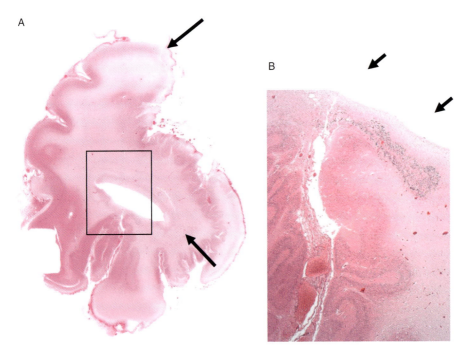

Fig. 52.4. (A) Section of occipital lobe. An area of polymicrogyria is seen between arrows. Here, the molecular layer at the surface in some areas dips into the underlying tissue to follow a festooned band of cortical cells, often irregular and continuous with clusters of immature non-migrated cells in the subcortical white matter. The area in the box, seen in higher power in (B), is a cleft extending through almost the full thickness of the brain wall (schizencephalic cleft or transmantle dysplasia?) (H&E ×1). (B) Higher-power image shows abnormally folded, polymicrogyric, cortex lining the cleft. Just beneath the ventricular wall (top of picture) a band of calcification (small arrows) marks an area of old necrosis of the periventricular white matter (H&E ×2).

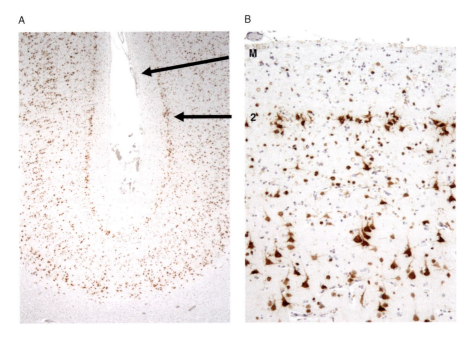

Fig. 52.5. Focal cortical dysplasia, female aged 53 years. (A) Dysplastic cortex in a sulcus (Neu N stain ×2), shown at higher power in (B) (×4). Note the lack of normal lamination. The molecular layer (layer 1) (M) is too cellular and an abnormal band of cells is seen in layer 2. Neurons are abnormally clustered.

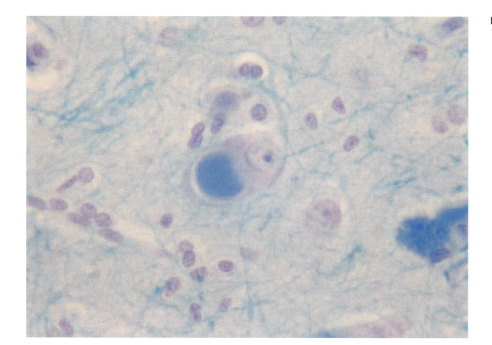

Fig. 52.6. Balloon cell. Focal cortical dysplasia 12 years with epilepsy (LBCV ×20).

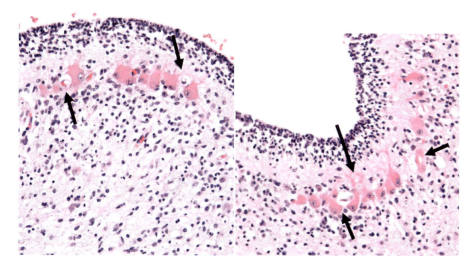

Fig. 52.7. Female fetus 35 weeks gestation. Cerebellar cortex showing dysplastic Purkinje cells. Some are binucleate, some have bizarre thickened dendrites (arrow), and some are apparently engulfing capillaries (short arrows). This was an isolated finding in this brain (H&E ×20).

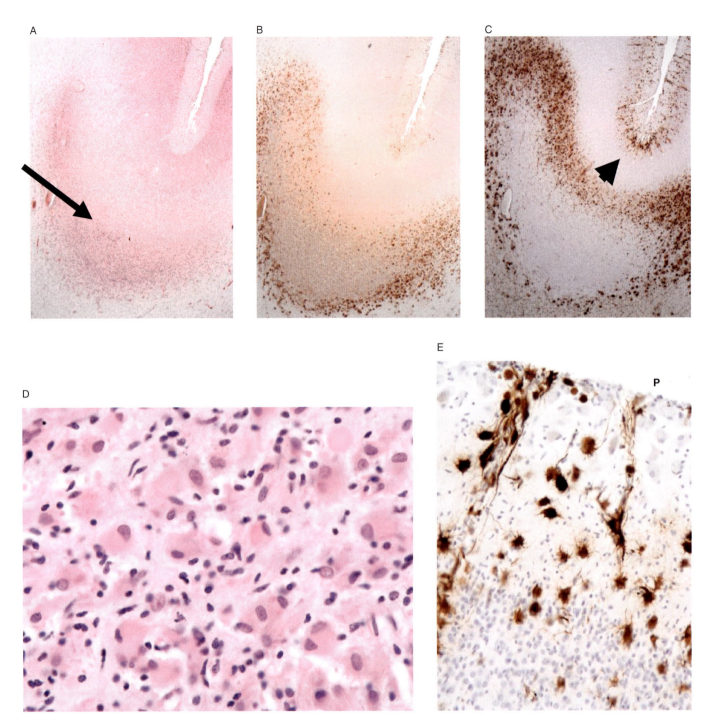

Fig. 52.8. Tuberous sclerosis: fetus 27 weeks gestation. (A) A large group of abnormal cells (arrow) is seen in a sulcus at the junction of the cortex with the white matter (H&E ×1). (B) Nestin stains most of the abnormal cells. (C) Vimentin stain shows only a proportion of the dysplastic cells at the edge of the mass. Note also a layer of abnormal cells in the superficial cortical layer (short arrow). (D) High-power image of the cells in the mass white matter shows two populations, large cells with abundant eosinophilic cytoplasm and small cells with dark oval nuclei (H&E ×20). (E) Vimentin-stained cortex shows only a proportion of the abnormal cells to stain. Note the vimentin-positive cells close to a blood vessel. Many vimentin-negative cells are collecting immediately beneath the pial surface (P) (x10).

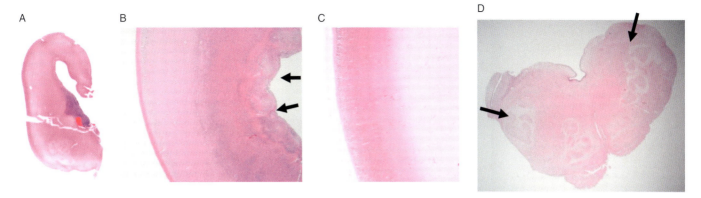

Fig. 52.9. Type 1 lissencephaly, fetus 24 weeks gestation. This fetus had a translocation (p13.3 to pter of chromosome 17 replaced b q27 to qter of chromosome 4). (A) Stained section of hemisphere (H&E). (B) The cerebral cortex is poorly cellular but with a clear marginal zone. The deep cortical border is indistinct and neurons are diffusely distributed in the subcortical white matter. There are prominent periventricular nodular heterotopias (arrows) (H&E ×2). (C) Normal fetal cortex at 25 weeks gestation. Even at this age the deep cortical border is well demarcated from the developing white matter, unlike the appearance in Type 1 lissencephaly (H&E ×2). (D) Olivary malformation with ectopic olivary tissue in the dorsolateral quadrants of the medulla representing incompletely migrated cells in the intramural rostral brainstem pathway (H&E ×1). Similar appearances were present in cousin at 21 weeks.

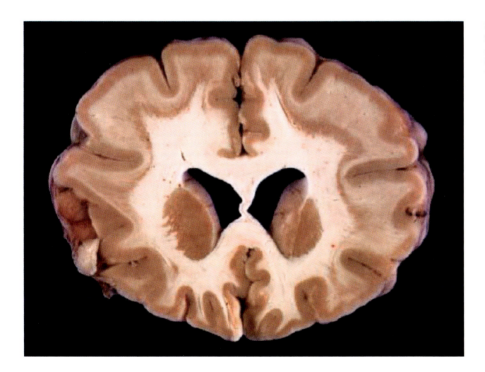

Fig. 52.10. Female 39 years. Fixed brain slice showing extensive double cortex malformation. A well-formed cortex is underlain by a less distinct band of cells which is clearly demarcated from the underlying white matter.

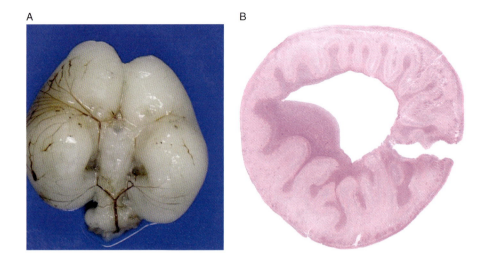

Fig. 52.11. Fetus 20 weeks gestation. (A) Inferior surface of the brain which is small, pale, and smooth. The cerebellar hemispheres are present but small. (B) Stained section of hemisphere shows large ventricle and a thin brain wall occupied by a bilayered band of cells which loops between the deep layer of the cortex to the lining of the lateral ventricle. Cores of germinal matrix extend between these loops. The bilayered band of cells consists of a densely cellular and a less cellular band. (H&E ×1).

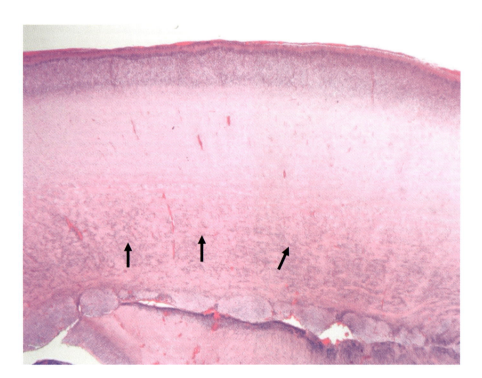

Fig. 52.12. Fetus 17 weeks gestation: an almost uninterrupted band of nodules of unmigrated cells (arrows) lines the ventricular wall. The overlying cortex appears to be forming normally (H&E ×2).

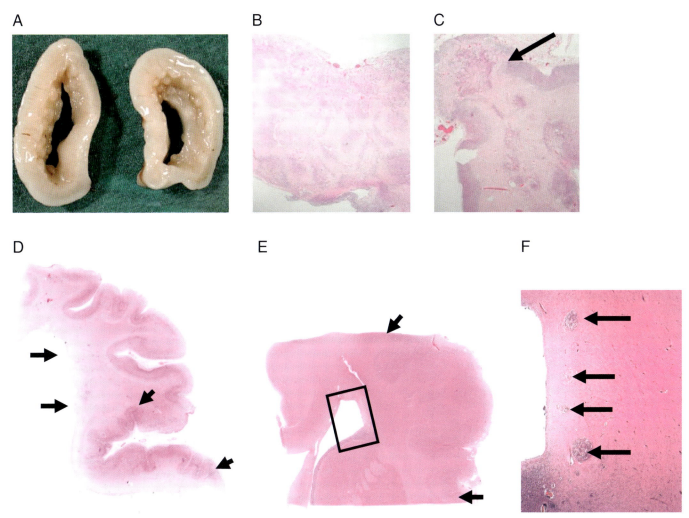

Fig. 52.13. Examples of three forms of periventricular heterotopia with dysplasia of the overlying cortex. (A)-(C) Fetus 20 weeks gestation. Section of fixed brain with multiple heterotopic neuronal nodules in the lining of the occipital horns of the lateral ventricles. This fetus had predominantly posterior BPNH. Clusters and columns of cells in the white matter and focal overmigration of cortical cells (arrow in C) into the leptomeninges associated with proliferation of connective tissue and blood vessels (B and C H&E ×4) (D) Term male infant; H&E-stained section of cerebral hemisphere shows large ventricle with multiple heterotopic neuronal nodules in the ventricular wall (arrows). There is extensive polymicrogyria in the overlying cortex, shown between short arrows. (E, F) Female fetus 36 weeks. H&E-stained section of cerebral hemisphere showing a large area of polymicrogyric cortex (between arrows). The box surrounds small nodules of heterotopic neurons in the periventricular region, shown in higher power (×1) in (F).

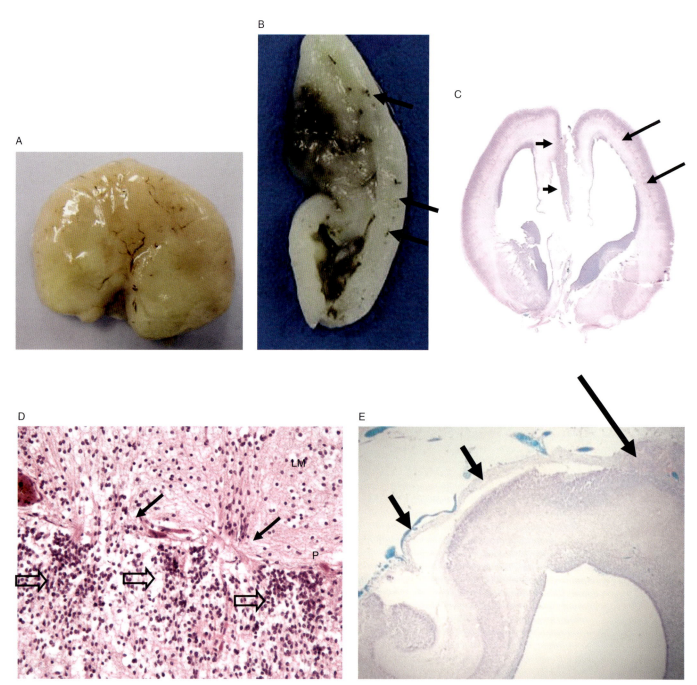

Fig. 52.14. Fetus 18 weeks gestation. (A) Whole brain surface: note the vertically oriented sylvian fissure and finely nodular cortical surface. (B) Coronal slice of the brain shows a line running through the mid part of the brain wall marked by large blood vessels (arrows). (C) Stained section at low power (×1) shows the line at the junction of normally formed cortex and the overmigration into the adherent leptomeninges. Note large ventricles and fusion between adjacent surfaces of medial frontal lobes (arrowheads). (D) A dense band of cells abuts the deep border of the pia (P); at irregular intervals gaps are seen (arrows) through which neurons are streaming into the leptomeninges (LM). Note the absence of a marginal layer which indicates that the original cortical band has not developed normally. Clusters of neurons abut directly on the pial remnants (open arrows) (H&E ×20). (E) Overmigration into the leptomeninges is seen over almost the entire cerebral hemispheres, but a notable exception is the medial temporal lobe and hippocampus. (D) Here the leptomeninges are normal and distinct from the underlying normal cortex (short arrows). As the cortex becomes abnormal so the meninges become adherent and buried in the thick abnormal cortical surface and infiltrated by immature neurons (long arrow; LBCV ×1).

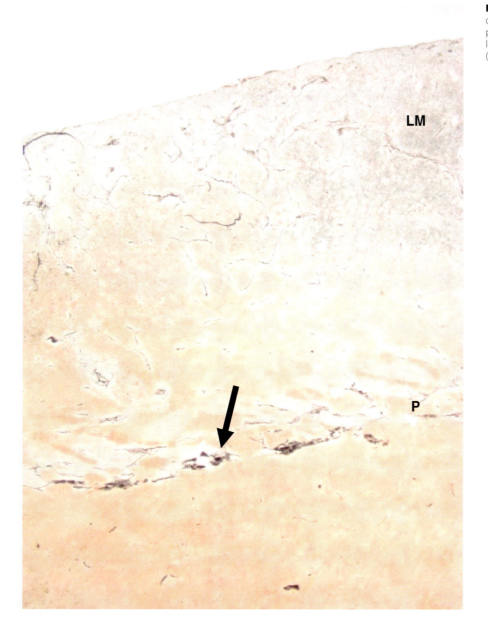

Fig. 52.15. Mature cobblestone cortex. The row of large blood vessels (arrow) denotes the original pial surface of the brain (P). Above it the thickened leptomeninges containing masses of neural tissue (pale golden stain) are seen Reticulin stain ×2.

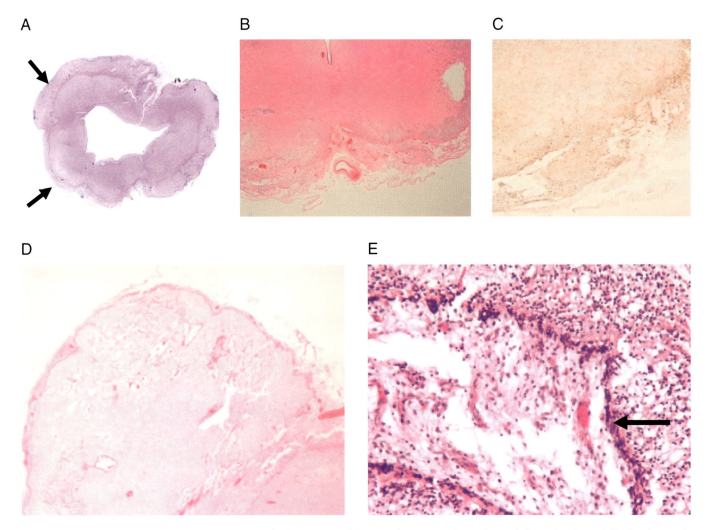

Fig. 52.16. Fetus 18 weeks gestation. (A) There is a band of pale tissue around the entire brainstem and over the cerebellar surface (arrows). The fourth ventricle is large. (B) The leptomeninges are thickened and contain masses of neurons and glial cells (H&E ×2). (C) Higher-power image (×4) stained with GFAP. (D) Fetal cerebellar hemisphere showing disorganized cortex containing many small cysts (H&E ×2). (E) Higher-power image (H&E ×10) shows a poorly formed cortical granule cell layer (arrow) with many cells straggling in the overlying leptomeninges.

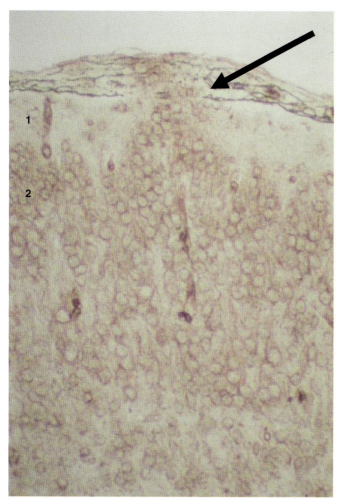

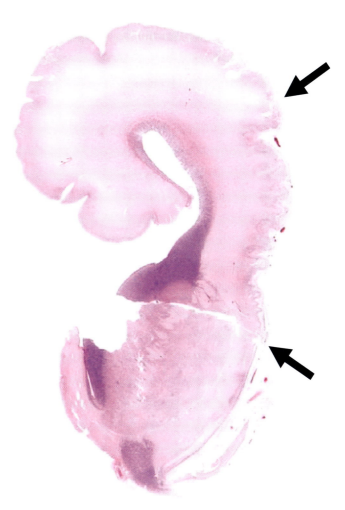

Fig. 52.17. Cortex of MARCKS-deficient mouse. There is a break in the pial basement membrane collagen through which neurons are migrating into the leptomeninges which are locally thickened. The border between layers 1 and 2 is well demarcated where the pia is intact (reticulin stain ×20).

Fig. 52.18. Fetus 18 weeks gestation. Stained section of cerebral hemisphere. Arrows mark an extent of abnormally folded cortex over the lateral aspect of the hemisphere destined to become the perisylvian region.

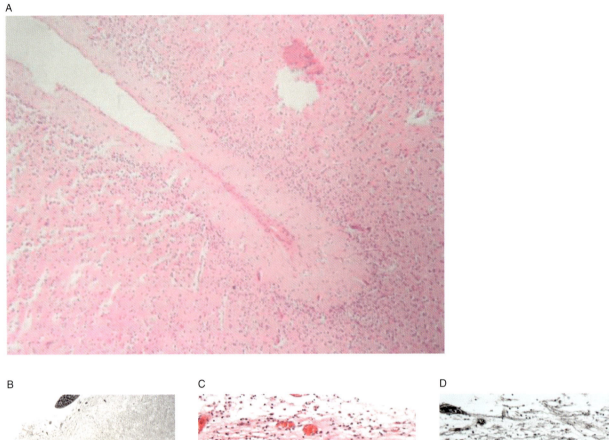

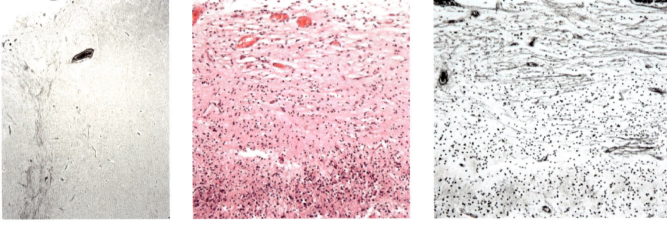

Fig. 52.19. (A) High-power image of the polymicrogyric cortex shows adhesion of adjacent gyri in the depth of a sulcus. In the fusing areas there were increased numbers of cells in the subpial surface of the cortex (H&E ×4). (B) Reticulin stain (×2) shows thickened and reduplicated layers of collagen of the pial basement membrane extending into a fold between gyri (arrows). (C, D) H&E and reticulin stains (×10) of the surface of the polymicrogyric cortex. There is an increase in reticulin fibres, seen running parallel to and embedded into the superficial cortical layers. Neurons, seen as black dots, are seen extending between these layers of basement membrane.

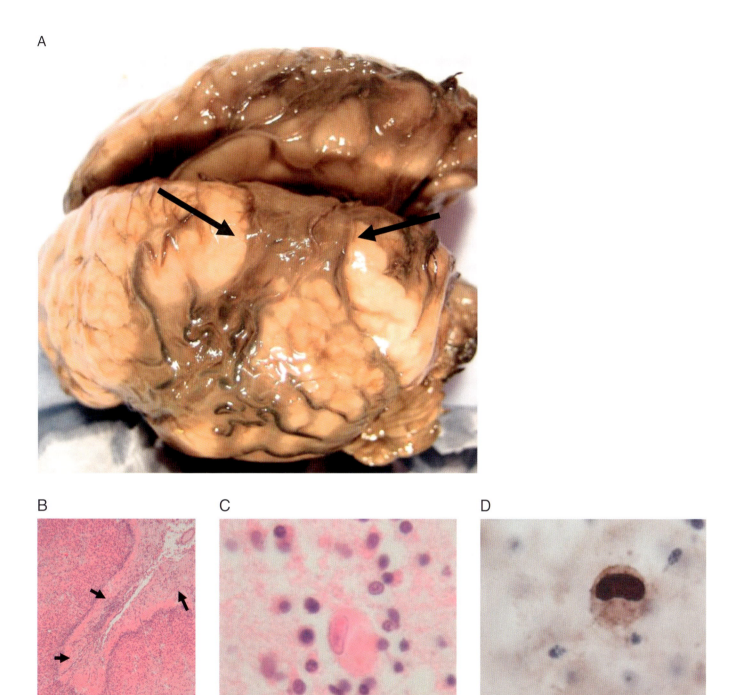

Fig. 52.20. Fetus 35 weeks gestation. (A) Macroscopic examination suggested perisylvian PMG (arrows). (B) Histology showed apparent fusion of adjacent gyri with excess small cells in the marginal and pial layers of the cortical surface (short arrows) (H&E ×4). (C) and (D) are higher-power images (×20) showing cells with intranuclear inclusions characteristic of cytomegalovirus (CMV). (D) Immunocytochemical stain for CMV.

A

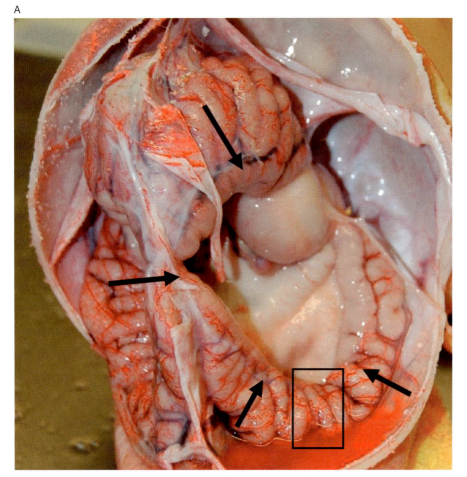

Fig. 52.21. Fresh brain at autopsy showing large old infarcts in middle cerebral artery territories bilaterally. That on the right side is indicated by arrows. The area in the box is shown at higher power in (B) (B) Luxol fast blue stained section of the edge of the infarcted area shown in (A). The edge of the lesion (arrows) has abnormally folded cortex with an irregular deep border indicating an origin before 28 weeks of gestation (×2). (C) Section of the brainstem showing secondary atrophy of the pyramidal tracts, which cannot be identified in the medulla (×1).

B   C

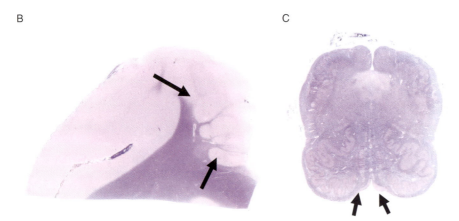

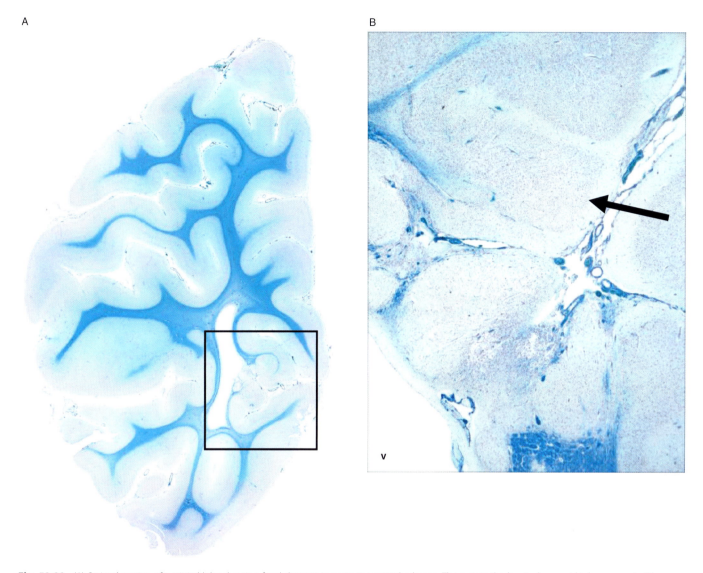

Fig. 52.22. (A) Stained section of occipital lobe showing focal damage in posterior watershed zone. The area in the box is shown at higher power in (B) (B) Almost complete cleft in the brain wall with scarring of the tissues beneath the ventricular lining (V). The cleft is lined by abnormally folded polymicrogyric cortex (arrow) (×2).

A

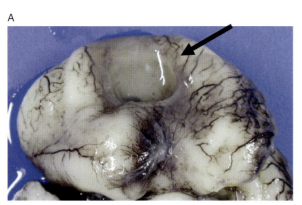

B

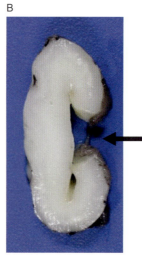

C

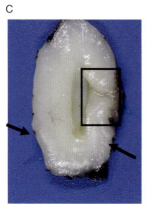

D

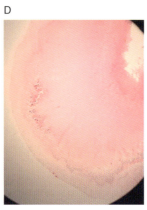

E

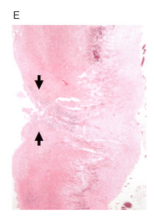

Fig. 52.23. Middle cerebral artery infarction in male fetus aged 23 weeks. (A) A central cystic area of infarction is seen in this lateral view of the cerebral hemisphere. (B) Coronal slice through the fixed brain shows the infarcted area where the brain wall is replaced by a thin membrane derived from the meninges. (C) The occipital pole, with small area of infarction and more widespread area of calicification and polymicrogyria (between arrows), seen in higher power in (D) (×1). The area in the box is seen in higher power in (E). Here the edge of the infarct shows a split extending almost to the germinal matrix of the ventricular lining and lined by masses of immature neurons which appear dark blue (short arrows (×2).

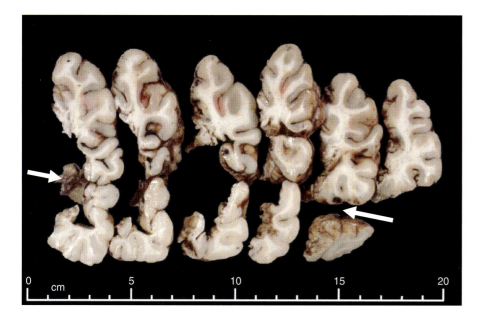

Fig. 52.24. Fixed slices of hemispherectomy specimen from child with old middle cerebral artery infarction. White arrows indicate the cystic cavity which is continuous with the lateral ventricle. The slice on the left shows the remnant of the membrane forming the wall of the cyst. The adjacent cortex has collapsed into the edge of the cavity giving the impression of gray matter lining a split in the brain wall.

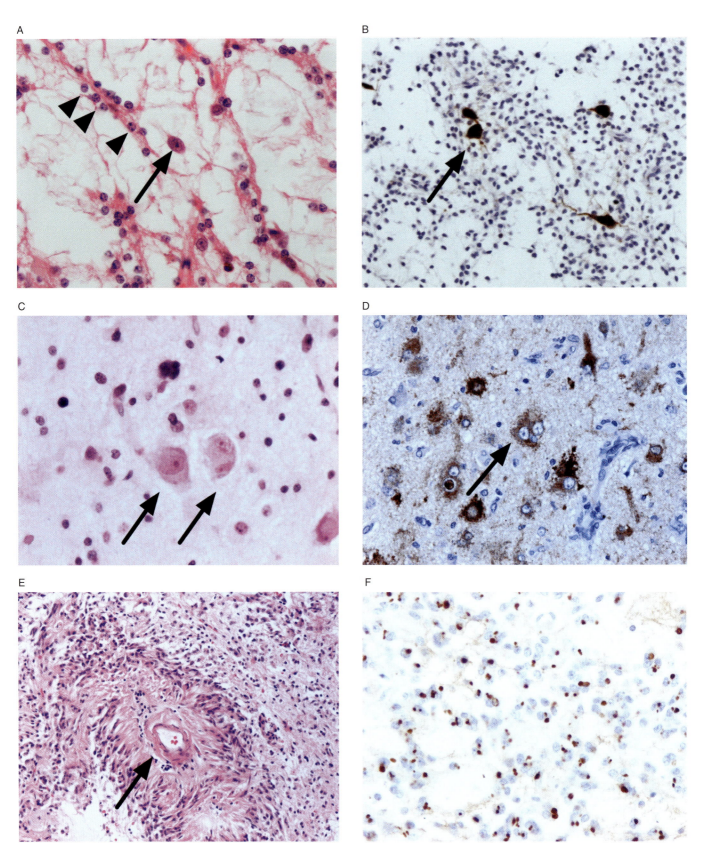

Fig. 63.1. Pathological features of dysembryoplastic neuroepithelial tumor (A and B), ganglioglioma (C and D), and angiocentric glioma (E and F). (A, B) The DNT consists of small round oligodendroglial-like cells arranged in columns separated by mucinous material (A: arrow heads). Scattered normally formed neurons are present in the tumor (A, B: arrows). (C, D) Dysplastic ganglion cells in a ganglioglioma (arrows), including some binucleate cells. The dysplastic cells show prominent staining for chromogranin (D). (E, F) Angiocentric glioma. The cells show a characteristic swirling pattern around blood vessels (E: arrow indicates the vessel lumen). They demonstrate evidence of ependymal differentiation, e.g., paranuclear dots of EMA staining (E). (A, C, E: hematoxylin and eosin; B: immunohistochemistry for the neuronal marker NeuN; DL: immunohistochemistry for chromogranin; F: immunohistochemistry for EMA.)

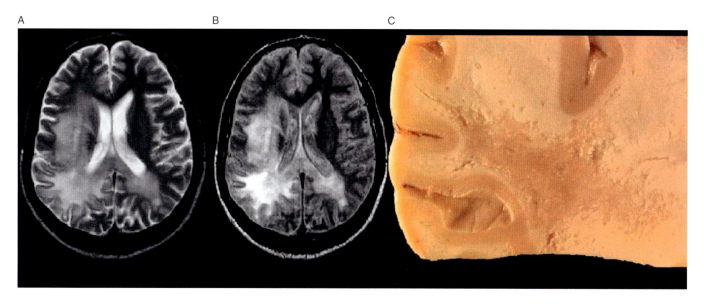

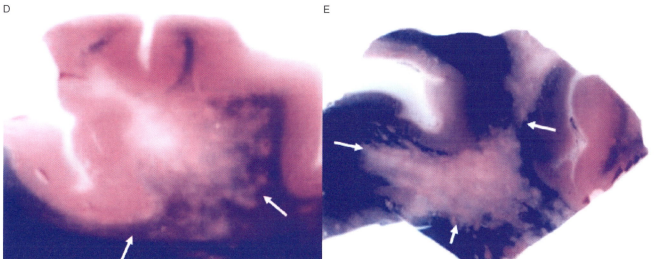

Fig. 74.3. (A,B) Axial MRI T2-weighted and fluid-attenuated inversion recovery (FLAIR) sequences revealing white-matter signal intensity changes in the parietal and frontal (right) and occipital (both sides) lobes without any mass effect; (C) demyelination of the white matter; (D,E) Luxol fast blue stain showing demyelination – these features are consistent with PML.

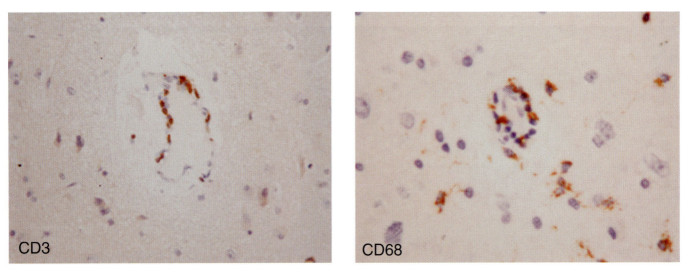

Fig. 81.2. Immunohistochemical study in a 31-year-old right-handed woman with RE. Immunohistochemistry showing sparse perivascular collection T cells (CD3 immunohistochemistry) and macrophages/microglia (CD68), which were also seen away from the blood wall. These changes are suggestive of RE.

Pyridoxine-dependent epilepsy

Sidney M. Gospe, Jr.

The causal disease

Definitions and epidemiology

Pyridoxine-dependent epilepsy (PDE) is a familial autosomal recessive disorder that results in intractable seizures presenting in newborns and older infants that come under control only after the administration of large doses of pyridoxine (vitamin B$_6$). Untreated, the disorder results in death from status epilepticus. This unfortunate scenario has been reported retrospectively in individuals who succumbed prior to the presentation and subsequent PDE diagnosis in a younger sibling (Haenggeli et al. 1991; Baxter 2001). Patients with PDE require lifelong supplementation with pyridoxine and generally do not need to be treated concomitantly with anticonvulsants. The disorder was first described in 1954 (Hunt et al. 1954), and through the 1990s about 100 cases were reported (Haenggeli et al. 1991; Gospe 1998, 2002; Baxter 2001). Published accounts over the past two decades have primarily concentrated on atypical clinical presentations (Bankier et al. 1983; Goutières and Aicardi 1985; Coker 1992; Bass et al. 1996), electroencephalographic (EEG) findings (Mikati et al. 1991; Shih et al. 1996; Nabbout et al. 1999; Naasan et al. 2009), neuroradiologic characteristics (Baxter et al. 1996; Shih et al. 1996; Gospe and Hecht 1998), longitudinal neurodevelopmental features (Baxter et al. 1996; Baynes et al. 2003; Basura et al. 2009), and most recently the biochemical and genetic basis of the disorder (Plecko et al. 2000, 2005, 2007; Mills et al. 2006; Bok et al. 2007; Kanno et al. 2007; Rankin et al. 2007; Salomons et al. 2007; Bennett et al. 2009; Gallagher et al. 2009; Sadilkova et al. 2009). While considered to be a rare cause of neonatal and infantile epilepsy, PDE is likely underrecognized. Only a few epidemiologic studies have been conducted (Baxter et al. 1996; Baxter 1999; Ebinger et al. 1999; Been et al. 2005; Basura et al. 2009). For example, a study in the United Kingdom and the Republic of Ireland reported a point prevalence of 1 in 687 000 for definite and probable cases (Baxter 1999), while a survey conducted in the Netherlands estimated a birth

incidence of 1 in 396 000 (Been et al. 2005). Despite a relatively recent increase in clinical recognition, PDE is probably underdiagnosed, and the incidence of this disorder is likely higher. This notion is supported by a study from a center in Germany where pyridoxine administration is part of a standard treatment protocol for neonatal seizures; this study reported a birth incidence of probable cases of 1 in 20 000 (Ebinger et al. 1999).

Clinical features

Pyridoxine-dependent epilepsy is due to an inborn error of metabolism where patients are dependent upon regular pharmacologic doses of pyridoxine; pyridoxine-deficiency is not present. The disorder may present in newborns within hours of birth as an epileptic encephalopathy which may mimic hypoxic–ischemic encephalopathy (Haenggeli et al. 1991; Baxter et al. 1996; Baxter 1999, 2001). In retrospect, some mothers may report having experienced fetal movements that likely represent intrauterine fetal seizures. Other cases may present with seizures at a later time during the first several weeks of life. Uncommonly, PDE may manifest after 2 months of age, and these are considered to be late-onset cases (Goutières and Aicardi 1985; Haenggeli et al. 1991; Coker 1992). In all circumstances, patients with PDE have clinical seizures which either recur serially or evolve into status epilepticus despite treatment with large doses of one or more conventional anticonvulsants. In most instances, the institution of either parenteral or enteral pyridoxine rapidly results in seizure control and improvement in the encephalopathy. Pyridoxine treatment must continue, or the epileptic encephalopathy will recur within days. However, atypical cases have been described, such as the late-onset cases, patients in whom seizures initially respond to anticonvulsants followed by a recurrence weeks to months later that then became intractable, and infants who do not respond to an initial large dose of pyridoxine but who do respond days later to a second trial (Bankier et al. 1983; Goutières and Aicardi 1985; Coker 1992; Bass et al. 1996; Baxter 2001). Patients with PDE have associated neurodevelopmental

The Causes of Epilepsy, eds. S. D. Shorvon, F. Andermann, and R. Guerrini. Published by Cambridge University Press. © Cambridge University Press 2011.

handicaps that may include cognitive, language, and motor features (Haenggeli *et al.* 1991; Baxter 2001; Basura *et al.* 2009). While it has been suggested that individuals who are diagnosed and treated early generally have a better outcome, this is not always the case (Haenggeli *et al.* 1991; Baxter 2001). The severity of the neurodevelopmental features of PDE likely has a multifactorial basis, which includes the time of clinical onset (fetal, vs. neonatal, vs. late-onset), the lag time to diagnosis and effective treatment, and phenotypic variation (Rankin *et al.* 2007; Basura *et al.* 2009).

Biochemical and genetic abnormalities and neuropathological findings

Mutations in the *ALDH7A1* gene which encodes the protein antiquitin, an aldehyde dehydrogenase that functions within the cerebral lysine catabolism pathway, have recently been demonstrated to be the molecular cause of PDE (Mills *et al.* 2006). Individuals who are homozygous or compound heterozygous for mutations in *ALDH7A1* have been described in many cases of patients with neonatal-onset PDE and in a few individuals with late-onset PDE (Mills *et al.* 2006; Kanno *et al.* 2007; Plecko *et al.* 2007; Rankin *et al.* 2007; Salomons *et al.* 2007; Bennett *et al.* 2009). Affected patients have elevations in α-aminoadipic semialdehyde (AASA) in plasma, urine, and cerebrospinal fluid (CSF) which persist even after years of effective treatment. Elevations of pipecolic acid (PA), an indirect biomarker, can also be detected in plasma and CSF, but have been demonstrated to normalize in some patients after effective long-term therapy (Plecko *et al.* 2000, 2005; Mills *et al.* 2006; Bok *et al.* 2007; Sadilkova *et al.* 2009). Accumulation of AASA results in an intracellular reduction in pyridoxal-5′-phosphate (PLP), the active vitamin B_6 co-factor (Mills *et al.* 2006). Seizures and encephalopathy likely are due to a concomitant imbalance of glutamic acid and γaminobutyric acid (GABA), excitatory and inhibitory neurotransmitters, respectively. Recently it was discovered that folinic acid-responsive seizures, another treatable neonatal epileptic encephalopathy with only a handful of cases reported, is also due to antiquitin deficiency. These patients also have elevated CSF levels of AASA and PA, which indicates that folinic acid-responsive seizures are identical to PDE (Gallagher *et al.* 2009). Pyridoxine-dependent epilepsy should be differentiated from an even less common inborn error of metabolism that results in intractable seizures due to a deficiency of pyridox(am)ine 5′-phosphate oxidase (PNPO). Seizures in infants with PNPO deficiency respond to PLP supplementation but not to pyridoxine (Hoffmann *et al.* 2007).

The neuropathologic features of PDE are not well established. The one reported autopsy study of an adolescent who died from status epilepticus secondary to pyridoxine non-compliance demonstrated reduced brain weight with sparse white matter in the cerebral hemispheres. Thalamic neuronal loss with gliosis, subependymal gliosis that resulted in aqueductal stenosis, and abnormal lobulation of the cerebellar folia

were also described. Of particular interest, glutamic acid concentrations were elevated and GABA concentrations were reduced in the frontal and occipital cortices (Lott *et al.* 1978).

Epilepsy in the disease
Clinical presentation, natural history, and seizure semiology

While it is possible that unrecognized phenotypes of PDE may present with only encephalopathy and developmental disability, our current understanding of this condition indicates that all patients present with lifelong anticonvulsant-resistant epileptic seizures. In diagnosed and treated patients, risk factors for seizures include the prescribed discontinuation of pyridoxine for clinical confirmation of pyridoxine dependency (see below), periodic non-compliance with pyridoxine supplementation, and intercurrent illness such as febrile respiratory disorders and gastroenteritis, of which the latter may lead to a temporary reduction in pyridoxine absorption.

The semiology of seizures in patients with PDE may be quite diverse. Affected neonates may present with encephalopathy and occasionally with abdominal symptoms such as emesis and distention, associated with recurrent partial motor seizures, generalized tonic seizures, or myoclonus, typically at some point leading to status epilepticus in untreated cases. Over time, for patients in whom PDE has not been diagnosed and treated, complex partial seizures, infantile spasms, and other myoclonic seizures as well as a mixed seizure pattern may develop. Late-onset cases may experience similar seizure types as well as generalized clonic seizures, atonic seizures, infantile spasms as an initial clinical presentation, and intermittent attacks of status epilepticus (Haenggeli *et al.* 1991; Baxter *et al.* 1996; Baxter 1999, 2001; Basura *et al.* 2009). In all cases, there is a high risk of status epilepticus occurring in patients who discontinue pyridoxine therapy. As such, patients with PDE require lifelong daily pyridoxine supplementation at pharmacologic doses.

Prognosis for seizure control in most patients with PDE is excellent, as long as parents and patients are compliant with pyridoxine supplementation, with only an occasional breakthrough seizure that may occur during an acute illness. Uncommonly, some patients treated appropriately with pyridoxine supplementation may continue to have recurrent seizures, and it has been suggested that in these circumstances a secondary cause of epilepsy, such as mesial temporal sclerosis, hydrocephalus, or other brain dysgenesis, may have developed (McLachlan and Brown 1995; Baxter 2001; Basura *et al.* 2009).

Neurodevelopmental features

A range of neurodevelopmental disabilities have been noted in patients with PDE. In particular, expressive language deficits are common, and affected patients have also been described with deficits in non-verbal cognitive skills, and delayed acquisition of motor skills with persistent mild reductions in tone (Haenggeli *et al.* 1991; Baxter 2001; Basura *et al.* 2009). Cerebral palsy and a significant intellectual handicap may develop in severely affected cases. Behavioral features characteristic of either obsessive–compulsive disorder or autistic spectrum disorder have been reported in some older individuals (Basura *et al.* 2009). It has been noted by several authors that early diagnosis and effective treatment of PDE results in a better neurodevelopmental outcome, and that individuals with late-onset PDE, in general, have a better prognosis (including a few cases with reportedly normal development) than early-onset cases. However, developmental outcome is most likely multifactorial and includes not only the times of clinical presentation, diagnosis, and treatment, but also long-term pyridoxine compliance, associated brain dysgenesis, and currently undiscovered associations between *ALDH7A1* genotype and neurodevelopmental phenotype (Haenggeli *et al.* 1991; Baxter 1999, 2001; Rankin *et al.* 2007; Basura *et al.* 2009).

Diagnostic tests

Clinical diagnosis

Classically, the diagnosis of PDE was made via clinical observation, where an infant with anticonvulsant-resistant seizures was offered a trial of pyridoxine that resulted in an often dramatic cessation of these events. The most convincing clinical demonstration of the effectiveness of pyridoxine therapy is to administer intravenous pyridoxine while the patient is actively experiencing seizures and is undergoing continuous EEG monitoring (Gospe 1998, 2002; Baxter 2001). In that situation, both clinical and electrographic evidence of pyridoxine's effectiveness may be demonstrated, generally within minutes of a single dose of 20–100 mg. In some circumstances, higher doses are required. Therefore, if a patient does not respond to an initial 100-mg dose, it is suggested that up to 500 mg of intravenous pyridoxine should be administered in sequential 100 mg doses every 5–10 min before concluding that the infant's seizures are not responsive to the vitamin. It is strongly recommended that this trial take place within an intensive care unit setting, as profound central nervous system depression has been noted in some patients with PDE after the initial treatment with pyridoxine (Bass *et al.* 1996; Gospe 1998; Baxter 2001). An alternate diagnostic approach is appropriate for patients who are experiencing frequent short anticonvulsant-resistant seizures. In this circumstance, oral pyridoxine (up to 30 mg/kg per day) should be prescribed; patients with PDE should have a resolution of clinical seizures within 3 to 7 days (Baxter 2001; Gospe 2002). As patients with PDE have a lifelong dependence on pyridoxine supplementation, the absolute clinical confirmation of the diagnosis is based on demonstrating continued control of seizures after the sequential withdrawal of all anticonvulsants, followed by seizure recurrence once pyridoxine is withdrawn, and regained control of seizures after pyridoxine is reintroduced. Clearly, many

parents and clinicians have been reluctant to take the step of withdrawing pyridoxine. Therefore, epidemiologic studies and case series have reported such instances as possible PDE cases (Baxter 1999, 2001; Basura *et al.* 2009). However, one needs to be careful in concluding that all patients treated in this fashion have PDE. Patients have been described with seizures that clinically respond to pyridoxine therapy, but in whom seizures do not recur once the vitamin is discontinued. The term pyridoxine-responsive seizures (PRS) has been coined to describe this particular condition (Baxter 1999, 2001). Therefore, some patients with possible PDE may actually have PRS.

Biochemical and genetic testing

The recent discovery of the biochemical and genetic bases of PDE has started to change our approach for the diagnosis of this disorder. In patients who have shown a clinical response to pyridoxine therapy, detection of elevated levels of PA in plasma samples, taken either prior to treatment or within several months after therapy has been initiated, can serve as indirect confirmatory evidence of PDE (Plecko *et al.* 2000, 2005). The demonstration of elevated levels of AASA in plasma, CSF, or urine would provide a more specific biochemical demonstration of the inborn error of metabolism that underlies PDE (Mills *et al.* 2006; Bok *et al.* 2007; Sadilkova *et al.* 2009). Genetic testing of patients with presumed PDE that demonstrates either homozygous or compound heterozygous mutations in the *ALDH7A1* gene will also provide an absolute confirmation of the disorder (Mills *et al.* 2006; Plecko *et al.* 2007; Rankin *et al.* 2007; Salomons *et al.* 2007; Bennett *et al.* 2009). In these circumstances, the withdrawal of pyridoxine to clinically confirm the diagnosis would not be necessary. Both biochemical and genetic testing is recommended, as a few individuals with elevated PA and/or AASA levels have not demonstrated mutations of one or both *ALDH7A1* alleles (Plecko *et al.* 2007; Bennett *et al.* 2009), and definite PDE patients treated for an extended period of time may have a normalization of PA levels (Plecko *et al.* 2005, 2007).

Electroencephalographic, neuroradiologic, and neuropsychologic findings

While several studies have reported EEG characteristics of patients with PDE, it is difficult to conclude that a specific pattern of EEG abnormalities exists (Mikati *et al.* 1991; Shih *et al.* 1996; Nabbout *et al.* 1999; Baxter 2001; Naasan *et al.* 2009). Investigations by EEG are typically performed in affected patients after several seizures have occurred and, more importantly, after the institution of anticonvulsant therapy, typically phenobarbital. Abnormal background activity together with a variety of paroxysmal features has been described including generalized and multifocal epileptiform activity, discontinuous patterns including burstsuppression, bursts of high-voltage slow waves, and hypsarrhythmia in patients with infantile spasms. In some untreated patients, as well as in many pyridoxine-treated patients, is it not uncommon for the interictal EEG to be normal or to demonstrate only minimal epileptiform activity. Therefore, it is important for clinicians to realize that a clinical diagnosis of PDE should not be made solely by examining the concurrent effects of pyridoxine administration on the interictal EEG. Clinical effectiveness, as well as biochemical and/or genetic confirmation of PDE, are necessary.

While patients with PDE may have normal findings on brain imaging studies, a variety of abnormal neuroradiologic features have been described in patients with PDE. While no pathognomonic features can be listed, certain abnormalities have been noted to be somewhat common including thinning of the isthmus of the corpus callosum, and mega cisterna magna, as well as degrees of cerebral atrophy in late-diagnosed or inadequately treated patients. Progressive hydrocephalus requiring neurosurgical intervention has also been described (Baxter et al. 1996; Shih et al. 1996; Gospe and Hecht 1998; Baxter 2001).

While the neurodevelopmental outcome of patients with PDE is variable and multifactorial, there is a suggestion of a characteristic neuropsychological profile. Presumably, most individuals with PDE have had psychological and educational testing performed either as part of their medical evaluation or through their school system. However, only a few cases have had their test scores reported in the literature. These formal psychometric assessments have shown a reduction in the cognitive/verbal IQ, particularly in measures of expressive language, together with a low normal motor/performance IQ (Baxter et al. 1996; Baxter 2001; Baynes et al. 2003; Basura et al. 2009).

Principles of management
Chronic pyridoxine maintenance therapy
Once a clinical diagnosis of PDE has been made, patients require lifelong pyridoxine supplements in order to prevent recurrent seizures. The recommended daily allowance for pyridoxine is 0.5 mg for infants and 2 mg for older children and adults, but patients with PDE generally require substantially higher (i.e., pharmacologic) doses. While the optimal dose of pyridoxine has not been firmly established, in most patients the daily administration of 50–200 mg (given once daily or in two divided doses) is generally effective in preventing seizures (Baxter 2001). Previously, it was not uncommon for patients to remain on the same amount of pyridoxine for many years, despite their continued growth that effectively reduced the mg/kg per day dose. A recent study of six children with PDE demonstrated that an increase in the daily pyridoxine dose resulted in an improvement in IQ scores, with the expressive language scores showing the least amount of improvement (Baxter et al. 1996; Baxter 2001). Additional improvement is generally not seen with doses higher than 15–18 mg/kg per day. As megavitamin therapy with pyridoxine has been reported

to result in a dorsal root ganglionopathy (Schaumburg et al. 1983), and sensory neuropathy has been reported in a few PDE patients (McLachlan and Brown 1995; Rankin et al. 2007), parents must be cautioned about the overzealous use of pyridoxine. It is recommended that patients with PDE receive daily supplements of approximately 15 mg/kg per day, with a maximum daily dose of 500 mg. As individuals with PDE are at an increased risk of seizure recurrence when experiencing a febrile illness, particularly gastroenteritis, the pyridoxine dose may be doubled for several days during this period. As folinic acid-responsive seizures have recently been demonstrated to be due to antiquitin deficiency, there may be an added benefit to supplement PDE patients with folinic acid, 3–5 mg/kg per day (Gallagher et al. 2009). Hypothetically, a reduced lysine diet may also be of benefit, but this has not been studied (Gallagher et al. 2009). Unless a secondary cause of seizures develops, patients with PDE do not require the concurrent use of anticonvulsants. However, due to the associated neurodevelopmental and behavioral features of the condition, some patients are prescribed certain anticonvulsants, specifically for their psychotropic effects, as well as neuroleptics and mood stabilizers (Basura et al. 2009). As deficits in expressive language are expected in PDE patients, these children should be offered early intervention services that focus on language. Older patients will benefit from special education and a variety of physical, occupational, and speech therapy services.

In utero and immediate postnatal pyridoxine prophylaxis for the fetus and neonate at risk for PDE
While the neurodevelopmental outcome of PDE patients is multifactorial, early diagnosis and treatment is clearly important. As PDE is an autosomal recessive disorder, there is a 25% recurrence risk in subsequent pregnancies. As such, it has been recommended that for at-risk pregnancies, mothers should take a daily pyridoxine dose of 50–100 mg during the last half of gestation (Baxter and Aicardi 1999; Baxter 2001). In some instances, affected newborns treated prenatally with pyridoxine followed by postnatal therapy had a better neurodevelopmental outcome when compared with their older affected siblings (Nabbout et al. 1999; Baxter 2001). However, this is not a universal occurrence, which suggests that genotype may play a role in the neurodevelopmental outcome of PDE (Rankin et al. 2007). For at-risk infants who received in utero followed by postnatal pyridoxine therapy, parents and healthcare providers have still been faced with the familiar dilemma of whether or not to withdraw pyridoxine supplementation in order to determine if the newborn will experience seizures, and therefore meet the clinical criteria for PDE. Once biochemical and ALDH7A1 gene testing become more clinically available, at-risk newborns treated prenatally with pyridoxine may be tested for PDE biomarkers and/or genotype, so that subsequent pyridoxine therapy may be either maintained or safely discontinued.

References

Bankier A, Turner M, Hopkins IJ (1983) Pyridoxine dependent seizures: a wider clinical spectrum. *Arch Dis Childh* **58**:415–18.

Bass NE, Wyllie E, Cohen B, Joseph SA (1996) Pyridoxine-dependent epilepsy: the need for repeated pyridoxine trials and the risk of severe electrocerebral suppression with intravenous pyridoxine infusion. *J Child Neurol* **11**:422–4.

Basura GJ, Hagland SP, Wiltse AM, Gospe SM Jr. (2009) Clinical features and the management of pyridoxine-dependent and pyridoxine-responsive seizures: review of 63 North American cases submitted to a patient registry. *Eur J Pediatr* **168**:697–704.

Baxter P (1999) Epidemiology of pyridoxine dependent and pyridoxine responsive seizures in the UK. *Arch Dis Childh* **81**:431–3.

Baxter P (2001) Pyridoxine dependent and pyridoxine responsive seizures. In: Baxter P (ed.) *Vitamin Responsive Conditions in Pediatric Neurology*. London: MacKeith Press, pp. 109–65.

Baxter P, Aicardi J (1999) Neonatal seizures after pyridoxine use. (Letter). *Lancet* **354**:2082–3.

Baxter P, Griffiths P, Kelly T, Gardner-Medwin D (1996) Pyridoxine-dependent seizures: demographic, clinical, MRI and psychometric features, and effect of dose on intelligence quotient. *Dev Med Child Neurol* **38**:998–1006.

Baynes K, Tomaszewski Farias S, Gospe SM Jr. (2003) Pyridoxine-dependent seizures and cognition in adulthood. *Dev Med Child Neurol* **45**:782–5.

Been JV, Bok JA, Andriessen P, Renier WO (2005) Epidemiology of pyridoxine-dependent seizures in The Netherlands. *Arch Dis Childh* **90**:1293–6.

Bennett CL, Chen Y, Hahn S, Glass IA, Gospe SM Jr. (2009) Prevalence of *ALDH7A1* mutations in 18 North American pyridoxine-dependent seizure (PDS) patients. *Epilepsia* **50**:1167–75.

Bok LA, Struys E, Willemsen MA, Been JV, Jakobs C (2007) Pyridoxine-dependent seizures in Dutch patients: diagnosis by elevated urinary alpha-aminoadipic semialdehyde levels. *Arch Dis Childh* **92**:687–9.

Coker S (1992) Postneonatal vitamin B_6-dependent epilepsy. *Pediatrics* **90**:221–3.

Ebinger M, Schutze C, Konig S (1999) Demographics and diagnosis of pyridoxine-dependent seizures. *J Pediatr* **134**:795–6.

Gallagher RC, Van Hove JL, Scharer G (2009) Folinic acid-responsive seizures are identical to pyridoxine-dependent epilepsy. *Ann Neurol* **65**:550–6.

Gospe SM Jr. (1998) Current perspectives on pyridoxine-dependent seizures. *J Pediatr* **132**:919–23.

Gospe SM Jr. (2002) Pyridoxine-dependent seizures: findings from recent studies pose new questions. *Pediatr Neurol* **26**:181–5.

Gospe SM Jr., Hecht ST (1998) Longitudinal MRI findings in pyridoxine-dependent seizures. *Neurology* **51**:74–8.

Goutières F, Aicardi J (1985) Atypical presentations of pyridoxine-dependent seizures: a treatable cause of intractable epilepsy in infants. *Ann Neurol* **17**:117–20.

Haenggeli C-A, Girardin E, Paunier L (1991) Pyridoxine-dependent seizures, clinical and therapeutic aspects. *Eur J Pediatr* **150**:452–5.

Hoffmann GF, Schmitt B, Windfuhr M (2007) Pyridoxal 5′-phosphate may be curative in early-onset epileptic encephalopathy. *J Inherit Metab Dis* **30**:96–9.

Hunt AD, Stokes J, McCrory WW, Stroud HH (1954) Pyridoxine dependency: report of a case of intractable convulsions in an infant controlled by pyridoxine. *Pediatrics* **13**:140–5.

Kanno J, Kure S, Narisawa A (2007) Allelic and non-allelic heterogeneities in pyridoxine dependent seizures revealed by *ALDH7A1* mutational analysis. *Mol Genet Metab* **91**:384–9.

Lott IT, Coulombe T, Di Paolo RV, Richardson EP, Levy HL (1978) Vitamin B_6-dependent seizures: pathology and chemical findings in brain. *Neurology* **28**:47–54.

McLachlan RS, Brown WF (1995) Pyridoxine-dependent epilepsy with iatrogenic sensory neuronopathy. *Can J Neurol Sci* **22**:50–1.

Mikati MA, Trevathan E, Krishnamoorthy KS (1991) Pyridoxine-dependent epilepsy: EEG investigation and long-term follow-up. *Electroencephalogn Clin Neurophys* **78**:215–21.

Mills PB, Struys E, Jakobs C (2006) Mutations in antiquitin in individuals with pyridoxine-dependent seizures. *Nat Med* **12**:307–9.

Naasan G, Yabroudi M, Rahi A, Mikati MA (2009) Electroencephalographic changes in pyridoxine-dependant epilepsy: new observations. *Epileptic Disord* **11**:293–300.

Nabbout R, Soufflet C, Plouin P, Dulac O (1999) Pyridoxine-dependent epilepsy: a suggestive electroclinical pattern. *Arch Dis Child Fetal Neonatal Ed* **81**:F125–9.

Plecko B, Stöckler-Ipsiroglu S, Paschke E, et al. (2000) Pipecolic acid elevation in plasma and cerebrospinal fluid of two patients with pyridoxine-dependent epilepsy. *Ann Neurol* **48**:121–5.

Plecko B, Hikel C, Korenke G-C, et al. (2005) Pipecolic acid as a diagnostic marker of pyridoxine-dependent epilepsy. *Neuropediatrics* **36**:200–5.

Plecko B, Paul K, Paschke E, et al. (2007) Biochemical and molecular characterization of 18 patients with pyridoxine-dependent epilepsy and mutations of the antiquitin (*ALDH7A1*) gene. *Hum Mutat* **28**:19–26.

Rankin PM, Harrison S, Chong WK, Boyd S, Aylett SE (2007) Pyridoxine-dependent seizures: a family phenotype that leads to severe cognitive deficits, regardless of treatment regime. *Dev Med Child Neurol* **49**:300–5.

Sadilkova K, Gospe SM Jr. Hahn SH (2009) Simultaneous determination of alpha-aminoadipic semialdehyde, piperideine-6-carboxylate and pipecolic acid by LC-MS/MS for pyridoxine-dependent seizures and folinic acid-responsive seizures. *J Neurosci Methods* **184**:136–41.

Salomons GS, Bok LA, Struys EA, et al. (2007) An intriguing "silent" mutation and a founder effect in antiquitin (*ALDH7A1*). *Ann Neurol* **62**:414–18.

Schaumburg H, Kaplan J, Windebank A, et al. (1983) Sensory neuropathy from pyridoxine abuse: a new megavitamin syndrome. *N Eng J Med* **309**:445–48.

Shih JJ, Kornblum H, Shewmon DA (1996) Global brain dysfunction in an infant with pyridoxine dependency: evaluation with EEG, evoked potentials, MRI, and PET. *Neurology* **47**:824–6.

Chapter

34

Rett syndrome and *MECP2* and *CDKL5* genotypes

Daniel G. Glaze

Rett syndrome (RTT, MIM 312750) is an X-linked neuro-developmental disorder which occurs in 1.09/10,000 females. Typical RTT is diagnosed based on a set of clinical criteria; atypical RTT, which can be milder or more severe than typical RTT, is diagnosed when some, but not all, of the typical RTT clinical criteria are present (Hagberg *et al.* 2002). Mutations in the gene encoding methyl-CpG-binding protein 2 (*MECP2*) cause the majority of cases of typical RTT and are identified in 93–97% (Neul *et al.* 2008; Glaze *et al.* 2009). A feature of RTT is the wide-ranging neurological manifestations. Among these seizures are reported to occur frequently. Cohorts from Australia, Europe, and the United States report seizures in 60–94% (Steffenburg *et al.* 2001; Jian *et al.* 2007; Glaze *et al.* 2009). Seizures represent a significant clinical problem in RTT and negatively impact on the quality of life of parents and care-givers of RTT individuals (Bahi-Buisson *et al.* 2008c).

Natural history of epilepsy

The National Institutes of Health (NIH) funded Rare Disease Network for Rett syndrome (clinicaltrials.gov, Identifier NCT00296764) is characterizing the clinical spectrum and natural history of RTT preparatory to the initiation of anticipated clinical trials. An initial report for enrollment from 2003 to 2009 included 602 patients (Glaze *et al.* 2009). Of these, 360 (60%) had a history of seizures. There were 528 patients with classic RTT and 315 had seizures (60%). Of the 74 with atypical RTT, 45 had seizures (61%). There was no significant difference in the occurrence of seizures in typical vs. atypical RTT. However, evaluation of the clinical description of the reported seizures by the RTT specialist physicians indicated only 48% (*n* = 291) were considered to have epileptic seizures. The majority of patients reported ethnicity/race as white (*n* = 512) for which 63% (323) seizures were reported. There were smaller numbers of other ethnic/race groups, however no significance difference in the occurrence of seizures was found for any of these groups.

Seizure onset in RTT appears to be later than in individuals with other neurodevelopmental disorders (Steffenburg *et al.*

2001). Seizures in RTT typically have onset after age 2 years, with a median age of seizure onset between 4 and 7 years, and as many as 70–80% beginning before 12 years (Steffenburg *et al.* 2001; Bahi-Buisson *et al.* 2008c; Jian *et al.* 2006; Glaze *et al.* 2009). Onset after age 20 years occurs only in a small number of RTT (Steffenburg *et al.* 2001; Glaze *et al.* 2009). In the USA Natural History study, the age range of the patients was 8 months to 64 years (Glaze *et al.* 2009). There appeared to be a significant age-related occurrence of seizures. A history of seizures was rarely reported before age 3 years and frequently reported between ages 5 and 15 years (60–80%) with a diminishing percentage after age 20 years. Similar findings have been reported in other patient cohorts. For RTT enrolled in the Australian Rett Syndrome Database, the mean age of onset was 48 months (Jian *et al.* 2006). For a French cohort, the mean age at first seizure was 7.3 years with a range of 1 to 24 years (Bahi-Buisson *et al.* 2008c).

MECP2 mutations and epilepsy

The NIH supported Natural History Study examined the relationship of *MECP2* mutations and epilepsy in RTT (Glaze *et al.* 2009). Mutations in *MECP2* were identified in 540 patients (90%) including 493 (93%) of the classic RTT. Seizures were reported in 317 (59%) of those with mutations and 41(73%) of those without a mutation. Those with mutations included 326 (60%) with one of the eight most common mutations (R106W, R133C, T158M, R168X, R255X, R270X, R294X, and R306C) and 51 (9%) with C-terminal deletions and 46 (8.5%) with large deletions (Fig. 34.1). When adjusted for age, seizures were reported significantly more frequently for those with a T158M mutation (74%, *p*-value < 0.050). No other significant differences were found for other mutations, though those RTT with R255X and R306C mutations tended to have a lower occurrence of seizures (49% each). In the Australian Rett Syndrome Database seizures occurred less frequently in those RTT individuals with R294X, R255X, and C-terminal mutations. (Jian *et al.* 2007). RTT individuals with R168X, R294X, and C-terminal *MECP2* mutations have been observed to be

The Causes of Epilepsy, eds. S. D. Shorvon, F. Andermann, and R. Guerrini. Published by Cambridge University Press. © Cambridge University Press 2011.

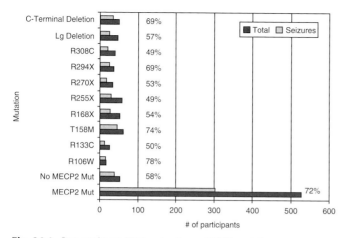

Fig. 34.1. Rett syndrome (RTT) and epilepsy: *MECP2* mutations.

less likely to have seizure onset before 4 years of age (Jian *et al.* 2006).

Character of seizures

Partial (simple and complex) and generalized seizures are reported to occur in RTT (Steffenburg *et al.* 2001; Glaze 2002). In a French cohort of 200 RTT individuals seizures were reported in 80% (Bahi-Buisson *et al.* 2008c). Of those with seizures, parents reported that 64% had generalized seizures, and of these 69% experienced a transient loss of consciousness and 54% were associated with cyanosis. Seizures were associated with falling in 44%. The median duration of seizures was 15 min with a range of 0.3 to 120 min. In nearly half, seizures were reported to occur both during the day and at night. Video-electroencephalogram (EEG) studies have been performed in RTT individuals with a history of seizures (Cooper *et al.* 1998; Glaze *et al.* 1998) Epileptic seizures included those associated with focal EEG seizure discharges in the occipital and central regions. These were associated with various clinical manifestations that included focal motor activity, staring, head turning, oxygen desaturation, and apnea. Generalized EEG seizure discharges were associated with absences (staring) episodes and flexor spasms. Events identified as seizures by parents but not associated with an EEG seizure discharge included episodes of twitching, jerking, head turning, falling forward, vacant or staring episodes, trembling, breath-holding, and hyperventilation.

Pathogenesis of seizures in RTT

Abnormalities in neuronal circuitry and synaptic plasticity are suggested by neurophysiological, neuropathological, and neurochemical studies (Glaze *et al.* 1998; Glaze 2002; Armstrong 2005; Johnston *et al.* 2005) Several studies of RTT animal models suggest that an imbalance between excitatory and inhibitory neurotransmission is responsible for the clinical manifestations of RTT including seizures (Dani *et al.* 2005; Asaka *et al.* 2006; Moretti *et al.* 2006; Medrihan *et al.* 2008; Zhang *et al.* 2008). Presumably, these alterations arise as a

consequence of the *MECP2* mutation, but the target genes that are dysregulated or overexpressed are largely unidentified.

The contribution of genotype to clinical seizures in RTT is complex. Specific *MECP2* mutations may influence the occurrence of seizures, as well as age of onset of seizures in RTT as noted above (Jian *et al.* 2006, 2007; Glaze *et al.* 2009) Other factors likely influence clinical manifestations and include the degree of X-chromosome inactivation, the type of mutation (i.e., missense), the location of the mutation (i.e., methyl binding domain), as well as background genetic and epigenetic factors. Missence mutations in the methyl-CpG-binding domain (MBD) of *MECP2* are associated with a more severe epileptic phenotype with early onset and drug resistant seizures (Nectoux *et al.* 2008). Early onset of seizures is reported to be linked to the combined *MECP2* mutations and brain-derived neurotrophic factor (BDNF) polymorphisms. It is suggested that the BDNF Met66 allele may protect against seizures in RTT. BDNF is one of the targets of MeCP2 and encodes a neurotrophic factor essential for neuronal survival, differentiation, and synaptic plasticity. BDNF knock-out animals are reported to have decreased seizure susceptibility; animals with BDNF overexpression have increased seizure susceptibility. It is suggested that BDNF contributes to epileptogenesis, and that the met-BDNF allele contributes to a decreased expression of BDNF resulting in decreased seizure susceptibility to seizures (Nectoux *et al.* 2008).

Prognosis

The occurrence of epilepsy was examined in the Natural History study (Glaze *et al.* 2009). Increased prevalence of seizures was significantly associated with a greater overall clinical severity, as well as, impairment of ambulation and hand use. While greater severity score for communication was observed, when adjusted for age there was not a significant difference in this parameter between the two groups. Head growth was not significantly different between the two groups. Similar findings were observed in the Australian Rett Syndrome Database. Not having gained the ability to walk and developmental problems in the first 10 months of age were associated with an almost twofold increased risk of seizures (Jian *et al.* 2006).

In the USA Natural History study, 36% of individuals with reported seizures had experienced no seizures during the 6 months prior to their initial evaluation; 27% had monthly seizures; 20% weekly seizures; and 11% daily seizures (Glaze *et al.* 2009). In respect to treatment of seizures, 20% were receiving no treatment, 37% one antiepileptic drug (AED) and 8% three or more AEDs. Alternative therapies included 13% using vagus nerve stimulator (VNS) and 12% receiving the ketogenic diet. The most commonly used AEDs were carbamazepine (37%), lamotrigine (33%), and levetiracetam (26%). Overall clinical severity scores increased ("greater severity") from those with seizures receiving no treatment, to those on any medication (higher severity scores) to those with VNS or ketogenic diet (highest severity scores) (Glaze *et al.* 2009).

The onset and occurrence of seizures appeared to diminish after puberty (Steffenburg *et al.* 2001; Glaze *et al.* 2009). A significant number of RTT individuals (36%) are reported to have been seizure-free for the previous 6 months (Glaze *et al.* 2009). However, the occurrence of seizures in RTT negatively impacts on family quality of life and is associated with greater clinical severity (Glaze *et al.* 2009). Seizures represent one of the major concerns of parents with RTT children (Bahi–Buisson *et al.* 2008c).

EEG and video-EEG monitoring

The EEG is invariably abnormal at some time during the course of RTT. There is no diagnostic EEG pattern, but certain characteristic EEG patterns have been described in RTT (Glaze *et al.* 1987; Glaze 2002). Three characteristic EEG changes have been reported. These are not specific or universally observed in all RTT individuals. First, there is a loss of expected developmental features including the occipital rhythm ("alpha") during wakefulness and non-rapid eye movement (NREM) sleep characteristics, with the appearance of generalized background slowing. Second, epileptiform abnormalities occur frequently. Initially, these are characterized by central–temporal spikes and/or sharp wave discharges more prominent during sleep. Later multifocal spikes and/or sharp waves and generalized spike and slow wave discharges are frequently recorded. Third, a pattern of rhythmic slow (theta) activity is frequently recorded in the central or frontal–central regions. While these EEG findings are characteristically seen in the majority of RTT individuals, there is variability in the EEG findings. For some older RTT girls and adults, the EEG may be minimally slow with expected awake and sleep characteristics and an absence of epileptiform abnormalities.

Video-EEG monitoring has been used to verify epileptic seizures in RTT (Cooper *et al.* 1998; Glaze *et al.* 1998) One study found about one-third of parent-reported seizure behaviors were associated with an EEG seizure discharge (Glaze *et al.* 1998). Epileptic seizures in RTT may be over-reported as result of the occurrence of clinical features including motor abnormalities (such as tone changes, involuntary movements) and autonomic dysfunction (including awake breathing dysrhythmia associated with vacant episodes) in the context of an abnormal EEG (epileptiform discharges without recording of EEG seizure discharge).

Management of seizures in RTT

There is no one best AED for treatment of seizures in RTT. Management follows standard practice parameters for treatment of epilepsy. Some patients may experience a single seizure or rare reoccurrence of brief seizures in their lifetime. In these cases a conservative approach of educating parents concerning seizure precautions and what to do in the case of prolonged or serial seizures and the possible judicious use of rectal diazepam may be considered. For those RTT with recurrent seizures (epilepsy), pharmacological therapy may be based on seizure type. Both generalized and partial seizures are reported in RTT, and a variety of AEDs have been used. Uncontrolled studies of small sample size have reported the efficacy of topiramate and lamotrigine (Kumandas *et al.* 2001; Goyal *et al.* 2004). In cases of epilepsy refractory to AEDs, non-pharmacological treatments including VNS and ketogenic diet may be useful (Wilfong and Schultz 2006). Three points concerning the treatment of epilepsy in RTT need to be emphasized. In addition to efficacy in treatment of seizures and potential side effects, AEDs may improve non-epileptic behaviors, such as anxiety and breathing dysrhythmia, commonly observed in RTT. Discontinuation of AEDs is warranted after a seizure-free period, especially in older teenage and adult RTT women. As noted above, not all paroxysmal behaviors in RTT are epileptic seizures and use of prolonged video-EEG monitoring may be helpful in making appropriate treatment choices.

Other RTT phenotype with epilepsy: *CDKL5* mutations

Mutations in the X-linked cyclin-dependent kinase-like 5 (*CDKL5*) gene have been reported in patients with severe neurodevelopmental disorders characterized by early-onset seizures, infantile spasms, and severe psychomotor impairment (Weaving *et al.* 2004; Archer *et al.* 2006). Mutations in *CDKL5* have been reported in individuals with a RTT-like phenotype including deceleration of head growth, stereotypies, and hand apraxia. Individuals with *CDKL5* mutations, in contrast to typical RTT, experience early-onset seizures and infantile spasms, and lack an early normal period followed by regression and do not demonstrate intense eye communication (Evans *et al.* 2005; Mari *et al.* 2005; Scala *et al.* 2005; Bahi-Buisson *et al.* 2008a). Early epilepsy with normal interictal EEG and severe hypotonia are reported to be key features identifying individuals with *CDKL5* mutations (Bahi-Buisson *et al.* 2008b). A changing epilepsy phenotype has been described in individuals with *CDKL5* mutations. Early onset of seizures at ages 1–10 weeks associated with normal interictal EEG was observed in almost all of the study sample of 12 patients. This was followed by an epileptic encephalopathy with infantile spasms and hypsarrthythmia in all individuals. Between 2.5 and 19 years of age, about half of individuals with *CDKL5* mutations are seizure-free, while the other half develop refractory epilepsy with tonic seizures and myoclonia (Bahi-Buisson *et al.* 2008b).

The pathogenesis of epilepsy in *CDKL5* mutations may be similar to that of *MECP2* mutations. In the mouse brain, Cdlk5 expression overlaps that of Mecp2 and its expression is unaffected by the loss of Mecp2 (Weaving *et al.* 2004). *CDKL5* is able to phosphorylate itself and to mediate MeCP2 phosphorylation, suggesting that they belong to the same molecular pathway (Mari *et al.* 2005).

References

Archer HL, Evans J, Edwards S, (2006) *CDKL5* mutations cause infantile spasms, early onset seizures, and severe mental retardation in female patients. *J Med Genet* 43:729–34.

Armstrong DD (2005) Neuropathology of Rett syndrome. *J Child Neurol* 20:747–53.

Asaka Y, Jugloff DG, Zhang L, Eubanks JH, Fitzsimonds RM (2006) Hippocampal synaptic plasticity is impaired in the Mecp2-null mouse model of Rett syndrome. *Neurobiol Dis* 21:217–27.

Bahi-Buisson N, Nectoux J, Rosas-Vargas H, *et al.* (2008a) Key clinical features to identify girls with *CDKL5* mutations. *Brain* 131:2647–61.

Bahi-Buisson N, Kaminska A, Boddaert N, (2008b) The three stages of epilepsy in patients with *CDKL5* mutations. *Epilepsia* 49:1027–37.

Bahi-Buisson N, Guellec I, Nabbout R, *et al.* (2008c) Parental view of epilepsy in Rett syndrome. *Brain Dev* 30:126–30.

Cooper RA, Kerr AM, Amos PM (1998) Rett syndrome: critical examination of clinical features, serial EEG and video-monitoring in understanding and management. *Eur J Paediatr Neurol* 2:127–35.

Dani VS, Chang Q, Maffei A, *et al.* (2005) Reduced cortical activity due to shift in the balance between excitation and inhibition in a mouse model of Rett syndrome. *Proc Natl Acad Sci USA* 102:12 560–15.

Evans JC, Archer HL, Colley JP, *et al.* (2005) Early onset seizures and Rett-like features associated with mutations in *CDKL5*. *Eur J Hum Genet* 13:1113–20.

Glaze DG (2002) Neurophysiology of Rett syndrome. *Ment Retard Dev Disabil Res Rev* 8:66–71.

Glaze DG, Frost JD, Zoghbi HY, Percy AK (1987) Rett syndrome: correlation of EEG characteristics with clinical staging. *Arch Neurol* 44:1053–6.

Glaze DG, Schultz RJ, Frost JD (1998) Rett syndrome: characterization of seizures versus non-seizures. *Electroencephalogr Clin Neurophysiol* 106:79–83.

Glaze D, Percy A, Skinner S, *et al.* (2009) Natural history of Rett syndrome: epilepsy. Abstract #753330, Pediatric Academic Societies' Annual Meeting, Baltimore Convention Center, Baltimore, MD, May 2–5.

Goyal M, O'Riordan MA, Wiznitzer M (2004) Effect of topiramate on seizures and respiratory dysrhythmia in Rett syndrome. *J Child Neurol* 19:588–91.

Hagberg B, Hanefield F, Percy A, Skjeldel O (2002) An update on clinically applicable diagnostic criteria in Rett syndrome. *Eur J Pediatr Neurol* 6:293–7.

Jian L, Nagarajan L, de Klerk N, *et al.* (2006) Predictors of seizure onset in Rett syndrome. *J Pediatr* 149:542–7.

Jian L, Nagarajan L, de Klerk N, *et al.* (2007) Seizures in Rett syndrome: an overview from a one-year calendar study. *Eur J Paediatr Neurol* 11:310–17.

Johnston MV, Blue ME, Naidu S (2005) Rett syndrome and neuronal development. *J Child Neurol* 20:759–63.

Kumandas S, Cakren H, Ciftci A, Ozturk M, Per H (2001) Lamotrigine in two cases of Rett syndrome. *Brain Devel* 23:240–2.

Mari F, Azimonti S, Bertani I (2005) *CDKL5* belongs to the same molecular pathway of MeCP2 and it is responsible for the early-onset seizure variant of Rett syndrome. *Hum Mol Genet* 14:1935–46.

Medrihan L, Tantalaki E, Aramuni G, *et al.* (2008) Early defects of GABAergic synapses in the brain stem of a MeCP2 mouse model of Rett syndrome. *J Neurophys* 99:112–21.

Moretti P, Levenson JM, Battaglia F, *et al.* (2006) Learning and memory and synaptic plasticity are impaired in a mouse model of Rett syndrome. *J Neurosci* 26:319–27.

Nectoux J, Bahi-Buisson N, Guellec I, *et al.* (2008) The p.Val66Met polymorphism in the BDNF gene protects against early seizures in Rett syndrome. *Neurology* 70:2145–51.

Neul JL, Fang P, Barrish J, *et al.* (2008) Specific mutations in methyl-CpG-binding protein 2 confer different severity in Rett syndrome. *Neurology* 70:1311–21.

Scala E, Ariani F, Mari F, *et al.* (2005) *CDKL5/STK9* is mutated in Rett syndrome variant with infantile spasms. *J Med Genet* 42:103–7.

Steffenburg U, Hagberg G, Hagberg B (2001) Epilepsy in a representative series of Rett syndrome. *Acta Paediatr* 90:34–9.

Weaving LS, Christodoulou J, Williamson SL, (2004) Mutations of *CDKL5* cause a severe neurodevelopmental disorder with infantile spasms and mental retardation. *Am J Hum Genet* 75:1079–93.

Wilfong AA, Schultz RJ (2006) Vagus nerve stimulation for treatment of epilepsy in Rett syndrome. *Dev Med Child Neurol* 48:683–6.

Zhang L, He J, Jugloff DG, Eubanks JH (2008) The MeCP2-null mouse hippocampus displays altered basal inhibitory rhythms and is prone to hyperexcitability. *Hippocampus* 18:294–309.

Chapter

35

Urea cycle disorders

Linda Huh and Kevin Farrell

The urea cycle disorders (UCD) are a group of rare congenital diseases caused by a deficiency of the enzymes or transport proteins required to remove ammonia from the body (Gropman *et al.* 2007). The clinical manifestations of these disorders are the result of acute or chronic hyperammonemia and include acute neurologic and gastrointestinal symptoms and signs. These disorders present either acutely in the neonatal period or as a chronic or acute intermittent problem in later childhood or adult life. There is a high mortality rate and considerable neurologic morbidity, particularly in patients who present in the neonatal period (Nassogne *et al.* 2005).

Hyperammonemia

Ammonia diffuses freely across the blood–brain barrier and is rapidly converted to glutamine within the astrocyte. The developing brain is much more susceptible to the deleterious effects of ammonia than the adult brain and the degree of elevation of ammonia influences the severity of the brain injury. Neuronal loss and altered synaptic growth occur as a result of alterations of amino acid pathways and neurotransmitter systems, cerebral energy metabolism, nitric oxide synthesis, oxidative stress, mitochondrial function, and signal transduction.

Ammonia is rapidly incorporated into glutamine, which is an organic osmolyte and is thought to cause astrocytic swelling and global cerebral edema (Gropman *et al.* 2007). Acute hyperammonemia also interferes with Na–K–ATPase activity and causes mitochondrial dysfunction, and free radical production. Furthermore, it leads to N-methyl-D-aspartate (NMDA)-receptor-mediated excitotoxicity, which can result in neuronal cell injury and ultimately apoptosis. In addition, acute hyperammonemia may increase the permeability of the blood–brain barrier resulting in depletion of the intermediates of cell energy metabolism. Finally, the effect on α-amino-3-hydroxy-5-methyl-isoxazolepropionic acid (AMPA)-receptor-mediated neurotransmission may adversely affect learning and memory.

Chronic hyperammonemia may induce changes in NMDA receptor-mediated neurotransmission and induction of astrocytosis. In developing rat models, ammonia exposure has been shown to inhibit axonal growth and disturb signaling transduction pathways. These potential mechanisms may underlie the cognitive impairment, behavioral difficulties, and epilepsy observed in older individuals with UCDs.

The cerebral white matter is particularly vulnerable to acute hyperammonemia. In addition to the white matter, acute hyperammonemia preferentially affects the basal ganglia, particularly the lentiform nuclei (Gropman *et al.* 2007). Neuropathologic studies in individuals with UCD have demonstrated multiple cystic lesions, ventricular dilatation with cerebral atrophy, necrosis of deep nuclei (caudate, putamen, thalamus, and hypothalamus), and abnormal myelination. Spongiform changes and gliosis are seen in the white matter with Alzheimer type II astrocytes. Extensive neuronal loss can be seen in the cortex, particularly the deep sulci of the insular and perirolandic regions, and hippocampus.

Individual urea cycle disorders

The urea cycle involves a series of enzymes and transporter proteins that facilitate the metabolism of ammonia. The two most proximal enzyme defects, carbamyl phosphate synthetase deficiency 1 (CPS 1) and ornithine transcarbamylase deficiency (OTC), account for 75% of reported cases and are associated with the highest risk for acute neurological injury (Nassogne *et al.* 2005; Gropman *et al.* 2007). Other enzymes involved include N-acetylglutamate synthetase (NAGS), arginosuccinate synthetase (ASS), arginosuccinate lyase (ASL), and arginase.

Severe deficiency or absence of enzyme activity results in the development of hyperammonemia and clinical signs in the first days of life. In patients with milder urea cycle enzyme deficiencies, the clinical presentation may occur much later, can be less severe, and can be precipitated by illness or stress. Patients with arginase deficiency may present during an episode of hyperammonemia but more commonly present with progressive spastic diplegia and normal blood ammonia.

The Causes of Epilepsy, eds. S. D. Shorvon, F. Andermann, and R. Guerrini. Published by CAMBRIDGE UNIVERSITY PRESS. © Cambridge University Press 2011.

Ornithine transcarbamylase deficiency has X-linked inheritance and the disease severity is particularly marked in boys (Nassogne *et al.* 2005). A full family history should include unexplained deaths in newborns and unexplained encephalopathies in maternal uncles. The other disorders are inherited in an autosomal recessive fashion.

Clinical features

Neonatal period

Just over half of the patients with UCD present on the first day of life with gastrointestinal signs followed by severe neurological distress (Nassogne *et al.* 2005). Altered conscious level, seizures, and motor dysfunction are the most common clinical features and seizures occur in approximately 50% of severely hyperammonemic neonates (Summar 2001). The clinical features may mimic neonatal infection. Approximately two-thirds have either CPS or OTC. The mortality rate is high in both disorders, particularly in boys with OTC, and the long-term neurologic outcome is poor in the survivors. The outcome for ASS deficiency appears more favorable.

Later onset

Approximately 40% of those presenting after the newborn period do so with an acute neurological crisis usually characterized by altered consciousness and, in one-third, status epilepticus. An acute neurological presentation after the newborn period is often precipitated by diet non-compliance, a febrile illness, surgery, or chemotherapy (Nassogne *et al.* 2005). Most of these children are found to have an OTC defect and there is a high mortality rate, particularly if there is delayed diagnosis and therefore delayed treatment.

Patients with partial urea cycle enzyme deficiencies may have a much later presentation, usually with hepatogastric, neurologic, or psychiatric symptoms. The combination of digestive and neurologic symptoms is characteristic of a UCD and half of such children have evidence of liver disease. Patients with only hepatogastric symptoms, e.g., anorexia, abdominal pain, and vomiting, tend to present earlier (average age 14 months) than those with neurologic symptoms (average age 4 years) or psychiatric symptoms (average age 8 years) (Nassogne *et al.* 2005). The neurologic symptoms can be chronic or acute relapsing and may involve altered consciousness, seizures, psychomotor retardation, and ataxia. The psychiatric symptoms include agitation, irritability, and confusion. The risk of permanent neurologic damage is much higher in late-onset UCD, that is not diagnosed and treated early in the course of the disease (Gropman *et al.* 2007). Both arginase deficiency and the hyperornithinemia–hyperammonemia–homocitrullinuria (HHH) syndrome, due to a defect on the ornithine transporter, differ clinically from the other UCDs in that the major neurological presentation is that of spastic diplegia/quadriplegia (Gropman *et al.* 2007).

Seizures and electroencephalography

Seizures in the neonate are a sign of acute hyperammonemia and occur in approximately 50% of severely hyperammonemic neonates (Summar 2001). The electroencephalographic (EEG) background may show burst suppression, diffuse high-voltage slow waves, and multifocal delta and theta activity during an acute hyperammonemic crisis (Brunquell *et al.* 1999; Nagata *et al.* 1991; Niedermeyer and Lopes da Silva 2005). Multifocal sharp waves, spikes, spike-and-wave complexes, and paroxysmal low-voltage fast activity are indicators of cortical irritability in acute hyperammonemia and electrographic seizures are not uncommon. The EEG abnormalities may parallel the clinical course with improvement in the background and resolution of the epileptiform discharges. Thus, the EEG may provide a useful adjunct to clinical assessment of efficacy of therapy.

Prolonged or recurrent intermittent hyperammonemia may alter synaptic growth and lead to neuronal loss (Cagnon and Braissant 2007). Thus, seizures in the context of normal ammonia levels in the older child or adult may represent remote symptomatic epilepsy due to prior brain injury. The prevalence of unprovoked seizures is not well documented. A recent abstract, based on a retrospective chart review over 30 years in one large center with a particular interest in UCD, described five patients who had either a single seizure or epilepsy (Zecavati *et al.* 2008). There are no characteristic electroclinical features of unprovoked seizures in children with UCD and video-EEG may be helpful in distinguishing seizures from other abnormal motor activity. EEGs performed during periods between attacks may range from normal to continued background abnormalities and epileptiform activity (Nagata *et al.* 1991). Abnormalities described include asymmetric background, diffuse or focal slowing (theta and delta waves), and focal or diffuse sharp waves, spikes, and spike-and-wave complexes.

Diagnostic tests

Hyperammonemia is always present in the symptomatic newborn with a UCD but fasting ammonia levels may be normal in the older child or adult. Measurement of blood ammonia after a protein load may help to establish the diagnosis in patients with normal baseline ammonia levels. Respiratory alkalosis has been demonstrated in approximately half of those presenting as newborns (Nassogne *et al.* 2005). Plasma amino acids and urinary orotic acid should be used to monitor response to treatment. Genetic confirmation of disease can now be made in the majority of individuals with a UCD and may be offered prenatally.

Reversible white matter changes in the deep sulci of the insular and peri-rolandic areas may be seen on magnetic resonance imaging (MRI) in acute hyperammonemia (Gropman *et al.* 2007). More severe neuroimaging abnormalities include diffuse edema with evolution to atrophy, extensive infarcts, watershed ischemia, and reversible cortical abnormalities.

Management

The acute management should be directed at decreasing the levels of ammonia and preventing a further hyperammonemic crisis. Provision of alternate nitrogen excretion pathways may be facilitated by the use of intravenous sodium benzoate and sodium phenylacetate (Enns *et al.* 2007). Hemodialysis and hemofiltration can be used to lower ammonia levels acutely while measures to reverse the catabolic state are implemented by infusion of glucose and insulin. The survival rate is higher in older children and in those with lower blood ammonia levels (Enns *et al.* 2007). Reducing the nitrogenous waste by means of a low nitrogen diet and prevention of endogenous metabolism through adequate nutrition are fundamental steps in both the acute and long-term management.

The treatment of seizures in the newborn period in these children usually includes phenobarbital with or without a benzodiazepine. The safe use of midazolam has been described in the management of acute symptomatic seizures in late-onset OTC (Schmidt *et al.* 2005).

Recurrent, unprovoked epileptic seizures may develop in patients with UCDs and prophylactic antiepileptic medication may be required. Valproic acid may cause hyperammonemia in individuals without a UCD, has precipitated hyperammonemic crises in those with a UCD, and should be avoided (Sewell *et al.* 1995; Oechsner *et al.* 1998). The mechanism is unknown but proposed mechanisms include: inhibition of *N*-acetylglutamate synthesis by inhibiting carbamoylphosphate sythetase; incrementation of mitochondrial glutamine transport; and reduction of ammonia metabolism by decreasing carnitine availability (Thakur *et al.* 2006). Levetiracetam and lamotrigine have been reported to be effective in individuals with known UCDs who developed epileptic seizures (Zecavati *et al.* 2008). However, no particular anticonvulsant has been shown to be more effective than another in individuals with UCD. Treatment of fever should involve ibuprofen rather than acetaminophen, which may exacerbate hepatic dysfunction.

References

Brunquell P, Tezcan K, DiMario FJ Jr. (1999) Electroencephalographic findings in ornithine transcarbamylase deficiency. *J Child Neurol* **14**:533–6.

Cagnon L, Braissant O (2007) Hyperammonemia-induced toxicity for the developing central nervous system. *Brain Res Rev* **56**:183–97.

Enns GM, Berry SA, Berry GT, *et al.* (2007) Survival after treatment with phenylacetate and benzoate for urea-cycle disorders. *N Eng J Med* **356**:2282–92.

Gropman AL, Summar M, Leonard JV (2007) Neurological implications of urea cycle disorders. *J Inher Metab Dis* **30**:865–79.

Nagata N, Matsuda I, Matsuura T, *et al.* (1991) Retrospective survey of urea cycle disorders. II. Neurological outcome in forty-nine Japanese patients with urea cycle enzymopathies. *Am J Med Genet* **40**:477–81.

Nassogne MC, Heron B, Touati G, Rabier D, Saudubray JM (2005) Urea cycle defects: management and outcome. *J Inher Metab Dis* **28**:407–14.

Niedermeyer E, Lopes da Silva F (eds.) (2005) *Electroencephalography: Basic Principles, Clinical Applications, and Related Fields*, 5th edn. Philadelphia, PA: Lippincott Williams and Wilkins.

Oechsner M, Steen C, Sturenburg HJ, Kohlschütter A (1998) Hyperammonaemic encephalopathy after initiation of valproate therapy in unrecognised ornithine transcarbamylase deficiency. *J Neurol, Neurosurg Psychiatry* **64**:680–2.

Schmidt J, Schroth M, Irouschek A, *et al.* (2005) Patients with ornithine transcarbamylase deficiency: anaesthesiological and intensive care management. *Der Anaesthesist* **54**:1201–8.

Sewell AC, Bohles HJ, Herwig J, Demirkol M (1995) Neurological deterioration in patients with urea cycle disorders under valproate therapy: a cause for concern. *Eur J Pediatrics* **154**:593–4.

Summar M (2001) Current strategies for the management of neonatal urea cycle disorders. *J Pediatr* **138**(Suppl):S30–9.

Thakur V, Rupar CA, Ramsay DA, Singh R, Fraser DD (2006) Fatal cerebral edema from late-onset ornithine transcarbamylase deficiency in a juvenile male patient receiving valproic acid. *Pediatr Crit Care Medi* **7**:273–6.

Zecavati N, Lichter-Konecki U, Singh R, *et al.* (2008) Seizures in urea cycle disorders: an under-recognized symptom in patients outside of the acute metabolic phase. Abstract, 58th Annual Meeting, American Society of Human Genetics. Available online at www.ashg.org/2008meeting/abstracts/fulltext/f22529.htm

Chapter

36

Wilson disease

J. M. Walshe

Definition

Wilson disease is a genetically determined, recessive disease carried on chromosome 13q14.3 mediating a P-type ATPase controlling the movement of copper through the cell membrane. There are now approaching 300 mutations of this gene. The incidence of the disease is believed to be 1 in 30 000.

It is now apparent that Wilson disease can present at almost any age. It is rare before the age of 7 or 8 and very rare after the age of 40 years. Before puberty presentation is usually with some variant of hepatic disease, acute or chronic. After puberty the presentation is more commonly of a movement disorder, often accompanied by a personality change. Less common presentations are hemolytic crises, bone and joint disease, or a major seizure. Abnormalities of renal function are common, e.g., hypercalcuria, aminoaciduria, and melli-turia, but seldom influence the presentation (Scheinberg and Sternlieb 1984)

Clinical features and pathology

Wilson disease should be considered as a possible diagnosis in any child who presents with liver disease particularly if it is subacute or chronic (Walshe 1987). Neurological presentation is almost invariably after puberty. The commonest presenting symptoms are changes in speech, drooling, or tremor of the arms. Tremor can be either parkinsonian, cerebellar in type, or in the younger teenagers it may be of choreic movement. As the disease progresses dystonia may predominate but it is uncommon as an early symptom (Walshe and Yealland 1992). The sensory nervous system is never involved. Personality changes are not uncommon as is a falling performance at school. Very occasionally the disease may present with a major seizure or with a severe psychiatric disturbance. The characteristic Kayser Fleischer rings in the cornea are always found in patients with neurological disease but less often in those with a hepatic presentation. Over a blue iris the rings are invariably brown in color, over a brown iris the rings may appear grey (Fig. 36.1). When in doubt the eye should be examined under a

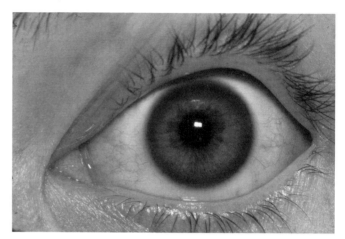

Fig. 36.1. Kayser Fleischer ring. This shows a brown ring as viewed over a blue iris. The pigment is densest in the top crescent where it is always first laid down. See color plate section.

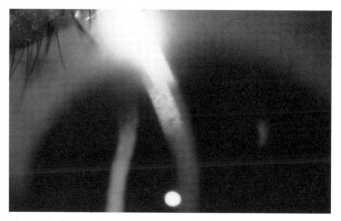

Fig. 36.2. Slit lamp photograph of a Kayser Fleischer ring showing the granular nature of the pigment in the inner layer of Descemet's membrane. See color plate section.

slit lamp: the pigment thus seen, is brown, granular, and located in Descemet's membrane. It needs an experienced ophthalmologist to give a certain opinion (Cairns and Walshe 1970) (Fig. 36.2).

The Causes of Epilepsy, eds. S. D. Shorvon, F. Andermann, and R. Guerrini. Published by Cambridge University Press. © Cambridge University Press 2011.

The pathogenesis of Wilson disease is an inability to excrete copper via the bile (Gibbs and Walshe 1980). The metal accumulates first in the liver, then, when binding sites are saturated, it overflows into other tissues, predominantly the brain, occasionally the kidneys. Thus whilst liver damage is always present it is not clear why some patients present with liver disease while others have a predominantly neurological illness, sometimes with remarkably little histological evidence of liver pathology. It is also not clear why the sensory nervous system escapes damage. Studies with radioactive copper have shown that in the early, presymptomatic stage, the liver takes up the metal avidly. As the disease progresses this changes, liver uptake is impaired, and copper can be shown to be more evenly spread throughout the body (Walshe and Potter 1977). In normal individuals a peak of biliary excretion can be demonstrated, but this is not found in patients.

Epilepsy in Wilson disease

A search of the literature has revealed only one systematic review of the incidence of epilepsy. This found an incidence of seizures in such patients as 6.2% in a series of 200 patients seen by the authors (Denning *et al.* 1988). This incidence is 10 times higher than that seen in the general population. In their monograph *Dégénérescence hépatolenticulaire* Boudin and Pepin (1959) consider "crises épileptiques" to be a serious late manifestation of Wilson disease and describe the electroencephalographic (EEG) changes involved, but give no figures for incidence. Scheinberg and Sternlieb's monograph refers to seizures which may be grand mal or complex and may be a presenting symptom, as is this author's experience (Scheinberg and Sternlieb 1984). They give no figures for the incidence of this complication of Wilson disease. There are a number of recent articles referring to single cases, either presenting with epilepsy or developing this after the start of therapy (Bladin 2005). Seizures can be grand mal, focal, or of the absence variety. The cause of seizures is almost certainly due to the toxic action of copper on the neuron. There has been a suggestion that seizures appearing for the first time after the start of treatment with penicillamine may be precipitated by penicillamine-induced pyridoxine deficiency but Denning *et al.* (1988) showed that this was extremely unlikely and others have shown that injection of a copper salt into the pigeon brain will result in the immediate onset of convulsions which can not be controlled by chelating agents (Peters and Walshe 1966). The onset of seizures after the start of treatment is most likely due to the mobilization of large amounts of copper, some of which is able to cross the blood–brain barrier.

Treatment is conventional as for other forms of epilepsy, but treatment of Wilson disease must be vigorously pursued with penicillamine or trientine (Walshe and Yealland 1993). Occasions arise when a change from one of these drugs to the other may be beneficial. The prognosis for cessation of seizures is usually good. In Denning *et al.* (1988) series 75% of patients, at 5 years, had been seizure-free for 2 years: but non-compliance with treatment must always be guarded against.

Diagnostic tests for Wilson disease

First and foremost it is necessary to bear in mind the possibility of Wilson disease, even though uncommon, as an underlying cause for a seizure. At this stage clinical examination may not be helpful though a search for evidence of hepatic or neurological abnormalities should be made. Kayser Fleischer rings may be present; they are always bilateral and appear first as a top crescent in the cornea; complete rings are evidence of established disease. The biochemical tests include serum ceruloplasmin, the copper-carrying protein in serum, serum copper, serum "free copper," and urine copper (see Table 36.1). Most routine laboratories can now perform these tests but use an immunonephelometric method for estimating serum ceruloplasmin which gives false high results making estimation of the "free copper" inaccurate (Walshe 2003). Great care must also be taken in urine collection as in routine wards contamination often occurs giving false high results which may suggest a diagnosis of Wilson disease when it does not exist. Magnetic resonance imaging (MRI) brain scans may show lesions in the basal ganglia, most commonly the putamen, also widening of the cerebral ventricles and cortical atrophy. White matter lesions are uncommon but tend to be associated with seizures. In the event of doubt a liver biopsy may be performed and should be subjected to both histological and chemical analysis. The earliest histological abnormalities are fatty changes in the hepatocytes, small cell infiltration in the portal tracts, and glycogen nuclei. Changes in the mitochondrial membrane are seen by electron microscopy (Sternlieb 1968). The levels of hepatic copper to be found in normals, heterozygotes and patients are given in Table 36.1. The ultimate test is to demonstrate a pair of abnormal *ATP7B* genes on chromosome 13. The common gene in Western Europe is His1069Gln but most patients are, in practice, compound heterozygotes and a complete search for all mutations can be very costly. Radiochemical investigations have now become largely redundant. They require specialist expertise and are very costly.

My policy, when investigating a potential patient, was to estimate first the serum ceruloplasmin and serum copper, from which the "free copper" can be calculated, also the 24-hour urine copper excretion. If these proved to be normal the diagnosis of Wilson disease could be ruled out. Problems arrive with individuals who are carriers of one abnormal gene. They never have signs or symptoms of Wilson disease but can give biochemical results in an intermediate range causing diagnostic doubt. In such cases resort must be had to liver biopsy or genetic analysis to prove, or disprove, the diagnosis.

The EEG, though it may help in confirming the epileptic nature of the seizure, is of no help in establishing the diagnosis of Wilson disease.

Table 36.1 Laboratory tests in patients with Wilson disease, heterozygotes and normal subjects[a]

	Normal subjects	Heterozygotes	Wilson disease
Serum copper μg/dl	90–140	50–140	10–100
Urine copper, μg/24 hrs	<30	<50	>80
Ceruloplasmin mg/dl	25–45	5–45	0–25
"Free copper" μg/dl	<10	<10	>10
Liver copper μg/g wet weight	<10	<45	>50

Note:
[a]It must be realized that there no absolutes in biological systems and these figures are no more than guidelines covering the great majority of cases.

Principles of management

The first principle and the sine qua non is correct and efficient management of the underlying Wilson disease; management of the seizures is strictly on conventional lines and is in no way different from that of idiopathic epilepsy. There is no recorded interaction between the two different sets of drugs used in this situation. Wilson disease is best managed at a specialist clinic. The patient should be seen by the same physician at every visit, not by a series of rotating registrars; it is essential to build rapport and trust between doctor and patient. My first choice of treatment is penicillamine, the starting dose for a new adult patient is 500 mg, three times daily before food. It was my practice to give also α-tocopherol 50 mg daily for the first month of treatment as a free radical scavenger.

Pyridoxine 50 mg once a week is only needed during a growth spurt, pregnancy, or intercurrent illness. About 25% of patients treated with penicillamine show an increase in symptoms after starting treatment. This can be worrying but is usually temporary. Rarely there is acute deterioration and this is an indication for immediate change of treatment to trientine, 600 mg three times daily before food. Improvement in Wilson disease can be expected after some months of treatment, it is never rapid and patience is required. In severely dystonic patients a course of British Anti-Lewisite (BAL) 200 mg daily by intramuscular injection into alternate buttocks, for 1 month, followed by a week's rest and then another month's course, may reverse the condition. Zinc sulphate has been used to block the absorption of copper from the gut (Schouwink 1961), but it is not an initial therapy and should never be used in combination with penicillamine or trientine as one combines with the other and both lose their effectiveness. Penicillamine can cause a number of immune reactions, the most serious being systemic lupus and immune complex nephritis and the development of these is an indication for a change of therapy to trientine. Trientine is largely free of toxic side effects but may induce iron deficiency anemia or sideroblastic anemia and occasionally gastrointestinal upsets. Zinc salts can cause sideroblastic anemia and when used in combination with trientine are very likely to do so. The prognosis for most patients with Wilson disease is excellent but the degree of recovery of the neurological deficit inevitably depends upon the amount of damage to the brain before treatment is started. A very small percentage of patients, perhaps around 1%, may follow a steadily downhill course irrespective of what treatment is given. The reason for this is not clear.

References

Bladin PF (2005) 'The epilepsies': Kinnier Wilson's landmark epileptology. *J Clin Neurosci* 12:863–72.

Boudin G, Pepin B (1959) *Dégénérescence hépatolenticulaire.* Paris: Masson.

Cairns JE, Walshe JM (1970) The Kayser Fleischer ring. *Trans Ophthalm Soc UK* 90:187–90.

Denning TR, Berrios GE, Walshe JM (1988) Wilson's disease and epilepsy. *Brain* 111:1139–55.

Gibbs K, Walshe JM (1980) Biliary excretion of copper in Wilson's disease. *Lancet* 2:538–9.

Peters RA, Walshe JM (1966) Studies on the toxicity of copper. The toxic action of copper in vitro and in vivo. *Proc Ry Soc Lond B* 166:273–84.

Scheinberg IH, Sternlieb I (1984) *Wilson's Disease.* Philadelphia, PA: WB Saunders.

Schouwink G (1961) *Hepatocerebraledegeneratie* (met een onderzoekvan de Zink-stofwisseling). Arnhem, the Netherlands: GW van der Wiel.

Sternlieb I (1968) Mitochondrial and fatty changes in hepatocytes of patients with Wilson's disease. *Gastroenterology,* 55:354–67.

Walshe JM, Potter G (1977) The pattern of the whole body distribution of radioactive copper (67Cu, 64Cu) in Wilson's disease and various control groups. *Q J Med* 46:445–62.

Walshe JM (1987) Wilson's disease presenting with features of hepatic dysfunction: a clinical clinical analysis of eighty-seven patients. *Q J Med* 70:253–63.

Walshe JM, Yealland M (1992) Wilson's disease: the problem of delayed diagnosis. *J Neurol Neurosurg Psychiatry* 55:92–6.

Walshe JM, Yealland M (1993) Chelation treatment of neurological Wilson's disease. *Q J Med* 86:297–304.

Walshe JM (2003) Wilson's disease: the importance of measuring caeruloplasmin non-immunologically. *Ann Clin Biochem* 40:115–21.

Chapter

37

Disorders of cobalamin and folate metabolism

Michael Shevell, David Watkins, and David Rosenblatt

Cobalamin deficiency

Causal disease

Cobalamin (vitamin B_{12}) is an essential co-factor for two intracellular reactions: (1) cytosolic methionine synthase-mediated conversion of homocysteine to methionine; and (2) mitochondrial methylmalonylCoA mutase-mediated conversion of methylmalonylCoA to succinylCoA (Watkins *et al.* 2008). Cobalamin is derived entirely from animal sources. Thus, cobalamin deficiency can occur in the context of dietary deprivation, as in a strictly vegan diet that is non-supplemented. Maternal lack of dietary cobalamin or subclinical pernicious anemia can lead to an infantile deficiency in the mother's offspring.

The absorption of dietary cobalamin requires the production by gastric parietal cells of cobalamin specific intrinsic factor (IF) that binds to cobalamin to form a cobalamin-intrinsic factor (Cbl-IF) complex. Specific distal ileum located enterocyte brush border receptors bind the Cbl-IF complex, which is then internalized through endocytosis. Lysosomal degradation releases the bound cobalamin, which is then coupled to transcobalamin II (TCII, TC) and released into the portal circulation for the systemic distribution of the bound complex (Watkins *et al.* 2009). The intracellular processing of the TCII–cobalamin complex and its distribution and interactions in lysosomal, cytosolic, and mitochondrial compartments are shown in Fig. 37.1.

Beyond dietary limitations, cobalamin deficiency may be inherited or acquired in origin. Genetically determined illnesses include disorders of cobalamin absorption, transport, and uptake that may involve: (1) deficient intrinsic factor (Tanner *et al.* 2005), (2) deficient enterocyte uptake of the Cbl-IF complex (Imerslund–Gräsbeck syndrome) (Gräsbeck 2006)[4], (3) deficient TCII availability (Hall 1992), and TC receptor deficiency (Quadros *et al.* 2009). Somatic cell complementation studies were utilized to define a number of inherited disorders of intracellular cobalamin metabolism (cblA–cblG) (Rosenblatt 2001). Three (cblA, cblB, cblD variant 2) involve isolated adenosylcobalamin formation resulting

in impaired succinylCoA synthesis, three (cblE, cblG, cblD variant 1) involve impaired methylcobalamin synthesis resulting in reduced methionine formation, and three (cblC, cblD, cblF) involve defective synthesis of both adenosylcobalamin and methylcobalamin, leading to both impaired succinylCoA and methionine formation. All of these inherited disorders, whether affecting absorption, transport, and uptake or the intracellular processing of cobalamin, are autosomal recessive in Mendelian inheritance.

Acquired disorders of cobalamin deficiency beyond the nutritional typically relate to disturbances affecting the gastrointestinal tract, specifically the gastric and ileal mucosa, the site of IF production and Cbl-IF complex endocytosis respectively (Shevell and Rosenblatt 1992). These disturbances include: (1) pernicious anemia, in which there is an auto-immune-mediated atrophic gastritis involving the production of autoantibodies against gastric parietal cells, (2) surgical resections and procedures involving the stomach (e.g., gastric bypass, gastrectomy) or ileum (e.g., ileal resection, ileostomy), (3) long-standing chronic gastritis (e.g., *Helicobacter pylori* infection), (4) malabsorption syndrome, (5) celiac disease, (6) proton pump inhibitor-use induced achlorhydria, (7) intestinal infection with the fish tapeworm (*Diphyllobothrium latum*) or the *Giardia* parasite.

Genetically determined and acquired disorders leading to relative cobalamin deficiency result in hematologic changes characterized by megaloblastic anemia. The genetically determined group of disorders is relatively rare, with those involving defects in intracellular cobalamin metabolism tending to lead to a more severe metabolic disturbance than those affecting the processes of cobalamin absorption, transport, and cellular uptake (Watkins *et al.* 2008). Clinically, feeding difficulties, hypotonia, and developmental delay are characteristic neurologic features of early-onset disorders, while those presenting later in the pediatric age group may be characterized by behavioral changes (e.g., delirium, psychosis), cognitive limitations, visual impairment related to retinal changes, long tract findings (e.g., spasticity, myelopathy), and gait disturbances (Whitehead 2006).

The Causes of Epilepsy, eds. S. D. Shorvon, F. Andermann, and R. Guerrini. Published by Cambridge University Press. © Cambridge University Press 2011.

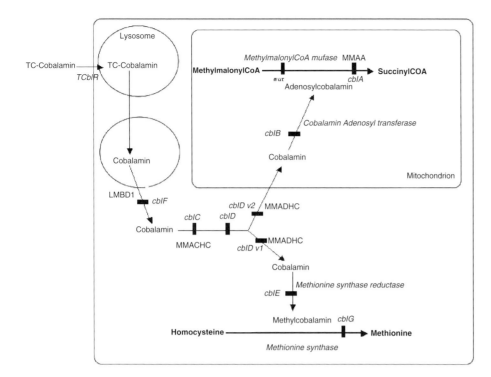

Fig. 37.1. Cobalamin metabolism in human cells. Cobalamin bound to transcobalamin (TC) is taken up by endocytosis mediated by the transcobalamin receptor (TCblR) and subsequently converted to the active coenzyme derivatives adenosylcobalamin (required for activity of the mitochondrial enzyme methylmalonylCoA mutase) and methylcobalamin (involved in activity of cytoplasmic methionine synthase). The steps affected by inborn errors of cobalamin metabolism (*cblA*–*cblG* and methylmalonylCoA mutase deficiency, *mut*) are indicated. MMAA, the product of the *MMAA* gene, affected in the *cblA* disorder; MMACHC, the product of the *MMACHC* gene, affected in the *cblC* disorder; MMADHC, the product of the *MMADHC* gene, affected in the *cblD*, *cblD* variant 1 (*cblD* v1), and *cblD* variant 2 (*cblD* v2) disorders; LMBD1, the product of the *LMBRD1* gene, affected in the *cblF* disorder. The *MMAB* gene encoding cobalamin adenosyltransferase is affected in the *cblB* disorder; the *MTRR* gene, encoding methionine synthase reductase, is affected in the *cblE* disorder; and the *MTR* gene, encoding methionine synthase reductase, is affected in the *cblG* disorder.

Acquired disorders of cobalamin deficiency occur far more frequently than genetically determined disorders and often result in a variety of neurologic syndromes (Healton *et al.* 1991; Shevell and Rosenblatt 1992). Those typically encountered include: (1) peripheral neuropathy, (2) myelopathy, reflecting involvement of corticospinal tracts and dorsal columns, (3) myeloneuropathy, (4) mental status changes including cognitive and executive function impairment, (5) optic neuropathy that affects central vision in the absence of optic atrophy, and (6) non-specific distal paresthesias without the objective findings of a neuropathy, either clinically or on nerve conduction studies.

Epilepsy in cobalamin deficiency

Seizures are recognized as an uncommon manifestation of cobalamin deficiency, especially in adults. The mechanisms of epileptogenesis are speculative, but several lines of evidence focus on the effects of homocysteine. Homocysteine is a sulfur-containing amino acid, and both it and its metabolic product (homocysteic acid) have been shown to induce seizures in immature and mature rats (Kubova *et al.* 1995; Mares *et al.* 1997). This epileptogenecity can be blocked, at least in immature rats, by both *N*-methyl-D-aspartate (NMDA) and non-NMDA glutamate receptor antagonists (Folbergrova *et al.* 2000). Furthermore, methylcobalamin through *S*-adenosylmethionine (SAM) is critically involved in central myelin synthesis (Surtees *et al.* 1991). Imperfectly myelinated central pathways may play a role in aberrantly generated and propagated seizure discharges. Finally, a protective effect in cultured cortical neurons against glutamate excitotoxicity has

been ascribed to methylcobalamin (Akaike *et al.* 1993). Despite the critical importance of homocysteine, West syndrome has been reported in isolated methylmalonic aciduria, where homocysteine levels are not expected to be elevated (Campeau *et al.* 2009).

Though rare in occurrence, seizures in the context of acquired cobalamin deficiency may take a variety of forms. These include: (1) de novo epileptic confusional status (ECS) with generalized continuous rhythmic epileptic sharp waves (Aguglia *et al.* 1995), (2) convulsive status and intractable seizures (Lee *et al.* 2005), (3) an association with apparent benign familial infantile seizures (Lundgren and Blennow 1999), (4) infantile spasms within the context of apparent West syndrome (Erol *et al.* 2007), and (5) focal motor seizures (Kumar 2004).

The cases of ECS, convulsive status, and intractable seizures arise in adults frequently in conjunction with other more typical neurologic syndromes associated with cobalamin deficiency such as myelopathy or neuropathy (Aguglia *et al.* 1995; Lee *et al.* 2005). These cases were responsive to acute management with appropriate anticonvulsants and longer-term remediation of the cobalamin deficiency through cobalamin supplementation. The infantile-onset seizures, whether spasms, benign familial infantile convulsions, or focal motor seizures, typically were encountered in the setting of a maternal vegan diet, and the resulting infantile lack of sufficient dietary cobalamin (Lundgren and Blennow 1999; Kumar 2004; Erol *et al.* 2007). Once again, supplemental exogenous cobalamin administered to the infants resulted in the resolution of seizures sufficient to discontinue anticonvulsant medication administration within a short time-frame. A normalization of varied abnormal electroencephalographic (EEG) findings was also noted in the above situations with exogenous cobalamin supplementation.

Early-onset cblC or cblD disorder, which results in both homocystinuria and methylmalonic aciduria, has been described in several reports to feature prominent seizures (Biancheri *et al.* 2002). These seizures may initially present as convulsive status epilepticus, but more typically are complex partial or focal clonic in semiology. On one occasion, epileptic ocular movements resulting in eyelid myoclonia which is more typically encountered in classical absence epilepsy has been described (Cogan *et al.* 1980). The seizures were in conjunction with other features of an inherited disorder of intracellular cobalamin processing, specifically feeding difficulties, failure to thrive, and developmental delay, together with a megaloblastic anemia and elevated levels in both serum and urine of homocysteine and methylmalonic acid. Focal and multifocal epileptiform abnormalities, sometimes assuming a diphasic spike or spike-and-wave configuration, were documented that were increased during sleep.

Diagnostic testing for cobalamin deficiency

Routine hematologic testing is utilized to detect indicators of a megaloblastic anemia that frequently occurs secondary to cobalamin deficiency (Watkins *et al.* 2008). Serum cobalamin levels can be reliably measured and can be supplemented by measurement of the metabolites homocysteine and methylmalonic acid. Disorders of absorption and transport can be further assessed by screening for intrinsic factor autoantibodies, as well as by the Schilling test which tests specifically for cobalamin absorption. The availability of the radioactive reagents required for the Schilling tests has limited its recent use in many centers. Suspected inherited disorders of cobalamin intracellular metabolism are diagnosed by measurement of serum and urine homocysteine and methylmalonic acid, as well as utilization of cultured skin fibroblasts to measure endogenous methylmalonyl CoA mutase and methionine synthase function and methylcobalamin and adenosylcobalamin synthesis, and to perform somatic cell complementation analysis to find the specific inherited disorder (i.e., *cblA–cblG*) affecting the patient. Where a specific diagnosis is suspected clinically, it is also possible to begin with sequencing the causal gene (e.g., *MMACHC* in *cblC*).

If neurologic symptoms are evident, relevant investigations include: (1) electromyography (EMG)/nerve conduction study (NCS) to evaluate a possible neuropathy, (2) somatosensory evoked responses (SER) to assess dorsal column integrity, (3) electroretinography (ERG)/visual evoked potential (VER) to assess retinal and optic nerve pathway function, and (4) neuroimaging (e.g. magnetic resonance imaging [MRI]) to detect and objectify central white matter changes in the spinal cord and brain (Healton *et al.* 1991; Shevell and Rosenblatt 1992). Needless to say, paroxysmal events that raise the possibility of coexisting seizures will necessitate EEG testing.

Management of cobalamin deficiency

Standard principles of antiepileptic drug selection apply to management of seizures within the context of disorders of cobalamin deficiency. Use of valproic acid, carbamazepine, and phenytoin has been shown in epileptic patients to lower serum cobalamin levels, thus caution should be employed with utilization of these specific agents or alternatives sought (Karabiber *et al.* 2003). Cobalamin deficiency itself is treated with pharmacologic intramuscular or oral doses of either hydroxycobalamin or cyanocobalamin (Watkins *et al.* 2008). Folate supplementation, in conjunction with prior adequate cobalamin treatment, will assist in the reversal of hematologic abnormalities, but it is essential not to treat cobalamin deficiency with folate alone. Specific antihelminthic (e.g., diatrizoic acid) or antiprotozoal (e.g., metronidizole) treatment should be utilized for documented fish tapeworm or *Giardia* infection. Additional modalities of adjunctive treatment for disorders of intracellular cobalamin metabolism can include dietary protein restriction and betaine supplementation. Efforts to correct the cobalamin deficiency will result in the stabilization or reversal of neurologic symptoms, but in the context of the genetically determined disorders this may be a function of the duration of neurologic symptoms prior to the initiation of corrective treatment. Thus early diagnosis and treatment leads to improved neurologic outcome in this specific population (Biancheri *et al.* 2002).

Folate deficiency
Causal disease

Like cobalamin, folate is entirely derived from exogenous dietary sources, but unlike cobalamin, folate is found in food derived from both plants and animals (Watkins *et al.* 2008). In that folate is typically ingested as polyglutamates, intestinal hydrolysis to a monoglutamate form is required prior to intestinal absorption. Both intestinal absorption and transport across the choroid plexus into the brain is mediated by specific transport proteins. The proton-coupled folate transporter (PCFT) is required for transport of folate across the intestinal wall and across the blood–brain barrier at the choroid plexus (Qiu *et al.* 2006); the latter process also appears to require folate receptor α (FRα) (Zhao and Goldman 2007; Steinfeld *et al.* 2009). Folate uptake by peripheral cells depends on folate receptors and the reduced folate carrier (RFC) (Matherly and Goldman 2003).

Intracellular folate functions as an essential co-factor in a myriad of complex reactions involving one-carbon transfers. Folates are implicated in the catabolism of serine, glycine, and histidine, and the synthesis of purines, pyrimidines (i.e., nucleotide biosynthesis), and methionine (Rosenblatt 2001; Watkins *et al.* 2008). The complexity of these reactions is evident in Fig. 37.2.

Mutations affecting the PCFT result in deficient uptake of folate at both the intestinal and choroid plexus levels and

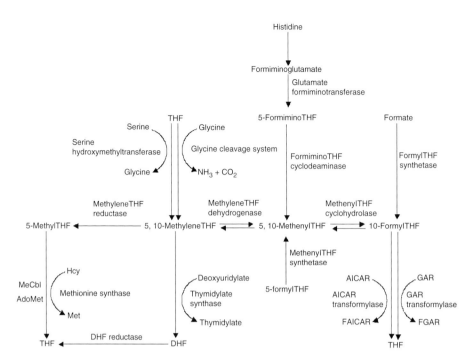

Fig. 37.2. Folate metabolism in human cells. One-carbon units are derived from breakdown of serine (catalyzed by serine hydroxymethyltransferase), glycine (the glycine cleavage system), and histidine (glutamate formiminotransferase). One-carbon units are utilized in conversion of homocysteine to methionine (cobalamin-dependent methionine synthase), synthesis of thymidine (thymidylate synthase), and in two steps in purine biosynthesis (GAR transformylase and AICAR transformylase). THF, tetrahydrofolate.

causes hereditary folate malabsorption (congenital malabsorption of folate) (Qiu *et al.* 2006; Watkins *et al.* 2009). This autosomal recessive disorder is characterized by early infantile megaloblastic anemia, failure to thrive, diarrhea, and progressive neurologic deterioration featuring frequently intractable seizures.

More recently, a disorder reflecting specific deficient transport of folate at the choroid plexus across the blood–brain barrier has been described (Ramaekers and Blau 2004). This disorder has been referred to as cerebral folate deficiency (CFD) or central nervous system (CNS) folate deficiency. Folate transport across the intestinal barrier appears to be intact as serum and red blood cell folate levels are within the normative range. Lumbar puncture reveals low levels of 5-methyltetrahydrofolate (MTHF) which is the active CNS folate metabolite. The folate receptor 1 protein appears to be non-functional due to: (1) aberrant post-translational processing of the protein, (2) the presence of irreversibly binding folate antagonists, (3) autoantibodies blocking the folate binding site, or (4) mutations in the *FOLR1* gene, which encodes FRα (Ramaekers and Blau 2004; Steinfeld *et al.* 2009). Affected children have early irritability and sleep disturbances that evolve into pronounced developmental delay, progressive visual loss (if untreated), dysmetric grasping, and profound dyskinesias characterized by ballistic movements and choreoathetosis. Early hypotonia is gradually replaced over time as an ascending paraparesis that eventually evolves into spastic quadriplegia. Autistic features are prominent, as is a mixed and frequently intractable seizure disorder (Moretti *et al.* 2008).

Secondary disorders of cerebral folate deficiency have been described in conjunction with Rett-like features (regardless of *MECP2* mutation status) (Ramaekers *et al.* 2003) and apparent

Aicardi–Goutieres syndrome (Blau *et al.* 2003). A secondary disorder of systemic folate deficiency related to defective intestinal transport has been documented in the context of celiac disease (Bye *et al.* 1993). A predilection for progressive bilateral occipital calcifications and seizures originating from the occipital cortex has been noted in this entity in several reports.

Two disorders of intracellular folate metabolism have been described. The first involves a rarely reported deficiency in the glutamate formimino transferase (GFT) enzyme disrupting histidine catabolism (Watkins *et al.* 2009). Cognitive, and in particular speech, limitations are clinically apparent, while imaging studies note cortical atrophy in more severely affected individuals. Seizures have been variably noted in this context and commented upon to a limited extent. The second disorder of intracellular folate metabolism is severe methylenetetrahydrofolate reductase (MTHFR) deficiency (Thomas and Rosenblatt 2005), caused by severe mutations in the *MTHFR* gene and inherited as an autosomal recessive trait. Whereas a common polymorphism in *MTHFR* confers enzymatic thermolability leading to relative hyperhomocysteinemia that has been implicated as a possible risk factor for vascular disease and neural tube defects (Frosst *et al.* 1995), severe MTHFR deficiency can lead to progressive neurologic deterioration including seizures in childhood and myelopathy, psychiatric illness, and cerebral vascular events in older affected individuals.

Epilepsy in folate deficiency

Seizures are frequently, but not invariably, noted in folate deficiency disorders attributed to both defects in folate absorption, transport, and uptake (i.e. hereditary malabsorption of folate, cerebral folate deficiency) and defects in intracellular metabolism (i.e., MTHFR deficiency). Unfortunately the literature rarely provides details on the specific type of seizures encountered, though frequently intractability is noted. In the largest series of children with cerebral folate deficiency (Ramaekers and Blau 2004), varied generalized seizures (i.e., absences, myoclonic–astatic, tonic–clonic) are specifically mentioned.

Epileptogenesis is likely related to disturbances in homocysteine metabolism (known to induce seizures in animal models) (Kubova et al. 1995; Mares et al. 1997), aberrations in central myelin synthesis (through inadequate formation of S-adenosyl methionine [SAM]) (Surtees et al. 1991), and intracranial structural changes (e.g., atrophy, calcifications) (Bye et al. 1993; Ramaekers and Blau 2004) that disrupt cortical pathways. Specific EEG changes in the context of disorders of folate deficiency have not been a subject of report to date.

Diagnostic testing for folate deficiency

Hematologic testing will reveal a megaloblastic anemia, which usually functions as the first clue to a possible folate deficiency in the clinical setting (Watkins et al. 2008). Serum and red blood cell folate levels can be determined. Serum amino acid profiles can detect alterations in intracellular homocysteine, methionine, serine, glycine, histidine, and glutamate (e.g., formiminoglutamate) metabolism that are dependent on folate mediated reactions. Cerebrospinal fluid MTHF can be measured to ascertain central folate status and indeed specialized testing is available to assess the functional status of the critical FRα protein that mediates folate transport across the choroid plexus and the blood–brain barrier (Ramaekers and Blau 2004). The intestinal absorption of orally administered and labeled folate can be used to assess the integrity of the intestinal absorption apparatus (Bye et al. 1993). Endoscopy and biopsy are prerequisites for accurate diagnosis of celiac disease (Bye et al. 1993). Neuroimaging studies will detect non-specific cerebral atrophy and the intracranial, particularly occipital, calcifications noted especially in folate deficiency.

Management of folate deficiency

Accurate diagnosis is essential and is rendered difficult by the relative rarity of folate deficiency entities and their non-specific symptomatology. Megaloblastic anemia, serum amino acid profile, and serum/red blood cell folate levels are important clues to diagnosis. More frequent measurement of MTHF on lumbar puncture in cases of unexplained progressive neurologic deterioration or intractable seizures would likely result in more cases of cerebral or CNS folate deficiency (CFD) being described (Ramaekers and Blau 2004).

Antiepileptic drug management is based on rational pharmacologic principles directed at best control of specific seizure types and the avoidance of unnecessary polypharmacy. Neurologic symptoms can be improved and indeed reversed, especially in younger patients, by the oral administration of folinic acid at a dose of 0.5–1 mg/kg per day (Watkins et al. 2008). Overdosing with folinic acid may have some neurotoxic effect, and thus both serum and cerebrospinal fluid folate levels should be periodically monitored to avoid such iatrogenic effects (Surtees 2001).

Acknowledgments

Alba Rinaldi provided the necessary secretarial assistance. MCH Foundation gave salary support for MS.

References

Aguglia U, Gambardella A, Oliveri R, et al. (1995) De novo epileptic confusional status in a patient with cobalamin deficiency. Metab Brain Dis 10:233–8.

Akaike A, Tamura Y, Sato Y, Yokota T (1993) Protective effects of a vitamin B$_{12}$ analog, methylcobalamin, against glutamate cytotoxicity in cultured cortical neurons. Eur J Pharmacol 241:1–6.

Biancheri R, Cerone R, Rossi A, et al. (2002) Early-onset cobalamin C/D deficiency: epilepsy and electroencephalographic features. Epilepsia 43:616–22.

Blau N, Bonafe L, Krägeloh-Mann I, et al. (2003) Cerebrospinal fluid pterns and folates in Aicardi–Goutieres syndrome: a new phenotype. Neurology 61:642–7.

Bye AME, Andermann F, Robitaille Y, et al. (1993) Cortical vascular abnormalities in the syndrome of celiac disease, epilepsy, bilateral occipital calcifications, and folate deficiency. Ann Neurol 34:399–403.

Campeau PM, Valayannopouolos V, Touati G, et al. (2009) Management of West syndrome in a patient with methylmalomnic aciduria. J Child Neurol (doi:10.1177/0883073809336119).

Cogan DG, Schulman J, Porter RJ, Mudd SH (1980) Epileptiform ocular movements with methylmalonic aciduria and homocysinuria. Am J Ophthalmol 90:251–3.

Erol I, Alehan F, Gümüs A (2007) West syndrome in an infant with vitamin B$_{12}$ deficiency in the absence of macrocytic anaemia. Dev Med Child Neurol 49:774–6.

Folbergrova J, Haugvicova R, Mares P (2000) Behavioral and metabolic changes in immature rats. Exp Neurol 161:336–45.

Frosst P, Blom HJ, Milos R (1995) A candidate genetic risk factor for vascular disease: a common methylenetetrahydrofolate reductase mutation causes thermoinstability. Nat Genet 10:111–13.

Gräsbeck R (2006) Imerslund–Gräsbeck syndrome (selective vitamin B$_{12}$ malabsorption with proteinuria). Orphanet J Rare Dis 1:17.

Hall CA (1992) The neurologic aspects of transcobalamin II deficiency. Br J Haematol 80:117–20.

Healton EB, Savage DG, Brust JCM, Garrett TJ, Lindenbaum J (1991) Neurologic aspects of cobalamin deficiency. Medicine 70:229–45.

Karabiber H, Sonmezgoz E, Ozerol E (2003) Effects of valporate and carbamazepine on serum levels of homocysteine, vitamin B$_{12}$ and folate. Brain Dev 25:113–15.

Kubova H, Folbergrova J, Mares P (1995) Seizures induced by homocysteine in rats during ontogenesis. *Epilepsia* **36**:750–6.

Kumar S (2004) Recurrent seizures: an unusual manifestation of vitamin B_{12} deficiency. *Neurology (India)* **52**:122–3.

Lee M, Chang HS, Wu HT, Weng HH, Chen CM (2005) Intractable epilepsy as the presentation of vitamin B_{12} deficiency in the absence of macrocytic anemia. *Epilepsia* **46**:1147–8.

Lundgren J, Blennow G (1999) Vitamin B_{12} deficiency may cause benign familial infantile convulsions: a case report. *Acta Pediatr* **88**:1158–60.

Mares P, Folbergrova J, Langmeir M, Haugvicova R, Kubova H (1997) Convulsant action of D,L-homocysteic acid and its stereo-isomers in immature rats. *Epilepsia* **38**:767–76.

Matherly LH, Goldman ID (2003) Membrane transport of folates. *Vitamins Hormones* **66**:403–56.

Moretti P, Peters SU, del Gaudio D, et al. (2008) Autistic symptoms, developmental regression, mental retardation, epilepsy, and dyskinesias in CNS folate deficiency. *J Autism Dev Disord* **38**:1170–7.

Qiu A, Jansen M, Sakaris A, et al. (2006) Identification of an intestinal folate transporter and the molecular basis for hereditary folate malabsorption. *Cell* **127**:917–26.

Quadros EV, Nakayama Y, Sequeira JM (2009) The protein and gene encoding the receptor for cellular uptake of transcobalamin bound cobalamin. *Blood* **113**:186–92.

Ramaekers VT, Blau N (2004) Cerebral folate deficiency. *Dev Med Child Neurol* **46**:843–51.

Ramaekers V, Hansen SI, Holm J, et al. (2003) Reduced folate transport to the CNS in female Rett patients. *Neurology* **61**:506–14.

Rosenblatt DS (2001) Inborn errors of folate and cobalamin metabolism. In: Carmel R, Jacobsen DW (eds.) *Homocysteine in Health and Disease*. Cambridge, UK: Cambridge University Press, pp. 244–58.

Shevell MI, Rosenblatt DS (1992) The neurology of cobalamin. *Can J Neurol Sci* **19**:472–86.

Steinfeld R, Grapp M, Kraetzner R, et al. (2009) Folate receptor alpha defect causes cerebral folate transport deficiency: a treatable neurodegenerative disorder associated with disturbed myelin metabolism. *Am J Med Genet* **85**:354–63.

Surtees R (2001) Cobalamin and folate responsive disorders. In: Baxter P (ed.) *Vitamin Responsive Conditions in Pediatric Neurology*. London: MacKeith Press, pp. 96–108.

Surtees R, Leonard J, Austin S (1991) Association of demyelination with deficiency of cerebrospinal-fluid S-adenosylmethionine in inborn errors of methyl-transfer pathway. *Lancet* **338**:1550–54.

Tanner SM, Li Z, Perko JD, et al. (2005) Hereditary juvenile cobalamin deficiency caused by mutations in the intrinsic factor gene. *Proc Natl Acad Sci USA* **102**:4130–3.

Thomas MA, Rosenblatt DS (2005) Severe methylenetetrahydrofolate reductase deficiency. In: Ueland PM, Rozen R (eds.) *MTHFR Polymorphisms and Disease*. Georgetown, TX: Landes Bioscience, pp. 54–70.

Watkins D, Shevell MI, Rosenblatt DS (2008) Vitamins: cobalamin and folate. In: Rosenberg RN, Prusiner SB, Mauro SD, Barchi RL, Nestler EJ (eds.) *The Molecular and Genetic Basis of Neurologic and Psychiatric Disease*, 4th edn. Philadelphia, PA: Lippincott, Williams and Wilkins, pp. 733–8.

Watkins D, Whitehead VM, Rosenblatt DS (2009) Megaloblastic anemia. In: Orkin SH, Ginsburg D, Nathan DA, Look AT, Fisher DE (eds.) *Nathan and Oski's Hematology of Infancy and Childhood*, 7th edn. Philadelphia, PA: WB Saunders, pp. 467–520.

Whitehead VM (2006) Acquired and inherited disorders of cobalamin and folate in children. *Br J Haematol* **134**: 125–36.

Yang YM, Ducos R, Rosenberg AJ, et al. (1985) Cobalamin malabsorption in three siblings due to abnormal intrinsic factor that is markedly susceptible to acid and proteolysis. *J Clin Invest* **76**:2057–65.

Zhao R, Goldman ID (2007) The molecular identity and characterization of a proton-coupled folate transporter: PCFT – biological ramifications and impact on the activity of pemetrexed. *Cancer Metastasis Rev* **26**:129–39.

Chapter 38

Other single-gene disorders

Vincent Navarro and Frédéric Sedel

Introduction

Epileptic seizures can occur in many inborn errors of metabolism (IEMs), usually as part of a larger clinical spectrum. However, seizures are rarely the initial or the main manifestations of IEM. The rare metabolic disorders described in this chapter merit attention from the clinicians for multiple reasons: (1) several of them may benefit from specific therapies, (2) certain antiepileptic drugs aggravate both seizures and the metabolic disorder, and (3) some of these IEMs may be underdiagnosed.

Most IEMs start in the neonatal or infantile period, though several of these diseases are first diagnosed in adults particularly when their phenotype is moderate with mild initial symptoms. The IEMs can be classified according to their pathogenesis (Table 38.1). Several IEMs responsible for epilepsy have been described in previous chapters. This chapter considers further IEMs, most of which are amenable to specific metabolic treatment. In all of the IEMs presented here, epileptic seizures tend to be associated with mental retardation.

Glucose transporter type 1 (GLUT-1) deficiency syndrome (De Vivo disease)

This disease is due to impaired glucose transport across the blood–brain barrier, due to mutations in the glucose transporter type 1 (GLUT-1) gene (Klepper 2004). It usually appears sporadically due to de novo mutations and may present with autosomal dominant inheritance. Failure to transport glucose through the blood–brain barrier is responsible for hypoglycorrhachia which may become symptomatic especially in the morning before eating. Fewer than 100 cases have been reported, but this disease is probably underdiagnosed. A variable clinical presentation probably depends on variation in residual function of GLUT-1. The most severe neurological phenotype, associated with a profound loss of GLUT-1 function, begins in infancy and consists of acquired microcephaly, epileptic encephalopathy, developmental retardation, spasticity, and ataxia. A milder phenotype, presumably associated

Table 38.1 Classification of epilepsies of metabolic origin according to their pathogenesis

Energy deficiency	Hypoglycemia (hyperinsulinism/ hyperammonemia [HI/HA], etc.), GLUT-1 deficiency, respiratory chain deficiency, creatine deficiency
Toxic effect	Aminoacidopathies, organic acidurias, urea cycle defects, HI/HA, homocystinuria
Impaired neuronal function	Storage disorders
Disturbance of neurotransmitter systems	Non-ketotic hyperglycinaemia, γ-aminobutyric acid (GABA) transaminase deficiency, succinic semialdehyde dehydrogenase deficiency (SSADH), HI/HA
Associated brain malformations	Peroxisomal disorders (Zellweger), O-glycosylation defects
Vitamin/co-factor dependency	Biotinidase deficiency, pyridoxine-dependent and pyridoxal phosphate-dependent epilepsy, folinic acid-responsive seizures, Menkes disease

Source: Modified from Wolf *et al.* (2005).

with a less severe loss of GLUT-1 function, is diagnosed in adults with normal intelligence or slight mental retardation and consists of intermittent symptoms: paroxysmal exertional dyskinesia or ataxia, lethargy, or confusion on waking that improves with sugar intake (Brockmann *et al.* 2001; Klepper *et al.* 2001; Suls *et al.* 2008).

Epilepsy is frequent in GLUT-1 deficiency. It is often the first symptom in the severe phenotype, with seizures first detected at about 6.5 months. Symptoms consist of chaotic ocular movements, episodes of cyanosis or apnea, and atonic seizures. Thereafter, myoclonic and generalized seizures are observed (Klepper 2004). Frequency of seizures varies between individuals and they may be associated with other paroxysmal

The Causes of Epilepsy, eds. S. D. Shorvon, F. Andermann, and R. Guerrini. Published by Cambridge University Press. © Cambridge University Press 2011.

manifestations. Seizures may be absent in 15–20% of patients with a mild "atypical" phenotype.

GLUT-1 deficiency is diagnosed from measurements of glucose in both blood and cerebrospinal fluid (CSF) after 4–6 hours fasting. A glucose CSF/blood ratio below 0.4 (normal > 0.6) is highly suggestive. The CSF glucose measurement may be a more reliable biomarker; typically CSF glucose is lower than 40 mg/L in the severe phenotype and 40–52 mg/L in the mild phenotype (De Vivo and Wang 2008). In addition, CSF lactate values are normal or low. Diagnosis should be confirmed by molecular analysis of the *GLUT-1* gene. If genetic studies are negative, glucose incorporation in erythroblasts should be examined. The electroencephalogram (EEG) in these patients may be normal or show epileptic focal or generalized abnormalities that typically worsen during fasting and improve after eating (Klepper and Leiendecker 2007).

A ketogenic diet is spectacularly effective in the management of GLUT-1 (Klepper 2004), but to our knowledge no data exist in adults. It may act in several ways and in particular circulating ketone bodies may be used by the brain as an alternative source of energy. A ketogenic diet is more effective in controlling seizures in patients with GLUT-1 deficiency than against paroxysmal manifestations and cognitive impairment (Klepper 2008).

Some antiepileptic drugs, including diazepam, phenobarbital, and sodium valproate, other drugs including theophyllin, tricyclic antidepressants, and androgens as well as alcohol, caffeine, and green tea, should be avoided since they inhibit GLUT-1. Without the ketogenic diet, seizures tend to resist antiepileptic drugs but neither carbamazepine nor phenytoin inhibit the glucose transporter.

Creatine synthesis or transport defects

Disorders of creatine metabolism include deficiencies in the arginine-glycine aminotransferase (AGAT), guanidinoacetate methyltransferase (GAMT), and X-linked brain creatine transporter (CRTR) (Cheillan *et al.* 2005). An AGAT deficiency has been reported in a few children. Few patients with GAMT deficiency surviving to adulthood have been described (Schulze *et al.* 2003; Caldeira Araujo *et al.* 2005). They have mental retardation, a severe language delay, behavioral problems, paraparesis, and rigidity. Male patients with an X-linked CRTR deficiency present a mild phenotype and heterozygotic women are either asymptomatic or have learning difficulties or autistic features.

In GAMT deficiency, various types of seizures including myoclonic, generalized tonic–clonic, partial, atypical absence, or astatic events occur frequently and are poorly controlled by antiepileptic drugs. In X-linked CRTR deficiency, seizures are rare and easily controlled with antiepileptic drugs.

These three deficits can be diagnosed from an absence of the normal creatine peak in brain proton magnetic resonance spectroscopy. Creatine and guanidinoacetate should then be measured in plasma and urine for a precise identification of the creatine metabolism defect.

Creatine supplements are effective in patients with defects of synthesis (GAMT and AGAT deficiencies) but usually ineffective in the creatine transporter defect. Dietary reduction of arginine and the addition of ornithine is also proposed in GAMT deficiency.

Succinic semialdehyde dehydrogenase deficiency

Succinic semialdehyde dehydrogenase (SSADH) catabolizes succinic semialdehyde produced from the catabolism of γ-aminobutyric acid (GABA) (Pearl *et al.* 2003). A deficiency results in accumulation of γ-hydroxybutyric acid.

The classical phenotype in patients with this deficiency includes a psychomotor retardation, hypotonia, and epilepsy with generalized tonic–clonic seizures or absence-like seizures. In 25% of cases, epilepsy begins in neonates. A few adults with mental retardation, psychotic features, behavioral disturbances, and generalized seizures have a SSADH deficiency (Gibson *et al.* 2003), and one patient, heterozygous for SSADH deficiency, has been reported with photosensitive absence epilepsy and myoclonias (Dervent *et al.* 2004).

This IEM is detected as an accumulation of γ-hydroxybutyrate in urinary organic acid chromatography. The EEG records show various patterns (Pearl *et al.* 2003).

The treatment of choice for this deficiency should be vigabatrin, which inhibits GABA transaminase, and so reduces γ-hydroxybutyric acid formation. However this drug may lead to GABA accumulation, aggravating absences and myoclonus. Good results have been obtained with benzodiazepines, lamotrigine, and carbamazepine (Gibson *et al.* 2003). Valproate inhibits SSADH and should be avoided.

Hyperinsulinism/hyperammonemia syndrome (HI/HA)

Hyperinsulinism/hyperammonemia syndrome (HI/HA) is a rare disorder resulting from missense mutations in glutamate dehydrogenase (GDH), which cause a gain of enzyme function (Stanley *et al.* 1998). Glutamate dehydrogenase oxidizes mitochondrial glutamate to α-ketoglutarate and ammonia. Overactivation of GDH depolarizes pancreatic β-cells, by increasing the ATP/ADP ratio which inactivates an ATP-sensitive potassium channel (K_{ATP}) and therefore initiates an enhanced insulin release. The phenotype is heterogeneous, such that the disease may be diagnosed in infants or sometimes in adults. Recurrent episodes of symptomatic hypoglycemia occur typically late in the first year of life. Mental retardation is frequent, and typically detected after repeated bouts of hypoglycemia. The hyperammonemia, up to two- to fivefold normal values, is asymptomatic.

Epilepsy is frequently associated with HI/HA (Raizen *et al.* 2005). Generalized tonic–clonic seizures are frequently associated with hypoglycemic episodes in the first year of life (Bahi-Buisson *et al.* 2008b). A childhood-onset non-hypoglycemic epilepsy was found in 14 of 22 patients with HI/HA. Atypical absences lasting more than 30 s were associated with eyelid myoclonia or myoclonic jerks. Myoclonic absence epilepsy with photosensitivity was reported in a family with dominant inheritance, while metabolic abnormalities varied in affected members (Bahi-Buisson et al. 2008a). Several hypotheses have been advanced to explain the pathophysiology of epilepsy in HI/HA: it may result from (1) acute hypoglycemia, or brain sequelae of hypoglycemic injuries, (2) hyperammonemia, (3) overactivity of GDH, resulting in a decrease of brain glutamate and therefore of brain GABA, or (4) neuronal depolarization due to K_{ATP} channel closure induced by the increased ATP/ADP ratio.

The diagnosis of HI/HA is suggested by the specific biochemical abnormalities and confirmed by genetic analysis.

Hyperinsulinemic hypoglycemia can be controlled by diazoxide and a protein-restricted diet. A subtotal pancreatectomy is sometimes required. Antiepileptic drugs should be adapted to the epileptic syndrome, while avoiding carbamazepine or drugs that aggravate myoclonic absences.

Developmental delay, epilepsy, neonatal diabetes syndrome (DEND)

This recently described syndrome is due to mutations in *Kir6.2*, a pore-forming subunit of the K_{ATP} channel (Shimomura et al. 2007; Shimomura 2009). This channel, expressed by neurons and pancreatic cells, is sensitive to the ATP/ADP ratio. Increased blood glucose raises the ATP/ADP ratio and normally closes the channel, resulting in a depolarization and insulin release from pancreatic cells. Mutations associated with the DEND syndrome alter channel closure and reduce insulin release. Typically severe diabetes is detected in the first 6 months. Several phenotypes are associated with different *Kir6.2* mutations: diabetes alone, DNED, or intermediate DNED. The more severe phenotype, DEND, is associated with developmental delay, muscle weakness, dysmorphic features, and epilepsy.

Patients with DEND present a severe neonatal-onset epileptic encephalopathy. Severe infantile spasms with hypsarrhythmia on the EEG have also been reported (Bahi-Buisson et al. 2007).

Diagnosis should proceed from a confirmed neonatal diabetes and be confirmed by genetic analysis.

Treatment with insulin is ineffective. Sulfonylurea, an oral hypoglycemic agent, closes the K_{ATP} channel permitting physiological insulin release and is reported to improve seizure control and developmental status (Shimomura et al. 2007; Slingerland et al. 2008).

Deficit in the biotin pathway: holocarboxylase synthetase deficiency and biotinidase deficiency

Both these enzymatic deficiencies disrupt the biotin cycle, disturbing gluconeogenesis, amino acid catabolism, and fatty acid synthesis, and resulting in lactate acidosis. Patients may present with an epileptic encephalopathy. Holocarboxylase synthetase (HCS) deficiency induces an early neonatal form with a metabolic coma, while patients with biotinidase deficiency tend to present later at 3 or more months after birth (Collins et al. 1994). Severe atopic dermatitis, alopecia, and severe hypotonia are suggestive of biotinidase deficiency.

Seizures occur in 25–50% of cases of HCS deficiency and eventually lead to myoclonic attacks. Pharmacoresistant myoclonic seizures occur in most patients with biotinidase deficiency (Salbert et al. 1993).

Biochemical diagnosis depends on the measurement of activity of these enzymes in lymphocytes.

Seizures are extremely well controlled by biotin supplements. Doses of 5–20 mg are needed in biotinidase deficiency and higher doses of 40–80 mg in HCS.

Non-ketotic hyperglycinemia

Non-ketotic hyperglycinemia (NKH) results from mutations in the subunits of the glycine cleavage enzyme that degrades the neurotransmitter glycine (Applegarth and Toone 2004). As well as operating as the major inhibitory transmitter in the spinal cord and brainstem, glycine binds to the excitatory glutamate N-methyl-D-aspartate (NMDA) receptor enhancing its actions (Thomson 1990). Excessive glycine binding to NMDA receptors contributes to seizures and excitotoxicity. Newborns present with coma, massive hypotonia, and signs of brainstem involvement (ophthalmoplegia, apnea). Surviving infants are severely retarded.

Neonates initially present segmental myoclonic jerks and hiccups. After 3 months, severe refractory epilepsy with myoclonic seizures emerges followed by infantile spasms. The EEG initially shows burst suppression, then hypsarrhythmia (Applegarth and Toone 2004).

An increased glycine concentration in urinary and plasma amino acid chromatography aids diagnosis of this syndrome, but it should be confirmed by enzymatic studies and genetic analysis. In some cases glycine increases in CSF alone resulting in a high CSF to plasma ratio (>0.08). False positivity of this ratio may result from valproate sodium treatment or contamination of CSF by blood cells.

No specific treatment is currently available for this syndrome. Neither a low glycine diet nor the glycine chelator sodium benzoate are effective, and the effects of NMDA antagonists, such as ketamine or dextrometorphan, are modest. Of the commonly used antiepileptic drugs, only sodium valproate should be avoided since it inhibits hepatic glycine cleavage systems.

Congenital disorders of glycosylation syndrome

The congenital disorders of glycosylation (CDG) syndrome covers a group of autosomal recessive diseases, resulting from

Table 38.2 Classification of epilepsies of metabolic origin according to age at onset

Neonatal period	Hypoglycemia, pyridoxine dependency, pyridoxine 5′-phosphate oxidase (PNPO) deficiency, non-ketotic hyperglycemia, organic acidurias, urea cycle defects, neonatal adrenoleukodystrophy, Zellweger syndrome, folinic acid-responsive seizures, holocarboxylase synthase deficiency, molybdenum co-factor deficiency, sulfite oxidase deficiency, SSADH, DEND
Infancy	Hypoglycemia (HI/HA), GLU-T1 deficiency, creatine deficiency, biotinidase deficiency, amino acidopathies, organic acidurias, congenital disorders of glycosylation, pyridoxine dependency, infantile form of neuronal ceroid lipofuscinosis (NCL1), GLUT-1 deficiency
Toddlers	Late infantile form of neuronal ceroid lipofuscinosis (NCL2), mitochondrial disorders including Alpers disease, lysosomal storage disorders, GLUT-1 deficiency
School age	Mitochondrial disorders, juvenile form of neuronal ceroid lipofuscinosis (NCL3), progressive myoclonus epilepsies, GLUT-1 deficiency
Adult	Mitochondrial disorders, homocystinuria, adult NCL (Kufs disease).

Source: Wolf *et al.* (2005).

Table 38.3 Classification of epilepsies of metabolic origin according to the type of seizures or epilepsy syndrome

Infantile spasms	Biotinidase deficiency, Menkes disease, mitochondrial disorders, organic acidurias, amino acidopathies, non-ketotic hyperglycemia
Epilepsy with myoclonic seizures	
Early myoclonic encephalopathy	Non-ketotic hyperglycinemia, pyridoxal phosphate deficiency, sulfite oxidase deficiency
Photosensitive myoclonic absence-like seizure	SSADH deficiency, HI/HA
Myoclonic seizures	Mitochondrial disorders, GLUT-1 deficiency, storage disorders, DEND, biotinidase deficiency
Progressive myoclonic epilepsies	Lafora disease, myoclonic epilepsy with ragged red fibers (MERRF), mitochonderial encephalopathy, lactic acidosis, and stroke-like episodes (MELAS), Unverricht–Lundborg disease, sialidosis, NCL
Epilepsy with myoclonic–astatic seizures	NCL2, creatine deficiency
Epilepsia partialis continua	Alpers disease, other mitochondrial disorders
Association of various types of seizures in the same patient (partial, atonic, myoclonic, spasms)	Pyridoxine dependent epilepsy, GAMT deficiency, GLUT-1 deficiency

Source: Wolf *et al.* (2005).

mutations in the enzymes responsible for protein glycosylation (Eklund and Freeze 2006). Seventy percent of the CDG syndrome result from a deficit in phosphomannomutase (CDG Ia). Mental retardation, cerebellar ataxia, strabismus, peripheral neuropathy, retinitis pigmentosa, cutaneous signs, and hepatic and digestive abnormalities are highly suggestive of CDG syndrome.

Epilepsy is rare in CDG Ia, but frequent in CDG Ic (Grunewald *et al.* 2000). There is also prominent neurological involvement including seizures in types Id, Ii, Ij, Ik, and Il as well as in types IIa and IIb (Eklund and Freeze 2006).

Diagnosis is based on isoelectric focusing of serum transferrin, dosage of the corresponding enzymes, and genetic analysis.

Specific treatments are available only for the CDG syndromes Ib and IIc, where there is no neurological involvement.

Other diseases

Other metabolic diseases, including cerebrotendinous xanthomatosis, metachromatic leukodystrophy, X-linked adrenoleukodystrophy, and α-methylacyl CoA racemase deficiency, are associated or may even present with epileptic seizures in children and adults (Esiri *et al.* 1984; Bostantjopoulou *et al.* 2000; Castelnovo *et al.* 2003; Thompson *et al.* 2008), but more specific signs are associated with the epilepsy.

Diagnostic approach
Features suggestive of IEM in epileptic patients

Inborn errors of metabolism are increasingly linked with epileptic syndromes even though the association remains rare. Epileptic patients, when an IEM is suspected, should have a complete clinical examination, EEG, brain magnetic resonance imaging (MRI) with proton magnetic resonance spectroscopy, ophthalmologic examination, and abdominal ultrasonography. Several clinical, radiological, or electrophysiological features point to an IEM in adults (Oguni 2005; Sedel *et al.* 2007): (1) the epileptic presentation does not match with classical epilepsy syndromes. Either the electroclinical presentation or the response to antiepileptic drugs may be atypical or the patient may present with an unusual mixture of generalized and partial epileptic manifestations such as myoclonus and partial seizures; (2) progressive myoclonic epilepsy; (3) association with cerebellar, pyramidal, or other neurological impairments, with movement disorders or with unexplained mental retardation; (4) association with disorders of other organs including the eyes, muscles, skin, and liver; (5) a family history suggestive of a genetic disease; (6) seizures related to eating, especially including fasting or protein-rich meals; (7) inefficacy or worsening with classical antiepileptic drugs; (8) unexplained status epilepticus; (9) MRI abnormalities suggestive of a defect in energy metabolism, such as basal ganglia lesions, or of a storage disease; (10) proton magnetic resonance spectroscopy abnormalities including a creatine peak decrease or lactate peak increase; and (11) EEG abnormalities including slowing of background activity, paroxysmal responses during intermittent photic stimulation at 1–6 Hz or improvement in EEG abnormalities after meals.

Table 38.4 Epilepsies amenable to metabolic treatment

GLUT-1 deficiency	Ketogenic diet
Co-factor-dependent epilepsy	Pyridoxine, pyridoxal phosphate, folinic acid, biotin
Homocystinuria	Folic acid, pyridoxin, vitamin B_{12}
GAMT deficiency	Creatine supplementation, arginine-restricted, ornithine-enriched diet
Phenylketonuria	Low-phenylalanine diet
Defects of serine biosynthesis	Serine supplementation
Defects in glycemia control (HI/HA, DEND, etc.)	Correction of the glycemia by oral drugs, or other specific measures

Source: Wolf *et al.* (2005).

Metabolic investigations in epileptic patients with suspected IEM

Exploration of metabolic diseases should be tailored to the individual patient to avoid multiple, unnecessary biological analyses and biopsies. The age of onset of the IEM-related epilepsy is particularly important (Table 38.2). The spectrum of IEM is smaller in adulthood than in children with epilepsy. Seizure semiology and EEG abnormalities, even if only moderately specific, help diagnoses, especially for progressive myoclonic epilepsy and epilepsy with myoclonic seizures (Table 38.3). Mental retardation and the involvement of other organs may be helpful pointers (Sedel *et al.* 2007).

Practical efforts should be made to identify the IEM that can benefit from tailored metabolic therapies (Table 38.4). A simple therapeutic trial with pyridoxine (15–30 mg/kg per day), pyridoxal phosphate (10–50 mg/kg per day), biotin (10–300 mg per day), and folinic acid (10–50 mg per day) for several days or weeks may be appropriate for children or adults

with pharmacologically refractory epilepsies or unexplained status epilepticus. Simple targeted examinations should be developed to diagnose epilepsies linked to IEM. Specific examinations for progressive myoclonic epilepsies are described in the relevant chapter. In the other syndromes, initial examinations might include fasting gblood glucose, ammonemia, plasma amino acid chromatography, urinary organic acid chromatography (especially for γ-hydroxybutyrate), blood and urine creatine and guanidinoacetate (and proton magnetic resonance spectroscopy), blood and CSF examination of glucose (with calculation of the blood/CSF ratio), lactate, folate, and amino acid chromatography (especially for serine and glycine), and homocysteinemia. Based on these results, specific genetic analyses should be performed.

Acknowledgment

The authors sincerely thank Richard Miles for his critical reading of the manuscript.

References

Applegarth DA, Toone JR (2004) Glycine encephalopathy (nonketotic hyperglycinaemia): review and update. *J Inherit Metab Dis* 27:417–22.

Bahi-Buisson N, Eisermann M, Nivot S, *et al.* (2007) Infantile spasms as an epileptic feature of DEND syndrome associated with an activating mutation in the potassium adenosine triphosphate (ATP) channel, *Kir6.2. J Child Neurol* 22:1147–50.

Bahi-Buisson N, El Sabbagh S, Soufflet C (2008a) Myoclonic absence epilepsy with photosensitivity and a gain of function mutation in glutamate dehydrogenase. *Seizure* 17:658–64.

Bahi-Buisson N, Roze E, Dionisi C, *et al.* (2008b) Neurological aspects of hyperinsulinism–hyperammonaemia syndrome. *Dev Med Child Neurol* 50:945–9.

Bostantjopoulou S, Katsarou Z, Michelakaki H, Kazis A (2000) Seizures as a presenting feature of late onset metachromatic leukodystrophy. *Acta Neurol Scand* 102:192–5.

Brockmann K, Wang D, Korenke CG, *et al.* (2001) Autosomal dominant GLUT-1 deficiency syndrome and familial epilepsy. *Ann Neurol* 50:476–85.

Caldeira Araujo H, Smit W, Verhoeven NM, *et al.* (2005) Guanidinoacetate

methyltransferase deficiency identified in adults and a child with mental retardation. *Am J Med Genet.* 133A:122–7.

Castelnovo G, Jomir L, Bouly S (2003) Cerebrotendinous xanthomatosis. *J Neurol Neurosurg Psychiatry* 74:1335.

Cheillan D, Cognat S, Vandenberghe N, Des Portes V, Vianey-Saban C (2005) Creatine deficiency syndromes. *Rev Neurol (Paris)* 161:284–9. (In French).

Collins JE, Nicholson NS, Dalton N, Leonard JV (1994) Biotinidase deficiency: early neurological presentation. *Dev Med Child Neurol* 36:268–70.

De Vivo DC, Wang D (2008) Glut1 deficiency: CSF glucose – how low is too low? *Rev Neurol (Paris)* **164**:877–80.

Dervent A, Gibson KM, Pearl PL, *et al.* (2004) Photosensitive absence epilepsy with myoclonias and heterozygosity for succinic semialdehyde dehydrogenase (SSADH) deficiency. *Clin Neurophysiol* **115**:1417–22.

Eklund EA, Freeze HH (2006) The congenital disorders of glycosylation: a multifaceted group of syndromes. *Neuro Rx* **3**:254–63.

Esiri MM, Hyman NM, Horton WL, Lindenbaum RH (1984) Adrenoleukodystrophy: clinical, pathological and biochemical findings in two brothers with the onset of cerebral disease in adult life. *Neuropathol Appl Neurobiol* **10**:429–45.

Gibson KM, Gupta M, Pearl PL, *et al.* (2003) Significant behavioral disturbances in succinic semialdehyde dehydrogenase (SSADH) deficiency (gamma-hydroxybutyric aciduria). *Biol Psychiatry* **54**:763–8.

Grunewald S, Imbach T, Huijben K, *et al.* (2000) Clinical and biochemical characteristics of congenital disorder of glycosylation type Ic, the first recognized endoplasmic reticulum defect in N-glycan synthesis. *Ann Neurol* **47**:776–81.

Klepper J (2004) Impaired glucose transport into the brain: the expanding spectrum of glucose transporter type 1 deficiency syndrome. *Curr Opin Neurol* **17**:193–6.

Klepper J (2008) Glucose transporter deficiency syndrome (GLUT1DS) and the ketogenic diet. *Epilepsia* **49**(Suppl 8):46–9.

Klepper J, Leiendecker B (2007) GLUT1 deficiency syndrome: 2007 update. *Dev Med Child Neurol* **49**:707–16.

Klepper J, Willemsen M, Verrips A, *et al.* (2001) Autosomal dominant transmission of GLUT1 deficiency. *Hum Mol Genet* **10**:63–8.

Oguni H (2005) Symptomatic epilepsies imitating idiopathic generalized epilepsies. *Epilepsia* **46**(Suppl 9):84–90.

Pearl PL, Novotny EJ, Acosta MT, Jakobs C, Gibson KM (2003) Succinic semialdehyde dehydrogenase deficiency in children and adults. *Ann Neurol* **54**(Suppl 6):S73–80.

Raizen DM, Brooks-Kayal A, Steinkrauss L, *et al.* (2005) Central nervous system hyperexcitability associated with glutamate dehydrogenase gain of function mutations. *J Pediatr* **146**:388–94.

Salbert BA, Pellock JM, Wolf B (1993) Characterization of seizures associated with biotinidase deficiency. *Neurology* **43**:1351–5.

Schulze A, Bachert P, Schlemmer H (2003) Lack of creatine in muscle and brain in an adult with GAMT deficiency. *Ann Neurol* **53**:248–51.

Sedel F, Gourfinkel-An I, Lyon-Caen O, *et al.* (2007) Epilepsy and inborn errors of metabolism in adults: a diagnostic approach. *J Inherit Metab Dis* **30**:846–54.

Shimomura K (2009) The KATP channel and neonatal diabetes. *Endocr J* **56**:165–75.

Shimomura K, Horster F, de Wet H, *et al.* (2007) A novel mutation causing DEND syndrome: a treatable channelopathy of pancreas and brain. *Neurology* **69**:1342–9.

Slingerland AS, Hurkx W, Noordam K, *et al.* (2008) Sulphonylurea therapy improves cognition in a patient with the V59M KCNJ11 mutation. *Diabet Med* **25**:277–81.

Stanley CA, Lieu YK, Hsu BY, *et al.* (1998) Hyperinsulinism and hyperammonemia in infants with regulatory mutations of the glutamate dehydrogenase gene. *N Engl J Med* **338**:1352–7.

Suls A, Dedeken P, Goffin K, *et al.* (2008) Paroxysmal exercise-induced dyskinesia and epilepsy is due to mutations in *SLC2A1*, encoding the glucose transporter GLUT1. *Brain* **131**:1831–44.

Thompson SA, Calvin J, Hogg S, *et al.* (2008) Relapsing encephalopathy in a patient with alpha-methylacyl-CoA racemase deficiency. *J Neurol Neurosurg Psychiatry* **79**:448–50.

Thomson AM (1990) Glycine is a coagonist at the NMDA receptor/channel complex. *Prog Neurobiol* **35**:53–74.

Wolf NI, Bast T, Surtees R (2005) Epilepsy in inborn errors of metabolism. *Epileptic Disord* **7**:67–81.

Down syndrome

Nadia Bahi-Buisson, Monika Eisermann, and Olivier Dulac

Down syndrome (DS) is caused by trisomy 21, and is one of the most common chromosomal disorders and etiology of congenital mental retardation. The syndrome is associated with a number of deleterious phenotypes, including learning disability, heart defects, early-onset Alzheimer disease, and childhood leukemia, many of which may generate epileptic seizures.

The diagnosis is made on the basis of the constellation of clinical features and confirmed by karyotype analysis. Non-disjunction of chromosome 21 during meiosis is the major cause of Down syndrome in 95% of individuals while about 4% have an unbalanced translocation and about 1% have mosaicism (with a less severe phenotype). A minimal percentage of DS patients have an intrachromosomal duplication around the 21q22.3 band which represents the critical region for DS. The frequency of non-disjunction and of associated aneuploidies increases with advancing maternal age, but they may occur at any maternal age. The mechanism for this meiotic error remains unknown. Most trisomy 21 pregnancies prove to be non-viable. Only one fourth of fetuses with trisomy 21 reach term and delivery.

The overall prevalence of DS is about 1 in 800 births. During the first trimester of pregnancy, detection includes the combination of high maternal levels of chorionic gonadotropin (hCG) and inhibin A, with low levels of α-fetoprotein and unconjugated estriol. Testing for this combination of markers, which is referred to as quadruple screening, has a detection rate of 80% for trisomy 21 at a positive screening rate of 5%.

Clinical features

Down syndrome is usually diagnosed at birth (or even prenatally) and is associated with well-known dysmorphic features, i.e., growth retardation, hypotonia, flat face with brachycephaly and upward slanted eyes, epicanthal folds, small ears, simian crease, and hypogonadism. These dysmorphic features become more prominent as the child grows older.

Table 39.1 Incidence of associated medical complications in persons with Down syndrome

Disorder	Incidence (%)
Mental retardation	>95
Growth retardation	>95
Early Alzheimer disease	Affects 75% by age 60
Congenital heart defects (atrioventricular canal defect, ventricular septal defect, atrial septal defect, patent ductus arteriosus, tetralogy of Fallot)	40
Hearing loss (related to otitis media with effusion or sensorineural)	40 to 75
Ophthalmic disorders (congenital cataracts, glaucoma, strabismus)	60
Epilepsy	5 to 10
Gastrointestinal malformations (duodenal atresia, Hirschsprung disease)	5
Hypothyroidism	5
Leukemia	1
Atlantoaxial subluxation with spinal cord compression	<1
Increased susceptibility to infection (pneumonia, otitis media, sinusitis, pharyngitis, periodontal disease)	Unknown
Infertility	>99% in men; anovulation in 30% of women

Major somatic malformations involve heart and gastro-intestinal tract, with tetralogy of Fallot, duodenal atresia, and annular pancreas being the most common.

Radiographic findings include narrowing of the cervical canal and subluxation of the atlantoaxis process, which can

The Causes of Epilepsy, eds. S. D. Shorvon, F. Andermann, and R. Guerrini. Published by Cambridge University Press. © Cambridge University Press 2011.

A

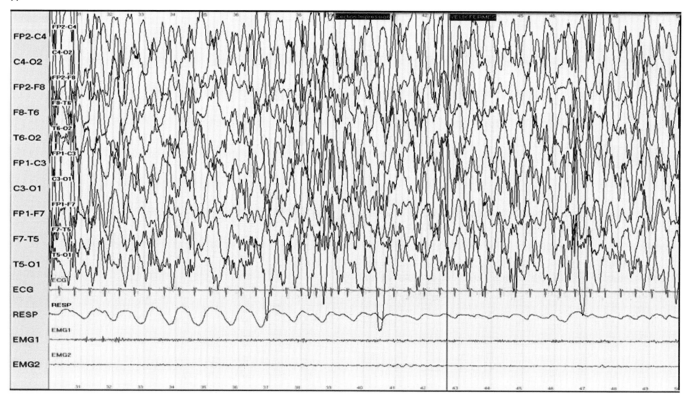

B

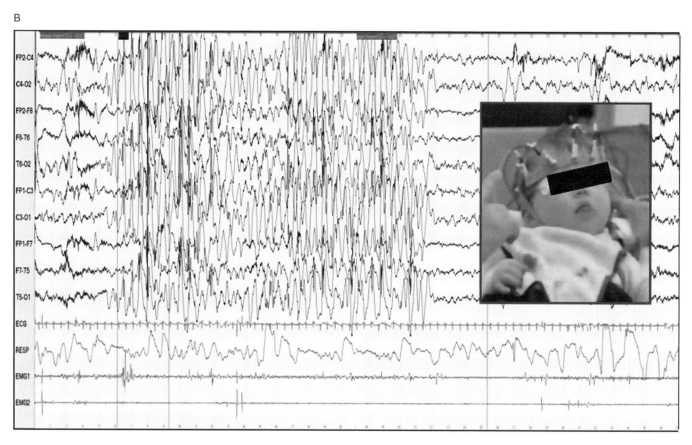

Fig. 39.1. (A) 11-month-old boy. Activation of occipital anomalies during slow wave sleep. Sensitivity 10 μV/mm, time constant 0.3 s, paper speed 15 mm/s. (B) Same infant: 11-month-old boy. Eye elevation and deviation to the right side associated with chewing and smacking movements associated with rhythmic high-voltage irregular spike–wave activity in the occipital areas during 16 s. Sensitivity 10 μV/mm, time constant 0.3 s, paper speed 15 mm/s. (C) Same infant: 11-month-old boy. Epileptic spasm with axial tonic attack, extension of both arms and upward eye deviation associated with diffuse electrodecremental event. Sensitivity 10 μV/mm, time constant 0.3 s, paper speed 15 mm/s.

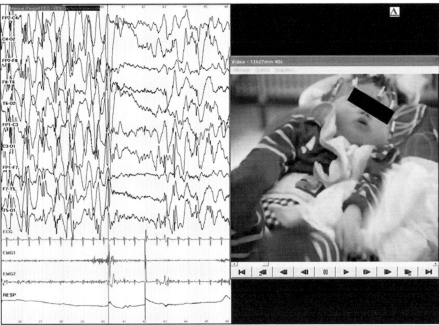

Fig. 39.1. (cont.)

lead to medullar and cervical cord compression. One-third of DS patients have 11 ribs, and multiple centers of ossification in the manubrium of the sternum are characteristic.

Down syndrome increases the risk of developing acute megakaryoblastic anemia (AMKL) and acute lymphoblastic leukemia (ALL). Approximately 10% of DS newborns present with transient myeloproliferative disorder (TMD), and 10–20% with TMD develop AMKL before 4 years of age.

Cognitive function in Down syndrome: learning disabilities and Alzheimer-like dementia

In addition to delayed psychomotor milestones, learning disabilities are a prominent feature in DS with a spectrum of severity ranging from mild to moderate mental retardation (Chapman and Hesketh 2000; Silverman 2007).

People with DS have a greatly increased risk of early-onset Alzheimer disease (AD). By the age of 60, between 50% and 70% of people with DS develop dementia. Cognitive characteristics of DS are summarized in Table 39.1.

Epilepsy in Down syndrome

Epileptic seizures occur in 5–10% of DS patients and prevalence increases with age. With regard to the onset of seizures, a bimodal distribution is characteristic with a higher prevalence of seizures before the age of 1 year and after the third decade of life.

Occasional seizures may express brain complication of cardiopathy. However, there is a lower incidence of febrile seizures compared with the general population.

Epilepsy presents in a large variety of forms in patients with DS, and it varies according to age. In the younger age group, primarily infantile spasms and tonic–clonic seizures with myoclonus are often observed whereas older patients tend to demonstrate simple or complex partial seizures as well as tonic–clonic seizures (Pueschel et al. 1991). Prognosis and therapeutic response vary according to the form of epilepsy and the course ranges from very benign and easily treatable forms to severe and refractory generalized epilepsies.

Infantile spasms are frequent. Prevalence is over 1% although often underestimated, and infantile spasms remain often unrecognized by carers if not properly informed about the possible occurrence of this seizure type. Although comorbidity, i.e. cardiopathy, may contribute to the genesis of infantile spasms, DS itself seems to be a determining factor with typical symmetric hypsarrhythmia on the electroencephalogram (EEG) (Figs. 39.1, 39.2). Delayed diagnosis may cause poorer response to therapy, and the incidence of pharmacoresistance combined with the development of autistic features is significantly increased when treatment lag exceeds 2 months (Eisermann et al. 2003). This contrasts with the overall prognosis being somewhat better than for the average patients with infantile spasms, especially those with symptomatic infantile spasms of other etiology. Indeed, they behave as cryptogenic infantile spasms. Furthermore, when treated early, there was a good response to vigabatrin in a large majority of patients, and the incidence of chronic epilepsy was found to be lower (Silva

A

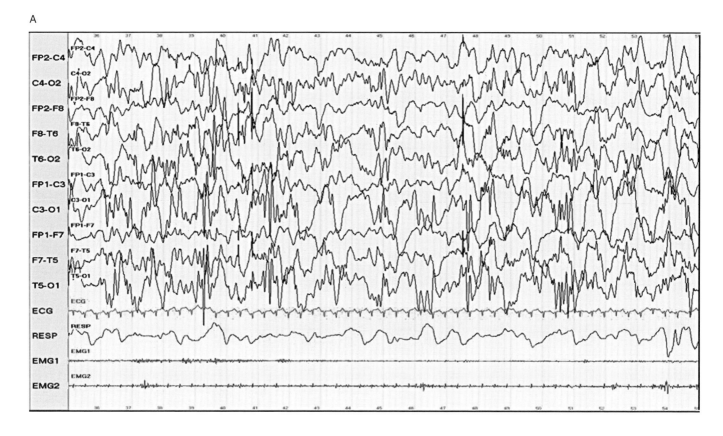

B

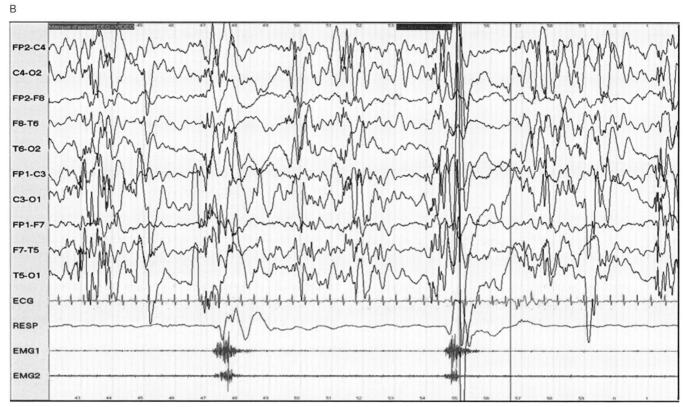

Fig. 39.2. (A) 5-month-old girl. Awake state. Eyes closed. Occipital spikes and slow waves predominating on the left side. Sensitivity 10 μV/mm, time constant 0.3 s, paper speed 15 mm/s. (B) Same infant: 5-month-old girl. Cluster of epileptic spasms. Sensitivity 10 μV/mm, time constant 0.3 s, paper speed 15 mm/s.

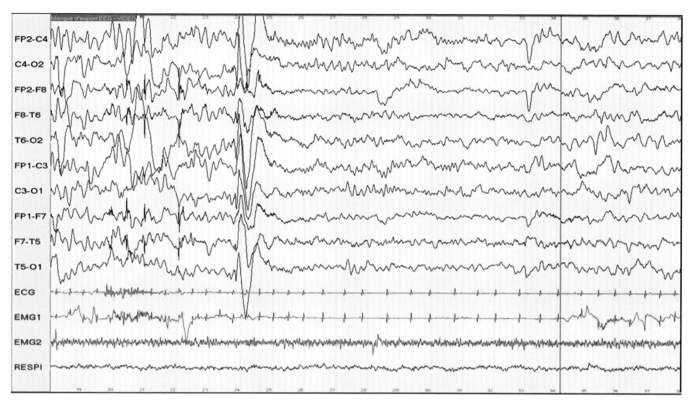

Fig. 39.3. Same infant as in Fig. 39.2: 18-month-old girl. Awake state. Subclinical diffuse slow wave with superimposed fast activity. Sensitivity 10 μV/mm, time constant 0.3 s, paper speed 15 mm/s.

et al. 1996) and neurodevelopmental outcome was better (Nabbout *et al.* 2001). In addition, it was possible to stop treatment without relapse after 6 months' vigabatrin treatment (Nabbout *et al.* 2001).

Children with DS may exhibit various seizures types, including myoclonic, atonic, tonic–clonic, and, rarely, partial seizures. Many seizure types can be found including massive myoclonus, atonic falls, and tonic spasms (Figs. 39.3, 39.4). Most characteristic and intriguing are reflex seizures which may present as generalized, particularly myoclonic, or focal. Various stimuli may be involved including light, noise, contact, and self-stimulation (Guerrini *et al.* 1990).

The Lennox–Gastaut syndrome (LGS) may also occur in DS around the age of 10 years. In most cases, the onset of LGS coincides with the onset of reflex seizures. In some cases with purely reflex seizures, the sensitivity to external stimuli abates and the electroclinical features of LGS appear thereafter. The course of LGS in DS is usually severe with marked mental deterioration and drug resistance. Finally, some DS patients also show generalized seizures that mimic those of idiopathic generalized epilepsy, with a benign course and good response to therapy.

At the other end of the spectrum, epilepsy is common in older patients, at the same age range as Alzheimer-like mental deterioration. Epilepsy in adults is mainly myoclonic, also called "senile myoclonic epilepsy in DS" (De Simone *et al.* 2006) or "late onset myoclonic epilepsy in DS – LOMEDS" (Möller *et al.* 2002).

The risk of early dementia does not seem to be increased in patients with childhood-onset epilepsy – in contrast to adult patients who develop epilepsy after the age of 35 and for which there is an increasing risk of early dementia (Puri *et al.* 2001).

Genetics and pathophysiology

The additional copy of chromosome 21 combined with imbalance in expression of chromosome 21 and non-chromosome 21 genes are proposed to result in the many phenotypes that characterize DS (Wiseman *et al.* 2009). Upregulation of dual-specificity tyrosine-(Y)-phosphorylation-regulated kinase 1A (*DYRK1A*) and regulator of calcineurin 1 (*RCAN1*) may dysregulate neuronal differentiation and the development of many cell types, leading to heart defects and abnormal learning and memory (Arron *et al.* 2006).

Recent work has also shed light on molecular mechanisms of brain dysfunction in DS. First, DS is associated with a reduction in brain volume, the size of the hippocampus and cerebellum being particularly affected. Abnormalities in cell-cycle length, apoptosis, and neocortical neurogenesis could account for alterations in short-term but not in long-term hippocampal-dependent learning (Weis *et al.* 1991; Aldridge *et al.* 2007).

Moreover, overexpression of *DYRK1A*, synaptojanin 1, and single-minded homologue 2 (*SIM2*), as well as neuronal

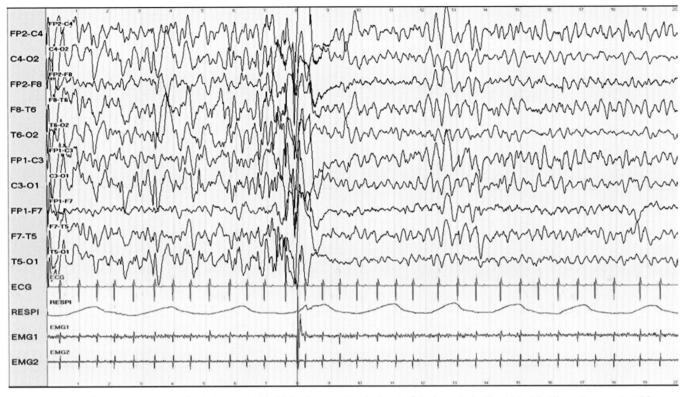

Fig. 39.4. Same infant as in Figs. 39.2 and 39.3: 21-month-old girl. Awake state. Mycolonic jerk of the lower limbs. Sensitivity 10 μV/mm, time constant 0.3 s, paper speed 15 mm/s.

channel proteins, such as G-protein-coupled inward-rectifying potassium channel subunit 2 (*GIRK2*) may contribute to learning disability in people with DS (Altafaj *et al.* 2001; O'Doherty *et al.* 2005; Voronov *et al.* 2008).

Therapy

There is no etiologic treatment for DS, but supportive care and treatment of associated conditions such as cardiac and gastrointestinal abnormalities are indicated.

Treatment of epilepsy does not require specific indications. Vigabatrin is effective and no worsening of epilepsy has been reported although these patients are prone to develop myoclonic seizures later in life. Steroids are indicated for infantile spasms and seem to be beneficial, based on retrospective data (Eisermann *et al.* 2003). Attention has been called on the potential benefit of pyridoxine on infantile spasms (N. Fejerman, personal communication). There is no contraindication reported to date for the classical antiepileptic compounds.

Course

Approximately one-third of patients die in infancy and 50% during the first 5 years from cardiac and respiratory infections. There is also a greater incidence of acute leukemia than in the general population, which also requires specific treatment.

References

Aldridge K, Reeves RH, Olson LE, *et al.* (2007) Differential effects of trisomy on brain shape and volume in related aneuploid mouse models. *Am J Med Genet* **143A**:1060–70.

Altafaj X, Dierssen M, Baamonde C, *et al.* (2001) Neurodevelopmental delay, motor abnormalities and cognitive deficits in transgenic mice overexpressing *Dyrk1A* (minibrain), a murine model of Down's syndrome. *Hum Mol Genet* **10**:1915–23.

Arron JR, Winslow MM, Polleri A, *et al.* (2006) NFAT dysregulation by increased dosage of *DSCR1* and *DYRK1A* on chromosome 21. *Nature* **441**:595–600.

Chapman RS, Hesketh LJ (2000) Behavioral phenotype of individuals with Down syndrome. *Ment Retard Dev Disabil Res Rev* **6**:84–95.

De Simone R, Daquin G, Genton P (2006) Senile myoclonic epilepsy in Down syndrome: a video and EEG presentation of two cases. *Epilept Disord* **8**:223–7.

Eisermann MM, DeLaRaillere A, Dellatolas G, *et al.* (2003) Infantile spasms in Down syndrome: effects of delayed anticonvulsive treatment. *Epilepsy Res* **55**:21–7.

Guerrini R, Genton P, Bureau M, *et al.* (1990) Reflex seizures are frequent in patients with Down syndrome and epilepsy. *Epilepsia* **31**:406–17.

Möller JC, Hamer HM, Oertel WH, Rosenow F (2002) Late-onset myoclonic epilepsy in Down's syndrome (LOMEDS). *Seizure* **11**(Suppl A):303–5.

Nabbout R, Melki I, Gerbaka B, Dulac O, Akatcherian C (2001) Infantile spasms in Down syndrome: good response to a short course of vigabatrin. *Epilepsia* **42**:1580–3.

O'Doherty A, Ruf S, Mulligan C, *et al.* (2005) An aneuploid mouse strain carrying human chromosome 21 with Down syndrome phenotypes. *Science* **309**:2033–7.

Pueschel SM, Louis S, McKnight P (1991) Seizure disorders in Down syndrome. *Arch Neurol* **48**:318–20.

Puri BK, Ho KW, Singh I (2001) Age of seizure onset in adults with Down's syndrome. *Int J Clin Pract* **55**:442–4.

Silva ML, Cieuta C, Guerrini R, *et al.* (1996) Early clinical and EEG features of infantile spasms in Down syndrome. *Epilepsia* **37**:977–82.

Silverman W (2007) Down syndrome: cognitive phenotype. *Ment Retard Dev Disabil Res Rev* **13**:228–36.

Voronov SV, Frere SG, Giovedi S, *et al.* (2008) Synaptojanin 1-linked phosphoinositide dyshomeostasis and cognitive deficits in mouse models of Down's syndrome. *Proc Natl Acad Sci USA* **105**:9415–20.

Weis S, Weber G, Neuhold A, Rett A (1991) Down syndrome: MR quantification of brain structures and comparison with normal control subjects. *AJNR Am J Neuroradiol* **12**:1207–11.

Wiseman FK, Alford KA, Tybulewicz LJ, *et al.* (2009) Down syndrome: recent progress and future prospects. *Hum Mol Genet* **18**(R1):R75–83.

Chapter

40

Fragile X syndrome

Irissa M. Devine and Carl E. Stafstrom

Definitions, genetics, and epidemiology

Fragile X syndrome is the most frequent cause of familial mental retardation and the second most common overall cause of mental retardation after Down syndrome. The prevalence of fragile X syndrome has not been uniformly defined, but is estimated to be approximately 1 in 4000 in males and 1 in 8000 in females (Crawford *et al.* 2001). Fragile X syndrome comprises one-fourth to one-third of patients with X-linked mental retardation.

Fragile X syndrome is an X-linked dominant disorder with reduced penetrance. It is named for the presence of an unstable chromosomal site on the long arm of chromosome X (Lubs 1969; Sutherland 1977). Typical fragile X syndrome is caused by a loss-of-function mutation of the gene *FMR1*, which is located at chromosome Xq27.3. The mutation leads to amplification of a CGG (cysteine-guanine-guanine) triplet nucleotide repeat in the 5′ untranslated region (exon 1) of *FMR1*. The result of this mutation is decreased or absent production of fragile X mental retardation protein (FMRP).

There are three categories of CGG repeats: unaffected (6–54 repeats), premutation (55–200 repeats), and full mutation (>200 repeats) (Debacker and Kooy 2007). The CGG repeats that cause fragile X syndrome lead to transcriptional silencing of the *FMR1* gene, which codes for FMRP; this is an RNA-binding protein that is expressed in a variety of tissues, but is most abundant in neurons. The presence of more than 200 CGG repeats leads to hypermethylation of the gene, causing reduced gene transcription, and thus a reduction or absence of FMRP synthesis. This lack of FMRP in turn causes the clinical features of fragile X syndrome.

The premutation category includes carrier females and transmitting males. Males with premutations are generally normal intellectually and phenotypically though some have mild mental impairment. About one-third of carrier females are mentally impaired or have social or emotional dysfunction. Individuals with premutations do not have decreased FMRP levels but rather increased production of *FMR1* mRNA. Some females with premutations have a syndrome of premature ovarian insufficiency (Murray 2000). Males with premutations may develop a neurodegenerative disorder known as the fragile X-associated tremor/ataxia syndrome (FXTAS) (Hagerman and Hagerman 2004), a disorder distinct from typical fragile X syndrome.

Clinical features, pathology, and physiology

Clinical features of fragile X syndrome vary widely, and include cognitive, behavioral, and morphologic signs and symptoms. Physical features vary to such a degree that abnormal behavior often leads to recognition of the syndrome. Phenotypically, individuals with fragile X syndrome may have a long, narrow face with prominent ears and forehead, protruding mandible, high arched palate, macroorchidism (after puberty), and hyperextensible joints. Neurobehavioral symptoms may include moderate to severe mental retardation, hyperactivity, social anxiety, sensory hypersensitivity, autism, gaze avoidance, socialization difficulties, stereotypic movements and behaviors such as hand flapping and rocking, poor motor coordination, delayed speech development, and echolalia. Heterozygous females typically present with only learning disabilities or difficulty with emotional regulation. In addition to the clinical features of the disease itself, concurrent medical problems that occur more frequently in patients with fragile X syndrome include strabismus, otitis media, sinusitis, gastroesophageal reflux disease, and seizures (Garber *et al.* 2008).

Anatomically, macroscopic brain structure is usually normal in fragile X syndrome, but brains of some affected individuals have been found to have an abnormally large caudate nucleus and decreased volume of the posterior cerebellar vermis (Wisniewski *et al.* 1991; Gothelf *et al.* 2008). Similar neuroanatomical findings are also seen in autism, which is seen in up to one-third of individuals with fragile X syndrome (Rogers *et al.* 2001; Belmonte and Bourgeron 2006). Functional implications of these observations are uncertain. Microscopically, dendritic spines are abnormally long, thin, and tortuous, hallmarks of dendritic immaturity associated with aberrant synaptic plasticity (Belmonte and

The Causes of Epilepsy, eds. S. D. Shorvon, F. Andermann, and R. Guerrini. Published by Cambridge University Press. © Cambridge University Press 2011.

Bourgeron 2006; Bassell and Warren 2008; Pfeiffer and Huber 2009). Similar dendritic pathology is found in *FMR1* knock-out mice (Comery *et al.* 1997). Knock-out mice have an *FMR1* gene deletion rather than an expanded CGG repeat as a cause of decreased FMRP, but the functional consequences are similar – abnormal dendrite structure and function, cognitive impairment especially in learning and memory, and neuronal hyperexcitability that might underlie seizure predisposition (see below).

FMRP plays a number of crucial roles in dendritic maturation and function (Pfeiffer and Huber 2009). It facilitates the transport of various mRNAs and translational regulation of mRNAs whose protein products are involved in synaptic development and plasticity. The absence of FMRP results in reduced ability to establish and maintain synaptic function required for learning and memory. FMRP knock-out mice display increased long-term depression (LTD) and aberrant long-term potentiation (LTP) (Huber *et al.* 2002; Wilson and Cox 2007; Pfeiffer and Huber 2009). Normally, activation of group I metabotropic glutamate receptors (e.g., mGluR5) leads to protein synthesis and LTD, a process antagonized by FMRP. In fragile X syndrome, without FMRP to perform this regulatory role, unchecked protein synthesis occurs, resulting in increased LTD; this altered synaptic plasticity is thought to underlie the cognitive deficiencies in fragile X syndrome (Dölen and Bear 2008). In FMRP knock-out mice, mGluR5 receptor inhibitors lead to increased protein translation, increased internalization of α-amino-3-hydroxy-5-methyl-isoxazolepropionic acid (AMPA) receptors, and abnormal synaptic function (Nakamoto *et al.* 2007). The high expression of FMRP in the hippocampus and neocortex could relate to a role in epilepsy when this protein is deficient in fragile X syndrome.

Epilepsy in fragile X syndrome

Since the first report of seizures in a patient with fragile X syndrome (Lubs 1969), it has been estimated that 10–25% of individuals with full-mutation fragile X syndrome develop seizures (Musumeci *et al.* 1988; Wisniewski *et al.* 1991; Sabaratnam *et al.* 2001; Berry-Kravis 2002; Incorpora *et al.* 2002). Seizures occur more frequently in fragile X syndrome than in the general population, but not more frequently than in males with developmental delays with unknown cause. Interestingly, the severity of epilepsy does not seem to correlate with the number of triplet repeats. However, one study showed that fragile X subjects with severe epilepsy had more pronounced facial dysmorphisms; it is unclear if this association is coincidental or causal (Incorpora *et al.* 2002).

A wide variety of seizure types is seen in fragile X syndrome (Wisniewski *et al.* 1991), but the most common seizure type is complex partial and the most common electroencephalogram (EEG) pattern is centrotemporal spikes (Berry-Kravis 2002; Incorpora *et al.* 2002). Mild background slowing is also seen commonly. Of 16 patients with fragile X syndrome and epilepsy, 12 exhibited partial seizures and 10 of those had an EEG with centrotemporal spikes (Berry-Kravis 2002). Therefore,

Table 40.1 Comparison between epilepsy in fragile X syndrome and benign childhood epilepsy with centrotemporal spikes (BCECTS)

	Fragile X syndrome	BCECTS
Seizure type	Mostly partial	Mostly partial
Seizure severity	Mild	Mild
Age range of seizure onset	6 m – 4 y	3–10 y
EEG findings	CTS	CTS
EEG findings in non-epileptic subjects	CTS in fragile X children without clinical seizures	CTS in siblings without clinical seizures
Cognitive/ behavioral abnormalities	Moderate to severe intellectual impairment	None to mild attentional and processing difficulties
Neuropathology	Mild atrophy Dendrite dysgenesis	Normal
Responsiveness to AEDs	Good	Good
Seizure prognosis	Most remit during childhood	Remit by adolescence

Notes:
BCECTS, benign childhood epilepsy with centrotemporal spikes; CTS, centrotemporal spikes; EEG, electroencephalogram; AEDs, antiepileptic drugs; m, months; y, years.

epilepsy in fragile X syndrome resembles benign childhood epilepsy with centrotemporal spikes (BCECTS or rolandic epilepsy) (Table 40.1). The peak age of seizure onset is 2 years, with most beginning between 6 months and 4 years of age (Berry-Kravis 2002). In addition to the relatively mild seizure phenotype, infrequent seizure occurrence, and typical remission during childhood, approximately one-fourth of individuals with fragile X syndrome have abnormal EEGs with centrotemporal spikes (sometimes only during sleep) but no clinical seizures (Musumeci *et al.* 1988, 1991; Wisniewski *et al.* 1991; Kluger *et al.* 1996; Sabaratnam *et al.* 2001; Berry-Kravis 2002; Incorpora *et al.* 2002). This electrographic finding represents an additional similarity between fragile X syndrome and BCECTS. Amongst fragile X individuals, this type of epilepsy has the best prognosis for seizure remission (Berry-Kravis 2002). In most cases, seizures disappear during childhood, suggesting an age-dependent, benign course, as in BCECTS.

Despite the similarities of clinical features and EEG findings in fragile X syndrome and BCECTS, it is also important to appreciate differences between these syndromes. Linkage analysis has excluded the fragile X site as a candidate gene for BCECTS (Rees *et al.* 1993). The two syndromes have a different genetic basis, cognitive profile, and associated clinical features. Not all authors have reported a benign course for seizures in fragile X syndrome; in one study, one-half of affected individuals continued to have seizures after age 20 and overall, seizures improved in only about 50% of patients (Sabaratnam *et al.* 2001). Therefore, epilepsy in fragile X syndrome can have a variable course.

There are numerous possible mechanisms for seizures and epilepsy in fragile X syndrome (Table 40.2), and this is an area of intense investigation (Qiu *et al.* 2008a; Hagerman and Stafstrom 2009). *FMR1* knock-out mice have increased susceptibility to audiogenic and kindled seizures (Musumeci *et al.*

Table 40.2 Possible mechanisms of epilepsy in fragile X syndrome

- Long, thin dendrites → increased flow of excitatory current (Huber *et al.* 2002)

- Excessive mGluR5 receptor activity → increased excitation (Chuang *et al.* 2005)

- Decreased GABA receptor subunits → decreased synaptic inhibition (D'Hulst and Kooy 2007)

- Increased internalization of AMPA receptors (Nakamoto *et al.* 2007)

- Decreased parvalbumin interneurons → decreased inhibition (Selby *et al.* 2007)

- Decreased excitatory drive onto inhibitory interneurons → decreased inhibition (Gibson *et al.* 2008)

- Increased glutamatergic neurons → aberrant excitation (Tervonen *et al.* 2009)

- Increased mGluR5-mediated excitatory current (Bianchi *et al.* 2009)

2000; Qiu *et al.* 2008b). Many of the pathophysiological features in fragile X syndrome that have been invoked to explain the cognitive deficits may contribute to the hyperexcitability underlying seizures as well. The involvement of mGluR5 receptor activation in both processes is indicated by the reduction of LTD, seizures, and behavioral abnormalities when these receptors are blocked or knocked out (Yan *et al.* 2005; Dölen *et al.* 2007). Absence of FMRP allows overactivation of metabotropic group 1 receptors, leading to persistent neuronal hyperexcitability via a voltage-gated cationic current (termed $I_{mGluR(V)}$) which mediates prolonged neuronal discharges (Bianchi *et al.* 2009). GABAergic function is also abnormal in fragile X syndrome, with downregulation of γ-aminobutyric acid (GABA) receptor subunits and altered GABA metabolic enzymes (D'Hulst and Kooy 2007; Curia *et al.* 2008; D'Hulst *et al.* 2009). A schematic of possible mechanisms is presented in Fig. 40.1. When considering the multiple potential mechanisms of epilepsy in fragile X syndrome, the mild nature of the seizures should be taken into account (Stafstrom 1999; Hagerman and Stafstrom 2009). The ultimate expression of pathophysiological mechanisms mediating hyperexcitability in fragile X syndrome must be modest in severity, since seizures in this disorder are usually not frequent or intractable.

Diagnostic tests for fragile X syndrome

The definitive diagnosis of fragile X syndrome is made by genetic testing and requires an alteration in the *FMR1* gene which can be detected by polymerase chain reaction (PCR) or

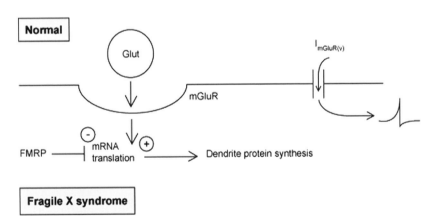

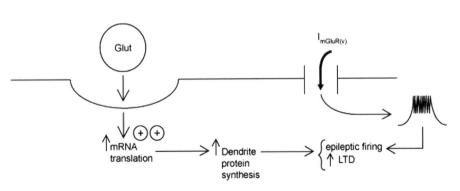

Fig. 40.1. Schematic of possible mechanisms for seizures in fragile X syndrome. In the normal case (top), glutamate activation of dendritic group I metabotropic receptors (mGluR) enables intracellular gene transcription leading to translation of dendritic proteins. This process is modulated by the fragile X mental retardation protein, FMRP, which keeps protein synthesis in check and prevents synaptic long-term depression. Activation of mGluR also activates a cation-mediated, voltage-activated non-inactivating inward current, $I_{mGluR(V)}$, which under normal conditions allows hippocampal CA3 neurons to fire in brief bursts (thin curved arrow). In fragile X syndrome (bottom), with absent FMRP, there is no inhibition of the downstream effects of mGluR activation, leading to excessive protein synthesis, LTD, and prolonged $I_{mGluR(V)}$ (thick curved arrow) which leads to epileptic firing. Concepts depicted here are derived from the work of several investigators (e.g., Dölen and Bear 2008; Bianchi *et al.* 2009).

Southern blot analysis. Polymerase chain reaction determines the number of CGG repeats; Southern blot analysis determines the methylation status and estimates the size of the full mutation (Garber *et al.* 2008). Most laboratories employ both methods. Combining these two tests results in a 99% sensitivity for detecting affected and carrier individuals, missing only those individuals who have fragile X syndrome due to a point mutation or deletion located outside the CGG repeat region. A positive *FMR1* test result is considered 100% specific for the disorder.

The American College of Medical Genetics recommends fragile X testing for individuals with mental retardation, developmental delay, or autism, especially when associated with other physical and behavioral characteristics of fragile X syndrome (see www.acmg.net/Pages/ACMG_Activities/stds-2002/fx.htm). Other indications for genetic testing include: (1) a family history of fragile X syndrome or a relative with undiagnosed mental retardation, (2) a family history of fragile X syndrome in patients seeking reproductive counseling, (3) prenatal testing in known *FMR1* mutation carriers, (4) individuals with prior cytogenetic testing inconsistent with a fragile X phenotype, (5) women with reproductive or fertility problems associated with increased follicle stimulating hormone levels especially if there is a family history of premature ovarian failure or undiagnosed mental retardation, and (6) individuals with new-onset tremor or cerebellar ataxia of unknown origin. Prenatal diagnosis can be made via amniocentesis or chorionic villus sampling.

Principles of seizure management of fragile X syndrome

There are few data regarding the optimal anticonvulsant treatment for seizures in fragile X syndrome, since most clinical studies have been quite small. Based on the mild severity and relatively rare occurrence of seizures in affected individuals, the question arises as to whether the seizures even require treatment. Certainly, treatment is warranted after a second seizure. The agent will depend upon seizure type. Since most seizures are partial in fragile X syndrome, carbamazepine has traditionally been used most often (Berry-Kravis 2002). For generalized seizures and in individuals who fail carbamazepine, valproic acid is a reasonable choice (Berry-Kravis 2002). Both of these medications have also been used for behavioral and emotional stabilization in seizure-free individuals with fragile X syndrome. Alternatively, lamotrigine has the advantage of fewer cognitive side effects. Phenobarbital tends to make behavior worse in young children, including those with fragile X syndrome. There are few data available regarding most of the new generation of anticonvulsants in fragile X syndrome.

The treatment of individuals with fragile X syndrome is mainly symptomatic and ideally involves a multidisciplinary team to address common comorbidities including anxiety, behavioral problems, attentional difficulties, and other psychiatric disorders (Hagerman *et al.* 2009). A multidisciplinary team can also assist with educational planning.

Conclusions

Seizures occur in many individuals with fragile X syndrome, and their specific characteristics (i.e., similarities to rolandic epilepsy) suggest that specific pathophysiological mechanisms are operative. The seizures are mild, infrequent, and tend to remit, features unlike those seen in many other mental retardation syndromes. The multiple pathophysiological processes that might underlie the hyperexcitability of the fragile X brain comprise specific targets for future innovative therapies such as decreasing mGluR activation or enhancing GABAergic function (Bear 2005; D'Hulst and Kooy 2007).

References

Bassell GJ, Warren ST (2008) Fragile X syndrome: loss of local mRNA regulation alters synaptic development and function. *Neuron* **60**:201–14.

Bear MF (2005) Therapeutic implications of the mGluR theory of fragile X mental retardation. *Genes Brain Behav* **4**:393–8.

Belmonte MK, Bourgeron T (2006) Fragile X syndrome and autism at the intersection of genetic and neural networks. *Nat Neurosci* **9**:1221–5.

Berry-Kravis E (2002) Epilepsy in fragile X syndrome. *Dev Med Child Neurol* **44**:724–8.

Bianchi R, Chuang S-C, Zhao W, Young SR, Wong RKS (2009) Cellular plasticity for group I mGluR-mediated epileptogenesis. *J Neurosci* **29**:3497–507.

Chuang SC, Zhao W, Bauchwitz R, *et al.* (2005) Prolonged epileptiform discharges induced by altered group 1 metabotropic glutamate receptor-mediated synaptic responses in hippocampal slices of a fragile X mouse model. *J Neurosci* **25**:8048–55.

Comery TA, Harris JB, Willems PJ, *et al.* (1997) Abnormal dendritic spines in fragile X knockout mice: maturation and pruning deficits. *Proc Natl Acad Sci USA* **94**:5401–4.

Crawford DC, Acuna JM, Sherman SL (2001) *FMR1* and the fragile X syndrome: human genome epidemiology review. *Genet Med* **3**:359–71.

Curia G, Papouin T, Seguela P, Avoli M (2009) Downregulation of tonic GABAergic inhibition in a mouse model of fragile X syndrome. *Cereb Cortex* **19**:1515–20.

D'Hulst C, Kooy RF (2007) The GABA$_A$ receptor: a novel target for treatment of fragile X? *Trends Neurosci* **30**:425–31.

D'Hulst C, Heulens I, Brouwer JR, *et al.* (2009) Expression of the GABAergic system in animal models for fragile X syndrome and fragile X associated tremor/ataxia syndrome (FXTAS). *Brain Res* **1253**:176–83.

Debacker K, Kooy RF (2007) Fragile sites and human disease. *Hum Mol Genet* **16**:R150–8.

Dölen G, Osterweil E, Rao BSS, *et al.* (2007) Correction of fragile X syndrome in mice. *Neuron* **56**:955–62.

Dölen G, Bear MF (2008) Role for metabotropic glutamate receptor 5 (mGluR5) in the pathogenesis of fragile X syndrome. *J Physiol* **586**:1503–8.

Garber KB, Visootsak J, Warren ST (2008) Fragile X syndrome. *Eur J Hum Genet* **16**:666–72.

Gibson JR, Bartley AF, Hays SA, Huber KM (2008) Imbalance of neocortical excitation and inhibition and altered UP states reflect network hyperexcitability in the mouse model of fragile X syndrome. *J Neurophysiol* **100**:2615–26.

Gothelf D, Furfaro JA, Hoeft F, *et al.* (2008) Neuroanatomy of fragile X syndrome is associated with aberrant behavior and the fragile X mental retardation protein (FMRP). *Ann Neurol* **63**:40–51.

Hagerman PJ, Hagerman RJ (2004) Fragile X-associated tremor/ataxia syndrome (FXTAS). *Ment Retard Dev Disabil Res Rev* **10**:25–30.

Hagerman PJ, Stafstrom CE (2009) Origins of epilepsy in fragile X syndrome. *Epilepsy Curr* **9**:108–12.

Hagerman RJ, Berry-Kravis E, Kaufmann WE, *et al.* (2009) Advances in the treatment of fragile X syndrome. *Pediatrics* **123**:378–89.

Huber KM, Gallagher SM, Warren ST, Bear MF (2002) Altered synaptic plasticity in a mouse model of fragile-X mental retardation. *Proc Natl Acad Sci USA* **99**:7746–50.

Incorpora G, Sorge G, Sorge A, Pavone L (2002) Epilepsy in fragile X syndrome. *Brain Dev* **24**:766–9.

Kluger G, Bohm I, Laub MC, Waldenmaier C (1996) Epilepsy and fragile X gene mutations. *Pediatr Neurol* **15**:358–60.

Lubs HA (1969) A marker X chromosome. *Am J Hum Genet* **21**:231–44.

Murray A (2000) Premature ovarian failure and the FMR1 gene. *Semin Reprod Med* **18**:59–66.

Musumeci SA, Colognola RM, Ferri R, *et al.* (1988) Fragile-X syndrome: a particular epileptogenic EEG pattern. *Epilepsia* **29**:41–7.

Musumeci SA, Ferri R, Elia M, *et al.* (1991) Epilepsy and fragile X syndrome: a follow-up study. *Am J Med Genet* **38**:511–13.

Musumeci SA, Bosco P, Calabrese G, *et al.* (2000) Audiogenic seizures susceptibility in transgenic mice with fragile X syndrome. *Epilepsia* **41**:19–23.

Nakamoto M, Nalavadi V, Epstein MP, *et al.* (2007) Fragile X mental retardation protein deficiency leads to excessive mGluR5-dependent internalization of AMPA receptors. *Proc Natl Acad Sci USA* **104**:15 537–42.

Pfeiffer BE, Huber KM (2009) The state of synapses in fragile X syndrome. *Neuroscientist* **15**:549–67.

Qiu LF, Hao Y-H, Li Q-Z, Xiong Z-Q (2008a) Fragile X syndrome and epilepsy. *Neurosci Bull* **24**:338–44.

Qiu LF, Lu TJ, Hu XL, *et al.* (2008b) Limbic epileptogenesis in a mouse model of fragile X syndrome *Cereb Cortex* **19**:1504–14.

Rees M, Diebold U, Parker K, *et al.* (1993) Benign childhood epilepsy with centrotemporal spikes and the focal sharp wave trait is not linked to the fragile X region. *Neuropediatrics* **24**:211–13.

Rogers SJ, Wehner DE, Hagerman RJ (2001) The behavioral phenotype in fragile X: symptoms of autism in very young children with fragile X syndrome, idiopathic autism, and other developmental disorders. *J Dev Behav Pediatr* **22**:409–17.

Sabaratnam M, Vroegop PG, Gangadharan SK (2001) Epilepsy and EEG findings in 18 males with fragile X syndrome. *Seizure* **10**:60–3.

Selby L, Zhang C, Sun QQ (2007) Major defects in neocortical GABAergic inhibitory circuits in mice lacking the fragile X mental retardation protein. *Neurosci Lett* **412**:227–32.

Stafstrom CE (1999) Mechanisms of epilepsy in mental retardation: insights from Angelman syndrome, Down syndrome and fragile X syndrome. In: Sillanpää M, Gram L, Johannessen SI, Tomson T (eds.) *Epilepsy and Mental Retardation.* Petersfield, UK: Wrightson Biomedical Publishing, pp. 7–40.

Sutherland GR (1977) Fragile sites on human chromosomes: demonstration of their dependence on the type of tissue culture medium. *Science* **197**:265–6.

Tervonen TA, Louhivuori V, Sun X, *et al.* (2009) Aberrant differentiation of glutamatergic cells in neocortex of mouse model for fragile X syndrome. *Neurobiol Dis* **33**:250–9.

Wilson BM, Cox CL (2007) Absence of metabotropic glutamate receptor-mediated plasticity in the neocortex of fragile X mice. *Proc Natl Acad Sci USA* **104**:2454–9.

Wisniewski KE, Segan SM, Miezejeski CM, Sersen EA, Rudelli RD (1991) The fra(X) syndrome: neurological, electrophysiological, and neuropathological abnormalities. *Am J Med Genet* **38**:476–80.

Yan QJ, Rammal M, Tranfaglia M, Bauchwitz RP (2005) Suppression of two major fragile X syndrome mouse model phenotypes by the mGluR5 antagonist MPEP. *Neuropharmacology* **49**:1053–66.

4p (Wolf–Hirschhorn) syndrome

Agatino Battaglia

The causal disease

Wolf–Hirschhorn syndrome (WHS) is a multiple congenital anomalies/intellectual disability disorder due to deletion, or loss of material, of the distal portion of the short arm of chromosome 4. The hallmark is represented by prenatal and postnatal growth deficiency, the "Greek warrior helmet appearance of the nose," deficits in neurological function (hypotonia and seizures), and variable degrees of intellectual deficits (Battaglia and Carey 2000; Rauch *et al.* 2001; Zollino *et al.* 2003; Fisch *et al.* 2008).

About 1 in 50 000 individuals is diagnosed with WHS, with a female preponderance of 2 : 1 (Lurie *et al.* 1980). In an UK epidemiological study, a minimum birth prevalence of 1 in 95 896 was found (Shannon *et al.* 2001).

Some 75% of individuals with WHS will have a de novo isolated deletion of the short arm of chromosome 4 (Lurie *et al.* 1980); about 12% will have either a ring 4 chromosome, mosaicism, or a sporadic unbalanced translocation. The remaining 13% will have the 4p deletion as the result of a parental chromosome translocation. In about 85% of de novo deletions, the origin of the deleted chromosome is paternal (Tupler *et al.* 1992; Dallapiccola *et al.* 1993), whereas in almost two-thirds of the translocations, the mother carries the rearrangement (Bauer *et al.* 1985). When an unbalanced translocation is identified, the parents are at increased risk of having another child with a chromosome abnormality (WHS or 4p trisomy with monosomy of the other involved chromosome, depending on the malsegregation of derivative chromosomes). With the refinement of cytogenetic techniques, cryptic translocations were increasingly described in WHS (Bauer *et al.* 1985; Altherr *et al.* 1991; Reid *et al.* 1996), most interestingly in familial cases. Over the last 20 years the minimal deleted region (WHSCR) has been progressively reduced to 165 kb (Estabrooks *et al.* 1992; Gandelman *et al.* 1992; Johnson *et al.* 1994; Somer *et al.* 1995; Wright *et al.* 1997). In 2003, Zollino *et al.* proposed a new critical region for WHS (WHSCR2). This region is contiguous distally with the currently defined critical region, and falls within a 300–600-kb interval in 4p16.3, between the loci D4S3327 and D4S98–D4S168.

The WHS clinical spectrum is complex and highly variable and, for this reason, it is thought that the disorder is a contiguous gene syndrome. More recently, the *WHSC1* gene has been related to the craniofacial characteristics, and *LETM1* gene to seizures (Battaglia *et al.* 2008, 2009; Zollino *et al.* 2008). From recent reviews, it seems that there might be a correlation between size of the deletion and severity of the clinical phenotype (Zollino *et al.* 2008). South *et al.* (2008) have recently shown that clinical variation may be explained by cryptic unbalanced translocations, where some expected clinical manifestations can be modified by the trisomic material.

Wolf–Hirschhorn syndrome is characterized by typical craniofacial features in infancy consisting of "Greek warrior helmet appearance" of the nose (the broad bridge of the nose continuing to the forehead), microcephaly, high forehead with prominent glabella, ocular hypertelorism, epicanthus, highly arched eyebrows, protruding eyes, short philtrum, downturned mouth, micrognathia, and poorly formed ears with pits/tags. All affected individuals have prenatal-onset growth deficiency followed by postnatal growth retardation and hypotonia with muscle underdevelopment. Developmental delay/intellectual disability of variable degree is present in all (Battaglia *et al.* 2008; Fisch *et al.* 2008). Other findings include skeletal anomalies (60–70%), varying from medically significant malformations to minor anomalies of limbs and skeleton; congenital heart defects (~50%); hearing loss (mostly conductive) (>40%), urinary tract malformations (25%), and structural brain abnormalities (33%).

Epilepsy in the disease

Seizures/epilepsy represent one of the main clinical challenges in 4p WHS. Seizures occur in 50% to 100% of infants and children with WHS (Guthrie *et al.* 1971; Centerwall *et al.* 1975; Stengel-Rutkowski *et al.* 1984; Battaglia and Carey 1999;

The Causes of Epilepsy, eds. S. D. Shorvon, F. Andermann, and R. Guerrini. Published by Cambridge University Press. © Cambridge University Press 2011.

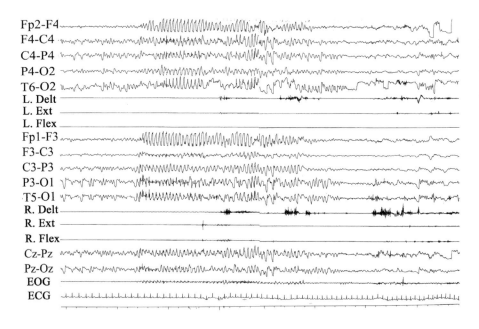

Fig. 41.1. Three-year-old female child with WHS. Awake. EEG showing an atypical absence characterized by diffuse rhythmic 2.5–3-Hz spike–wave, ill-defined, complexes, reaching up to 300 μV, lasting 19 ss. This child had 15 such episodes, lasting up to 25 ss, during a 50-min video-EEG-polygraphic recording. Amplitude 150 μV/cm; Speed 1 s/1.5 cm. (From Battaglia et al. 2009, with permission.)

Battaglia *et al.* 1999a, b). The author's study of 87 individuals in Italy and the USA documented seizures in 93% of affected children. Age at onset varies between the neonatal period and 36 months of age with a peak incidence around 6 to 12 months of age. Seizures are either unilateral clonic or tonic, with or without secondary generalization, or generalized tonic–clonic from the onset. The latter is the only seizure pattern in almost 40% of individuals (Battaglia *et al.* 2009). Seizures are frequently triggered by fever, even low-grade fever, in three-fourths of the children; can occur in clusters; and last over 15 min. Other risk factors are mainly represented by respiratory or urinary tract infections; and apparently, by tiredness and excitement in a few cases (Battaglia *et al.* 2008). Unilateral or generalized clonic or tonic–clonic status epilepticus occurs in about 50% of children, particularly during the first 3 years of life, in spite of adequate pharmacotherapy. One-third of children develop daily and long-lasting atypical absences by age 1 to 6 years, often accompanied by a mild myoclonic component involving the eyelids and, less frequently, the eyeballs and the upper limbs (Fig. 41.1).

Epilepsy is well controlled in most WHS individuals (80%). Phenobarbital has been reported as the most effective drug against tonic-clonic seizures. Valproate (VPA) alone or associated with ethosuximide (ESM) succeeds in treating the atypical absences. Only in a minority of cases (10%) atypical absences require the association of VPA, ESM, and a benzodiazepine, in order to be controlled (Battaglia *et al.* 2009).

Epilepsy improves with age in all patients. In a recent study, 55% of individuals, for whom such information was available, were seizure-free. Seizures tend to stop between ages 1 year 9 months and 13 years (Battaglia *et al.* 2009). In a previous study, about 20% of individuals had discontinued antiepileptic drugs (Battaglia *et al.* 2001).

Diagnostic tests for the disease

About 30–40% of the deletions will not be detected by karyotype (Battaglia *et al.* 2006). Therefore, fluorescence in situ hybridization (FISH) with cosmid probes from the WHS critical region (WHSCR), or comparative genomic hybridization microarray (aCGH) are necessary to confirm the diagnosis. Both tests have a detection rate of >95%, and are clinically available.

It is always recommended to perform state-of-the-art karyotypes on the parents of a child with WHS, in search of a possible translocation or other less common rearrangements. In an apparently de novo deletion (where parental chromosomes are normal), whole chromosome painting of chromosome 4 of both parents or aCGH is advisable to exclude a cryptic unbalanced translocation (Altherr *et al.* 1991; Reid *et al.* 1996). However, it is worth bearing in mind that aCGH analysis does not identify unbalanced translocations involving the acrocentric p-arms (South *et al.* 2008).

The distinctive electroencephalographic (EEG) abnormalities, observed in almost all individuals during waking and sleep, can direct the epileptologist/neurologist toward the right diagnosis (Battaglia *et al.* 1996, 2001, 2009). These distinctive findings include: (1) frequent, ill-defined, diffuse or generalized, high-amplitude sharp element spike–wave complexes at 2–3.5 Hz occurring in bursts lasting up to 25 s (often associated with atypical absences: Fig. 41.1), activated by slow wave sleep; and (2) frequent high-amplitude spikes, polyspikes/wave complexes at 4–6 Hz, over the posterior third of the head, often triggered by eye closure (not strictly related to seizures; also seen for many years after seizures have stopped; not affected by antiepileptic treatment).

Brain magnetic resonance imaging (MRI) should be performed in all individuals with seizures, since malformation of the cerebral cortex may modify prognosis and management.

A systematic study of cognitive–behavioral aspects of children with WHS has just begun. A preliminary report on 12 such cases shows that: (1) socialization score is significantly higher than mean communication score; (2) there is a relative strength in verbal and quantitative reasoning, and relative weakness in abstract/visual reasoning and short-term memory. This neuropsychological pattern differs from that observed in other subtelomeric microdeletion syndromes (Fisch *et al.* 2008).

Principles of management

A waking/sleeping video-EEG-polygraphic study (including electrooculogram [EOG], electrocardiogram [ECG], surface electromyogram [EMG]) is recommended in infancy and childhood, in order to achieve the best characterization of seizures. This is of paramount importance when parents/guardians or professionals report the occurrence of "staring spells" or "eye-tics". On most occasions, these episodes are shown to be atypical absences.

Regular follow-up of seizure status and pharmacotherapy is essential.

Clonic or tonic–clonic seizures are usually effectively controlled by phenobarbital.

Clonic or tonic–clonic status epilepticus can be effectively controlled by intravenous benzodiazepines such as diazepam or midazolam. On occasion it may be necessary to add intravenous phenytoin.

Absence or myoclonic status epilepticus can be effectively controlled by intravenous benzodiazepines.

In the author's experience the atypical absences are well controlled by valproic acid, alone or associated with ethosuccimide. Only rarely, the addition of a benzodiazepine, such as clobazam or clonazepam, may be needed. Carbamazepine can severely worsen the electroclinical picture.

Management of respiratory and urinary tract infection are the same as in any individual. An approach to reduce seizures triggered by fever consists in reducing the frequency of febrile illness in infancy and childhood. Vaccination against common infancy and childhood infectious illness is to be encouraged.

References

Altherr MR, Bengtsson U, Elder FF, et al. (1991) Molecular confirmation of Wolf–Hirschhorn syndrome with a subtle translocation of chromosome 4. *Am J Hum Genet* **49**:1235–42.

Battaglia A, Carey JC (1999) Health supervision and anticipatory guidance of individuals with Wolf–Hirschhorn syndrome. *Am J Med Genet* **89**:111–15.

Battaglia A, Carey JC (2000) Update on the clinical features and natural history of Wolf–Hirschhorn syndrome (WHS): experience with 48 cases. *Am J Hum Genet* **6**:127.

Battaglia A, Carey JC, Thompson JA, Filloux F (1996) EEG studies in the Wolf–Hirschhorn (4p-) syndrome. *EEG Clin Neurophysiol* **99**:324.

Battaglia A, Carey JC, Cederholm P, et al. (1999a) Natural history of Wolf–Hirschhorn syndrome: experience with 15 cases. *Pediatrics* **103**:830–36.

Battaglia A, Carey JC, Cederholm P, et al. (1999b) Storia naturale della sindrome di Wolf–Hirschhorn: esperienza con 15 casi. *Pediatrics* **11**:236–42.

Battaglia A, Carey JC, Wright TJ (2001) Wolf–Hirschhorn (4p-) syndrome. *Adv Pediatr* **48**:75–113.

Battaglia A, Carey JC, Wright TJ (2006) Wolf–Hirschhorn syndrome. In: *GeneReviews* at *GeneTests*: Medical Genetics Information Resource. Available on line at www.genetests.org.

Battaglia A, Filippi T, Carey JC (2008) Update on the clinical features and natural history of Wolf–Hirschhorn (4p-) syndrome: experience with 87 patients and recommendations for routine health supervision. *Am J Med Genet* **148C**:246–51.

Battaglia A, Filippi T, South ST, Carey JC (2009) Spectrum of epilepsy and electroencephalogram patterns in Wolf–Hirschhorn syndrome: experience with 87 patients. *Dev Med Child Neurol* **51**:373–80.

Bauer K, Howard-Peebles PN, Keele D, Friedman JM (1985) Wolf–Hirschhorn syndrome owing to 1:3 segregation of a maternal 4;21 translocation. *Am J Med Genet* **21**:351–6.

Centerwall WR, Thompson WP, Allen IE, Foubes TC (1975) Translocation 4p- syndrome. *Am J Dis Child* **129**:366–70.

Dallapiccola B, Mandich P, Bellone E, et al. (1993) Parental origin of chromosome 4p deletion in Wolf–Hirschhorn syndrome. *Am J Med Genet* **47**:921–4.

Estabrooks LL, Lamb AN, Kirkman HN, Callanan RP, Rao KW (1992) A molecular deletion of distal chromosome 4p in two families with a satellited chromosome 4 lacking the Wolf–Hirschhorn syndrome phenotype. *Am J Hum Genet* **51**:971–8.

Fisch GS, Battaglia A, Parrini B, Youngbloum J, Simensen R (2008) Cognitive–behavioral features of children with Wolf–Hirschhorn syndrome: preliminary report of 12 cases. *Am J Med Genet* **148C**:252–6.

Gandelman K-Y, Gibson L, Meyn MS, Yang-Feng TL (1992) Molecular definition of the smallest region of deletion overlap in the Wolf–Hirschhorn syndrome. *Am J Hum Genet* **51**:571–8.

Guthrie RD, Aase JM, Asper AC, Smith D (1971) The 4p- syndrome. *Am J Dis Child* **122**:421–5.

Johnson VP, Altherr MR, Blake JM, Keppen LD (1994) FISH detection of Wolf–Hirschhorn syndrome: exclusion of D4F26 as critical site. *Am J Med Genet* **52**:70–4.

Lurie IW, Lazjuk CL, Ussova I, Presman EB, Gurevich DB (1980) The Wolf–Hirschhorn syndrome. I. Genetics. *Clin Genet* **17**:375–84.

Rauch A, Schellmoser S, Kraus C, et al. (2001) First known microdeletion within the Wolf–Hirschhorn-syndrome critical region refines genotype phenotype correlation. *Am J Med Genet* **99**:338–42.

Reid E, Morrison N, Barron L (1996) Familial Wolf–Hirschhorn syndrome resulting from a cryptic translocation: a clinical and molecular study. *J Med Genet* **33**:197–202.

Shannon NL, Maltby EL, Rigby AS, Quarrell OWJ (2001) An epidemiological study of

Wolf–Hirschhorn syndrome: life expectancy and cause of mortality. *J Med Genet* **38**:674–9.

Somer M, Peippo M, Keinanen M (1995) Controversial findings in two patients with commercially available probe D4S96 for the Wolf–Hirschhorn syndrome. *Am J Hum Genet* **57A**:127.

South ST, Hannes F, Fisch GS, Vermeesch JR, Zollino M (2008) Pathogenic significance of deletions distal to the currently described Wolf–Hirschhorn syndrome critical regions on 4p16.3. *Am J Med Genet* **148C**:270–4.

Stengel-Rutkowski S, Warkotsch A, Schimanek P, Stene J (1984) Familial Wolf's syndrome with a hidden 4p deletion by translocation of an 8p segment: unbalanced inheritance from a maternal translocation (4;8)(pl5.3;p22) – case report, review and risk estimates. *Clin Genet* **25**:500–21.

Tupler R, Bortotto L, Buhler E, *et al.* (1992) Paternal origin of de novo deleted chromosome 4 in Wolf–Hirschhorn syndrome. *J Med Genet* **29**:53–5.

Wright TJ, Ricke DO, Denison K, *et al.* (1997) A transcript map of the newly defined 165kb Wolf–Hirschhorn syndrome critical region. *Hum Mol Genet* **6**:317–24.

Zollino M, Lecce R, Fischetto R (2003) Mapping the Wolf–Hirschorn syndrome phenotype outside the currently accepted WHS critical region and defining a new critical region, WHSCR-2. *Am J Hum Genet* **72**:590–7.

Zollino M, Murdolo M, Marangi G, *et al.* (2008) On the nosology and pathogenesis of Wolf–Hirschhorn syndrome: genotype–phenotype correlation analysis of 80 patients and literature review. *Am J Med Genet* **148C**:257–69.

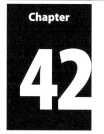

Inverted duplicated chromosome 15 (isodicentric chromosome 15)

Agatino Battaglia

The causal disease

The idic(15) (isodicentric chromosome 15) or inv dup(15) (inverted duplicated chromosome 15) syndrome is a complex neurogenetic condition characterized by early central hypotonia, developmental delay and intellectual disability, epilepsy, and autistic or autistic-like behavior. The latter is characterized by lack of social interaction, non-functional use of objects, primordial type of exploration, stereotypies, absent or very poor echolalic language, limited comprehension, and poor intention to communicate. Physically, there are only minor anomalies (Battaglia *et al.* 1997; Battaglia 2005, 2008).

Incidence at birth is estimated to be 1 in 30 000 with a sex ratio of almost 1 (Schinzel and Niedrist 2001). However, due to dysmorphic features being absent or subtle and to the rarity of major malformations, chromosome analysis may not be thought to be indicated, and a number of individuals probably remain undiagnosed.

The chromosome region 15q11–q13 is prone to genomic rearrangements, due to the presence of repeated DNA elements (Christian *et al.* 1999; Makoff and Flomen 2007). The rearrangements include deletions leading to either Angelman syndrome (AS) or Prader–Willi syndrome (PWS), according to parental origin (Lalande 1996); translocations; inversions; and supernumerary marker chromosomes (SMCs) formed by the inverted duplication of proximal chromosome 15. Interstitial duplications, triplications, and balanced reciprocal translocations may also occur (Browne *et al.* 1997). Idic(15) or inv dup(15) is the most common of the heterogeneous group of the SMCs. Two cytogenetic types of SMCs(15) have been identified, with different phenotypic consequences (Maraschio *et al.* 1988; Leana-Cox *et al.* 1994; Crolla *et al.* 1995; Huang *et al.* 1997). One is a metacentric or submetacentric and heterochromatic chromosome, smaller or similar to a G group chromosome, not containing the PWS/AS critical region, and the cytogenetic description is dic(15)(q11). This can be familial or de novo, and is the most common SMC accounting for about 70% of all small SMCs. Most individuals with this aberration show a normal

phenotype (Cheng *et al.* 1994), although exceptions have been reported (Hou and Wang 1998). The second type of SMC(15) is as large as, or larger than, a G group chromosome and has 15q euchromatin. It includes the PWS/AS critical region (Robinson *et al.* 1993; Blennow *et al.* 1995), and the cytogenetic description is dic(15)(q12 or q13). Most dic(15)(q12 or q13) derives from the two homologous maternal chromosomes at meiosis, and is reportedly associated with increased mean maternal age at conception, similar to other aneuploidies. The presence of a large SMC(15) results in tetrasomy 15p and partial tetrasomy 15q. However, considerable structure heterogeneity has recently been described (Wang *et al.* 2008). The large SMCs(15) are associated with an abnormal phenotype, which constitutes the idic(15) syndrome (Flejter *et al.* 1996; Battaglia *et al.* 1997). Large SMCs (15), which include the PWS/AS critical region, or idic(15), are nearly always sporadic.

Maternally derived cytogenetic mosaicism with a normal cell line has been described in a small subset of individuals (Crolla *et al.* 2005; Loitzsch and Bartsch 2006); and one patient with a mosaic paternally derived inv dup(15), showing a mild PWS phenotype, has been recently reported (Saitoh *et al.* 2007).

Idic(15) syndrome is characterized by a distinct neurobehavioral phenotype including moderate to profound developmental delay/intellectual disability, absent or very poor speech, hypotonia, epilepsy, and an autism spectrum disorder (ASD) (Gillberg *et al.* 1991; Robinson *et al.* 1993; Webb 1994; Crolla *et al.* 1995; Battaglia *et al.* 1997; Webb *et al.* 1998; Battaglia 2005). Sitting is usually achieved between 10 and 20 months of age, and independent walking between 2 and 3 years (Robinson *et al.* 1993; Battaglia *et al.* 1997). Immediate and delayed echolalia with pronoun reversal can be present. Comprehension is limited to the context and accompanied by the gesture. Intention to communicate is often absent or very poor (Battaglia *et al.* 1997; Battaglia 2005). The idic(15) distinct behavior disorder has been described as autistic or autistic-like. A strong association between autistic features and idic(15) was reported by Rineer *et al.* (1998), and the individuals described by Borgatti *et al.* (2001) met the clinical criteria for the diagnosis

The Causes of Epilepsy, eds. S. D. Shorvon, F. Andermann, and R. Guerrini. Published by Cambridge University Press. © Cambridge University Press 2011.

of autistic disorder by The *Diagnostic and Statistical Manual of Mental Disorders* 4th edition (DSM IV). Idic(15) children have gaze avoidance from very early on; shun body contact; stare at people as looking through them. They can be fascinated by certain sounds, by water, or by spinning or any glittering objects, and usually prefer being left alone, lying on the back just looking at their fingers and taking bizarre postures. Symbolic play is, on most occasions, never acquired. No interest towards peers and no appropriate social interactions are usually observed. Outbursts of shouting or aggressiveness are triggered by thwarting situations. Non-functional use of objects with a primordial type of exploration is also observed. Stereotypies are frequently seen, including hand flapping, hand wringing, and hand clapping over plane surfaces, finger biting, head turning, spinning him/herself for long periods of time. Hyperactivity has been reported in a number of instances (Gillberg *et al.* 1991; Battaglia *et al.* 1997; Battaglia 2005).

Muscle hypotonia, associated with joint hyperextensibility and drooling, is observed in most individuals. Other physical findings include minor facial dysmorphisms, such as downslanting palpebral fissures, epicanthal folds, deep-set eyes, low-set and/or posteriorly rotated ears, highly arched palate, broad nose, anteverted nares; fifth finger clinodactyly and unusual dermatoglyphics; partial second–third toe syndactyly (Battaglia *et al.*, 1997: Schinzel and Niedrist 2001;). Brachycephaly, frontal bossing, synophrys, broad nose, short philtrum, cleft palate, prominent mandible in adults, brachydactyly, and areas of increased and reduced skin pigmentation can be occasionally observed. Major malformations are seldom reported (Centerwall and Morris 1975; Schreck *et al.* 1977; Schinzel 1981; Robinson *et al.* 1993; Blennow *et al.* 1995; Crolla *et al.* 1995; Battaglia *et al.* 1997; Qumsiyeh *et al.* 2003). Feeding difficulties are observed in the neonatal period (Dennis *et al.* 2006). Growth is retarded in about 20–30% of the patients. Microcephaly is seen in fewer than 20% of individuals, while macrocephaly in fewer than 3%. Hypogonadism is reported in about 20% (Webb 1994; Schinzel and Niedrist 2001). Although puberty is reportedly normal in most individuals (Schinzel 2001), pubertal disorders, such as central precocious puberty or ovarian dysgenesis, have been observed in three girls (Grosso *et al.* 2001).

Pregnancies and birth weights are mostly normal. Mean parental/maternal ages at birth of the probands were markedly advanced (Connor and Gilmore 1984; Webb *et al.* 1998). Brain neuroimaging (computed tomography [CT] and magnetic resonance imaging [MRI]) does not show abnormal findings in most cases (Battaglia *et al.* 1997; Borgatti *et al.* 2001).

Epilepsy in idic(15)

Epilepsy represents one of the main clinical challenges in idic (15) individuals. It occurs with a wide variety of seizures, with onset between ages 6 months and 9 years (Gillberg *et al.* 1991; Crolla *et al.* 1995; Bingham *et al.* 1996; Battaglia *et al.* 1997;

Webb *et al.* 1998). Infantile spasms associated with an hypsarrhythmic electroencephalogram (EEG) have been reported in several patients (Robinson *et al.* 1993; Crolla *et al.* 1995; Bingham *et al.* 1996; Webb *et al.* 1998). Typical Lennox–Gastaut syndrome or Lennox–Gastaut-like syndrome was observed in four idic(15) patients with seizure onset between ages 4 and 8 years (Battaglia *et al.* 1997). Complex partial and myoclonic seizures were reported in a number of other individuals (Gillberg *et al.* 1991). Drug-resistant myoclonic absence-like seizures induced by emotionally gratifying stimuli (kissing, viewing of pleasant or funny events) have been observed in a 9-year-old boy (Aguglia *et al.* 1999). A mild, adult-onset, generalized epilepsy with absence seizures and occasional head drops and generalized tonic–clonic seizures has also been occasionally reported, with a good outcome (Chifari *et al.* 2002). Benign epilepsy with centrotemporal spikes with a benign evolution has been observed in another idic(15) individual (Gobbi *et al.* 2002).

Seizures tend to be difficult to control and/or drug resistant in many patients (Gillberg *et al.* 1991; Robinson *et al.* 1993; Crolla *et al.* 1995; Mignon *et al.* 1996; Battaglia *et al.* 1997).

Diagnostic tests for the disease

Standard cytogenetics must be associated with fluorescent in situ hybridization (FISH) analysis, using probes both from proximal chromosome 15 and from the PWS/AS critical region (Luke *et al.* 1994; Webb *et al.* 1998). Molecular studies, such as microsatellite analysis on parental DNA or methylation analysis on the proband DNA, are also needed in order to detect the parent-of-origin of the idic(15) chromosome (Luke *et al.* 1994; Webb *et al.* 1998). During recent years, array comparative genomic hybridization (aCGH) has provided a powerful approach to detect the duplication and its extent (Wang *et al.* 2004).

Prenatal diagnosis has frequently been reported (Miny *et al.* 1986). Cells obtained by chorionic villus sampling (CVS) at approximately 12 weeks' gestation, or amniocentesis, performed at approximately 15–18 weeks' gestation, can be analyzed by a combination of cytogenetic (G–C banding, FISH), and molecular (methylation analysis) methods.

Very little is known about the EEG characteristics in idic(15) syndrome, mainly due to the poor description of these findings, and total lack of serial EEG studies (Gillberg *et al.* 1991; Crolla *et al.* 1995; Bingham *et al.* 1996; Webb *et al.* 1998; Battaglia 2005). In 1997 Battaglia *et al.* described in detail the EEG abnormalities in four such individuals. All EEGs were abnormal, showing: (1) slow background activity; (2) absence or poverty of the rhythmic activities usually elicited over the posterior third of the brain, on eye closure; (3) multifocal discharges with variable hemispheric predominance; (4) frequent, large amplitude, generalized paroxysms, lasting 2 to 20 s, characterized by slow sharp element spike–wave complexes, mostly accompanied by atypical absences; (5) frequent generalized bursts of fast rhythms during slow wave sleep in two of the four patients, accompanied by tachypnea and/or by an upward rotation of the eyes, and/or by tonic fits; (6) disruption of the usual sleep structure. Other EEG findings include generalized rhythmic 3.5–4-Hz spike-and-wave discharges, lasting 4–6 s (Chifari *et al.* 2002), and spikes, polyspikes, and ill-defined polyspike/wave complexes, with variable hemispheric predominance (Battaglia 2008).

Although brain neuroimaging (CT/MRI) is reportedly normal in most idic(15) individuals (Battaglia *et al.* 1997; Borgatti *et al.* 2001), brain MRI should be performed in all those having seizures, since a malformation of the cerebral cortex may modify prognosis and management.

A formal and careful developmental evaluation by a specialist should be performed at intervals appropriate for planning early intervention, including physical, occupational, and speech therapies, and for educational and vocational planning.

Principles of management

A waking/sleeping video-EEG-polygraphic recording (including electrooculogram [EOG], electrocardiogram [ECG], polyneurogram [PNG], surface electromyogram [EMG] is recommended in infancy and childhood, in order to achieve the best characterization of seizures, and detect subtle seizures. This is of the utmost importance for the first choice pharmacotherapy.

Regular follow-up of the seizure status and pharmacotherapy is essential.

In the author's experience, the most helpful drug treatment is represented by the association of valproate and/or carbamazepine with lamotrigine. Valproate is the first-choice drug for atypical absences; whereas carbamazepine can be chosen whenever tonic seizures are the most frequent.

Management of upper respiratory tract infections is the same as in any individual. Vaccination against common infancy and childhood infectious illness is to be encouraged.

References

Aguglia U, Le Piane E, Gambardella A, *et al.* (1999) Emotion-induced myoclonic absence-like seizures in a patient with inv-dup(15) syndrome: a clinical, EEG, and molecular genetic study. *Epilepsia* 40:1316–19.

Battaglia A (2005) The inv dup(15) or idic(15) syndrome: a clinically recognisable neurogenetic disorder. *Brain Devel* 27:365–9.

Battaglia A (2008) The inv dup(15) or idic(15) syndrome (Tetrasomy 15q). *Orphanet Journal Rare Diseases* 3:30. Available online at www.ojrd.com/content/3/1/30

Battaglia A, Gurrieri F, Bertini E, *et al.* (1997) The inv dup(15) syndrome: a clinically recognizable syndrome with altered behavior, mental retardation and epilepsy. *Neurology* 48:1081–6.

Bingham PM, Spinner NB, Sovinsky L, Zackai EH, Chance PF (1996) Infantile spasms associated with proximal duplication of chromosome 15q. *Pediatr Neurol* 15:163–5.

Blennow E, Nielsen KB, Telenius H, *et al.* (1995) Fifty probands with extra structurally abnormal chromosomes characterized by fluorescence in situ hybridization. *Am J Med Genet* 55:85–94.

Borgatti R, Piccinelli P, Passoni D, *et al.* (2001) Relationship between clinical and genetic features in "inverted duplicated chromosome 15" patients. *Pediatr Neurol* 24:111–16.

Browne CE, Dennis NR, Maher E, *et al.* (1997) Inherited interstitial duplications of proximal 15q: genotype–phenotype correlations. *Am J Hum Genet* 61:1342–52.

Centerwall WR, Morris JP (1975) Partial D15 trisomy: a case and general review. *Hum Hered* 25:442–52.

Cheng SD, Spinner NB, Zackai EH, Knoll JH (1994) Cytogenetic and molecular characterization of inverted duplicated chromosomes 15 from 11 patients. *Am J Hum Genet* 55:753–9.

Chifari R, Guerrini R, Pierluigi M, *et al.* (2002) Mild generalized epilepsy and developmental disorder associated with large inv dup (15). *Epilepsia* 43:1096–100.

Christian SL, Fantes JA, Mewborn SK, Huang B, Ledbetter D (1999) Large genomic duplicons map to sites of instability in the Prader–Willi/Angelman syndrome chromosome region (15q11–q13). *Hum Mol Genet* 8:1025–37.

Connor JM, Gilmore DH (1984) An analysis of the parental age effect for inv dup (15). *J Med Genet* 21:213–14.

Crolla JA, Harvey JF, Sitch FL, Dennis NR (1995) Supernumerary marker 15 chromosomes: a clinical, molecular and FISH approach to diagnosis and prognosis. *Hum Genet* 95:161–70.

Crolla JA, Youings SA, Ennis S, Jacobs PA (2005) Supernumerary marker chromosomes in man: parental origin, mosaicism and maternal age revisited. *Eur J Hum Genet* 13:154–60.

Dennis NR, Veltman MWM, Thompson R, *et al.* (2006) Clinical findings in 33 subjects with large supernumerary marker(15) chromosomes and 3 subjects with triplication of 15q11–q13. *Am J Med Genet* 140A:434–41.

Flejter WL, Bennet-Barker PE, Ghaziuddin M, *et al.* (1996) Cytogenetic and molecular analysis of inv dup(15) chromosomes observed in two patients with autistic disorder and mental retardation. *Am J Med Genet* 61:182–7.

Gillberg C, Steffenburg S, Wahlstrom J, *et al.* (1991) Autism associated with marker chromosome. *J Am Acad Child Adolesc Psychiat* 30:489–94.

Gobbi G, Genton P, Pini A, Gurrieri F, Livet MO (2002) Epilepsies and chromosomal disorders. In: Roger J, Bureau M, Dravet C, Genton P, Tassinari CA, Wolf P (eds.) *Epileptic Syndromes in Infancy, Childhood and Adolescence*, 3rd edn. Eastleigh, UK: John Libbey, pp. 431–55.

Grosso S, Balestri P, Anichini C, *et al.* (2001) Pubertal disorders in inv dup(15) syndrome. *Gynecol Endocrinol* 15:165–9.

Hou JW, Wang TR (1998) Unusual features in children with inv dup(15) supernumerary marker: a study of genotype–phenotype correlation in Taiwan. *Eur J Pediatr* 157:122–7.

Huang B, Crolla JA, Christian SL, *et al.* (1997) Refined molecular characterization of the breakpoints in small inv dup (15) chromosomes. *Hum Genet* 99:11–17.

Lalande M (1996) Parental imprinting and human disease. *Ann Rev Genet* **30**:173–95.

Leana-Cox J, Jenkins L, Palmer CG, *et al.* (1994) Molecular cytogenetic analysis of inv dup (15) chromosomes, using probes specific for the Prader–Willi/Angelman syndrome region: clinical implications. *Am J Hum Genet* **54**:748–56.

Loitzsch A, Bartsch O (2006) Healthy 12-year-old boy with mosaic inv dup(15) (q13). *Am J Med Genet* **140A**:640–3.

Luke S, Verma RS, Giridharan R, Conte RA, Macera MJ (1994) Two Prader–Willi/Angelman syndrome loci present in an isodicentric marker chromosome. *Am J Med Genet* **51**:232–3.

Makoff AJ, Flomen RH (2007) Detailed analysis of 15q11–q14 sequence corrects errors and gaps in the public access sequence to fully reveal large segmental duplications at breakpoints for Prader–Willi, Angelman, and inv dup(15) syndromes. *Genome Biol* **8**:R114.

Maraschio P, Cuocco C, Gimelli G, Zuffardi O, Tiepolo L (1988) Origin and clinical significance of inv dup (15). In: Danil A (ed.) *The Cytogenetics of Mammalian Autosomal Rearrangements*. New York: Alan R. Liss pp. 615–34.

Mignon C, Malzac P, Moncla A, *et al.* (1996) Clinical heterogeneity in 16 patients with inv dup(15) chromosome: cytogenetic and molecular studies, search for an imprinting effect. *Eur J Hum Genet* **4**:88–100.

Miny P, Basaran S, Kuwertz E, Holzgreve W, Pawlowitzki IH (1986) Inv dup (15): prenatal diagnosis and postnatal follow-up. *Prenat Diagn* **6**:303–06.

Qumsiyeh MB, Rafi SK, Sarri C, *et al.* (2003) Double supernumerary isodicentric chromosomes derived from 15 resulting in partial hexasomy. *Am J Med Genet* **116A**: 356–9.

Rineer S, Finucane B, Simon EW (1998) Autistic symptoms among children and young adults with isodicentric chromosome 15. *Am J Med Genet* **81**:428–33.

Robinson WP, Binkert F, Gine R, *et al.* (1993) Clinical and molecular analysis of five inv dup (15) patients. *Eur J Hum Genet* **1**:37–50.

Saitoh S, Hosoki K, Takano K, Tonoki H (2007) Mosaic paternally derived inv dup (15) may partially rescue the Prader–Willi syndrome phenotype with uniparental disomy. *Clin Genet* **72**:378–80.

Schinzel A (1981) Particular behavioral symptomatology in patients with rarer autosomal chromosome aberrations. In: Schmid W, Nielsen J (eds.) *Human Behavior and Genetics*. Amsterdam: Elsevier/North Holland, pp. 195–210.

Schinzel A (2001) *Catalogue of Unbalanced Chromosome Aberrations in Man*. Berlin: Walter de Gruyter.

Schinzel A, Niedrist D (2001) Chromosome imbalances associated with epilepsy. *Am J Med Genet* **106C**:119–24.

Schreck RR, Breg WR, Erlanger BF, Miller OJ (1977) Preferential derivation of abnormal human G-group-like chromosomes from chromosome 15. *Hum Genet* **36**:1–12.

Wang NJ, Liu D, Parokonny AS, Schanen NC (2004) High-resolution molecular characterization of 15q11–q13 rearrangements by array comparative genomic hybridization (array CGH) with detection of gene dosage. *Am J Hum Genet* **75**:267–81.

Wang NJ, Parokonny AS, Thatcher KN, *et al.* (2008) Multiple forms of atypical rearrangements generating supernumerary derivative chromosome 15. *BMC Genet* **9**:2.

Webb T (1994) Inv dup (15) supernumerary marker chromosomes. *J Med Genet* **31**:585–94.

Webb T, Hardy CA, King M, *et al.* (1998) A clinical, cytogenetic and molecular study of ten probands with inv dup (15) marker chromosomes. *Clin Genet* **53**:34–43.

Chapter

Ring chromosome 20

43

Geneviève Bernard and Frederick Andermann

The causal disease

Definitions

Ring chromosome 20 is a rare chromosomal abnormality and a rare cause of intractable epilepsy. As its name implies, the genetic abnormality consists of one of the two chromosomes 20 being shaped as a ring.

Ring chromosome 20 syndrome was first described as an epileptic syndrome in 1972 by several unrelated groups (Atkins *et al.* 1972; De Grouchy *et al.* 1972; Faed *et al.* 1972; Uchida and Lin 1972). Atkins and co-workers (1972) reported a 7-year-old male with 94% ring 20 chromosome [r(20)] who had his first seizure at the age 6 years. He developed frequent generalized tonic–clonic seizures. His electroencephalogram (EEG) was characterized by continuous sharp and multiple spike and slow wave complexes in both hemispheres. Faed and co-workers (1972) reported an 11-year-old male with seizure onset at age 4 and episodes of alteration of consciousness accompanied by automatic behavior and mood abnormality. His karyotype revealed 60% r(20). De Grouchy and colleagues (1972) reported a 6-month-old male with seizure onset at the age of 3 months. The karyotype revealed 100% r(20). He died at age 7 months. Finally, Uchida and Lin (1972) reported a 23-year-old female with seizure onset at age 10, absence-like attacks, and generalized tonic–clonic seizures. Her karyotype revealed 22% r(20).

Epidemiology

Even though they represent rare causes of epilepsy, genetic disorders and chromosomal abnormalities have been shown to represent 2–3% of all cases of epilepsy (Berkovic 1997). The exact prevalence of ring chromosome 20 syndrome is unknown. It is certainly a rare cause of epilepsy; about 60 cases have been reported in the literature (Jacobs *et al.* 2008) but it is believed that the disorder is probably underdiagnosed.

Pathology and physiology

The pathophysiology is poorly understood. It is known that the formation of the ring chromosome is associated with loss of telomeric material on both arms of the chromosome. In the case of the ring chromosome 20, these telomeric or terminal deletions have been demonstrated by cytogenetic techniques (Brandt *et al.* 1993). The most commonly accepted pathophysiological hypothesis is that the deleted regions (p13 and q13) of chromosome 20 contain important genes, and that their loss leads to the development of epilepsy with or without other clinical manifestations. Among the genes located in these regions, two have already been shown to cause epileptic syndromes and represent potential candidates: *KCNQ2* and *CHRNA4* (Serrano-Castro *et al.* 2001). They are both located on the telemetric region of the long arm of chromosome 20 (20q). The gene *KCNQ2* encodes for the voltage-gated potassium channel KQT-like subfamily member 2 and is known to be responsible for benign familial neonatal convulsions type 1. The gene *CHRNA4* encodes for the α4-subunit of the neuronal nicotinic acetylcholine receptor and is known to cause autosomal dominant nocturnal frontal lobe epilepsy type 1. This has led to the hypothesis that patients with ring chromosome 20 have nocturnal frontal lobe seizures because this gene is deleted. In summary, the deletion of one or both of the genes would put this epileptic syndrome into the group of disorders called channelopathies.

Another pathophysiological hypothesis was proposed by Biraben *et al.* (2004). They demonstrated reduced dopamine uptake in the putamen and caudate nuclei in patients with ring chromosome 20 syndrome, using ^{18}F-fluoro-l-dopa positron emission tomography (PET) studies. They postulated that dopaminergic reduction leads to impaired seizure interruption.

The brain pathology of one case was reported in the literature (Jacobs *et al.* 2008). This patient had ring chromosome 20 in 100% of the lymphocytes studied. His brain pathology did not reveal any abnormality. No other pathological studies have been reported but abnormalities have been suspected on magnetic resonance imaging (MRI) in a minority of patients; mainly focal atrophy and focal cortical dysplasia (Inoue *et al.* 1997). Functional studies and EEG of some patients were

The Causes of Epilepsy, eds. S. D. Shorvon, F. Andermann, and R. Guerrini. Published by Cambridge University Press. © Cambridge University Press 2011.

described to show focal abnormalities, most of the time associated with normal brain MRI.

Clinical features

The cardinal clinical features of ring chromosome 20 are epilepsy, often intractable, mild to moderate cognitive impairment, and behavior disorder. Typically there is no significant dysmorphism. Less commonly, mild dysmorphic features are present, such as microcephaly, growth delay, strabismus, high arched palate, micrognathia, downslanting palpebral fissures, and ear abnormalities.

The most consistent clinical feature described is epilepsy. Seizure onset is typically at around 3 to 5 years of age. The epilepsy generally progresses in severity and becomes refractory to antiepileptic medications. Concomitantly, patients typically present cognitive regression. As the epilepsy progresses, they develop episode(s) of non-convulsive status epilepticus. A significant number of patients develop behavior disorder. Etiological diagnosis is often delayed because most patients do not have dysmorphic features.

For most patients described in the literature, the genetic abnormality consisted of mosaicism. Some authors studied and established a clear relationship between the severity of the clinical features and the degree of mosaicism (Nishiwaki et al. 2005). More precisely, dysmorphic features, degree of mental retardation or cognitive slowing, and age at seizure onset are related to the percentage of abnormal lymphocytes. However, the severity of the epilepsy does not seem to correlate well with the degree of mosaicism (Inoue et al. 1997).

Epilepsy in the disease

As mentioned above, the only consistent clinical feature of this syndrome is epilepsy. Seizures are reported in 76–100% of patients (Canevini et al. 1998; Kobayashi et al. 1998). Seizure onset ranges from the first day of life to 14 years, with a mean age of onset at 4.5 years (Inoue et al. 1997).

Typical seizure types are short-lasting partial motor seizures and episodes of non-convulsive status epilepticus. These are characterized by a prolonged confusional state and clouding of consciousness, which may fluctuate, with or without mutism, inattentiveness, perseveration, slowness of response, and an expressionless face. Throughout the course, seizures become more frequent and prolonged, lasting between 10 and 50 min. Other seizure types may occur, e.g., nocturnal frontal lobe seizures (Augustijn et al. 2001), generalized tonic–clonic seizures, and complex partial seizures with fear and in some cases hallucinations.

Seizures are typically resistant to all antiepileptic drugs and the prognosis for seizure control is poor. However, only a few studies have looked at long-term prognosis (Kobayashi et al. 1998, Roubertie et al. 2000, Augustijn et al. 2001, De Falco et al. 2006). De Falco and colleagues (2006) reported a patient

who was followed for 25 years; with time, they observed worsening of both clinical and EEG features.

Diagnostic tests for the disease
Genetic tests

This disorder is typically sporadic. To date, only one family with more than one affected member has been described: a phenotypically normal mother with ring chromosome 20 who had two symptomatic children (Back et al. 1989).

The diagnosis is made by karyotype analysis. Since the majority of patients are mosaic, at least 100 mitoses should be examined when the diagnosis is strongly suspected. It is of note that the mosaicism is typically post-zygotic. The karyotype result will be reported as the presence of a ring chromosome 20 in a certain percentage of mitoses studied; the other chromosome 20 as well as the remaining chromosomes are normal.

Electroencephalogram studies

The EEG may help in suggesting the diagnosis. Typical EEG features are seen on both the interictal and ictal EEG. One of the most characteristic EEG findings, when the patient is in non-convulsive status epilepticus, consists of high-amplitude rhythmic slow delta activity (2–3 Hz) with superimposed spikes or spike-and-wave discharges, maximally seen over both frontal regions. These spikes are described as being less "spiky" and of lower amplitude compared with those found in typical absence status. The other seizure types (e.g., generalized tonic–clonic seizures and motor seizures) do not show any typical EEG abnormality other than the EEG changes known to be associated with the specific seizure type.

The interictal EEG shows typical abnormalities consisting of background slowing with diffuse 1–3 Hz-slow waves, often predominating over both frontal regions, with intermingled sharp waves and spikes (Inoue et al. 1997; Augustijn et al. 2001). Sometimes, the interictal EEG shows slowing in the theta range; again, a non-specific finding. Polyspikes and waves during non rapid eye movement (REM) sleep have also been described. Rarely, the EEG may show some lateralizing features or be clearly lateralized (Inoue et al. 1997). With time, the EEG background deteriorates (Inoue et al. 1997, De Falco et al. 2006). Sometimes, the interictal EEG may be normal or may show unilateral or bilateral sharp and slow waves without specific features.

Neuroimaging

Neuroimaging, including high-resolution MRI and other imaging techniques, is typically normal. Occasional cases are reported with focal abnormalities on MRI such as cortical dysplasia or focal atrophy (Inoue et al. 1997). On the other hand, it is not unusual to have focal single photon emission computed tomography (SPECT) abnormalities (Inoue et al. 1997).

Neuropsychological evaluations

It is well recognized that patients with ring chromosome 20 syndrome have cognitive slowing and behavioral difficulties (Inoue *et al.* 1997; Alpman *et al.* 2005). The degree of cognitive slowing correlates with the degree of mosaicism (Nishiwaki *et al.* 2005). The spectrum of IQ is wide, including patients with moderate to severe mental retardation, with IQ scores as low as 47 and patients with normal IQ (Inoue *et al.* 1997).

Principles of management

It is very well known that this epilepsy syndrome is refractory to antiepileptic medications. Only one case of seizure control by antiepileptic medications has been reported (Lancman *et al.* 1993). There are no specific antiepileptic drugs recommended for these patients but occasional good results have been obtained with a combination of valproate and lamotrigine (Vignoli *et al.* 2009).

In this syndrome, there seems to be no place for resective surgery; this was performed in one patient with ring chromosome 20 and focal cortical dysplasia with no improvement in seizure control (Inoue *et al.* 1997).

Reports on vagal nerve stimulation are somewhat contradictory. Chawla *et al.* (2002) and Parr *et al.* (2006) reported a 6-year-old and an 8-year-old patient who underwent vagal nerve stimulator implantation. Both showed improvement in seizure control. The patient reported by the second group showed improvement both in terms of ambulation and social interaction. Alpman *et al.* (2005), on the other hand, reported a patient who did not respond to this modality of treatment.

References

Alpman A, Serdaroglu G, Cogulu O, *et al.* (2005) Ring chromosome 20 syndrome with intractable epilepsy. *Dev Med Child Neurol* **47**:343–6.

Atkins L, Miller WL, Salam M (1972) A ring-20 chromosome. *J Med Genet* **9**:377–80.

Augustijn PB, Parra J, Wouters CH, *et al.* (2001) Ring chromosome 20 epilepsy syndrome in children: electroclinical features. *Neurology* **57**:1108–11.

Back E, Voiculescu I, Brunger M, Wolff G (1989) Familial ring (20) chromosomal mosaicism. *Hum Genet* **83**:148–54.

Berkovic SF (1997) Genetics of epilepsy syndromes. In: Engel J Jr., Pedley TA (eds.) *Epilepsy: A Comprehensive Textbook*. Philadelphia, PA: Lippincott-Raven, pp. 217–24.

Biraben A, Semah F, Ribeiro MJ, *et al.* (2004) PET evidence for a role of the basal ganglia in patients with ring chromosome 20 epilepsy. *Neurology* **63**:73–7.

Brandt CA, Kierkegaard O, Hindkjaer J, *et al.* (1993) Ring chromosome 20 with loss of telomeric sequences detected by multicolour PRINS. *Clin Genet* **44**:26–31.

Canevini MP, Sgro V, Zuffardi O, *et al.* (1998) Chromosome 20 ring: a chromosomal disorder associated with a particular electro-clinical pattern. *Epilepsia* **39**:942–51.

Chawla J, Sucholeiki R, Jones C, Silver K (2002) Intractable epilepsy with ring chromosome 20 syndrome treated with vagal nerve stimulation: case report and review of the literature. *J Child Neurol* **17**:778–80.

De Falco FA, Olivieri P, De Falco A, *et al.* (2006) Electroclinical evolution in ring chromosome 20 epilepsy syndrome: a case with severe phenotypic features followed for 25 years. *Seizures* **15**:449–53.

De Grouchy J, Plachot M, Sebaoun M, Bouchard R (1972) Chromosome F en anneau (46,XY,Fr) chez un garçon multimalformé. *Ann Genet* **15**:121–6.

Faed M, Morton HG, Robertson J (1972) Ring F chromosome mosaicism (46, XY,20r–46,XY) in an epileptic child without apparent haematological disease. *J Med Genet* **9**:470–3.

Inoue Y, Fujiwara T, Matsuda K, *et al.* (1997) Ring chromosome 20 and nonconvulsive status epilepticus: a new epileptic syndrome. *Brain* **120**:939–53.

Jacobs J, Bernard G, Andermann E, Dubeau F, Andermann F (2008) Refractory and lethal status epilepticus in a patient with ring chromosome 20 syndrome. *Epilept Disord* **10**(4):1–6.

Kobayashi K, Inagaki M, Sasaki M, *et al.* (1998) Characteristic EEG findings in ring 20 chromosome as a diagnostic clue. *Electroencephalogr Clin Neurophysiol* **107**:258–62.

Lancman ME, Penry JK, Asconape JJ, Brotherton TA (1993) Number 20 ring chromosome: a case with complete seizure control. (Letter.) *J Child Neurol* **8**:186–7.

Nishiwaki T, Hirano M, Kumazawa M, Ueno S (2005) Mosaicism and phenotype in ring chromosome 20 syndrome. *Acta Neurol Scand* **111**:205–8.

Parr JR, Pang K, Mollett A, *et al.* (2006) Epilepsy responds to vagus nerve stimulation in ring chromosome 20 syndrome. *Dev Med Child Neurol* **48**:80.

Roubertie A, Petit J, Genton P (2000) Chromosome 20 en anneau: un syndrome épileptique identifiable. *Rev Neurol (Paris)* **156**:149–53.

Serrano-Castro PJ, Aguilar-Castillo MJ, Olivares-Romero J, Jiménez-Machado R, Molina-Aparicio MJ (2001) Ring chromosome 20: an epileptic channel disorder? *Rev Neurol* **32**:237–41.

Uchida IA, Lin CC (1972) Ring formation of chromosomes Nos. 19 and 20. *Cytogenetics* **11**:208–15.

Vignoli A, Canevini MP, Darra F, *et al.* (2009) Ring chromosome 20 syndrome: a link between epilepsy onset and neuropsychological impairment in three children. *Epilepsia* **50**:2420–7.

Chapter

Hemimegalencephaly

M. Scott Perry and Michael Duchowny

Introduction

Hemimegalencephaly is a rare congenital brain malformation characterized by excessive growth of one cerebral hemisphere frequently associated with hemiparesis, hemianopia, psychomotor retardation, and refractory epilepsy. Hemimegalencephaly often presents in early infancy with either cerebral hemisphere affected, and occurs in every ethnic group and both genders (Flores-Sarnat 2002). Between one and three cases per 1000 children with epilepsy and up to 14% of those with abnormalities of cortical development have hemimegalencephaly (DiRocco et al. 2006).

The etiology of hemimegalencephaly is unknown, and it differs from other forms of cerebral dysgenesis, in that it fails to correspond to any normal stage of human brain development (Flores-Sarnat 2002). Hemimegalencephaly is most often regarded as a disturbance of neuronal migration that occurs early in gestation. However, an abnormality of neuroepithelial cell lineage has recently been suggested as the primary cause, with the migratory disturbance and cellular proliferation existing as secondary features (Flores-Sarnat 2003). This is supported by the discovery of several genes that influence body symmetry and cellular proliferation early in gestation, thus suggesting hemimegalencephaly is a genetically programmed developmental disorder (Flores-Sarnat 2002, 2003).

Grossly, the affected hemisphere is enlarged and malformed (agyria, polymicrogyria, pachygyria, lissencephaly), with involvement of the entire hemisphere or individual lobes interspersed with apparently normal brain (DiRocco et al. 2006). In general, the posterior regions of the affected hemisphere are more clearly involved. Histologically, the cortex lacks normal lamination; there are prominent heterotopic giant neurons organized abnormally within the cortical layers and ectopically present within the white matter (Flores-Sarnat, 2003; DiRocco et al. 2006). Pathologically, there are no distinct characteristics to differentiate the various subtypes and associated syndromes of hemimegalencephaly, thus suggesting hemimegalencephaly may be a common result of several genetic disorders (Flores-Sarnat 2003).

Three subtypes of hemimegalencephaly are presently recognized. In the isolated form, unilateral hemispheric enlargement is the sole manifestation. The rarest type, regarded as "total" hemimegalencephaly, is characterized by unilateral enlargement of the brainstem and cerebellum, in addition to the ipsilateral cerebral hemisphere. The syndromic form, a finding in several well-recognized disorders, is associated with somatic hemihypertrophy, cutaneous manifestations, or systemic involvement (Flores-Sarnat 2002).

In epidermal nevus syndrome, affected patients present with diverse cutaneous lesions, linear nevus sebaceous of Jadassohn being most common. Ipsilateral hemifacial hypertrophy is often associated, along with skeletal and ocular abnormalities. Proteus syndrome is characterized by unilateral or generalized somatic hypertrophy with hyperpigmentation of the skin and skeletal involvement. Klippel–Trénaunay–Weber syndrome is less frequently associated with hemimegalencephaly and presents with hemicorporal hypertrophy with vascular nevi. Hypomelanosis of Ito consists of a linear area of depigmentation either ipsilateral or contralateral to the cerebral malformation. Other common neurocutaneous disorders such as neurofibromatosis type I and tuberous sclerosis are rarely associated with hemimegalencephaly.

Macrocephaly or cranial asymmetry may be noted at birth, though normocephaly is frequently encountered. Subsequent rapid enlargement of head circumference has been reported within the first months of life concordant with progressive growth of the cerebral hemisphere. Clinical signs of increased intracranial pressure are absent (Laurence 1964). Global developmental retardation is common, and a spectrum of language delay is often present, with some affected individuals learning to speak simple sentences while others demonstrate a total lack of speech. Varying degrees of hemiparesis occur contralateral to the hemimegalencephalic hemisphere, though some patients have no focal motor deficit (Flores-Sarnat 2002). Hemianopia is invariably present, but may be difficult to document conclusively in young infants.

The Causes of Epilepsy, eds. S. D. Shorvon, F. Andermann, and R. Guerrini. Published by Cambridge University Press. © Cambridge University Press 2011.

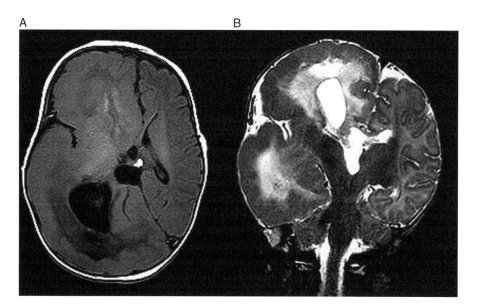

Fig. 44.1. (A) Axial T1-weighted (TR = 600 ms/TE = 10ms) and (B) coronal T2-weighted (TR = 54167 ms/TE = 117 ms) MR images of a 2-week-old neonate with right hemisphere hemimegalencephaly. Note the diffuse enlargement of the right hemisphere with midline shift towards the left, in addition to extensive right cerebral cortical thickening and colpocephaly.

Epilepsy manifestations

More striking than the associated physical manifestations of hemimegalencephaly is the frequent relentless progression of early-onset seizures towards catastrophic epilepsy. Epilepsy occurs in up to 93% of patients with hemimegalencephaly, and seizures often begin within the first days of life; seizure onset after 6 months of age is rare (Vigevano *et al.* 1996). Partial seizures, seldom with secondary generalization, are the most frequent initial seizure type, often presenting as contralateral hemibody motor seizures, eye deviation, or oral automatisms. Tonic seizures, infantile spasms, and myoclonic seizures may also be encountered. Seizures are generally frequent, often occurring daily, and are notoriously refractory to antiepileptic drugs.

Hemimegalencephaly may be the primary etiology of several epilepsy syndromes. In Ohtahara syndrome, tonic seizures, frequently asymmetric, present early in association with a burst suppression pattern. West syndrome (infantile spasms with hypsarrhythmia) is another frequently encountered epilepsy type with infantile spasms present in up to 50% of patients with hemimegalencephaly (Dulac *et al.* 1994). Many patients evolve to the Lennox–Gastaut syndrome after the first year of life or rarely to epilepsia partialis continua (Flores-Sarnat 2002; DiRocco *et al.* 2006).

Diagnosis

The diagnosis of hemimegalencephaly is made definitively by magnetic resonance imaging (MRI) examination; however, early detection using postnatal cranial ultrasound and computed tomography (CT) is possible (Lam *et al.* 1992). There are no significant differences in the neuroimaging findings of the three subtypes of hemimegalencephaly (Flores-Sarnat 2002). The most frequent radiological correlates of hemimegalencephaly include marked cerebral asymmetry due to enlargement of one hemisphere, dysplastic cortex, and ventricular deformation (Fig. 44.1). The affected ventricle may demonstrate straightening of the frontal horn, minimal to extreme dilation of the lateral ventricle, or colpocephaly. A variety of neuronal migration disorders including pachygyria, polymicrogyria, and other dysplastic features are often present and produce distinct cortical MRI changes characterized by thickened gyri with poor gray/white matter differentiation.

Functional imaging characteristics using positron emission tomography (PET) and single photon emission computed tomography (SPECT) have also been reported (Konkol *et al.* 1990; Rintahaka *et al.* 1993; Alfonso *et al.* 1998; Soufflet *et al.* 2004). In a single study of eight patients with hemimegalencephaly and refractory epilepsy, cerebral hypometabolism was present within the affected hemisphere, though evidence of cortical hypometabolism within the opposite hemisphere was present in some patients, and suggested a poorer prognosis for seizure freedom following hemispherectomy (Rintahaka *et al.* 1993).

Brain SPECT imaging most often reveals hypoperfusion of the malformed hemisphere in the interictal state and hyperperfusion during the ictus. The perfusion patterns are widespread, but similar despite different electroencephalogram (EEG) and seizure patterns (Konkol *et al.* 1990; Alfonso *et al.* 1998). Soufflet *et al.* (2004) demonstrated a progressive hyperperfusion within the normal hemisphere using SPECT over the first 2 years of life which was consistent with evolution of interictal EEG abnormalities within the normal hemisphere over the same time. Hyperperfusion normalized following hemispherectomy and resolution of EEG abnormalities suggesting that early intervention is important to avoid future dysfunction of the uninvolved hemisphere.

The EEG findings in hemimegalencephaly are varied, but often fit within three commonly reported patterns which may have value for the prognosis of neurodevelopmental outcome

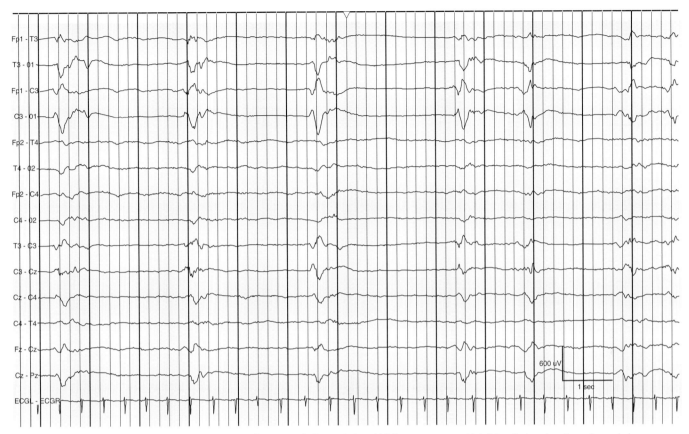

Fig. 44.2. EEG pattern of left hemispheric triphasic complexes recorded in a 10-day-old full-term neonate with left hemisphere hemimegalencephaly and neonatal seizures (neonatal AP bipolar montage, sensitivity 30 µV/mm).

(Paladin *et al.* 1989). The first is a burst-suppression pattern that typically appears at birth or in the first months of life and is often associated with infantile spasms. The EEG demonstrates bursts of alpha-like activity interspersed with quiescent phases over the affected hemisphere, while the unaffected hemisphere demonstrates the high-amplitude polymorphic polyspikes more typically encountered in burst suppression (Paladin *et al.* 1989). Outcome in this pattern is not well defined and appears to relate primarily to resolution of the associated seizures.

Another pattern of triphasic complexes with an initial small negative spike followed by large-amplitude positive spike and slow wave is present in the first days to weeks of life and is associated with poor psychomotor development (Paladin *et al.* 1989) (Fig. 44.2). Still other children may demonstrate an asymmetric high amplitude "alpha-like" activity which is non-reactive and predominates over the affected hemisphere (Paladin *et al.* 1989). This pattern tends to develop later in infancy and is associated with more favorable developmental outcome, in that children often learn to walk and speak (Paladin *et al.* 1989).

Management

Seizure control is the primary goal of management in most children with hemimegalencephaly. The choice of antiepileptic medication rests largely on the seizure type present in each case. Corticosteroids, vigabatrin, valproic acid, and topiramate are often used in children with infantile spasms, while almost every other available antiepileptic medication has been used for partial onset seizures. Multiple drug regimens and frequent substitutions are common, as the high seizure frequency in hemimegalencephaly allows rapid determination of medical intractability.

Hemispherectomy is the therapeutic option of choice for intractable epilepsy. Early intervention is favored to reduce the high morbidity, mortality, and neurodevelopmental regression associated with catastrophic epilepsy (Flores-Sarnat 2002; Obeid *et al.* 2008). Significant reduction in seizure frequency is obtained in the majority of patients after hemispherectomy with at least 60% achieving seizure control (DiRocco *et al.* 2006; Obeid *et al.* 2008). The selection of surgical candidates is not absolute, as the postsurgical outcome of patients with hemimegalencephaly is not as favorable as those with other hemispheric syndromes such as Sturge–Weber and Rasmussen encephalitis (Soufflet *et al.* 2004).

Specific attention to the function and structure of the uninvolved cerebral hemisphere is of utmost importance as the "uninvolved" hemisphere may not be functionally normal. Contralateral cortical malformations are a relative contraindication for hemispherectomy (Obeid *et al.* 2008). Glucose hypometabolism in the unaffected hemisphere on PET suggests an underlying structural lesion that may be associated with a less favorable outcome (Rintahaka *et al.* 1993). Electroencephalographic abnormalities inevitably progress to involve the contralateral hemisphere; thus careful determination of unilateral seizure onset is necessary. These EEG findings may resolve in the unaffected hemisphere following hemispherectomy performed early in the course of the disease (Soufflet *et al.* 2004).

Anatomic or functional hemispherectomy have been employed in patients with hemimegalencephaly and both show similar rates of postoperative seizure-freedom (DiRocco *et al.* 2006). Patients with hemimegalencephaly constitute a higher-risk population because of the technical challenges associated with operating on a megalencephalic hemisphere. Hemorrhage is the most important intraoperative risk and is further complicated by the large size and consistency of the malformed hemisphere making access to the vasculature difficult (DiRocco *et al.* 2006). Postoperative hydrocephalus is another common complication, which is predominantly present in children operated on during the first year of life (DiRocco *et al.* 2006).

Although the outcome following hemispherectomy for hemimegalencephaly is not as favorable as for other hemispheric diseases, developmental prognosis is improved compared to the dismal prognosis of unoperated hemimegalencephalic patients with catastrophic epilepsy. While fully normal development is unlikely even after complete seizure-freedom, motor development often stabilizes or improves, and cognitive skills progress (DiRocco *et al.* 2006). Unfavorable outcomes may be related to prolonged history of epilepsy, poor preoperative development, or involvement of the contralateral hemisphere.

References

Alfonso I, Papazian O, Litt R, Villalobos R, Acosta JI (1998) Similar brain SPECT findings in subclinical and clinical seizures in two neonates with hemimegalencephaly. *Pediatr Neurol* **19**:132–4.

DiRocco C, Battaglia D, Pietrini D, Piastra M, Massimi L (2006) Hemimegalencephaly: clinical implications and surgical treatment. *Childs Nerv Syst* **22**:852–66.

Dulac O, Chugani HT, Bernardina BD (1994) *Infantile Spasms and West Syndrome*. Philadelphia, PA: WB Saunders.

Flores-Sarnat L (2002) Hemimegalencephaly. I. Genetic, clinical, and imaging aspects. *J Child Neurol* **17**:373–84.

Flores-Sarnat L (2003) Hemimegalencephaly. II. Neuropathology suggests a disorder of cellular lineage. *J Child Neurol* **18**:776–85.

Konkol RJ, Maister BH, Wells RG, Sty JR (1990) Hemimegalencephaly: clinical, EEG, neuroimaging, and IMP-SPECT correlation. *Pediatr Neurol* **6**:414–18.

Lam AH, Villanueva AC, de Silva M (1992) Hemimegalencephaly cranial sonographic findings. *J Ultrasound Med* **11**:241–4.

Laurence KM (1964) A new case of unilateral megalencephaly. *Dev Med Child Neurol* **6**:585–90.

Obeid M, Wyllie E, Rahi AC, Mikati MA (2008) Approach to pediatric epilepsy surgery: state of the art. II. Approach to specific epilepsy syndromes and etiologies. *Eur J Paediatr Neurol* **13**:115–27.

Paladin F, Chiron C, Dulac O, Plouin P, Ponsot G (1989) Electroencephalographic aspects of hemimegalencephaly. *Dev Med Child Neurol* **31**:377–83.

Rintahaka PJ, Chugani HT, Messa C, Phelps M (1993) Hemimegalencephaly: evaluation with positron emission tomography. *Pediatr Neurol* **9**:21–8.

Soufflet C, Bulteau C, Delalande O, *et al.* (2004) The nonmalformed hemisphere is secondarily impaired in young children with hemimegalencephaly: a pre- and postsurgery study with SPECT and EEG. *Epilepsia* **45**:1375–82.

Vigevano F, Fusco L, Granata T (1996) Hemimegalencephaly: clinical and EEG characteristics. In: Guerrini R, Andermann F, Canapichi R, Roger J, Zifkin B, Pfanner P (eds.) *Dysplasias of Cerebral Cortex and Epilepsy*. Philadelphia, PA: Lippincott-Raven, pp. 285–94.

Focal cortical dysplasia and related variants

Ruben I. Kuzniecky

Introduction

Since its original description more than 35 years ago by Taylor (Taylor *et al.* 1971), focal cortical dysplasia (FCD) has now evolved to encompass a number of associated disorders. Although these disorders may share a number of pathologic substrates they may not necessarily share similar underlying pathophysiologic mechanisms and origin. This fact underscores the little progress we have made since recognizing that FCD is an important cause of intractable epilepsy (Kuzniecky *et al.* 1988; Palmini *et al.* 1991; Cotter *et al.* 1999; Becker *et al.* 2002; Bingaman 2004; Fauser *et al.* 2004; Bast *et al.* 2006; Kuzniecky 2006).

The development of the human brain is a complex process that begins with the formation of the notochord and continues after birth. Any disruption of the normal mechanisms responsible for the formation of the cerebral structure will result in a malformation due to abnormal cortical development (MCD). A wide variety of genetic and environmental factors can cause a disturbance in these developmental processes and can therefore lead to an abnormality in the mature brain (Barkovich *et al.* 2005). Focal cortical dysplasia is a definable disorder among the MCD and as such it should be recognized and diagnosed accordingly.

Pathology

Focal cortical dysplasia is characterized by the presence of abnormal cortical organization of different degrees with or without the presence of large abnormal cells (Taylor *et al.* 1971). These changes are often restricted to a small or larger cortical area but in most patients do not involve an entire hemisphere or lobe. The specific histological features include loss of the normal cortical lamination with abnormal pyramidal cell orientation, altered dendritic arborizations, cytomegalic cells, and larger pale cells termed balloon cells. Focal cortical dysplasia is classified into two or more types depending on a classification scheme that we proposed several decades ago (Kuzniecky 1994; Palmini *et al.* 2004). It is the presence of balloon cells that differentiates FCD type I

(without balloon cells) from FCD type II (with balloon cells) and that leads to the distinction in the most used classification scheme. This distinction is based on the possible pathophysiologic processes underlying this malformation (see below).

Pathophysiology and animal models

The pathologic hallmarks of FCD are: (1) cortical dyslamination, (2) dysmorphic cells, and (3) balloon cells. Although several animal models of FCD have been proposed none captures all the features seen in patients. The uterine irradiation rat model causes abnormal lamination but in general lacks the focal nature and the presence of large dysmorphic cells (Roper 1998). Similarly, other models such as the one induced by methylazoxymethanol acetate (MAM) and the neonatal freeze lesions (Hablitz and DeFazio 2000) do not share all the pathologic abnormalities seen in FCD. Finally, *TSC2* mutants such as the Eker rat are better models of tuberous sclerosis than of FCD as no consistent demonstrable cortical focal lesions are seen in these animals (Yeung 2002).

We have recently proposed that FCD can be viewed mechanically as a disorder of abnormal gyral formation. At the end of migration (20–24 weeks gestational age), the cortical surface is still predominantly smooth. However, during the second half of gestation multiple fissures develop driven by the need to accommodate a larger neuronal volume (cells and axons). A model based on the mechanical properties of the cerebral cortex, combined with the mechanical characteristics of the axial and glial bundles pulling radially, results in the development of convolutions. Taking into consideration this model (Hua and Crino 2003), one can hypothesize that a focal injury to the developing brain during proliferation can induce a focal lesion. This hypothesis is supported by the finding of unrelated clonal cell lineages in FCD (Hua and Crino 2003). Alternatively, a somatic mutation in one of the neuronal progenitor cells can explain the wedge-like extension of FCDs because clonally related neurons share the same distribution (Ware *et al.* 1999). There are many examples of single-gene defects

The Causes of Epilepsy, eds. S. D. Shorvon, F. Andermann, and R. Guerrini. Published by Cambridge University Press. © Cambridge University Press 2011.

that lead to abnormal cortical development, but most cases of human FCD can be attributed to a combination of environmental and genetic factors.

The molecular mechanisms mediating epileptogenesis in FCD are not well understood despite the fact that FCD is one of nature's best models for intrinsic epileptogenicity. Experimental data suggest that in some animal models there are decreased numbers of GABAergic interneurons whereas in other models, an increased glutamatergic dysfunction has been reported (Avoli *et al.* 1999). The role of abnormal astrocytes is another possible source for increased excitation and epilepsy as glia are crucial in the enzymatic conversion of glutamate (Lurton *et al.* 2002).

Clinical and electroencephalographic features

Patients with FCD have a heterogeneous clinical picture that can present in almost any type and at any age. Yet while there are no clinical features that are specific for FCD as a whole, there are some factors that create a strong suspicion that an FCD may underlie the epilepsy; these factors include an association with developmental delay and static focal neurologic deficits, frequent seizures from an early onset, or focal status epilepticus. While such features may create suspicion, it must be emphasized that none of them is specific for an FCD.

The severity of seizures in patients with FCD also varies enormously. There are some individuals with large FCD who have relatively few seizures. On the other hand, there are some individuals with relatively small FCD who have very severe and intractable epilepsy. The mechanism of seizure generation in these abnormalities is complex and generally poorly understood.

The clinical manifestations of patients with cortical FCD are variable. More often than not, seizures begin in the first decade of life but usually after age 2 to 3 years. However, seizures may be the presenting clinical problem in the second decade or thereafter. We have encountered patients with seizure onset in the sixth decade. Simple or pure motor seizures, complex partial seizures, or secondary generalized attacks are common. Interestingly, seizures often occur in clusters, but generalized status epilepticus is rare, except in patients with FCD involving the central region. Epilepsia partialis continua and intractable focal myoclonus has been reported (Kuzniecky *et al.* 1988).

In our experience, the majority of patients have extratemporal cortical dysplasia with the pre- and postcentral region being the most frequently affected. This anatomical localization is shared with other MCD such as polymicrogyria (Kuzniecky *et al.* 1991). It is possible that both of these MCD share genes crucial to the development of the central cortex or that the central cortical area is vulnerable to injury resulting in a focal lesion.

Focal cortical dysplasia involving the temporal lobe has also been recognized (Kuzniecky *et al.* 1991) and it may have a different clinical pattern from the above, more common, extratemporal pattern. These patients may present at any age with temporal lobe seizures. The pathology is often FCD type I with a paucity of balloon cells and the age of onset tends to be later than in the previous group. Although pure cortical localization is seen in some patients, involvement of both medial and lateral neocortical structures is common.

Electroencephalographic features

The interictal scalp electroencephalogram (EEG) may demonstrate focal ictal-like activity over the dysplastic lesions, underscoring their high epileptogenicity. However, there is no clear correlation between the interictal EEG and imaging features in FCD.

In patients with FCD EEG studies have reported continuous epileptiform discharges (CEDs) in FCD and these EEG findings correlate with greater surgical success (Palmini *et al.* 1995). The intrinsic hyperexcitability of abnormal cortex in FCD has been confirmed in numerous studies using in vitro recordings and drug applications. Increased intrinsic excitability has been observed by paired pulse stimulation experiments. In addition, fast propagation from neocortex to mesial temporal regions occurs.

Ictal EEG studies have suggested that FCD is a neural network disorder with secondary ictal zones. Intraictal activation is typical of FCD and can be contiguous or at a distance from the primary epileptogenic area (Duchowny 2009).

Imaging features

Most FCD are amenable to diagnosis by brain magnetic resonance imaging (MRI) alone as computed tomography (CT) scan is insensitive and positron emission tomography (PET) studies are non-specific for the pathology. The classical MRI findings consist of abnormal gyral thickening and abnormal gyral architecture with or without underlying T2-weighted gray and/or white matter changes. Focal increased signal changes on T2-weighted images involving the gray–white matter junction and subcortical white matter and to a lesser degree the cortex are observed. Blurring of the gray–white matter junction and focal cortical thickening are however the hallmarks. These abnormalities can be circumscribed in nature but can be extensive, involving more than one gyrus or lobe. High-resolution MRIs with thin slices and multiplanar reconstruction are often necessary to make the diagnosis (Barkovich *et al.* 2001) (Fig. 45.1). A number of variations have been reported such as transmantle cortical dysplasia and bottom of the sulcus FCD where the abnormality is very small and restricted to the bottom of the sulcus. These entities are further described below.

Transmantle cortical dysplasia (TCD) was described by us a few years ago as a subtype of FCD (Barkovich *et al.* 1997). These patients have onset of epilepsy from infancy to early adulthood and share clinical and EEG findings with patients with typical FCD. Pathology shows similar findings to those with Taylor's FCD but the imaging findings differentiate this

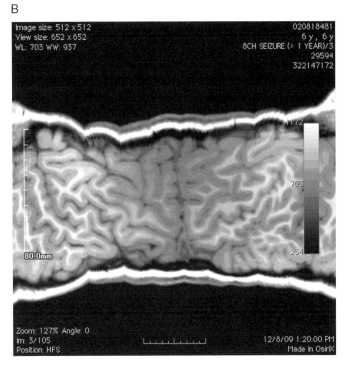

Fig. 45.1. (A) Axial T2-weighted MRI image shows an area of cortical thickness in the right parietal region consistent with FCD. The lesion extends into the adjacent white matter. (B) T1-weighted manipulation shows the abnormal gyration on the same area with more accuracy.

entity from classical FCD. In TCD, the imaging abnormality extends from the ventricle to the cerebral cortex. Signal abnormality extends radially inward toward the lateral ventricle from the cortical surface on T2-weighted or fluid-attenuated inversion recovery (FLAIR) imaging. The lesions are most often small but a few patients have large abnormalities with abnormal cortical gyration. It is thought that this particular malformation stems from a disorder affecting the radial–glial neuronal unit.

Bottom of the sulcus FCD (BOSD) is another subtype of FCD. This entity is clinically important because it appears to be a highly focal epileptogenic lesion, and has an excellent prognosis for seizure control following focal resection. The most common imaging findings are typical of FCD as previously described. In these patients the lesions are very small and can be restricted to the bottom of the sulcus. A recent study showed this localization in 70% of patients. A characteristic feature of BOSD is the funnel-shaped structure directed towards the ependymal surface (Fig. 45.2), present in most cases. Partial volume effect could sometimes make this hard to see even if present. In some patients a focal widening of the subarachnoid space can be appreciated (Fig. 45.3). The pathological features of a few resection specimens have been identical to those of typical FCD.

The major problem with these lesions is that they are often small, subtle, and easily missed on initial examination of the images. Diagnosis is aided by having images with good signal-to-noise ratio so that the blurring of the gray–white matter

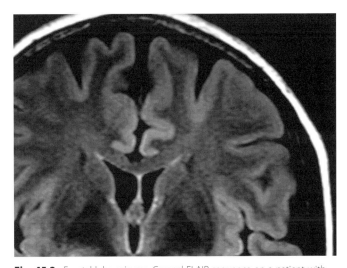

Fig. 45.2. Frontal lobe seizures. Coronal FLAIR sequence on a patient with transmantle cortical FCD. Note the abnormal sulcus with area of thickness and underlying white matter changes extending towards the ventricle.

junction at the bottom of the sulcus can be properly appreciated as well as the increased signal intensity of the cortex and underlying white matter on T2-weighted images.

The extent and the localization in BOSD distinguishes it from TCD or other FCDs. The absence of gross gyration abnormalities is also typical of BOSD. Furthermore, the postsurgical outcome appears to be excellent since the lesions are often very small and surgically accessible.

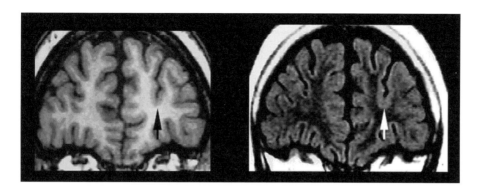

Fig. 45.3. Frontal lobe seizures in a 6-year-old child. The coronal T1-weighted and FLAIR images show a small bottom of the sulcus FCD (arrows). The underlying white matter appears normal.

Some disorders, such as FCD without balloon cells and microdysgenesis, usually require histopathological study before a final classification is established (Barkovich *et al.* 2005).

Future directions

There are two main challenges facing workers in the FCD field today. The first is how can we improve the detection of these lesions in patients with focal epilepsy. It is likely that a large percentage of patients with cryptogenic focal epilepsy have various forms of FCD or related malformations. The second challenge is the management of these patients, in particular the surgical treatment strategies.

Advances in MRI are likely to incrementally improve the detection of FCD. First are techniques based on improved imaging hardware. New sequences such as susceptibility-weighted imaging (SWI) and perfusion–diffusion imaging may provide evidence of focal dysfunction. Surface coils or multichannel coils can provide increased sensitivity in the detection of FCD (Goyal *et al.* 2004). Increased field strength at 3 and 7 T has demonstrated improved signal-to-noise ratio and resolution with smaller voxel size. Improved contrast can

also be seen. Second are postprocessing techniques such as voxel-based morphometry, which uses statistical parametric mapping (SPM) to detect abnormal tissue comparing patients and controls (Woermann *et al.* 1999). In addition, cortical curvature and cortical thickness measurements have been applied to small groups of patients with FCD with encouraging results. This last methodology is particularly appealing since FCDs are cortically based lesions with thicker cortex. Finally, studies looking at diffusion tensor imaging have shown abnormal tracts as would be expected in patients with FCD.

Postsurgical outcome has been reported to be variable among series (Park *et al.* 2006; Kral *et al.* 2007). Patients with small lesions that can be resected in toto have a much better chance to be seizure-free. The challenge is the structural and functional identification of the entire lesion. This is often very difficult even when combining all imaging and electrophysiologic data. The ultimate problem is that often the lesions involve essential cortex and surgery will result in unacceptable neurologic morbidity. New surgical treatment options that combine network disconnection or disruption and augmentation such as electrical stimulation are being developed.

References

Avoli M, Bernasconi A, Mattia D, *et al.* (1999) Epileptiform discharges in the human dysplastic neocortex: in vitro physiology and pharmacology. *Ann Neurol* 46:816–26.

Bast T, Ramantani G, Seitz A, *et al.* (2006) Focal cortical dysplasia: prevalence, clinical presentation and epilepsy in children and adults. *Acta Neurol Scand* 113:72–81.

Becker AJ, Urbach H, Scheffler B, *et al.* (2002) Focal cortical dysplasia of Taylor's balloon cell type: mutational analysis of the *TSC1* gene indicates a pathogenic relationship to tuberous sclerosis. *Ann Neurol* 52:29–37.

Bingaman WE (2004) Surgery for focal cortical dysplasia. *Neurology* 62(6 Suppl 3):S30–4.

Barkovich AJ, Kuzniecky R, Jackson G, Guerrini R, Dobbyns W. A developmental and genetic classification for malformations of cortical development. *Neurology* 65: 1873–87.

Barkovich AJ, Kuzniecky RI, Dobyns WB (2001) Radiologic classification of malformations of cortical development. *Curr Opin Neurol* 14:145–9.

Barkovich AJ, Kuzniecky R, Bollen AW, *et al.* (1997) Focal transmantle dysplasia: a specific malformation of cortical development. *Neurology* 49:1148–52.

Caviness V (1989) Normal development of the cerebral cortex. In: Evrard P, Minkowski A (eds.) *Developmental Neurobiology*. New York: Raven Press, pp. 1–10.

Cotter DR, Honavar M, Everall I (1999) Focal cortical dysplasia: a neuropathological and developmental perspective. *Epilepsy Res* 36:155–64.

Duchowny M (2009) Clinical, functional, and neurophysiologic assessment of dysplastic cortical networks: implications for cortical functioning and surgical management. *Epilepsia* 50:19–27.

Fauser S, Schultze-Bonhage A, Honegger J, *et al.* (2004) Focal cortical dysplasias: surgical outcome in 67 patients in relation to histological subtypes and dual pathology. *Brain* 127:2406–18.

Goyal M, Bangert BA, Lewin JS, *et al.* (2004) High-resolution MRI enhances identification of lesions amenable to surgical therapy in children with intractable epilepsy. *Epilepsia* **45**:954–9.

Hablitz JJ, DeFazio RA (2000) Altered receptor subunit expression in rat neocortical malformations. *Epilepsia* **41**(Suppl 6):S82–5.

Hua Y, Crino PB (2003) Single cell lineage analysis in human focal cortical dysplasia. *Cereb Cortex* **13**:693–9.

Kral T, Von Lehe M, Podlogar M, *et al.* (2007) Focal cortical dysplasia: long-term seizure outcome after surgical treatment. *J Neurol Neurosurg Psychiatry* **78**:853–6.

Kuzniecky R, Berkovic S, Andermann F, *et al.* (1988) Focal cortical myoclonus and rolandic cortical dysplasia: clarification by magnetic resonance imaging. *Ann Neurol* **23**:317–25.

Kuzniecky RI (1994) Magnetic resonance imaging in developmental disorders of the cerebral cortex. *Epilepsia* **35**(Suppl 6):S44–56.

Kuzniecky RI (2006) Malformations of cortical development and epilepsy. I. Diagnosis and classification scheme. *Rev Neurol Dis* **3**:151–62.

Kuzniecky R, Morawetz R, Faught E, *et al.* (1995) Frontal and central lobe focal dysplasia: clinical, EEG and imaging features. *Dev Med Child Neurol* **37**:159–66.

Kuzniecky R, Garcia JH, Faught E, *et al.* (1991) Cortical dysplasia in temporal lobe epilepsy: magnetic resonance imaging correlations. *Ann Neurol* **29**:293–8.

Lurton D, Yacubian EM, Sanabria EG, *et al.* (2002) Immunohistochemical study of six cases of Taylor's type focal cortical dysplasia: correlation with electroclinical data. *Epilepsia* **43**(Suppl 5):217–19.

Palmini A, Andermann F, Olivier A, *et al.* (1991) Focal neuronal migration disorders and intractable partial epilepsy: results of surgical treatment. *Ann Neurol* **30**:750–7.

Palmini A, Gambardella A, Andermann F (1995) Intrinsic epileptogenicity of human dysplastic cortex as suggested by corticography and surgical results. *Ann Neurol* **37**:476–87.

Palmini A, Najm I, Avanzini G, *et al.* (2004) Terminology and classification of the cortical dysplasias. *Neurology* **62** (6 Suppl 3):S2–8.

Park CK, Kim SK, Wang KC, *et al.* (2006) Surgical outcome and prognostic factors of pediatric epilepsy caused by cortical dysplasia. *Childs Nerv Syst* **22**:586–92.

Roper SN (1998) In utero irradiation of rats as a model of human cerebrocortical dysgenesis: a review. *Epilepsy Res* **32**:63–74.

Taylor DC, Falconer MA, Bruton CJ, *et al.* (1971) Focal dysplasia of the cerebral cortex in epilepsy. *J Neurol Neurosurg Psychiat* **34**:369–87.

Ware ML, Tavazoie S, Reid C, *et al.* (1999) Coexistence of widespread clones and large radial clones in early embryonic ferret cortex. *Cereb Cortex* **9**:636–45.

Woermann FG, Sisodiya SM, Free SL, *et al.* (1999) Voxel-by-voxel comparison of automatically segmented cerebral gray matter: a rater-independent comparison of structural MRI in patients with epilepsy. *Neuroimage* **10**: 373–84.

Yeung RS (2002) Tuberous sclerosis as an underlying basis for infantile spasm. *Int Rev Neurobiol* **49**:315–32.

Chapter 46

Agyria–pachygyria band spectrum

Elena Parrini and Renzo Guerrini

Lissencephaly (LIS) (derived from the Greek words *lissos* meaning smooth and *enkephalos* meaning brain) is a neuronal migration disorder characterized by absent (agyria) or decreased (pachygyria) convolutions, producing a smooth cerebral surface (Friede 1989). Several different types of LIS have been recognized. The most common, known as classical LIS or type 1 LIS, features a very thick cortex (10–20 mm vs. the normal 4 mm) and no other major brain malformations. The cytoarchitecture consists of four primitive layers, including an outer marginal layer which contains Cajal–Retzius neurons (layer 1), a superficial cellular layer, which contains numerous large and disorganized pyramidal neurons (layer 2) corresponding to the true cortex, a variable cell-sparse layer (layer 3), and a deep cellular layer (composed of medium and small neurons) which extends through more than half the width of the mantle (layer 4) (Golden and Harding 2004) (Fig. 46.1).

Subcortical band heterotopia (SBH) is a related disorder in which there are bilateral bands of gray matter interposed in the white matter, between the cortex and the lateral ventricles (Barkovich 2000) (Fig. 46.2). This may appear as a solid band of heterotopic tissue or as numerous islands of radially oriented gray matter separated by white matter. Pyramidal cells in the heterotopic band may be smaller than normal compared to those in the overlying cortex, which usually appears structurally normal, with the exception of shallow sulci (Golden and Harding 2004).

Genetic basis and diagnosis

Two major genes have been associated with classical LIS and SBH. The *LIS1* gene (OMIM* 601545) on chromosome 17p13.3 is responsible for the autosomal dominant form of LIS (Reiner *et al.* 1993), while the doublecortin gene (*DCX* or *XLIS*) (OMIM* 300121) is X-linked (des Portes *et al.* 1998; Gleeson *et al.* 1998). Although either gene can result in either LIS or SBH, most cases of classical LIS are due to deletions or mutations of *LIS1* (Mei *et al.* 2008), whereas most cases of SBH

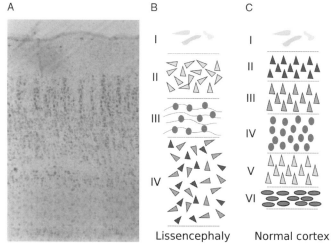

Fig. 46.1. (A) Histopathological section from a patient with lissencephaly. Scheme of (B) cortical layering in classical lissencephaly (four non-organized layers) and (C) normal cortical laminar organization (six layers).

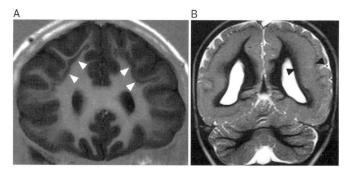

Fig. 46.2. Brain MRI: coronal sections of the brain of two young women with different mutations of the *DCX* gene. Beneath the cortex, and separated from it by a thin layer of white matter, there is a subcortical laminar (band) heterotopia showing the same signal intensity as the cortex (white arrowheads). Patient in (B) is more severely affected, as shown by the degree of simplification of the cortical pattern and the thickness of the heterotopic band (black arrowheads).

The Causes of Epilepsy, eds. S. D. Shorvon, F. Andermann, and R. Guerrini. Published by Cambridge University Press. © Cambridge University Press 2011.

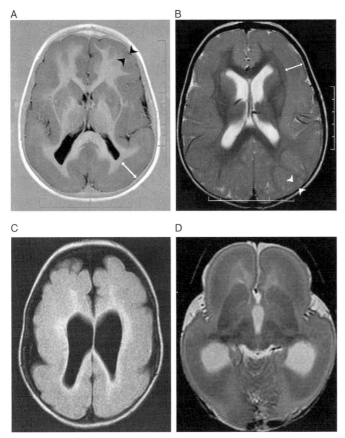

Fig. 46.3. Brain MRI of four different patients: axial sections. (A) Classical lissencephaly in a boy with *LIS1* gene mutation; (B) lissencephaly in a girl with *DCX* mutation. In (A), there is a posterior > anterior malformative gradient with relative preservation of the gyral pattern and almost normal cortical thickness in the anterior brain; cortical thickness is around 6 mm in the frontal lobes (two black arrowheads; normal cortical thickness = 4 mm) and around 3 cm in the posterior brain (white arrow). In (B), there is a typical anterior > posterior malformative pattern; cortical thickness is around 2 cm in the frontal lobes (white arrow) and around 4 mm in the posterior brain (two white arrowheads). (C) Lissencephaly in a patient with Miller–Dieker syndrome; the gyral pattern is simplified more severely in the posterior brain and the cortex is thickened. (D) Severe diffuse lissencephaly with relatively small frontal lobes in a boy with *DCX* mutation.

are due to mutations of *DCX* (Matsumoto *et al.* 2001). *LIS1*-related LIS is more severe in the posterior brain regions (posterior > anterior [p > a] gradient) (Fig. 46.3A), whereas *DCX*-related LIS is more severe in the anterior brain (anterior > posterior [a > p] gradient) (Fig. 46.3B).

The *LIS1* gene is closely related to p > a isolated LIS syndrome (ILS). About 60% of patients with p > a ILS carry genomic alterations or mutations involving *LIS1* (Uyanik *et al.* 2007; Mei *et al.* 2008). Most mutations (84%) are truncating (Cardoso *et al.* 2002). Small genomic deletions and duplications of *LIS1* occur in almost 50% of patients (Mei *et al.* 2008). The type and position of mutations of *LIS1* do not appear to correlate with the phenotype (Uyanik *et al.* 2007). A simplified gyral pattern in the posterior brain, with underlying SBH, has been associated with mosaic mutations of *LIS1* (Sicca *et al.* 2003). Miller–Dieker syndrome (MDS) is caused by deletion of *LIS1* and contiguous genes and features

severe p > a LIS (Fig. 46.3C), accompanied by distinct dysmorphic facial features and additional malformations. Deletion of two additional genes, *CRK* and *YWHAE*, telomeric to *LIS1*, may contribute to the most severe LIS grade and dysmorphic features (Cardoso *et al.* 2003).

All reported *LIS1* alterations are de novo. Nevertheless, if a *LIS1* mutation is found, it is appropriate to perform mutation analysis on both parents. Given the theoretical risk of germline mosaicism in either parent (which has never been demonstrated for *LIS1*), a couple with a child with lissencephaly is usually given a 1% recurrence risk (Guerrini and Carrozzo 2001).

Mutations in the DCX gene classically cause the SBH phenotype in females and X-linked lissencephaly (XLIS) in males. Females with *DCX* mutations have anteriorly predominant band/pachygyria of variable severity. However, women harboring missense mutations have been described, exhibiting normal brain magnetic resonance imaging (MRI) with or without epilepsy (Guerrini *et al.* 2003). Favorable X-inactivation skewing or mutations with mild functional consequences are likely to explain these milder phenotypes. Mutations of *DCX* have been found in all reported pedigrees, including families in which females have SBH and males have LIS, and in approximately 80% of sporadic females and 25% of sporadic males with SBH (Matsumoto *et al.* 2001; D'Agostino *et al.* 2002). Genomic deletions of the *DCX* gene have been identified in females with sporadic SBH and in males with X-linked lissencephaly (Mei *et al.* 2007) (Fig. 46.3D). Maternal germline or mosaic *DCX* mutations may occur in about 10% of cases of either SBH or XLIS (Gleeson *et al.* 2000a). Hemizygous males with *DCX* mutations have classical LIS, but rare boys with missense *DCX* mutations with an anteriorly predominant SBH have also been described (Pilz *et al.* 1999; Guerrini *et al.* 2003; D'Agostino *et al.* 2002).

When a mutation in the *DCX* gene is found in a boy with LIS, mutation analysis of *DCX* should be extended to the proband's mother, even if her brain MRI is normal (Guerrini *et al.* 2003). If the mother is a mutation carrier, the mutation will be transmitted according to Mendelian inheritance. If the mother is not a carrier, she can still be at risk of germline mosaicism; the risk of transmitting the mutation might roughly be estimated at around 5% (Gleeson *et al.* 2000b). For this reason, a prenatal diagnosis is indicated in every pregnancy of a woman who has a child with features of XLIS with a *DCX* mutation.

Three rarer forms of lissencephaly–pachygyria have been identified in recent years. One form, due to mutations of the *TUBA1A* gene, exhibits characteristics that are partially overlapping with the lissencephaly–SBH spectrum (Poirier *et al.* 2007). A second form, X-linked lissencephaly with absent corpus callosum and ambiguous genitalia (XLAG), results from mutations of the *ARX* gene (Kato *et al.* 2004). A third, recessive form, results from homozygous mutations of the *RELN* gene (Hong *et al.* 2000). Lissencephaly due to *ARX* and *RELN* mutations exhibits particular features that set them out of the classical lissencephaly spectrum.

Pathogenesis

The *LIS1* gene encodes a 45-kDa protein (PAFAH1B1), which functions as a regulatory subunit of platelet-activating factor acetylhydrolase (PAF-AH) (Hirotsune *et al.* 1998). PAFAH1B1 heterozygous mutant mice show a dose-dependent histopathological disorganization of cortical lamination as well as hippocampal and cerebellar cortical defects (Hirotsune *et al.* 1998). SiRNA knock-down of Lis1 in rat cortical slice cultures resulted in defects in migration, interkinetic nuclear migration, and ventricular zone/intermediate zone defects in cell division (Tsai *et al.* 2005). It has been proposed that LIS1 colocalizes with microtubules and promotes their stabilization in vitro (Sapir *et al.* 1997); however, no evidence of LIS1 colocalization with microtubules has been found in vivo (Faulkner *et al.* 2000). Further, LIS1 also interacts with NUDEL and mNudE to regulate cytoplasmic dynein motor function and location within the cell. Loss of function of either NUDEL, LIS1 or dynein impact on the microtubule network that couples the centrosome and nucleus, leading to a defect in nuclear translocation, cell migration, and positioning during cortical development (Wynshaw-Boris and Gambello 2001). The LIS1/NUDEL pathway has also been linked to the Reelin/Cdk5/p35 pathway. Recently, it has been demonstrated that Lis1 is essential for precise control of mitotic spindle orientation in neuroepithelial stem cells (Yingling *et al.* 2008).

The *DCX* gene encodes a 40-kDa microtubule-associated protein (DCX) which is expressed in migrating neuroblasts (Gleeson *et al.* 2000b). The DCX protein contains two tandem conserved repeats. Each of the repeats binds to tubulin and both repeats are necessary for microtubule polymerization and stabilization. Disrupting DCX function through RNAi in a rat model resulted in SBH (Bai *et al.* 2003). Dcx and Dclk2 (a homolog of DCX)-null mice display frequent spontaneous seizures that originate in the hippocampus, with most animals dying in the first few months of life. Both Dcx and Dclk2 are coexpressed in developing hippocampus and, in their absence, there is dosage-dependent disrupted hippocampal lamination associated with a cell-autonomous simplification of pyramidal dendritic arborizations leading to reduced inhibitory synaptic tone. These data suggest that hippocampal dysmaturation and an insufficient receptive field for inhibitory input may underlie the epilepsy in double cortex syndrome (Kerjan *et al.* 2009).

Phenotype

Classical LIS is rare, with a prevalence of about 12 per 1 000 000 births (de Rijk-van Andel *et al.* 1991). Patients with severe LIS have early developmental delay, early diffuse hypotonia, later spastic quadriplegia, and eventual severe or profound mental retardation. Patients with less severe cortical malformations have moderate mental and motor impairment and may have a normal life-span. In patients with MDS, classical LIS is accompanied by distinct dysmorphic facial features, including prominent forehead, bitemporal hollowing, flattened ear helices, mild hypertelorism, epicanthic folds, short nose and anteverted nares, prominent lateral nasal folds and round philtrum. Additional malformations may be observed. Affected children have severe psychomotor delay, epilepsy, and feeding problems.

Seizures occur in over 90% of LIS children, with onset before 6 months in about 75% of cases. About 80% of children have infantile spasms, although the electroencephalogram (EEG) does not show typical hypsarrhythmia (Guerrini and Filippi 2005). Most LIS children will subsequently continue to have epileptic spasms in association with multiple seizure types. The EEG shows diffuse, high-amplitude, fast rhythms, which are considered to be highly specific for this malformation.

The main clinical manifestations of SBH are mental retardation and epilepsy (Barkovich *et al.* 1994). Epilepsy is present in almost all patients and is intractable in about 65% of cases. About 50% of these epilepsy patients have focal seizures, and the remaining 50% have generalized epilepsy, often within the spectrum of Lennox–Gastaut syndrome. Those with more severe MRI abnormalities have significantly earlier seizure onset and are more likely to develop Lennox–Gastaut syndrome (Guerrini and Filippi 2005).

Depth electrode studies have demonstrated that epileptiform activity can originate directly from the heterotopic neurons, with nearly constant simultaneous involvement of the "true" cortex (Mai *et al.* 2003). Callosotomy has been associated with worthwhile improvement in drop attacks in a few patients (Palmini *et al.* 1991; Landy *et al.* 1993). Epilepsy surgery for focal seizures yields poor results in most patients (Bernasconi *et al.* 2001). Functional impairment of the cortex overlying the heterotopia is variable. Positron emission tomography (PET) studies suggest that the laminar heterotopia has the same metabolic activity as normal cortex (Lee *et al.* 1994) and that cerebral cortex overlying the heterotopia can either retain its expected map of functional activation or show extensive reorganization (Richardson *et al.* 1998).

TUBA1A-related lissencephaly

Mutations in the *TUBA1A* gene (mapping to chromosome 12q12–214; OMIM: *602529) have recently been identified in sporadic patients with LIS. The clinical and anatomic spectrum of severity of *TUBA1A*-related LIS appears to be wide, ranging from perisylvian cortical thickening, in the less severe form, to posteriorly predominant pachygyria in the most severe, associated with dysgenesis of the anterior limb of the internal capsule and mild to severe cerebellar hypoplasia. In addition, patients with *TUBA1A* mutations share a common clinical phenotype that consists of congenital microcephaly, mental retardation, and diplegia/tetraplegia (Poirier *et al.* 2007; Bahi Buisson *et al.* 2008). Only de novo heterozygous missense mutations in the *TUBA1A* gene have been identified so far (Poirier *et al.* 2007; Bahi Buisson *et al.* 2008).

A mutant mouse was generated with abnormalities in the laminar architecture of the hippocampus and cortex,

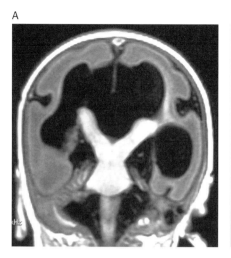
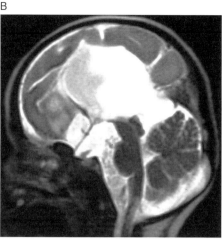

Fig. 46.4. Brain MRI: coronal section (A) and sagittal section (B) of a boy with X-linked lissencephaly, corpus callosum agenesis, and ambiguous genitalia (XLAG) due to the mutation of the *ARX* gene.

accompanied by impaired neuronal migration (Keays *et al.* 2007). This animal had a mutation in the *guanosine triphosphate (GTP) binding pocket of a-1 tubulin (Tuba1)*. Human *TUBA1A* is highly homologous to the mouse and rat *Tuba1* gene. The pattern of expression of *TUBA1A* is limited to early-born post-mitotic migrating neurons throughout development, and to specific neurogenic regions in the adult brain (Keays *et al.* 2007).

X-linked lissencephaly with absent corpus callosum and ambiguous genitalia

X-linked lissencephaly with absent corpus callosum and ambiguous genitalia (XLAG) is a severe malformation syndrome that is only observed in boys (Fig. 46.4). Affected patients show lissencephaly with p < a gradient, absent corpus callosum, moderate increase of the cortical thickness (only 6–7 mm), atrophic striatal and thalamic nuclei, postnatal microcephaly, neonatal-onset epilepsy, hypothalamic dysfunction including deficient temperature regulation, chronic diarrhea, and ambiguous genitalia with micropenis and cryptorchidism. Most XLAG patients die within 1 year after birth (Okazaki *et al.* 2008).

Brain neuropathology reveals an abnormally laminated three-layered cortex containing exclusively pyramidal neurons, with a thick molecular layer consisting of small- or medium-sized sparse neurons, a subsequent cell-dense layer with an increased number of small-sized neurons, and a third layer containing sparse cells without myelinated fibers (Bonneau *et al.* 2002).

Mutations of the X-linked *aristaless*-related homeobox gene (*ARX*) (OMIM *300382) were identified in individuals with XLAG and in some female relatives. Females carrying *ARX* mutations usually have normal cognition and may either have a normal brain MRI scan, or show partial or complete agenesis of the corpus callosum. Mild mental retardation and epilepsy have been reported in rare carriers (Kato *et al.* 2004).

The ARX protein is expressed in the ganglionic eminence and subventricular zone during early development. Its major functions are thought to be the regulation of proliferation and tangential migration of GABAergic interneurons and the regulation of radial migration of pyramidal neurons (Friocourt *et al.* 2008). Earlier studies have indicated that the murine *Arx* gene is specifically expressed in the GABAergic neural lineages, where it controls both the specification and migration of these neurons (Colombo *et al.* 2004). However, more recent studies have evidenced that *Arx*-null mice show deficient tangential migration and abnormal differentiation of GABAergic inter-neurons in the ganglionic eminence and neocortex as well as misplacement of radially migrating pyramidal cells, which normally do not express *Arx*. The mechanism by which *Arx* regulates the fate of pyramidal neurons (proliferation defect versus radial migration defect) is still unknown (Friocourt *et al.* 2008).

The *ARX* gene product has two functional domains, an *aristaless* domain and a *prd*-like homeodomain; mutations that affect these two domains lead to XLAG. Non-conservative missense mutations near the C-terminal *aristaless* domain caused unusually severe XLAG with microcephaly and mild cerebellar hypoplasia. Mutations in the homeodomain are largely premature termination mutations; missense mutations are usually less common. Among these, non-conservative missense mutations are associated with less severe XLAG, while conservative substitutions cause Proud syndrome (agenesis of the corpus callosum with abnormal genitalia). Mutations of *ARX* are also associated with non-malformative phenotypes including X-linked infantile spasms, Partington syndrome, dyskinetic quadriparesis with status dystonicus (Guerrini *et al.* 2007) and X-linked non-syndromic mental retardation (Gécz *et al.* 2006).

Autosomal recessive lissencephaly with cerebellar hypoplasia

Lissencephaly with cerebellar hypoplasia (LCH) is associated with severe abnormalities of the cerebellum, hippocampus, and brainstem. It was mapped to chromosome 7q22, and mutations were identified in the *RELN* gene (OMIM: *600514) (Hong *et al.* 2000; Ross *et al.* 2001) (Fig. 46.5).

Table 46.1 Additional phenotypes associated with the lissencephaly–SBH spectrum but not belonging to the subgroup of the type 1 lissencephalies

Syndrome	Clinical features associated with lissencephaly/pachygyria	Locus (gene)	OMIM accession number[a]
Baraitser–Winter syndrome	Eye coloboma, ptosis, hypertelorism, epicanthic folds, broad nasal bridge, long philtrum, thin upper lip, telecantus, short stature	Possibly autosomal recessive	–
Walker–Warburg syndrome (HARD+/– E syndrome)	Congenital muscular dystrophy, congenital retinal non-attachment with or without microphthalmia and persistent hyperplastic primary vitreous	9q34.1 (*POMT1*) 14q24.3 (*POMT2*) 9q31 (*FKTN*) 19q13.3 (*FKRP*) 22q12.3–q13.1 (*LARGE*)	236670
Muscle–eye–brain disease (MEB)	Congenital muscular dystrophy, congenital hypotonia and muscle weakness, severe visual failure, uncontrolled eye movements, myopia	19q13.3 (*FKRP*) 1p34–p33 (*POMGNT1*)	253280
Fukuyama congenital muscular dystrophy (FCMD)	Generalized muscle weakness, hypotonia, speech defect	9q31 (*FKTN*)	253800
Lissencephaly and bone dysplasia	Craniofacial edema and arthrogryposis, epiphyseal stippling of cervical vertebrae, feet, and sacrum; shortened metacarpal bones and hypoplastic phalanges	Supposed autosomal recessive	601160
Neu–Laxova syndrome (NLS)	Severe subcutaneous edema, atrophic muscles, camptodactyly, syndactyly of toes and fingers, hypoplastic genitalia, hypertelorism, protruding eyes	Unknown	256520
Lissencephaly with cleft palate and cerebellar hypoplasia	Cleft palate	Unknown	604382
Craniotelencephalic dysplasia	Frontal bone protrusion, encephalocele, craniosynostosis, septooptic dysplasia	Unknown	218670
Muscular dystrophy with severe central nervous system atrophy and absence of large myelinated fibers	Hypertelorism, telecanthus, small and posteriorly angulated ears, micrognathia and high-arched palate, severe hypotonia, muscle weakness	Unknown	601170

Note:
[a]OMIM (Online Mendelian Inheritance in Man): www.ncbi.nlm.nih.gov/omim/

A

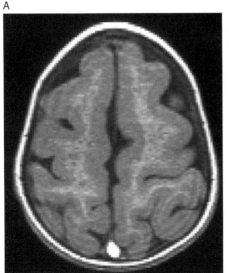

B

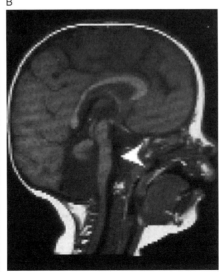

Fig. 46.5. Brain MRI scans of two patients from a family with lissencephaly with cerebellar hypoplasia (LCH) type b and a mutation in the *RELN* gene. (A) Axial section: the cortex is thickened and the gyral pattern is simplified. (B) Sagittal section: the cerebellum is severely reduced in size, with hypoplasia of the inferior vermis and of the hemispheres. The pons (arrowhead) is reduced in size. (Reprinted by permission from Nature Publishing Group Publishers Ltd., (from Hong *et al.* *Nature Genet* 2000 **26**:93–6.)

Patients exhibit dysmorphic facial features and generalized seizures. The *RELN* gene encodes a large (388-kDa) extracellular matrix protein that acts on migrating cortical neurons by binding to the very-low-density lipoprotein receptor (VLDLR), the apolipoprotein E receptor 2, and α3-β1 integrin and cadherin-related receptors (CNRs) (Hiesberger *et al.* 1999). In mice, *Reln* mutations cause cerebellar hypoplasia, abnormal cerebral cortical neuronal migration, and abnormal axonal connectivity. Neurons in affected mice fail to reach their correct location in the developing brain, disrupting the organization of the cerebellar and cerebral cortices and other laminated regions. In this animal model, the cortical layering appears inverted (D'Arcangelo 2006). Thus, Reln is thought to control cell–cell interactions critical for cell positioning in the brain.

Nine additional phenotypes have been associated with the LIS–SBH spectrum, although they do not belong to the type 1 LIS subgroup. Clinical features and associated genes or loci, if at all identified, are reported in Table 46.1.

Acknowledgments

This work was supported in part by a grant from the EU Sixth Framework Thematic Priority Life Sciences, Genomics and Biotechnology for Health, contract number LSH-CT-2006–037315 (EPICURE) (to RG).

References

Bahi-Buisson N, Poirier K, Boddaert N, *et al.* (2008) Refinement of cortical dysgeneses spectrum associated with *TUBA1A* mutations. *J Med Genet* **45**:647–53.

Bai J, Ramos RL, Ackman JB, *et al.* (2003) RNAi reveals doublecortin is required for radial migration in rat neocortex. *Nat Neurosci* **6**:1277–83.

Barkovich AJ (2000) Congenital malformations of the brain and skull. In: Barkovich A (ed.) *Pediatric Neuroimaging*. Philadelphia, PA: Lippincott William and Wilkins, pp. 251–90.

Barkovich AJ, Guerrini R, Battaglia G, *et al.* (1994) Band heterotopia: correlation of outcome with magnetic resonance imaging parameters. *Ann Neurol* **36**:609–17.

Bernasconi A, Martinez V, Rosa-Neto P, *et al.* (2001) Surgical resection for intractable epilepsy in "double cortex" syndrome yields inadequate results. *Epilepsia* **42**:1124–9.

Bonneau D, Toutain A, Laquerrière A, *et al.* (2002) X-linked lissencephaly with absent corpus callosum and ambiguous genitalia (XLAG): clinical, magnetic resonance imaging, and neuropathological findings. *Ann Neurol* **51**:340–9.

Cardoso C, Leventer RJ, Dowling JJ, *et al.* (2002) Clinical and molecular basis of classical lissencephaly: mutations in the *LIS1* gene (PAFAH1B1). *Hum Mutat* **19**:4–15.

Cardoso C, Leventer RJ, Ward HL, *et al.* (2003) Refinement of a 400-kb critical region allows genotypic differentiation between isolated lissencephaly, Miller–Dieker syndrome, and other phenotypes secondary to deletions of 17p13.3. *Am J Hum Genet* **72**:918–30.

Colombo E, Galli R, Cossu G, Gécz J, Broccoli V (2004) Mouse orthologue of *ARX*, a gene mutated in several X-linked forms of mental retardation and epilepsy, is a marker of adult neural stem cells and forebrain GABAergic neurons. *Dev Dyn* **231**:631–9.

D'Agostino MD, Bernasconi A, Das S, *et al.* (2002) Subcortical band heterotopia (SBH) in males: clinical, imaging and genetic findings in comparison with females. *Brain* **125**:2507–22.

D'Arcangelo G (2006) Reelin mouse mutants as models of cortical development disorders. *Epilepsy Behav* **8**:81–90.

des Portes V, Francis Pinard JM, Desguerre Moutard ML, *et al.* (1998) Doublecortin is the major gene causing X-linked subcortical laminar heterotopia (SCLH). *Hum Mol Genet* **7**:1063–70.

de Rijk-van Andel JF, Arts WF, Hofman A, Staal A, Niermeijer MF (1991) Epidemiology of lissencephaly type I. *Neuroepidemiology* **10**:200–4.

Faulkner NE, Dujardin DL, Tai CY, *et al.* (2000) A role for the lissencephaly gene *LIS1* in mitosis and cytoplasmic dynein function. *Nat Cell Biol* **2**:784–91.

Friede RL (1989) *Developmental Neuropathology*. New York: Springer-Verlag.

Friocourt G, Kanatani S, Tabata H, *et al.* (2008) Cell-autonomous roles of ARX in cell proliferation and neuronal migration during corticogenesis. *J Neurosci* **28**:5794–805.

Gécz J, Cloosterman D, Partington M (2006) *ARX*: a gene for all seasons. *Curr Opin Genet Develop* **16**:308–16.

Gleeson JG, Allen KM, Fox JW, *et al.* (1998) Doublecortin, a brain-specific gene mutated in human X-linked lissencephaly and double cortex syndrome, encodes a putative signaling protein. *Cell* **92**:63–72.

Gleeson JG, Minnerath S, Kuzniecky RI, *et al.* (2000a) Somatic and germline mosaic mutations in the doublecortin gene are associated with variable phenotypes. *Am J Hum Genet* **67**:574–81.

Gleeson JG, Luo RF, Grant PE, *et al.* (2000b) Genetic and neuroradiological heterogeneity of double cortex syndrome. *Ann Neurol* **47**:265–9.

Golden AJ, Harding BN (2004) *Pathology and Genetics: Developmental Neuropathology*. Basel: ISN Neuropath Press.

Guerrini R, Carrozzo R (2001) Epilepsy and genetic malformations of the cerebral cortex. *Am J Med Genet* **106**:160–73.

Guerrini R, Filippi T (2005) Neuronal migration disorders, genetics, and epileptogenesis. *J Child Neurol* **20**:287–99.

Guerrini R, Moro F, Andermann E, *et al.* (2003) Nonsyndromic mental retardation and cryptogenic epilepsy in women with doublecortin gene mutations. *Ann Neurol* **54**:30–7.

Guerrini R, Moro F, Kato M, *et al.* (2007) Expansion of the first polyA tract of *ARX* causes infantile spasms and status dystonicus. *Neurology* **69**:427–33.

Hiesberger T, Trommsdorff M, Howell BW, *et al.* (1999) Direct binding of Reelin to VLDL receptor and ApoE receptor 2 induces tyrosine phosphorylation of disabled-1 and modulates tau phosphorylation. *Neuron* **24**:481–9.

Hirotsune S, Fleck MW, Gambello MJ, *et al.* (1998) Graded reduction of Pafah1b1 (Lis1) activity results in neuronal migration defects and early embryonic lethality. *Nat Genet* **19**:333–9.

Hong SE, Shugart YY, Huang DT, *et al.* (2000) Autosomal recessive lissencephaly with cerebellar hypoplasia is associated with human RELN mutations. *Nat Genet* **26**:93–6.

Kato M, Das S, Petras K, *et al.* (2004) Mutations of *ARX* are associated with striking pleiotropy and consistent genotype–phenotype correlation. *Hum Mutat* **23**:147–59.

Keays DA, Tian G, Poirier K, *et al.* (2007) Mutations in alpha-tubulin cause abnormal neuronal migration in mice and lissencephaly in humans. *Cell* **128**:45–57.

Kerjan G, Koizumi H, Han EB, *et al.* (2009) Mice lacking doublecortin and doublecortin-like kinase 2 display altered hippocampal neuronal maturation and spontaneous seizures. *Proc Natl Acad Sci USA* **106**:6766–71.

Landy HJ, Curless RG, Ramsay RE, *et al.* (1993) Corpus callosotomy for seizures associated with band heterotopia. *Epilepsia* **34**:79–83.

Lee N, Radtke RA, Gray L, *et al.* (1994) Neuronal migration disorders: positron emission tomography correlations. *Ann Neurol* **35**:290–7.

Mai R, Tassi L, Cossu M, *et al.* (2003) A neuropathological, stereo-EEG, and MRI study of subcortical band heterotopia. *Neurology* **60**:1834–8.

Matsumoto N, Leventer RJ, Kuc JA, *et al.* (2001) Mutation analysis of the *DCX* gene and genotype/phenotype correlation in subcortical band heterotopia. *Eur J Hum Genet* **9**:5–12.

Mei D, Parrini E, Pasqualetti M, *et al.* (2007) Multiplex ligation-dependent probe amplification detects *DCX* gene deletions in band heterotopia. *Neurology* **68**:446–50.

Mei D, Lewis R, Parrini E, *et al.* (2008) High frequency of genomic deletions and duplications in the *LIS1* gene in lissencephaly: implications for molecular diagnosis. *J Med Genet* **45**:355–61.

Okazaki S, Ohsawa M, Kuki I, *et al.* (2008) *Aristaless*-related homeobox gene disruption leads to abnormal distribution of GABAergic interneurons in human neocortex: evidence based on a case of X-linked lissencephaly with abnormal genitalia (XLAG). *Acta Neuropathol* **116**:453–62.

Palmini A, Andermann F, Olivier A, Tampieri D, Robitaille Y (1991) Focal neuronal migration disorders and intractable partial epilepsy: results of surgical treatment. *Ann Neurol* **30**:750–7.

Pilz DT, Kuc J, Matsumoto N, *et al.* (1999) Subcortical band heterotopia in rare affected males can be caused by missense mutations in *DCX* (XLIS) or *LIS1*. *Hum Mol Genet* **8**:1757–60.

Poirier K, Keays DA, Francis F, *et al.* (2007) Large spectrum of lissencephaly and pachygyria phenotypes resulting from de novo missense mutations in tubulin alpha 1A (*TUBA1A*). *Hum Mutat* **28**:1055–64.

Reiner O, Carrozzo R, Shen Y, *et al.* (1993) Isolation of a Miller–Dieker lissencephaly gene containing G protein beta-subunit-like repeats. *Nature* **364**:717–21.

Richardson MP, Koepp MJ, Brooks DJ, *et al.* (1998) Cerebral activation in malformations of cortical development. *Brain* **121**:1295–304.

Ross ME, Swanson K, Dobyns WB (2001) Lissencephaly with cerebellar hypoplasia (LCH): a heterogeneous group of cortical malformations. *Neuropediatrics* **32**:256–63.

Sapir T, Elbaum M, Reiner O (1997) Reduction of microtubule catastrophe events by LIS1, platelet-activating factor acetylhydrolase subunit. *EMBO J* **16**:6977–84.

Sicca F, Kelemen A, Genton P, *et al.* (2003) Mosaic mutations of the *LIS1* gene cause subcortical band heterotopia. *Neurology* **61**:1042–6.

Tsai JW, Chen Y, Kriegstein AR, Vallee RB (2005) *LIS1* RNA interference blocks neural stem cell division, morphogenesis, and motility at multiple stages. *J Cell Biol* **170**:935–45.

Uyanik G, Morris-Rosendahl DJ, Stiegler J, *et al.* (2007) Location and type of mutation in the *LIS1* gene do not predict phenotypic severity. *Neurology* **69**:442–7.

Wynshaw-Boris A, Gambello MJ (2001) *LIS1* and dynein motor function in neuronal migration and development. *Genes Dev* **15**:639–51.

Yingling J, Youn YH, Darling D, *et al.* (2008) Neuroepithelial stem cell proliferation requires LIS1 for precise spindle orientation and symmetric division. *Cell* **132**:474–86.

Chapter 47

Agenesis of the corpus callosum

Dorothy Jones-Davis, Yolanda Lau, and Elliott H. Sherr

Introduction

The corpus callosum is the largest white matter tract in the brain, composed of 200 million axons that connect the two cerebral hemispheres. Most of these connections are homotopically organized; a small subset may be organized in a more complex, or "heterotopic" fashion (Wahl *et al.* 2009). Disrupted formation of the corpus callosum is the second most common central nervous system birth defect, occurring in approximately 1 in 3000 live births (Glass *et al.* 2008). Clinically, individuals with agenesis of the corpus callosum (ACC) can present with a wide range of deficits, from mild cognitive and behavioral deficits in the autism spectrum (Badaruddin *et al.* 2007), to severe epilepsy, mental retardation, and cerebral palsy (Paul *et al.* 2007). The mechanisms that underlie this disruption in patients are mostly not understood. However, evidence gleaned from mouse models (primarily inactivation or knock-outs of single genes) suggest that ACC can occur from disruption of multiple developmental steps (Richards *et al.* 2004). These begin with the birth and specification of commissural neurons and extend through the precise axonal guidance mechanisms necessary for midline crossing and the precise coordination of commissural connectivity. Because of the complexity of these developmental processes, it follows that ACC can be caused by either complete disruption of any one of these mechanisms, or by an interplay of milder disruptions of multiple developmental steps. This complexity makes prediction of clinical outcomes difficult at this stage of knowledge, but there are some general principles that can be discerned from studies of large cohorts of ACC individuals, and we can comment on outcomes in specific known syndromes. Indeed, with the upcoming advances in clinical genetic sequencing (and other modes of genetic analysis), we anticipate that the next edition of this book will have considerably more precise information about prognosis and the likelihood of epilepsy in given scenarios.

Epilepsy and the general ACC cohort

The incidence of epilepsy in patients with ACC and its related syndromes ranges from 25% to 62% ((Taylor and David 1998; Shevell 2002; Schell-Apacik *et al.* 2008). This is a difficult percentage to assess accurately, given the ascertainment bias of each cohort. Some of the cohorts are hospital-based and will be biased toward a more clinically affected population. To address this and other issues, we have enrolled perhaps the largest cohort of ACC individuals. However, this method recruits families that are interested in participating in our research, which is clearly a different bias than the hospital-based populations. Given those inherent limitations, we recently sent questionnaires to all 300+ families in our study and received seizure (and other clinical) information back from 130 families (Y. Lau and E. Sherr, unpublished data). We did the analysis of the overall cohort and then we repeated the analysis, having removed individuals specifically with Aicardi syndrome. This specific disorder (see below) is always associated with epilepsy, usually intractable. Any analysis of ACC individuals would then have to take this into consideration when devising predictive tools. When including Aicardi syndrome patients, 53/130 (40.8%) of the cohort had seizures. Nine individuals (6.9%) had had seizures in the past but were now seizure-free and 28 patients (21.5%) had intractable epilepsy (Fig. 47.1).

A quick inspection of Fig. 47.1 demonstrates that the difference between the "include" and "exclude" Aicardi syndrome cohorts are the 17 Aicardi syndrome patients with intractable epilepsy. This does not change the number of non-Aicardi syndrome patients with a history of seizures, but it does shift the percentage of the overall group with seizures from 41% to 32%. It even more dramatically shifts the percentage of patients with intractable epilepsy from 21.5% to 9.7%. Therefore, by analogy to other cohorts, it is critically important to understand who is represented in any cohort and at what percentage. Ideally, we would wish to acquire these data for a true population-based cohort, but this level of clinical information is currently not available.

We also assessed whether certain associated brain magnetic resonance imaging (MRI) findings would help predict whether epilepsy was more or less likely (Table 47.1). As in the overall incidence of seizures, we also compared the cohort in which we

The Causes of Epilepsy, eds. S. D. Shorvon, F. Andermann, and R. Guerrini. Published by Cambridge University Press. © Cambridge University Press 2011.

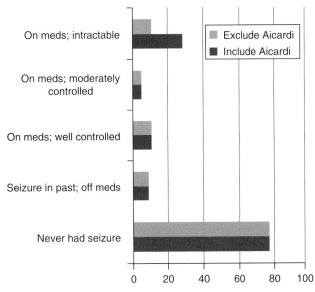

Fig. 47.1. Relative percentages of seizure severity in ACC individuals. The full cohort (*n* = 130) includes all ACC individuals, including those with Aicardi syndrome (dark gray bars). The cohort with Aicardi patients removed is displayed with light gray bars (*n* = 113).

Table 47.1 Correlations of MRI findings to likelihood of seizures

	Include Aicardi (*n* = 130)		Exclude Aicardi (*n* = 131)	
	Chi-Squared	*p*-value	Chi-squared	*p*-Value
Absent anterior commissure	11	0.81	10.4	0.85
Abnormal brainstem	8	0.79	10.7	0.56
Cortical malformations	22.9	0.0035	10	0.26
Colpocephaly	4.3	0.36	5.7	0.22
Corpus callosum type	8.5	0.39	4.5	0.81
Cysts	16.1	0.041	15.1	0.058
Gender	20.4	0.0004	2.5	0.64
Abnormal myelination	14.3	0.074	7.2	0.52
Polymicrogyria	13.5	0.0091	8.7	0.07
Periventricular heterotopia	34.8	0.0001	10.4	0.034
Probst bundles	8.2	0.41	6.3	0.61
Subcortical heterotopia	14.2	0.0068	12.3	0.016
Ventricle size	7.2	0.51	5.4	0.71
White matter volume	13.3	0.87	13.8	0.84

included Aicardi syndrome patients (*n* = 17; total = 130) to the cohort in which Aicardi syndrome patients were specifically excluded (total = 113). In both groups, the presence of periventricular heterotopia and subcortical heterotopia significantly correlated with an increased risk of having seizures. In the group that included Aicardi syndrome patients, the overall presence of cortical malformations and polymicrogyria were also significantly correlated, as were the presence of interhemispheric cysts and gender (*p* = 0.0004). The latter would be expected, as all patients with Aicardi syndrome are females (except for case reports of Klinefelter syndrome males: Hopkins *et al.* 1979). Both the presence of cysts and polymicrogyria nearly reach statistical significance in the group without Aicardi syndrome patients as well. Interestingly, the type of corpus callosum malformation (absent versus partial) did not correlate with seizure severity, nor did other features of abnormal brain development. It has been previously reported that the type of callosal anomaly does not predict the presence of seizures (Taylor and David 1998) and in one series (Shevell 2002), the presence of epilepsy predicted an overall poorer prognosis, a finding that is not unexpected.

These findings suggest that the presence of other malformations besides the absent corpus callosum may be key to determining whether ACC individuals have seizures and of what type and severity. However, these associated findings must not explain the whole association with epilepsy, as some cases of ACC alone also have epilepsy. For example, in our cohort, 68/130 individuals do not have cortical malformations (which include periventricular nodular heterotopia and subcortical heterotopia). Of these 68 individuals, 14 (20.5%) have an active seizure disorder.

A review of the Online Mendelian Inheritance in Man database (OMIM: www.ncbi.nlm.nih.gov/omim/) indicates that approximately 24 syndromes feature both ACC and epilepsy as symptoms. These syndromes probably represent a small percentage of the total group of individuals with ACC. As an example, Aicardi syndrome patients make up only about 1% of the total and this may be one of the largest subgroups except for chromosomal anomalies (Glass *et al.* 2008). Below we have highlighted a subset of these syndromes to provide additional context for understanding the link between ACC and epilepsy.

Epilepsy and specific ACC syndromes
Aicardi syndrome

First described in 1965 by the French neurologist Jean Aicardi, Aicardi syndrome is a presumed X-linked syndrome, as it is seen only in females and Klinefelter syndrome (XXY) males (Aicardi 2005). It is characterized by a trio of features, including callosal agenesis (ACC), chorioretinal lacunae, and infantile spasms. In most Aicardi syndrome patients, infantile spasms begin by 3 months of age, developing into other medically refractory seizure types as the child matures. Asynchronous multifocal epileptiform abnormalities with burst suppression are the characteristic electroencephalo-graphic (EEG) finding of these patients (Fariello *et al.* 1977). Other brain abnormalities that have been characterized include cerebellar and retinal migration defects, as well as cortical migrational defects such as subcortical and periventricular heterotopias and polymicrogyria. In addition, patients with Aicardi syndrome also frequently exhibit mental retardation. The cause for the intractable seizures is unknown, but may relate to the presence of the other malformations (Hopkins *et al.* 2008). It is also possible that these severe seizures are caused by a underappreciated reduction in white matter microstructural organization. We conducted diffusion tensor imaging with tractography to analyze the white matter organization in Aicardi syndrome patients. In addition to the aforementioned cortical defects, we also found that the cortico-cortical white matter tracts were either absent or severely diminished in Aicardi syndrome (E. Sherr, unpublished data).

ARX-related disorders: X-linked lissencephaly with abnormal genitalia (XLAG), ACC with abnormal genitalia (ACC/AG; Proud syndrome)

Homeobox transcription factors are crucial for appropriate development and patterning in the cerebral cortex (Bienvenu *et al.* 2002). The *ARX* gene is a homeobox gene that has been shown to be crucial in forebrain, pancreatic, and testicular development (Gecz *et al.* 2006). Given this important role in development, mutation of the homeobox domain protein ARX has emerged as a key cause of of X-linked developmental disorders, especially those characterized by a loss of the corpus callosum and epilepsy. A conservative mutation in the homeodomain of the ARX protein was shown to cause agenesis of the corpus callosum and lissencephaly with abnormal genitalia (XLAG). To date, *ARX* mutations have also been shown to cause X-linked West syndrome (X-linked infantile spasms) as well as Partington syndrome (mental retardation, ataxia, and dystonia) (Sherr 2003).

Clinically, patients with XLAG are genotypic males presenting with a number of neurological impairments, including an anterior-to-posterior gradient of lissencephaly, a moderately thickened three-layer (versus the normal five-layer) cortex, gliotic and spongy white matter, ACC, disorganized basal ganglia, microcephaly, hypothalamic dysfunction (temperature instability, hypothermia), hippocampal dysplasia, absent olfactory bulbs, enlarged third ventricle, and intractable tonic–clonic and myoclonic sezures from birth. Interestingly, these seizures likely result from a lack of birth and migration of inhibitory neurons from the medial ganglionic eminence (Kato and Dobyns 2005). It is interesting to speculate that other causes of ACC may also affect interneuron migration through related or parallel signaling pathways. Females with heterozygous inactivation of *ARX* also exhibit symptoms of neurological impairment, including mental retardation, epilepsy, and ACC (Bonneau *et al.* 2002).

Andermann syndrome

Andermann syndrome, also known as peripheral neuropathy associated with agenesis of the corpus callosum (ACCPN), was first described as an autosomal dominant disorder by Andermann and colleagues in 1972 (Larbrisseau *et al.* 1984). Affected children present in the first few years of life with delayed development, and hallmark facial characteristics such as hypertelorism, blepharoptosis, facial diplegia, hypoplastic maxilla, prominent chin, narrow forehead, low hairline, large ears, open mouth with protruding fissured tongue, and high arched palate (Uyanik *et al.* 2006). Of particular interest to this chapter, many affected individuals also present with full ACC (although some may have partial ACC) and seizures. Other symptoms of Andermann syndrome include hypotonia, amyotrophy, scoliosis, psychomotor retardation, and hallucinosis. As the children age, symptoms of this debilitating disorder deteriorate, and motor function declines until the patient is ultimately bedridden.

A genome-wide scan identified the Andermann locus on chromosome 15q, an area previously linked to juvenile myoclonic epilepsy and familial rolandic epilepsy (Casaubon *et al.* 1996). Ultimately the Andermann gene was identified as being *KCC3*, a potassium–chloride (K^+–Cl^-) co-transporter (Howard *et al.* 2002). Mutations in *KCC3* have since been shown to cause Andermann syndrome. It is likely that these same mutations, through an imbalance of potassium–chloride (K^+–Cl^-) transport, and therefore, an imbalance in excitation and inhibition, explain the seizures manifested in this disorder. In fact, a *KCC3* knock-out mouse generated by Boettger exhibited a reduced flurothyl seizure threshold and aberrant spike–wave activity that was reminiscent of the EEG activity of Andermann syndrome patients (Boettger *et al.* 2003). Interestingly, *KCC3* is expressed along white matter tracts, with a particularly high expression in the corpus callosum (Pearson *et al.* 2001). This expression pattern suggests that the ACC noted in patients with *KCC3* mutations might in fact be a result of aberrant *KCC3* expression and perhaps the absence of important KCC3 protein–protein interactions that mediate white matter tract development.

Mowat–Wilson syndrome

Hirschsprung disease, or congenital aganglionic megacolon, is characterized by a loss of ganglionic cells in the distal colon and rectum, resulting in an enlargement of the colon, and bowel obstruction. Patients exhibit chronic constipation. This congenital malformation can be associated with many other birth defects (Amiel *et al.* 2008).

In 1998, Mowat and colleagues reported six children with distinct facial features, mental retardation, and several other congenital anomalies including microcephaly (Mowat *et al.* 1998). Four of the six children had Hirschsprung disease, and the Mowat–Wilson group deemed this apparent new syndrome as a more severe variant of the disease. In 2003, Wilson and colleagues characterized a full spectrum of symptoms for these patients, including distinct facial features, Hirschsprung disease, genitourinary defects, congenital heart defects, eye defects (microphthalmia, Axenfeld anomaly), and growth retardation, as well as a host of neurological abnormalities (Wilson *et al.* 2003). The latter include mental and motor retardation, microcephaly, severe speech impediment, agenesis or hypogenesis of the corpus callosum, and seizures. In this study, ACC presented in only 4/17 patients examined with MRI, and hypogenesis presented in only 1/17 patients. Seizures were more frequent with 73% (17/23) of individuals presenting with epilepsy at varying ages. Zweier found a slightly higher percentage of patients exhibiting seizures (82%) and ACC (35%), but in both studies, patients displayed a variety of seizure types: tonic–clonic, absence, focal, and complex partial seizures. No one seizure type was characteristic of the syndrome, but most seizures were difficult to control (Zweier *et al.* 2003).

An autosomal dominant disorder, Mowat–Wilson, is caused by de novo mutations or deletions within the *ZFHX1B* (ZEB2) gene. Although seizure severity or severity of other symptoms did not seem to be correlated with the size of deletion, Zweier found that one patient with a larger deletion (~11 Mb) had neonatal epilepsy that resulted in death. Notably, this deletion spanned the region containing the calcium channel β4-subunit (CACNB4), in which some mutations have been shown to cause idiopathic generalized epilepsy and juvenile myoclonic epilepsy (Escayg *et al.*, 2000).

Microphthalmia with linear skin defects

Symptoms of microphthalmia with linear skin defects syndrome (MLS) include severe microphthalmia, corneal opacities, and irregular linear areas of erythematous skin hypoplasia of the head and neck. Patients also exhibit ACC, retinal lacunae, infantile seizures, mental retardation, and skeletal (costovertebral) abnormalities. Male lethality indicates that the syndrome is X-linked, and studies show that the syndrome stems from unbalanced translocations of the X chromosome, resulting in monosomy from Xpter to Xp22 or terminal deletion of the Xp22.3 region, suggesting that the gene(s) responsible for the syndrome are found in this area (Lindsay *et al.* 1994). Taking a candidate gene approach, it was found that the sole gene that is fully located within this area is the mitochondrial holocytochrome c-type synthase (*HCCS*) gene and was confirmed by point mutations within the same gene (Wimplinger *et al.* 2006).

It is unclear how the loss of the *HCCS* gene might contribute to epilepsy. It is known that cytochrome *c* is involved in the process of oxidative phosphorylation, and that a deficit of cytochrome *c* oxidase leads to strokes, seizures, and lactic acidosis (MELAS) (Pavlakis *et al.* 1984)). Furthermore, in addition to involvement of cytochrome *c* in the process of oxidative phosphorylation, cytochrome *c* is released from mitochondria in response to apoptosis. Holocytochrome c-type synthase ultimately gives rise to cytochrome *c*, and the involvement of that protein in apoptosis has been hypothesized

to cause the variable yet severe phenotype noted in MLS patients (Wimplinger *et al.* 2006).

Sakoda complex

In 1979, Sakoda *et al.* first described a condition that was marked by a trio of symptoms: sphenoethmoidal encephalomeningocele (SEEM), ACC, and cleft lip and/or palate (Sakoda *et al.* 1979). This condition was later termed Sakoda complex by Tada and Nakamura (1985), who had reported a case associated with microphthalmia. In 1998, Ehara *et al.* reported a Japanese male patient with Sakoda complex who also had other accompanying symptoms (Ehara *et al.* 1998). After reviewing this case and 21 other similar cases that included additional symptoms such as intractable epilepsy, bilateral anophthalmia, cortical dysgenesis, severe mental retardation, hemiparesis, microcephalus, short stature, hemivertebrae, and optic disk dysplasia, he ranked patients into four levels based on disease severity and symptom presentation. These were (from least severe to most severe): (1) basal encephalomeningocele with ACC; (2) Sakoda complex; (3) Sakoda complex with optic disk dysplasia (including morning glory syndrome); and (4) Sakoda complex with bilateral anophthalmia, cortical dysgenesis, severe psychomotor and mental retardation, and neonatal-onset intractable epilepsy. Ehara *et al.* (1998) suggest that the mental retardation and intractable epilepsy are resultant from cortical dysgenesis, whereas Dempsey *et al.* (2007) suggest genetic causality (an X-linked inheritance pattern) for the entire complex, perhaps suggesting disruption of a common developmental gene. However, to date, the specific cause of the complex and of the accompanying symptoms are as yet unknown.

Periventricular nodular heterotopia (PVNH)

Periventricular nodular heterotopia (PVNH) is an X-linked disorder characterized by the presence of bilateral heterotopic areas of cortex in the lateral ventricles in an otherwise normotopic cortex. The disorder is embryonic lethal for males. In addition to the heterotopic cortex, females with PVNH exhibit an association with agenesis of the corpus callosum (Guerrini and Marini 2006) and childhood onset focal epilepsy with that ranges from mild to intractable (Guerrini and Carrozzo 2001). Information from our cohort shows that about 15% of the ACC patients have PVNH. It is not known how many patients with PCNH have ACC. Guerrini and Carrozzo (2001) report that 88% of PVNH patients also have partial epilepsy. In treatable cases, seizures are usually treated with carbamazepine. In 1998, electrophysiological recordings from Kothare *et al.* demonstrated epileptogenic discharges from nodules, suggesting that the cause of epilepsy in these patients is aberrant electrical activity from the heterotopic cortex (Kothare *et al.*, 1998). However, Guerrini and Carrozzo (2001) found that there was no correlation between the extent and severity of the heterotopic area and the severity of the seizures.

Filamin-A is a gene that is highly expressed in the developing cortex, and is required for normal neuronal migration. Mutations in the gene encoding filamin-A (*FLNA*) were shown to cause PVNH, by preventing normal neuronal migration of cortical neurons (Fox *et al.* 1998).

Temtamy syndrome

Temtamy syndrome is characterized by craniofacial dysmorphism, iris coloboma, mild mental retardation, and agenesis of the corpus callosum (Temtamy *et al.* 1996). Additionally, Li and colleagues described a sibling pair that also had intractable epilepsy, suggesting a spectrum for the disorder (Li *et al.*, 2007). Homozygosity mapping by these investigators excluded the genes *ASXL2*, *ZNF462*, and *VAX1* (ones implicated in previous work with ACC and coloboma formation: Bertuzzi *et al.* 1999; Ramocki *et al.* 2003; Talisetti *et al.* 2003) as causative and the family structure was too small to identify a linked locus. Gene identification awaits ascertainment of additional families.

1q44 deletion syndrome

In 2001, De Vries *et al.* identified a male child with deletion of the distal end of chromosome 1q (De Vries *et al.* 2001). The child presented with dysmorphic facial features, visual and speech impairment, short stature, partial ACC, and seizures. Three groups, led by Black, Dobyns, and Sherr, reported multiple patients with ACC, cerebellar malformations, acquired microcephaly and seizures, all with de novo deletions of 1q44 (Boland *et al.* 2007). This was consistent except for one patient who had a de novo reciprocal balanced translocation t(1;13)(q44;q32) that was within the critical region defined by mapping patients with overlapping deletion intervals. One gene in that interval, *AKT3*, when inactivated in mouse models, leads to a thin corpus callosum. Subsequently, Van Bon and colleagues (2008) identified 11 patients with a similar constellation of symptoms as well as microcephaly. Ten of the patients had full or partial ACC, and nine of the 11 patients had epilepsy, most of which were successfully managed by antiepileptic drugs. However, in this series there is one patient without a deletion of *AKT3*, thus suggesting that another adjacent gene may also be important for callosal formation (van Bon *et al.* 2008).

Summary

In summary, agenesis of the corpus callosum is a common developmental brain anomaly that can frequently be associated with epilepsy. It is also seen in children with mental retardation and autism. Recent work in studying large cohorts of ACC individuals is providing insight into the diversity of causes which lead to ACC, which will provide important insight into mechanisms and outcomes.

References

Aicardi J (2005) Aicardi syndrome. *Brain Dev* **27**:164–71.

Amiel J, Sproat-Emison E, Garcia-Barcelo M (2008) Hirschsprung disease, associated syndromes and genetics: a review. *J Med Genet* **45**:1–14.

Badaruddin DH, Andrews GL, Bolte S, *et al.* (2007) Social and behavioral problems of children with agenesis of the corpus callosum. *Child Psychiat Hum Dev* **38**:287–302.

Bertuzzi S, Hindges R, Mui SH, O'Leary DD, Lemke G (1999) The homeodomain protein vax1 is required for axon guidance and major tract formation in the developing forebrain. *Genes Dev* **13**:3092–105.

Bienvenu T, Poirier K, Friocourt G, *et al.* (2002) *ARX*, a novel Prd-class-homeobox gene highly expressed in the telencephalon, is mutated in X-linked mental retardation. *Hum Mol Genet* **11**:981–91.

Boettger T, Rust MB, Maier H, *et al.* (2003) Loss of K-Cl co-transporter KCC3 causes deafness, neurodegeneration and reduced seizure threshold. *Embo J* **22**:5422–34.

Boland E, Clayton-Smith J, Woo VG, *et al.* (2007) Mapping of deletion and translocation breakpoints in 1q44 implicates the serine/threonine kinase AKT3 in postnatal microcephaly and agenesis of the corpus callosum. *Am J Hum Genet* **81**:292–303.

Bonneau D, Toutain A, Laquerriere A, *et al.* (2002) X-linked lissencephaly with absent corpus callosum and ambiguous genitalia (XLAG): clinical, magnetic resonance imaging, and neuropathological findings. *Ann Neurol* **51**:340–9.

Casaubon LK, Melanson M, Lopes-Cendes I, *et al.* (1996) The gene responsible for a severe form of peripheral neuropathy and agenesis of the corpus callosum maps to chromosome 15q. *Am J Hum Genet* **58**:28–34.

De Vries BB, Knight SJ, Homfray T, *et al.* (2001) Submicroscopic subtelomeric 1qter deletions: a recognizable phenotype? *J Med Genet* **38**:175–8.

Dempsey MA, Torres-Martinez W, Walsh LE (2007) Two cases further delineating the Sakoda complex. *Am J Med Genet* **143A**:370–6.

Ehara H, Kurimasa A, Ohno K, Takeshita K (1998) New syndrome with the Sakoda complex, bilateral anophthalmia, and cortical dysgenesis. *Pediatr Neurol* **18**:445–51.

Escayg A, De Waard M, Lee DD, *et al.* (2000) Coding and noncoding variation of the human calcium-channel beta4-subunit gene *CACNB4* in patients with idiopathic generalized epilepsy and episodic ataxia. *Am J Hum Genet* **66**:1531–9.

Fariello RG, Chun RW, Doro JM, Buncic R, Prichard JS (1977) EEG recognition of Aicardi's syndrome. *Arch Neurol* **34**:563–66.

Fox JW, Lamperti ED, Eksioglu YZ, *et al.* (1998) Mutations in filamin 1 prevent migration of cerebral cortical neurons in human periventricular heterotopia. *Neuron* **21**:1315–25.

Gecz J, Cloosterman D, Partington M (2006) *ARX*: a gene for all seasons. *Curr Opin Genet Dev* **16**:308–16.

Glass HC, Shaw GM, Ma C, Sherr EH (2008) Agenesis of the corpus callosum in California 1983–2003: a population-based study. *Am J Med Genet* **146A**:2495–500.

Guerrini R, Carrozzo R (2001) Epileptogenic brain malformations: clinical presentation, malformative patterns and indications for genetic testing. *Seizure* **10**:532–43; quiz 544–7.

Guerrini R, Marini C (2006) Genetic malformations of cortical development. *Exp Brain Res* **173**:322–33.

Hopkins B, Sutton VR, Lewis RA, Van Den Veyver I, Clark G (2008) Neuroimaging aspects of Aicardi syndrome. *Am J Med Genet* **146A**:2871–8.

Hopkins IJ, Humphrey I, Keith CG, *et al.* (1979) The Aicardi syndrome in a 47, XXY male. *Aust Paediatr J* **15**:278–80.

Howard HC, Mount DB, Rochefort D, *et al.* (2002) The K-Cl cotransporter *KCC3* is mutant in a severe peripheral neuropathy associated with agenesis of the corpus callosum. *Nat Genet* **32**:384–92.

Kato M, Dobyns WB (2005) X-linked lissencephaly with abnormal genitalia as a tangential migration disorder causing intractable epilepsy: proposal for a new term, "interneuronopathy". *J Child Neurol* **20**:392–7.

Kothare SV, Vanlandingham K, Armon C, *et al.* (1998) Seizure onset from periventricular nodular heterotopias: depth-electrode study. *Neurology* **51**:1723–7.

Larbrisseau A, Vanasse M, Brochu P, Jasmin G (1984) The Andermann syndrome: agenesis of the corpus callosum associated with mental retardation and progressive sensorimotor neuronopathy. *Can J Neurol Sci* **11**:257–61.

Li J, Shivakumar S, Wakahiro M, *et al.* (2007) Agenesis of the corpus callosum, optic coloboma, intractable seizures, craniofacial and skeletal dysmorphisms: an autosomal recessive disorder similar to Temtamy syndrome. *Am J Med Genet* **143A**:1900–5.

Lindsay EA, Grillo A, Ferrero GB, *et al.* (1994) Microophthalmia with linear skin defects (MLS) syndrome: clinical, cytogenetic, and molecular characterization. *Am J Med Genet* **49**:229–34.

Mowat DR, Croaker GD, Cass DT, *et al.* (1998) Hirschsprung disease, microcephaly, mental retardation, and characteristic facial features: delineation of a new syndrome and identification of

a locus at chromosome 2q22–q23. *J Med Genet* **35**:617–23.

Paul LK, Brown WS, Adolphs R, *et al.* (2007) Agenesis of the corpus callosum: genetic, developmental and functional aspects of connectivity. *Nat Rev Neurosci* **8**:287–99.

Pavlakis SG, Phillips PC, Dimauro S, De Vivo DC, Rowland LP (1984) Mitochondrial myopathy, encephalopathy, lactic acidosis, and strokelike episodes: a distinctive clinical syndrome. *Ann Neurol* **16**:481–8.

Pearson MM, Lu J, Mount DB, Delpire E (2001) Localization of the K(+)-Cl(−) cotransporter, KCC3, in the central and peripheral nervous systems: expression in the choroid plexus, large neurons and white matter tracts. *Neuroscience* **103**:481–91.

Ramocki MB, Dowling J, Grinberg I, *et al.* (2003) Reciprocal fusion transcripts of two novel Zn-finger genes in a female with absence of the corpus callosum, ocular colobomas and a balanced translocation between chromosomes 2p24 and 9q32. *Eur J Hum Genet* **11**:527–34.

Richards LJ, Plachez C, Ren T (2004) Mechanisms regulating the development of the corpus callosum and its agenesis in mouse and human. *Clin Genet* **66**:276–89.

Sakoda K, Ishikawa S, Uozumi T, *et al.* (1979) Sphenoethmoidal meningoencephalocele associated with agenesis of corpus callosum and median cleft lip and palate: Case report. *J Neurosurg* **51**:397–401.

Schell-Apacik CC, Wagner K, Bihler M, *et al.* (2008) Agenesis and dysgenesis of the corpus callosum: clinical, genetic and neuroimaging findings in a series of 41 patients. *Am J Med Genet* **146A**:2501–11.

Sherr EH (2003) The *ARX* story (epilepsy, mental retardation, autism, and cerebral malformations): one gene leads to many phenotypes. *Curr Opin Pediatr* **15**:567–71.

Shevell MI (2002) Clinical and diagnostic profile of agenesis of the corpus callosum. *J Child Neurol* **17**:896–900.

Tada M, Nakamura N (1985) Sphenoethmoidal encephalomeningocele

and midline anomalies of face and brain. *Hokkaido Igaku Zasshi* **60**:48–56.

Talisetti A, Forrester SR, Gregory D, *et al.* (2003) Temtamy-like syndrome associated with translocation of 2p24 and 9q32. *Clin Dysmorphol* **12**:175–7.

Taylor M, David AS (1998) Agenesis of the corpus callosum: a United Kingdom series of 56 cases. *J Neurol Neurosurg Psychiatry* **64**:131–4.

Temtamy SA, Salam MA, Aboul-Ezz EH, *et al.* (1996) New autosomal recessive multiple congenital abnormalities/mental retardation syndrome with craniofacial dysmorphism absent corpus callosum, iris colobomas and connective tissue dysplasia. *Clin Dysmorphol* **5**:231–40.

Uyanik G, Elcioglu N, Penzien J, *et al.* (2006) Novel truncating and missense mutations of the *KCC3* gene associated with Andermann syndrome. *Neurology* **66**:1044–8.

Van Bon BW, Koolen DA, Borgatti R, *et al.* (2008) Clinical and molecular characteristics of 1qter microdeletion syndrome: delineating a critical region for corpus callosum agenesis/hypogenesis. *J Med Genet* **45**:346–54.

Wahl M, Strominger Z, Jeremy RJ, *et al.* (2009) Variability of homotopic and heterotopic callosal connectivity in partial agenesis of the corpus callosum: a 3T diffusion tensor imaging and Q-ball tractography study. *AJNR Am J Neuroradiol* **30**:282–9.

Wilson M, Mowat D, Dastot-Le Moal F, *et al.* (2003) Further delineation of the phenotype associated with heterozygous mutations in *ZFHX1B*. *Am J Med Genet* **119A**:257–65.

Wimplinger I, Morleo M, Rosenberger G, *et al.* (2006) Mutations of the mitochondrial holocytochrome c-type synthase in X-linked dominant microphthalmia with linear skin defects syndrome. *Am J Hum Genet* **79**:878–89.

Zweier C, Temple IK, Beemer F, *et al.* (2003) Characterisation of deletions of the ZFHX1B region and genotype–phenotype analysis in Mowat–Wilson syndrome. *J Med Genet* **40**:601–5.

Chapter

48

Polymicrogyria and schizencephaly

Renzo Guerrini and Carmen Barba

The causal disease

The term polymicrogyria defines an excessive number of abnormally small, and partly fused, cortical gyri, that produce an irregular cortical surface (Barkovich *et al.* 2005). Polymicrogyria has been ever more recognized since the advent of magnetic resonance imaging (MRI). Its pathogenesis is not understood; brain pathology demonstrates an abnormally developed thin cortical ribbon, with loss of neurons in middle and deep cortical layers (Englund *et al.* 2005), variably associated with an unlayered cortical structure (Fig. 48.1A, B). There is causal heterogeneity. A variety of intrinsic, genetically determined mechanisms have been associated with polymicrogyria (Golden and Harding 2004). However, autopsy observations in fetuses demonstrate that acquired disruption of cortical development is also possible, acting from the third to fifth month of gestation and interfering with the later stages of neuronal migration and causing postmigrational destruction (Friede 1989; Golden and Harding 2004).

Polymicrogyria is a common cortical malformation and is associated with a wide spectrum of anatomic patterns (Table 48.1). It can appear as an isolated manifestation or be associated with multiple different conditions including metabolic disorders, especially Zellweger syndrome, or intrauterine hypoperfusion or infection, especially with cytomegalovirus, toxoplasma, and syphilis (Golden and Harding 2004), fetal alcohol syndrome (Reinhardt *et al.* 2010), and be part of multiple congenital anomalies/mental retardation syndromes. Affected patients may have a wide spectrum of clinical problems other than those attributable to the polymicrogyria. Polymicrogyria has been related to mutations of several genes including *SRPX2* (Roll *et al.* 2006), *PAX6* (Glaser *et al.* 1994), *TBR2* (Baala *et al.* 2007), *KIAA1279* (Brooks *et al.* 2005), *RAB3GAP1* (Aligianis *et al.* 2005), *COL18A1* (Sertie *et al.* 2000), and copy-number variations (Guerrini and Parrini 2010) (Table 48.2). The anatomic spectrum caused by mutations of the *TUBA1A* and *TUBB2B* genes is still poorly known due to the paucity of reported

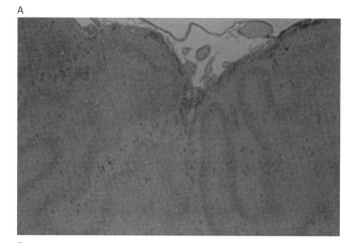

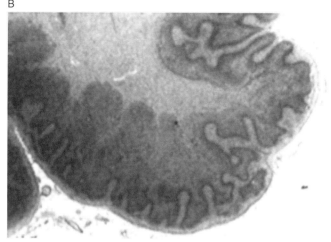

Fig. 48.1. (A) Unlayered polymicrogyria in Aicardi syndrome. Contiguous microgyri are fused. As a consequence the cortical surface at the molecular layer is smooth. (B) Magnification of the transition from unlayered to "four-layered" microgyri in a child with perisylvian polymicrogyria associated with more widespread areas of polymicrogyric cortex.

cases and their apparent heterogeneity, but appears to be wide and includes lissencephaly and polymicrogyria (Jaglin *et al.* 2009).

The Causes of Epilepsy, eds. S. D. Shorvon, F. Andermann, and R. Guerrini. Published by Cambridge University Press. © Cambridge University Press 2011.

Table 48.1 Classification of the polymicrogyria and schizencephalies

(1) Unilateral polymicrogyria

    (a) Unilateral hemispheric polymicrogyria

    (b) Unilateral focal–regional polymicrogyria

(2) Bilateral polymicrogyria syndromes

    (a) Bilateral generalized polymicrogyria

    (b) Bilateral frontal polymicrogyria

    (c) Bilateral perisylvian polymicrogyria (BPP)

        (i) Autosomal dominant (22q11.2 and others)

        (ii) X-linked (Xq28)

        (iii) Autosomal recessive

    (d) Bilateral frontoparietal with white matter and cerebellar dysplasia (recessive GPR56)

    (e) Bilateral parasagittal and mesial parieto-occipital polymicrogyria

    (f) Bilateral lateral parietal polymicrogyria

(3) Schizencephaly (polymicrogyria with clefts, open or closed lips)

    (a) Isolated schizencephaly

    (b) Septo-optic dysplasia – schizencephaly syndrome

    (c) Other rare schizencephaly syndromes

(4) Polymicrogyria or schizencephaly as part of multiple congenital anomaly/mental retardation syndromes

    (a) Adams–Oliver syndrome

    (b) Aicardi syndrome

    (c) Arima syndrome

    (d) Oculocerebrocutaneous (Delleman) syndrome

    (e) Galloway–Mowat syndrome

    (f) Micro syndrome

    (g) Thanatophoric dysplasia

Source: Modified from Barkovich *et al.* (2005).

Table 48.2 Genes and loci associated with polymicrogyria

Condition	Gene	Locus	Reference
X-linked, autosomal dominant			
Rolandic seizures, oromotor dyspraxia	SRPX2	Xq22	Roll *et al.* (2006)
Agenesis of the corpus callosum, microcephaly and polymicrogyria	TBR2	3p21	Baala *et al.* (2007)
Aniridia plus	PAX6	11p13	Glaser *et al.* (1994)
Polymicrogyria		1p36.3-pter	Ribeiro *et al.* (2007)
Microcephaly, polymicrogyria		1q44-qter	Zollino *et al.* (2003)
Facial dysmorphism and polymicrogyria		2p16.1–p23	Dobyns *et al.* (2008)
Microcephaly, hydrocephalus, and polymicrogyria		4q21–q22	Nowaczyk *et al.* (1997)
Polymicrogyria		21q2	Yao *et al.* (2006)
DiGeorge syndrome and polymicrogyria		22q11.2	Robin *et al.* (2006)
Autosomal recessive			
Bilateral frontoparietal cobblestone malformation (previously polymicrogyria)	GPR56	16q13	Piao *et al.* (2005)
Goldberg–Shprintzen syndrome	KIAA1279	10q21.3	Brooks *et al.* (2005)
Micro syndrome	RAB3GAP1	2q21.3	Aligianis *et al.* (2005)
Knobloch syndrome	COL18A1	21q22.3	Sertie *et al.* (2000)

Overall, mutations of known genes or consistent association with copy-number variations account for only a small minority of cases of polymicrogyria and in the great majority of cases the cause remains unknown. Bilateral symmetric polymicrogyria syndromes, involving discrete homologous cortical areas (Barkovich *et al.* 1999), strongly suggest a causative role of regionally expressed developmental genes, although etiologic and genetic heterogeneity make the search for specific causative genes particularly difficult. Developmental studies are available for only *PAX6* and *TBR2*. The mouse homologs of these two genes, plus the mouse *Tbr1* gene are expressed sequentially by radial glia (*Pax6*), intermediate progenitor cells (*Tbr2*), and postmitotic neurons (*Tbr1*) in the developing neocortex. Disruption of this pathway can lead to loss or altered fate of large cortical neurons (Englund *et al.* 2005). *SRPX2* is a ligand for urokinase-type plasminogen activator receptor (uPAR) and as other *SRPX2*-associated proteins, is involved in proteolytic remodeling of the extracellular matrix. How these changes may determine an increased epileptogenesis has not been defined yet (Royer-Zemmour *et al.* 2008). The *SRPX2* gene maps to band Xq23, and does not account for X-linked forms of perisylvian polymicrogyria that map to Xq27 and Xq28.

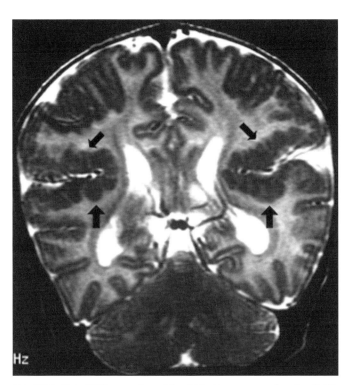

Fig. 48.2. Brain MRI in a newborn. T2-weighted image, coronal section (1.5 T). Bilateral perisylvian polymicrogyria (arrows) is visible as thin undulated cortex.

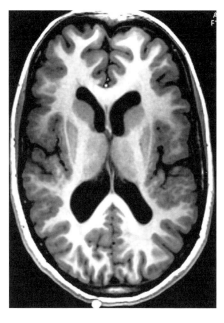

Fig. 48.3. Brain MRI in a newborn. T2-weighted image, axial section (3 T). Bilateral perisylvian polymicrogyria, more severe on the left, is visible as irregular, thickened cortex.

The imaging appearance of polymicrogyria varies with the age of the patient (Takanashi and Barkovich 2003). In newborns and young infants, the polymicrogyric cortex is very thin, with multiple, very small undulations (Fig. 48.2). After myelination, polymicrogyria appears as slightly thick cortex with a somewhat irregular cortex–white matter junction. The pial surface may appear paradoxically smooth, due to fusion of the molecular layer (cortical layer 1) across adjacent microgyri (Fig. 48.1A). Polymicrogyria can be localized to a single gyrus, involve portions of a hemisphere, be bilateral and asymmetrical, bilateral and symmetrical, or diffuse. Sometimes polymicrogyria is associated with deep clefts that may extend through the entire cerebral mantle to communicate with the lateral ventricle; this malformation complex is defined as *schizencephaly*.

The spectrum of clinical manifestations associated with polymicrogyria ranges from normal individuals with only selective impairment of cognitive functions (Galaburda *et al.* 1985) to patients with severe encephalopathies and intractable epilepsy (Guerrini *et al.* 2008). The extent and location of the cortical abnormality influence the severity of neurologic manifestations but probably not that of epilepsy. The most frequently observed polymicrogyria syndromes include bilateral perisylvian polymicrogyria, bilateral frontal and frontoparietal polymicrogyria, bilateral parasagittal parieto-occipital polymicrogyria, unilateral multilobar polymicrogyria, and diffuse polymicrogyria. Schizencephaly is less frequent than polymicrogyria without cleft and is variably associated with a polymicrogyric area in the contralateral hemisphere.

Bilateral perisylvian polymicrogyria (Figs. 48.2, 48.3) involves bilaterally the gray matter bordering the lateral fissure which, in typical cases, is shallow and almost vertical and in continuity with the central or postcentral sulcus. The cortical abnormality is most often symmetric, but of variable extent. The clinical features are often distinctive, with prominent oromotor dysfunction (Guerrini *et al.* 1992b; Kuzniecky *et al.* 1993). Speech production impairment ranges from mild dysarthria to complete absence of speech. Almost all patients have intellectual disability and most have epilepsy. Familial cases have been reported with possible autosomal recessive, autosomal dominant, and X-linked inheritance, although X-linked inheritance appears most frequent (Guerreiro *et al.*, 2000). A locus for X-linked bilateral perisylvian polymicrogyria maps to Xq28 (Villard *et al.* 2002). Mutations of the *SRPX2* gene have been associated with bilateral perisylvian polymicrogyria, which is regularly accompanied by oral and speech dyspraxia, but also with oral and speech dyspraxia and seizures in individuals with normal brain MRI (Roll *et al.* 2006). Bilateral perisylvian polymicrogyria has also been associated with chromosome 22q11.2 deletions (Robin *et al.* 2006) and with twin-to-twin transfusion syndrome with death of the co-twin between the 10th and 18th week of gestation (Van Bogaert *et al.* 1996).

Bilateral parasagittal parieto-occipital polymicrogyria (Fig. 48.4A, B) has been reported in sporadic patients with partial epilepsy and mild cognitive slowing (Guerrini *et al.* 1997). There is no genetic mechanism known for this abnormality. In some patients perisylvian polymicrogyria extends posteriorly to involve the parieto-occipital cortex, the sylvian fissure being prolonged across the entire hemispheric convexity up to the mesial surface of the hemispheric convexity.

Bilateral frontal polymicrogyria has been described in children with developmental delay, mild spastic quadriparesis

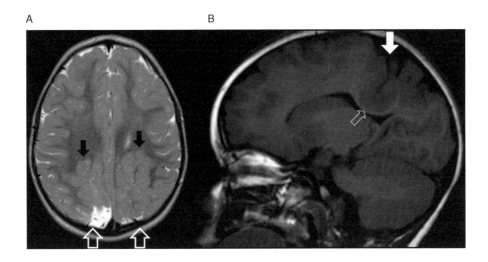

Fig. 48.4. Brain MRI in a newborn (1.5 T). (A) T2-weighted image, axial section showing bilateral infoldings of irregular thickened cortex at the parieto-occipital junction (arrows). (B) T1-weighted image, sagittal section showing a deep infolding of cortex reaching the ventricular wall (arrows).

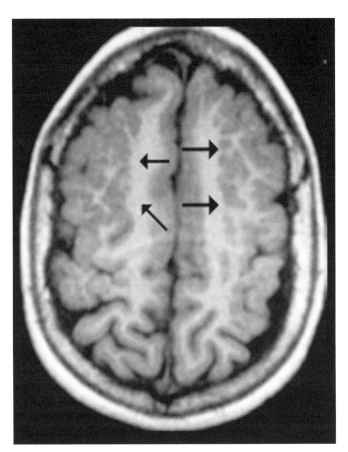

Fig. 48.5. Brain MRI. T1-weighted image, axial section. Bilateral frontal polymicrogyria (arrows).

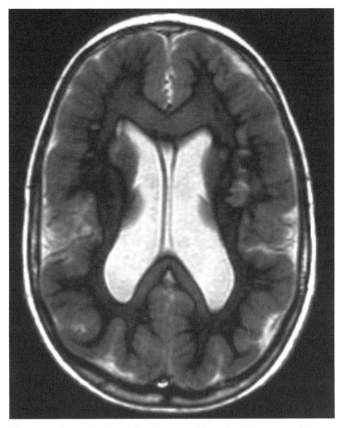

Fig. 48.6. Brain MRI. T2-weighted image, axial section. Fifteen-year-old girl with bilateral frontoparietal polymicrogyria, *GPR56* gene mutation and Lennox–Gastaut syndrome. There is increased cortical thickness, simplified gyral pattern, and multiple patchy areas of increased signal intensity are seen in the white matter.

and epilepsy (Guerrini *et al.* 2000) (Fig. 48.5). *Bilateral frontoparietal polymicrogyria* has been reported in consanguineous and non-consanguineous families with recessive pedigrees and has been associated with mutations of the *GPR56* gene (Piao *et al.* 2004). The topography of the cortical abnormality, as well as the pattern of expression of mouse *Gpr56*, suggests that *GPR56* regulates cortical patterning. The imaging characteristics of bilateral frontoparietal

polymicrogyria (myelination defects, cerebellarcortical dysplasia with cysts, frequent involvement of the medial aspects of the cerebral hemispheres) (Fig. 48.6) resemble those of the cobblestone malformative spectrum (muscle–eye–brain disease and Fukuyama congenital muscular dystrophy) that are also associated with *N*-glycosylation defects in the developing brain (Jin *et al.* 2007). Therefore, it has been suggested that

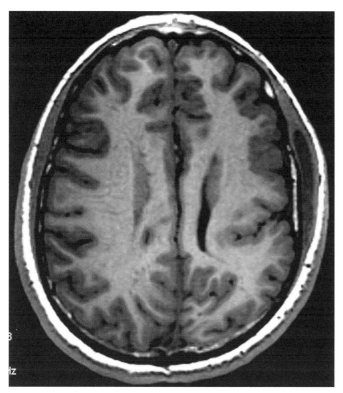

Fig. 48.7. Brain MRI. T1-weighted image, axial section. Young man with mild right hemiparesis and a history of focal seizures and atypical absences. Polymicrogyria affecting the left hemisphere with irregular cortical folding in the perisylvian and perirolandic cortex.

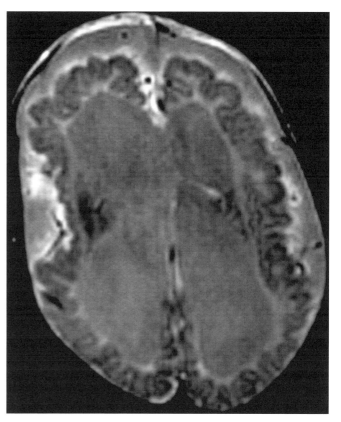

Fig. 48.8. Brain MRI. T2-weighted image, axial section. Child with severe spastic quadriparesis, profound developmental delay, and intractable seizures. Scan shows a severe malformation with ventricular dilatation and diffusely abnormal gyral pattern with numerous small microgyri covering the entire cortical surface.

this disorder might be best classified as a cobblestone malformation (Barkovich *et al.* 2005; Guerrini *et al.* 2008).

Unilateral perisylvian or hemispheric polymicrogyria (Fig. 48.7) is accompanied by a combination of seizures (75%), mild to moderate hemiparesis (75%), and mild to moderate mental retardation (70%). Hemiparesis is typically associated with prominent mirror movements of the affected limb (Guerrini *et al.* 1996). This feature has been attributed to ipsilateral cortical representation of the sensorimotor hand area (Maegaki *et al.* 1995). In patients with interictal electroencephalographic (EEG) abnormalities and seizures involving the motor cortex, hemiparesis may worsen with worsening of interictal epileptiform abnormalities or of seizures. Age at seizure onset and epilepsy severity are quite variable.

Generalized polymicrogyria (Fig. 48.8) is often accompanied by microcephaly and severe–profound cognitive and motor delay, as well as epilepsy. It is likely that, rather than a distinct syndrome (Chang *et al.* 2004), generalized polymicrogyria, whether symmetric or asymmetric, is the expression of a variety of largely unknown genetic and environmental factors.

Aicardi syndrome is exclusively observed in females, with the exception of two reported males with two X chromosomes (Aicardi 1996) and is thought to be caused by an X-linked gene with lethality in the hemizygous male. However, the genetic basis is still unknown. Clinical features include severe mental

retardation, infantile spasms, and chorioretinal lacunae. Neuropathological findings are consistent with a neuronal migration disorder and include diffuse unlayered polymicrogyria with fused molecular layers (Fig. 48.1A), agenesis of the corpus callosum, and nodular heterotopias in the periventricular or subcortical region (Fig. 48.9). Microgyri are packed and usually not visible at MRI.

Schizencephaly is a cortical malformation characterized by clefts in the cerebral mantle, surrounded by polymicrogyric cortex (Ferrer 1984). Both polymicrogyria and schizencephaly have been reported in the same family (Muntaner *et al.* 1997) and both may occur with prenatal cytomegalovirus infection (Barkovich and Lindan 1994) or with vascular problems related to twinning (Barth and van der Harten 1985). It has been suggested that considering their frequent association and shared causative factors, polymicrogyria and schizencephaly should be classified together (Barkovich *et al.* 2005). The schizencephalic fissures are unilateral or bilateral and produce an abnormal full thickness communication between the ventricle(s) and pericerebral subarachnoid space(s). The walls of the clefts may be widely separated (open-lip schizencephaly) (Fig. 48.10), or closely apposed (closed-lip schizencephaly) (Fig. 48.11) and may be located in any region of the

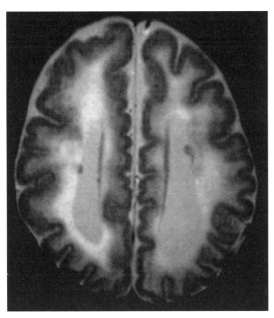

Fig. 48.9. Brain MRI. T2-weighted image, axial section. Girl with Aicardi syndrome. Note the simplified gyral pattern with poor gray–white matter delimitation, agenesis of the corpus callosum, and dilated ventricles with small subependymal nodules of gray matter heterotopia.

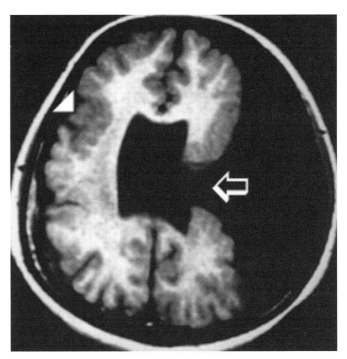

Fig. 48.10. Brain MRI. T1-weighted image, axial section. Twelve-year-old boy with focal epilepsy and spastic quadriparesis, more severe on the right. Left-sided open-lip schizencephaly, lined by polymicrogyric cortex (empty arrow). Contralateral patchy area of polymicrogyria (white triangle).

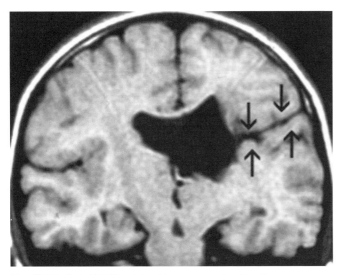

Fig. 48.11. Brain MRI. T1-weighted image, coronal section. Young man with mild right hemiparesis and focal epilepsy. Left-sided closed-lip schizencephaly, lined by polymicrogyric cortex (arrows).

hemispheres, but are by far most frequent in the central and perisylvian area (Friede 1989; Barkovich and Kjos 1992). Bilateral clefts are usually symmetric in location, but not necessarily in size. Unilateral clefts, especially if large, may be associated with a localized focus of polymicrogyria in the contralateral cortex (Friede 1989). Schizencephaly is associated with agenesis of septum pellucidum in about 30% of cases and agenesis or hypoplasia of corpus callosum in about 70% of cases. An association between unilateral or bilateral clefts, agenesis of septum pellucidum, and optic nerve atrophy

(so called septo-optic dysplasia) may be observed in 6–25% of patients (Barkovich and Kjos 1992; Granata *et al.* 1999; Denis *et al.* 2000). Schizencephaly has been associated with several environmental factors including maternal trauma, substance abuse, viral infection (particularly cytomegalovirus), twin–twin transfusion syndrome, and other vascular disorders (Barkovich and Kjos 1992; Curry *et al.* 2005). Several sporadic patients and two siblings of both sexes harboring germline mutations in the homeobox gene *EMX2* have been described but involvement of this gene has not been confirmed in large series (Merello *et al.* 2008). Experimental models do not support a causal relationship between *EMX2* mutations and schizencephaly. Heterozygous $Emx2^+$/knock-out mice show a normal phenotype, whereas knockout mice with homozygous *Emx2* deletions exhibit severe developmental defects of the urogenital system and structural alterations of the olfactory bulbs and hippocampal dentate gyrus, but do not have clefts in the cerebral cortex (Pellegrini *et al.* 1996; Yoshida *et al.* 1997).

It is difficult to establish at which time during embryonic development schizencephaly originates. There is no agreement as to whether it should be classified as a defect originating early, with localized fault in neuronal proliferation. The presence of polymicrogyric cortex, however, is the hallmark of a disorder of cortical layering that extends through late cortical organization.

Clinical findings include focal seizures present in most patients (81% of cases in one large review), usually beginning before age 3 years if bilateral clefts are present. Bilateral clefts are usually associated with severe neurological abnormalities whereas unilateral schizencephaly is usually accompanied by hemiparesis or just detected after seizure onset in otherwise neurologically normal individuals. Patients with bilateral schizencephaly usually exhibit spastic quadriparesis, often associated with apraxia, pseudobulbar paralysis, and microcephaly (Granata *et al.* 2005). The report of quadriparesis in a few patients with unilateral cleft has been attributed to subtle cortical abnormality in the contralateral cortex. Cognitive level is normal in 30% to 80% of patients with a unilateral cleft, whereas it is moderately to severely impaired in most patients with bilateral clefts (Barkovich and Kjos 1992; Denis *et al.* 2000). Abnormal speech development has been reported in up to 52% of unilateral schizencephaly patients, whereas delay in language development is observed in 95–100% of bilateral cases.

Epilepsy in the disease

Epilepsy, motor impairment, and disorders of higher cortical functions are the most common clinical manifestation of polymicrogyria. Diffuse polymicrogyria, involving most of the brain, usually causes resistant generalized or multifocal epilepsy. Polymicrogyria involving a discrete region of one hemisphere is often detected after brain MRI, prompted by onset of focal seizures at school age or later in otherwise healthy individuals. In one large series (Guerrini *et al.* 1996), unilateral polymicrogyria was accompanied by partial motor seizures (73%), atypical absences (47%), generalized tonic–clonic seizures (27%), and complex partial seizures (20%). Epilepsy could be classified as partial in 80% of patients and generalized in 20%. Interictal EEG findings in most patients suggested epileptogenesis from lager areas than expected from MRI. Extensive polymicrogyria involving a whole hemisphere or with multilobar distribution (*unilateral hemispheric polymicrogyria*) has been associated with a specific clinical syndrome, including seizures, hemiparesis, and mild to moderate cognitive impairment (Guerrini *et al.* 1998). Patients have continuous generalized EEG discharges during slow-wave sleep and suffer from partial motor, atonic, and atypical absence seizures with cognitive deterioration (epilepsy with continuous spikes and waves during sleep [CSWS] or electrical status epilepticus during sleep [ESES]). The condition is usually detected between ages 2 and 10 years and may last for months to years, before epilepsy invariably remits. The course is not different from that seen in patients with the same epilepsy syndrome but no apparent brain abnormality. Bilateral perisylvian polymicrogyria has been consistently associated with atypical absences, tonic or atonic drop attacks, and tonic–clonic seizures, often presenting as Lennox–Gastaut-like syndromes (Guerrini *et al.* 1992b; Kuzniecky *et al.* 1993). A minority of patients with bilateral perisylvian polymicrogyria have partial seizures and a small number of patients may present with infantile spasms (Kuzniecky *et al.* 1994a, b). Bilateral fronto-parietal polymicrogyria has also been consistently associated with intractable epilepsy in the majority of patients, mainly manifested by partial seizures, atypical absences (Piao *et al.* 2004) or full-blown Lennox–Gastaut syndrome (Parrini *et al.* 2009).

Specific electroclinical features of Aicardi syndrome include early onset infantile spasms and partial seizures. Hypsarrhythmia is observed in a minority of children (Aicardi 1996). Interictal EEG abnormalities, which include a burst suppression EEG, are typically asymmetric and asynchronous (split brain EEG). Seizures and EEG patterns change little, if at all, over time and epilepsy is almost always resistant.

In addition to the above anatomoclinical syndromes, polymicrogyria has been linked with a wide spectrum of anatomic patterns of distribution and epilepsy phenotypes. Diffuse epileptogenesis is frequently encountered, even with seemingly limited abnormalities (Guerrini *et al.* 1992a). Intracranial recordings have confirmed observations obtained non-invasively that large epileptogenic networks are often observed, extending well beyond the limits of the visible abnormality even when polymicrogyria is limited to a focal region (Guerrini *et al.* 1992a; Chassoux *et al.* 2008).

Epileptogenicity of polymicrogyria and its mechanisms are not known but a considerable number of patients do not have epilepsy. Experimental models produced by localized freezing suggest widespread functional disruption, with downregulation of different γ-aminobutyric acid GABA$_A$ receptor subunits extending far beyond the visualized abnormality (Redecker *et al.* 2000).

Epilepsy is present in 36–65% of patients with schizencephaly and is refractory to antiepileptic drugs in 9–38% of them (Barkovich and Kjos 1992; Packard *et al.* 1997; Denis *et al.* 2000). In two series (Granata *et al.* 1999; Denis *et al.* 2000), epilepsy was more frequently associated with unilateral schizencephaly, in comparison with bilateral cases, in which seizure intractability was less frequent. Other authors (Barkovich and Kjos 1992; Packard *et al.* 1997) have pointed out that bilateral open-lip schizencephaly implies an earlier age at seizure onset and more frequent drug-resistance. Severity and type of seizures does not seem to correlate with the topography of the schizencephalic cleft (Leventer *et al.* 2008).

Diagnostic tests

Using computed tomography (CT) and low-field-strength MRI, polymicrogyria is difficult to discern and may only appear as thickened cortex. The only role for CT in the evaluation of polymicrogyria is to assess for evidence of calcification, which is seen in polymicrogyria resulting from congenital cytomegalovirus infection. Using high-quality 1.5 T MRI with appropriate age-specific protocols, it is now possible to reliably differentiate polymicrogyria from other malformations of cortical development. Polymicrogyric cortex often appears mildly thickened (6–10 mm) on imaging due to cortical overfolding rather than true cortical thickening. With better imaging (such as inversion recovery) using thin contiguous slices microgyri and microsulci may be appreciated. Diffusely abnormal white matter signal should raise the question of an in utero infection or a peroxisomal disorder. Other developmental anomalies may also be seen including ventricular enlargement or dysmorphism and abnormalities of the corpus callosum and cerebellum, although the patterns and prevalence of these associated brain malformations are poorly documented. In spite of progress in neuroimaging, polymicrogyria may still be difficult to recognize in its full extent; polymicrogyria apparently unilateral on MRI may turn out to be bilateral and extensive on microscopic examination of the brain (Guerrini *et al.* 1992a).

Polymicrogyria should be differentiated from cobblestone cortex ("type II lissencephaly"). This differentiation is difficult, both by imaging and by pathologic examination. By MRI, the mild cortical thickening and irregularity of the cortical–white matter junction observed in the frontal lobes in Fukuyama congenital muscular dystrophy and in muscle–eye–brain disease is very difficult to distinguish from polymicrogyria (Barkovich 1998). Even pathologists have provided different descriptions, with some considering unlayered polymicrogyria in the frontal lobes as part of the malformation complex in Fukuyama congenital muscular dystrophy (Takada *et al.* 1988) and others considering overmigration of cells beyond the external glial limitans to be identical to that observed in muscle–eye–brain disease, which is classified as cobblestone cortex (Leyten *et al.* 1991; Haltia *et al.* 1997) (see Chapter 52).

Polymicrogyria should also be differentiated from polygyria, a macroscopically hyperconvoluted cortex, most often associated with hydrocephalus, in which cortical layering and histology is normal (Golden and Harding 2004). Ulegyria, a peculiar pattern of ischemic cortical damage, typical of watershed areas, is often confused with polymicrogyria. In ulegyria, the cortex of the crest of gyri is preserved while the depth of sulci is preferentially damaged. As a consequence, cortical gyri often have a mushroom-like morphological pattern and the depth of sulci appears as overfolded.

Electroencephalography in polymicrogyria and schizencephaly shows variable patterns of abnormality, which are more widely distributed than expected from an estimate of the extent of the macroscopic structural abnormality. It is not unusual to observe multifocal bilateral spikes or diffuse discharges even in patients with a circumscribed area of polymicrogyria. Generalized spike-and-wave or multifocal discharges with a centroparietal emphasis are often observed (Guerrini *et al.* 1992a). The characteristics of the EEG, however, are much influenced by the associated epilepsy syndrome.

Genetic analysis and counseling in polymicrogyria is still problematic, considering anatomic and etiologic heterogeneity. Identified genes account for only a small number of patients with very rare syndromes. Isolated perisylvian polymicrogyria, in the absence of a clustering of clinical manifestations suggestive for a specific syndrome, should be investigated with chromosome analysis, comparative genomic hybridization (CGH) array or with fluorescent in situ hybridization (FISH) analysis to rule out chromosome 22q11.2 deletions (Robin *et al.* 2006). The yield appears to be higher when the polymicrogyria is asymmetric. In view of the causal heterogeneity of perisylvian polymicrogyria, including the potential for recessive and X-linked inheritance, parents of an affected child should be given 25% recurrence risk. The possibility of X-linked inheritance should be discussed in the case of a male offspring, with a recurrence risk of up to 50%. Mutations of *KIAA1279* have been found in patients with Goldberg–Shprintzen syndrome, which consists of mental retardation, microcephaly, polymicrogyria, and Hirschsprung disease (Brooks *et al.* 2005). Mutations of *GPR56* have been consistently associated with bilateral frontoparietal polymicrogyria (Piao *et al.* 2004; Parrini *et al.* 2009). Mutations of the *TUBB2B* gene have been associated with asymmetric polymicrogyria (Jaglin *et al.* 2009) but genotype–phenotype correlations need to be clarified.

Regrettably, while several causal genes for polymicrogyria have now been discovered, they only account for a small minority of cases and clinical testing is available for only a few. Current information regarding clinical testing is available at the GeneReviews–GeneTests website (www.genereviews.org/ or www.genetests.org/). For other genes, testing can sometimes be performed in research laboratories. When results are obtained from a research laboratory, they should be confirmed in a clinical laboratory as a custom diagnostic test (Barkovich *et al.* 2005).

Although schizencephaly is usually sporadic, familial occurrence has been reported and a specific genetic origin is possible in some cases. The possible pattern(s) of inheritance of schizencephaly is still unclear and molecular study of the *EMX2* gene in an individual with schizencephaly is probably useless.

Principles of management

Many patients with polymicrogyria have severe disability and need comprehensive medical care and rehabilitation (Turkelson and Martin 2009). Epilepsy is often resistant to drugs. Patients who develop infantile spasms, Lennox–Gastaut syndrome, or epilepsy with CSWS should be treated according to drug treatment strategies for these syndromes. In a narrow subset of patients with focal epilepsy curative treatment using a surgical approach is possible.

In diffuse forms of polymicrogyria, frequent involvement of most of the brain usually gives rise to severe cognitive impairment with generalized or multifocal epilepsies, which cannot be operated on. Even less diffuse forms of polymicrogyria are frequently characterized by multiple uncontrolled seizure types with likely involvement of eloquent cortex in the epileptogenic zone and poor delimitation of the abnormal cortex. Consequently, surgical treatment of epilepsy is applicable to a limited number of patients in whom remission of epilepsy is not expected (Guerrini *et al.* 1997) and large resections are feasible (Chassoux *et al.* 2008). An integrated fMRI, somatosensory eroked potentials and motor evoked potentials approach for assessing functional organization in the malformed cortex may reduce the need for invasive recordings in patients who can collaborate in these investigations (Barba *et al.* 2010). Functional studies suggest variability in cortical representation, probably in relation to both the severity of anatomic disruption and the involved modality. Magnetic source imaging studies show that the somatosensory function remains localized in the polymicrogyric rolandic cortex, as long as the anatomy is not distorted by a schizencephalic cleft, in which case function is located in the hemisphere ipsilateral to stimulation, in the expected anatomic locations (Burneo *et al.* 2004). Studies with fMRI indicate that the polymicrogyric language and motor areas tend to preserve functionality in the expected sites (Araujo *et al.* 2006). Combined fMRI and transcranial magnetic stimulation studies in patients with polymicrogyria and hemiparesis suggest that ipsilateral corticospinal projections from the contralesional hemisphere to the paretic hand, corticospinal projections to the paretic hand originating in the

polymicrogyric cortex, and bilateral motor representation are all possible (Staudt *et al.* 2004; Guzzetta *et al.* 2007). Generalization of findings to the entire population of patients with polymicrogyria may be inappropriate, however, in view of its high degree of histopathologic variability (Guerrini *et al.* 1992a) and causal heterogeneity.

Selected patients with schizencephaly have been treated with surgery for epilepsy (Leblanc *et al.* 1996). Resections were guided using intraoperative electrocorticography (ECoG) and, where necessary, by depth electrode exploration. Resection caused no deficit and produced worthwhile seizure reduction in all patients, though none remained seizure-free. In planning surgical treatment, careful clinical, neurophysiological, and functional imaging studies are necessary, in order to assess the degree of functional activity of the tissue surrounding the cleft (Lee *et al.* 1999). In patients with bilateral lesions resective surgery is unwise and callosotomy must be considered when tonic or atonic drop attack seizures occur.

References

Aicardi J (1996) Aicardi syndrome. In: Guerrini R, Andermann F, Canapicchi R, Roger J, Zifkin BG, Pfanner P (eds.) *Dysplasias of Cerebral Cortex and Epilepsy*. Philadelphia, PA: Lippincott-Raven, pp. 211–16.

Aligianis IA, Johnson CA, Gissen P (2005) Mutations of the catalytic subunit of *RAB3GAP* cause Warburg Micro syndrome. *Nat Genet* **37**:221–3.

Araujo D, de Araujo DB, Pontes-Neto OM, *et al.* (2006) Language and motor fMRI activation in polymicrogyric cortex *Epilepsia* **47**:589–92.

Baala L, Briault S, Etchevers HC, *et al.* (2007) Homozygous silencing of T-box transcription factor EOMES leads to microcephaly with polymicrogyria and corpus callosum agenesis. *Nat Genet* **39**:454–6.

Barba C, Montanaro D, Cincotta M, Giovannelli F, Guerrini R (2010) An integrated fMRI, SEPs and MEPs approach for assessing functional organization in the malformed sensorimotor cortex. *Epilepsy Res* **89**:66–71.

Barkovich AJ (1998) Neuroimaging manifestations and classification of congenital muscular dystrophies. *AJNR Am J Neuroradiol* **19**:1389–96.

Barkovich AJ, Kjos BO (1992) Schizencephaly: correlation of clinical findings with MR characteristics. *AJNR Am J Neuroradiol* **13**:85–94.

Barkovich AJ, Lindan CE (1994) Congenital cytomegalovirus infection of the brain: imaging analysis and embryologic considerations. *AJNR Am J Neuroradiol* **15**:703–15.

Barkovich AJ, Hevner R, Guerrini R (1999) Syndromes of bilateral symmetrical polymicrogyria. *AJNR Am J Neuroradiol* **20**:1814–21.

Barkovich AJ, Kuzniecky RI, Jackson GD, Guerrini R, Dobyns WB (2005) A developmental and genetic classification for malformations of cortical development. *Neurology* **65**:1873–87.

Barth PG, van der Harten JJ (1985) Parabiotic twin syndrome with topicalisocortical disruption and gastroschisis. *Acta Neuropathol* **67**:345–9.

Brooks AS, Bertoli-Avella AM, Burzynski GM, *et al.* (2005) Homozygous nonsense mutations in *KIAA1279* are associated with malformations of the central and enteric nervous systems. *Am J Hum Genet* **77**:120–6.

Burneo JC, Bebin M, Kuzniecky RI, Knowlton RC (2004) Cortical reorganization in malformations of cortical development: a magnetoencephalographic study. *Neurology* **63**:1818–24.

Chang BS, Piao X, Giannini C, *et al.* (2004) Bilateral generalized polymicrogyria (BGP): a distinct syndrome of cortical malformation. *Neurology* **62**:1722–8.

Chassoux, F, Landre E, Rodrigo S, *et al.* (2008) Intralesional recordings and

epileptogenic zone in focal polymicrogyria. *Epilepsia* **49**:51–64.

Curry CJ, Lammer EJ, Nelson V, Shaw GM (2005) Schizencephaly: heterogeneous etiologies in a population of 4 million California births. *Am J Med Genet* **137A**:181–9.

Denis D, Chateil JF, Brun M, *et al.* (2000) Schizencephaly: clinical and imaging features in 30 infantile cases. *Brain Dev* **22**:475–83.

Dobyns WB, Mirzaa G, Christian SL, *et al.* (2008) Consistent chromosome abnormalities identify novel polymicrogyria loci in 1p36.3, 2p16.1–p23.1, 4q21.21–q22.1, 6q26–q27, and 21q2. *Am J Med Genet* **146A**:1637–54.

Englund C, Fink A, Lau C, *et al.* (2005) *Pax6, Tbr2, and Tbr1* are expressed sequentially by radial glia, intermediate progenitor cells, and postmitotic neurons in developing neocortex. *J Neurosci* **25**:247–51.

Ferrer I (1984) A Golgi analysis of unlayered polymicrogyria. *Acta Neuropathol* **65**:69–76.

Friede RL (1989) *Developmental Neuropathology*. New York: Springer-Verlag.

Galaburda AM, Sherman GF, Rosen GD, Aboitiz F, Geschwind N (1985) Developmental dyslexia: four consecutive patients with cortical anomalies. *Ann Neurol* **18**:222–33.

Glaser T, Jepeal L, Edwards JG, *et al.* (1994) *PAX6* gene dosage effect in a family with congenital cataracts, aniridia, anophthalmia and central nervous system defects. *Nat Genet* 7:463–71.

Golden JA, Harding BN (2004) *Pathology and Genetics: Developmental Neuropathology.* Basel: ISN Neuropath Press.

Granata T, D'Incerti L, Freri E, *et al.* (1999) Schizencephaly: clinical and genetic findings in a case series. In: Spreafico R, Avanzini G, Andermann F (eds.) *Abnormal Cortical Development and Epilepsy.* London: John Libbey, pp. 181–9.

Granata T, Freri E, Caccia C, *et al.* (2005) Schizencephaly: clinical spectrum, epilepsy, and pathogenesis. *J Child Neurol* 20:313–18.

Guerreiro MM, Andermann E, Guerrini R, *et al.* (2000) Familial perisylvian polymicrogyria: a new familial syndrome of cortical maldevelopment. *Ann Neurol* 48:39–48.

Guerrini R, Parrini E (2010) Neuronal migration disorders. *Neurobiol Dis* 38:154–66.

Guerrini R, Dravet C, Raybaud C, *et al.* (1992a) Epilepsy and focal gyral anomalies detected by magnetic resonance imaging: electroclinico-morphological correlations and follow-up. *Dev Med Child Neurol* 34:706–18.

Guerrini R, Dravet C, Raybaud C, *et al.* (1992b) Neurological findings and seizure outcome in children with bilateral opercular macrogyric-like changes detected by MRI. *Dev Med Child Neurol* 34:694–705.

Guerrini R, Dravet C, Bureau M, *et al.* (1996) Diffuse and localized dysplasias of cerebral cortex: clinical presentation, outcome, and proposal for a morphologic MRI classification based on a study of 90 patients. In: Guerrini R, Andermann F, Canapicchi R, Roger J, Zifkin BG, Pfanner P (eds.) *Dysplasias of Cerebral Cortex and Epilepsy.* Philadelphia, PA: Lippincott-Raven, pp. 255–69.

Guerrini R, Dubeau F, Dulac O, *et al.* (1997) Bilateral parasagittal parietooccipital polymicrogyria and epilepsy. *Ann Neurol* 41:65–73.

Guerrini R, Genton P, Bureau M, *et al.* (1998) Multilobar polymicrogyria, intractable drop attack seizures, and sleep-related electrical status epilepticus. *Neurology* 51:504–12.

Guerrini R, Barkovich AJ, Sztriha L, Dobyns WB (2000) Bilateral frontal polymicrogyria: a newly recognized brain malformation syndrome. *Neurology* 54:909–13.

Guerrini R, Dobyns WB, Barkovich JA (2008) Abnormal development of the human cerebral cortex: genetics, functional consequences and treatment options. *Trends Neurosci.* 31:153–6.

Guzzetta A, Bonanni P, Biagi L, *et al.* (2007) Reorganization of the somatosensory system after early brain damage. *Clin Neurophysiol* 118:1110–21.

Haltia M, Leivo I, Somer H, *et al.* (1997). Muscle–eye–brain disease: a neuropathological study. *Ann Neurol* 41:173–80.

Jaglin XH, Poirier K, Saillour Y, *et al.* (2009) Mutations in the beta-tubulin gene *TUBB2B* result in asymmetrical polymicrogyria. *Nat Genet* 41:746–52.

Jin Z, Tietjen I, Bu L, *et al.* (2007) Disease associated mutations affect GPR56 protein trafficking and cell surface expression. *Hum Mol Genet* 16:1972–85.

Kuzniecky R, Andermann F, Guerrini R, CBPS Study Group (1993) Congenital bilateral perisylvian syndrome: study of 31 patients. *Lancet* 341:608–12.

Kuzniecky RI, Andermann F, CBPS Study Group (1994a) The congenital bilateral perisylvian syndrome: imaging findings in a multicenter study. *AJNR Am J Neuroradiol* 15:139–44.

Kuzniecky R, Andermann F, Guerrini R (1994b) The epileptic spectrum in the congenital bilateral perisylvian syndrome. *Neurology* 44:379–85.

Leblanc R, Meyer E, Zatorre R, Klein D, Evans A (1996) Functional imaging of cerebral arteriovenous malformations with a comment on cortical reorganization. *Neurosurg Focus* 15:e4.

Lee HK, Kim JS, Hwang YM, *et al.* (1999) Location of the primary motor cortex in schizencephaly. *AJNR Am J Neuroradiol* 20:163–6.

Leventer RJ, Guerrini R, Dobyns WB (2008) Malformations of cortical development and epilepsy. *Dialogues Clin Neurosci* 10:47–62.

Leyten QH, Renkawek K, Renier WO, *et al.* (1991) Neuropathological findings in muscle–eye–brain disease: neuropathological delineation of MEB-D from congential muscular dystrophy of the Fukuyama type. *Acta Neuropathol* 83:55–60.

Maegaki Y, Yamamoto T, Takeshita K (1995) Plasticity of central motor and sensory pathways in a case of unilateral extensive cortical dysplasia: investigation of magnetic resonance imaging, transcranial magnetic stimulation, and short-latency somatosensory evoked potentials. *Neurology* 45:2255–61.

Merello E, Swanson E, De Marco P, *et al.* (2008) No major role for the *EMX2* gene in schizencephaly. *Am J Med Genet* 146A:1142–50.

Muntaner L, Pérez-Ferrón J, Herrera M, *et al.* (1997) MRI of a family with focal abnormalities of gyration. *Neuroradiology* 39:605–8.

Nowaczyk MJ, Teshima IE, Siegel-Bartelt J, Clarke JT (1997) Deletion 4q21/4q22 syndrome: two patients with de novo 4q21.3q23 and 4q13.2q23 deletions. *Am J Med Genet* 69:400–5.

Packard AM, Miller VS, Delgado MR (1997) Schizencephaly: correlations – Septo-optic dysplasia schizencephaly: radiographic and clinical features. *Neurology* 48:1427–34.

Parrini E, Ferrari AR, Dorn T, Walsh CA, Guerrini R (2009) Bilateral frontoparietal polymicrogyria, Lennox–Gastaut syndrome, and *GPR56* gene mutations. *Epilepsia* 50:1344–53.

Pellegrini M, Mansouri A, Simeone A, Boncinelli E, Gruss P (1996) Dentate gyrus formation requires *Emx2*. *Development* 122:3893–98.

Piao X, Chang BS, Bodell A, *et al.* (2005) Genotype-phenotype analysis of human frontoparietal polymicrogyria syndrome. *Ann Neurol* 58:680–7.

Piao X, Hill RS, Bodell A, *et al.* (2004) G protein-coupled receptor dependent development of human frontal cortex. *Science* 303:2033–6.

Redecker C, Luhmann HJ, Hagemann G, Fritschy JM, Witte OW (2000) Differential downregulation of GABA$_A$ receptor subunits in widespread brain regions in the freeze-lesion model of focal cortical malformations. *J Neurosci* 20:5045–53.

Reinhardt K, Mohr A, Gärtner J, Spohr HL, Brockmann K (2010). Polymicrogyria in fetal alcohol syndrome. *Birth Defects Res A Clin Mol Teratol* 88:128–31.

Ribeiro MDC, Gama de Sousa S, Freitas MM, Carrilho I, Fernandes I (2007) Bilateral perisylvian polymicrogyria and chromosome 1 anomaly. *Pediatr Neurol* 36:418–20.

Robin NH, Taylor CJ, McDonald-McGinn DM, *et al.* (2006) Polymicrogyria and deletion 22q11.2 syndrome: window to the etiology of a common cortical malformation. *Am J Med Genet* **140A**:2416–25.

Roll P, Rudolf G, Pereira S, *et al.* (2006) *SRPX2* mutations in disorders of language cortex and cognition. *Hum Mol Genet* **15**:1195–207.

Royer-Zemmour B, Ponsole-Lenfant M, Gara H, *et al.* (2008) Epileptic and developmental disorders of the speech cortex: ligand/receptor interaction of wild-type and mutant *SRPX2* with the plasmin- ogen activator receptor uPAR. *Hum Mol Genet* **17**:3617–30.

Sertie AL, Sossi V, Camargo AA, *et al.* (2000) Collagen XVIII, containing an endogenous inhibitor of angiogenesis and tumor growth, plays a critical role in the maintenance of retinal structure and in neural tube closure (Knobloch syndrome). *Hum Mol Genet* **9**:2051–8.

Staudt M, Krägeloh-Mann I, Holthausen H, Gerloff C, Grodd W (2004) Searching for motor functions in dysgenic cortex: a clinical transcranial magnetic stimulation and functional magnetic resonance imaging study. *J Neurosurg* **101**:69–77.

Takada K, Nakamura H, Takashima S (1988) Cortical dysplasia in Fukuyama congenital muscular dystrophy: a Golgi and angioarchitectonic analysis. *Acta Neuropathol* **76**:170–8.

Takanashi J, Barkovich A (2003) The changing MR imaging appearance of polymicrogyria: a consequence of myelination. *AJNR Am J Neuroradiol* **24**:788–93.

Turkelson SL, Martin C (2009) Management of the child with polymicrogyria. *J Neurosci Nurs* **41**:251–60.

Van Bogaert P, Donner C, David P, *et al.* (1996) Congenital bilateral perisylvian syndrome in a monozygotic twin with intra-uterine death of the co-twin. *Dev Med Child Neurol* **38**:166–71.

Villard L, Nguyen K, Cardoso C, *et al.* (2002) A locus for bilateral perisylvian polymicrogyria maps to Xq28. *Am J Hum Genet* **70**:1003–8.

Yao G, Chen XN, Flores-Sarnat L, *et al.* (2006) Deletion of chromosome 21 disturbs human brain morphogenesis. *Genet Med* **8**:1–7.

Yoshida M, Suda Y, Matsuo I, *et al.* (1997) Emx1 and Emx2 functions in development of dorsal telencephalon. *Development* **124**:101–11.

Zollino M, Colosimo C, Zuffardi O, *et al.* (2003) Cryptic t(1;12)(q44;p13.3) translocation in a previously described syndrome with polymicrogyria, segregating as an apparently X-linked trait. *Am J Med Genet* **117A**:65–71.

Chapter

49

Periventricular nodular heterotopia

Rahul Rathakrishnan, Yahya Aghakhani, and François Dubeau

The causal disease

Definition

Normal cortical development involves postmitotic neuronal migration from the ventricular zone into the cortical plate and subsequent differentiation into the layers that define the cerebral cortex (Lu and Sheen 2005). Neuronal heterotopia are collections of gray matter located in abnormal position within the cerebral hemispheres, likely to be due to a primary failure of radial migration of neurons from the ventricular zone to the cortex. They can be found anywhere from the subependyma along the lateral ventricles to the cortical mantle (Barkovich and Kuzniecky 2000). We usually distinguish two types of heterotopia: the *laminar* or band heterotopia, or "double cortex," and the *nodular* heterotopia that can be periventricular (or subependymal) or subcortical. Periventricular heterotopia arises from abnormal initiation of neuronal migration (Pang *et al.* 2008). This disruption affects a subpopulation of neurons and occurs late during the migration period, close to the 16th gestational week, by which time most neuroblasts would have normally completed the process (Raymond *et al.* 1994; Lu and Sheen 2005; Pang *et al.* 2008). They are typically nodular but can be linear or have a ribbon-like appearance (Parrini *et al.* 2006). The periventricular nodular heterotopia (PNH) are located along the walls of the lateral ventricles, sparing the third and fourth ventricles (Dubeau *et al.* 1995; Battaglia and Granata 2007). They usually protrude into the lumen of the ventricles, and are either uni- or bilateral, symmetrical or asymmetrical, diffuse and contiguous, or scattered and isolated. The nodules sometimes predominate in the anterior aspect of the lateral ventricles but are often more prominent posteriorly along the trigones and temporal and occipital horns (d'Orsi *et al.* 2004; Leventer *et al.* 2008). Periventricular nodular heterotopia is a frequent type of malformation of cortical development (MCD) and can be sporadic or familial (Kothare *et al.* 1998; Guerrini and Carrozzo 2001; Montenegro *et al.* 2006; Battaglia and Granata 2007; Pang *et al.* 2008; Cardoso *et al.* 2009). Electrophysiological

studies revealed that they are capable of generating normal and epileptic activity (Francione *et al.* 1994; Dubeau *et al.* 1995; Kothare *et al.* 1998; Aghakhani *et al.* 2005; Battaglia *et al.* 2006; Battaglia and Granata 2007; Leventer *et al.* 2008; Valton *et al.* 2008). Histologically, the nodules contain normal-appearing neurons with an abnormal position and synaptic organization. They are interconnected between themselves and also with the overlying cortex (Dubeau *et al.* 1995; Thom *et al.* 2004; Battaglia and Granata 2007; Leventer *et al.* 2008; Pang *et al.* 2008).

Pathophysiology

A common mechanism to all gray matter heterotopia is the failure of radial migration of neurons from their origin in the periventricular zone to the cortex. This is most likely due to disruption of radial glial organization that facilitates this process (Rakic 1978, 1995; Tassi *et al.* 2005). The nodular masses contain neuronal and glial cells surrounded by myelinated fibers, some of which penetrate the nodules (Dubeau *et al.* 1995; Thom *et al.* 2004; Battaglia and Granata 2007; Leventer *et al.* 2008; Pang *et al.* 2008). Normal pyramidal neurons with randomly oriented apical dendrites are located within these nodules (Thom *et al.* 2004; Battaglia and Granata 2007). This is possibly due to the disrupted maturation of Cajal-Retzus cells within the heterotopia that secrete the protein reelin which plays an integral part in forming normal cortical architecture (Thom *et al.* 2004). Gammma-aminobutyric acid (GABA)-ergic interneurons are also seen within the nodules. These are less organized and mature than their cortical counterparts (Thom *et al.* 2004).

Periventricular nodular heterotopia may represent the only visible malformation or be part of a more complex developmental disorder (Parrini *et al.* 2006; Battaglia and Granata 2007). Also of interest is the frequent association of PNH with anomalies of the hippocampal formation (Dubeau *et al.* 1995; Battaglia *et al.* 2005; Montenegro *et al.* 2006; Parrini *et al.* 2006; Battaglia and Granata 2007). In the surgical series by Li *et al.*

The Causes of Epilepsy, eds. S. D. Shorvon, F. Andermann, and R. Guerrini. Published by Cambridge University Press. © Cambridge University Press 2011.

(1997) involving 10 epileptic patients with PNH, six had evidence of hippocampal sclerosis. A study by Montenegro *et al.* (2006) reported that 30% of patients with PNH also have hippocampal abnormalities on magnetic resonance imaging (MRI): volumetric analysis revealed hippocampal atrophy and on visual analysis the hippocampal malformation showed abnormalities of shape or position. A recent neuropathological study revealed histological evidence of heterotopic nodules in the temporal lobes of patients who underwent surgery for pharmacoresistant epilepsy. These nodules were not detected on presurgical MRI scans (Meroni *et al.* 2009). In all the cases, focal cortical dysplasia and hippocampal sclerosis were also found, lending support to the theory of a common malformative process that leads to these multiple abnormalities.

Genetic and acquired factors can explain the occurrence of this migrational disorder. Advances in genetic studies reveal that several genes may be involved in PNH. The one that has been best described is filamin A (FLNA). Mutations in the *FLN1* gene (filamin A or FLNA) on chromosome Xq28 account for 50% of the so-called "classical PNH," i.e., with bilateral and symmetrically distributed nodules. In this type of PNH, the incidence of the mutation is 100% in familial cases and 26% in sporadic ones (Lu and Sheen 2005; Montenegro *et al.* 2006; Pang *et al.* 2008; Cardoso *et al.* 2009). Filamin A is a large (280 kDa) cytoplasmic phosphoprotein with a structure that facilitates binding to membrane receptors (Meyer *et al.* 1997; Bellanger *et al.* 2000). The protein also stabilizes the cytoskeleton and may be required for the neuronal attachment onto radial glial scaffolding, enabling the migration of the maturing neurons (Battaglia and Granata 2007; Pang *et al.* 2008). The X-linked dominant transmission causes expression almost exclusively in females due to the effect of random X-inactivation (Guerrini *et al.* 2004; Lu and Sheen 2005; Battaglia and Granata 2007). Males who inherit the mutation via this mechanism suffer high prenatal mortality from multiorgan involvement (Battaglia and Granata 2007; Leventer *et al.* 2008). Mutations in *FLNA* represent only 9% of all men with PNH (Guerrini *et al.* 2004). Mild missense mutations and somatic mosaicism account for the minority of males who have this mutation (Guerrini *et al.* 2004; Leventer *et al.* 2008). Also, mutations of this gene have been described in association with Ehlers–Danlos syndrome and a unilateral pattern of PNH (Parrini *et al.* 2006) as well as conditions without associated PNH such as the oro-palatal-digital syndrome, Melnick–Needles syndrome, and fronto-metaphyseal dysplasia (Lu and Sheen 2005).

A less common mutation associated with PNH is found in the *ARFGEF2* (ADP-ribosylation factor guanine exchange factor 2) gene on chromosome 20. It is inherited as an autosomal recessive disorder and codes for the protein brefeldin-inhibited GEF2 (BIG2). The result is defective vesicle trafficking of filamin A from the interior of the cells to the surface (Lu and Sheen 2005; Pang *et al.* 2008). The phenotype is more severe than the X-linked *FLN1* mutation and consists of bilateral PNH, microcephaly, developmental delay, and early-onset refractory epilepsy (Parrini *et al.* 2006).

Other genetic anomalies that have been reported in sporadic cases include duplications in the distal regions of chromosome 5p, causing non-contiguous PNH and subcortical heterotopia; translocation of chromosomes 1 and 6, associated with PNH and polymicrogyria; and translocation of chromosome 2p24 and 9q32, associated with agenesis of the corpus callosum and ocular colobomas (Leeflang *et al.* 2003; Lu and Sheen 2005; Neal *et al.* 2006; Parrini *et al.* 2006; Battaglia and Granata 2007; Pang *et al.* 2008; Cardoso *et al.* 2009). An unidentified mutation with linkage to the *FLN1* locus causing PNH and hydrocephalus has also been discovered (Lu and Sheen 2005; Battaglia and Granata 2007). Recently, deletions involving the 5q chromosome in three unrelated patients with bilateral PNH restricted to the temporal horns of the lateral ventricles, early-onset epilepsy, significant mental retardation and developmental delay were reported (Cardoso *et al.* 2009). Clearly the full spectrum of genetic culprits of this disorder has not yet been fully uncovered (Battaglia and Granata 2007). A summary of recent discoveries is presented in Table 49.1.

Finally, acquired insults occurring during important phases of neurogenesis, such as ischemia, irradiation, and infection, may also affect neuronal migration in utero (Lu and Sheen 2005; Pang *et al.* 2008). Prenatal injuries probably play an important role particularly in unilateral and more focal cases of PNH (Battaglia *et al.* 2005; Battaglia and Granata 2007). Heterotopia may result from the contribution of both genetic and epigenetic mechanisms (Battaglia and Granata 2007).

Epilepsy in the disease
Prevalence

Periventricular nodular heterotopia is the most common clinically encountered heterotopia and makes up 15–20% of all cortical dysgenesis series (Raymond *et al.* 1994; Dubeau *et al.* 1995; Li *et al.* 1997; Tassi *et al.* 2005; Battaglia and Granata 2007). Bilateral PNH is more common in females (Raymond *et al.* 1994; Dubeau *et al.* 1995; Guerrini and Carrozzo 2001; Battaglia *et al.* 2006) and this is likely related to the X-linked transmission of the FLNA mutations and the resulting high prenatal mortality in males (Guerrini and Carrozzo 2001; Battaglia *et al.* 2006). However for reasons that are as yet unclear the gender distribution also applies to PNH not associated with this particular anomaly (Raymond *et al.* 1994; Dubeau *et al.* 1995).

The prevalence of this disorder in the general community is not known (Tassi *et al.* 2005). The collection of epidemiological data is complicated by multiple factors. First, cases can be clinically asymptomatic (for instance, despite frequently causing refractory seizures, epilepsy starts later compared to other dysgeneses such as focal cortical dysplasia or polymicrogyria and is often much less severe) and PNH is incidentally detected during neuroimaging performed for other reasons (Barkovic and Kuzniecky 2000). Second, PNH can be part of complex brain malformations involving the archi- or

Table 49.1 Summary of current genetic associations of PNH

Region	Gene	Phenotype
Xq28	*FLNA*	Predominantly female with normal to borderline intelligence; systemic manifestations include coagulopathy, cardiovascular abnormalities, Ehlers–Danlos syndrome, and frontometaphyseal dysplasias
20q13.1	*ARFGEF2*	Microcephaly; profound developmental delay and spastic quadriparesis
1p36 (deletion)	Uncertain	Dysmorphism; developmental delay; hearing loss in first year; congenital Duane syndrome
7q11.23 (deletion)	Uncertain	Williams syndrome; congenital Duane syndrome; language developmental delay
5p15 (duplication and trisomy)	Uncertain	Normal to mildly impaired mental development; dysmorphism; cardiac defects (atrial septal defects, tricuspid regurgitation)
5q14 (deletion)	Uncertain	Mental developmental delay; dysmorphism
t(1; 6) (p12; p12.2)	Interruption of mannosidase alpha (*MAN1A2*) and glutathione S-transferase (*GSTA2*)	Infantile spasms and myoclonic seizures; dysmorphism
t(2;9) (p24; q32)	Disruption of *KIAA1803* and *ASXL2*	Hearing loss; dysmorphism; hemangiomas

allocortex, which causes difficulty in classification (Battaglia and Granata 2007; Battaglia *et al.* 2006). Third, the incidence of PNH may be underreported if only radiological criteria for diagnosis are used. Improving imaging techniques have increased the detection rate of PNH, although some heterotopic nodules still escape radiological detection (Meroni *et al.* 2009). Finally, PNH appears to have less impact on brain functioning. Many subjects have normal or near-normal IQ

and neurological examinations, which again are factors that may render PNH more difficult to detect (Pang *et al.* 2008; Battaglia and Granata 2007).

Epilepsy syndromes

Periventricular nodular heterotopia often has no apparent impact on brain function except to cause epilepsy. The majority of patients with PNH (80–90%) have seizures or epilepsy (Dubeau *et al.* 1995; Aghakhani *et al.* 2005; Battaglia *et al.* 2006; Battaglia and Granata 2007; Leventer *et al.* 2008; Pang *et al.* 2008). It is not clear exactly why epilepsy occurs and the apparent heterogeneity of the lesions may possibly underline a variety of epileptogenic mechanisms. This will be discussed further in the following sections. Approximately 2% of adult patients with refractory epilepsy have PNH (d'Orsi *et al.* 2004; Tassi *et al.* 2005). The majority of patients have localization-related epilepsy though some present with semiologies and electroencephalographic (EEG) features suggestive of generalized epilepsy syndromes (Raymond *et al.* 1994). The proportion of patients with epileptic manifestations is smaller and the age at onset of seizures usually late compared to other MCD types (Battaglia *et al.* 2006; Parrini *et al.* 2006; Battaglia and Granata 2007). Prognosis of the epileptic disorder depends on type of PNH, and is worsened by the presence of other brain anomalies (Tinuper *et al.* 2003).

Mechanisms of epileptogenesis

Although gray matter heterotopia has a definite association with epilepsy, the mechanisms underlying the generation of seizures or interictal spiking remain unknown. Abnormal cellular representation and connectivity of interneurons in heterotopia may explain or contribute to epileptogenicity of PNH. Rudimentary laminar patterns and random poorly organized interneurons within the heterotopia have been observed (Thom *et al.* 2004). The existence of immature GABAergic circuitry, alterations in the NMDA and calcium/calmodulin-dependent kinase II complex, and limited neuropeptide Y susceptibility contribute to the potential excitatory and epileptogenic nature of the nodules themselves (Aghakhani *et al.* 2005; Battaglia and Granata 2007).

The histological, electrophysiological, and functional imaging evidence suggests a degree of connectivity between the nodules and overlying cortex (Dubeau *et al.* 1995; Aghakhani *et al.* 2005; Tassi *et al.* 2005; Natsume *et al.* 2008; Meroni *et al.* 2009). Their connections with adjacent or distant structures may play a role in amplification and synchronization of epileptiform discharges, explaining the widespread epileptogenic areas often seen. Such a network may provide a number of loops, within the PNH and between PNH and overlying cortex, to produce a seizure (Hannan *et al.* 1999; Aghakhani *et al.* 2005; Valton *et al.* 2008). Finally, PNH is often associated with a structural disorganization of the overlying neocortex or of distant areas such as the hippocampal formation, which may allow the cerebral cortex to act as a primary epileptogenic substrate (Hannan *et al.* 1999; Aghakhani *et al.* 2005; Tassi *et al.* 2005; Meroni *et al.* 2009).

Classification

Several groups have advocated a subclassification of PNH using radiological grounds, based on contiguity and symmetry of nodules, or the clinical and genetic associations. Parrini and colleagues (2006) proposed a classification based on anatomical distribution of the heterotopia and associated malformations; 54% of the 182 patients they studied had classical bilateral symmetrical PNH. The rest of the group was divided into 14 subtypes that included patients with bilateral PNH associated with a variety of anatomical findings (11 subtypes) and patients with unilateral diffuse PNH, diffuse bilateral linear PNH, or with PNH with ribbon-like aspect.

Perhaps the best method is indeed to employ a combination of these factors. This method of classification provides a framework to allow us to recognize the patterns of epilepsy likely to be encountered and may be useful to guide selection of patients with medically intractable epilepsy for surgical treatment. It also provides information regarding other systemic features that have been associated with the particular subtype of PNH (Battaglia and Granata 2007).

Bilateral symmetrical PNH

In this type, multiple and contiguous nodules of gray matter line the ventricular walls symmetrically (Battaglia and Granata 2007) though in some cases there can be a predilection for the peritrigonal or frontal regions (Battaglia *et al.* 2006). Often described as the "classical" PNH, mutations in the *FLN1* gene are responsible in a significant number of cases and hence a definite female preponderance exists (Parrini *et al.* 2006). In addition, patients frequently have mega cisterna magna, mild-to-moderate cerebellar hypoplasia, thin corpus callosum, and asymmetrical hippocampal formations (Battaglia and Granata 2007). Filamin A plays a role in vascular development and blood coagulation (Battaglia and Granata 2007). Up to 20% of patients may have additional cardiovascular and hematological disorders such as aortic insufficiency, patent ductus arteriosus, and idiopathic thrombocytopenia (Parrini *et al.* 2006). The majority of patients are neurologically normal, however. Some patients have mild mental retardation (Guerrini *et al.* 2004) and subtle impairments in reading ability such as dyslexia (Rakic 1978; Lu and Sheen 2005). Focal and refractory epilepsy develops in the second decade of life though the seizures themselves are relatively infrequent (Battaglia *et al.* 2006; Parrini *et al.* 2006). Generalized tonic–clonic seizures are easily controlled with medication and status epilepticus is not seen in this group (Battaglia *et al.* 2006).

Bilateral asymmetrical PNH

In this type, the nodules while bilateral, are clearly asymmetrical and coalescent (Tassi *et al.* 2005; Battaglia *et al.* 2006).

There appears to be a right-sided preponderance that may be related to the later completion of neuroblast migration on that side during development (Raymond *et al.* 1994). They frequently show a cortical extension. Mutations in *FLN1* are rarely observed though the female preponderance remains (Battaglia and Granata 2007). The presence of mildly abnormal neurological or cognitive function occurs in approximately 40% of patients (Battaglia *et al.* 2006). Focal epilepsy is seen in all such patients and is often medically refractory (Battaglia *et al.* 2006).

Bilateral focal PNH

Here, the nodules are isolated, non-confluent, and small. This group appears to be unrelated to the *FLN1* mutation and is more commonly seen in males (Battaglia and Granata 2007). Up to 70% of patients have normal cognition though the remainder can have significant mental retardation, particularly in association with ventricular enlargement (Battaglia *et al.* 2006). Non-specific facial dysmorphisms are occasionally seen. The epilepsy, which presents itself by the second decade of life, is often easily controlled (Battaglia *et al.* 2006).

Unilateral PNH with no cortical involvement

These nodules are unilateral and often extend into the white matter but not to the neocortex (Battaglia and Granata 2007). The right side appears to be preferentially involved, possibly via the same mechanism as for bilateral asymmetrical PNH (Raymond *et al.* 1994). Whilst there is no direct extension of the nodules into the cortex, neocortical malformations of varying degrees are seen in up to 30% of cases (Battaglia *et al.* 2006). In one surgical series, cortical abnormalities such as abnormal thickness, ventricular enlargement, lobar atrophy, and polygyria were detected in all patients with unilateral PNH (Tassi *et al.* 2005). A minority of patients have mild mental retardation; focal seizures occur frequently and can be medically refractory, but generalized convulsions are rare (Battaglia *et al.* 2006).

Unilateral PNH with cortical involvement

Large heterotopic nodules extend into the neocortical region occasionally with involvement of entire lobes and hemispheres (Dubeau *et al.* 1995; Barkovic and Kuzniecky 2000; Battaglia *et al.* 2006; Battaglia and Granata 2007). The extent of the cortical involvement determines the severity of the neurological and mental deficits but not the severity of the epilepsy (Battaglia *et al.* 2006). Frequent and refractory focal seizures are however the common pattern in this group (Battaglia and Granata 2007).

Outside this classification group there are patients who have PNH in conjunction with other complex malformations such as schizencephaly and polymicrogyria and it is debatable if such patients should even be considered as having "pure" PNH (Battaglia and Granata 2007). Patients in any of these subgroups may have additional brain anomalies such as mega cisterna magna, thinning of the corpus callosum, or malformations and asymmetry of the hippocampi occurring in varying degrees though these remain most common in the bilateral symmetrical group (Battaglia *et al.* 2006). In addition, the association of some forms of PNH with a wide spectrum of systemic anomalies complicates the issue. It is unclear if different anomalies affect the characteristics of their epilepsies and the relationship of such abnormalities to the severity of the epilepsy has not been firmly established (Barkovic and Kuzniecky 2000; Leventer *et al.* 2008). Whilst no classification system of this disorder can neatly categorize all the different phenotypes, the one above is also useful to guide the selection of patients for surgical evaluation, which has been a major advance in the management of patients who have epilepsy as a result of PNH (see subsequent sections)

Diagnostic tests

Neuroimaging

Magnetic resonance imaging

The MRI appearance of PNH is quite characteristic and has been extensively reviewed elsewhere (Dubeau *et al.* 1995; Barkovic and Kuzniecky 2000; Tassi *et al.* 2005; Battaglia *et al.* 2006; Battaglia and Granata 2007). The nodules are ovoid, isointense to mature gray matter, and protrude slightly into the ventricular lumen, resulting in an irregular ventricular wall (Barkovic and Kuzniecky 2000). These can be uni- or bilateral, symmetrical or asymmetrical, diffuse or very localized, and contiguous or non-contiguous. The nodules may line the external walls of the lateral ventricles or be localized to either temporal or occipital horns and peritrigonal regions (d'Orsi *et al.* 2004; Leventer *et al.* 2008). In symmetrical and bilateral PNH, the cortex appears normal though mild cortical atrophy has been described (Tassi *et al.* 2005). In unilateral cases with cortical involvement, radial bands isointense with gray matter are seen extending from the nodules to the cortex. The cortical rim has been described as polygyric and reduced in thickness (Lu and Sheen 2005). When associated with FLNA mutations PNH involves the frontal horns and ventricular bodies with minimal extension to the temporo-occipital regions (Cardoso *et al.* 2009). Brain computerized tomography (CT) would usually demonstrate the malformation in cases of diffuse and contiguous PNH but can miss more subtle and focal types. There are no calcifications. As mentioned earlier, hippocampal abnormalities have been associated with PNH. In addition, PNH may occur with other developmental anomalies (as in the case of bilateral symmetrical disease). Hence neuroimaging findings may not be entirely homogenous in all cases of PNH.

Functional studies

Fluoro-deoxy-glucose positron emission tomography (FDG-PET) and single positron emission computerized tomography (SPECT) have shown that the metabolic activity and perfusion to the nodules are identical to that of the overlying cortex,

indicating a degree of functional connectivity between the two regions (Meyer *et al.* 1997; Barkovic and Kuzniecky 2000). The use of α-[^{11}C]methyl-l-tryptophan PET has yielded interesting results. Increased tracer uptake has been demonstrated in epileptogenic tissue and reflects localized alteration in tryptophan metabolism. Recently, Natsume and colleagues (2008) demonstrated similar abnormalities in the neocortical regions overlying the heterotopias without involvement of the nodules themselves. They proposed that this pattern may either be due to a compensatory phenomenon that reduces cortical excitability via a serotonin-mediated mechanism or be reflective of increased epileptogenicity via an increased kynurenine pathway.

The development of simultaneous EEG-fMRI has allowed the co-registration of epileptiform activity with fMRI (Tyvaert *et al.* 2008). In two distinct studies (Kobayashi *et al.* 2006; Tyvaert *et al.* 2008), we demonstrated inconsistent blood-oxygen-dependent level (BOLD) changes in the heterotopia during interictal spiking but clear maximal activations in the neocortex overlying or surrounding the malformations during seizures. Our results suggest that the heterotopia seem to be part of a complex circuitry involving the lesion and the surrounding and distant cerebral cortex. While the role of the nodules in the onset of seizures is not conclusive, the findings again support the notion that some connectivity exists between the nodules and the neocortex.

Scalp electroencephalography

Unlike what has been described in focal cortical dysplasia, no diagnostic EEG patterns or signatures have been reported in cases of PNH. However, regardless of their different anatomic features, PNH cases seem to share common electrophysiologic features (Battaglia *et al.* 2006). Most patients will have a consistently normal background with normal sleep architecture and photic driving (d'Orsi *et al.* 2004; Battaglia *et al.* 2006). In cases of bilateral uninodular or bilateral asymmetrical PNH, the photic driving may be more prominent in the hemisphere with more extensive disease. In unilateral PNH, the photic response can be confined to that hemisphere alone (d'Orsi *et al.* 2004; Battaglia *et al.* 2006). This finding suggests that functional connections exist between neocortical areas responsible for the photic response and the nodules themselves (Battaglia *et al.* 2006). Focal interictal abnormalities are present in most patients and can be bilaterally asynchronous (Battaglia *et al.* 2006). In unilateral PNH these abnormalities may be restricted to the ipsilateral hemisphere though the multifocal nature may persist (Battaglia *et al.* 2006). In the same study, ictal EEG abnormalities at the onset and postictal changes were always recorded on the EEG leads exploring the brain regions where PNH was located though a more precise identification of the seizure onset was rare using surface EEG alone. There have also been reports of generalized 3–4-Hz spike–wave discharges resembling those in the primary generalized epilepsies (Raymond *et al.* 1994; Battaglia and Granata 2007).

Intracranial electroencephalography

Intracranial EEG using depth electrodes has been pivotal in showing that gray matter heterotopia can generate electrical activity. Human studies using acute or chronic intracranial EEG recordings showed that heterotopia can generate normal EEG activity, spikes, and ictal discharges (Francione et al. 1994; Kothare et al. 1998; Aghakhani et al. 2005; Scherer et al. 2005; Tassi et al. 2005; Stefan et al. 2007; Valton et al. 2008), usually synchronous with, but sometimes independent from, the surrounding allo- or neocortex. These studies demonstrated connectivity between nodules and the overlying cortical regions (Aghakhani et al. 2005; Scherer et al. 2005; Valton et al. 2008; Wagner et al. 2009), a concept that has influenced the significant change in the management of the epilepsy in patients with PNH. As with EEG/fMRI, depth electrode studies first showed that interictal epileptic activity can be generated by nodular heterotopia, but seizures are more likely to be generated by the overlying cortex.

Both in humans and animal models, heterotopic nodules consist of a large number of cells, some grouped in small clusters of neurons randomly organized and others arranged in a pattern suggestive of cortical lamination (Hannan et al. 1999). This neuronal substrate can probably generate synchronous discharges, but only small potentials that may be difficult to capture even with closely located electrode contacts. Patients with PNH and epilepsy represent a heterogeneous group and epileptic activity probably results from complex interactions between this malformation and the neocortex. Sometimes it seems that the heterotopia need to be removed to stop the epileptogenic process, but at other times they appear to have no role in the epileptic network. Intracranial recordings provided a definite role for the hippocampus and neocortex in the generation and propagation of epileptic activity. However, the connections of the gray matter heterotopia with adjacent and distant structures may facilitate amplification and synchronization of epileptic discharges that may explain the widespread epileptogenicity often observed in patients with PNH (Francione et al. 1994; Aghakhani et al. 2005; Scherer et al. 2005; Tassi et al. 2005; Battaglia et al. 2006; Battaglia and Granata 2007; Catenoix et al. 2008; Valton et al. 2008).

Genetic testing

Considering the increasingly heterogenous genetic pattern of this disorder, the yield of genetic testing is uncertain and would depend on the classification of the heterotopia, its phenotype, and the presence of an identifiable pedigree. Hence, female patients with bilateral symmetrical PNH and a dominant X-linked pattern of inheritance would likely be positive for mutations of *FLNA* (Guerrini and Carrozzo 2001). Patients with PNH as part of a more complex congenital disorder with either neurological or extraneurological manifestations should also be considered for appropriate genetic testing though this still remains in the research domain (see Table 49.1).

Neuropsychological evaluation

The majority of patients with PNH in the absence of other anomalies have normal IQ, no motor defect, and no focal deficits. Neuropsychological testing is useful to identify specific domains of deficiency in patients who display signs of neurological developmental delay. Recently, subtle impairments in reading speed and comprehension akin to developmental dyslexia in patients with bilateral PNH and grossly normal intelligence have been discovered (Chang et al. 2005). This association appears to be independent of the severity of the epilepsy and is not specific to any particular genetic form of PNH. Also, several studies have demonstrated that heterotopic gray matter, in patients with nodular or band heterotopia, may be involved during specific cognitive tasks which argues again for a functional relationship between the malformation and cortex and also raises concerns about potential deficits after surgical removal (Preul et al. 1997; Pinard et al. 2000; Spreer et al. 2001; Scherer et al. 2005; Jirsh et al. 2006).

Principles of management

The phenotypes of PNH vary significantly with the degree of the heterotopia and the association with other developmental brain anomalies that might occur (Parrini et al. 2006; Pang et al. 2008). Hence the severity of the epilepsy and the response to antiepileptic drugs can differ among individual patients (Pang et al. 2008). No class of anticonvulsants has been shown to be particularly efficacious in treating epilepsy caused by this disease. A significant proportion of patients are medically refractory. Beyond the use of vagal nerve stimulation as a palliative procedure, it was previously thought that patients with PNH were not candidates for epilepsy surgery (Battaglia and Granata 2007; Pang et al. 2008; Valton et al. 2008). An early surgical series involving 10 patients with PNH reported Engel class III and IV outcomes in 89% patients who were followed up for more than 12 months (Li et al. 1997). It should be noted that these patients had had temporal lobe surgery and only one patient had had part of a nodule studied using intracranial EEG (Li et al. 1997).

There is now mounting evidence that the surgical approach may be highly beneficial in selected cases (Battaglia and Granata 2007; Aghakhani et al. 2005; Tassi et al. 2005; Meroni et al. 2009). This is the result of the increasing use of stereo-EEG with detailed sampling of the nodules and the surrounding cortical regions (Battaglia and Granata 2007). This technique is crucial in accurate localization of the seizure generators and the resection of these areas appears to have significant impact on surgical outcome (Aghakhani et al. 2005). Those with unilateral and focal nodules appear to have better surgical outcomes though it is important to sample the nodules and the surrounding regions (Dubeau et al. 1995; Aghakhani et al. 2005). If the nodules are involved, they should be removed along with the surrounding cortex. Patients with diffuse bilateral disease are less likely to do as well as they are more likely to have bilateral epileptiform discharges (Dubeau *et al.* 1995; Battaglia *et al.* 2006). Bilateral multiple or contiguous PNH are often associated with more widespread epileptogenesis, in which case classical surgical approaches are unlikely to be effective.

Whilst most reports of good surgical outcome follow the careful evaluation using depth electrodes examining the nodules and surrounding regions, there may be a role in using a combination of other methods. In one case (Stefan *et al.* 2007), a combination of perioperative electrocorticography and magnetic source imaging (MSI) enabled a resection of neocortex from which the majority of the epileptogenic activity was arising. Whilst involvement of the region in close proximity to the nodules was detected using both these modalities, the nodule was not resected due to its close proximity to the visual pathways. The result was an Engel class I outcome at 18 months follow-up. However, it is unclear in this situation if indeed the generator was removed or if this was a more advanced disconnection surgery.

A technique that might be useful in the future is the use of radiofrequency thermocoagulation guided by SEEG (Catenoix *et al.* 2008). Whilst at present the outcomes are not as good as surgical resection, it does appear that this technique might be beneficial in patients with PNH in whom the epileptogenic nodule has been clearly identified but located in a region unsuitable for resective surgery. In the series recently reported by Catenoix and colleagues, two patients with PNH who were not surgical candidates had a 50% seizure reduction during follow-up at 28 and 72 months, respectively (Catenoix *et al.* 2008). Further development of this technique may yield an additional therapeutic option that may be offered to patients with PNH.

References

Aghakhani Y, Kinay D, Gotman J, *et al.* (2005) The role of periventricular nodular heterotopia in epileptogenesis. *Brain* 128:641–51.

Barkovich AJ, Kuzniecky RI (2000) Gray matter heterotopia. *Neurology* 55:1603–8.

Battaglia G, Chiapparini L, Franceschetti S, *et al.* (2006) Periventricular nodular heterotopia: classification, epileptic history, and genesis of epileptic discharges. *Epilepsia* 47:86–97.

Battaglia G, Franceschetti S, Chiapparini L, *et al.* (2005) Electroencephalographic recordings of focal seizures in patients affected by periventricular nodular heterotopia: role of the heterotopic nodules in the genesis of epileptic discharges. *J Child Neurol* 20:369–77.

Battaglia G, Granata T (2007) Periventricular nodular heterotopia. *Handbk Clin Neurol* 87:177–89.

Bellanger JM, Astier C, Sardet C, *et al.* (2000) The Rac1- and RhoG-specific GEF domain of trio targets filamin to remodel cytoskeletal actin. *Nat Cell Biol* 2:888–92.

Cardoso C, Boys A, Parrini E, *et al.* (2009) Periventricular heterotopia, mental retardation, and epilepsy associated with 5q14.3–q15 deletion. *Neurology* 72:784–92.

Catenoix H, Mauguière F, Guénot M, *et al.* (2008) SEEG-guided thermocoagulations: a palliative treatment of nonoperable partial epilepsies. *Neurology* 71:1719–26.

Chang BS, Ly J, Appignani B, *et al.* (2005) Reading impairment in the neuronal migration disorder of periventricular nodular heterotopia. *Neurology* 64:799–803.

Dubeau F, Tampieri D, Lee N, *et al.* (1995) Periventricular and subcortical nodular heterotopia: a study of 33 patients. *Brain* 118:1273–87.

d'Orsi G, Tinuper P, Bisulli F, *et al.* (2004) Clinical features and long-term outcome of epilepsy in periventricular nodular heterotopia: simple compared with plus forms. *J Neurol Neurosurg Psychiatry* 75:873–8.

Francione S, Kahane P, Tassi L, *et al.* (1994) Stereo-EEG of interictal and ictal electrical activity of a histologically proved heterotopic gray matter associated with partial epilepsy. *Electroencephalogr Clin Neurophysiol* 90:284–90.

Guerrini R, Carrozzo R (2001) Epileptogenic brain malformations: clinical presentation, malformative patterns and indications for genetic testing. *Seizure* 10:532–43.

Guerrini R, Mei D, Sisodiya S, *et al.* (2004) Germline and mosaic mutations of *FLN1* in men with periventricular nodular heterotopia. *Neurology* 63:51–6.

Hannan AJ, Servotte S, Katsnelson A, *et al.* (1999) Characterization of nodular neuronal heterotopia in children. *Brain* 122:219–38.

Jirsh JD, Bernasconi N, Villani F, *et al.* (2006) Sensorimotor organization in double cortex syndrome. *Hum Brain Mapp* 27:535–43.

Kobayashi E, Bagshaw AP, Grova C, Gotman J, Dubeau F (2006) Grey matter heterotopia: what EEG–fMRI can tell us about epileptogenicity of neuronal migration disorders. *Brain* 129:366–74.

Kothare SV, VanLandingham K, Armon C, *et al.* (1998) Seizure onset from periventricular nodular heterotopias: depth-electrode study. *Neurology* 51:1723–7.

Leeflang EP, Marsh SE, Parrini E, *et al.* (2003) Patient with bilateral periventricular nodular heterotopia and polymicrogyria with apparently balanced reciprocal translocation t(1;6)(p12;p12.2) that interrupts the mannosidase alpha, class 1A, and glutathione S-transferase A2 genes. *J Med Genet* 40:e128.

Leventer RJ, Guerrini R, Dobyns WB (2008) Malformations of cortical development and epilepsy. *Dialogues Clin Neurosci* 10:47–62.

Li LM, Dubeau F, Andermann F, *et al.* (1997) Periventricular nodular heterotopia and intractable temporal lobe epilepsy: poor outcome after temporal lobe resection. *Ann Neurol* 41:662–8.

Lu J, Sheen V (2005) Periventricular heterotopia. *Epilepsy Behav* 7:143–9.

Meroni A, Galli C, Bramerio M, *et al.* (2009) Nodular heterotopia: a neuropathological study of 24 patients undergoing surgery for drug-resistant epilepsy. *Epilepsia* 50:116–24.

Meyer S, Zuerbig S, Cunningham C, *et al.* (1997) Identification of the region in actin-binding protein that binds to the cytoplasmic domain of glycoprotein IB. *J Biol Chem* 272:2914–19.

Montenegro MA, Kinay D, Cendes F, *et al.* (2006) Patterns of hippocampal abnormalities in malformations of cortical development. *J Neurol Neurosurg Psychiatry* 77:367–71.

Natsume J, Bernasconi N, Aghakhani Y, *et al.* (2008) Alpha-[11C]methyl-L-tryptophan uptake in patients with periventricular nodular heterotopia and epilepsy. *Epilepsia* **49**:826–31.

Neal J, Apse K, Sahin M, Walsh CA, Sheen VL (2006) Deletion of chromosome 1p36 is associated with periventricular nodular heterotopia. *Am J Med Genet* **140A**:1692–5.

Pang T, Atefy R, Sheen V (2008) Malformations of cortical development. *Neurologist* **14**:181–91.

Parrini E, Ramazzotti A, Dobyns WB, *et al.* (2006) Periventricular heterotopia: phenotypic heterogeneity and correlation with Filamin A mutations. *Brain* **129**:1892–906.

Pinard JM, Feydy A, Carlier R, *et al.* (2000) Functional MRI in double cortex: functionality of heterotopia. *Neurology* **54**:1531–3.

Preul MC, Leblanc R, Cendes F, *et al.* (1997) Function and organization in dysgenic cortex: case report. *J Neurosurg* **87**:113–21.

Rakic P (1978) Neuronal migration and contact guidance in the primate telencephalon. *Postgrad Med J* **54**:25–40.

Rakic P (1995) Radial versus tangential migration of neuronal clones in the developing cerebral cortex. *Proc Natl Acad Sci USA* **92**:11 323–7.

Raymond AA, Fish DR, Stevens JM, *et al.* (1994) Subependymal heterotopia: a distinct neuronal migration disorder associated with epilepsy. *J Neurol Neurosurg Psychiatry* **57**:1195–202.

Scherer C, Schuele S, Minotti L, *et al.* Intrinsic epileptogenicity of an isolated periventricular nodular heterotopia. *Neurology* **65**:495–6.

Spreer J, Martin P, Greenlee MW, *et al.* (2001) Functional MRI in patients with band heterotopia. *Neuroimage* **14**:357–65.

Stefan H, Nimsky C, Scheler G, *et al.* (2007) Periventricular nodular heterotopia: a challenge for epilepsy surgery. *Seizure* **16**:81–6.

Tassi L, Colombo N, Cossu M, *et al.* (2005) Electroclinical, MRI and neuropathological study of 10 patients with nodular heterotopia, with surgical outcomes. *Brain* **128**:321–37.

Thom M, Martinian L, Parnavelas JG, Sisodiya SM (2004) Distribution of cortical interneurons in grey matter heterotopia in patients with epilepsy. *Epilepsia* **45**:916–23.

Tinuper P, d'Orsi G, Bisulli F, *et al.* (2003) Malformation of cortical development in adult patients. *Epilept Disord* **5**:S85–90.

Tyvaert L, Hawco C, Kobayashi E, *et al.* (2008) Different structures involved during ictal and interictal epileptic activity in malformations of cortical development: an EEG–fMRI study. *Brain* **131**:2042–60.

Valton L, Guye M, McGonigal A, *et al.* (2008) Functional interactions in brain networks underlying epileptic seizures in bilateral diffuse periventricular heterotopia. *Clin Neurophysiol* **119**:212–23.

Wagner J, Elger CE, Urbach H, Bien CG (2009) Electric stimulation of periventricular heterotopia: participation in higher cerebral functions. *Epilepsy Behav* **14**:425–8.

Chapter

50

Microcephaly

M. Elizabeth Ross

Microcephaly

Definitions and epidemiology

Microcephaly (MIC) is defined as an occipital–frontal circumference (OFC) that is 2 standard deviations below the mean (–2 SD) or smaller with respect to normative growth curves for age. This is generally termed microcephaly vera or "true" microcephaly when the OFC is congenitally small ($\leq$ –2 SD at birth). However, this definition is not helpful for establishing a syndromic or genetic form of microcephaly. There is a distinction between borderline microcephaly at –2 SD that might be acquired and microcephaly of $\leq$ –3 SD at birth or $\leq$ –4 SD in later childhood, which is far more likely to have a genetic basis. In addition, it is becoming clear that some forms of genetically caused microcephaly become apparent postnatally, starting at –1 to –2 SD at birth and falling further off the normative curve in infancy. Despite its striking variety of presentations, microcephaly as a whole is very common, having prevalence as high as 1% worldwide. The complexity of the disorder is reflected in the numerous gene associations that are coming to light, a few of which are provided in Table 50.1. Although once thought to be diagnostically intractable because of the disorder's heterogeneity and often sporadic nature, the genetic causes of microcephaly are emerging as technologies including comparative genome hybridization (CGH) to detect copy-number variation (CNV) and autozygosity mapping are enabling mutation detection in individuals and single consanguineous families.

Clinical features of microcephaly

Despite the phenotypic heterogeneity, useful microcephaly classifications are emerging (Table 50.1). Virtually all forms of microcephaly display some degree of simplification of the cortical gyral pattern, with fewer gyri and shallow sulci.

Congenital microcephalies

Microcephalic cortex without other distinguishing features is termed microcephaly with simplified gyri (MSG). Features of MSG include fewer gyri with comparatively shallow sulci,

normal to slight thinning of cortical gray matter, foreshortened frontal lobes, often with sloping forehead. Microcephaly of the MSG1 type is a relatively benign malformation in which the OFC is often –4 SD or smaller, but the brain is nevertheless rather well formed. Affected individuals are comparatively high functioning, able to walk, run, and acquire language and some level of self-care. Seizures are uncommon or easily controlled in MSG1 and the lifespan is near normal. At least six primary microcephaly loci (MCPH1–6) have been mapped, for which four genes have been identified (Cox *et al.* 2006).

Microcephaly of the MSG2 type is characterized by a more pronounced simplification of the cortical gyral pattern, with normal to thinned cortical gray matter. This is undoubtedly a diverse group that awaits further subclassification. Most cases are thought to be autosomal recessive, though CNV analyses will likely uncover sporadic autosomal dominant mutations as well. While MSG2 children are more neurologically impaired than those with MSG1, the range of impairment is very broad, so that prognosis for MSG2 infants cannot be made with great accuracy. Significant cognitive impairment is almost certain, but MSG2 children may develop a surprising level of motor function, capacity for social interaction, and rudimentary communication skills. Poorer prognosis may be inferred from additional features when present, such as brainstem hypoplasia or enlarged extra-axial spaces that imply loss of brain volume after a certain point in development.

Lethal microcephaly is a particularly severe category of MSG in which children succumb within the first year postnatally. First encountered in the Amish, MCPHA infants display severe microcephaly, with almost total absence of the cranial vault, and metabolic abnormalities including α-ketoglutaric aciduria due to a mutation in the deoxynucleotide transmembrane carrier, SCL25A19, important for mitochondrial function (Rosenberg *et al.* 2002). Infants are irritable but overt seizures have been noted in fewer than 50% of cases. Children have feeding difficulties and problems with thermoregulation. Most die by 5 to 6 months of age. Another severe microcephaly has been recognized in Omani families, characterized by OFC of –4 to –8 SD, marked cortical simplification and brainstem hypoplasia,

The Causes of Epilepsy, eds. S. D. Shorvon, F. Andermann, and R. Guerrini. Published by Cambridge University Press. © Cambridge University Press 2011.

Table 50.1 Microcephaly genes in humans

Microcephaly type	Locus name	Gene/Interval	Reference
Microcephaly vera			
Microcephaly with simplified gyri (MSG1)	MCPH1	microcephalin	Jackson *et al.* (1998)
	MCPH2	19q13.1–q13.2	Roberts *et al.* (1999)
	MCPH3	*CDK5RAP2*	Bond *et al.* (2005)
	MCPH4	15q15–q21	Jamieson *et al.* (1999)
	MCPH5	*ASPM*	Bond *et al.* (2002)
	MCPH6	*CENPJ*	Bond *et al.* (2005)
Microcephaly with simplified gyri (MSG2)	Autosomal recessive MSG2	*unk*[a]	Peiffer *et al.* (1999); Dobyns (2002)
Lethal microcephaly	MCPHA (Amish)	*SCL25A19*	Rosenberg *et al.* (2002)
	Neonatal lethal microcephaly	*unk*[a]	Rajab *et al.* (2007)
Microcephaly with intrauterine growth retardation (MIC-IUGR)	MIC–osteodyspastic primordial dwarfism I (MOPD1) (severe MR, MIC, and malformation)	*unk*[a]	Sigaudy *et al.* (1998)
	Seckel syndrome (moderate MR, MSG1)	*ATR*	O'Driscoll *et al.* (2003); Willems *et al.* (2010)
	MOPD2 (high functioning, MSG1)	*PCN*	Griffith *et al.* (2008); Rauch *et al.* (2008)
Microcephaly with other brain malformation	MIC and periventricular heterotopia	*ARFGEF2*[a]	Sheen *et al.* (2004)
	MIC and lissencephaly, ACC, Cb hypoplasia	*TUBA1A*[a]	Morris-Rosendahl *et al.* (2008)
	MIC and pontocerebellar hypoplasia (Barth syndrome)	*unk*[a]	Barth *et al.* (1982)
	MIC and lissencephaly (Norman–Roberts syndrome)	*unk*[a]	
	MIC and holoprosencephaly	*SIX3*	Wallis *et al.* (1999)
Microcephaly with diffuse polymicrogyria		*EOMES (Tbr2)*[a]	Baala *et al.* (2007)
	Warburg micro syndrome, with microphthalmia	*RAB3GAP*[a]	Aligianis *et al.* (2005)
Postnatal microcephaly			
Microcephaly with agenesis of the corpus callosum	Variety of gene deletion syndromes	Deletion involving *AKT3*[a]	Boland *et al.* (2007)
Microlissencephaly (microcephaly/lissencephaly)	XLAG	*ARX*[a]	Kitamura *et al.* (2002)
Microcephaly with brainstem and cerebellar hypoplasia	X-Linked MR with Cb hypoplasia	*CASK*[a] (seizures in childhood)	Najm *et al.* (2008)
Microcephaly with asymmetric polymicrogyria	MAP	*TUBB2B*[a]	Jaglin *et al.* (2009)
Microcephaly with calcification	AGS1	*TREX1/DNaseIII*	Crow *et al.* (2006a)
	AGS2	*RNASEH2B*[a]	Crow *et al.* (2006b)
	AGS3	*RNASEH2C*[a]	Crow *et al.* (2006b)

Table 50.1 (cont.)

Microcephaly type	Locus name	Gene/Interval	Reference
	AGS4	*RNASEH2A*[a]	Crow *et al.* (2006b)
	AGS5	*unk*[a]	
	Pseudo-TORCH	*unk*[a]	Briggs *et al.* (2008a)
	CRMCC	*unk*[a]	Briggs *et al.* (2008b)
	CALC-MIC	2q35–q36.3	Rajab *et al.* (2009)
Microcephaly with X-linked mental retardation	Rett syndrome	*MeCP2*[a] (seizures in childhood)	Amir *et al.* (1999)
Developmental encephalopathy with Rett-like features		*FOXG1*[a]	Jacob *et al.* (2009)
	Angelman syndrome	*UBE3A*[a]	Dan (2009)

Note:
[a]Commonly associated with epilepsy.

marked irritability and tremulousness, respiratory difficulties and death by 4 to 6 postnatal weeks (Rajab *et al.* 2007).

A distinctive category of microcephaly is coupled with significant intrauterine growth retardation (MIC-IUGR), in which affected individuals have an average adult height of 100 cms (3.25 feet) and an OFC of –6 to –8 SD, comparable to a 3-month-old infant (40 cm). There are at least three forms of MIC-IUGR. The first, microcephalic osteodysplastic primordial dwarfism type I (MOPDI), is characterized by short limbs and neck, multiple skeletal anomalies, and microcephaly with features of other cortical dysplasia including agenesis of the corpus callosum (ACC), heterotopia, and gyral abnormalities; the few reported cases were lethal within the first postnatal year due to infection (Sigaudy *et al.* 1998). Seckel syndrome, sometimes referred to incorrectly as MOPDII, encompasses an MSG1-like brain and moderate to mild mental retardation, but is distinguished from MSG1 by unusually small stature. MOPDII is a syndrome that should be reserved for MIC-IUGR in which MSG is subtle and cognitive function is normal or near normal (Griffith *et al.* 2008; Rauch *et al.* 2008). There are a variety of skeletal anomalies that accompany MOPDII (Hall *et al.* 2004). However, blurring of the diagnostic boundary between Seckel syndrome and MOPDII persists, so that in practical terms, the two conditions are becoming part of the same spectrum attributed to loss-of-function mutations in a centrosomal associated protein (Willems *et al.* 2010).

A large subset of microcephaly is accompanied by other brain malformation types (Table 50.1). Examples include microcephaly with periventricular heterotopia associated with a loss-of-function mutation in ARFGEF2 (Sheen *et al.* 2004), or microcephaly with lissencephaly, ACC, and cerebellar hypoplasia caused by mutation in the microtubule subunit TUBA1A (Bahi-Buisson *et al.* 2008; Morris-Rosendahl *et al.* 2008). These mixed phenotypes imply that the causative genes have functions that overlap several critical stages of brain formation, such as proliferation and migration and axon extension or guidance.

Because of its prominence and frequent association with epilepsy, the combination of microcephaly with polymicrogyria

(MIC-PMG) deserves its own category. Several causative gene mutations have been identified for this phenotype, including the Tbr2 transcription factor (also known as EOMES or eomesodermin), in which patients display MIC with diffuse PMG, enlarged ventricles, ACC/dysgenesis, and cerebellar hypoplasia (Baala *et al.* 2007). Children with Warburg micro syndrome (WMS) have microcephaly with widespread PMG, corpus callosum thinning, and also microphthalmos, microcornea, congenital cataracts, and hypothalamic hypogenitalism. This syndrome has been associated with loss-of-function mutation in the *RAB3GAP* gene encoding RAB3 GTPase activating protein (Aligianis *et al.* 2005).

Postnatal microcephalies

An important distinction has recently been recognized between congenital microcephaly, which is eminently apparent at birth, and postnatal microcephaly which advances in the first year or two after birth (Table 50.1). In the latter condition, the OFC at birth is small but at about –2 SD, it may be overlooked as an MIC syndrome. However, microcephaly in this category progresses postnatally, so that the OFC can reach –6 SD or smaller after 1 to 2 years of age, reflecting a more brain-specific mechanism than generalized growth retardation. An example is microcephaly with ACC and cerebellar vermis hypoplasia associated with mutations in AKT3, in which half of patients had a birth OFC of –2 SD or larger, while all measured –2 to –4 SD smaller (–2.5 to –7 SD) after 1 to 5 years. Additional examples are found in X-linked postnatal microcephaly with mental retardation (MR) and pontocerebellar hypoplasia due to disruption of the CASK calcium/calmodulin dependent serine kinase (Najm *et al.* 2008) and in microcephaly with asymmetric polymicrogyria (MAP) due to mutation in microtubule subunit TUBB2B (Jaglin *et al.* 2009). In both conditions, patients displayed borderline microcephaly (approx –1 to –2 SD) at birth, becoming severe after 1 year (–3 to –8 SD at time of last examination).

Similar patterns of postnatal microcephaly have been recognized in forms with brain calcifications and in Rett syndrome. The former group includes five loci for Aicardi–Gutières syndrome (AGS1–5), a severe autosomal recessive encephalopathy for which four responsible genes have been identified (Rice *et al.* 2007). The AGS subtypes usually present with a normal to small OFC at birth and progress to moderate to severe microcephaly associated with mutations in genes involved in nucleotide degradation. The typical AGS presentation is one of subacute onset in the neonatal period, or within the first year, of irritability, inconsolable crying, loss of developmental skills, and frequently intermittent sterile fevers, cerebrospinal fluid lymphocytosis and elevated cerebrospinal fluid α-interferon. Seizures occur in at least 50% of AGS patients and hepatosplenomegaly with liver function abnormalities may occur in some.

Three additional postnatal microcephaly with extensive brain calcification phenotypes are pseudo-TORCH (Briggs *et al.* 2008a), cerebromicroangiopathy with calcifications and cysts (CRMCC) (Briggs *et al.* 2008b), and microcephaly with calcifications (CALC-MIC) (Rajab *et al.* 2009). Pseudo-TORCH mimics the neonatal infectious encephalopathy with severe postnatal microcephaly, lissencephaly/polymicrogyria, and seizures but TORCH titers are negative. Both CRMCC and CALC-MIC conditions display less severe postnatal microcephaly, delayed growth, and osteopenia. However CRMCC patients show signs of microangiopathy, including retinopathy due to abnormal retinal vascular permeability and telangectasia and a prominent leukoencephalopathy in which a brain biopsy in one patient showed astrocytosis and small cerebral vessel calcification (Crow *et al.* 2004).

Rett syndrome is an X-linked condition with sporadic occurrence that classically presents in girls who are seemingly normal until age 6–18 months when they cease to acquire developmental skills, display decelerating head growth, and autistic features of lost eye contact and social regression, motor incoordination, and loss of purposeful hand movement. Seizures are common in early childhood, but frequency diminishes after age 10 years as the electroencephalogram (EEG) progressively shows. One gene, for methyl-CpG binding protein 2 (MeCP2), has been associated with the disorder and accounts for 70–90% of sporadic and 50% of familial cases (Shahbazian and Zoghbi 2002).

Several syndromes involving a complex neurodevelopmental encephalopathy and postnatal microcephaly with Rett-like features have been characterized. One such syndrome has been found in association with single-gene deletion of the transcription factor FOXG1 (Jacob *et al.* 2009). This parallels findings of reduced brain volume and brain disorganization in mice bearing a single allele disrupting the mouse Foxg1 (Eagleson *et al.* 2007). Another is Angelman syndrome, caused by mutation – often deletion – of the ubiquitin ligase gene, *UBE3A*, on chromosome 15. This is an imprinted chromosomal region with complex effects, so that Angelman syndrome is associated with maternal transmission while

Table 50.2 Microcephaly candidate genes (indicated by mouse models)

Microcephaly type	Mouse genes	Reference
Microcephaly with interneuronopathy (MSG2?)	cyclin D2	Glickstein et al. (2007)
	Nkx2.1	Butt et al. (2008)
	uPAR	Powell et al. (2003)
Cell proliferation (MSG2?)	Insm1	Farkas et al. (2008)
	Citron Kinase	Sarkisian et al. (2001)
	Nde1	Feng and Walsh (2004)
Cell proliferation (MSG1?)	Cyclin D1	Glickstein et al. (2009)
Apoptosis (lethal MIC?)	Dicer	Davis et al. (2008)
	Rac1	Chen et al. (2009)
Cell proliferation/survival (MIC with cerebellar hypoplasia and white matter disease)	Nijmegen breakage syndrome – Nibrin (Nbs1) mutation	Assaf et al. (2008)

Prader–Willi syndrome is associated with paternal transmission of the chromosome 15 alterations (Dan, 2009; Van Buggenhout *et al.*, 2009)

Pathophysiology of microcephaly

The special nature of brain growth is first indicated by the fact that OFC is relatively independent of body size. Thus, in certain forms of dwarfism such as achondroplasia (Rousseau *et al.* 1996), an individual with short stature may nevertheless have an OFC that falls within the normal range, while as noted above, there are examples of microcephaly in which stature is preserved or only slightly reduced. Therefore, one should not discount an OFC of –2 SD or smaller when the subject is also small in stature – this is microcephaly regardless of the accompanying height or body mass. At the molecular level, in addition to the genes listed in Table 50.1, there are a number of genes that have been found when inactivated in the mouse to cause microcephaly and these make excellent candidates for microcephaly genes in humans (Table 50.2). Functional analyses of these human and mouse genes indicate three major mechanistic routes to microcephaly, notably reduced neural cell proliferation, enhanced cell death, or a combination of reduced neuritogenesis and reduced cell survival.

Neural progenitor proliferation

The special growth characteristics of brain derive from its several modes of neural proliferation during embryogenesis (Kriegstein *et al.* 2006; Bystron *et al.* 2008; Pontious *et al.* 2008). Two particular modes of neural progenitor division in the developing cerebral cortex are symmetric and asymmetric. In asymmetric divisions, radial glial progenitors in the ventricular zone (VZ) give rise to a post-mitotic neuron and a radial glial daughter that re-enters the cell cycle. In another type of asymmetric division, one daughter becomes an intermediate progenitor (IPC), moving to a secondary proliferative population in the subventricular zone (SVZ) where it will divide again, without the radial processes characteristic of the VZ. In symmetric divisions of the SVZ, IPCs divide to produce two identical daughters that exit the cell cycle to become two neurons or two glia, then subsequently migrate to their final cortical position. Gene alterations that selectively affect these transit amplifying divisions of the SVZ will result in microcephaly, while sparing other organ systems. This is exemplified by the microcephaly encountered in cyclin D2 knock-out mice (Glickstein *et al.*, 2007, 2009). Inactivation of this G1-active cell cycle protein reduces IPC divisions in developing cortex leading to marked microcephaly, but body size and mass of these cyclin-D2-deficient mice is entirely normal. Similarly, mice lacking the Tbr2 transcription factor show a deficit in IPCs, resulting in microcephaly (Sessa *et al.* 2008). As indicated above, hypomorphic Tbr2 mutation underlies a phenotype of microcephaly with polymicrogyria in humans (Baala *et al.* 2007). Further studies of the conditional knock-out mouse models affecting Tbr2, cyclin D2, and insulinoma-associated 1 protein (Insm1) (Farkas *et al.* 2008), all of which impact intermediate progenitor cell expansion, are expected to illuminate steps leading to microcephaly with other brain malformations like polymicrogyria.

Neural progenitor proliferation can be disturbed in a surprising range of events. Cell cycle progression can be impaired by alterations early in the cell cycle – via trophic factors influencing G1–S phase progression, such as fibroblast growth factors (FGFs), WNTs or sonic hedgehog (SHH), or direct participants in the cell cycle machinery, such as G1-phase active cyclins D2 or D1 that couple with cyclin dependent kinases 4 or 6 to advance cells through G1–S. Interestingly, cyclin D2 loss of function produces a profound microcephaly in mice by reducing neural expansion through diminished intermediate progenitor divisions, while cyclin D1 loss of function results in significant body runting, but brain size is relatively spared (Glickstein *et al.* 2009). The comparatively mild reduction in brain size of cyclin D1 knock-out mice is likely due to the persistence of cyclin D2 expression which promotes expansion of the neural progenitor pool.

A number of the genes currently associated with primary microcephaly affect later aspects of the cell cycle, such as the G2–M transit or M-phase progression itself. Thus far, all of these MSG1 genes have been associated with abnormalities of cell cycle checkpoint regulation and the mitotic spindle/centrosome apparatus (Bond and Woods 2006; O'Driscoll *et al.* 2006). For example, MCPH1 protein contains two BRCT domains that are common in DNA damage response genes and MCPH1 has a role in the ATR-dependent DNA damage response pathway (reviewed in O'Driscoll *et al.* 2006). MCPH1 also has an effect on mitotic entry and chromosome condensation. CDK5 regulatory subunit associated protein 2 (CDK5RAP2), abnormal spindle-like microcephaly related (ASPM), and centromere protein J (CENPJ) are all centrosome-associated proteins, though they serve somewhat distinct roles in the regulation of mitosis (reviewed in Cox *et al.* 2006a).

Two genes have been associated with MIC-IUGR. The first, a DNA damage response gene called ataxia–telangiectasia and Rad3-related (ATR), is most appropriately ascribed to Seckel syndrome (O'Driscoll *et al.* 2003). A second gene encoding a centrosomal protein, pericentrin (PCNT), is most appropriately ascribed to MOPDII. PCNT is a centrosome-associated protein which anchors both structural and regulatory proteins important for spindle function and chromosomal segregation in mitosis. Cells lacking PCNT display disorganized mitotic spindles and abnormal chromosomal segregation. Significantly, PCNT has recently been shown to participate in ATR-dependent checkpoint signaling in response to DNA damage, for the first time linking DNA damage pathways and centrosomal regulation (Griffith *et al.* 2008). The centrosomal localization and abnormal cell cycle checkpoint features of the ATR/PCNT mutations are also found in other genes associated with MSG1 type microcephaly, including MCPH1, CDK5RAP2, ASPM, and CENPJ, suggesting significant mechanistic overlap in these MIC-IUGR and MCPH brain phenotypes.

The citron kinase defect cloned in the *Flathead* rat mutant indicates that proteins required for cytokinesis, or the final cleavage of a dividing cell into two daughter cells, are likely to underlie certain human microcephalies as well. The protein is particularly important for cytokinesis of neuronal precursors (LoTurco *et al.* 2003). Citron kinase is a downstream effector of the small GTPase, RhoA, and co-localizes with RhoA in the cleavage furrow and mid-body of dividing cells completing M-phase (Shandala *et al.*, 2004).

An unexpected consequence of some disturbances of neural cell proliferation is selective loss of inhibitory interneurons, providing at least one mechanism for epileptogenesis in microcephalic patients. For example, mice lacking cyclin D2 are microcephalic due to generalized deficit in neuron numbers, but they also display a selective, more severe loss of medial ganglionic eminence (MGE) derived, parvalbuminergic interneurons in cortex and hippocampus (Glickstein *et al.* 2007). This deficit is accompanied by increased fast frequency background on the awake EEG, loss of high-amplitude inhibitory postsynaptic potentials, and lowered seizure threshold to certain epileptic drugs. Disproportionate deficits in interneurons are seen as well in the urokinase-type plasminogen activator receptor (uPAR) mouse which is predisposed to seizures (Powell *et al*. 2003).

Unlike cyclin D2 null mice, those lacking cyclin D1 display normal cell densities of all interneuron subtypes yet examined (Glickstein *et al*. 2007). Cyclin D1 knock-out mice have a less severe microcephaly than those lacking cyclin D2 and cyclin D1 mutants are significantly runted. Cyclin D1 knock-out mice do not have spontaneous seizures, but they display lowered seizure threshold to kainate-induced, but not pentyle-netetrazol (PTZ)-induced, seizures compared to wild-type siblings (Koeller *et al*. 2008). The biological reason for this susceptibility to excitotoxic effects is not known, but presumably there is some alteration of synaptic function in these cyclin D1 deficient mice.

Progenitor cell signaling and protein trafficking

The cell-signaling side of the equation is exemplified in microcephalic mice that bear a loss-of-function mutation in the uPAR gene, encoding a multifunctional protein that interacts with integrins to alter cell proliferation, adhesion, and migration (Ossowski and Aguirre-Ghiso 2000; Powell *et al*. 2003). Several human microcephaly and postnatal microcephaly syndromes with features of cortical malformation are associated with intracellular signaling proteins. These include congenital microcephaly with heterotopia due to mutations in the ADP ribosylation factor guanine nucleotide exchange factor 2 (ARFGEF2) gene which encodes brefeldenA-inhibited GEF2 (*BIG2*). This small GTPase effector protein is required for proper intracellular trafficking of E-cadherin and β-catenin through the trans-Golgi network to localize at the inner plasma membrane (Sheen *et al*. 2004). These functions place ARFGEF2 in a position to influence both neural proliferation and migration in developing cortex.

Cell signaling is undoubtedly affected as well in Warburg micro syndrome associated with mutations in *RAB3GAP* (Aligianis *et al*. 2005). The RAB GTPases are essential components of vesicular protein trafficking and Rab3 is known to regulate exocitic release of neurotransmitters and hormones. It has been postulated that the WMS mutations in *RAB3GAP* interfere with exocytic release of ocular and neuroepithelial trophic factors. Dysfunction of *RAB3GAP* might also interfere with the cycling of cellular adhesion molecules like L1 and so could disrupt migration to produce the polymicrogyria that accompanies microcephaly in this syndrome.

The theme of impaired signaling continues in postnatal microcephalies, as exemplified by MIC with ACC seen in a human 1q43–q44 deletion syndrome that involves AKT3 (Boland *et al*. 2007) and by microcephaly with brainstem and cerebellar hypoplasia due to inactivation of CASK (Najm *et al*. 2008). AKT3 is an important serine-threonine kinase in the insulin-like growth factor 1 (IGF1) and PI3K intracellular signaling pathway. Inactivation of Akt3 in the mouse produces a very similar phenotype of postnatal microcephaly, and defects of corpus callosum. The mechanism of postnatal microcephaly may involve effects both on cell proliferation through IGF1 signaling and cell survival. Exposure of Akt3

$(EX4)^{-/-}$ mouse hippocampal neurons in primary culture to either glutamate or staurosporine leads to increased apoptosis compared to wild-type controls (Tschopp *et al*. 2005), suggesting that cell death may contribute to the microcephaly phenotype in humans. CASK is a calcium-calmodulin dependent protein kinase of the membrane-associated guanylate kinase (MAGUK) family, localized in neuronal synapses to regulate ion-channel protein trafficking, and membrane targeting and function. CASK has been identified as part of large pre- and postsynaptic signaling complexes (Hong and Hsueh 2006; Samuels *et al*. 2007). Interestingly, CASK is not only a scaffolding protein that participates in signaling events at the synapse, it also interacts in the nucleus with transcription factors including Tbr1 and a nucleosome assembly protein, CINAP, to modulate expression of neuronal proteins like Reelin and NMDAR subunit NR2B (Hsueh 2006). Thus CASK is positioned to affect both embryonic brain development and postnatal events including elaboration of neurites and growth of the neuropil that constitutes a significant part of human brain growth in the first two postnatal years.

Cytoskeletal regulation in progenitor proliferation and neuronal migration

Mutations in several tubulin genes encoding microtubule components underscore the importance of this cytoskeletal system for neural proliferation and brain organization. Microtubules are formed through a complex cascade of protein-folding steps regulated by molecular chaperones (prefoldin-, cytosolic chaperonin-, and tubulin-specific chaperones) that facilitate the formation of tubulin α/β heterodimers, which then polymerize into microtubules. Mutations associated with congenital microcephaly with lissencephaly ACC and cerebellar hypoplasia (TUBA1A) (Morris-Rosendahl *et al*. 2008) or postnatal microcephaly with lissencephaly/asymmetric polymicrogyria (TUBB2B) (Jaglin *et al*. 2009) interfere with functional domains of these tubulin proteins. For example, mutations have been detected that prevent guanine trinucleotide binding to the guanosine triphosphate pocket or that prevent specific binding of the tubulin subunit with its folding and chaperone proteins, thereby interfering with tubulin α/β heterodimerization and microtubule polymerization. Thus, depending on the expression pattern of the particular tubulin subunit, these mutations may disrupt microtubule dynamics needed for cell proliferation and neuronal/glial migration either during embryogenesis or in the postnatal period. Altered microtubule dynamics are also likely to underlie agenesis or dysgenesis of long axonal projections such as in the corpus callosum, since axon projection depends on the precise regulation of microtubule polymerization and depolymerization in the axon shaft.

Transcription factors, fate determination, and microcephaly

Several microcephaly-associated genes have been found among transcription factors known for their role in cortical patterning. These include SIX3 mutations causing microcephaly with holoprosencephaly (Wallis *et al.* 1999). The microcephaly aspect of this phenotype is likely related to downstream targets of the SIX3 transcription factor that function in the SHH and WNT pathways impacting neural progenitor proliferation as well as fate determination. Additional examples of transcription factors associated with microcephaly are found in Tbr2, discussed above, and *ARX*. The *aristaless* homeobox gene on X (*ARX*) is of interest for its remarkable pleiotropy, with mutations involving missense substitutions, frameshifts, and expansions of polyalanine tracts in the transcript. These changes relate to phenotypes ranging from severe microcephaly with XLAG (lissencephaly and abnormal genitalia), to non-syndromic mental retardation, dystonia, or autism in the absence of overt brain malformation (Kato *et al.* 2004; Guerrini *et al.* 2007). This range of effects and *ARX* expression patterns in brain suggest that this paired domain homeobox protein functions in fetal neural patterning and proliferation/cell survival as well as having a role in the function of mature neurons. A consistent finding in *ARX* mutant mouse models and patient neuropathology is a deficit in interneurons derived from the ganglionic eminences. Thus, deficits in GABAergic neurotransmission likely underlie the severe epilepsy (including infantile spasms) and dystonia in *ARX* patients.

Apoptosis, neuritogenesis, and postnatal microcephaly

Disruption of neural progenitor proliferation is but one path leading to microcephaly. Another is increased cell death starting during either the fetal or postnatal period. Impaired cell survival is a likely factor in microcephaly of the Amish type (MCPHA), in which a nuclear mitochondrial deoxynucleotide carrier protein malfunction interferes with transport across the inner mitochondrial membrane (Rosenberg *et al.* 2002). This could impact both neural proliferation and promote oxidative stress, reducing cell survival. The association of microcephaly with ATR-mediated DNA damage pathways in primary microcephaly and in Seckel syndrome also implies that reduced cell survival contributes to the small OFCs in these conditions. However, since MCPH and Seckel syndromes lack evidence for significant ongoing neurodegeneration, the effects on cell survival are likely to be at least relatively limited to a particular developmental stage. Neural cell survival is also thought to be impaired in the postnatal microcephaly associated with AGS due to deficits in DNA degradation (TREX1 mutations in AGS1) or RNA degradation (RNASEH2 subunits mutated in AGS2, 3, and 4). These enzymes have a role in removing nucleotides released during apoptosis and it is hypothesized that impaired nucleotide removal stimulates an autoimmune response that causes AGS symptoms (Rice *et al.* 2007).

Several mouse models underscore the potential for accelerated apoptosis to underlie microcephaly. Conditional inactivation of small GTPase Rac1 at around E14.5 induces cell cycle exit and increased apoptosis in telencephalon to result in microcephalic mice (Chen *et al.* 2009). Similarly, conditional postnatal inactivation of Dicer, required for processing of microRNAs, leads to microcephaly accompanied by marked

activation of caspase-3 and increased apoptosis of cortical cells as well as reduced dendritic arborization (Davis *et al.* 2008).

In postnatal microcephaly, processes that expand the brain size in the postnatal period are particularly affected. These include neuronal and glial migration to their final positions in cerebral cortex, extension of neurites (neuritogenesis), axon extension/growth cone guidance, and formation of synapses. These are mechanistic targets in microcephaly associated with AKT3, CASK, TUBB2B, and MeCP2 mutations. For example, CASK is a molecular scaffold protein of the MAGUK family which upon phosphorylation by CDK5 is localized to neuronal synapses and especially to postsynaptic densities of dendritic spines (Samuels *et al.* 2007), where it regulates trafficking and function of ion-channel proteins. Interestingly, CASK also translocates to the nucleus where it binds and co-activates transcription factor Tbr1, regulating expression of neuronal migration protein, reelin (Hsueh *et al.* 2000). Thus, CASK is well positioned to impact brain size, organization, and synaptic function underlying epilepsy. TUBB2B, whose expression peaks postnatally, has been investigated using in utero electroporation methods, and interference with this tubulin isotype produces neuronal migration defects (Jaglin *et al.* 2009). TUBB2B-deficient cells become hung up in the VZ/SVZ of embryonic rat brain, while in human brain, asymmetric polymicrogyria appears as early as 27 weeks' gestation, and heterotopic neurons are seen in white matter on magnetic resonance imaging (MRI). Gene expression changes resulting from interference with DNA methylation due to mutation in MeCP2 which binds methylated DNA has significant effects on postnatal brain growth as well as synaptogenesis, likely impacting brain size through effects on the developing neuropil (Shahbazian and Zoghbi 2002). In fact, neuropathological studies support slowed neurodevelopment rather than neurodegeneration as responsible for the reduced OFCs in Rett syndrome patients (Armstrong 2001). Neurites in those studies were reduced in length and complexity compared to age matched controls. Recent studies in mouse models demonstrate striking effects of mutant MeCP2 expression on dendritic spine number and morphology (Chapleau *et al.* 2009).

Epilepsy in microcephaly
Frequency and risk factors for epilepsy in microcephaly

Seizures are a manifestation of microcephaly that occurs with variable frequency, according to the clinical syndrome and causative gene. The degree of OFC reduction is not in itself a reliable predictor of whether seizures are likely to occur in a microcephalic individual. The most significant risk factors for seizures are the extent of structural simplification, diencephalic/brainstem hypoplasia, and presence of accompanying cortical malformation. Seizures are uncommon (probably around 10% of cases or fewer) in microcephaly of the MSG1 type (MCPH1–6, Seckel syndrome, MOPDII), in which brain is small but cortex is rather well organized. When seizures do occur in those conditions, they are readily controlled with antiepileptic drugs (AEDs).

As noted above, the MSG2 phenotype encompasses a heterogeneous group, but seizures are relatively more common in MSG2 than MSG1 (perhaps around 25–30% of MSG2 cases overall). As a general rule, seizures are more likely as the cortex is increasingly simplified, probably reflecting the severity of brain disorganization. In addition, animal models of microcephaly, like cyclin D2 knock-out mice, reveal that reductions in OFC linked to proliferation defects can be accompanied by disproportionately more severe reductions in interneuron populations, predisposing to epilepsy due to loss of inhibitory GABAergic input to the cortex (Glickstein et al. 2007).

Seizures are common in patients with microcephaly forms that include features of neuronal migration defects, such as microcephalies with heterotopia, lissencephaly, or ACC/callosal dysgenesis. This is likely due primarily to disturbances of normal neuronal function accompanied by altered cytoskeletal function (TUBA1A and ARFGEF2 mutations), or altered intracellular signaling (AKT3 mutations), and not solely to displacement of neurons. In the case of ARX mutations, seizures are the consequence of altered cell fate, with a marked deficit in GABAergic interneurons, as well as migrational deficits (Kato and Dobyns 2005). Microcephaly with polymicrogyria, including WMS (RAB3-GAP mutation), EOMES (Tbr2) mutation, and MAP (TUBB2B mutation) carries the same exceptionally high risk for epilepsy (affecting 80% or more cases) as polymicrogyria with OFC values in the normal range.

Mutations affecting neuronal function, such as those in CASK or MeCP2 genes, also confer an increased propensity to seize. In these cases, there is significant evidence for impaired dendritogenesis, synaptogenesis, and synaptic dysfunction during postnatal cortical development (Armstrong 2001; Najm et al. 2008; Chapleau et al. 2009). In the case of CASK mutations, the gene product has a direct role in synaptic function as well as indirect impact through regulation of protein expression including the glutamate receptor subunit, NR2B (Hsueh 2006; Huang and Hsueh 2009). The impact of MeCP2 on dendritogenesis and synapses is indirect, through its role as a methyl-CpG binding protein affecting DNA methylation patterns and chromatin remodeling. FOXG1 heterologous mutation has recently been associated with a complex developmental encephalopathy with Rett-like features (MR, stereotypic behaviors, seizures in infancy, postnatal microcephaly: –2SD at birth, –4SD at 3 years) (Jacob et al. 2009). This suggests that FOXG1 expression changes might be one of the outcomes of the epigenetic effects of MeCP2 contributing to the Rett syndrome phenotype. Mutations in the ubiquitin ligase complex related (UB3A) gene which cause Angelman syndrome when the chromosome 15 locus is inherited through the mother also produce postnatal microcephaly, severe developmental delay, epilepsy, and behavioral features that include stereotypies and "happy" disposition (Van Buggenhout et al.

2009). Despite the tantalizing possible relationship between imprinting of the UB3A locus and MeCP2-regulated methylation, no evidence for UB3A expression changes has been found in mouse models that inactivate MeCP2.

Types of epilepsy, specific characteristics, treatment, and prognosis

Relatively little is known about the specific types of epilepsy referable to a particular microcephaly type. However, available information indicates seizure types roughly correlate with the underlying malformation. Most seizure presentations in microcephaly are generalized tonic–clonic or a mixed picture of complex partial and generalized motor types. Cryptogenic West syndrome or infantile spasms occur in microcephalies associated with interneuron deficits and are especially encountered in patients with ARX mutations. Infantile spasms with hypsarrhythmia have also been encountered in patients with periventricular nodular heterotopia due to ARFGEF2 mutation. Frontal predominant triphasic delta waves are a particularly characteristic feature of interictal EEG recordings in Angelman syndrome, though a range of seizure types are encountered, including atypical absence and myoclonic epilepsies. Focal seizures are less common, but may occur in microcephalic patients with focal heterotopia. Seizures are common among those with polymicrogyria, though the underlying mechanism is not necessarily obvious. Polymicrogyria associated with impaired intracellular protein trafficking such as with RAB3GAP mutations could certainly impact neuronal excitability, but the mechanism leading to epilepsy in the setting of Tbr2 inactivation is less apparent. One possibility is that loss of Tbr2 function impacts neuronal–glial fate determination and a resulting imbalance between neuronal and glial population numbers alters the extracellular ionic milieu.

In terms of treatment, AED selection is guided by individual seizure phenotype and EEG pattern, but medications enhancing GABA transmission may tend to be more effective than other agents. The earlier the age of onset of seizures, the more likely they will be refractory to treatment.

Diagnostic tests for microcephaly

The first-line diagnostic test for microcephaly is an accurate measurement of OFC obtained in the delivery room and repeated at each postnatal office visit. After the first few months, tracking the OFC may be overlooked. However the ability to distinguish between congenital microcephaly and postnatal microcephaly will be helpful in prioritizing the possible etiologies. An essential test for the appropriate diagnostic classification of microcephaly is the MRI, looking for basic patterns discussed above. This will permit determination of the degree of gyral simplification and the presence of any accompanying malformation of cortex, corpus callosum, subcortical structures, brainstem, or cerebellum. The possibility of acquired microcephaly due to intrauterine or perinatal infection from toxoplasmosis, rubella, cytomegalovirus, or herpes virus should be ruled out with TORCH titers. This is especially important in those cases involving polymicrogyria, calcification, early epilepsy, retinopathy, or other symptoms associated with AGS. Metabolic screening for aminoaciduria, altered pterin compound levels, organic acids, may be helpful for characterizing MSG phenotypes such as MCPHA and could identify rare treatable disorders like tetrahydrobiopterin (BH4) deficiency (Longo 2009).

Genetic testing for microcephaly is not yet widely available. However, among the MSG1 primary microcephaly phenotypes, ASPM appears to account for a significant proportion of cases – perhaps as much as 40% of MCPH (Cox *et al.* 2006). It is therefore likely that clinical testing for ASPM will be among the first to be available for routine diagnostics. Testing for MeCP2 mutations is likely to be available in the near future as well.

Principles of management

The management of patients with microcephaly is similar to that required for those with any brain malformation. Careful monitoring of the individual growth curve and review of the child's caloric intake should provide indication of when support measures like feeding-tube placement should be considered to optimize nutrition. Evaluation by physical and speech therapists should be sought to provide guidance regarding developmental-stage-appropriate activities to maximize acquisition of motor, cognitive, and communication skills. The possibility of seizures should be discussed with parents, who should be questioned regarding symptoms such as unusual startle responses, staring, posturing, or shaking episodes that could indicate seizures in their child.

The management of epilepsy when it occurs should be guided by the type of seizure encountered and these principles are discussed in detail elsewhere in this volume. Therapy with AEDs is the first line of management. Monotherapy is always preferred over treatment with multiple AEDs, as it carries a lower risk of untoward side effects and greater likelihood of sustainable, adequate control. Seizure types such as West syndrome or infantile spasms that often accompany interneuronopathy are more likely to respond to medications that promote GABA transmission. Depakote may therefore be prescribed at an earlier age than typical in the general pediatric population. Use of vigabatrin is more problematic in this microcephaly population since tunnel vision, a potential side effect of the medication, might be difficult to detect early in these children and could have a significant impact on quality of life. Microcephaly has diffuse effects on brain structure, and epilepsy, when it occurs in this setting, is therefore unlikely to be amenable to surgical ablation methods. However, in rare instances in which focal heterotopias are present that can be associated with localized EEG evidence for epileptiform activity, surgical intervention may be considered.

References

Aligianis IA, Johnson CA, Gissen P, *et al.* (2005) Mutations of the catalytic subunit of RAB3GAP cause Warburg Micro syndrome. *Nat Genet* 37:221–3.

Amir RE, Van den Veyver IB, Wan M, *et al.* (1999) Rett syndrome is caused by mutations in X-linked MECP2, encoding methyl-CpG-binding protein 2. *Nat Genet* 23:185–8.

Armstrong DD (2001) Rett syndrome neuropathology review 2000. *Brain Dev* 23(Suppl 1):S72–6.

Assaf Y, Galron R, Shapira I, *et al.* (2008) MRI evidence of white matter damage in a mouse model of Nijmegen breakage syndrome. *Exp Neurol* 209:181–91.

Baala L, Briault S, Etchevers HC, *et al.* (2007) Homozygous silencing of T-box transcription factor EOMES leads to microcephaly with polymicrogyria and corpus callosum agenesis. *Nat Genet* 39:454–6.

Bahi-Buisson N, Poirier K, Boddaert N, *et al.* (2008) Refinement of cortical dysgeneses spectrum associated with TUBA1A mutations. *J Med Genet* 45:647–53.

Barth PG, Mullaart R, Stam FC, Slooff JL (1982) Familial lissencephaly with extreme neopallial hypoplasia. *Brain Dev* 4:145–51.

Boland E, Clayton-Smith J, Woo VG, *et al.* (2007) Mapping of deletion and translocation breakpoints in 1q44 implicates the serine/threonine kinase AKT3 in postnatal microcephaly and agenesis of the corpus callosum. *Am J Hum Genet* 81:292–303.

Bond J, Woods CG (2006) Cytoskeletal genes regulating brain size. *Curr Opin Cell Biol* 18:95–101.

Bond J, Roberts E, Mochida GH, *et al.* (2002) ASPM is a major determinant of cerebral cortical size. *Nat Genet* 32:316–20.

Bond J, Roberts E, Springell K, *et al.* (2005) A centrosomal mechanism involving CDK5RAP2 and CENPJ controls brain size. *Nat Genet* 37:353–5.

Briggs TA, Wolf NI, D'Arrigo S, *et al.* (2008a) Band-like intracranial calcification with simplified gyration and polymicrogyria: a distinct "pseudo-TORCH" phenotype. *Am J Med Genet* 146A:3173–80.

Briggs TA, Abdel-Salam GM, Balicki M, *et al.* (2008b) Cerebroretinal microangiopathy with calcifications and cysts (CRMCC). *Am J Med Genet* 146A:182–90.

Butt SJ, Sousa VH, Fuccillo MV, *et al.* (2008) The requirement of Nkx2–1 in the temporal specification of cortical interneuron subtypes. *Neuron* 59:722–32.

Bystron I, Blakemore C, Rakic P (2008) Development of the human cerebral cortex: Boulder Committee revisited. *Nat Rev Neurosci* 9:110–22.

Chapleau CA, Calfa GD, Lane MC, *et al.* (2009) Dendritic spine pathologies in hippocampal pyramidal neurons from Rett syndrome brain and after expression of Rett-associated MECP2 mutations. *Neurobiol Dis* 35:219–33.

Chen L, Melendez J, Campbell K, Kuan CY, Zheng Y (2009) Rac1 deficiency in the forebrain results in neural progenitor reduction and microcephaly. *Dev Biol* 325:162–70.

Cox J, Jackson AP, Bond J, Woods CG (2006) What primary microcephaly can tell us about brain growth. *Trends Mol Med* **12**:358–66.

Crow YJ, McMenamin J, Haenggeli CA, *et al.* (2004) Coats' plus: a progressive familial syndrome of bilateral Coats' disease, characteristic cerebral calcification, leukoencephalopathy, slow pre- and post-natal linear growth and defects of bone marrow and integument. *Neuropediatrics* **35**:10–19.

Crow YJ, Hayward BE, Parmar R, *et al.* (2006a) Mutations in the gene encoding the 3′-5′ DNA exonuclease TREX1 cause Aicardi–Goutieres syndrome at the AGS1 locus. *Nat Genet* **38**:917–20.

Crow YJ, Leitch A, Hayward BE, *et al.* (2006b) Mutations in genes encoding ribonuclease H2 subunits cause Aicardi–Goutieres syndrome and mimic congenital viral brain infection. *Nat Genet* **38**:910–16.

Dan B (2009) Angelman syndrome: current understanding and research prospects. *Epilepsia* **50**:2331–9.

Davis TH, Cuellar TL, Koch SM, *et al.* (2008) Conditional loss of Dicer disrupts cellular and tissue morphogenesis in the cortex and hippocampus. *J Neurosci* **28**:4322–30.

Dobyns WB (2002) Primary microcephaly: new approaches for an old disorder. *Am J Med Genet* **112**:315–17.

Eagleson KL, Schlueter McFadyen-Ketchum LJ, *et al.* (2007) Disruption of Foxg1 expression by knock-in of cre recombinase: effects on the development of the mouse telencephalon. *Neuroscience* **148**:385–99.

Farkas LM, Haffner C, Giger T, *et al.* (2008) Insulinoma-associated 1 has a panneurogenic role and promotes the generation and expansion of basal progenitors in the developing mouse neocortex. *Neuron* **60**:40–55.

Feng Y, Walsh CA (2004) Mitotic spindle regulation by Nde1 controls cerebral cortical size. *Neuron* **44**:279–93.

Glickstein SB, Monaghan JA, Koeller HB, Jones TK, Ross ME (2009) Cyclin D2 is critical for intermediate progenitor cell proliferation in the embryonic cortex. *J Neurosci* **29**:9614–24.

Glickstein SB, Moore H, Slowinska B, *et al.* (2007) Selective cortical interneuron and GABA deficits in cyclin D2-null mice. *Development* **134**:4083–93.

Griffith E, Walker S, Martin CA, *et al.* (2008) Mutations in pericentrin cause Seckel syndrome with defective ATR-dependent DNA damage signaling. *Nat Genet* **40**:232–6.

Guerrini R, Moro F, Kato M, *et al.* (2007) Expansion of the first PolyA tract of ARX causes infantile spasms and status dystonicus. *Neurology* **69**:427–33.

Hall JG, Flora C, Scott CI Jr., Pauli RM, Tanaka KI (2004) Majewski osteodysplastic primordial dwarfism type II (MOPD II): natural history and clinical findings. *Am J Med Genet* **130A**:55–72.

Hong CJ, Hsueh YP (2006) CASK associates with glutamate receptor interacting protein and signaling molecules. *Biochem Biophys Res Commun* **351**:771–6.

Hsueh YP (2006) The role of the MAGUK protein CASK in neural development and synaptic function. *Curr Med Chem* **13**:1915–27.

Hsueh YP, Wang TF, Yang FC, Sheng M (2000) Nuclear translocation and transcription regulation by the membrane-associated guanylate kinase CASK/LIN-2. *Nature* **404**:298–302.

Huang TN, Hsueh YP (2009) CASK point mutation regulates protein–protein interactions and NR2b promoter activity. *Biochem Biophys Res Commun* **382**:219–22.

Jackson AP, McHale DP, Campbell DA, *et al.* (1998) Primary autosomal recessive microcephaly (MCPH1) maps to chromosome 8p22-pter. *Am J Hum Genet* **63**:541–6.

Jacob FD, Ramaswamy V, Andersen J, Bolduc FV (2009) Atypical Rett syndrome with selective FOXG1 deletion detected by comparative genomic hybridization: case report and review of literature. *Eur J Hum Genet* **17**:1577–81.

Jaglin XH, Poirier K, Saillour Y, *et al.* (2009) Mutations in the beta-tubulin gene *TUBB2B* result in asymmetrical polymicrogyria. *Nat Genet* **41**:746–52.

Jamieson CR, Govaerts C, Abramowicz MJ (1999) Primary autosomal recessive microcephaly: homozygosity mapping of MCPH4 to chromosome 15. *Am J Hum Genet* **65**:1465–9.

Kato M, Dobyns WB (2005) X-linked lissencephaly with abnormal genitalia as a tangential migration disorder causing intractable epilepsy: proposal for a new term, "interneuronopathy." *J Child Neurol* **20**:392–7.

Kato M, Das S, Petras K, *et al.* (2004) Mutations of ARX are associated with striking pleiotropy and consistent genotype-phenotype correlation. *Hum Mutat* **23**:147–59.

Kitamura K, Yanazawa M, Sugiyama N, (2002) Mutation of ARX causes abnormal development of forebrain and testes in mice and X-linked lissencephaly with abnormal genitalia in humans. *Nat Genet* **32**:359–69.

Koeller HB, Ross ME, Glickstein SB (2008) Cyclin D1 in excitatory neurons of the adult brain enhances kainate-induced neurotoxicity. *Neurobiol Dis* **31**:230–41.

Kriegstein A, Noctor S, Martinez-Cerdeno V (2006) Patterns of neural stem and progenitor cell division may underlie evolutionary cortical expansion. *Nat Rev Neurosci* **7**:883–90.

Longo N (2009) Disorders of biopterin metabolism. *J Inherit Metab Dis* **32**:333–42.

LoTurco JJ, Sarkisian MR, Cosker L, Bai J (2003) Citron kinase is a regulator of mitosis and neurogenic cytokinesis in the neocortical ventricular zone. *Cereb Cortex* **13**:588–91.

Morris-Rosendahl DJ, Najm J, Lachmeijer AM, *et al.* (2008) Refining the phenotype of alpha-1a Tubulin (TUBA1A) mutation in patients with classical lissencephaly. *Clin Genet* **74**:425–33.

Najm J, Horn D, Wimplinger I, *et al.* (2008) Mutations of CASK cause an X-linked brain malformation phenotype with microcephaly and hypoplasia of the brainstem and cerebellum. *Nat Genet* **40**:1065–7.

O'Driscoll M, Jackson AP, Jeggo PA (2006) Microcephalin: a causal link between impaired damage response signalling and microcephaly. *Cell Cycle* **5**:2339–44.

O'Driscoll M, Ruiz-Perez VL, Woods CG, Jeggo PA, Goodship JA (2003) A splicing mutation affecting expression of ataxia-telangiectasia and Rad3-related protein (ATR) results in Seckel syndrome. *Nat Genet* **33**:497–501.

Ossowski L, Aguirre-Ghiso JA (2000) Urokinase receptor and integrin partnership: coordination of signaling for cell adhesion, migration and growth. *Curr Opin Cell Biol* **12**:613–20.

Peiffer A, Singh N, Leppert M, Dobyns WB, Carey JC (1999) Microcephaly with simplified gyral pattern in six related children. *Am J Med Genet* **84**:137–44.

Pontious A, Kowalczyk T, Englund C, Hevner RF (2008) Role of intermediate progenitor cells in cerebral cortex development. *Dev Neurosci* **30**:24–32.

Powell EM, Campbell DB, Stanwood GD, *et al.* (2003) Genetic disruption of cortical interneuron development causes region- and GABA cell type-specific deficits, epilepsy, and behavioral dysfunction. *J Neurosci* **23**:622–31.

Rajab A, Manzini MC, Mochida GH, Walsh CA, Ross ME (2007) A novel form of lethal microcephaly with simplified gyral pattern and brain stem hypoplasia. *Am J Med Genet* **143A**:2761–7.

Rajab A, Aldinger KA, El-Shirbini HA, Dobyns WB, Ross ME (2009) Recessive developmental delay, small stature, microcephaly and brain calcifications with locus on chromosome 2. *Am J Med Genet* **149A**:129–37.

Rauch A, Thiel CT, Schindler D, *et al.* (2008) Mutations in the pericentrin (PCNT) gene cause primordial dwarfism. *Science* **319**:816–19.

Rice G, Patrick T, Parmar R, *et al.* (2007) Clinical and molecular phenotype of Aicardi–Goutieres syndrome. *Am J Hum Genet* **81**:713–25.

Roberts E, Jackson AP, Carradice AC, *et al.* (1999) The second locus for autosomal recessive primary microcephaly (MCPH2) maps to chromosome 19q13.1–13.2. *Eur J Hum Genet* **7**:815–20.

Rosenberg MJ, Agarwala R, Bouffard G, *et al.* (2002) Mutant deoxynucleotide carrier is associated with congenital microcephaly. *Nat Genet* **32**:175–9.

Rousseau F, Bonaventure J, Legeai-Mallet L, *et al.* (1996) Clinical and genetic heterogeneity of hypochondroplasia. *J Med Genet* **33**:749–52.

Samuels BA, Hsueh YP, Shu T, *et al.* (2007) Cdk5 promotes synaptogenesis by regulating the subcellular distribution of the MAGUK family member CASK. *Neuron* **56**:823–37.

Sarkisian MR, Frenkel M, Li W, Oborski JA, LoTurco JJ (2001) Altered interneuron development in the cerebral cortex of the *flathead* mutant. *Cereb Cortex* **11**:734–43.

Sessa A, Mao CA, Hadjantonakis AK, Klein WH, Broccoli V (2008) Tbr2 directs conversion of radial glia into basal precursors and guides neuronal amplification by indirect neurogenesis in the developing neocortex. *Neuron* **60**:56–69.

Shahbazian MD, Zoghbi HY (2002) Rett syndrome and MeCP2: linking epigenetics and neuronal function. *Am J Hum Genet* **71**:1259–72.

Shandala T, Gregory SL, Dalton HE, Smallhorn M, Saint R (2004) Citron Kinase is an essential effector of the Pbl-activated Rho signalling pathway in Drosophila melanogaster. *Development* **131**:5053–63.

Sheen VL, Ganesh VS, Topcu M, *et al.* (2004) Mutations in ARFGEF2 implicate vesicle trafficking in neural progenitor proliferation and migration in the human cerebral cortex. *Nat Genet* **36**:69–76.

Sigaudy S, Toutain A, Moncla A, *et al.* (1998) Microcephalic osteodysplastic primordial dwarfism Taybi–Linder type: report of four cases and review of the literature. *Am J Med Genet* **80**:16–24.

Tschopp O, Yang ZZ, Brodbeck D, *et al.* (2005) Essential role of protein kinase B gamma (PKB gamma/Akt3) in postnatal brain development but not in glucose homeostasis. *Development* **132**:2943–54.

Van Buggenhout G, Fryns JP (2009) Angelman syndrome (AS, MIM 105830). *Eur J Hum Genet* **17**:1367–73.

Wallis DE, Roessler E, Hehr U, *et al.* (1999) Mutations in the homeodomain of the human SIX3 gene cause holoprosencephaly. *Nat Genet* **22**:196–8.

Willems M, Geneviève D, Borck G, *et al.* (2010) Molecular analysis of Pericentrin gene (PCNT) in a series of 24 Seckel/MOPD II families. *J Med Genet* **47**:797–802.

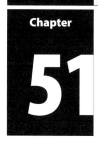

Arachnoid cysts

Concezio Di Rocco and Gianpiero Tamburrini

Definition, pathogenesis, and epidemiology

Definition and pathogenesis

Congenital arachnoid cysts (AC) are also called leptomeningeal cysts. This term excludes secondary "arachnoid" cysts (i.e., post-traumatic, post-infectious, etc.), lined with diseased or inflammatory arachnoidal membranes, and glio-ependymal cysts, lined with glial tissue and epithelial cells.

True AC are developmental lesions that arise from the splitting or duplication of the arachnoid membrane (thus they are in fact intra-arachnoid cysts). The etiology of these lesions has long been the subject of debate. The most accepted theory is that they develop from a minor aberration in the development of the arachnoid mater from around week 15 of gestation onward, when the cerebrospinal fluid (CSF) is generated to gradually replace the extracellular ground substance between the external and the internal arachnoid membrane (endomeninx) (Di Rocco 1996). The malformative hypothesis is supported by the common location of arachnoid cysts at the level of normal arachnoid cisterns, their occasional occurrence in siblings, the presence of accompanying anomalies of the venous architecture (i.e., the absence of the sylvian vein), and the association with other congenital anomalies (agenesis of the corpus callosum and Marfan syndrome).

Specific problems in the definition of the pathogenesis concern intraventricular AC. For some authors, they represent a kind of "internal" meningocele; for others, they derive from the arachnoid layer and are transported along with the vascular mesenchyme when it invaginates through the choroidal fissure (Di Rocco 1996; Eskandari *et al.* 2005).

Epidemiology

Congenital AC have been reported to account for roughly 1% of atraumatic intracranial mass lesions. This relatively old figure is the result of a correlation between data obtained from the clinical experience in the era before computed tomography (CT) and magnetic resonance imaging (MRI) (0.7–2% of space-occupying lesions), and those obtained from autopsy observations (0.1–0.5% of incidental autoptic findings) (Helland *et al.* 2007); recent MRI studies in healthy subjects suggest that this rate is higher, approximating 1.5–2.0% (Weber *et al.* 2006). Intracranial AC are nearly always sporadic and single. They occur two or three times more often in males than in females and three to four times more often on the left side of the brain than on the right. The bilateral occurrence of more or less symmetrical cysts has been reported, although rarely, in normal as well as in neurologically impaired children. In the latter instance, especially in patients with bitemporal cysts, the differential diagnosis should be made with lesions resulting from perinatal hypoxia or metabolic diseases.

According to the information provided by large mixed series (i.e., including both children and adults), 6–90% of patients belong to the pediatric age group; it is recognized that the largest proportion of infantile cases occur during the first 2 years of life (Wester 1999).

The most common location for AC is within the middle cranial fossa, 30–50% of lesions being found there. Another 10% occur over the cerebral convexity, 9–15% in the suprasellar region, 5–10% in the quadrigeminal plate cistern, 10% in the cerebellopontine angle, and 10% in the midline posterior fossa (Di Rocco 1996; Beldzinska *et al.* 2002). The anatomical classification and topographic distribution of the different types of AC are summarized in Table 51.1. Because most of the reports on the relationship between AC and epilepsy are centered on sylvian AC we will specifically deal only with the clinicoradiological features of this location, briefly reporting in the section on "Epilepsy and arachnoid cysts" the epileptological findings in children with cysts located in other intracranial sites.

General clinical and imaging features

Sylvian fissure cysts

Sylvian fissure cysts alone account for about half of adult and one-third of pediatric cases. Their most accepted classification is the one of Galassi and colleagues who divided sylvian fissure

The Causes of Epilepsy, eds. S. D. Shorvon, F. Andermann, and R. Guerrini. Published by Cambridge University Press. © Cambridge University Press 2011.

Table 51.1 Anatomical classification and topographical distribution of intracranial arachnoid cysts

Location	Percentage distribution
Supratentorial	
Sylvian fissure	30–50
Sellar region	9–15
Cerebral convexity	4–15
Interhemispherical fissure	5–8
Quadrigeminal plate	5–10
Infratentorial	
Median	9–17
Cerebellar hemisphere	5–11
Cerebellopontine angle	4–10
Retro-clival	0.5–3

cysts into three types, depending on their size and apparent communication (metrizamide CT study) with the normal CSF spaces (Galassi *et al.* 1982).

Sylvian fissure cysts can manifest clinically at any age, but they become symptomatic more frequently in children and adolescents than in adults, and in most series infants and toddlers account for about a quarter of the cases. The diagnosis is frequently incidental. In symptomatic patients, the symptoms are often non-specific, headache being the most common complaint. Among focal signs, mild proptosis and contralateral motor weakness may be noted in advanced cases. Seizures and signs of increased intracranial pressure (ICP) represent the clinical onset in about 20–35% of patients. When signs of increased ICP appear acutely they are usually the consequence of an abrupt increase in the cyst volume, because of subdural or intracystic bleeding.

Mental impairment is found in only 10% of the cases; however, developmental delay and behavioral abnormalities are common in children with large lesions and are nearly constant and severe in patients with bilateral cysts (Wester and Hugdhal 1995; Fewel *et al.* 1996; Gosalakkal 2002; Zaatreh *et al.* 2002; Raeder *et al.* 2005).

A localized bulging of the skull and/or asymmetrical macrocrania are characteristic features in half of the patients. In these cases CT reveals an outward bulging and thinning of the temporal squama and anterior displacement of the lesser and greater wings of the sphenoid bone. Cysts appear as well-defined lesions between the dura and the distorted brain, with the same density of CSF and without contrast enhancement. Cerebral ventricles are usually of normal size or minimally dilated (Galassi *et al.* 1982; Eskandary *et al.* 2005). Studies with MRI show lesions to have hypointensity on T1-weighted and hyperintensity on T2-weighted images. Scanning of the vascular structures is useful in order to define the arteries and veins

in relation to the cyst wall. Cine-flow sequences have been recently employed as substitutes for metrizamide CT in order to define the presence or absence of communication between the cysts and the subarachnoid spaces (Hoffman *et al.* 2000; Yildiz *et al.* 2005, 2006). This may be particularly important in asymptomatic patients, as in patients with non-specific clinical symptoms. In this context, further information that might indicate the need for surgery may be provided by ICP monitoring (Di Rocco *et al.* 2003; Tamburrini *et al.* 2004, 2005; Helland and Wester 2007). Perfusion MRI sequences and single photon emission computed tomography (SPECT) studies have also been proposed; the latter may help to evaluate brain perfusion around the cyst walls (Kim DS *et al.* 1999; Sgouros and Chapman 2001; Hund-Georgiadis *et al.* 2002; Germanò *et al.* 2003; Martinez-Lage *et al.* 2006).

Arachnoid cysts and epilepsy

The incidence of epilepsy in AC patients has been reported to be between 7.5% and 42.4%; conversely MRI screening studies in epileptic patients have showed that AC are incidentally found in up to 2% of the cases. The frequency of seizures is greater in children than adults and their initiation seems not to be related to the size of the AC (Ozisik *et al.* 2008). The most common type of AC presenting with epilepsy are sylvian AC, seizures being the clinical onset in 20–35% of these patients (Tamburrini *et al.* 2008). This common association has prompted many neurosurgeons to utilize the semiology of the seizures and the topography of interictal electroencephalographic (EEG) anomalies in epileptic subjects harboring this kind of lesion, to verify the coincidence of the epileptogenic area with this location and with the characteristics of the cyst (Koch *et al.* 1995, 1998; Arroyo and Santamaria 1997; Kramer *et al.* 1998; Morioka *et al.* 1998; Kawamura *et al.* 2002; Yalcin *et al.* 2002; Kobayashi *et al.* 2003; Sztriha and Guruaj 2005). However none of these studies has been able to show a definite association and, whatever the surgical technique adopted, the role of surgical treatment on the control of seizures remains uncertain.

In 1998 Koch *et al.* (1998) reviewed the world's medical literature dealing with surgically treated sylvian ACs in epileptic patients adding six personal cases. They found a correlation between a reduction of cysts' size as documented on postoperative neuroradiological examinations and seizures outcome. Sixty of a total of 76 patients had a reduction in size of their AC, with 76.6% experiencing seizures improvement. This rate fell to 50% when the postoperative AC size was unchanged. In the previous year Arroyo and Santamaria (1997) had reported that only three of the 12 patients with sylvian AC presenting with seizures in their series had temporal lobe epilepsy, and developmental pathologies (namely focal heterotopias) far from the AC could be found in 25% of the cases (3/12 cases). Based on these results the authors emphasized that the dissociation between structural and functional pathology is particularly likely in patients with AC and a comprehensive preoperative evaluation in such cases is of utmost importance. These considerations have been confirmed in many further single case reports and clinical series (Kramer et al. 1998; Morioka et al. 1998; Kawamura et al. 2002; Yalcin et al. 2002; Kobayashi et al. 2003; Sztriha and Guruaj 2005). Prolonged surface EEG recordings are still regarded as the essential tool in improving the location of the seizure focus. In a series of 21 patients with sylvian AC and seizures, Yalcin et al. (2002) found that only five had seizures types (partial seizures) which could be clinically related with the presence of the AC; repeated EEG recordings further improved the location of the seizure focus demonstrating an association with the AC site in only one case. As in other forms of symptomatic epilepsy further details in the diagnostic work-out of these patients could be achieved by intracranial EEG recordings; however the positioning of depth electrodes arrays near to the AC cavity might be difficult, especially if we consider subdural electrodes. A technical improvement in this context has been recently suggested by Kushen and Frim (2007); gelatine foam padding was used to fill the AC cavity in two children and succeeded in conforming the grids to the adjacent concave temporal lobe surface.

In a recent international survey that was conducted by our unit on the management of a Type II sylvian AC, participants were asked what they should have done if the child presented with temporal seizures as the only clinical symptom (Tamburrini et al. 2008).

All the investigators asked for one or more further diagnostic examinations, 77.7% of them indicating an EEG evaluation and 33.3% a SPECT study, in order to clarify if a correlation could exist among the presence of the AC and the seizures, confirming the belief that the indication for surgical treatment in children with sylvian AC cannot be established only on the clinical evidence of epilepsy at diagnosis.

More than 30% of the participants would have asked for a SPECT study, the hypoperfusion of brain structures surrounding the cyst being considered as suggestive for a correlation between seizures and the presence of the AC. In fact, cerebral SPECT has been only occasionally used for evaluating AC, most papers in the literature consisting of anecdotal case reports. Sgouros and Chapman (2001) documented a global preoperative regional cerebral blood flow (rCBF) reduction (^{99m}Tc-hexamethylpropyleneamineoxime SPECT scans) in three children affected by sylvian fissure AC with non-specific symptoms. After successful surgical excision of the cyst, the perfusion defects disappeared. This was associated with general improvement of pre-existing non-specific symptoms. Germanò et al. (2003) came to similar conclusions comparing pre and post-surgical SPECT studies in two of seven children with AC that showed normalization of rCBF after cyst shunting. In their series of 11 patients Martinez-Lage et al. (2006) demonstrated impaired brain perfusion in 70% of symptomatic patients, with a normalization of rCBF in all the four cases who underwent surgery. Conversely in a previous report from our institution (Tamburrini et al. 2005) based on 11 patients who underwent

contemporary measurement of rCBF and prolonged ICP monitoring, SPECT studies proved more sensitive than ICP monitoring in children with unspecific clinicoradiologic correlation. However, uncertain results were achieved in children in whom the clinical findings were regarded as typical of this type of lesion; we attributed this last result to a limit of the methodology which was based on a comparison of rCBF between the two hemispheres, a difference which could be less significant in cases of larger cysts influencing the rCBF in both temporal lobes.

A further attempt to determine if a correlation might exist among seizures and AC is the investigation using magnetic resonance spectroscopy (MRS) of Hajek et al. (1997). They reported two patients affected by AC; MRS study showed increased glutamate and aspartate peaks in the cyst fluid; one of the patients also showed a moderate increase in glutamate in the epileptogenic cerebral tissue adjacent to the cyst, with no increase in the excitatory amino acid levels in the non-epileptic cerebral tissue. On these grounds they suggested that the relative increase of excitatory amino acids in the cyst fluid and adjacent cerebral tissue might explain the development and continuation of epileptogenesis in some cases and that, reducing the levels of these excitatory amino acids, performing a cysto-subarachnoid communication or shunting might make it easier to control seizures by decreasing the levels of excitatory amino acids. However, it should be pointed out that both of their patients had associated epileptogenic pathologies (one a Rasmussen encephalitis and the second a mesiotemporal ganglioglioma) which certainly might have influenced both the levels of excitatory amino acids and the results of surgical treatment, which included the removal of the epileptogenic tissue. In a more recent study Ozisik et al. (2008), evaluated the levels of N-acetylaspartate (NAA), creatine (Cr), choline (Cho), and myoinositol (MI) in 12 patients with AC, of whom six were affected by temporal cysts and the remaining six by a posterior fossa cyst. Levels of NAA, Cr, Cho, and MI were dosed in tissues adjacent to the AC and in the symmetrical brain area of the contralateral hemisphere. No difference was found in the NAA/Cr, Cho/Cr, and MI/Cr ratios among the affected and normal sides, which confirms the absence of any association among AC and epilepsy.

Concerning supratentorial AC located in other regions, away from the sylvian fissure, only occasional papers in the literature have dealt with their possible association with the seizures. Epilepsy is a common finding in children with inter-hemispheric fissure cysts but in almost all cases is related to the presence of associated cerebral developmental anomalies such as agenesis of the corpus callosum or holoprosencephaly. Seizures have also been reported as a possible manifestation in patients with cerebral convexity cysts, but as is the case with sylvian cysts, the relationship between the presence of the cyst and the clinical evidence of seizures is considered uncertain. If surgery is contemplated, a strict preoperative evaluation is advised in all cases (Agarwal et al. 1997; Lewis et al. 2002). The possibility of seizures being the presenting sign in children with isolated posterior fossa cysts has also been raised by recent, though occasional, case reports, possibly justified by the recognized modulator effect of the cerebellum and the brainstem on cerebral epileptiform activity (Ozisik *et al.* 2008). Recio *et al.* (2007) reported focal seizures in two patients with posterior fossa AC. The EEG focus was identified in the left temporal lobe in one case and in the left occipital lobe in the other. Gan *et al.* (2008) presented a child with quadrigeminal cistern AC and seizures resistant to medical treatment, where the seizures were dramatically improved by cyst decompression. As for sylvian AC, Ozisik *et al.* (2008) were not able to find any relationship between the presence of an AC in the posterior fossa and modifications of MRS peaks, in six patients presenting with epilepsy, again confirming that this association could be considered coincidental.

Principles of management

There are essentially three surgical options for the management of AC, to be considered alone or in combination:

(1) cyst marsupialization through open craniotomy
(2) endoscopic cyst marsupialization
(3) Cyst shunting, both intraventricular or extrathecal.

Open cyst marsupialization is considered the preferable surgical procedure. Successful open fenestration rates vary from 75% to 100%; moreover, a substantial reduction in the earlier morbidity rates has been reported in recent series and surgical mortality has been reduced to almost nil (Tamburrini *et al.* 2008). Two issues concerning open surgery should be pointed out:

(1) Total excision of the AC membranes is no longer considered worthwhile; large windows in a bipolar fashion are sufficient to allow CSF pulsations through the cyst cavity and reduce the risk of harming the adjacent cortex. A more focal cyst opening might also prevent CSF escape into the subdural space and the development of postoperative subdural hygromas.
(2) All vessels either traversing the cyst cavity or lying in the cyst membrane represent the normal vasculature and are therefore to be preserved.

Pure endoscopic cyst marsupialization has been proposed as an alternative to open fenestration in recent years and is considered as the gold standard in children with selective cyst locations (e.g., sellar and suprasellar cysts and intraparaventricular locations). Endoscopy has also been used to assist open surgery in children with sylvian fissure AC, in order to reduce the extension of the surgical approach. Alternating results of pure endoscopic techniques have been reported, with success rates ranging between 45% and 100% (Choi *et al.* 1999; Godano *et al.* 2004; Cinalli *et al.* 2007; Elhammady *et al.* 2007).

Cyst extrathecal diversions are obviously safer, but are accompanied by a high incidence of additional surgical procedures (around 30%) and the stigma of lifelong shunt dependency (Lena *et al.* 1996; Kim *et al.* 2002). As previously stated no difference has been described among different surgical techniques concerning results on the control of seizures, this last again generally appearing as scarcely influenced by surgery in most series.

References

Agarwal HS, Rane S, Nanavati RN, Udani RH (1997) Interhemispheric arachnoid cyst with agenesis of corpus callosum. *Indian Pediatr* **34**:737–40.

Arai H, Sato K, Wachi A, Okuda O, Takeda N (1996) Arachnoid cysts of the middle cranial fossa: experience with 77 patients who were treated with cystoperitoneal shunting. *Neurosurgery* **39**:1108–13.

Arroyo S, Santamaria J (1997) What is the relationship between arachnoid cysts and seizure foci? *Epilepsia* **38**:1098–102.

Beldzinska MM, Ostrowska ED (2002) Presentation of intracranial arachnoid cysts in children: correlation between localization and clinical symptoms. *Med Sci Monit* **8**:462–5.

Beltramello A, Mazza C (1985) Spontaneous disappearance of a large middle fossa arachnoid cyst. *Surg Neurol* **24**:181–3.

Choi JU, Kim DS, Huh R (1999) Endoscopic approach to arachnoid cyst. *Childs Nerv Syst* **15**:285–91.

Cinalli G, Spennato P, Ruggiero C, *et al.* (2007) Complications following endoscopic intracranial procedures in children. *Childs Nerv Syst* **23**:633–44.

Di Rocco C (1996) Arachnoid cysts. In: Youmans JR, (ed.) *Neurological Surgery*. Philadelphia, PA: WB Saunders, pp. 967–94.

Di Rocco C, Tamburrini G, Caldarelli M, Velardi F, Santini P (2003) Prolonged ICP monitoring in sylvian arachnoid cysts. *Surg Neurol* **60**:211–18.

Elhammady MS, Bhatia S, Ragheb J (2007) Endoscopic fenestration of middle fossa arachnoid cysts: a technical description and case series. *Pediatr Neurosurg* **43**:209–15.

Eskandary H, Sabba M, Khajehpour F, Eskandari M (2005) Incidental findings in brain computed tomography scans of 3000 head trauma patients. *Surg Neurol* **63**:550–3.

Fewel ME, Levy ML, McComb JG (1996) Surgical treatment of 95 children with 102 intracranial arachnoid cysts. *Pediatr Neurosurg* **25**:165–73.

Galassi E, Tognetti F, Gaist G, *et al.* (1982) CT scan and metrizamide CT cisternography in arachnoid cysts of the middle cranial fossa: classification and pathophysiological aspects. *Surg Neurol* **17**:363–9.

Gan YC, Connolly MB, Steinbok P (2008) Epilepsy associated with a cerebellar arachnoid cyst: seizure control following fenestration of the cyst. *Childs Nerv Syst* **24**:125–34.

Germanò A, Caruso G, Caffo M, *et al.* (2003) The treatment of large supratentorial arachnoid cysts in infants with cyst-peritoneal shunting and Hakim programmable valve. *Childs Nerv Syst* **19**:166–73.

Godano U, Mascari C, Consales A, Calbucci F (2004) Endoscope-controlled microneurosurgery for the treatment of intracranial fluid cysts. *Childs Nerv Syst* **20**:839–41.

Gosalakkal JA (2002) Intracranial arachnoid cysts in children: a review of pathogenesis, clinical features and management. *Ped Neurol* **26**:93–8.

Hajek M, Do KQ, Duc C, Boesiger P, Wieser HG (1997) Increased excitatory amino acid levels in brain cysts of epileptic patients. *Epilepsy Res* **28**:245–54.

Helland CA, Wester K (2007) Intracystic pressure in patients with temporal arachnoid cysts: a prospective study of preoperative complaints and postoperative outcome. *J Neurol Neurosurg Psychiatry* **78**:620–3.

Hoffman KT, Hosten N, Meyer BU, *et al.* (2000) CSF flow studies of intracranial cysts and cyst-like lesions achieved using reversed fast imaging with steady-state precession MR sequences. *AJNR Am J Neuradiol* **21**:493–502.

Hund-Georgiadis M, von Cramon Y, Kruggel F, Preul C (2002) Do quiescent arachnoid cysts alter CNS functional organization? A fMRI and morphometric study. *Neurology* **52**:1935–9.

Kawamura T, Morioka T, Nishio S, *et al.* (2002) Temporal lobe epilepsy associated with hippocampal sclerosis and a contralateral middle fossa arachnoid cyst. *Seizure* **11**:60–2.

Kim DS, Choi JU, Huh R, Yun PH, Kim DI (1999) Quantitative assessment of cerebrospinal fluid hydrodynamics using phase-contrast cine-MR in hydrocephalus. *Childs Nerv Syst* **15**:461–7.

Kim SK, Cho BK, Chung YN, Kim HS, Wang KC (2002) Shunt dependency in shunted arachnoid cyst a reason to avoid shunting. *Pediatr Neurosurg* **37**:178–85.

Kobayashi E, Bonilha L, Li LM, Cendes F (2003) Temporal lobe hypogenesis associated with arachnoid cyst in patients with epilepsy. *Arq Neuropsiquiatr* **61**:327–9.

Koch CA, Voth D, Kraemer G, Schwarz M (1995) Arachnoid cysts: does surgery improve epileptic seizures and headaches? *Neurosurg Rev* **18**:173–81.

Koch CA, Moore JL, Voth D (1998) Arachnoid cysts: how do postsurgical cyst

size and seizure outcome correlate? *Neurosurg Rev* **21**:14–22.

Kramer U, Nevo Y, Reider-Grosswasser I (1998) Neuroimaging of children with partial seizures. *Seizure* **7**:115–18.

Kushen MC, Frim D (2007) Placement of subdural electrode grids for seizure focus localization in patients with a large arachnoid cyst: technical note. *Neurosurg Focus* **22**:E5.

Lena G, Erdincler P, Van Calenbergh F, Genitori L, Choux M (1996) Arachnoid cysts of the middle cranial fossa in children: a review of 75 cases, 47 of which have been operated in a comparative study between membranectomy with opening of cisterns and cystoperitoneal shunt. *Neurochirurgie* **42**:29–34.

Lewis AJ, Simon EM, Barkovich AJ, *et al.* (2002) Middle interhemispheric variant of holoprosencephaly: a distinct cliniconeuroradiologic subtype. *Neurology* **59**:1860–5.

Martinez-Lage JF, Valenti JA, Piqueras C, *et al.* (2006) Functional assessment of intracranial arachnoid cysts with TC99 m-HMPAO SPECT a preliminary report. *Childs Nerv Syst* **22**:1091–7.

Morioka T, Nishio S, Ishibashi H, Fukui M (1998) What is the relationship between arachnoid cysts and seizure foci? (Letter.) *Epilepsia* **49**:804–5.

Ozisik HI, Sarac K, Ozcan C (2008) Single-voxel Magnetic Resonance Spectroscopy of brain tissue adjacent to arachnoid cysts of epileptic patients. *Neurologist* **14**:382–9.

Raeder MB, Helland CA, Hugdhal K, Wester K (2005) Arachnoid cysts cause cognitive deficits that improve after surgery. *Neurology* **64**:60–2.

Recio MV, Gallagher MJ, McLean MJ, Abou-Khalil B (2007) Clinical features of epilepsy in patients with cerebellar structural abnormalities in a referral center. *Epilepsy Res* **76**:1–5.

Sgouros S, Chapman S (2001) Congenital middle fossa arachnoid cysts may cause global brain ischaemia: a study with ^{99}Tc-hexamethylpropyleneamineoxime single photon emission computerized tomography scans. *Pediatr Neurosurg* **35**:188–94.

Sztriha L, Guruaj A (2005) Hippocampal dysgenesis associated with temporal lobe hypoplasia and arachnoid cyst of the middle cranial fossa. *J Child Neurol* **20**:926–30.

Tamburrini G, Di Rocco C, Velardi F, Santini P (2004) Prolonged intracranial pressure (ICP) monitoring in non-traumatic pediatric neurosurgical diseases. *Med Sci Monit* **10**:MT53–T63.

Tamburrini G, Caldarelli M, Massimi L, *et al.* (2005) Prolonged ICP monitoring combined with SPECT studies in children with sylvian fissure arachnoid cysts. *Childs Nerv Syst* **21**:840.

Tamburrini G, Dal Fabbro M, Di Rocco C (2008) Sylvian fissure arachnoid cysts: a survey on their diagnostic workout and practical management. *Childs Nerv Syst* **24**:593–604.

Weber F, Knopf H (2006) Incidental findings in magnetic resonance imaging of the brains of healthy young men. *J Neurol Sci* **240**:81–4.

Wester K, Hugdhal K (1995) Arachnoid cysts of the temporal fossa: impaired preoperative cognition and postoperative improvement. *J Neurol Neurosurg Psychiatry* **59**:293–8.

Wester K (1999) Peculiarities of intracranial arachnoid cysts: location sidedness and sex distribution in 126 consecutive patients. *Neurosurgery* **45**:775–9.

Yalcin DA, Oncel C, Kaymaz A, Kuolu N, Forta H (2002) Evidence against association between arachnoid cysts and epilepsy. *Epilepsy Res* **49**:255–60.

Yildiz H, Erdogan C, Yalcin R, *et al.* (2005) Evaluation of communication between intracranial arachnoid cysts and cisterns with phase-contrast cine MR imaging. *AJNR Am J Neuroradiol* **26**:145–51.

Yildiz H, Yazici Z, Hakyemez B, Erdogan C, Parlak M (2006) Evaluation of CSF flow patterns of posterior fossa cystic malformations using CSF flow MR imaging. *Neuroradiology* **48**:595–605.

Zaatreh MM, Bates E, Hooper SR, *et al.* (2002) Morphometric and neuropsychologic studies in children with arachnoid cysts. *Ped Neurol* **26**:134–8.

Malformations of human cerebral cortex

Waney Squier

Introduction

Brain imaging has become the standard means of defining patterns of malformation in patients presenting with epilepsy. The availability, safety, and increasing resolution of brain scans has facilitated the scanning of large numbers of patients and screening families. Modern imaging techniques are of a resolution and sophistication that allow the anatomical fine detail of the brain to be identified and are now increasingly employed to examine the developing brain in utero. Brain scanning has proved invaluable for correlation of phenotype with genotype and has revealed the genetic basis of many brain malformation syndromes, in particular the lissencephalies.

However, imaging cannot achieve the resolution needed to identify the cellular architecture of malformations. Examination of the mature brain by imaging, or even by microscopy, shows the malformation together with any secondary changes, such as atrophy and damage resulting from seizures and therapy. In order to understand fully the nature of brain malformation we need to unravel the particular developmental processes that have been disrupted; something which is only possible by examination of the very early developing brain in fetal life. Fetal studies show that a specific malformation, e.g., polymicrogyria or cobblestone cortex, may be the end point of disruption of one of a number of developmental pathways and may have more than one etiology.

Special considerations in the examination of human fetal brains

Examination of human fetal brain samples is constrained by unavoidable artifact due to intrauterine death and periods of delay prior to delivery but that does not outweigh the enormous value of this material in understanding human brain development. All of the cases described are from an archive collected over many years within the regulations appropriate to the period and are described here within the terms of the UK Human Tissue Act. The majority of cases studied within the last 10 years, and all since 2006, have the express consent of

the parents for use in teaching and research. Behind every one of these cases lies the personal tragedy of the loss of a baby. I owe my gratitude to those parents who at a time of loss have consented to the study of their baby's brain. Their contribution to our understanding is enormous and all who read this book are indebted to those parents and families.

A case study

This case is presented as a preface to the chapter for its exceptional educational value; it is a rare example of a well-described injury following a single timed insult. This single insult has resulted in a multitude of malformations, each the result of disruption of a pathway active at the time of the insult. Each of the malformations is illustrated here and will be described in more detail in the appropriate section below.

I am deeply indebted to the parents for consent to use the brain for medical education and research.

The mother of this baby was involved in a road traffic accident at 24 weeks of gestation. She suffered abdominal bruising. Post-injury fetal movements were normal, as was initial ultrasound brain scan and a repeat at 28 weeks. At 30 weeks fetal magnetic resonance imaging (MRI) scan showed reduction in supratentorial brain volume and prominent extra-axial spaces. There was a suggestion of bilateral "porencephalic cysts" and bilateral subdural hemorrhage was seen.

The pregnancy was terminated 12 weeks after the injury. The baby's development was consistent with gestational age. No abnormality was found outside the brain and the placenta showed no evidence of infarction or hemorrhage associated with the trauma at 24 weeks. There was no evidence of direct traumatic injury to the baby.

The brain weighed 199 g (expected weight at 35 weeks 291 g) (Fig. 52.1). There was bilateral infarction of middle cerebral artery territory, sparing the majority of the frontal, temporal, and occipital lobes.

Coronal slices showed bilateral loss of tissue in the mid part of each hemisphere through the full thickness of the brain wall, in middle cerebral artery territory. The adjacent cortex showed

The Causes of Epilepsy, eds. S. D. Shorvon, F. Andermann, and R. Guerrini. Published by Cambridge University Press. © Cambridge University Press 2011.

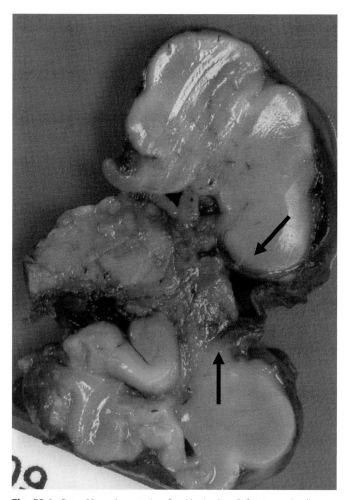

Fig. 52.1. Fetus 32 weeks gestation: fixed brain slice. Softening and collapse of the tissues in the middle cerebral artery territory are indicated by arrows. A large cystic cavity is covered by thickened and hemorrhagic meninges. See color plate section.

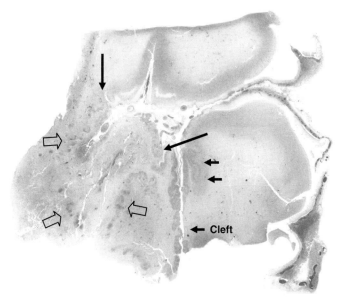

Fig. 52.2. Stained section of mid part of cerebral hemisphere. (Original magnification ×1). The area of infarction is indicated by long arrows. Note an area of polymicrogyria at the junction with normal cortex (short arrows) and a cleft lined by abnormal cortex extending deep into the brain from the surface. Groups of immature unmigrated neurons are seen in the white matter of the damaged area (open arrows). See color plate section.

no obvious macroscopic abnormality. The corpus callosum had formed and was preserved. The hippocampus was normal. The frontal and occipital lobes showed focal cortical abnormality in watershed zones consisting of small areas of excessive folding of the neuronal layer visible with the naked eye. The hindbrain appeared relatively well preserved.

Histology of the cerebral hemispheres showed, apart from necrosis, failure of neuronal migration with subcortical heterotopia, polymicrogyria, overmigration into the leptomeninges, transmantle dysplasia, and schizencephaly. There was middle cerebral artery infarction as well as watershed zone damage. The clinical features and the pattern of infarction indicate that the brain damage resulted from fetal cerebral ischemia following trauma, rather than direct trauma to the baby or the brain.

Undermigration, overmigration, and polymicrogyria

Although cortical neuronal migration is said to be complete by 20–23 weeks in the human brain, in this case clusters of

incompletely migrated cells and overmigrated cells in the leptomeninges were observed following damage at 24 weeks.

Polymicrogyria

The junction of damaged and normal cortex was abrupt, but in some areas associated with abnormal festooning of the cortical neuronal band. Similar cortical festooning was seen in the lining of the schizencephalic cleft (Fig 52.2).

Schizencephaly

In one area a cleft extended from the cortex into the deep white matter, lined by abnormally folded and nodular cortex (Fig. 52.3). The deepest part of this cleft was very close to the ventricular wall. Had the baby survived this cleft would be most likely to have appeared as "schizencephaly" lined by abnormal cortex.

Watershed damage

In the occipital and frontal lobes areas of excessive folding of the neuronal band were identified. These are notable for being in watershed territories, the inferolateral border of the occipital cortex (Fig. 52.4). This demonstrates that watershed damage can occur as early as 24 weeks and is not restricted to late gestation.

Transmantle dysplasia

In the occipital lobe a further malformation was seen. Abnormally folded cortex extended through almost the full thickness

A

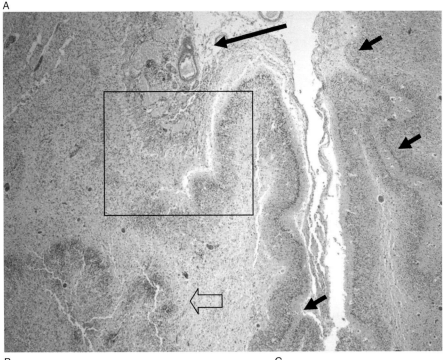

B

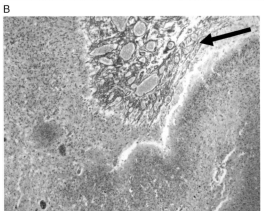

C

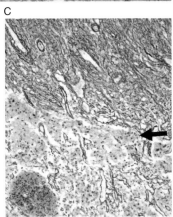

Fig. 52.3. (A) Necrotic cortex (arrow) with loss of nerve cells and proliferation of blood vessels and surface connective tissue; area in box is shown at higher magnification in (B). The open arrow indicates groups of immature cells in the white matter which have failed to migrate to the cortex. Three short arrows mark abnormal areas of cortex bordering the infarcted area; this is developing polymicrogyria (hematoxylin and eosin [H&E] stain original magnification ×2). (B) Extensive proliferation of capillaries (arrow) in the leptomeninges overlying the necrotic cortex (reticulin stain ×4). (C) Higher-power image showing nuclei of cortical neurons which appear as black dots in the cortex and extending between the new capillaries in the leptomeninges. Note many new capillaries in the cortex. An arrow marks the border of cortex and the leptomeninges (reticulin ×10). See color plate section.

of the brain wall to the ventricular lining where focal mineralization indicates old periventricular necrosis (or periventricular leuckomalacia). If the brain had developed to maturity this area might have appeared as schizencephaly or "transmantle dysplasia" on MRI scans.

The brainstem showed early cystic breakdown and extensive pyknosis in the corticospinal tracts.

This case holds an important lesson for our understanding of cortical malformation. A spectrum of malformative patterns, including failed migration to the cortex, overmigration from the cortical surface, abnormal cortical folding, and watershed damage can all originate from a single insult at 24 weeks, indicating that all of the disrupted developmental processes were still in progress at that time.

The remainder of this chapter is an overview of a range of cortical malformations as seen in their earliest stages, in fetal life. They are grouped according to the developmental process which has been disrupted in their origin.

Failure of neuroblast proliferation, growth, and differentiation

Focal cortical dysplasia and tuberous sclerosis

These are lesions restricted to a small region of the cortex and thought to result from early abnormalities in cell growth and proliferation. They are characterized by disorganization of cortical lamination and the presence of cells of abnormal morphology (Palmini *et al.* 2004), specifically balloon cells and dysmorphic or cytomegalic neurons which result from very early dysregulation of cell growth (Crino 2005) (Fig. 52.5).

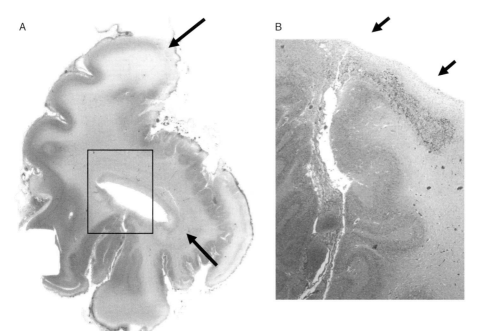

Fig. 52.4. (A) Section of occipital lobe. An area of polymicrogyria is seen between arrows. Here, the molecular layer at the surface in some areas dips into the underlying tissue to follow a festooned band of cortical cells, often irregular and continuous with clusters of immature non-migrated cells in the subcortical white matter. The area in the box, seen in higher power in (B), is a cleft extending through almost the full thickness of the brain wall (schizencephalic cleft or transmantle dysplasia?) (H&E ×1). (B) Higher-power image shows abnormally folded, polymicrogyric, cortex lining the cleft. Just beneath the ventricular wall (top of picture) a band of calcification (small arrows) marks an area of old necrosis of the periventricular white matter (H&E ×2). See color plate section.

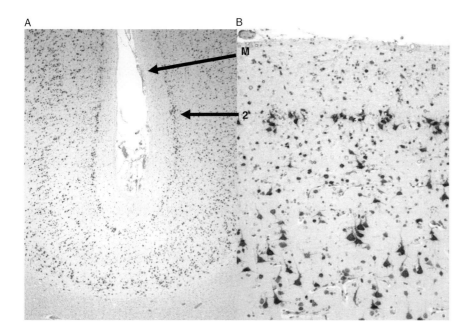

Fig. 52.5. Focal cortical dysplasia, female aged 53 years. (A) Dysplastic cortex in a sulcus (Neu N stain ×2), shown at higher power in (B) (×4). Note the lack of normal lamination. The molecular layer (layer 1) (M) is too cellular and an abnormal band of cells is seen in layer 2. Neurons are abnormally clustered. See color plate section.

Several subtypes are described:

- Type 1 "architectural dysplasia," is characterized by abnormal lamination and distribution of cortical neurons.
- Type II may be described as "cytoarchitectural dysplasia"; in type IIa the dysplastic cortex contains dysmorphic neurons and in type IIb dysmorphic neurons and balloon cells. (Fig. 52.6). Few fetal examples have been described. An unusual fetal cerebellar cortical dysplasia is shown in Figure 52.7.

Similar abnormal cells are seen in tuberous sclerosis; both the giant cells of tuberous sclerosis (TS) and balloon cells express proteins indicating a mixed glial and astrocytic lineage (Fig. 52.8). Both also express phopho-S6, a protein involved in ribosomal protein translation and regulation of cell growth (Crino 2005); in TS mutations of specific genes *TSC1* or *TSC2* are implicated. Tuberous sclerosis is associated with both malformations and benign neoplasms, including subependymal nodules of abnormal cells (Boer *et al.* 2008).

349

Abnormal cells, throughout the cortex and collecting in the subpial zone, frequently close to vessels of the marginal layer, represent a developing tuber. Both cytomegaly and disordered neuronal migration are manifest.

Disorders of neuronal migration

Undermigration syndromes

Malformations resulting from undermigration may be generalized, as in type 1 lissencephaly and subcortical band (double cortex) syndromes, or focal as represented by subcortical and periventricular heterotopias.

Type 1 lissencephaly

Type 1 lissencephaly is characterized by a more or less smooth brain surface with coarse, if any, gyration (Fig. 52.9). The cortex is thick with poor lamination and an indistinct deep border with the underlying white matter. There may be associated

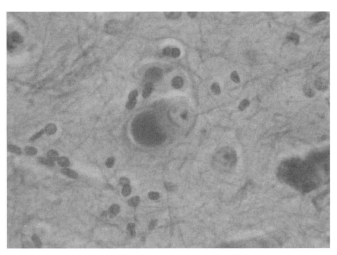

Fig. 52.6. Balloon cell. Focal cortical dysplasia 12 years with epilepsy (LBCV ×20). See color plate section.

periventricular heterotopia. The hindbrain is variably, and usually only mildly, malformed (Berkovich 2009).

Double cortex syndrome

This syndrome is classified with the lissencephalies, and is identified pathologically by incompletely migrated neurons which form a thick band underlying, and to some extent following, the contour of a relatively well-formed overlying cortex (Fig. 52.10).

Undulating band heterotopia

This malformation has not been well described. Jissendi-Tchofo *et al.* (2009) describes two cases of undulating band heterotopia which could not be further determined by MRI. A single pathological study was reported by Hori (1983). These authors showed loss of double cortin in the neurons of the subcortical band, suggesting that this malformation is a form of double cortex syndrome. I have seen three fetal cases have been identified with a bizarre looping double cortex, the upper layer forming a simple cortical plate, the lower forming sinuous bands and loops in the subcortical tissues (Fig. 52.11). Two fetuses were female, one male. None of these cases had significant malformation outside the head.

In these very unusual cases the deep band shows pronounced and orderly folding as early as 20 weeks, well before the period in which cortical folding normally begins. The signals responsible for premature folding are quite unknown.

Periventricular heterotopia

Nodules of unmigrated neurons may be seen as discrete nodules or form an almost continuous band beneath the lining of the lateral ventricles.

Many different syndromes are described with predominant collections in one or another region of the ventricular lining (Wieck *et al.* 2005) (Fig. 52.12). In many cases there

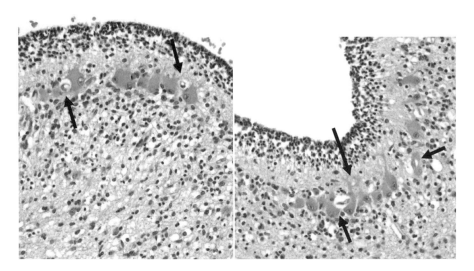

Fig. 52.7. Female fetus 35 weeks gestation. Cerebellar cortex showing dysplastic Purkinje cells. Some are binucleate, some have bizarre thickened dendrites (arrow), and some are apparently engulfing capillaries (short arrows). This was an isolated finding in this brain (H&E ×20). See color plate section.

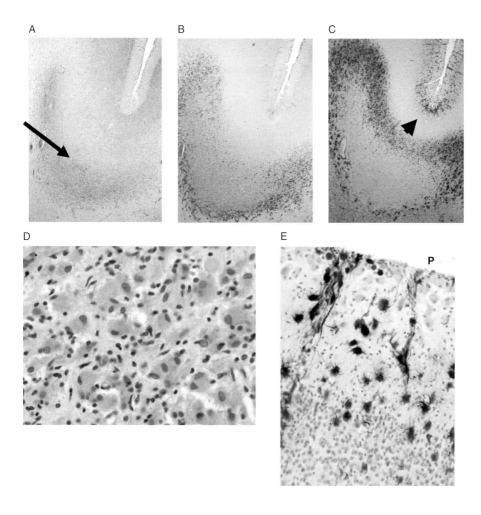

Fig. 52.8. Tuberous sclerosis: fetus 27 weeks gestation. (A) A large group of abnormal cells (arrow) is seen in a sulcus at the junction of the cortex with the white matter (H&E ×1). (B) Nestin stains most of the abnormal cells. (C) Vimentin stain shows only a proportion of the dysplastic cells at the edge of the mass. Note also a layer of abnormal cells in the superficial cortical layer (short arrow). (D) High-power image of the cells in the mass white matter shows two populations, large cells with abundant eosinophilic cytoplasm and small cells with dark oval nuclei (H&E ×20). (E) Vimentin-stained cortex shows only a proportion of the abnormal cells to stain. Note the vimentin-positive cells close to a blood vessel. Many vimentin-negative cells are collecting immediately beneath the pial surface (P) (x10). See color plate section.

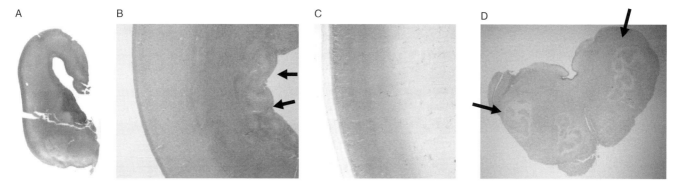

Fig. 52.9. Type 1 lissencephaly, fetus 24 weeks gestation. This fetus had a translocation (p13.3 to pter of chromosome 17 replaced by q27 to qter of chromosome 4). (A) Stained section of hemisphere (H&E). (B) The cerebral cortex is poorly cellular but with a clear marginal zone. The deep cortical border is indistinct and neurons are diffusely distributed in the subcortical white matter. There are prominent periventricular nodular heterotopias (arrows) (H&E ×2). (C) Normal fetal cortex at 25 weeks gestation. Even at this age the deep cortical border is well demarcated from the developing white matter, unlike the appearance in Type 1 lissencephaly (H&E ×2). (D) Olivary malformation with ectopic olivary tissue in the dorsolateral quadrants of the medulla representing incompletely migrated cells in the intramural rostral brainstem pathway (H&E ×1). Similar appearances were present in a cousin at 21 weeks. See color plate section.

is associated malformation of the overlying cortex. This has typically been described as polymicrogyria, but several different patterns of associated cortical malformation may be seen. Three cases are illustrated (Fig. 52.13); in one the

heterotopic nodules were found predominately in the posterior horns of the lateral ventricles, in the other two bilateral periventricular nodular heterotopia (BPNH) was more widely dispersed.

These three examples show that failure of neuronal migration with periventricular heterotopias may be associated with very different patterns of disruption of the overlying cortex.

Overmigration syndromes

Widespread overmigration is the basis of cobblestone malformation (type 2 lissencephaly), usually associated with dystroglycanopathies. However, similar widespread disruption of the cortical surface is also seen in the malformations associated with *TUBB2B*, *GPR56*, and *MARCKS* mutations (Blackshear *et al.* 1997, Li *et al.* 2008, Jaglin and Chelly 2009). Less extensive, focal overmigration in the cerebral cortex (sometimes called "brain warts") may be an incidental finding and is described in a number of syndromes, such as fetal alcohol syndrome.

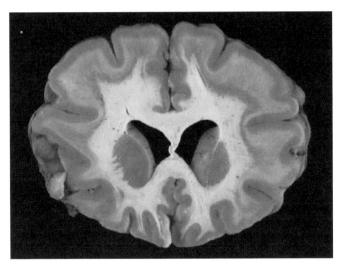

Fig. 52.10. Female 39 years. Fixed brain slice showing extensive double cortex malformation. A well-formed cortex is underlain by a less distinct band of cells which is clearly demarcated from the underlying white matter. See color plate section.

Cobblestone cortex (type 2 lissencephaly)

Most reports of lissencephalies have described MRI appearances of the mature and adult brain. The typical cortical malformation is defined radiologically by a thick (>7 mm) cortex with a smooth outer surface, irregular deep surface with nodules of gray matter in the subcortical white matter, but a range of associated cerebral malformations may be seen, including polymicrogyria, pachygyria, and lissencephaly as well as cerebellar cysts and hindbrain dysplasia (Clement *et al.* 2008).

Examination of the mature brain with cobblestone malformation shows a virtually smooth surface with superficial grooves but no true gyri. The cerebellum has a multinodular, cauliflower-like surface. It is by examination of fetal cases that the development of this malformation can be understood. The developing cortex shows striking abnormality from as early as 18 weeks of gestation (Fig. 52.14). A band of pial remnants and blood vessels is found in the middle of the brain wall and running parallel to the brain surface. Beneath these remnants are masses of immature nerve cells forming a simple cortical plate. Unlike the normal cortical plate there is no molecular (or marginal) layer, but neurons of the presumptive cortical plate abut directly against the pial basement membrane.

With increasing fetal age the gaps become more numerous and the residual neuronal band loses its continuity and is represented only by groups of neurons beneath residual vascular fragments of the pial surface. The outer part of the wall contains clusters of immature neurons intermingled with proliferated blood vessels and connective tissue of the leptomeninges. As development proceeds the neurons mature and settle as rounded masses, separated by bands of collagen and large blood vessels (Fig. 52.15).

Fetuses with severe cobblestone malformation may show other patterns of cortical dysplasia. Fusion of the medial frontal lobes is common with microscopic bridges of connective tissue

A

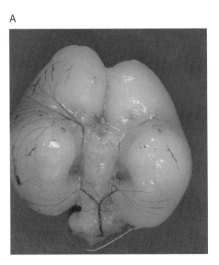

B

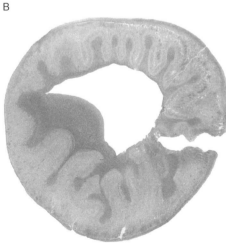

Fig. 52.11. Fetus 20 weeks gestation. (A) Inferior surface of the brain which is small, pale, and smooth. The cerebellar hemispheres are present but small. (B) Stained section of hemisphere shows large ventricle and a thin brain wall occupied by a bilayered band of cells which loops between the deep layer of the cortex to the lining of the lateral ventricle. Cores of germinal matrix extend between these loops. The bilayered band of cells consists of a densely cellular and a less cellular band. (H&E ×1). See color plate section.

containing immature cells between the adjacent medial frontal lobe surfaces. The medial frontal cortex may also show a festooned or undulating neuronal band characteristic of polymicrogyria (Fig. 52.14C).

Cobblestone malformation is commonly associated with disruptions of hindbrain development. The brainstem is typically surrounded by a thick band of connective tissue which may give it a rounded appearance. This band is composed of thickened fibrous leptomeninges with proliferation of collagen, and frequent bridges to the surface of the brainstem (Fig. 52.16). Glio-neuronal ectopia containing morphologically

differentiated neurons are readily identified in the brainstem meninges (Saito et al. 2003).

The developing cerebellar hemispheres show mild thickening of the leptomeninges with small clusters of granule cells within them. The external granule cell layer is thin or incomplete and "ragged." In later development there may be extensive disorganization of the cerebellar cortex.

Hindbrain malformation is inconsistent and milder in type 1 (classic and variant) lissencephalies with LIS-1 mutations than in cobblestone lissencephaly (Barkovich et al. 2009).

Bilateral frontoparietal "polymicrogyria"

This localized cortical malformation, associated with GPR56 mutation, shares similar MRI appearances with dystroglycanopathies (Clement et al. 2008). While human fetal pathology has not yet been described, the mouse model indicates that there are subtle differences between the development of this malformation and cobblestone malformation associated with dystroglycanopathies (Hu et al. 2007). In the mouse GPR56 model the sequence of events is of formation of a normal cortex, followed by the appearance of breaks in the pial basement membrane through which cells migrate (Li et al. 2008). This is unlike the sequence of events in human or mouse cobblestone malformation where the original cortex appears to lack a marginal zone. These subtle differences suggest that it may be too soon to reclassify GPR56 malformation as a cobblestone malformation as suggested by Li et al. (2008). Hypoplasia of the brainstem and cerebellum has been described by MRI in patients with bilateral frontoparietal polymicrogyria, but no histological studies are reported (Koirala et al. 2009).

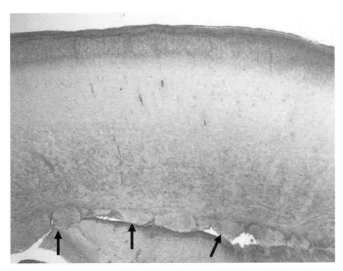

Fig. 52.12. Fetus 17 weeks gestation: an almost uninterrupted band of nodules of unmigrated cells (arrows) lines the ventricular wall. The overlying cortex appears to be forming normally (H&E ×2). See color plate section.

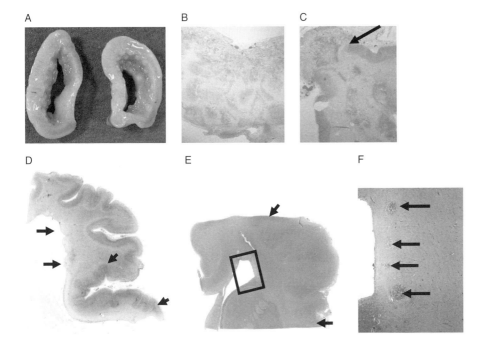

Fig. 52.13. Examples of three forms of periventricular heterotopia with dysplasia of the overlying cortex. (A)-(C) Fetus 20 weeks gestation. Section of fixed brain with multiple heterotopic neuronal nodules in the lining of the occipital horns of the lateral ventricles. This fetus had predominantly posterior BPNH. Clusters and columns of cells in the white matter and focal overmigration of cortical cells (arrow in C) into the leptomeninges associated with proliferation of connective tissue and blood vessels (B and C H&E ×4) (D) Term male infant; H&E-stained section of cerebral hemisphere shows large ventricle with multiple heterotopic neuronal nodules in the ventricular wall (arrows). There is extensive polymicrogyria in the overlying cortex, shown between short arrows. (E, F) Female fetus 36 weeks. H&E-stained section of cerebral hemisphere showing a large area of polymicrogyric cortex (between arrows). The box surrounds small nodules of heterotopic neurons in the periventricular region, shown in higher power (×1) in (F). See color plate section.

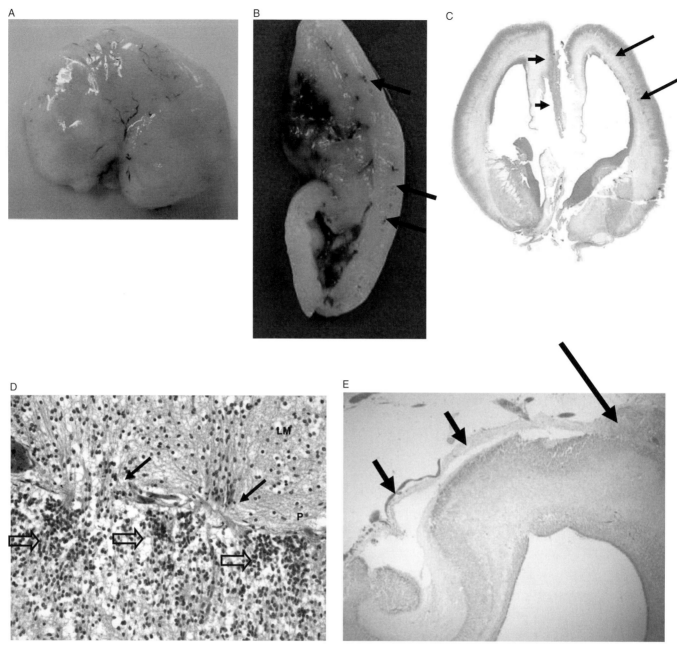

Fig. 52.14. Fetus 18 weeks gestation. (A) Whole brain surface: note the vertically oriented sylvian fissure and finely nodular cortical surface. (B) Coronal slice of the brain shows a line running through the mid part of the brain wall marked by large blood vessels (arrows). (C) Stained section at low power (×1) shows the line at the junction of normally formed cortex and the overmigration into the adherent leptomeninges. Note large ventricles and fusion between adjacent surfaces of medial frontal lobes (arrowheads). (D) A dense band of cells abuts the deep border of the pia (P); at irregular intervals gaps are seen (arrows) through which neurons are streaming into the leptomeninges (LM). Note the absence of a marginal layer which indicates that the original cortical band has not developed normally. Clusters of neurons abut directly on the pial remnants (open arrows) (H&E ×20). (E) Overmigration into the leptomeninges is seen over almost the entire cerebral hemispheres, but a notable exception is the medial temporal lobe and hippocampus. (D) Here the leptomeninges are normal and distinct from the underlying normal cortex (short arrows). As the cortex becomes abnormal so the meninges become adherent and buried in the thick abnormal cortical surface and infiltrated by immature neurons (long arrow; LBCV ×1). See color plate section.

MARCKS deficiency

A similar sequence of events is seen in the MARCKS-deficient mouse (Blackshear *et al.* 1997) where cortex and basement membrane are normal at E9.5 but by E13 basement membrane defects are apparent and cells are seen in the subarachnoid space (Fig. 52.17). At focal gaps in the basement membrane neurons from layer 2 are seen in the molecular layer and entering the leptomeninges. Where the pial–glial barrier is intact orderly lamination and a distinct border between cortical layers 1 and 2 is maintained.

TUBB2B mutation

Mutations in the *TUBB2B* gene are associated with polymicrogyria and overmigration of neurons into the leptomeninges (Jaglin 2009).

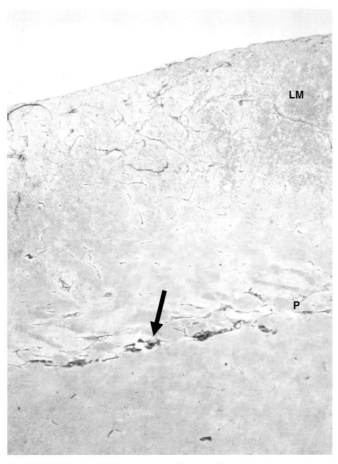

Fig. 52.15. Mature cobblestone cortex. The row of large blood vessels (arrow) denotes the original pial surface of the brain (P). Above it the thickened leptomeninges containing masses of neural tissue (pale golden stain) are seen Reticulin stain ×2. See color plate section.

The pathology of "cobblestone" lissencephalies indicates two sites of developmental disruption; the pial–glial boundary of the cerebral cortex and the surface migration pathways of the hindbrain. Basement membrane proteins are involved at both sites but there are reasons to consider that different factors are operating at each site. First, there are patients who have involvement of only one site. Clement *et al.* (2008) demonstrated patients with cerebral cortical abnormalities in the absence of brainstem pathology and conversely there are rare cases with isolated brainstem involvement (Ichofue 2009).

Polymicrogyria

This term implies the presence of too many gyri, which also appear too small. The malformation can only be definitively diagnosed microscopically, although there are no clear diagnostic criteria. Polymicrogyria (PMG) is generally recognized by the presence of many small gyri with fused surfaces with such microscopic features as disordered lamination, an intracortical fiber plexus, and fusion of gyral surfaces. Two- and four-layered and unlayered forms are described (Friede 1989). There is considerable overlap between these types and both are commonly encountered in the same case.

Polymicrogyria is considered to occur before 28 weeks of gestation (Barth 1987, 1992) and results from a number of insults including vascular insufficiency, infections, and genetic syndromes.

We have identified PMG in fetuses as early as 18 weeks of gestation; Fig. 52.18 shows an example where abnormally folded cortex was seen in the future perisylvian region

A
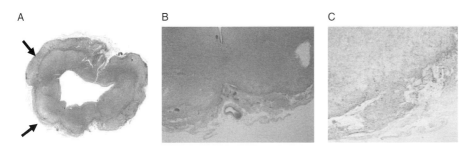

D
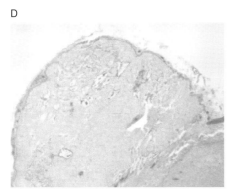

E
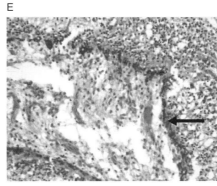

Fig. 52.16. Fetus 18 weeks gestation. (A) There is a band of pale tissue around the entire brainstem and over the cerebellar surface (arrows). The fourth ventricle is large. (B) The leptomeninges are thickened and contain masses of neurons and glial cells (H&E ×2). (C) Higher-power image (×4) stained with GFAP. (D) Fetal cerebellar hemisphere showing disorganized cortex containing many small cysts (H&E ×2). (E) Higher-power image (H&E ×10) shows a poorly formed cortical granule cell layer (arrow) with many cells straggling in the overlying leptomeninges. See color plate section.

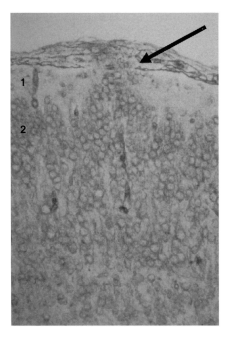

Fig. 52.17. Cortex of MARCKS-deficient mouse. There is a break in the pial basement membrane collagen through which neurons are migrating into the leptomeninges which are locally thickened. The border between layers 1 and 2 is well demarcated where the pia is intact (reticulin stain ×20). See color plate section.

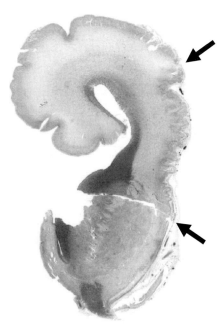

Fig. 52.18. Fetus 18 weeks gestation. Stained section of cerebral hemisphere. Arrows mark an extent of abnormally folded cortex over the lateral aspect of the hemisphere destined to become the perisylvian region. See color plate section.

A

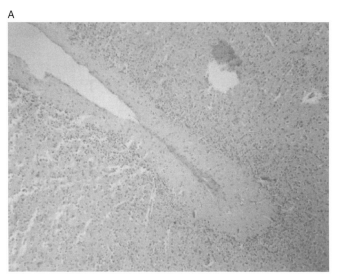

Fig. 52.19. (A) High-power image of the polymicrogyric cortex shows adhesion of adjacent gyri in the depth of a sulcus. In the fusing areas there were increased numbers of cells in the subpial surface of the cortex (H&E ×4). (B) Reticulin stain (×2) shows thickened and reduplicated layers of collagen of the pial basement membrane extending into a fold between gyri (arrows). (C, D) H&E and reticulin stains (×10) of the surface of the polymicrogyric cortex. There is an increase in reticulin fibres, seen running parallel to and embedded into the superficial cortical layers. Neurons, seen as black dots, are seen extending between these layers of basement membrane. See color plate section.

B

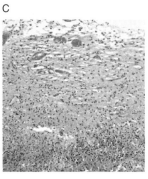

C

D

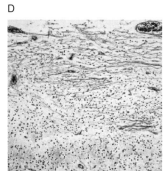

A

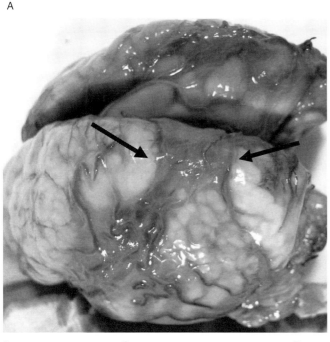

Fig. 52.20. Fetus 35 weeks gestation. (A) Macroscopic examination suggested perisylvian PMG (arrows). (B) Histology showed apparent fusion of adjacent gyri with excess small cells in the marginal and pial layers of the cortical surface (short arrows) (H&E ×4). (C) and (D) are higher-power images (×20) showing cells with intranuclear inclusions characteristic of cytomegalovirus (CMV). (D) Immunocytochemical stain for CMV. See color plate section.

B

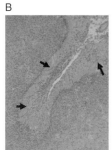

C

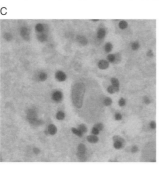

D

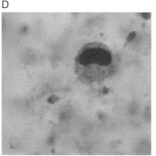

bilaterally. This case illustrates abnormal folding of the cortical neuronal band many weeks before cortical folding would normally be expected to occur and brings into question how and when the cues for cortical folding operate.

Studies in fetuses show that polymicrogyria develops by a number of pathways and shows many different patterns. In Fig. 52.18 there is simple folding of the cortical neuronal band. Figure 52.19 illustrates two other patterns, both seen in association with heterotopic periventricular nodules. In the case illustrated in Fig. 52.19A adjacent gyri appear to be zipping up in regions where there is an increased number of residual cells of the subpial layer, but normal surface layers. Figure 52.19B shows abnormal adhesion of adjacent gyri in association with thickening of the surface basement membrane collagen, proliferation of surface blood vessels, and overmigration of cortical neurons into the leptomeninges. This appearance has been described in *TUBB2B* mutation (Jaglin and Chelly 2009). Yet another subtle variation is seen in polymicrogyria associated with cytomegalovirus (CMV) infection (Fig. 52.20).

Destructive lesions

Most intrauterine ischemic lesions occur in the territory of a major cerebral artery, most commonly the middle cerebral arteries (Dekaban 1965; Richman *et al.* 1974; Mercuri *et al.* 2002). The major arterial supply to the brain is developed by three months of intrauterine life. Watershed infarcts are considered to be typical of the term brain (Huang and Castillo 2008), but rare examples of watershed damage in earlier development are described (Guerrini *et al.* 1997).

Figure. 52.21 illustrates a focal cortical lesion in the occipital watershed zone between the middle and posterior arterial territories. This baby suffered brain damage following amniocentesis injury. In addition to scarring of the midbrain, thought to be the direct result of trauma from the amniocentesis needle, there was more widespread pathology due to generalized ischemia associated with the amniocentesis injury (Squier *et al.* 2000, case 4) (Fig. 52.22). This illustrates that watershed damage may indeed occur as early as 16 weeks of gestation.

A

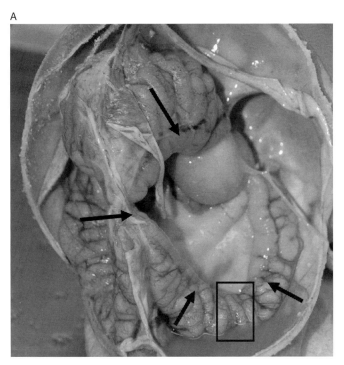

Fig. 52.21. Fresh brain at autopsy showing large old infarcts in middle cerebral artery territories bilaterally. That on the right side is indicated by arrows. The area in the box is shown at higher power in (B) (B) Luxol fast blue stained section of the edge of the infarcted area shown in (A). The edge of the lesion (arrows) has abnormally folded cortex with an irregular deep border indicating an origin before 28 weeks of gestation (×2). (C) Section of the brainstem showing secondary atrophy of the pyramidal tracts, which cannot be identified in the medulla (×1). See color plate section.

B   C

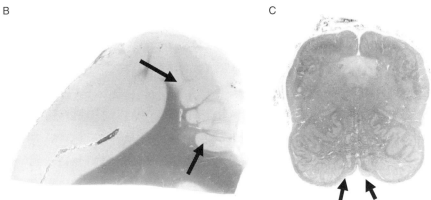

Schizencephaly

Schizencephaly is defined as a cleft in the brain wall extending through the full thickness from the ventricle to the leptomeningeal surface and typically lined by dysplastic cortex.

It was first proposed as a malformation resulting from primary failure of development of a small focus of the germinal matrix (Yakovlev and Wadsworth 1946). Familial cases are rarely described, more frequently this malformation is sporadic and results from focal infarction of the brain (Fig. 52.23). Intrauterine insults have been described, e.g., road traffic accidents, amniocentesis injury and abdominal trauma (Mancini *et al.* 2001).

Bilateral cases are more common than unilateral (Curry *et al.* 2005) and most involve middle (Fig. 52.24) or, less commonly, anterior cerebral artery territory. Cases have been identified on ultrasound scans in utero from as early as 18 weeks of gestation (Ceccherini *et al.* 1999), but not earlier, and pathological descriptions do not exist before this age.

Conclusion

Pathological studies have shown that disruptions of several different developmental pathways may lead to the same malformation and, conversely, that the same disruptions are common to diverse malformations. This is perhaps not surprising when we consider the heterogeneity of causes for some common malformations, for example polymicrogyria, schizencephaly, and porencephaly. It does, however, lead to complications in classification of cortical malformation and warns of the difficulties of classification systems based on MRI diagnosis which cannot accurately reflect the underlying malformative process.

A

B

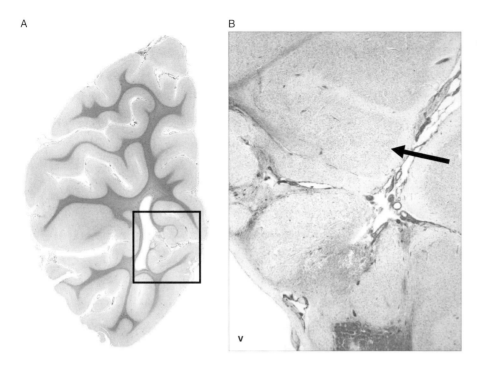

Fig. 52.22. (A) Stained section of occipital lobe showing focal damage in posterior watershed zone. The area in the box is shown at higher power in (B) (B) Almost complete cleft in the brain wall with scarring of the tissues beneath the ventricular lining (V). The cleft is lined by abnormally folded polymicrogyric cortex (arrow) (×2). See color plate section.

A

B

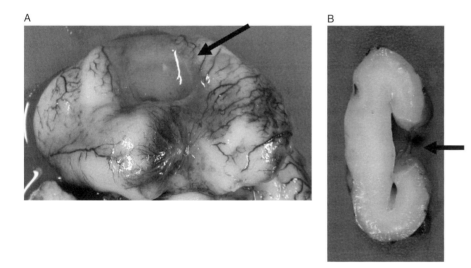

Fig. 52.23. Middle cerebral artery infarction in male fetus aged 23 weeks. (A) A central cystic area of infarction is seen in this lateral view of the cerebral hemisphere. (B) Coronal slice through the fixed brain shows the infarcted area where the brain wall is replaced by a thin membrane derived from the meninges. (C) The occipital pole, with small area of infarction and more widespread area of calicification and polymicrogyria (between arrows), seen in higher power in (D) (×1). The area in the box is seen in higher power in (E). Here the edge of the infarct shows a split extending almost to the germinal matrix of the ventricular lining and lined by masses of immature neurons which appear dark blue (short arrows (×2). See color plate section.

C

D

E

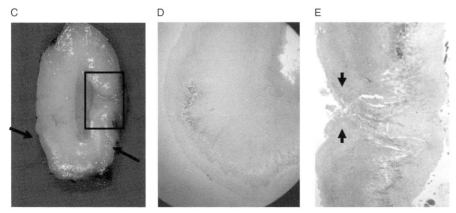

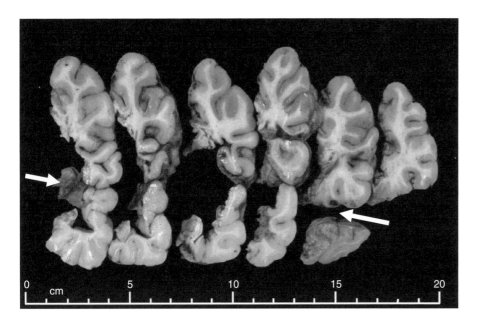

Fig. 52.24. Fixed slices of hemispherectomy specimen from child with old middle cerebral artery infarction. White arrows indicate the cystic cavity which is continuous with the lateral ventricle. The slice on the left shows the remnant of the membrane forming the wall of the cyst. The adjacent cortex has collapsed into the edge of the cavity giving the impression of gray matter lining a split in the brain wall. See color plate section.

References

Barkovich AJ, Millen KJ, Dobyns WB (2009) A developmental and genetic classification for midbrain–hindbrain malformations. *Brain* **132**:3199–230.

Barth PG (1987) Disorders of neuronal migration. *Can J Neurol Sci* **14**:1–16.

Barth PG (1992) Migrational disorders of the brain. *Curr Opin Neurol Neurosurg* **5**:339–43.

Blackshear PJ, Silver J, Nairn AC, *et al.* (1997) Widespread neuronal ectopia associated with secondary defects in cerebrocortical chondroitin sulfate proteoglycans and basal lamina in MARCKS-deficient mice. *Exp Neurol* **145**:46–61.

Boer K, Troost D, Jansen F, *et al.* (2008) Clinicopathological and immunohistochemical findings in an autopsy case of tuberous sclerosis complex. *Neuropathology* **28**:577–90.

Ceccherini AF, Twining P, Variend S (1999) Schizencephaly: antenatal detection using ultrasound. *Clin Radiol* **54**:620–2.

Clement E, Mercuri E, Godfrey C, *et al.* (2008) Brain involvement in muscular dystrophies with defective dystroglycan glycosylation. *Ann Neurol* **64**:573–82.

Crino PB (2005) Molecular pathogenesis of focal cortical dysplasia and hemimegalencephaly. *J Child Neurol* **20**:330–6.

Curry CJ, Lammer EJ, Nelson V, Shaw GM (2005) Schizencephaly: heterogeneous etiologies in a population of 4 million California births. *Am J Med Genet* **137A**:181–9.

Dekaban A (1965) Large defects in cerebral hemispheres associated with cortical dysgenesis. *J Neuropathol Exp Neurol* **24**:521–30.

Friede RL (1989) *Developmental Neuropathology*, 2nd edn. Berlin: Springer-Verlag.

Guerrini R, Dubeau F, Dulac O, *et al.* (1997) Bilateral parasagittal parietooccipital polymicrogyria and epilepsy. *Ann Neurol* **41**:65–73.

Herman L, Rico S (1999) Schizencephaly: presentation in a 6-week-old boy with fetal death of co-twin. *Int Pediatr* **14**:32–4.

Hori A (1983) A brain with two hypophyses in median cleft face syndrome. *Acta Neuropathol* **59**:150–4.

Hu H, Yang Y, Eade A, Xiong Y, Qi Y (2007) Breaches of the pial basement membrane and disappearance of the glia limitans during development underlie the cortical lamination defect in the mouse model of muscle–eye–brain disease. *J Comp Neurol* **501**:168–83.

Huang BY, Castillo M (2008) Hypoxic–ischemic brain injury: imaging findings from birth to adulthood. *Radiographics* **28**:417–39.

Jaglin XH, Chelly J (2009) Tubulin-related cortical dysgeneses: microtubule dysfunction underlying neuronal migration defects. *Trends Genet* **25**:555–66.

Jissendi-Tchofo P, Kara S, Barkovich AJ (2009) Midbrain–hindbrain involvement in lissencephalies. *Neurology* **72**:410–18.

Koirala S, Jin Z, Piao X, Corfas G (2009) GPR56-regulated granule cell adhesion is essential for rostral cerebellar development. *J Neurosci* **29**:7439–49.

Li S, Jin Z, Koirala S, *et al.* (2008) GPR56 regulates pial basement membrane integrity and cortical lamination. *J Neurosci* **28**:5817–26.

Mancini J, Lethel V, Hugonenq C, Chabrol B (2001) Brain injuries in early foetal life: consequences for brain development. *Dev Med Child Neurol* **43**:52–5.

Mercuri E, Rutherford M, Barnett A, *et al.* (2002) MRI lesions and infants with neonatal encephalopathy: is the Apgar score predictive? *Neuropediatrics* **33**:150–6.

Palmini A, Najm I, Avanzini G, *et al.* (2004) Terminology and classification of the cortical dysplasias. *Neurology* **62**(6 Suppl 3):S2–8.

Richman DP, Stewart RM, Caviness VS Jr. (1974) Cerebral microgyria in a 27-week fetus: an architectonic and topographic analysis. *J Neuropathol Exp Neurol* **33**:374–84.

Saito Y, Kobayashi M, Itoh M, *et al.* (2003) Aberrant neuronal migration in the brainstem of Fukuyama-type congenital muscular dystrophy. *J Neuropathol Exp Neurol* **62**:497–508.

Squier M, Chamberlain P, Zaiwalla Z, *et al.* (2000) Five cases of brain injury following amniocentesis in mid-term pregnancy. *Dev Med Child Neurol* **42**:554–60.

Wieck G, Leventer RJ, Squier WM, *et al.* (2005) Periventricular nodular heterotopia with overlying polymicrogyria. *Brain* **128**:2811–21.

Yakovlev PI, Wadsworth RC (1946) Schizencephalies: a study of the congenital clefts in the cerebral mantle. I. Clefts with fused lips. *J Neuropathol Exp Neurol* **5**:116–30.

Chapter

53

Hippocampal sclerosis

Fernando Cendes and Márcia Elisabete Morita

The causal factors

Definitions

The terms "Ammon's horn sclerosis," "hippocampal sclerosis," and "mesial temporal sclerosis" are often used as synonymous. The term "sclerosis" is originally a macroscopic and descriptive one: it indicates shrinkage and induration of the structure. Hippocampal sclerosis (HS) is a histological term that indicates selective neuronal loss with secondary astroglial proliferation that affects various sectors of the hippocampus to a different degree: the most vulnerable to damage are the sectors cornu ammonis CA1, CA3, and endfolium (sector CA4), while the granule cells of the dentate gyrus, sector CA2, and subiculum are the most resistant (Fig. 53.1). The amygdala, uncus, and parahippocampal gyrus are often involved as well; thus, according to some authors, the term mesial temporal sclerosis would be more appropriate (Gloor 1997; Thom 2009). This cell loss, if sufficiently pronounced, will appear in magnetic resonance imaging (MRI) scans as a reduced volume or shrinkage of the hippocampus, often associated with changes in signal intensity. Therefore the MRI scan provides a marker for a known histopathological process (Van Paesschen *et al.* 1997) (Fig. 53.2).

Hippocampal sclerosis has been recognized as the most commonly encountered pathological substrate of mesial temporal lobe epilepsy (MTLE) (Wieser 2004). It is present in 60–70% of patients with MTLE who undergo surgery for treatment of medically refractory seizures (Falconer 1974). Other structural lesions can also cause temporal lobe epilepsy (TLE), such as hamartomas, glial tumors, vascular and congenital malformations, and gliotic lesions due to trauma or infections.

Epidemiology

Epilepsy affects approximately 1.0–2.0% of the population (Hauser *et al.* 1996). Epilepsies can be classified as generalized or localization-related (partial or focal) (ILAE 1989). Temporal lobe epilepsy is the most frequent form of partial epilepsy in adults (Hauser *et al.* 1996); however, the incidence of HS or MTLE in the general population is unknown, since most studies are based on surgical series. Nevertheless, HS contributes to a major part of partial seizures in adults which are often resistant to antiepileptic drugs. In one hospital-based study, half of patients seen in the epilepsy outpatient clinic had TLE, and half of these had MRI evidence of HS (Semah *et al.* 1998). In a recent series of 84 patients with well-controlled partial seizures, MRI volumetry showed hippocampal atrophy indicating mild HS in 39 (46%) patients (Cardoso *et al.* 2006). In surgical series, 60–70% of patients have HS (Babb and Brown 1987).

Pathogenesis of hippocampal sclerosis

Studies of the relationship between seizures and HS spans more than 150 years (Meencke 2009). The pathological condition was initially described by early neuropathologists based on postmortem material (Bouchet and Cazauvieilh 1825). Only later was the potential importance of this lesion in epilepsy recognized (Gloor 1997; Thom 2009). Autopsy and neuroimaging studies indicate that patients with MTLE with HS often have bilateral asymmetric hippocampal damage, with one side showing HS and the other side with varying degrees of hippocampal damage, ranging from mild non-specific neuronal loss to well-characterized milder HS (Gloor 1997; Meencke 2009).

Since first histological descriptions, the question of whether HS is a cause or consequence of seizures has been raised (Gloor 1997; Cendes 2005). This is a controversial issue, and as in many other biological issues, the answer is most likely to lie in between.

Different lesions involving hippocampus have been extensively studied in different types of animal models, each having features of cell loss and plasticity similar to those observed in surgical specimens of patients with MTLE with HS (Schwartzkroin 1993; Gloor 1997). By comparing these models, different conclusions may emerge regarding the role of discrete or intense cell loss, mossy fiber sprouting, and other histochemical features (Franck and Schwartzkroin 1985; Gloor 1997). In spite of these differences, it is clear that the

The Causes of Epilepsy, eds. S. D. Shorvon, F. Andermann, and R. Guerrini. Published by Cambridge University Press. © Cambridge University Press 2011.

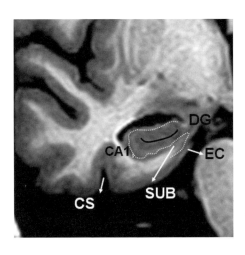
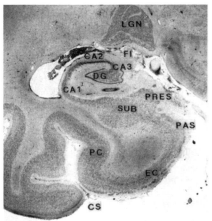

Fig. 53.1. The medial temporal region (MRI illustration and histological detail) at the level of the posterior tip of uncus illustrating the hippocampal subfields and related structures. CA1, CA2, and CA3 indicate sectors cornu Ammonis 1, 2, and 3; CS, collateral sulcus; DG, dentate gyrus; EC, entorhinal cortex; FI, fimbria; LGN, lateral geniculate nucleus; PRES, presubiculum; SUB, subiculum.

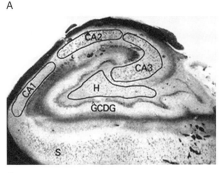
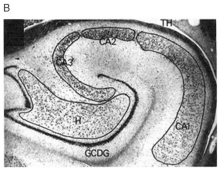
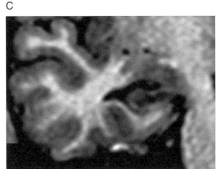
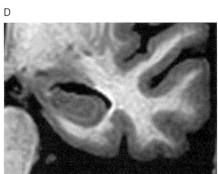

Fig. 53.2. Typical histology picture and MRI (T1-weighted image) from hippocampal sclerosis (A and C) and from a normal hippocampus (B and D). Note the relative sparing of subfield CA2 as opposed to the intense cell loss in CA1 and CA3 in (A) as compared to (B). (C) An atrophic hippocampus with loss of internal structure and hypointense T1 signal. (Panels A and B were modified from Van Paesschen et al. [1997].)

clinical manifestation of MTLE depends on a critical combination of these morphological changes. However, there is also evidence that even if complete HS is produced experimentally, seizures may not develop (Schwartzkroin 1993). These findings, in addition to several others (Cendes 2005), may indicate that HS and seizures are signs and symptoms of a complex underlying pathological process, and that they may evolve concomitantly. While HS may be produced by seizures (in particular during status epilepticus), the development of MTLE as a syndrome does not depend solely on cell loss or plasticity in the hippocampus. This would be a gross oversimplification that cannot account for common associated features, as for example, the high incidence of depression in MTLE (Kanner 2006).

Hippocampal sclerosis has all the hallmarks of an inert lesion acquired in the remote past and seems to be both a cause and a consequence of seizures: a cause as supported by evidence, discussed below, that HS may come before the development of seizures, and a consequence as supported by clinical and experimental evidence indicating progressive neuronal damage and synaptic reorganization secondary to seizures (Mathern et al. 2002; Cendes 2005).

The mechanisms underlying the development of HS remain undetermined. The condition most likely has different causes in different individuals, and may result from complex interactions among genetic and environmental factors.

Initial precipitating injury

In the early 1950s Penfield defended the hypothesis that HS was caused by transtentorial herniation of the mesial temporal lobe during birth. This herniation would cause an ischemic lesion termed incisural sclerosis that with time would cause epilepsy (Earle *et al.* 1953). Meyer and Falconer (1954) stated that in addition to a history of difficult birth, there were other factors related to HS, including head trauma and, in particular, prolonged febrile seizures (FS) in early childhood; this became known as Meyer's hypothesis. However, population-based studies have not shown a significant relationship between FS early in life and subsequent MTLE (Cendes 2005). The interpretation of these observations remains controversial. One possibility is that the early FS damages the hippocampus and is therefore a cause of HS. Another possibility is that the child has a prolonged FS because the hippocampus has previously been damaged due to a prenatal or perinatal insult or to a genetic predisposition. The first interpretation would favor the hypothesis that more frequent seizures would cause more severe HS, and the second would be in favor of more severe HS causing more severe seizures. In either hypothesis, a cross-sectional, retrospective analysis would result in a positive correlation between seizure frequency and degree of HS, thus not solving the enigma of cause or consequence (Cendes 2005).

Recent studies have shown that prolonged and focal FS can produce acute hippocampal injury that evolves to hippocampal atrophy and that complex FS can actually originate in the temporal lobes in some children. Although there is a high incidence of complex FS among patients with mesial temporal sclerosis in retrospective studies, it is still not clear whether complex FS are an epiphenomenon or a causative factor (Mathern *et al.* 2002).

Chemoanatomical studies have shown that the vulnerable sectors of the hippocampus are rich in kainate (endfolium and sector CA3) and N-methyl-D-aspartate (NMDA) receptors (sector CA1) (Schwartzkroin 1993; Gloor 1997). Activation of NMDA receptors and of a subclass of kainate receptors leads to considerable Ca^{2+} influx into postsynaptic neurons and if, as is the case in prolonged seizures, these neurons are not protected by Ca^{2+}-binding proteins, they may become irreversibly damaged and die. In the human hippocampus, the principal cells of the vulnerable sector, i.e., the endfolium, sectors CA3 and CA1, contain virtually no Ca^{2+}-binding proteins (calbindin or parvalbumin), while the relatively resistant structures such as the dentate granule cells and sector CA2 are rich in calbindin (Gloor 1997). The destruction of neurons in the vulnerable sectors of the hippocampus that characterizes HS, may thus be the consequence of two of their chemoanatomical features: (1) the high content of the type of glutamate receptors that promotes Ca^{2+} entry into the neuron during a seizure, and (2) their lack of protection against Ca^{2+} overload due to their virtual lack of Ca^{2+}-binding proteins. A similar profile of hippocampal vulnerability to seizures presumably caused by the same pathogenetic mechanism is also seen in some experimental models of epilepsy (Schwartzkroin 1993; Gloor 1997).

This pathogenetic explanation fails, however, to account for the cause of the frequent unilaterality of HS. It is possible that both prolonged FS (which have commonly a unilateral predominance) and the ensuing damage have been primed by some pre-existing hippocampal damage.

Genetic predisposition appears to be an important causal factor in patients with HS and antecedent prolonged FS (Berkovic and Scheffer 1998; Kobayashi *et al.* 2001, 2002). Recent clinical and molecular genetic studies show that there is some specificity in the types of epilepsy that follow FS, rather than FS being a non-specific marker of a lowered seizure threshold. The relationship between FS and later development of epilepsy is frequently genetic and there are a number of syndrome-specific genes for FS (Berkovic and Scheffer 1998).

Recent evidence from experimental and clinical studies also provides data suggesting the importance of innate immunity in the etiology and pathogenesis of MTLE. The presence of inflammatory processes, indicated, for example, by the presence of highly upregulated chemokines genes in chronic MTLE (van Gassen *et al.* 2008) may directly and indirectly affect neuronal excitability. Early upregulation of chemokines, for instance after a viral infection, trauma, FS, tumors, or other infections, may be a common pathway linking initial precipitating injuries (IPIs) in the etiology of MTLE. There has been evidence of a possible role of complement activation and other inflammatory pathway involvement in both experimental and human MTLE (Aronica *et al.* 2007; van Gassen *et al.* 2008). Indeed recent studies indicate that the role of viral infection in the etiology of MTLE might be underestimated (Donati *et al.* 2003).

Falconer and Taylor (1968) developed the concept that HS is both a cause and also a consequence of epileptic seizures, which has been supported by more recent investigations (Cendes 2005; Meencke 2009). In fact, by expanding the concept of IPI to include any significant medical event likely to injure the brain before the onset of seizures, such as prolonged FS, trauma, hypoxia, and intracranial infection, studies of surgical series of MTLE have found a strong association between HS and IPI (Mathern *et al.* 2002). These studies support the concept that HS is likely an acquired pathology, and most of the neuronal loss occurs with the IPI; however, ongoing frequent seizures do cause additional progressive hippocampal damage (Mathern *et al.* 2002; Cendes 2005; Bonilha *et al.* 2006).

Familial mesial temporal lobe epilepsy

Studies in familial MTLE are also important for better understanding of the pathogenesis of HS.

Signs of HS were present in MRI scans of subjects with familial MTLE (Kobayashi *et al.* 2001; Andrade-Valenca *et al.* 2008) and in some asymptomatic family members (Kobayashi *et al.* 2001, 2002). These findings alone suggest that hippocampal abnormalities associated with HS are not the sole consequence of repeated seizures and that genetically determined mechanisms might play an important role in the development of hippocampal damage, which may be hereditary, at least in these familial cases (Kobayashi *et al.* 2001).

Most affected individuals with familial MTLE have a benign clinical course, and in some families all affected members have good seizure control or remit after a short period of seizures. However, as in patients with non-familial MTLE, some affected family members may have poor seizure control and require surgical treatment. Although MRI signs of HS, including hippocampal atrophy and hyperintense T2-weighted signal, are more frequent and more pronounced in patients with refractory seizures, these changes are also observed in patients with a good clinical outcome, and even in asymptomatic family members. These are strong indicators that genetic factors play a role in the genesis of hippocampal pathology in patients with familial MTLE. While the pattern of inheritance is autosomal dominant with incomplete penetrance, the genetic background in familial MTLE does not imply a more widespread structural abnormality on MRI.

The presence of HS in both affected and asymptomatic family members in familial MTLE suggests that the hippocampus abnormalities themselves could be inherited, and not necessarily lead to epilepsy (Kobayashi et al. 2002). The phenotype would then be dependent on interaction with other modifying factors. These data together with the existence of a number of syndrome-specific genes for FS emphasize the importance of genetic factors as one of the causes of HS.

Available qualitative pathology from surgical specimens obtained from operated familial MTLE patients showed the typical pattern of HS: selective neuronal loss in CA1, CA3, and CA4 with relative preservation of CA2, and variable involvement of the amygdala and parahippocampal region (Kobayashi et al. 2003). The observation of HS in operated Familial MTLE patients who became seizure-free suggests that HS represents the epileptogenic substrate, at least in some of these families, analogous to what is observed in non-familial or "sporadic" cases. One study looked further into hippocampal cell densities and intensity of supragranular mossy fiber staining in postoperative tissues from patients with familial and sporadic MTLE (Andrade-Valenca et al. 2008). Patients with familial MTLE present most histological findings comparable to patients with sporadic MTLE; however, mossy fiber sprouting was less pronounced in patients with familial MTLE, suggesting that they respond differently to plastic changes plausibly induced by cell loss, neuronal deafferentation, or epileptic seizures when compared to sporadic MTLE (Andrade-Valenca et al. 2008).

Most likely, familial MTLE will be found to have a major gene leading to hippocampal abnormalities, and the phenotype could be influenced by additional genetic and environmental modifying factors, including known and unknown IPIs or unidentified environmental injuries.

Magnetic resonance imaging studies

It has been widely accepted, based on large series of surgical patients, that there is a strong correlation between HS and the severity of the epilepsy. Hippocampal sclerosis identified by MRI has been associated with poor medical control of seizures by Semah et al. (1998). However, the findings of MRI abnormalities in patients with good outcome or seizure remission, indicates that MTS is found not only in patients with medically refractory TLE (Kobayashi et al. 2001). Evidence for this has already been hinted at in the literature, including descriptions

of sporadic patients with HS (Kim et al. 1999). Furthermore, there is upcoming MRI evidence of MTS acquired in adulthood (Briellmann et al. 2001) not necessarily associated with poor seizure control (Kobayashi et al. 2002; Cardoso et al. 2006).

Neuropathological studies

Recent molecular neuropathological studies focusing on developmental aspects of hippocampal organization revealed two intriguing findings in HS specimens of MTLE patients who underwent surgery: (1) the persistence of Cajal-Retzius cells in HS patients points towards an early insult and an altered Reelin signaling pathway and (2) increased neurogenesis in and abnormal architectural organization of the dentate granule cell layer can be observed in young patients with early hippocampal seizure onset (Blumcke et al. 2002, 2009). These findings suggest a developmental malformation of the hippocampus (inherited or acquired) that in association with other subsequent injury during life (e.g., trauma, infection, FS) could develop ongoing seizures, then resulting in the full-blown neuropathological features of HS (Blumcke et al. 2002).

There seems to be in association with neuronal loss, presence of aberrant axons, and synaptic reorganization in human HS. Studies have described synaptic reorganization of the mossy fibers system (the axons of the dentate granule neurons). Mossy fiber sprouting is characterized by the formation of novel, aberrant synaptic contacts of mossy fibers onto the proximal dendrites of the hippocampal dentate granule neurons. This aberrant circuitry is probably related to epileptogenesis by changes in excitatory and inhibitory processes (Blumcke et al. 2002; Sutula 2004).

Laboratory studies

Some laboratory studies have provided significant data for understanding the epileptogenesis in HS. Some studies suggest that the affected hippocampus has some important functional differences when compared to the "normal" hippocampus, for example structural changes such as sprouting, neurotransmitter and receptor changes, modification in ion channels, water channels, changes in mitochondrial and glial function, and also signs of inflammatory processes (Aronica et al. 2007; van Gassen et al. 2008; Blumcke et al. 2009; Meencke 2009; Thom 2009).

Pathophysiology: progression

Studies have shown progression of neuronal damage and dysfunction in patients with MTLE and HS (Cendes 2005). However, it is still unclear why, when, and how neuronal damage and dysfunction occur in these patients. Seizure frequency is considered the most important factor for progression of damage and dysfunction in MTLE with HS. Nevertheless, it is possible, for example, that not all types of seizures do cause harm, or yet that some individuals are more resistant to seizure-induced damage than others (Schwartzkroin 1993; Gloor 1997; Brandt et al. 2004; Cendes 2005). Genetic background, age, and type of initial brain insult, and other environmental factors, most likely interact in a number of ways, making it difficult to determine what are the exact mechanisms of ongoing brain damage in MTLE (Cendes 2005).

Furthermore, mechanisms that are responsible for, or influence, the development of an epileptic condition differ from those that actually precipitate acute epileptic seizures. Another complication is the fact that seizure-related damage may be expressed in a number of ways, and does not necessarily represent neuronal loss or atrophy. For example, many patients with MTLE who do not respond well to treatment have progressive memory loss and signs of diffuse cognitive impairment, as well as progressive increase of bilateral epileptiform discharges (Morrell 1989; Gloor 1997). These observations suggest that focal epileptic discharges may lead to neuronal dysfunction remote from the seizure focus.

Epilepsy and hippocampal sclerosis
Risk factors

As discussed above, familial history seems to be one of the risk factors for HS, as well as prolonged FS and other brain injuries in early childhood, although these factors have been described mostly in surgical series (Cendes 2005) and have not been clearly confirmed in population-based studies (Camfield et al. 1994).

Type of epilepsy
Clinical presentation

The natural history of MTLE with HS is classically described as a latent period between IPI and/or onset of seizures, although the IPI is often not identifiable. Seizures may be initially well controlled for some time before they become medically refractory. However, not all patients with MTLE and HS become refractory and it is not uncommon to encounter patients without a typical history, particularly in the familial forms (Wieser 2004).

The first habitual seizures usually occur in late childhood or early adolescence. The initial ictal event may be a generalized convulsion or a complex partial seizure. Complex partial seizures are usually preceded by an aura, typically involving epigastric rising sensation associated with an emotional disturbance such as fear. Other psychic (e.g., déjà vu) and autonomic symptoms (e.g., flushing, pallor, tachycardia) are also seen, and some patients can have olfactory or gustatory sensations. Auras typically occur in isolation (simple partial seizures), as well as in association with complex partial seizures (Cendes et al. 2002a).

The complex partial seizure commonly begins with a motionless stare and oroalimentary automatisms (e.g., lip smacking, chewing) with a progressive clouding of consciousness. Gestural automatisms, as well as reactive automatisms that can be ictal or postictal, are also common. When posturing of one extremity occurs, it is contralateral to the side of ictal onset. Hand automatisms are frequent and tend to be ipsilateral to the HS, mainly when associated with a contralateral dystonic posturing. Verbal automatisms may be present in seizures originating in the non-dominant hemisphere. There is transient postictal disorientation and, with onset in the language-dominant hemisphere, there may also be some degree of postictal aphasia. Postictal nose-wiping may occur, usually with the hand ipsilateral to the seizure onset. Patients are frequently amnesic of the ictal phase, even though they may make semi-appropriate responses during the seizure. The aura, however, is usually remembered.

Seizures typically last 1 to 2 min and are relatively stereotyped in a given patient. Patients may recall occasional auras years before they experienced the first habitual complex partial seizure. Precipitating factors include stress, sleep deprivation, and, in women, hormonal changes associated with the menstrual cycle. Secondary generalization as well as status epilepticus are infrequent, but may occur (Cendes et al. 2002a).

There are no definitive characteristics that distinguish complex partial seizures in MTLE with HS from complex partial seizures generated in the anterior portion of the temporal lobe. The classic presentation as described above may be similar to ictal symptoms described by patients with mesio temporal lesions other than HS or without any detectable MRI abnormalities. For this reason, the accurate diagnosis of MTLE is based on a constellation of signs and symptoms and diagnostic tests (Wieser 2004).

Seizures that begin with primary visual, auditory, or focal somatosensory auras, focal, or violent motor behaviors and extratemporal electroencephalogram (EEG) spikes do not fill clinical criteria for MTLE with HS (Cendes et al. 2002a; Wieser 2004).

Diagnostic principles

The diagnosis of MTLE requires a constellation of signs and symptoms, but the most important is the presence of characteristic seizure semiology (Wieser 2004). The accurate recognition of MTLE with HS is usually based on MRI findings, EEG and video-EEG, neuropsychological tests, and sometimes positron emission tomography (PET) and single photon emission computed tomography (SPECT).

Neurologic examination is usually normal except for facial asymmetry and memory deficits, which are material-specific for the side of ictal onset (Jones-Gotman and Smith 2006).

Diagnostic tests
Genetic tests

There is no genetic test available yet for diagnosis of HS.

Histological tests

Histopathological hallmarks include segmental loss of pyramidal neurons, granule cell dispersion, reactive gliosis, and axonal sprouting of surviving neurons. The neuronal loss and gliosis involve hippocampal sectors CA1, CA3, hilus, and dentate gyrus, in addition to granule cell dispersion, with relative sparing of CA2 and subiculum (Thom 2009). The neuronal damage often involves also the amygdala, uncus, and parahippocampal gyrus.

Neurophysiological test

Interictal electroencephalography

Interictal EEG findings in patients with MTLE typically include unilateral or bilaterally independent mesial temporal spikes, best seen with basal (sphenoidal, inferior temporal) derivations.

Temporal intermittent rhythmic delta activity appears to have a localizing value of the epileptogenic zone in MTLE, unlike intermittent rhythmic delta activity in other brain regions (Cendes *et al.* 2002a).

Ictal electroencephalography

Ictal EEG recordings usually reveal a characteristic ictal pattern consisting of regular well-lateralized rhythmic 5–9-Hz activity in one anterior-mid and infero-mesial temporal region, before the first clinical manifestations, or within 30 s (delayed focal onset), with or without contralateral propagation.

Ictal discharges may be confined to the medial temporal structures for a few seconds or even longer, without evident EEG changes on scalp recordings. This may be followed by a fast propagation of ictal discharges to the ipsilateral or contralateral temporal neocortex, or it may propagate to both hemispheres in a diffuse fashion. In these circumstances, the scalp EEG record may miss the initial (truly localizing) seizure discharges. Thus, ictal scalp EEG recordings may have limited localizing value when the first clinical manifestations clearly precede the first EEG changes. This false localization phenomenon may be associated with severe hippocampal damage (Mintzer *et al.* 2004).

Intracranial recordings

Although diagnosis of MTLE with HS and identification of the side of ictal onset for surgical therapy is now possible in the majority of patients using non-invasive investigation (Diehl and Luders 2000), when the side of mesial temporal ictal onset is unclear, or there remains a possibility of neocortical ictal onset, additional long-term monitoring with intracranial electrodes is appropriate. Most centers utilize depth electrodes for this purpose, but subdural strips or grids and foramen ovale electrodes can also be used (Cendes *et al.* 2002a).

Biochemical tests

There are no biochemical markers for HS.

Immunological tests

There are no immunological tests available. However, there are recent investigations towards immunological aspects in MTLE as discussed above (Aronica *et al.* 2007; van Gassen *et al.* 2008).

Table 53.1 Imaging of hippocampal sclerosis

Magnetic resonance imaging (MRI)
Detects most MTS
Abnormalities highly specific to MTS
Insensitive to epileptogenicity
Magnetic resonance spectroscopy (MRS)
Detects metabolic changes in mild to severe MTS
Interictal ^{18}F-fluorodeoxyglucose positron emission tomography (FDG PET)
Detects metabolic changes in mild to severe MTS
Highly sensitive to epileptogenicity, not specific to MTS
Ictal single photon emission computed tomography (SPECT)
Highly sensitive to epileptogenicity, not specific to MTS

Neuroimaging

A summary of neuroimaging findings of HS is presented in Table 53.1.

Magnetic resonance imaging

High-resolution MRI is a highly sensitive and specific non-invasive method to diagnose HS in vivo. Images need to be optimized for the evaluation of features indicating hippocampal pathology. Coronal slices are mandatory and they need to be obtained on a plane perpendicular to the long axis of the hippocampus guided by a sagittal scout image. The slices need to be thin to allow appreciation of fine details of the different portions of hippocampal anatomy. Ideally, the slice thickness should be 3 mm or less, and never more than 5 mm. To evaluate volume, shape, orientation, and internal structure, high resolution T1-weighted images, particularly with inversion recovery (IR), are essential. T2-weighted or fluid attenuation inversion recovery (FLAIR) images are important to assess qualitatively the signal intensity.

Visual discrimination of a normal from an abnormal hippocampus is straightforward when one is clearly normal and the other is grossly abnormal, but the visual binary paradigm breaks down in the presence of symmetric bilateral disease or mild unilateral disease. In this case volumetric MRI can be used to detect mild unilateral disease or bilateral hippocampal volume loss. Most radiologists can detect visually a side-to-side asymmetry ratio of 80% or less.

A majority of patients with HS undergoing presurgical evaluation will have a clear-cut unilateral atrophic hippocampus with increased T2-weighted signal and a normal appearing contralateral hippocampus (Fig. 53.3). Therefore, qualitative visual analysis is quite sensitive, especially if the MR images are carefully and properly acquired (Kuzniecky *et al.* 1997).

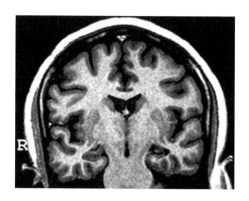 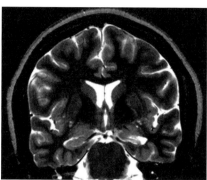

Fig. 53.3. T1-weighted inversion recovery and T2-weighted coronal MRI from a patient with left HS who underwent selective amygdalohippocampectomy and became seizure-free. Observe the atrophy, loss of internal structure, hypointense signal on T1-weighted, and hyperintense signal on T2-weighted image.

In surgically treated MTLE–HS the usual hippocampal abnormalities are:

- Atrophy (detected with MRI in 90–95% of cases in which HS is found in resected tissue)
- Loss of internal architecture (in 60–95%)
- T2-weighted increase (in 80–85%)
- T1-weighted decrease (in 10–95%).

The commonly occurring extrahippocampal abnormalities are:

- Atrophy-signal alterations of the ipsilateral amygdala, temporal neocortex, temporal lobe white matter, fornix, mamillary body, insula, thalamus, or basal frontal cortex
- Atrophy-signal alterations of the contralateral hippocampus (less severe than ipsilateral hippocampal alterations)
- Dilatation of the ipsilateral or contralateral temporal horn of the lateral ventricle (often a "falsely lateralizing" finding, in that temporal horn dilatation often is more severe on the side contralateral to the sclerotic hippocampus). Diffuse hemispheric atrophy can occur ipsilaterally in MTLE–HS, but is rare.

More detailed high-resolution MRI analyses reveals a network of gray matter atrophy that involves mesial temporal and other structures interconnected with the limbic system, including amygdala, entorhinal, perirhinal and parahippocampal cortices, and thalamus.

Proton magnetic resonance spectroscopy

Proton magnetic resonance spectroscopy (MRS) studies have shown focal reductions of N-acetylaspartate (NAA) signal in MTLE with HS, including patients with normal MRI. Both single-voxel and multivoxel [^{1}H]MRS have high sensitivity for detecting low NAA indicative of neuronal dysfunction in focal epilepsies. Decreases in NAA correlate strongly with EEG abnormalities and severity of cell loss, and may be a more sensitive measure than structural MRI. However, the NAA decrease is often more widespread than the epileptogenic focus (Cendes *et al.* 2002b).

Proton MRS studies have shown recovery of relative NAA either ipsilaterally or contralaterally after successful temporal lobe removal. This suggests that structural or functional changes associated with seizure activity may lead to depression of NAA in the ipsilateral and contralateral temporal lobe (Cendes *et al.* 2002b).

Positron emission tomography and single photon emission computed tomography

The same temporal lobe with HS is usually hypometabolic on interictal [^{18}F]flurorodeoxyglucose (FDG) PET with an area that involves the mesial structures, the pole, and part of the lateral cortex, which is helpful and reliable in localizing temporal lobe foci for surgical treatment (Wieser 2004).

The area of decreased flumazenil binding, as assessed by [^{11}C]flumazenil-PET, is often smaller than that of glucose hypometabolism, since it is thought to largely reflect an underlying neuronal loss (Koepp *et al.* 1997).

Logistical and other difficulties (such as high cost and the need for a local cyclotron for PET) limit accessibility to these techniques and they are not routinely used in most institutions.

Ictal and early postictal SPECT scans are also helpful in localizing the epileptogenic focus in patients with TLE (Velasco *et al.* 2002).

Interictal SPECT may reveal an area of temporal hypoperfusion, but it is not reliable and should be performed only for the purpose of comparison with ictal SPECT, particularly by using ictal–interictal subtraction images co-registered to MRI (O'Brien *et al.* 1998). True ictal injections almost always show hyperperfusion of the whole temporal lobe with hypoperfusion of the surrounding cortex.

Neuropsychological tests

Neuropsychological evaluation commonly demonstrates memory dysfunction, which is material-specific according to the hemisphere involved and has been correlated to the degree of HS as measured by postoperative histopathology and by hippocampal volumetry. Verbal memory is mostly affected with left-sided HS, whereas visuospatial memory is more affected with right HS (Jones-Gotman and Smith 2006).

Principles of management

Therapeutic principles

Treatment is based on the patient's response to antiepileptic drugs (AEDs) since some patients, especially those with familial MTLE, may have good seizure control with low doses of any of the AEDs indicated for partial epilepsies.

Treatment should start with a first-line AED in monotherapy, the dose of which is increased until seizure freedom or the occurrence of side effects such as tiredness, dizziness, diplopia, or gait disturbance. No data are available showing superiority of one AED over another, so that those drugs with fewer side effects should be preferred (Glauser et al. 2006).

The choice of first AED will determine the subsequent strategy and should be made with an element of forethought. The list includes phenytoin, carbamazepine, sodium valproate, lamotrigine, oxcarbazepine, topiramate, or levetiracetam (Kwan and Brodie 2004).

Seizures usually respond well for several years. Once seizures return very high levels of AED may be effective, but usually high-dose monotherapy results in intolerable side effects and fails to control disabling seizures (Cendes et al. 2002a; Kwan and Brodie 2004).

When monotherapy fails, combinations can be useful, but interactions and side effects should be considered and monitored carefully.

Carbamazepine and/or phenytoin as monotherapy are appropriate medications for management of MTLE. Higher serum levels than those used for generalized convulsions may be necessary, and medication should be increased until seizures stop or unacceptable side effects occur. Oxcarbazepine has an efficacy similar to that of carbamazepine, but some patients may tolerate higher dosages with fewer side effects, and in some cases this can make a difference in seizure control. Valproate, topiramate, lamotrigine, levetiracetam, or other broad-spectrum AEDs are sometimes of benefit when carbamazepine and phenytoin fail. A combination of drugs may be helpful for some patients, in particular clobazam associated with carbamazepine or phenytoin. When seizures become refractory to medical treatment, they are unlikely to remit spontaneously. With a long duration of uncontrolled seizures, increasing memory problems and other behavioral disturbances are usually reported. This sequence of events is a further suggestion that MTLE with HS may be a progressive epileptic disorder.

Surgical management

Definitions for medical intractability may vary among centers, but it usually includes failure to achieve seizure control with two or more AEDs with adequate dosage and posology. The decision as to when one should perform surgery may be more difficult and controversial. Delaying surgery, however, while running through a range of AED monotherapies and combination options may worsen the long-term prognosis (Yoon et al. 2003).

Because of the psychosocial consequences of disabling epilepsy in adolescence and early adulthood, patients who may have MTLE with HS should be referred to epilepsy centers as soon as it is apparent that control cannot be achieved with first-line medication. Surgery is worth considering because the long-term postoperative prognosis is very good (McIntosh et al. 2004). Patients with MTLE and unilateral HS are excellent candidates for surgical treatment, with a 60–80% chance of becoming free of disabling seizures (Wiebe et al. 2001). However, the frequency of complete seizure freedom drops to 47% in 5 years and 41% in 10 years of follow-up (McIntosh et al. 2004).

The presurgical evaluation should be made considering clinical factors, EEG, preoperative MRI, neuropsychological evaluation, and often functional imaging with either PET or SPECT as discussed above (Wieser 2004).

The choice of whether to perform an anterior temporal lobectomy or to take a more selective approach depends on the surgical teams. Whether this influences the postoperative neuropsychological outcome is still uncertain.

While outcome following a temporal lobectomy is most often thought of in terms of postoperative seizure control, the most common serious cognitive complication of surgery is a postoperative decline in verbal memory following a dominant temporal lobectomy. The clear link between functional and anatomic integrity has lead to the evaluation of hippocampal volumetric measurements as a means of predicting postoperative memory decline. Patients at greatest risk for a decline in verbal memory following a dominant left temporal lobectomy are those with bilaterally symmetric severe hippocampal atrophy. Patients at next greatest risk are those with a volumetrically normal hippocampus (i.e., no atrophy). Patients with less risk for a postoperative verbal memory are those with significant unilateral left hippocampal atrophy.

There are a number of other postoperative issues that occur infrequently, which include visual field problems, double vision, word-finding problems, and other, usually subtle, neuropsychological concerns. In several cases, these problems are transitory. In addition, postoperative psychiatric disturbances may occur, including de novo psychiatric symptoms. Depression, anxiety, and psychosis are the most frequently reported postsurgical psychiatric disturbances (Foong and Flugel 2007). Whilst there are no absolute psychiatric contraindications to surgery, certain pre-existing psychiatric conditions may need careful consideration as there may be a risk of postsurgical psychiatric complications. A history of postictal psychosis, which is often associated with bilateral independent ictal foci and diffuse brain damage, has been associated with poor postsurgical seizure outcome (Alper et al. 2008).

References

Alper K, Kuzniecky R, Carlson C, et al. (2008) Postictal psychosis in partial epilepsy: a case-control study. *Ann Neurol* **63**:602–10.

Andrade-Valenca LP, Valenca MM, Velasco TR, et al. (2008) Mesial temporal lobe epilepsy: clinical and neuropathologic findings of familial and sporadic forms. *Epilepsia* **49**:1046–54.

Aronica E, Boer K, Van Vliet EA, et al. (2007) Complement activation in experimental and human temporal lobe epilepsy. *Neurobiol Dis* **26**:497–511.

Babb TL, Brown WJ (1987) Pathological findings in epilepsy. In: Engel J Jr. (ed.) *Surgical Treatment of the Epilepsies*. New York: Raven Press, pp. 511–40.

Berkovic SF, Scheffer IE (1998) Febrile seizures: genetics and relationship to other epilepsy syndromes. *Curr Opin Neurol* **11**:129–34.

Blumcke I, Thom M, Wiestler OD (2002) Ammon's horn sclerosis: a maldevelopmental disorder associated with temporal lobe epilepsy. *Brain Pathol* **12**:199–211.

Blumcke I, Kistner I, Clusmann H, et al. (2009) Towards a clinico-pathological classification of granule cell dispersion in human mesial temporal lobe epilepsies. *Acta Neuropathol* **117**:535–44.

Bonilha L, Rorden C, Appenzeller S, et al. (2006) Gray matter atrophy associated with duration of temporal lobe epilepsy. *Neuroimage* **32**:1070–9.

Bouchet C, Cazauvieilh JB (1825) De l'épilepsie considéré dans ses rapports avec l'aliénation mentale. *Arch Gen Med* **9**:510–42.

Brandt C, Ebert U, Loscher W (2004) Epilepsy induced by extended amygdala-kindling in rats: lack of clear association between development of spontaneous seizures and neuronal damage. *Epilepsy Res* **62**:135–56.

Briellmann RS, Newton MR, Wellard RM, Jackson GD (2001) Hippocampal sclerosis following brief generalized seizures in adulthood. *Neurology* **57**:315–17.

Camfield P, Camfield C, Gordon K, Dooley J (1994) What types of epilepsy are preceded by febrile seizures? A population-based study of children. *Dev Med Child Neurol* **36**:887–92.

Cardoso TA, Coan AC, Kobayashi E, et al. (2006) Hippocampal abnormalities and seizure recurrence after antiepileptic drug withdrawal. *Neurology* **67**:134–6.

Cendes F (2005) Progressive hippocampal and extrahippocampal atrophy in drug resistant epilepsy. *Curr Opin Neurol* **18**:173–7.

Cendes F, Kahane P, Brodie MJ, Andermann F (2002a) The mesio-temporal lobe epilepsy syndrome. In: Roger J, Bureau M, Dravet C, Genton P, Tassinari CA, Wolf P (eds.) *Epileptic Syndromes in Infancy, Childhood and Adolescence*, 3rd edn. Eastleigh, UK: John Libbey, pp. 513–30.

Cendes F, Knowlton RC, Novotny E, et al. (2002b) Magnetic resonance spectroscopy in epilepsy: clinical issues. *Epilepsia* **43**:32–9.

Diehl B, Luders HO (2000) Temporal lobe epilepsy: when are invasive recordings needed? *Epilepsia* **41**(Suppl 3):S61–74.

Donati D, Akhyani N, Fogdell-Hahn A, et al. (2003) Detection of human herpesvirus-6 in mesial temporal lobe epilepsy surgical brain resections. *Neurology* **61**:1405–11.

Earle K, Baldwin M, Penfield W (1953) Incisural sclerosis and temporal lobe seizures produced by hippocampal herniation at birth. *AMA Arch Neurol Psychiatry* **69**:27–42.

Falconer MA (1974) Mesial temporal (Ammon's horn) sclerosis as a common cause of epilepsy: etiology, treatment, and prevention. *Lancet* **2**:767–70.

Falconer MA, Taylor DC (1968) Surgical treatment of drug-resistant epilepsy due to mesial temporal sclerosis: etiology and significance. *Arch Neurol* **19**:353–61.

Foong J, Flugel D (2007) Psychiatric outcome of surgery for temporal lobe epilepsy and presurgical considerations. *Epilepsy Res* **75**:84–96.

Franck JE, Schwartzkroin PA (1985) Do kainate-lesioned hippocampi become epileptogenic? *Brain Res* **329**:309–13.

Glauser T, Ben-Menachem E, Bourgeois B, et al. (2006) ILAE treatment guidelines: evidence-based analysis of antiepileptic drug efficacy and effectiveness as initial monotherapy for epileptic seizures and syndromes. *Epilepsia* **47**:1094–120.

Gloor P (1997) *The Temporal Lobe and Limbic System*. New York: Oxford University Press.

Hauser WA, Annegers JF, Rocca WA (1996) Descriptive epidemiology of epilepsy: contributions of population-based studies from Rochester, Minnesota. *Mayo Clin Proc* **71**:576–86.

International League Against Epilepsy (1989) Commission on classification and terminology: proposal for revised classification of epilepsies and epileptic syndromes. *Epilepsia* **30**:389–99.

Jones-Gotman M, Smith ML (2006) Neuropsychological profiles. *Adv Neurol* **97**:357–66.

Kanner AM (2006) Epilepsy, suicidal behavior, and depression: do they share common pathogenic mechanisms? *Lancet Neurol* **5**:107–8.

Kim WJ, Park SC, Lee SJ, et al. (1999) The prognosis for control of seizures with medications in patients with MRI evidence for mesial temporal sclerosis. *Epilepsia* **40**:290–3.

Kobayashi E, Lopes-Cendes I, Guerreiro CA, et al. (2001) Seizure outcome and hippocampal atrophy in familial mesial temporal lobe epilepsy. *Neurology* **56**:166–72.

Kobayashi E, Li LM, Lopes-Cendes I, Cendes F (2002) Magnetic resonance imaging evidence of hippocampal sclerosis in asymptomatic, first-degree relatives of patients with familial mesial temporal lobe epilepsy. *Arch Neurol* **59**:1891–4.

Kobayashi E, D'Agostino MD, Lopes-Cendes I, et al. (2003) Outcome of surgical treatment in familial mesial temporal lobe epilepsy. *Epilepsia* **44**:1080–4.

Koepp MJ, Richardson MP, Labbe C, et al. (1997) ^{11}C-flumazenil PET, volumetric MRI, and quantitative pathology in mesial temporal lobe epilepsy. *Neurology* **49**:764–73.

Kuzniecky RI, Bilir E, Gilliam F, et al. (1997) Multimodality MRI in mesial temporal sclerosis: relative sensitivity and specificity. *Neurology* **49**:774–8.

Kwan P, Brodie MJ (2004) Drug treatment of epilepsy: when does it fail and how to optimize its use? *CNS Spectr* **9**:110–19.

Mathern GW, Adelson PD, Cahan LD, Leite JP (2002) Hippocampal neuron damage in human epilepsy: Meyer's hypothesis revisited. *Progr Brain Res* **135**:237–51.

McIntosh AM, Kalnins RM, Mitchell LA, et al. (2004) Temporal lobectomy: long-term seizure outcome, late recurrence and risks for seizure recurrence. *Brain* **127**:2018–30.

Meencke HJ (2009) Clinical neuropathology of the epilepsies in the 100 years of

371

the ILAE (1909–2009). *Epilepsia* 50(Suppl 3):8–16.

Meyer A, Falconer MA (1954) Pathological findings in temporal lobe epilepsy. *J Neurol Neurosurg Psychiatry* 17:276–85.

Mintzer S, Cendes F, Soss J, *et al.* (2004) Unilateral hippocampal sclerosis with contralateral temporal scalp ictal onset. *Epilepsia* 45:792–802.

Morrell F (1989) Varieties of human secondary epileptogenesis. *J Clin Neurophysiol* 6:227–75.

O'Brien TJ, So EL, Mullan BP, *et al.* (1998) Subtraction ictal SPECT co-registered to MRI improves clinical usefulness of SPECT in localizing the surgical seizure focus. *Neurology* 50:445–54.

Schwartzkroin PA (1993) *Epilepsy: Models, Mechanisms, and Concepts.* Cambridge, UK: Cambridge University Press.

Semah F, Picot MC, Adam C, *et al.* (1998) Is the underlying cause of epilepsy a major prognostic factor for recurrence? *Neurology* 51:1256–62.

Sutula TP (2004) Mechanisms of epilepsy progression: current theories and perspectives from neuroplasticity in adulthood and development. *Epilepsy Res* 60:161–71.

Thom M (2009) Hippocampal sclerosis: progress since Sommer. *Brain Pathol* 19:565–72.

van Gassen KL, De WM, Koerkamp MJ, *et al.* (2008) Possible role of the innate immunity in temporal lobe epilepsy. *Epilepsia* 49:1055–65.

Van Paesschen W, Revesz T, Duncan JS, King MD, Connelly A (1997) Quantitative neuropathology and quantitative magnetic resonance imaging of the hippocampus in temporal lobe epilepsy. *Ann Neurol* 42:756–66.

Velasco TR, Wichert-Ana L, Leite JP, *et al.* (2002) Accuracy of ictal SPECT in mesial temporal lobe epilepsy with bilateral interictal spikes. *Neurology* 59:266–71.

Wiebe S, Blume WT, Girvin JP, Eliasziw M (2001) A randomized, controlled trial of surgery for temporal-lobe epilepsy. *N Engl J Med* 345:311–18.

Wieser HG (2004) ILAE Commission Report: Mesial temporal lobe epilepsy with hippocampal sclerosis. *Epilepsia* 45:695–714.

Yoon HH, Kwon HL, Mattson RH, Spencer DD, Spencer SS (2003) Long-term seizure outcome in patients initially seizure-free after resective epilepsy surgery. *Neurology* 61:445–50.

Chapter

54

Neonatal seizures and postneonatal epilepsy – causes

Eli M. Mizrahi and Kevin E. Chapman

The causal diseases

Seizure occurrence may be the most frequent sign of central nervous system (CNS) dysfunction in the newborn, heralding the onset of disorders that may lead to long-term sequelae. Accurate diagnosis and management are critical to minimizing the potential associated adverse impact such as developmental delay, neurological impairment, and postneonatal epilepsy. Neonatal seizures are typically acute reactive events and while they are typically considered as a single group of disorders, they are the manifestation of a heterogeneous group of etiologies, causes, and risk factors (Chapman *et al.* 2010; Mizrahi 2010). Long-term outcome is most often related to the underlying cause of the seizures.

Diagnosis may be challenging due to the wide range of age-dependent paroxysmal clinical and electroencephalographic (EEG) manifestations. Seizures are based upon the stage of brain maturation which, in turn, is most often defined clinically by the age of the infant, whether preterm or term. The most useful method is by assigning conception age (CA): the gestational age (duration of pregnancy prior to birth) plus the chronologic age (legal age of the infant). The neonatal period is defined as the first 28 days of life of a term infant or up to 44 weeks CA.

Neonatal seizures are usually considered of epileptic origin, although some may be generated by non-epileptic mechanisms (Mizrahi and Kellaway 1987). During the following discussion, the term "neonatal seizures" will refer to the entire group of these events and assume them to be of epileptic origin. However, when necessary, some distinctions will be specified based upon pathophysiology.

Epilepsy in this period
Neonatal seizures

Neonatal seizures occur in from 1.5 to 5.5 in 1000 newborns. The International League Against Epilepsy (ILAE) describes most neonatal seizures as "acute reactive" and "symptomatic"

(ILAE 1989). There is much discussion as to whether such seizures constitute the condition of "epilepsy" or just the transient occurrence of seizures of epileptic origin. Some neonatal seizures are self-limited or easily controlled with antiepileptic drugs (AEDs) or etiologic-specific therapy, making the designation of "epilepsy" not relevant. However, for other infants, seizures may begin in the neonatal period and either persist beyond the first month of life or resolve and then recur in various forms after a latent period (Watanabe *et al.* 1999). For these infants, the designation of epilepsy is more certain.

Some neonatal seizure types share features with those of older children including clonic activity; tonic activity; myoclonus; and epileptic spasms. Other features are relatively unique to the neonatal period and age-dependent: fragmentation; disorganization; unusual patterns of migration; and simultaneous but asynchronous of involvement in multiple brain regions. Some of these differences are based on the mechanisms of epileptogenesis and the state of early development in the immature brain.

There are a number of classification methods. Neonatal seizures may be classified by clinical features: focal clonic (unifocal and multifocal), focal tonic, myoclonic, spasms, generalized tonic and motor automatisms (also referred to as "subtle seizures") (Mizrahi and Kellaway 1998) (Table 54.1). Clinical seizures may consist of a single type of movement or a sequence of behaviors. With a sequence of behaviors, the seizure is classified according to its predominant feature. Paroxysmal changes in heart rate, respiration, and blood pressure have also been reported as manifestations of neonatal seizures, although they are rare as isolated epileptic events. If they do occur, they most often are in association with motor manifestations of seizures. Seizures may also be classified according to their pathophysiology: epileptic or non-epileptic. Those of epileptic origin are: focal clonic, focal tonic, some types of myoclonic seizures, and spasms. Those that may be considered non-epileptic in origin include some types of myoclonic events, generalized tonic posturing and motor automatisms such as oral–buccal–lingual movements, movements

The Causes of Epilepsy, eds. S. D. Shorvon, F. Andermann, and R. Guerrini. Published by Cambridge University Press. © Cambridge University Press 2011.

Table 54.1 Classification of neonatal seizures based on electroclinical findings

Clinical seizures with a consistent electrocortical signature (pathophysiology: epileptic)
Focal clonic
Unifocal
Multifocal
Hemiconvulsive
Axial
Focal tonic
Asymmetrical truncal posturing
Limb posturing
Sustained eye deviation
Myoclonic
Generalized
Focal
Spasms
Flexor
Extensor
Mixed extensor/flexor
Clinical seizures without a consistent electrocortical signature (pathophysiology: presumed non-epileptic)
Myoclonic
Generalized
Focal
Fragmentary
Generalized tonic
Flexor
Extensor
Mixed extensor/flexor
Motor automatisms
Oral–buccal–lingual movements
Ocular signs
Progression movements
Complex purposeless movements
Electrical seizures without clinical seizure activity

Source: From Mizrahi and Kellaway (1998).

of progression, and some ocular signs (Mizrahi and Kellaway 1998). Neonatal seizures may also be classified according to the relationship between clinical and electrographic events: electroclinical seizures, with a temporal overlap of the clinical seizure and the electrographic seizure; electrical only events with EEG seizures without clinical events; and clinical only seizures in the absence of EEG seizure activity. There are also neonatal epileptic syndromes which will be discussed below.

Postneonatal epilepsy

Neonatal seizures are associated with significant long-term sequelae. Approximately 25% of those with neonatal seizures die, and of the survivors about 40% have abnormal neurological examinations and 50% have developmental delay. Approximately 25% experience postneonatal epilepsy, although this varies and is dependent upon the underlying disorder (Ellenberg and Nelson 1988; Ronen *et al.* 1993; Ortibus *et al.* 1996; Mizrahi *et al.* 2001; Plouin and Anderson 2005; Pisani *et al.* 2008). Pisani and colleagues found that 80% of neonates with postneonatal epilepsy had more than one seizure type including: focal/multifocal clonic, tonic, and myoclonic. Watanabe *et al.* (1999) found the frequency and type of postneonatal seizures varied with neonatal epileptic syndrome, with the more severe neonatal disorders evolving to age-dependent epileptic encephalopathies.

Diagnostic tests for the diseases

The assessment for an underlying cause of neonatal seizures begins at the time of seizure recognition since etiologic-specific therapy is most effective in minimizing long-term sequelae. Diagnostic testing is based upon potential etiologic and risk factors within the clinical setting. While the evaluation of each infant is individualized, some common concerns are addressed for virtually all neonates with seizures. The main categories of etiological factors of neonatal seizures include hypoxic–ischemic encephalopathy, CNS infections, structural brain abnormalities, and metabolic disturbances. Some are discussed in some detail below, while a more comprehensive list is provided in Table 54.2. Etiologies can also be categorized as either acute or chronic. Diagnostic testing (Table 54.3) is directed towards understanding the relative importance and presence or absence of these main categories of etiological factors. As these factors become more apparent or are excluded, more detailed evaluations may be required to address the rarer causes of neonatal seizures. It should also be noted that often there may be multiple coexisting causes found. In other cases, there may be only associated risk factors identified or no specific causes may be identified despite a comprehensive evaluation. It is critical to search for an etiologic factor since etiologic-specific therapy can both prevent further injury and successfully control seizures. Finally, not all etiologic factors may be successfully treated, but their elucidation provides important information concerning other aspects of management and determination of prognosis.

Electroencephalography

While the EEG may not be diagnostic for the cause of seizures, its discussion is necessary because of its value in the diagnosis

Table 54.2 Etiologies of neonatal seizures

Acute	Chronic
Acute neonatal encephalopathy (includes classic hypoxic–ischemic encephalopathy, both ante- and intrapartum)	Isolated cerebral dysgenesis, e.g., lissencephaly, hemimegalencephaly
Arterial ischemic stroke	Cerebral dysgenesis associated with inborn errors of metabolism
Sinovenous thrombosis	Chronic infection (TORCH [toxoplasmosis, other infections, rubella, cytomegalovirus, and herpes simplex] syndromes)
Extracorporeal membrane oxygenation	Neurocutaneous syndromes:
Congenital heart disease	Incontinentia pigmenti (Bloch Sulzberger syndrome)
Vein of Galen malformation	Hypomelanosis of Ito
Giant arteriovenous malformation	Sturge–Weber syndrome
Hypertensive encephalopathy	Tuberous sclerosis
Intracranial hemorrhage (subdural subarachnoid, intraventricular, intraparenchymal)	Linear sebaceous nevus (epidermal nevus syndrome)
Trauma (intrapartum and non-accidental)	Genetic conditions
Infections (sepsis, meningitis, encephalitis)	22q11 microdeletion
Transient, simple metabolic disorders	ARX (aristaless-related homeobox) mutations
Inborn errors of metabolism (including pyridoxine-dependent seizures)	Specific very early onset epilepsy syndromes
Intoxication	Fifth-day fits (benign neonatal convulsions)
	Benign familial neonatal seizures
	Early myoclonic encephalopathy
	Early infantile epileptic encephalopathy
	Migrating partial seizures of infancy

Source: From Chapman *et al.* (2010).

Table 54.3 Data to determine the etiology of neonatal seizures

Clinical	Complete history, general physical and neurologic examinations, eye examination
Neuroimaging	Computerized tomographic or magnetic resonance imaging
Blood tests	Arterial blood gases and pH
	Sodium, glucose, calcium, magnesium, ammonia, lactate and pyruvate, serum amino acids
	Comprehensive "neogen" panel[a]
	TORCH (toxoplasmosis, other infections, rubella, cytomegalovirus, and herpes simplex) titers
	Biotin
Urine tests	Reducing substances, sulfites, organic acids
	Toxicologic screen
Cerebrospinal fluid tests	Red and white blood cell counts
	Glucose and protein
	Culture
	Neurotransmitter profile[b]

Notes:
[a]Varies by US states.
[b]In the proper clinical context.
Source: Chapman *et al.* (2010).

of seizures themselves and eventual management of affected neonates (Mizrahi *et al.* 2003). Interictal EEG sharp wave activity is typically not considered an indicator of potential epileptogenesis. However, sharp waves may be present on neonatal EEG as normal activity (developmental elements or randomly occurring, low or moderate in voltage sharp waves present in transitional or light sleep) or as abnormal waves which suggest focal injury or when multifocal suggest diffuse dysfunction. The interictal background activity may provide information concerning the extent and type of CNS dysfunction and provide some insight to prognosis. Infants with initial normal background activity are less likely to eventually experience seizures than those with persistent diffuse background abnormalities (Laroia *et al.* 1998). An EEG with normal background activity recorded within the first 24 hours of life may suggest a good outcome, while EEG background activity with persistent or slowly resolving abnormal features in serial recordings suggests a poorer outcome (Holmes and Lombroso 1993).

The morphology, frequency, and voltage of epileptic seizure discharges vary widely (Mizrahi *et al.* 2003). Seizure discharges may be consistent from event to event, or may change within an individual seizure or between seizures in an individual infant or among infants. While the minimum duration of an electrographic seizure has been defined as 10 s, the duration of seizure discharges may also vary. The electrical events are predominantly focal and well circumscribed, most frequently arising from the central or centrotemporal region of one hemisphere and less commonly from the occipital, frontal, or midline central regions. While seizures may arise focally and remain confined to that region, they may also spread to other regions. This may appear as a gradual widening of the focal area, by an abrupt change from a small regional focus to involvement of the entire hemisphere (such as that found in hemiconvulsive seizure), or by migration of the electrical seizure from one area of a hemisphere to another or from one hemisphere to another. The seizures may also be multi-focal. There are some ictal patterns that are unique to the neonatal period. Seizure discharges of the depressed brain are typically low in voltage, long in duration, and highly localized. They may be unifocal or multifocal and show little tendency to spread or modulate. Alpha seizure activity is characterized by a sudden appearance of paroxysmal, rhythmic activity of the alpha frequency (8–12 Hz) typically in the temporal or central region. Both patterns are usually associated with severe encephalopathy, depressed and undifferentiated EEG back-ground, no clinical seizures, and a poor prognosis.

Etiologic-specific diagnostic tests

Acute causes

Hypoxic–ischemic encephalopathy

The most common neurological condition associated with neonatal seizures is "acute neonatal encephalopathy" charac-terized by depressed mental status (lethargy or coma), seizures, axial and appendicular hypotonia with an overall reduction in spontaneous motor activity, and clear evidence of bulbar dys-function including poor sucking and swallowing, and an inex-pressive face (Durham et al. 2000). Some of these infants may be diagnosed with hypoxic–ischemic encephalopathy (HIE) which entails a group of clinical and laboratory findings and within the context of a sentinel hypoxic event. The clinical and laboratory findings include: evidence of metabolic acidosis in fetal umbilical cord arterial blood obtained at delivery (pH value less than 7 and base deficit greater than 12 mmol/L); early onset of severe or moderate neonatal encephalopathy in infants born at 34 or more weeks of gestation; subsequent cerebral palsy of the spastic quadriplegic or dyskinetic type; and exclusion of other identifiable etiologies such as trauma, coagulation disorders, infectious conditions, or genetic dis-orders (ACOG 2003). There should also be a sudden and sustained fetal bradycardia or the absence of fetal heart rate variability; persistent, late, or variable decelerations; Apgar scores of 0 to 3 after 5 mins; and in most, multisystem involve-ment within 72 hr of birth. Examples of multisystem malfunc-tion include acute renal tubular necrosis, elevated values of liver function tests, necrotizing enterocolitis from bowel ische-mia, and depressed blood cell lines (e.g., thrombocytopenia).

Diagnostic testing –– The diagnosis of these disorders is based upon history, clinical examination, pH values of fetal umbilical cord blood, Apgar scores, and assessment of multiorgan function (kidney, liver, lung, cardiac). These tests are critical for meeting the recommended guidelines for the diagnosis of HIE (ACOG 2002). Early neuroimaging studies, particularly magnetic resonance imaging (MRI) with diffusion imaging, should show acute diffuse abnormalities consistent with hypoxia/ischemia.

Neonatal and perinatal stroke

Perinatal stroke is defined as a cerebrovascular event occurring between 28 weeks of gestation and 7 days of age. The incidence is 1 in 4000 live births. Infants may present with acute appear-ance of neonatal seizures, hypotonia, feeding difficulties, and, rarely, hemiparesis (Clancy et al. 1985; Perlman et al. 1994). Alternatively there may be a later discovery of stroke through the gradual appreciation of a congenital hemiparesis or the onset of a partial seizure disorder in an infant apparently healthy at birth. Risk factors include congenital heart defects (CHDs), blood and lipid disorders, infection, placental dis-orders, vasculopathy, trauma, dehydration, and extracorporeal membrane oxygenation (ECMO). Cerebral sinovenous throm-bosis may present with seizures and other non-specific CNS signs such as lethargy although infrequently frank hemiparesis (deVeber et al. 2001). The sagittal and transverse sinuses are most commonly involved, but multiple sinus thromboses also occur. While ECMO is an effective therapy for newborn infants with life-threatening respiratory failure, a high propor-tion of survivors have MRI-identified focal parenchymal brain lesions, often announced by seizures during ECMO. Cerebral hemorrhage and infarction have been reported in 28–52% of ECMO-treated infants (Lago et al. 1995). Congenital heart defects enhance the risk for neonatal seizures secondary to strokes. Ischemic strokes can arise preoperatively or post-operatively and may occur from multiple mechanisms includ-ing right-to-left intracardiac shunting or embolization during cardiac catheterization.

Diagnostic testing –– There are a number of neuroimaging techniques applicable to the neonatal setting and their use is dependent upon mobility of the infant and suspected etiologic entity. Head ultrasound (HUS) may be performed at the bed-side, but may provide a limited examination for acute focal ischemia. Computed tomography (CT) requires infant trans-portation and may not identify infarctions early in their course. Infant transportation is also required for MRI and this may be the most logistically difficult of these techniques. However, MRI with diffusion imaging is superior to HUS and CT imaging for identification of acute focal ischemia. Assessment should also be directed towards the underlying cause of the stroke including the search for cardiac defects, coagulopathies, systemic infection, and other risk factors.

Intracranial hemorrhage

This group of disorders is diverse and may be the direct cause of seizures in up to 15% of patients (Volpe 2008). There are five types including: intraparenchymal hemorrhage, subarachnoid hemorrhage, subdural hemorrhage, cerebellar hemorrhage, and intraventricular hemorrhage. Depending on the extent and location of the hemorrhage, they may only present with signs of increased intracranial pressure or brainstem abnormalities. The seizures associated with subarachnoid hemorrhage and HIE may occur on the first postnatal day, while the seizures associated with uncomplicated subarachnoid hemorrhage, intraventricular hemorrhage, and subdural hemorrhage typically occur after the second day of life.

Diagnostic testing –– Head ultrasound may provide a rapid, bedside limited examination that may be helpful in identifying hemorrhage. Computed tomography may provide limited resolution, but is helpful in identifying calcifications, skull fractures, and hemorrhage. Magnetic resonance imaging provides greatest resolution, but may miss skull fractures in suspected cases of non-accidental trauma. Abnormal findings in the cerebrospinal fluid may also suggest the diagnosis.

Acute CNS infection

Central nervous system infections are important etiologic factors of neonatal seizures because they are both associated with significant morbidity and mortality and are also potentially treatable. Early treatment may limit adverse outcome. A wide variety of infections may be found including bacterial and viral which may give rise to meningitis, encephalitis, and sepsis (see Chapters 67, 68 and 69). In addition, CNS infections may be complicated by intracranial hemorrhage, effusions, infarctions, and metabolic disturbances.

Diagnostic testing –– All neonates with seizure typically undergo a thorough evaluation for potential presence of infection. This includes: lumbar puncture and blood and urine cultures. Some infants are treated empirically with antiviral agents and antibacterial agents acutely while test results are being analysed.

Transient metabolic etiologies

The most frequently identified transient metabolic causes of neonatal seizures are hypoglycemia, hypocalcemia, and hypomagnesemia. In addition, hyponatremia, hypernatremia, and acute hyperbilirubinemia (acute kernicterus) may be factors. Some of these factors may coexist. In addition, there are specific causes of hypoglycemia, that are not transient, that should be investigated including prematurity, maternal diabetes, nesidioblastosis, galactosemia, defects of gluconeogenesis, glycogen storage diseases, respiratory chain defect, and glucose transporter type 1 syndrome (GLUT1 deficiency) (De Vivo *et al.* 1991).

Diagnostic testing –– This includes specific serum assays for the suspected metabolic etiology. The presence of hypoglycemia may be urgent and rapid testing may be applied at the bedside while waiting for the results of the full assay. When investigating for glucose transporter deficiency a lumbar puncture is required and is best performed in consultation with a metabolic specialist.

Inborn errors of metabolism

This is a complex group of rare disorders. However, diagnosis is important for prognostic value as well as some emerging therapies. These disorders may induce severe acute encephalopathy with seizures and include: maple-syrup urine disease, non-ketotic hyperglycinemia, ketotic hyperglycinemia (such as proprionic and methylmalonic acidemias) and the urea-cycle abnormalities (such as carbamoylphosphate synthetase deficiency, orthnithine carbamyl transferase deficiency, citrullinemia, and arginosuccinic acidemia) (see Chapters 31 and 35).

In addition there are a group of metabolic deficiencies that may be benign when recognized and treated. Biotinidase deficiency may produce alopecia, seborrheic dermatitis, developmental delay, hypotonia, and ataxia. Seizures may begin as early as the first week of life. Oral administration of free biotin daily is the treatment. Pyridoxine-dependent seizures (Coker 1992) usually arise between birth and 3 months of age, although atypical cases have been reported up to 3 years. The diagnosis is made when seizures immediately cease and epileptiform EEG activity disappears within a few hours of the intravenous administration of 50 to 100 mg of pyridoxine. Lifelong therapy with pyridoxine 50 to 100 mg per day is necessary (see Chapter 33). Folinic acid-responsive neonatal seizures may appear in term infants during the first few hours or days of life (Torres *et al.* 1999). It has been reported that seizures may cease and the EEG pattern improved after the administration of 2.5 mg of folinic acid twice daily (see Chapter 29).

Diagnostic testing –– The diagnosis of disorders of amino acid metabolism and urea cycle defects requires some degree of clinical suspicion. Clinical examination and, in some instance, the finding of a modified hypsarrhythmia with suppression burst on EEG may suggest these disorders. Laboratory testing is directed towards specific disorders. These include serum assays of ammonia, lactate and pyruvate, and amino acids and the testing of urine for reducing substances, sulfites and organic acids. Cerebrospinal fluid may be tested for neurotransmitter profile. For biotinidase deficiency, blood levels may be obtained. For both pyridoxine-dependent seizures and folinic acid-responsive seizures, diagnosis is made by sequential empirical treatment, typically with initial administration of pyridoxine.

Chronic causes

Some neonatal seizures result from long-standing disorders. They are considered "long-standing" because of their presumed developmental or genetic origin. These disorders include cerebral dysgenesis, neurocutaneous syndromes, genetic disorders, or very early onset epilepsy in association with well-defined epileptic syndromes.

Cerebral dysgenesis

Cerebral dysgenesis may occur in isolation or in association with other disorders such as inborn errors of metabolism, genetic disorders, or other neurocutaneous syndromes. Those that occur in isolation include focal cortical dysplasia (see Chapter 45), hemimegalencephaly (see Chapter 44), schizencephaly, and lissencephaly (although the later may also be associated with specific genetic findings) (see Chapter 48). Both cerebral dysgenesis and inborn errors of metabolism may coexist (Tharp 2002) so that the finding of dysgenesis should prompt the investigation of other conditions. Similarly, some cerebral dysgenesis may be associated with or be the manifestations of an underlying genetic condition or syndrome, also prompting a more thorough evaluation.

Diagnostic testing -- The definitive diagnostic test for cerebral dysgenesis in the neonate is MRI, although if the infant cannot be transported to the radiology suite, HUS may provide some initial, although limited information. In addition, when clinically indicated an evaluation for inborn errors of metabolism, neurocutaneous syndromes or genetic evaluation may be warranted.

TORCH infections

Chronic TORCH (toxoplasmosis, other infections, rubella, cytomegalovirus, and herpes virus) infections can be identified by ophthalmologic changes, microcephaly, periventricular calcifications on neuroimaging, and appropriate serological blood tests. Congenital infections acquired before the fourth month of gestation may cause an acquired form of migration defect and give rise to "dysgenetic" patterns on CT or MRI scanning.

Diagnostic testing -- Clinical and ophthalmologic examination, CT and MRI, and appropriate TORCH titers are part of the evaluation of infants suspected of these infections.

Neurocutaneous syndromes

There are a number of neurocutaneous syndromes that may be associated with neonatal seizures. Familial incontinentia pigmenti is a mixed syndrome of different mosaicisms with a distinctive pattern of hyperpigmentation and dermal scarring. The cause is a mutation in the *NEMO* (NFκB essential modulator) gene located on Xq28 (Nelson 2006). There is also the sporadic syndrome of hypomelanosis of Ito, which maps to Xp11, with cutaneous lesions appearing as areas of hypopigmentation. Tuberous sclerosis (see Chapter 24) may generate neonatal seizures through associated cortical tubers or secondary to embolic strokes caused by intracardiac tumors. In the neonate, the classic neurocutaneous signs of tuberous sclerosis are often not apparent, except for hypomelanotic macules noted at or soon after birth; however, these may be evident only on skin examination under a Wood's lamp. The disorders of linear sebaceous nevi have distinctive raised, waxy, sometimes verrucous nevi on the scalp or face, associated with hemihypertrophy, hemimegalencephaly, and neonatal seizures. Sturge–Weber syndrome is a sporadic syndrome featuring the distinctive facial "port-wine stain" and associated vascular anomaly over the cortical surface and may manifest with neonatal seizures (see Chapter 26).

Diagnostic testing -- Clinical examination, including a detailed dermatological evaluation, and, in some instances, family history suggest these diagnoses. Genetic testing and neuroimaging may be useful for diagnosis of some of the neurocutaneous syndromes.

Epilepsy syndromes of early infantile onset

The International League Against Epilepsy (ILAE) has designated four epileptic syndromes which may occur in the neonatal period (ILAE 1989).

Benign neonatal convulsions

This syndrome is characterized by focal clonic seizures or, rarely, focal tonic seizures in an otherwise normal neonate with no family history of neonatal seizures. Infants are typically full term with a history of a normal pregnancy, labor, and delivery. Seizures usually occur between the fourth and sixth day of life and are typically brief (1 to 3 min) although, rarely, the seizures can be prolonged. The seizure disorder is self-limited (24 to 48 hr), although, rarely, it can also be prolonged. The background EEG is typically normal although it has also been reported that up to 60% of affected neonates show an interictal EEG pattern referred to as *theta pointu alternant*. This is a discontinuous, asynchronous pattern which is non-reactive, focal, rhythmic 4–7-Hz activity, at times mixed with sharp waves. Treatment for this disorder is controversial, but most are treated with phenobarbital. The prognosis is generally good although the incidence of postneonatal epilepsy – 0.5% of patients – is slightly higher than those without neonatal seizures (Plouin and Anderson 2005).

Diagnostic testing -- This diagnosis is often one of exclusion in infants who are neurologically normal with new-onset focal clonic seizures. Clinical examination, history, and seizure characterization are the cornerstones of diagnosis. All other potential etiologies must be excluded. The interictal EEG may be helpful, although the *theta pointu alternant* pattern is only suggestive, but not diagnostic.

Benign familial neonatal convulsions

This syndrome is characterized by focal clonic or focal tonic seizures, a family history of neonatal seizures, and no neurological findings (Quattlebaum 1979) (see Chapter 7). There is an autosomal dominant pattern of inheritance with incomplete penetrance. Potassium channel genes have been associated with this disorder: BFNC type I has a defective gene *KCNQ2* at chromosomal locus 20q13.3 with an aberrant α-subunit of a voltage-gated potassium channel (Cooper and Jan 1998). Type II has an abnormal *KCNQ3* gene, located on 8q24, and also codes for an aberrant α-subunit of a voltage-gated potassium channel. A form of BFNC with myokymia (Dedek *et al.* 2001) has been reported as a separate mutation of *KCNQ2*, also on 20q13.3.

The seizures may be brief, but can recur for up to 2–3 months of age, when they will remit spontaneously. The interictal EEG is typically normal although *theta pointu alternant* pattern may also occur. While the outcome is generally good, there is a higher incidence of postneonatal seizures in affected infants later in life, ranging from 11% to 16% (Ronen *et al.* 1993). It has been reported that phenobarbital therapy is often successful.

Diagnostic testing -- The key to this diagnosis is a positive family history. In addition, as with the syndrome of benign neonatal convulsions, clinical examination, seizure characterization, and lack of other etiological factors are necessary to make the diagnosis of BFNC. While genetic testing is available, it often does not have immediate clinical utility.

Early myoclonic encephalopathy

Early myoclonic encephalopathy (EME) is characterized by erratic, fragmentary myoclonus in the first month of life and with the eventual development of both focal seizures and infantile spasms (Aicardi and Goutières 1978). Early on there is a periodic, suppression burst pattern on EEG. Affected infants are typically neurologically abnormal either at birth or at the onset of clinical seizures and most often are hypotonic and poorly responsive. Metabolic etiologies may include: non-ketotic hyperglycinemia, proprionic acidemia, D-glyceric acidemia, and methylmalonic acidemia. Other causes may include: familial, cerebral malformations, and cryptogenic etiologies. Therapy is typically symptomatic, directed towards the specific inborn error of metabolism. Antiepileptic drugs or hormonal therapy may be utilized for infantile spasms although they may not be particularly effective. The outcome for infants with EME is reportedly poor, consistent with etiology, and there is a high incidence of death within the first few years of life. Some survivors may remain in a vegetative state while others have significant developmental delay.

Diagnostic testing -- Clinical examination and seizure characterization are initial points of reference in the evaluation of infants suspected of EME. The EEG may be helpful with the finding of a periodic, suppression burst pattern. With increasing clinical concern about this diagnosis, assessment for inborn errors of metabolism should be undertaken.

Early infantile epileptic encephalopathy

Early infantile epileptic encephalopathy (EIEE) is characterized by onset in early infancy; tonic spasms; suppression burst EEG background; severe psychomotor retardation; medically intractable seizures; poor prognosis; and evolution to West syndrome (i.e., infantile spasms, retardation, hypsarrhythmia on EEG) (Ohthara *et al.* 1992). There have been a number of etiologic factors associated with this syndrome. Most symptomatic infants have structural brain abnormalities such as porencephaly, cerebral atrophy, or dygenesis. Specific metabolic disorders are not typically seen. These infants are often treated with hormonal therapy (typically adrenocorticotropic hormone) with the emergence of West syndrome. Other AEDs have been utilized, also with limited success, including

Table 54.4 Comparison of early myoclonic encephalopathy (EME) and early infantile epileptic encephalopathy (EIEE)

	EME	EIEE
Age of onset	Neonatal period	Within first 3 months
Neurologic status at onset	Abnormal at birth or at seizure onset	Always abnormal, even prior to seizure onset
Characteristic seizure type	Erratic or fragmentary myoclonus	Tonic spasm
Additional seizure types	Massive myoclonus, simple partial seizures, infantile spasms (tonic)	Focal motor seizures, hemiconvulsions, generalized seizures
Background EEG	Suppression burst	Suppression burst
Etiology	Inborn errors of metabolism, familial, cryptogenic	Cerebral dysgenesis, anoxia, cryptogenic
Natural course	Progressive impairment	Static impairment
Incidence of death	Very high, occurring in infancy	High, occurring in infancy, childhood or adolescence
Status of survivors	Vegetative state	Severe mental retardation, quadriplegia, bedridden
Long-term seizure evolution	Infantile spasms	West syndrome, Lennox–Gastaut syndrome

Sources: Based on data from Aicardi (1997) and Ohtahara *et al.* (1992); from Mizrahi and Clancy (2000).

clonazepam, nitrazepam, valproate, and pyridoxine. The prognosis for those with EIEE is poor in terms of developmental delay and neurological impairment although there are some long-term survivors. There are both similarities and differences between early EIEE and EME (Table 54.4) suggesting to some that the two syndromes may actually represent a continuum of one (Djukic *et al.* 2006), while others consider them distinct.

Diagnostic testing -- Clinical examination and seizure characterization will raise the possibility of this disorder. In addition, the EEG will demonstrate a suppression burst pattern. Because of the high incidence of associated structural brain abnormalities, MRI or other neuroimaging is an essential part of the evaluation.

Principles of management

Management is first directed towards stabilization of the infant's airway and circulatory system. If a treatable cause of the seizure has been found, etiologic-specific therapy is given and maintained. The decision to initiate AED therapy is dependent upon seizure frequency, duration, and type. Phenobarbital is most often given as the first-line AED; first as a loading dose followed by additional boluses titrated to response, tolerance, and serum levels. After phenobarbital, phenytoin is the first-line AED most often used (now fosphenytoin).

Benzodiazepines are frequently used as alternative second-line AEDs, although more often they are given following phenobarbital and in place of phenytoin. These AEDs include diazepam and lorezapam. Midazolam has been used more frequently, either in bolus form or as a continuous infusion in cases of otherwise medically refractory seizures (Sheth *et al.*

1996). Other second-line or adjuvant AEDs have been utilized either intravenously or orally with variable success including clonazepam, carbamazepine, primidone, valproate, vigabatrin, lamotrigine, and leveracitam. More recently lidocaine as been investigated as an acute AED with promising results in infants with seizures otherwise refractory to standard AEDs (Hellström-Westas *et al.* 1988; Boylan *et al.* 2004). When necessary, phenobarbital or phenytoin are given in maintenance doses and serum levels are monitored. Due to the high incidence of electromechanical dissociation, confirmation of seizure control with a repeat EEG is recommended.

There are no well-established criteria for discontinuation of maintenance AED therapy. Some advocate a short duration of therapy of 1 week while others recommend 12 months following the latest seizure. Another schedule recommends 2 weeks of therapy beyond the last clinical seizure along with a seizure-free EEG.

References

ACOG (American College of Obstetricians and Gynecologists' Task Force on Neonatal Encephalopathy and Cerebral Plan, the American College of Obstetricians and Gynecologist, the American Academy of Pediatrics) (2003) *Neonatal Encephalopathy and Cerebral Palsy: Defining the Pathogenesis and Pathophysiology.* Washington, DC: American College of Obstetricians and Gynecologists.

Aicardi J, Goutières F (1978) Encéphalopathie myoclonique néonatale. *Rev Electroencephalogr Neurophysiol Clin* **8**:99–101.

Boylan GB, Rennie JM, Chorley G, *et al.* (2004) Second-line anticonvulsant treatment of neonatal seizures: a video-EEG monitoring study. *Neurology* **10**:486–8.

Chapman KE, Mizrahi EM, Clancy RR (2010) Neonatal seizures. In: Wyllie E, Cascino GD, Gidal B, Goodkin H (eds.) *Wyllie's Treatment of Epilepsy: Principles and Practice*, 5th edn. Philadelphia, PA: Lippincott Williams and Wilkins, pp. 405–27.

Clancy RR, Legido A (1987) The exact ictal and interictal duration of electroencephalographic neonatal seizures. *Epilepsia* **28**:537–41.

Clancy R, Malin S, Laraque D, Baumgart S, Younkin D (1985) Focal motor seizures heralding stroke in full-term neonates. *Am J Dis Child* **139**:601–6.

Coker SB (1992) Post-neonatal vitamin B6-dependent epilepsy. *Pediatrics* **90**:221–3.

Cooper EC, Jan LY (1998) Ion channel genes and human neurological disease: recent progress prospects and challenges. *Proc Natl Acad Sci USA* **96**:4759–66.

Dedek K, Kunath B, Kananura C, *et al.* (2001) Myokymia and neonatal epilepsy caused by a mutation in the voltage sensor of the *KCNQ2* K^+ channel. *Proc Natl Acad Sci USA* **98**:12 272–7.

deVeber G, Andrew M, Adams C, *et al.* (2001) Cerebral sinovenous thrombosis in children. *N Engl J Med* **345**:417–23.

De Vivo DC, Trifiletti RR, Jacobson RI, *et al.* (1991) Defective glucose transport across the blood–brain barrier as a cause of persistent hypoglycorrhachia, seizures and developmental delay. *N Engl J Med* **325**:703–9.

Djukic A, Lado FA, Shinnar S, Moshé SL (2006) Are early myoclonic encephalopathy (EME) and the Ohtahara syndrome (EIEE) independent of each other? *Epilepsy Res* **70**:68–76.

Dreyfus-Brisac C, Monod N (1964) Electroclinical studies of status epilepticus and convulsions in the newborn. In: Kellaway P, Petersén I (eds.) *Neurological and Electroencephalographic Correlative Studies in Infancy*. New York: Grune and Stratton, pp. 250–72.

Durham SR, Clancy RR, Leuthardt E, *et al.* (2000) CHOP Infant Coma Scale ("infant face scale"): a novel coma scale for children less than two years of age. *J Neurotrauma* **17**:729–37.

Ellenberg JH, Nelson KB (1988) Cluster of perinatal events identifying infants at high risk for death or disability. *J Pediatr* **113**:546–52.

Hellström-Westas L, Westgren U, Rosen I, Svenningsen NW (1988) Lidocaine for treatment of severe seizures in newborn infants. I. Clinical effects and cerebral electrical activity monitoring. *Acta Paediatr Scand* **77**:79–84.

Holmes GL, Lombroso CT (1993) Prognostic value of background patterns in the neonatal EEG. *J Clin Neurophysiol* **10**:323–52.

International League Against Epilepsy (1989) Commission on Classification and Terminology: Proposal for revised clinical and classification of epilepsies and epileptic syndromes. *Epilepsia* **30**:389–99.

Kellaway P, Hrachovy RA (1983) Status epilepticus in newborns: a perspective on neonatal seizures. *Adv Neurol* **34**:93–9.

Kellaway P, Mizrahi EM (1987) Neonatal seizures. In: Luders H, Lesser RP (eds.) *Epilepsy: Electroclinical Syndromes*. New York: Springer-Verlag, pp. 13–47.

Lago P, Rebsamen S, Clancy RR, *et al.* (1995) MRI, MRA and neurodevelopmental outcome following neonatal ECMO. *Pediatr Neurol* **12**:294–304.

Laroia N, Guillet R, Burchfiel J, McBride MC (1998) EEG background as predictor of electrographic seizures in high-risk neonates. *Epilepsia* **39**:545.

Mizrahi EM (2010) Neonatal seizures. In: Panayiotopoulos CP (ed.) *The Atlas of Epilepsies*. London: Springer-Verlag, in press.

Mizrahi EM, Clancy RR (2000) Neonatal seizure: early-onset seizure syndromes and their consequences for development. *Ment Retard Dev Disabil Res Rev* **6**:229–41.

Mizrahi EM, Kellaway P (1987) Characterization and classification of neonatal seizures. *Neurology* **37**:1837–44.

Mizrahi EM, Kellaway P (1998) *Diagnosis and Management of Neonatal Seizures.* Philadelphia, PA: Lippincott-Raven.

Mizrahi EM, Clancy R, Dunn JK, *et al.* (2001) Neurologic impairment, developmental delay and post-natal seizures two years after video-EEG documented seizures in near-term and full-term neonates: report of the Clinical Research Centers for Neonatal Seizures. *Epilepsia* **102**:47.

Mizrahi EM, Hrachovy RA, Kellaway P (2003) *Atlas of Neonatal Electroencephalography,* 3rd edn. Philadelphia, PA: Lippincott Williams and Wilkins, pp. 189–240.

Nelson DL (2006) NEMO, NFκB signalling and incontinentia pigmenti. *Curr Opin Genet Dev* **16**:282–8.

Ohtahara S, Yamatogi Y (2003) Epileptic encephalopathies in early infancy with suppression-burst. *J Clin Neurophysiol* **20**:499–509.

Ohtahara S, Ohstsuka Y, Yamatogi Y, Oka E, Inoue H (1992) Early-infantile epileptic encephalophatty with suppression-bursts. In: Roger J, Bureau M, Dravet C, Dreifuss FE, Perret A, Wolf PI (eds.) *Epileptic Syndromes in Infancy, Childhood and Adolescence*, 2nd edn. London: John Libbey, pp. 25–34.

Ortibus EL, Sum JM, Hahn JS (1996) Predictive value of EEG for outcome and epilepsy following neonatal seizures. *Electroencephalogr Clin Neurophysiol* **98**:175–85.

Perlman JM, Rollins NK, Evans D (1994) Neonatal stroke: clinical characteristics and cerebral blood flow velocity measurements. *Pediatr Neurol* **11**:281–4.

Phelan JP, Korst LM, Ahn MO, Martin GL (1998) Neonatal nucleated red blood cell and lymphocyte counts in fetal brain injury. *Obstet Gynecol* **91**:485–9.

Pisani F, Barilli AL, Sisti L, Bevilacqua G, Seri S (2008) Preterm infants with video-EEG confirmed seizures: outcome at 30 months of age. *Brain Dev* **30**:20–30.

Plouin P, Anderson VE (2005) Benign familial and non-familial neonatal seizures. In: Roger J, Bureau M, Dravet C, Genton P, Tassinari CA, Wolf P (eds.) *Epileptic Syndromes in Infancy, Childhood and Adolescence*, 4th edn. Montrouge, France: John Libbey Eurotext, pp. 3–16.

Quattlebaum TG (1979) Benign familial convulsions in the neonatal period and early infancy. *J Pediatr* **95**:257–9.

Ronen GM, Rosales TO, Connolly ME, Anderson VE, Leppert M (1993) Seizure characteristics in chromosome 20 benign familial neonatal convulsions. *Neurology* **43**:1355–60.

Scher MS, Aso K, Berggarly ME, *et al.* (1993) Electrographic seizures in pre-term and full-term neonates: clinical correlates, associated brain lesions, and risk for neurologic sequelae. *Pediatrics* **91**:128–34.

Sheth RD, Buckley DJ, Gutierrez AR, *et al.* (1996) Midazolam in the treatment of refractory neonatal seizures. *Clin Neuropharm* **19**:165–70.

Tharp BR (2002) Neonatal seizures and syndromes. *Epilepsia* **43**:2–10.

Torres OA, Miller VS, Buist NM, Hyland K (1999) Folinic acid-responsive neonatal seizures. *J Child Neurol* **14**:529–32.

Volpe JJ (1973) Neonatal seizures. *N Engl J Med* **289**:413–16.

Volpe JJ (2008) *Neurology of the Newborn*, 5th edn. Philadelphia, PA: WB Saunders.

Watanabe K, Miura K, Natsume J, *et al.* (1999) Epilepsies of neonatal onset: seizure type and evolution. *Dev Med Child Neurol* **41**:318–22.

Chapter

55

Cerebral palsy

Sameer M. Zuberi and Andreas Brunklaus

The causal disease

Definitions and epidemiology

Cerebral palsy (CP) affects between 2 and 3 per 1000 live births and is thought to be the most common cause of serious physical disability in childhood (SCPE 2000). The definition and classification of cerebral palsy is not straightforward and remains an area of debate and controversy. Martin Bax's elegant 1964 definition describes cerebral palsy as "a dynamic disorder of posture and movement caused by a non-progressive defect or lesion of the developing brain." A developmental perspective is key to understanding cerebral palsy and one of its strongest associations, epilepsy.

William Little in his 1843 lecture to the Orthopaedic Institution of London on "The deformities of the human frame" noted that epilepsy could adversely affect the already vulnerable child with CP. Recent studies have emphasized that epileptic seizures can impact on behavior and cognition, and impair the ability to thrive, learn, and develop in individuals with CP (Carlsson *et al.* 2008). Optimal seizure management is therefore very important to allow an individual to achieve their full developmental potential and improve their quality of life.

The brain continues to develop into adult life but epidemiological studies of CP tend to use the term infancy or 1, 2, or 4 years of postnatal life as cut-offs for research purposes. In reality an 8-month fetus, a 6-month-old infant, and a 3-year-old child could each suffer a left middle cerebral artery territory infarction for different reasons and could all reasonably be said to have CP. However, with the technologies and knowledge available to the twenty-first-century physician, it is not satisfactory to simply say a child has cerebral palsy. The CP should be qualified in terms of the nature of the motor impairment, the etiology, and any associated problems.

A recent international workshop on definition and classification of cerebral palsy emphasized this point (Rosenbaum *et al.* 2007):

Cerebral palsy (CP) describes a group of permanent disorders of the development of movement and posture, causing activity

limitations, that are attributed to non-progressive disturbances that occurred in the developing fetal or infant brain. The motor disorders of cerebral palsy are often accompanied by disturbances of sensation, perception, cognition, communication, and behavior; by epilepsy, and by secondary musculoskeletal problems.

Pathology, physiology, and clinical features

In a study of 217 cases of CP a single etiology was identified in 66% cases with a further 16% having two major causes of the brain lesion (Shevell *et al.* 2003). The figure of 82% with defined etiologies will increase as further metabolic and genetic lesions are described. The manifestations of CP are the result of the injury to the brain and its subsequent repair processes. This will be influenced by many interacting processes, including the nature of the primary injury (e.g., inflammation, ischemia), the stage of brain development, the nutritional status of the child, and the degree of secondary injury. These causal pathways interact in complex ways to produce the final outcome (Stanley *et al.* 2000). For example ischemia, with or without cytokine-mediated inflammation in the premature infant, may result in periventricular leukomalacia and a spastic diplegic CP, whereas a short-duration but profound hypoxic–ischemic insult at term may result in basal ganglia injury with sparing of the cerebral cortex resulting in a dyskinetic/athetoid CP (Shapiro 2004).

Clinically CP is best classified using both the etiology of the injury and the topography of the motor disorder. The etiologies of CP can be grouped into prenatal, perinatal, and postnatal causes (Table 55.1). Stroke, infection, and inflammation are important etiologies in all groups. Despite the common misconception to the contrary it is important to acknowledge that only 10–12% of CP is likely to be associated with intrapartum asphyxia (Shevell *et al.* 2003).

A widely used topographical classification of CP has been formulated by the Surveillance of Cerebral Palsy in Europe group. This divides CP into spastic, dyskinetic, and ataxic subtypes. The spastic subtype is further divided into unilateral

The Causes of Epilepsy, eds. S. D. Shorvon, F. Andermann, and R. Guerrini. Published by Cambridge University Press. © Cambridge University Press 2011.

Table 55.1 Risk factors associated with cerebral palsy

Prenatal
Congenital infections
Stroke
Toxemia
Placental abruption, uterine/placental dysfunction
Chromosomal abnormalities
Cerebral malformations, malformation of cortical development
Perinatal
Hypoxic–ischemic encephalopathy
Kernicterus
Trauma
Perinatal infection
Periventricular leukomalacia in very preterm children
Postnatal
Infection
Post-infectious/immune-mediated encephalopathy
Trauma (non-accidental and accidental head injury)
Stroke
Hydrocephalus

Table 55.2 Classification of cerebral palsy subtypes

Subtype (frequency)[a]	Motor component	Common etiologies
Unilateral spastic (32%)	Persisting increased muscle tone in one or more limbs	Vascular, polyventricular leukomalacia, cerebral dysgenesis, asphyxia
Hemiplegic Bilateral spastic (57%)	Persisting increased muscle tone in one or more limbs	Diplegia: polyventricular leukomalacia, hemorrhage asphyxia, toxins
Diplegic or tetraplegic		Tetraplegia: asphyxia, polyventricular leukomalacia, cerebral dysgenesis, hemorrhage, infection
Dyskinetic (7%)	Dystonic: reduced activity and increased tone	Asphyxia, toxins
Dystonic or choreo-athetotic	Choreo-athetotic: increased activity and decreased tone	
Ataxic (4%)	Generalized hypotonia and ataxia	Cerebral dysgenesis

Note:
[a]Beckung *et al.* (2008).

and bilateral types (SCPE 2000). Table 55.2 lists the CP subtypes with frequencies, main motor components, and underlying etiologies. The spastic subtypes are most clearly linked with vascular territory/ischemic lesions identified on brain imaging. Dyskinetic CP, characterized by athetosis, implies a primary basal ganglia injury. Many children will have mixed dyskinetic and spastic CP but in these children the dyskinesia is primarily dystonic in nature.

The term ataxic cerebral palsy is not one that I use with confidence. It is a diagnostic label often employed when the physician hasn't really made a diagnosis. Most of these children have genetic or metabolic disorders. Children with Angelman syndrome are commonly mislabeled as having ataxic cerebral palsy.

Epilepsy in cerebral palsy
Frequency of epilepsy in cerebral palsy

In a recent literature review Odding *et al.* reported that the overall epilepsy prevalence in CP was 22–40% and was highest among the group with tetraplegia (19–36%) and hemiplegia (28–35%) and lower among the diplegic (14%), dyskinetic/athetoid (8–13%), and ataxic groups (13–16%) (Odding *et al.* 2006). Of children with tetraplegic cerebral palsy and severe

learning disability 94% have epilepsy. Carlsson *et al.* (2003) found that seizure onset tended to be earlier in children with tetraplegic CP starting at a median age of 6 months, whereas the onset in diplegic and hemiplegic CP was later at 1 year, and 2 years 6 months respectively. The occurrence of epilepsy varied with etiology. Children with CP due to central nervous system (CNS) malformation, infection, and gray matter damage were more likely to have epilepsy than those with CP due to white matter damage (Carlsson *et al.* 2003).

Risk factors

Factors associated with an in increased risk of developing epilepsy in children with CP include low birth weight, perinatal asphyxia, periventricular leukomalacia (PVL), neonatal seizures, microcephaly, developmental delay, severity of CP, and abnormal neuroimaging (Kulak and Sobaniec 2003; Venkateswaran and Shevell 2008).

Several studies have shown a higher than expected frequency of epilepsy in first-degree relatives of children with CP, emphasizing the importance of background genetic predisposition in individuals with lesional epilepsies (Arpino *et al.* 1999; Kulak & Sobaniec 2003).

Types of epilepsy, specific characteristics, and treatment and prognosis

All seizure types can occur in individuals with CP. The predominant type is focal seizures or focal seizures evolving into secondary generalized tonic–clonic (GTC) seizures. Even when children with CP present with generalized seizures, electroencephalogram (EEG) recordings confirm that the majority have a focal onset. Epilepsy syndromes including subtypes of idiopathic generalized epilepsy may present in children with CP as in the general population. It is therefore important to classify the epilepsy syndrome correctly in order to choose the appropriate treatment (Aksu 1990; Carlsson et al. 2003).

Gururaj et al. (2003) compared the course of epilepsy among 56 children with and 50 children without CP. This study demonstrated that seizures start significantly earlier in the CP group, with up to 79% developing epilepsy in the first year of life and only 9% presenting after their fifth birthday. The earlier the onset of epilepsy, the higher the seizure frequency tends to be. The principal seizure types among individuals with CP were partial (39%), GTC (32%), myoclonic (14%), and infantile spasms (5%). The risk of status epilepticus was eight times greater among the CP group: 34% compared to 4% in controls (Gururaj et al. 2003). The majority of individuals with hemiplegic CP tend to have focal seizures, whereas other CP forms can present with a mixture of different seizure types.

Treatment success will often depend on the underlying etiology. Carlson et al. (2003) found that after 6 years of follow-up children with white matter damage had a 58% chance of becoming seizure-free compared to a 15% chance of seizure freedom in a group including children with CP due to a CNS malformation, CNS infection, and gray matter damage. Overall, good seizure control – defined as seizure freedom for at least 12 months – can be achieved in up to one-third of all children with CP and the chance of becoming seizure-free will increase with time and continues to improve beyond childhood (Odding et al. 2006).

More than half of all affected children are on two or more antiepileptic drugs (AEDs) and are likely to remain on medication in the long term. Discontinuation of medication after 2 years of seizure freedom can only be achieved in a minority of cases and relapse rates in the first 12 months are reported to be as high as 62%, more so in spastic hemiplegia and less in other CP types (Delgado et al. 1996).

More than 70% of individuals with spastic tetraplegia have intractable epilepsy despite polytherapy. Infantile spasms and myoclonic seizures are common in this group and typically refractory to treatment (Gururaj et al. 2003). Seizure control in children with hemiplegic CP and spastic diplegia can be achieved in up to 73% and 83% respectively (Kulak and Sobaniec 2003).

The incidence of epilepsy in pure dyskinetic CP is relatively low. If an individual with this subtype presents with frequent epileptic seizures the clinician should ensure adequate neuroimaging and consider the possibility of a neurometabolic disorder. The incidence of CP in children with tetraplegia and mixed spastic dystonic CP is high.

Reflex epilepsies including startle epileptic seizures and eating epilepsy occur in tetraplegic and hemiplegic CP. Startle seizures are induced by sudden unexpected stimuli such as sound or touch and result in brief mainly generalized tonic or myoclonic seizures. Seizure frequency is usually high (>10 per day) and can sometimes progress to status epilepticus (Tibussek et al. 2006).

It is important to consider electrical status epilepticus in sleep (ESES) as a possibility in a child or adolescent with CP who has regression of cognitive function. Recent reports suggest that up to one-third of children presenting with ESES have underlying structural brain anomalies. Cognitive deterioration evolves into permanent deficit in up to one-half of these patients (Dorris et al. 2005; Kramer et al. 2008).

Odding et al. (2006) found evidence that when epileptic seizures are frequent, already impaired cognitive abilities are further compromised. Poorly controlled epilepsy can affect the motor performance of ambulant children so they lose skills and become non-ambulant, and their quality of life diminishes. In non-ambulant children refractory seizures can affect posture thus increasing the risk of scoliosis.

Diagnostic tests for cerebral palsy

A correct diagnosis allows implementation of adequate treatment strategies, guidance on how to manage complications, and prognostic information. Risks of recurrence can be assessed, thus aiding genetic counseling, and further unnecessary investigations can be avoided.

There are a number of diseases that are characterized by a movement disorder and epilepsy and can therefore mimic CP (Table 55.3). The major challenge for the clinician is to identify disorders with specific treatments, disorders with risks of recurrence, and progressive neurological disorders. This is primarily done through a meticulous history, including family history, and examination. Clinical examination in the epilepsy clinic is unlikely to help diagnose epilepsy but it is invaluable in diagnosing the cause of the epilepsy. Some disorders are very slowly progressive therefore serial video recordings by the parent and physician can be very helpful. Significant variability in symptoms may be a clue to dopa-responsive dystonia or glucose transporter (GLUT1) deficiency. The latter is an important treatable cause of a motor disorder and epilepsy and can be diagnosed with a fasting lumbar puncture and appropriate genetic investigations (Wang et al. 2005). Treatable disorders also include serine biosynthetic disorders and guanidinoacetate N-methyltransferase (GAMT) deficiency. It has been estimated that 5% of CP cases have an identifiable underlying genetic or metabolic etiology; however, this is likely to be an underestimate and the figure will be greater as new

Table 55.3 Inherited metabolic and genetic disorders

Metabolic disorders masquerading as cerebral palsy
Glutaric aciduria (type 1)
Lesch–Nyhan syndrome
3-Methyl-glutaconic aciduria
Pyruvate dehydrogenase deficiency
Argininemia
Cytochrome oxidase deficiency
Succinic semialdehyde dehydrogenase deficiency
Female carriers of ornithine transcarbamylase deficiency
Other neurological disorders imitating cerebral palsy
Dopa-responsive dystonia
Hereditary spastic paraplegia
Ataxia telangiectasia
Disorders with cerebral palsy and epilepsy
Pelizaeus–Merzbacher disease
Aicardi–Goutière syndrome
Serine biosynthesis deficiency
GAMT deficiency
GLUT1 deficiency syndrome

genetic techniques such as array comparative genomic hybridization (CGH) identify microchromosomal lesions, and new metabolic disorders are described (Mantovani 2007).

Role of neuroimaging

The majority of CP etiologies can be established based on a detailed history, examination, and neuroimaging without the need for other investigations. Magnetic resonance imaging (MRI) is the imaging modality of choice and if there is any doubt about potential metabolic etiologies proton magnetic resonance spectroscopy (MRS) should be performed at the same time. The major concern relating to neuroimaging in early childhood is the need to sedate or anesthetize the child in order to obtain good-quality images and whether this can be justified; for example in a child with a non-progressive congenital hemiplegia. Unless there is an obvious cause for an individual's motor impairment our view is that, with informed consent from carers, an anesthetic is justified. Neuroimaging patterns are not always specific and lesions that appear at first sight ischemic or inflammatory in origin may also be caused by a variety of genetic or neurometabolic disorders. If clinical signs progress imaging may need to be repeated.

A meta-analysis of MRI studies including 682 children with all forms of CP showed abnormalities in an average of 89% of cases (Russman and Ashwal 2004). The yield varied depending on the type of CP, with ataxic CP being the lowest at 75% and all other types of CP reaching a 94–100% yield of diagnosis. Russman and Ashwal (2004) also demonstrated that MRI was helpful in determining the timing of the injury, indicating that the injury was prenatal in 37% of cases, perinatal in 35%, and postnatal in 4% of cases.

The American Academy of Neurology has recommended that neuroimaging should be performed in all children unless an etiological cause for the CP has already been obtained through previous imaging, e.g., in the neonatal period (Ashwal et al. 2004).

Role of electroencephalography

The EEG should be interpreted with caution in individuals with structural brain lesions such as in CP. Underlying structural defects are highly likely to produce slow wave abnormalities, sharp waves and spike–wave complexes on the surface EEG. Kulak and Sobaniec (2003) reported abnormal EEG recordings in 74% of individuals with CP who did not have epilepsy. This figure rose to 93% in those with CP and epilepsy.

The American Academy of Neurology has recommended that "an EEG should be obtained when a child with CP has a history or examination features suggesting the presence of epilepsy or an epileptic syndrome, but not to determine the etiology of CP" (Ashwal et al. 2004).

We think a more pragmatic case-by-case approach is justified. If a child presents with left-sided focal epileptic seizures and has a left hemiplegia with a known MRI lesion suggesting a right middle cerebral artery infarct then an interictal EEG is unlikely to add useful information. If the same child presents with absences then an EEG can be justified. If the child presents with epileptic seizures, cognitive decline, and/or new behavioral problems then a 24-hr ambulatory or video-EEG to capture sleeping and waking rhythms and look for ESES is justified. If the epilepsy proves refractory to treatment then an EEG to capture events, ideally video-EEG, is justified.

Children with CP and learning difficulties may present with behavioral stereotypies and movement disorders that may be difficult to classify and an EEG with video recording can be helpful in this situation.

Differential diagnosis of epilepsy in cerebral palsy

Individuals with CP can have all the non-epileptic paroxysmal phenomena that occur in the general population; however, they are more likely to have a mixture of both epileptic and non-epileptic events (Stephenson 1990; Zuberi 2008). Common phenomena such as vasovagal syncope, breath-holding attacks, and reflex anoxic seizures can occur in this group. The incidence of learning disability and communication disorders is high in individuals with CP; therefore behavioral stereotypies including hand-flapping, repetitive vocalizations, and compulsive valsalvas are frequently seen.

When a child with CP has an increase in seizure frequency, and particularly when the nature of the events change, the possibility of non-epileptic phenomena should be considered. There is a high incidence of psychological morbidity in adolescents with hemiplegia, and pseudoseizures can present in this group (Goodman & Graham 1996).

Dyskinesia should not be difficult to distinguish from epileptic seizures except in the context of a child with mixed spastic and dystonic tetraplegic CP who has paroxysmal attacks of dyskinesia caused by painful gastroesophageal reflux – the Sandifer syndrome (Werlin et al. 1980). These events can involve facial dyskinesia, torsional dystonia of the neck and trunk, dystonic extension of limbs and head, and eye deviation. A trial of anti-reflux therapy can be justified to aid diagnosis.

Forced cramped synchronized movements are episodes of extension at the knees and flexion of the hips which can mimic epileptic spasms (Ferrari et al. 2002). They may be the first sign of an evolving spastic diplegia.

Easily reproducible clonus should not be a diagnostic difficulty but differentiating epileptic and non-epileptic myoclonus may require video-EEG. Non-epileptic startle as a response to a sudden unexpected stimulus, particularly noise and touch, is frequently observed in individuals with tetraplegia and less commonly hemiplegia.

Sleep starts, also known as hypnic or hypnagogic jerks, are non-epileptic jerks or spasms, which can occur in all individuals in the early stages of light sleep but they are more common in the neurologically impaired (Fusco et al. 1999).

Principles of management

The basic principles of treatment of epilepsy in CP are similar to those for the general population including using particular medications for specific seizure types and syndromes. If the family and individual choose treatment then AEDs, dietary treatments, surgical treatments, and vagal nerve stimulator (VNS) treatment are all options that should be available. The evidence base for specific treatment options in CP is not of high quality; therefore the opinions expressed here are largely of the first author and based on clinical experience.

The choice for early treatment rather than a "wait and see" approach can be influenced by the strong likelihood of recurrent epileptic seizures and lower chance of spontaneous remission than the general population. A single AED should be commenced in the lowest possible dose to achieve control with a plan for incremental increase if necessary. Treatment with two AEDs is common. Treatment with three may occur when improved control is achieved as one AED is gradually replacing another and a family decides they do not want to change that particular combination. The risks of side effects increase with polypharmacy and should be balanced against trying to seek seizure freedom when that is not a realistic prospect.

When epileptic seizures begin in the first year of life they often accompany features of the developing motor disorder such as dystonia or myoclonus. Small doses of nitrazepam may be effective for both problems. Clinical experience, but little evidence, suggests that vigabatrin may be effective in children who have malformations of cortical development. This should be balanced against the known side effect of this medication on visual fields. West syndrome can present at a few months in infants who have a brain injury from a hypoxic–ischemic encephalopathy at term. Vigabatrin, steroids, and adrenocorticotropic hormone are the treatments of choice in most European countries for children with and without CP.

Lesional focal epileptic seizures are the commonest seizure type in CP. Carbamazepine is usually the first-line medication but sodium valproate, lamotrigine, and oxcarbazepine as well as many other AEDs are reasonable options. Valproate should be used with caution in infants particularly if there is any suspicion of an undiagnosed metabolic disorder.

Myoclonic seizures may be responsive to sodium valproate, benzodiazepines, and levetiracetam. Conversely, carbamazepine, phenytoin, and vigabatrin have the potential to aggravate epileptic myoclonus. Startle seizures respond best to benzodiazepines (clobazam/clonazepam), carbamazepine, and lamotrigine (Manford et al. 1996; Faught 1999).

Rescue medication (along with a written plan) should be prescribed for individuals with prolonged seizures or clusters of seizures. Buccal or nasal midazolam is our first-line rescue medication. If a diagnosis of ESES is made we may commence a regular night-time dose of clobazam followed by repeat 24-hr EEG and repeat neuropsychological evaluation.

Recent reports suggest that bone health in individuals with epilepsy and CP might be affected by the enzyme-inducing AEDs phenytoin, phenobarbitone, and carbamazepine as well as valproate (Sheth et al. 1995; Verrotti et al. 2002). It is reasonable to consider vitamin D and calcium supplementation in non-ambulant children who may be at highest risk of osteopenia and fractures.

The ketogenic diet should be regarded as a treatment option earlier rather than waiting for the individual to have tried multiple AEDs. If the child is gastrostomy-fed then liquid preparations of the diet with added vitamins and mineral supplements are available and straightforward to administer. Computer programs, increasing numbers of recipes, and peer support from parent groups make the diet much less of a challenge for families than in the past.

Epilepsy surgery can have a good outcome particularly for children with hemiplegia. Surgery does not necessarily harm the motor performance of children (van Empelen et al. 2005). In certain conditions such as Sturge–Weber syndrome it may prevent progression of the epileptic encephalopathy.

If seizures are poorly controlled it may be more difficult for the family to obtain respite care. To ensure the best possible outcome it is imperative to achieve optimal seizure control and recognize the family's needs, and for the physician to work closely within a multidisciplinary team of allied professionals.

References

Aksu F (1990) Nature and prognosis of seizures in patients with cerebral palsy. *Dev Med Child Neurol* **32**:661–8.

Arpino C, Curatolo P, Stazi MA, Pellegri A, Vlahov D (1999) Differing risk factors for cerebral palsy in the presence of mental retardation and epilepsy. *J Child Neurol* **14**:151–5.

Ashwal S, Russman BS, Blasco PA, *et al.* (2004) Practice parameter: diagnostic assessment of the child with cerebral palsy. *Neurology* **62**:851–63.

Bax MCO (1964) Terminology and classification of cerebral palsy. *Dev Med Child Neurol* **6**:295–307.

Beckung E, Hagberg G, Uldall P, *et al.* (2008) Probability of walking in children with cerebral palsy in Europe. *Pediatrics* **121**: e187–e192.

Carlsson M, Hagberg G, Olsson I (2003) Clinical and etiological aspects of epilepsy in children with cerebral palsy. *Dev Med Child Neurol* **45**:371–6.

Carlsson M, Olsson I, Hagberg G, Beckung E (2008) Behavior in children with cerebral palsy with and without epilepsy. *Dev Med Child Neurol* **50**:784–9.

Delgado MR, Riela AR, Mills J, Pitt A, Browne R (1996) Discontinuation of antiepileptic drug therapy after two seizure-free years in children with cerebral palsy. *Pediatrics* **97**:192–7.

Dorris L, Zuberi SM, Wilson M, O'Regan ME (2005) Electrical status epilepticus during slow sleep (ESES): an important cause of childhood dementia. *Epilepsia* **46**(Suppl 1):151.

Faught E (1999) Lamotrigine for startle-induced seizures. *Seizure* **8**:361–3.

Ferrari F, Cioni G, Einspieler C, *et al.* (2002) Cramped synchronized general movements in preterm infants as an early marker for cerebral palsy. *Arch Pediatr Adolesc Med* **156**:460–7.

Fusco L, Pachatz C, Cusmai R, Vigevano F (1999) Repetitive sleep starts in neurologically impaired children: an unusual non-epileptic manifestation in otherwise epileptic subjects. *Epilept Disord* **1**:63–7.

Goodman R, Graham P (1996) Psychiatric problems in children with hemiplegia: cross sectional epidemiological survey. *Br Med J* **312**:1065–9.

Gururaj AK, Sztriha L, Bener A, Dawodu A, Eapen V (2003) Epilepsy in children with cerebral palsy. *Seizure* **12**:110–14.

Kramer U, Sagi L, Goldberg-Stern H, *et al.* (2008) Clinical spectrum and medical treatment of children with electrical status epilepticus in sleep (ESES). *Epilepsia* **50**:1517–24.

Kulak W, Sobaniec W (2003) Risk factors and prognosis of epilepsy in children with cerebral palsy in north-eastern Poland. *Brain Dev* **27**:499–506.

Little WJ (1843) Course of lectures on the deformities of the human frame. *Lancet* **41**:318–22.

Manford MR, Fish DR, Shorvon SD (1996) Startle provoked epileptic seizures: features in 19 patients. *J Neurol Neurosurg Psychiatry* **61**:151–6.

Mantovani JF (2007) Classification of cerebral palsy: clinical genetic perspective. *Dev Med Child Neurol* **49**(Suppl 109):26–7.

Odding E, Roebroeck ME, Stam HJ (2006) The epidemiology of cerebral palsy: incidence, impairments and risk factors. *Disabil Rehab* **28**:183–91.

Rosenbaum P, Paneth N, Leviton A, *et al.* (2007) A report: the definition and classification of cerebral palsy April 2006. *Dev Med Child Neurol.* **49**(Suppl 109):8–14.

Russman BS, Ashwal S (2004) Evaluation of the child with cerebral palsy. *Semin Pediatr Neurol* **11**:47–57.

Shapiro BK (2004) Cerebral palsy: a reconceptualization of the spectrum. *J Pediatr* **145**:S3–7.

Sheth RD, Wesolowski CA, Jacob JC, *et al.* (1995) Effect of carbamazepine and valproate on bone mineral density. *J Pediatr* **127**:256–62.

Shevell MI, Majnemer A, Morin I (2003) Etiologic yield of cerebral palsy: a contemporary case series. *Pediatr Neurol* **28**:352–9.

Stanley F, Blair E, Alberman E (2000) *Cerebral Palsies: Epidemiology and Causal Pathways.* London: MacKeith Press.

Stephenson JBP (1990) *Fits and Faints.* London: MacKeith Press.

Surveillance of Cerebral Palsy in Europe (2000) Surveillance of cerebral palsy in Europe (SCPE): a collaboration of cerebral palsy surveys and registers. *Dev Med Child Neurol* **42**:816–24.

Tibussek D, Wohlrab G, Boltshauser E, Schmitt B (2006) Proven startle-provoked epileptic seizures in childhood: semiologic and electrophysiologic variability. *Epilepsia* **47**:1050–8.

van Empelen R, Jennekens-Schinkel A, Gorter JW, *et al.* (2005) Dutch Collaborative Epilepsy Surgery Programme: epilepsy surgery does not harm motor performance of children and adolescents. *Brain* **128**:1536–45.

Venkateswaran S, Shevell MI (2008) Comorbidities and clinical determinants of outcome in children with spastic quadriplegic cerebral palsy. *Dev Med Child Neurol* **50**:216–22.

Verrotti A, Greco R, Latini G, Morgese G, Chiarelli F (2002) Increased bone turnover in prepubertal, pubertal, and postpubertal patients receiving carbamazepine. *Epilepsia* **43**:1488–92.

Wang D, Pascual JM, Yang H, *et al.* (2005) Glut-1 deficiency syndrome: clinical, genetic, and therapeutic aspects. *Ann Neurol* **57**:111–18.

Werlin SL, D'Souza BJ, Hogan WJ, Dodds WJ, Arndorfer RC (1980) Sandifer syndrome: an unappreciated clinical entity. *Dev Med Child Neurol* **22**:374–8.

Zuberi SM (2008) The differential diagnosis of epilepsy. In: Prasher VP, Kerr MP (eds.) *Epilepsy and Intellectual Disabilities.* London: Springer-Verlag, pp. 61–84.

Chapter

56

Vaccination and immunization

Simon D. Shorvon

Vaccination is one of medicine's most successful interventions. It has eradicated some very serious diseases and hugely reduced the levels of others. In England for instance, small-pox deaths fell from 196 per million in 1850–69 to 26 per million in 1885–94 after only 20 years of a vaccination campaign (Glynn and Glynn 2005), and this disease which was the scourge of the world has now been completely abolished. Similar extraordinary successes are recorded for polio and measles.

Perhaps surprisingly, then, throughout its history, there has been public concern about its safety – a concern frankly disproportionate in terms of risk/benefit when compared to public reaction about other therapies. The reasons are complex, and include fear of coercion (especially by politicians, scientists, and the pharmaceutical industry), a feeling that vaccination is unnatural and spiritually polluting, that side effects are not recognized, that commercial greed is the real driver of vaccination campaigns, and even that vaccination is a devious political plot (Cohen 1976; Allen 2007; Shorvon and Berg 2008). The most feared side effect is encephalopathy and the resulting long-term brain damage and epilepsy. The chances of this happening are very small.

Epilepsy can be caused by vaccination as a leading symptom of vaccine-induced encephalopathy and febrile seizures can also occur as a result of vaccine-induced fever. The vaccine most studied is the pertussis vaccine and it is this vaccine which has been most linked to cases of post-vaccination encephalopathy.

Pertussis vaccination

In the pre-vaccination era, pertussis (whooping cough) was a highly prevalent and sometimes fatal disease. In the USA, for instance, between 1922 and 1931, about 17 million cases of whooping cough were reported and there were 73 000 deaths. It was estimated to cause encephalopathy, with epilepsy a prominent feature, at a frequency of 0.08–0.8 per 1000 cases – in other words, about 1 case per 1200–12 000

infections (US Institute of Medicine 1991; Committee on Infectious Diseases 1996; Geier and Geier 2002). The risk of encephalopathy following pertussis is highest in neonates and infants.

Vaccine preparation was begun as early as 1906, and early vaccines carried a significant risk of encephalopathy and were optional and not widely taken up. In 1942, the first modern whole-cell vaccine, which was combined with vaccines against diphtheria and tetanus, was produced (the DTP or DPT vaccine). It was effective and by the mid-1960s, compulsory vaccination was practiced in several countries. The endotoxin in the early whole-cell vaccines resulted in an immediate minor, but to parents alarming, febrile reaction in most children, and in some a febrile seizure. It was then reported that a more severe *vaccine-related encephalopathy* might occur, resulting in severe epilepsy, mental regression, and lifelong disability. These reports of vaccine-induced encephalopathy caused serious public alarm and this prompted the setting up of the National Childhood Encephalopathy Study (NCES) in 1976 in Britain. The NCES was the first and is still the largest prospective case–control study aimed at assessing the risk of vaccine-induced encephalopathy. The study attempted, through active surveillance, to ascertain all children who were admitted to hospital with a severe childhood brain disease and to establish whether there was a temporal association with pertussis vaccination. The children were compared to two randomly selected controls matched for age, sex, and area of residence. Outcome was assessed up to 18 months, and there were 5.4 million child–years of observation after over 2 million doses of DTP vaccine. A total of 1182 children were ascertained who developed neurological disease and 39 (3.3%) had done so within 7 days of a DTP vaccination, and an attributable risk of a serious neurologic disorder within 7 days of DTP vaccination was calculated to be 1 in 110 000 vaccinations (Alderslade *et al.* 1981). In the original report (Miller *et al.* 1981), seven of the 39 had died or were seriously permanently brain-damaged, and it was concluded that the rate of permanent neurological deficit after immunization was 1 per 330 000 immunizations (Miller *et al.* 1985). The study authors pointed out that most

The Causes of Epilepsy, eds. S. D. Shorvon, F. Andermann, and R. Guerrini. Published by Cambridge University Press. © Cambridge University Press 2011.

cases of neurological disease occurring after vaccination were due to other causes. However, neurological disturbance (including mild reactions) in the first 72 hr after DTP vaccination was 2.4 times more frequent than in non-vaccinated children. The methodology of the study, and its findings, has been the subject of considerable contention and criticism (Scheifele 1988; Griffith 1989; Marcuse and Wentz 1990).

A number of smaller (but still large-scale) studies have been carried out but have failed to show any association. Gale *et al.* (1994), for instance, in a prospective active surveillance program in a population of 218 000 children under the age of 2 years, ascertained 424 cases of neurological illness. Each child was matched to two population control children by birth date, gender, and county of birth. The estimated odds ratio (OR) for onset of serious acute neurological illness within 7 days for young children exposed to DTP vaccine was 1.1 (95% confidence interval [CI], 0.6 to 2.0). The odds ratio for encephalopathy or complicated seizures was 3.6 (95% CI, 0.8 to 15.2). No elevated risk was observed for non-febrile seizures (OR, 0.5; 95% CI, 0.2 to 1.5). It was concluded that there was no statistically significant increased risk of onset of serious acute neurological illness in the 7 days after DTP vaccine exposure for young children. Similarly, a retrospective case–control study (Ray *et al.* 2006) amongst 2 197 000 children, ascertained a total of 452 encephalopathy cases of whom 49 had received DTP in the previous 60 days. Of these 49, 15 (31%) were of known non-vaccine cause. Six cases of encephalopathy were exposed to DTP within 7 days of onset which corresponds roughly to an all-cause incidence of 1 in 370 000, which was not statistically different from the risk in controls.

The type of vaccine also influences risk, and this applies to vaccination against pertussis as to other diseases. Initially, whole-cell vaccines (wP) which contain endotoxin were used, and cause a relatively high frequency of minor reactions. The acellular vaccines (aP) comprise detoxified pertussis antigens, produced by genetic recombinant technology (the polyvalent vaccines containing up to five antigens), and in these the rate of adverse reactions, particularly febrile reactions, is lower. Whether severe reactions differ is not known and these vaccines are likely to be less efficacious.

Current UK guidelines are that acellular pertussis vaccine should be given (in an injection combined with diphtheria, tetanus, *Haemophilus influenzae* type B, and inactivated polio vaccines) at 2, 3, and 4 months of age and then a booster (given with inactivated polio vaccine) at between 3 years 4 months and 5 years of age. Existing epilepsy or a stable neurological condition are not considered contraindications.

Berkovic *et al.* (2006) published the findings which further complicate the picture. In a study of childhood encephalopathy, 14 patients were identified who had developed the encephalopathy within 72 hr of pertussis vaccination and of these 11 had the phenotype of severe myoclonic epilepsy of infancy (SMEI or Dravet syndrome) (Dravet *et al.* 2005) (see Chapter 10); and 10 of the 11 had mutations in the *SCN1A*

gene which are typical of SMEI (Claes *et al.* 2001; Harkin *et al.* 2007). The authors concluded that many cases of apparent vaccine encephalopathy were cases of SMEI which became manifest by coincidence or because of a fever induced by the vaccine. In other words, these "post-vaccine cases" had in actual fact no causal relationship with vaccination, but had an inherent genetic encephalopathy. It has also been proposed (Shorvon and Berg 2008) on the basis of the Australian findings that the encephalopathy following pertussis may in some cases have a similar basis (and if this were the case, then the currently accepted estimate of the risk of pertussis-induced encephalopathy may also be too high). This has not been studied but would be important to do so.

The following conclusions were drawn from the data by Shorvon and Berg (2008):

(1) Pertussis (whooping cough) can be followed by encephalopathy in neonates and young children, and the attributable risk of encephalopathy due to pertussis is currently estimated to be between 1 in 1200–12 000 infections. This is much higher than any estimate of the risk of DTP vaccination, which is a rare event. Even the worst estimates suggest a frequency of fewer than 3 per million vaccinations, and most estimates are substantially less than this figure.

(2) The likelihood exists that some of these cases of encephalopathy, like that of the alleged vaccine, are not due to whooping cough per se but the coincidental onset of SMEI.

(3) Pertussis vaccination is a highly effective means to prevent a disabling and sometimes deadly disease. It provides excellent protection to the young children vaccinated and also "herd immunity" which is vital in the protection of neonates and infants who are those most at risk from serious consequences of the condition. Adding booster doses to older children is increasingly advocated for this purpose, and in countries where vaccination rates are high and where booster doses are administered, rates of pertussis are very low indeed.

(4) A not uncommon side effect of vaccination is fever (especially after the whole-cell vaccine), and if febrile seizures occur, these may be mediated via fever rather than by a direct cerebral action of the vaccine itself. Studies have suggested that vaccine-induced febrile seizures are no more frequent than febrile seizures due to any other cause of fever and carry the same relatively benign consequences as any other febrile seizure (Jackson *et al.* 2002). The rate of non-febrile seizures associated with vaccination is very low (an example estimate is 1 per 116 976 vaccinations in the study of Jackson *et al.* (2002).

For all these reasons, it seems the risk of non-vaccination is greatly outweighed by the risk of vaccination. Furthermore, any child in the future suspected of having a vaccine-induced encephalopathy (or epilepsy) should be tested for SMEI before the diagnosis can be accepted.

Epilepsy after other vaccinations

As the research into pertussis vaccination demonstrates, assessing the frequencies of rare complications after any vaccination can be very difficult. Much depends on the age of the population being vaccinated, the type of vaccine (the latter point is important, as vaccine technology has progressively improved), and the risks of not vaccinating (to the individual and to the society), and adequate statistics are generally not available. Large numbers of patients are required to be followed to obtain accurate data and this is an enormous undertaking. The live vaccines and the vaccines prepared from infective neural tissue are perhaps the vaccines that carry the greatest risk. The cellular vaccines, and also vaccines with high levels of endotoxin, are said to be generally less safe than the acellular vaccines although evidence on these points is weak especially where seizures are a rare side effect, largely because of the absence of sufficiently powered comparisons. The risks also probably vary according to manufacturer and to the quantity and type of adjuvant which further complicates assessment. The earlier smallpox vaccines carried a risk of death or severe complications (including encephalopathy) of about 1 in 14 000 vaccinations according to an official UK report in 1896 (cited in Glynn and Glynn 2005), but the risk of encephalopathy (almost always with epilepsy) after modern smallpox vaccination with the smallpox vaccine is much less and estimated to be in the region of 3–12 cases per million (Pankhurst 1965).

The vaccines with the greatest risk are those for Japanese encephalitis, smallpox, pertussis (but see above), measles, and rabies – but as will be clear, associations may not be causal, and the evidence is generally poor. Case reports exist of epilepsy, autism, and cerebral palsy developing after measles–mumps–rubella (MMR) and measles vaccines. The MMR vaccine particularly has been the subject of intense public debate and legal dispute, much as was the case with the pertussis vaccines, regarding the risk of autism and learning disability following vaccination, but the current orthodoxy is that there is no excess risk. In 1996, a similar public rumpus erupted concerning the risk of multiple sclerosis following hepatitis B vaccination, although now no such risk is felt to exist.

Other vaccines are reported to have been followed by seizures – sometimes febrile seizures and occasionally encephalopathy, but no case–control studies exist and it is often impossible to say whether these reports are simply coincidental or reflect any risk at all. It is very difficult to "prove a negative" and when adverse reactions are rare, it will take many years before rare events can be definitively shown not to be associated with any newly licensed products. A list of what information there is concerning convulsions following vaccinations is given in Table 56.1.

Table 56.1 Some vaccines which have been associated with the occurrence of post-vaccination epileptic or febrile seizures

Diphtheria/tetanus/pertussis (DTP)	See text
Pertussis	See text
Diphtheria	Rare
Diphtheria/tetanus (DT)	Very rare
Haemophilus influenzae type b (Hib)	Rare
Hepatitis B	Very rare (probably none)
H1N1 virus ("swine flu")	Very rare
Influenza	Very rare
Japanese B encephalitis	Encephalopathy in 1–2.3 vaccinees per million Neurological events in 1 in 5000–50 000 vaccinations
Measles	Febrile convulsions 1 in 1000 doses (higher in predisposed children)
Measles–mumps–rubella (MMR)	Encephalopathy in fewer than 1 in 3 million
Meningococcus	Very rare
Mumps	Meningoencephalitis in 1 in 1.8 million doses (Jeryl Lynn strain); 1 in 300 000 doses (Urabe Am 9 strain)
Poliomyelitis	Rare
Pneumococcus	Very rare
Rabies	Rare
Smallpox	Encephalopathy in 3–13 per million
Tic-borne encephalitis	Febrile seizures rare
Yellow fever	Encephalopathy in less than 4 per million vaccinations

Note:
These associations are usually registered on the basis of post-marketing surveillance, and it is likely that some associations are co-incidental rather than causal.

References

Alderslade R, Bellman MH, Rawson NSB, Ross EM, Miller DL (1981) *The National Childhood Encephalopathy Study: A Report on 1000 Cases of Serious Neurological Disorders in Infants and Young Children*. London: Her Majesty's Stationery Office.

Allen A (2007) *Vaccine: The Controversial Story of Medicine's Greatest Lifesaver*. New York: WW Norton.

Berkovic SF, Harkin L, McMahon JM, *et al.* (2006) De-novo mutations of the sodium channel gene *SCN1A* in alleged vaccine encephalopathy: a retrospective study. *Lancet Neurol* 5:488–92.

Claes L, Del-Favero J, Ceulemans B, *et al.* (2001) De novo mutations in the sodium-channel gene *SCN1A* cause severe myoclonic epilepsy of infancy. *Am J Hum Genet* **68**:1327–32.

Cohen R (1976) Science as fiction makes skeptical fan. *Washington Post*, November 14.

Committee on Infectious Diseases (1996) The relationship between pertussis vaccine and central nervous system sequelae: continuing assessment. *Pediatrics* **97**:279–81.

Dravet C, Bureau M, Oguni H, *et al.* (2005) Severe myoclonic epilepsy in infancy (Dravet syndrome). In: Roger J, Bureau M, Dravet C, Genton P, Tassinari CA, Wolf P (eds.) *Epileptic Syndromes in Infancy, Childhood and Adolescence*, 4th edn. Montrouge, France: John Libbey Eurotext, pp. 89–113.

Gale JL, Thapa PB, Wassilak SG, *et al.* (1994) Risk of serious acute neurological illness after immunization with diphtheria–tetanus–pertussis vaccine: a population-based case-control study. *J Am Med Ass* **271**:37–41.

Geier D, Geier M (2002) The true story of pertussis vaccination: a sordid legacy? *J Hist Med* **57**:249–84.

Glynn I, Glynn J (2005) *The Life and Death of Smallpox*. London: Profile books.

Griffith AH (1989) Permanent brain damage and pertussis vaccination: is the end of the saga in sight? *Vaccine* **7**:199–210.

Harkin LA, McMahon JM, Iona X, *et al.* (2007) The spectrum of *SCN1A*-related infantile epileptic encephalopathies. *Brain* **130**:843–52.

Jackson LA, Carste BA, Malais D, Froeschle J (2002) Retrospective population-based assessment of medically attended injection site reactions, seizures, allergic responses and febrile episodes after acellular pertussis vaccine combined with diphtheria and tetanus toxoids. *Pediatr Inf Dis J* **21**:781–6.

Marcuse EK, Wentz KR (1990) The NCES reconsidered: summary of a 1989 workshop. *Vaccine* **8**:531–5.

Miller DL, Ross EM, Alderslade R, Bellman MH, Rawson NS (1981) Pertussis immunisation and serious acute neurological illness in children. *Br Med J* **282**:1595–9.

Miller D, Wadsworth J, Diamond J, *et al.* (1985) Pertussis vaccine and whooping cough as risk factors in acute neurological illness and death in young children. *Dev Biol Stand* **61**:389–94.

Pankhurst R (1965) The history and traditional treatment of smallpox in Ethiopia. *Med Hist* **9**:343–55.

Ray P, Hayward J, Michelson D, *et al.* (2006) Encephalopathy after whole-cell pertussis or measles vaccination: lack of evidence for a causal association in a retrospective case-control study. *Pediatr Inf Dis J* **25**:768–73.

Scheifele DW (1988) Pertussis vaccine and encephalopathy after the Loveday trial. *Can Med Ass J* **139**:1045–6.

Shorvon S, Berg A (2008) Pertussis vaccination and epilepsy: an erratic history, new research and the mismatch between science and social policy. *Epilepsia* **49**:219–25.

US Institute of Medicine (1991) *Adverse Effects of Pertussis and Rubella Vaccines*. Washington, DC: National Academy Press.

Open head injury

Flavio Giordano, Barbara Spacca, and Lorenzo Genitori

Definitions and epidemiology

Open head injuries (OHIs) are the result of an impact with an outside force that breaches the skin, the skull vault, and/or the cranial base and the dura mater with involvement of the brain in various degree (Cooper and Golfinos 2000). The main causes of OHIs are missile wounds in war or a civilian setting, road accidents, and sharp and semi-sharp objects (Krieger et al. 2007).

Open head injuries may be classified according to the dynamics of trauma into perforating and penetrating: perforating injuries occur when an object enters and exits the skull, while penetrating injuries occur when the object does not exit the cranial vault (Dutcher et al. 2001). They are also distinguished according to the agent in low-velocity (arrow, nail, stab, etc.) and high-velocity wounds (gunshot wounds). The gunshot wounds are also subdivided in low (civilian handguns,

air guns) and high velocity (rifles, military weapons, shrapnel shell) (Harrington and Apostolides 2000) (Fig. 57.1).

Open head injuries are more common in war than in a civilian setting; therefore most of the knowledge on early and late complications and outcomes come from reports on perforating and penetrating brain injuries sustained during military service (Eftekhar et al. 2009). On the other hand, although the frequency of admission to emergency departments is increased because of firearms diffusion, the true incidence of OHIs is difficult to quantify in the civilian setting. In the USA, nearly 1 million people every year experience an OHI; 70% of them die at the scene or soon after injury (Kaufman 1995). Over the past years OHIs due to gunshot wounds in the civilian setting have been raised to an incidence as high as 8.4 in 100 000 (Sosin et al. 1989) with an overall mortality of 92% (Siccardi et al. 1991). Even if high-velocity gunshot

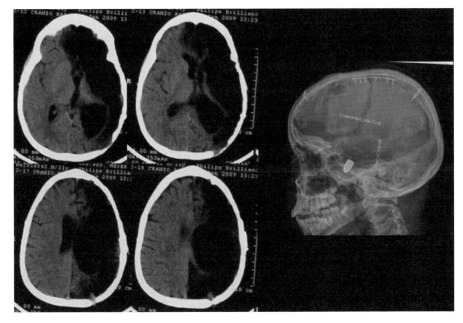

Fig. 57.1. Sequelae of civilian gunshot wound. The computed tomography (CT) scan shows a hemispheric leukoporoencephaly (left side). The bullet has not been removed because it was entrapped into the skull base inside the cavernous sinus (right side).

The Causes of Epilepsy, eds. S. D. Shorvon, F. Andermann, and R. Guerrini. Published by Cambridge University Press. © Cambridge University Press 2011.

wounds are becoming more common in metropolitan areas, low-velocity gunshot wounds are still the first cause for OHIs (Harrington and Apostolides 2000).

Pathology, physiology, and clinical features

Although missile and road traffic accident (non-missile) (Fig. 57.2) OHIs are probably the most frequent causes, a large variety of objects has been described in penetrating brain injury: arrows, screwdrivers, plugs, chopsticks, dinner forks, knives, scissors, pencils, toys, toy-weapons, and many other (Krieger *et al.* 2007) (Fig. 57.3). The entry site, the type of penetrating object, its velocity, and its trajectory define the involvement both of the external layers of the cranium and the brain with nerve and vessels that corresponds to the first head injury. The clinical condition at presentation in terms of Glasgow Coma Scale (GCS) depends on the first brain lesion and associated injuries. Retained foreign bodies are a frequent complication that raise the risk of infection and the genesis of epileptogenic scar (Cooper and Golfinos 2000).

Two types of mechanism for brain damages are described in OHIs: primary and secondary. The first is due to missile physics and kinetic energy which leads to tissue destruction, cavitation, and shock-wave formation (Dutcher *et al.* 2001). The kinetic energy translated to the brain mainly depends on missile velocity, hence the destroying effect is directly related to missile velocity which is partially absorbed on impact by the skin and the skull (Dutcher *et al.* 2001). If the velocity is below 275 m/s, the damage is only due to tearing and shearing forces; if the velocity is higher than 275 m/s, the volume of damaged brain is increased by cavitation and shock-waves (Liau *et al.* 1996). Military weapons have non-deformable full-metal jacket bullets with high perforating effect and very high velocity (730–975 m/s) which produce dramatic tissue cavitation (Cooper 1993); moreover, their shock-wave and cavitation energy raise intracranial pressure to 60–100 mm Hg (Crockard *et al.* 1977). Bullets used with civilian firearms have a velocity less than 300 m/s, so they usually cause penetrating OHIs (Cooper 1993);

these bullets are often destroyed and deformed in the so-called "mushroom" effect, and finally transformed into multiple small fragments projected in a wide diameter leading to many secondary bullet tracts with low velocity but with higher amount of tissue destroyed (Dutcher *et al.* 2001). In these cases, the risk of small retained foreign bodies is higher, and these may result in late infections and seizures (Fig. 57.4).

The secondary mechanisms of brain damage are the results of cell death, infections, and biochemical cascade that includes hypoxia–ischemia damage, release of excitatory amino acids, and excitotoxicity phenomena. The first pathological event is direct tissue destruction and cavitation with disruption of brain architecture, followed by vasogenic edema, swelling of astrocytes (cyotoxic edema), hemorrhage, perivascular bleeding, and hypoxia–ischemia (Allen *et al.* 1983; Cooper 1993). All these events lead to raised intracranial pressure as shown in an experimental model by Allen and colleagues (Allen *et al.* 1983). Furthermore, Crockard and colleagues analyzed in a primate model the early effects of missile injury showing that the damage is rapidly followed both by raised intracranial pressure

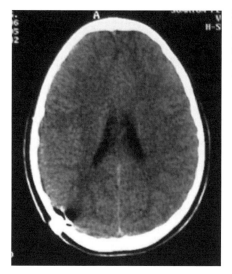

Fig. 57.3. Open head injury due to a stone thrown with a sling. The foreign object is stuck in the calvarium. No brain lesions are visible.

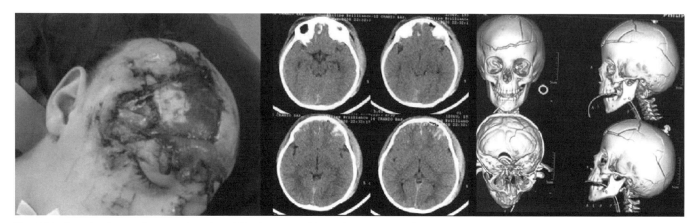

Fig. 57.2. Open head injury due to road accident: diffuse laceration of the scalp with retained foreign bodies and outflow of brain tissue (left side). The CT scan shows diffuse and comminuted fractures extended to skull base. Frontal lobe hemorrhagic contusions coexist (right side).

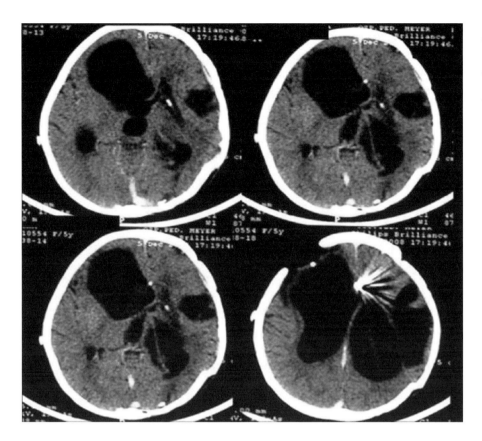

Fig. 57.4. Sequelae of civilian gunshot wound due to military weapon (AK-47). Bilateral diffuse leukoporoencephaly is present along with post-traumatic hydrocephalus. Some small fragments of the bullet are retained inside the brain. The patient suffers from late severe drug-resistant epilepsy.

and by hypoxia–ischemia in brain and brainstem; all these findings were closely linked to mortality (Crockard *et al.* 1977). The secondary effects of hypoxia–ischemia are increased intracellular calcium influx and excitotoxic release of glutamate and aspartate (Choi 1988) leading to the excitotoxic cascade (Choi and Rothman 1990) as tested by microdialysis titration by Goodman *et al.* (1996) in human brain after gunshot. The same excitotoxic neurotransmitters may activate different gene pathways linked to secondary brain damage (Dutcher *et al.* 1998). The deposition of iron from catabolyzed hemoglobin acts as a causative factor starting the cascade of lipid peroxidation of cell-membrane arachidonic acid (Temkin *et al.* 1996) which finally leads to elevation of intracellular calcium levels. The rising calcium level causes excitotoxic damage with neuronal death, reactive gliosis, and finally a glial scar that becomes the center of the hyperexcitable focus (Willmore *et al.* 1986). According to previous theories described by Willmore *et al.* (1986), iron deposition along with vasogenic edema, hypoxic–ischemic neuronal damage, axonal sprouting, and synaptic disassembly are crucial for post-traumatic epileptogenesis. More recent studies underline the role of destruction of the blood–brain barrier as demonstrated in some experimental models; the exposure of animal cortical surface to low levels of albumin induces extravasation of plasma proteins leading to early activation of astrocytes and long-lasting hypersynchronization (Seiffert *et al.* 2004). Albumin itself seems to play a significant role in neurotoxicity phenomena and in some degenerative diseases (Hooper 2005). Recent investigations have demonstrated

the involvement of thrombin (Lee *et al.* 1997) and some pro-inflammatory cytokines, like interleukin-1β, in mechanisms of direct neurotoxicity and excitotoxicity (Vezzani *et al.* 2004).

Besides the concept of an anatomically damaged astroglia, new reports have ruled out the hypothesis of a functionally damaged astroglia. Samuelsson and colleagues have demonstrated in a rat model of post-traumatic epilepsy that the excitotoxic effect of higher extracellular glutamate depends on deranged synaptic release, as well as on a reduced reuptake due to abnormal and downregulated cellular carriers such as the astrocytic glutamate transporter protein (GLUT-1) (Samuelson *et al.* 2000).

Epilepsy in open head injury: frequency, risk factors, types of epilepsy, treatment, and prognosis

Post-traumatic seizures are classified as immediate (within hours after injury), early (within the first 7 days), and late (beyond the first week after injury) (Pagni 1990).

Immediate seizures are usually generalized and they do not always correspond to true epilepsy but represent an acute response to brain injury (Majkowski 1991).

Early post-traumatic seizures are reported in 2.2–8.9% of cases (Rish and Caveness 1973; Salazar *et al.* 1985a) and are associated with a higher risk of late seizures, as reported by Weiss who found that 75% of patients with early seizures developed late epilepsy (Weiss *et al.* 1983). The series of Iran–Iraq war OHIs described by Aarabi and colleagues confirm these observations (Aarabi *et al.* 2000). In other series, a 25–50% incidence is reported for late epilepsy after early post-traumatic seizures (Caveness *et al.* 1979). Early seizures are more common in children younger than 5 years old. The incidence reduces with age: 9.4% up to 5 years, 3.3% in children from 6 to 15 years old, 5.1% in people aged 16 to 25 years, and 1.5–4.1% in adults 26 years old or older (Jennet and Lewin 1960).

The diagnosis of "post-traumatic epilepsy" requires at least two seizures after head injury (Temkin *et al.* 1996). The peak incidence of late seizures is 1 month after trauma though late epilepsy may start more than 20 years after injury (Rasmussen 1969). Post-traumatic epilepsy does not persist in all cases: 5 to 10 years after trauma, half of the patients no longer have seizures. Remissions are more difficult in patients affected by frequent seizures (Weiss and Caveness 1972).

Post-traumatic seizures are usually partial at onset even if secondary generalization may be rapid enough to simulate generalized seizures from onset. About 25% of seizures are focal, 50% focal with secondary generalization, while 25% are generalized (Caveness *et al.* 1979).

In military OHIs, early and late post-traumatic epilepsy account for 20% and 53% of the cases respectively (Temkin *et al.* 1996). The study of Vietnam veterans made by Salazar and colleagues found an incidence of late epilepsy in 35–50% of survivors with a risk of late epilepsy increased 25-fold for the following 10–15 years (Salazar *et al.* 1985b). According to more recent analysis on survivors of the Iran–Iraq war, the risk of persistent late seizures after 16 and 21 years rises to 70% and 86% respectively (Eftekhar *et al.* 2009). Few data are available about the incidence of seizures after civilian OHIs: one paper reports a 10–35% incidence (Benzel *et al.* 1991).

On a general point of view, the risk factors for post-traumatic seizures are prolonged loss of consciousness, depressed skull fractures, hematomas and hemorrhagic contusions, and focal neurological impairment (Pagni 1990).

Risk factors for late epilepsy are divided according to wound profile and clinical condition (Aarabi, 2000). The highest risk for late epilepsy occurs after missile wounds because of brain volume loss and dural lacerations. Additional risk factors are focal neurological signs, intracranial hematoma, and retained metallic and bone fragments (Salazar *et al.* 1985a). The closer the lesion to the central sulcus (Adeloye and Odeku 1971), the higher the risk of late epilepsy. As shown by wounded soldiers, motor and speech deficits are additional significant risk factors for developing late-onset epilepsy (Salazar *et al.* 1985b; Aarabi *et al.* 2000).

The number of damaged brain lobes may be a predictive factor to evaluate the volume of brain loss (Weiss *et al.* 1983). Tangential and through-and-through injury are adjunctive risk factors (Adeloye and Odeku 1971) as well as wound infection and intracranial sepsis (Ascroft 1941), that seem to raise the risk of late epilepsy to 68.4% (Aarabi *et al.* 2000), while brain abscess does not (Salazar *et al.* 1985a). A recent magnetic resonance imaging (MRI) study on OHIs showed that patients with gliosis (T1–T2-weighted hyperintense signal) around hemosiderin deposit (T1–T2-weighted hypointense signal) are at higher risk for refractory seizure (Kumar *et al.* 2003).

The level of consciousness on admission (as measured by Glasgow Coma Scale) is also significantly associated with the risk of late epilepsy: the lower the GCS, the higher the risk of epilepsy after OHI (Weiss *et al.* 1986; Aarabi *et al.* 2000). In adults, a persistent low GCS score (3 to 8) along with diffuse cerebral edema, acute subdural hematoma, prolonged loss of consciousness, and depressed skull fracture are associated with a higher incidence of post-traumatic epilepsy. The Glasgow Outcome Score is highly predictive for late epilepsy: almost 40–46% of patients with moderate to severe disability developed epilepsy as compared to 7.4% of patients with no or mild deficit (Aarabi *et al.* 2000). These predictive factors are not completely confirmed in children (Krieger *et al.* 2007).

Antiepileptic drugs (AEDs) should be administered to all patients with OHI, in both early and late post-injury phases, especially if a significant loss of brain tissue has occurred (Nagib *et al.* 1986). Temkin and colleagues demonstrated with a randomized trial that phenytoin is effective in preventing early seizures and it should be administered for the first week to all patients who have suffered a severe injury with high risk of seizures; however, its effectiveness to prevent late seizures is not proven (Temkin *et al.* 1990). Phenytoin has a prophylactic role and its use is not recommended beyond 7 days after injury. At that time, if late post-traumatic epilepsy occurs, different AEDs should be preferred (D'Ambrosio and Perucca 2004). Carbamazepine, phenytoin, and valproate have been suggested as first-choice treatment of both complex partial seizures and secondarily generalized seizures (Mattson *et al.* 1992).

Discontinuation of AEDs should be considered on an individual basis, according to Krieger *et al.* (2007), 3 to 6 months later if the patient is seizure-free. On the other hand, some authors like Kaufman (1995) suggest maintaining phenytoin therapy for at least 1 year because significant brain parenchyma damage is linked to a high risk of late epilepsy. There does not seem to be a clear efficacy in patients younger than 16 years (Young *et al.* 2004). Other AEDs may be considered, such as phenobarbital for toddlers and very young children, and valproate for older children (Krieger *et al.* 2007). Keeping in mind the physiopathologic process leading to post-traumatic epilepsy, new drugs acting to reduce lipid peroxidation, neuroprotectors (antioxidants), glutamic receptor blockers, and inhibitors of apoptosis by caspase inhibition should be investigated in the future to reduce the risk.

Management of open head injury and correlated post-traumatic epilepsy

In the acute phase of OHI the first goals are patient resuscitation and stabilization with immediate neurosurgical management that must include evaluation of location, size and appearance of the wounds, GCS score, intracranial pressure control, and neuroprotection (Krieger *et al.* 2007). Medical and surgical management on admission are driven by the result of the first injury but, among survivors, both first and second injuries are responsible for the outcome in terms of disability and epilepsy. Open head injuries are often associated with very high morbidity and mortality, especially in the adult population. The lower the GCS on admission, the worse the outcome. In children, morbidity and mortality are lower, due to greater cerebral compliance and incomplete differentiation of eloquent areas. According to our experience, these specific features of pediatric population together with OHIs localized in the anterior brain regions correlates with better prognosis in children.

According to Kaufman (1995), surgery is mandatory to debride and close scalp wounds and to remove foreign objects, in order to avoid late complications like infections and seizures. Timing of surgery is essential for a low rate of complications. Early surgery is suggested after OHIs to close the scalp wound with the aim of preventing infection and/or inadequate perfusion of the cranial vault. Although the most effective way to prevent post-traumatic epilepsy is that of preventing head trauma, its occurrence may be reduced by minimizing the development of meningocerebral scars and reactive gliosis through a complete debridement of damaged brain tissue and preventing complications such as edema, hemorrhage, and infection (Caveness *et al.* 1979). During surgery, the necrotic brain must be removed to prevent further hemorrhage and scarring and to reduce mass effect. Secondary cerebral scars are often responsible for late epilepsy in these cases. Microsurgical treatment of cerebral lesion with high magnification allows better control of the quality of the scar. With early surgery, the main goals are to remove the larger and easier-to-reach objects, to remove hematomas, and to control the bleeding. None of the studies demonstrated that extensive brain debridement and removal of hematomas and of deep located foreign bodies correlated with a better outcome, though it is assumed that retained fragments raise the risk of late seizures and aneurysm formation (Aarabi 1995). If the OHI is due to an object only partially penetrating into the brain with part of it protruding outside the skull (e.g., fish-hook, scissors, piece of wood), it is mandatory not to cut the visible part of the penetrating object that could otherwise be sucked into the brain. The patient will be intubated and operated on with the entire penetrating object in situ. Microsurgical accurate dissection of the object inside the brain will allow efficient removal without adjunctive lesions to the adjacent parenchyma.

Watertight closure of the dura mater is mandatory to prevent cerebral swelling, brain herniation, leptomeningeal cyst development, and secondary growing fracture which especially in children is a frequent cause of late epilepsy. If a growing fracture is suspected, it is mandatory to operate as soon as possible to minimize the risks of late epilepsy. The procedure consists of closing the dural defect with autologous

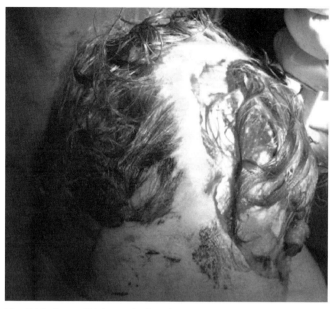

Fig. 57.5. Severe OHI due to dog bite. The aims of surgery are complete debridment of necrotic tissue, removal of foreign objects, and complete reconstruction of the vault by mantaining an adequate vascularization of the flap.

or synthetic material. The dural defect is always much bigger than the bone defect; accurate planning of the surgical bone flap is therefore important in performing both dural and bone reconstruction. In children, autologous bone is tolerated better than synthetic. Custom-made prostheses made of various kinds of materials are suitable for the adult population.

Reconstruction of the cranial vault is possible immediately during the surgical procedure. Depressed skull fractures require wiring or plating of different fragments and immediate repositioning. Non-autologous materials are not suitable in these cases. In the absence of mass effect lesions, deep reconstruction of skull vault and base and of its layers may be delayed waiting for cerebral edema to reduce; leaking of the cerebrospinal fluid (rhinorrhea and/or otorrhea) is not a contraindication to delayed reconstruction. In selected cases (e.g., dog bite lesions) when the risk of diffuse infection is high, immediate and complete reconstruction is mandatory (Fig. 57.5).

During recovery from the acute phase, immediate and early seizures must be prevented to avoid a rise in intracranial pressure. After the acute phase of OHI, post-traumatic epilepsy is to be treated as all the other forms of symptomatic partial-onset epilepsy. Carbamazepine and valproate are first-choice drugs for partial and secondarily generalized seizures (Mattson *et al.* 1992). New drugs such as gabapentin, lamotrigine, levetiracetam, oxcarbazepine, tiagabine, topiramate, and zonisamide are also effective.

If drug-resistant post-traumatic epilepsy occurs, epilepsy surgery is to be considered. Besides tailored resection of leukomalacic and gliotic lesions, palliative surgery, such as hemispherotomy, corpus callosotomy, and vagal nerve stimulation (VNS), may be useful in selected cases.

The authors' series in a pediatric population

From 1994 to 2008, we observed 33 cases of OHIs out of a total number of 1058 children admitted for head injuries (3.12%). There were 18 males, 15 females; mean age was 9.7 years (range 3 months to 17.4 years). The main causes were road accidents (18 cases; 56.2%) and gunshot wounds (6 cases; 18.2%), followed by falls (4 cases; 12.5%), sharp objects (2 cases; 6.2%), sport-related events (2 cases; 6.2%), and dog-bite (1 case; 3.3%).

All patients received first aid support with resuscitation and stabilization at the scene of trauma and were transported to our department afterwards. On admission, a full neurological examination was carried out with direct inspection of the wounds to evaluate the size and type of lesion and detect retained foreign bodies. A complete radiological diagnostic work-up was performed in all cases by computed tomography (CT) scan. Nineteen cases (57.6%) were severe injuries with GCS less than 10. Nine cases (27.3%) were mild head injuries (GCS 14–15), while five children (15.1%) experienced a moderate head injury (GCS 11–13). In ten patients the direct inspection revealed retained foreign bodies.

The fracture was limited to the vault in 22 cases and extended to the skull base in 12 children. The fractures of the vault were comminuted and extended to multiple sutures in 16 cases. Linear fractures were especially located in the fronto-orbital region (14 cases), followed by the parietal (2 cases) and temporal region (1 case). In 16 subjects the fractures were depressed. Different types of hemorrhagic complications were observed: epidural hematoma (8), acute subdural hematoma (12), subarachnoid hemorrhage (19), and cerebral contusions (27) that were multiple in 12 cases, frontal and basofrontal (9), temporal (2), parietal (3), and cerebellar (1).

All cases of severe OHIs (GCS ≤ 10) received AED prophylaxis with phenobarbital and phenytoin in toddlers and children respectively. In mild and moderate OHIs the prophylaxis was given if the patient was considered at high risk of early post-traumatic seizures or had immediate post-traumatic seizures, and in presence of previous history of epilepsy. The AEDs were administered for the whole duration of hospitalization.

Surgery consisted of immediate debridement with removal of necrotic brain tissue and foreign objects along with reconstruction of skull base and vault in the same step in 18 patients. Surgical reconstruction was delayed by no more than 48 hr in 15 cases of fronto-orbitary fractures extended to the paranasal sinuses. In one case of gunshot wound the bullet was not removed because it was located inside the cavernous sinus at the skull base. One child wounded by perforating gunshot died (3%) 12 hr after surgery. Surgical morbidity occurred in 12 patients (37.5%) in the form of meningitis (4), wound infections (2), pituitary impairment (2), nasal cerebrospinal fluid leakage (2), and osteomyelitis (1). Five patients developed post-traumatic hydrocephalus (15.6%) treated as first choice by ventricular peritoneal shunting of cerebrospinal fluid. Seven patients underwent late surgery for cranioplasty (21.3%).

Mean follow-up after surgery was 16 months (range 4 months to 5 years). At last neurological examination the Glasgow Outcome Score (GOS) was 5 in 16 cases (48.5%), 4 in 7 (21.2%), 3 in 6 (18.2%). Three children (9.1%) were in persistent vegetative state (GOS 2). There was only one death in the series (GOS 1) (3%). As far as epilepsy is concerned, 17 among survivors did not develop post-traumatic epilepsy (53.1%). Twelve patients (37.5%) had late post-traumatic epilepsy with good control of seizures by AED therapy, while three patients developed drug-resistant epilepsy (9.4%).

According to our experience, severe OHIs (GCS ≤ 10), multiple brain contusions especially located in temporal and frontobasal lobes, wound infection and meningitis seem to be the most influencing risk factors for post-traumatic epilepsy. These findings are confirmed by several reports in the literature (Salazar *et al.* 1985a; Aarabi *et al.* 2000; Eftekhar *et al.* 2009).

References

Aarabi B (1995) Management of traumatic aneurysm caused by high velocity missile head wounds. *Neursurg Clin N Am* 6:775–97.

Aarabi B, Taghipour M, Haghnegahdar A, *et al.* (2000) Prognostic factors in the occurrence of posttraumatic epilepsy after penetrating head injury suffered during military service. *Neurosurg Focus* 8:E1

Adeloye A, Odeku EL (1971) Epilepsy after missile wounds of the head. *J Neurol Neurosurg Psychiatry* 34:98–103.

Allen I, Kirk J, Maynard R, *et al.* (1983) An ultrastructural study of experimental high velocity penetrating head injury. *Acta Neuropathol* 59:277–82.

Ascroft PB (1941) Traumatic epilepsy after gunshot wounds of the head. *Br Med J* 1:739–44.

Benzel EC, Day WT, Kesterton L, *et al.* (1991) Civilian craniocerebral gunshot wounds. *Neurosurgery* 29:67–71.

Caveness WF, Meirowsky AM, Rish BL, *et al.* (1979) The nature of posttraumatic epilepsy. *J Neurosurg* 50:545–53.

Choi D (1988) Calcium-mediated neurotoxicity: relationship to specific channel type and role in ischemic damage. *Trends Neurosci* 11:465–9.

Choi D, Rothman S (1990) The role of glutamate neurotoxicity in hypoxic-ischemic neuronal death. *Ann Rev Neurosci* 13:171–82.

Cooper P (1993) *Head Injury*, 3rd edn. Baltimore, MD: Williams and Wilkins.

Cooper PR, Golfinos JG (2000) *Head Injury*, 4th edn. New York: McGraw Hill.

Crockard A, Brown F, Calica A, *et al.* (1977) Physiological consequences of experimental missile injury and use of data analysis to predict survival. *J Neurosurg* 46:784–94.

D'Ambrosio R, Perucca E (2004) Epilepsy after head injury. *Curr Opin Neurol* 17:731–5.

Dutcher S, Underwood B, Walker P, *et al.* (1998) Patterns of heat-shock protein 70 biosynthesis following human traumatic brain inury. *J Neurotrauma* 15:411–20.

Dutcher S, Sood S, Ham S, Canady A (2001) Skull fractures and penetrating brain injury. In: McLone D (ed.) *Pediatric Neurosurgery*, 4th edn. Philadelphia, PA: WB Saunders, pp. 573–83.

Eftekhar B, Sahraian MA, Nouralishai B, *et al.* (2009) Prognostic factors in the persistence of posttraumatic epilepsy after penetrating head injuries sustained in war. *J Neurosurg* **110**:319–26.

Goodman JC, Valadka AB, Gopinath SP, *et al.* (1996) Lactate and excitatory aminoacids measured by microdialysis are decreased by pentobarbital coma in head-injured patients. *J Neurotrauma* **13**:549–56.

Harrington T, Apostolides P (2000) Penetrating brain injury. In: Cooper PR, Golfinos JG (eds.) *Head Injury*, 4th edn. New York: McGraw Hill, pp. 349–59.

Hooper C, Taylor DL, Pocock JM (2005) Pure albumin is a potent trigger of calcium signalling and proliferation in microglia but not in macrophages or astrocytes. *J Neurochem* **92**:1363–76.

Jennett WB, Lewin W (1960) Traumatic epilepsy after closed head injuries. *J Neurol Neurosurg Psychiatry* **23**:295–301.

Kaufman HH (1995) Care and variations in the care of patients with gunshot wounds to the brain. *Neurosurg Clin N Am* **6**:727–34.

Krieger MD, Bowen IE, McComb G (2007) Penetrating craniocerebral injuries. In: Albright AL, Pollack IF, Adelson PD (eds.) *Principles and Practice of Pediatric Neurosurgery*, 2nd edn. New York: Georg Thieme.

Kumar R, Gupta RK, Husain M, *et al.* (2003) Magnetization transfer MR imaging in patients with post-traumatic epilepsy. *AJNR Am J Neuroradiol* **24**:218–24.

Lee KR, Dury I, Vitarbo E, Hoff J (1997) Seizures induced by intracerebral injection of thrombin: a model of intracerebral hemorrhage. *J Neurosurg* **87**:73–8.

Liau L, Bergsneider M, Becker D (1996) Pathology and pathophysiology of head injury. In: Youmans J, Becker D (eds.) *Neurological Surgery*, 4th edn.

Philadelphia, PA: WB Saunders, pp. 1549–68.

Majkowski J (1991) Posttraumatic epilepsy. In: Dam M, Gram L (eds.) *Comprehensive Epileptology*. New York: Raven Press, pp. 281–8.

Mattson RH, Cramer JA, Collins JF, *et al.* (1992) A comparison of valproate with carbamazepine for the treatment of complex partial seizures and secondarily generalized tonic–clonic seizures in adults. *N Engl J Med* **327**:765–71.

Nagib MG, Rockswold GL, Sherman RS, *et al.* (1986) Civilian gunshot wounds to the brain: prognosis and management. *Neurosurgery* **18**:533–7.

Pagni CA (1990) Post-traumatic epilepsy: incidence and prophylaxis. *Acta Neurochirurgica Suppl* (*Wien*) **50**:38.

Rasmussen T (1969) Surgical therapy of post-traumatic epilepsy. In: Walker AE, Caveness WF, Critchley M (eds.) *The Late Effects of Head Injury*. Springfield, IL: Charles C. Thomas, pp. 277–305.

Rish BL, Caveness WF (1973) Relation of prophylactic medication to the occurrence of early seizures following cranio-cerebral trauma. *J Neurosurg* **38**:155–8.

Salazar AM, Amin D, Vance SC, *et al.* (1985a) Epilepsy after penetrating head injury: anatomic correlates. *Neurology* **35**(Suppl 1):230.

Salazar AM, Jabbari B, Vance SC, *et al.* (1985b) Epilepsy after penetrating head injury. I. clinical correlates: a report of the Vietnam Head Injury Study. *Neurology* **35**:1406–14.

Samuelson C, Kumlien E, Flink R (2000) Decreased cortical levels of astrocytic glutamate transport protein GLT-1 in a rat model of posttraumatic epilepsy. *Neurosci Lett* **289**:185–8.

Seiffert E, Dreier JP, Ivens S, *et al.* (2004) Lasting blood–brain disruption induces epileptic focus in the rat somatosensory cortex. *J Neurosci* **24**:7829–36.

Siccardi D, Cavaliere R, Pau A (1991) Penetrating craniocerebral missile injuries in civilians: a retrospective

analysis of 314 cases. *Surg Neurol* **35**:455–60.

Sosin D, Sacks J, Smith S (1989) Head-injury associated death in the United States from 1979–1986. *J Am Med Ass* **262**:2251–5.

Temkin NR, Dikmen SS, Wilensky AJ, *et al.* (1990) A randomized double-blind study of phenytoin for the prevention of post-traumatic seizures. *N Engl J Med* **323**:497–502.

Temkin NR, Haglund MM, Winn RH (1996) Post-traumatic seizures. In: Youmans JR (ed.) *Neurological Surgery* 4th edn. Philadelphia, PA: WB Saunders, pp. 1834–9.

Temkin NR, Dikmen SS, Anderson GD, *et al.* (1999) Valproate therapy for prevention of posttraumatic seizures: a randomized trial. *J Neurosurg* **91**:593–600.

Vezzani A, Moneta D, Richichi C, *et al.* (2004) Functional role of proinflammatory and anti-inflammatory cytokines in seizures. *Adv Exp Med Biol* **548**:123–33.

Walker AE, Jablon S (1961) *A Follow-Up Study of Head Wounds in World War II*. Washington, DC: US Government Printing Office.

Weiss GH, Caveness WF (1972) Prognostic factors in the persistence of posttraumatic epilepsy. *J Neurosurg* **37**:164–9.

Weiss GH, Feeney DM, Caveness WF, *et al.* (1983) Prognostic factors for the occurrence of post-traumatic epilepsy. *Arch Neurol* **40**:7–10.

Weiss GH, Salazar AM, Vance SC, *et al.* (1986) Predicting posttraumatic epilepsy in penetrating injury. *Arch Neurol* **43**:771–3.

Willmore LJ, Triggs WJ, Gray JD (1986) The role of induced hippocampal peroxidation in acute epileptogenesis. *Brain Res* **382**:422–6.

Young KD, Okada PJ, Sokolove PE, *et al.* (2004) A randomized, double-blind, placebo-controlled trial of phenytoin for the prevention of early post-traumatic seizures in children with moderate to severe blunt head injury. *Ann Emerg Med* **43**:435–46.

Chapter

58

Closed head injury

Manuel Murie-Fernandez, Jorge G. Burneo, and Robert W. Teasell

Traumatic brain injury

Despite the lack of standard definitions for the severity of head injury, classification is usually based on the level of altered consciousness experienced by the patient following injury. The most common measures of traumatic brain injury (TBI) severity include the Glasgow Coma Scale (GCS), the duration of loss of consciousness (LOC), and the duration of post-traumatic amnesia (PTA). According to these three measures and the presence or absence of a skull fracture, brain contusion, or intracerebral hematoma, patients can be classified as having "mild," "moderate," or "severe" TBI (Annagers *et al.* 1980) (Table 58.1).

Epidemiology of traumatic brain injury

Traumatic brain injury is one of the leading causes of death and lifelong disability in North America. Traumatic brain injuries are three times more common in men (Greenwald *et al.* 2003). In Western developed countries incidence figures for TBI are estimated to be at around 180–250 per 100 000 people (Bruns and Hauser 2003). The estimated incidence of TBI doubles between the ages of 5 and 14 years and peaks in both males and females during adolescence and early adulthood. However, older TBI victims usually show a greater severity of injury, and higher mortality rates (Frey 2003).

Evidence suggests that the predominant causes of TBI vary with age. Overall, motor vehicle and related transportation accidents comprise the most common cause of TBI, accounting for more than 50% of all head injuries by some estimates.

The resulting neurologic impairments from closed head injuries have a wide range of severity: from severe paralysis and major mental impairment and with up to 50% experiencing subtle cognitive impairments (Jensen 2009). Seizures are a common consequence of TBI (Gupta and Gupta 2006) and post-traumatic epilepsy (PTE) plays a significant role in the inability of head injury survivors to return to their pre-existing lifestyles and employment.

Table 58.1 Definitions of injury severity

Mild	Moderate	Severe
PTA < 30 min	If there is a skull fracture	Documented brain contusion or intracerebral hematoma
GCS 13–15	PTA 30 min–24 hr	
LOC < 15 min	GCS 9–12	
No skull fracture	LOC < 6 hr	PTA > 24 hr
		GCS between 3 and 8
		LOC > 6 hr

GCS, Glasgow Coma Scale; LOC, loss of consciousness; PTA, post-traumatic amnesia.

Traumatic brain injury is recognized as a major cause of acquired epilepsy, and can exacerbate seizure severity in individuals with pre-existing epilepsy (Jensen 2009).

Post-traumatic seizure

Post-traumatic seizure (PTS) is defined as an initial or recurrent seizure episode not attributable to another obvious cause after penetrating or non-penetrating TBI (Frey 2003). The term post-traumatic seizure is preferred to post-traumatic epilepsy because the former encompasses both single and recurrent events.

Post-traumatic seizures are usually divided into three categories: immediate, early seizures, and late seizures (Lowestein 2009). Immediate are those that occur at the time of or minutes after impact (some groups include in this category the seizures occurring within the first 24 hr of injury). Early seizures are those occurring while the patient is still suffering from the direct effects of the head injury, a period commonly defined as 1 week after head injury. Late seizures are usually defined as seizures occurring after the first week of injury.

Epidemiology of post-traumatic seizures

Traumatic brain injury accounts for 20% of symptomatic epilepsy in the general population and 5% of all epileptic cases (Hauser *et al.* 1991). In young adults TBI is the leading cause of symptomatic epilepsy. The overall incidence of late seizures, following non-penetrating TBI among hospitalized patients, is 4–7% (Annagers *et al.* 1980). However, the incidence of PTS is much higher on rehabilitation units (as high as 17%) reflecting the severity of the injury in this population (Armstrong *et al.* 1990).

Patients with severe TBI can have up to 29-fold increased risk of developing epilepsy compared to the general population. The incidence of immediate seizures following TBI is 1–4%, early seizures 4–25%, and late post-traumatic seizures 9–42% (Annegers *et al.* 1998; Asikainen *et al.* 1999). Approximately 80% of individuals with PTE experience their first seizure within the first 12 months post-injury and more than 90% before the end of the second year (da Silva *et al.* 1990). However, the risk still is increased more than 10 years after the trauma-causing event (Christensen *et al.* 2009)

Clinical seizure types

Post-traumatic seizures may present across the spectrum of simple to complex seizures, including generalized and secondarily generalized seizures. Overall the most frequent seizures are focal or partial complex seizures (Haltiner *et al.* 1997). Most early seizures are found to be of the generalized tonic–clonic type, whereas with late post-traumatic seizures, the seizure types are more variable. Mesial temporal lobe epilepsy after TBI appears to be relatively uncommon (although most experienced epileptologists have seen apparent cases) and may have a predilection for children (Diaz-Arrastia *et al.* 2000), perhaps related to the increased vulnerability of the hippocampus to TBI in younger patients. Fortunately, clinically apparent status epilepticus is an infrequent complication of PTS.

Pathophysiology

Epileptogenesis is defined as the process whereby the non-epileptic brain is transformed into one that generates unprovoked seizures. In addition, epileptogenesis refers to the development of brain tissue capable of generating chronic, recurrent, spontaneous behavioral and/or electrographic seizures. The process may start with an initial insult that may or may not involve acute seizure activity, but that may lead to later development of epilepsy. In the case of TBI, this latency can be up to several years (Lowestein 2009).

Head trauma of sufficient severity to cause focal deficits results in injury to brain tissue in a pattern determined by mechanical effects initiated by the traumatic injury. Depending on the severity of the mechanical force of injury, it may result in isolated changes in the traumatic area or distant sequelae that depend upon variables such as acceleration with translational or rotational forces, shearing injury to fiber tracts and blood vessels, and contusion (Gennarelli *et al.* 1982).

Early seizures are likely have a different pathogenesis than late seizures; early PTS are thought to be due to mechanical damage to neurons, related to extravasated blood (Gupta and Gupta 2006), brain swelling, perioperative events from cerebral manipulation or stress from general anaesthesia, and metabolic factors.

The precise mechanisms of epileptogenesis in late PTS are poorly understood. However, many structural, physiologic, and biochemical changes take place in the brain following head trauma. Understanding these changes will allow better understanding of epileptogenesis after head trauma (Gupta and Gupta 2006).

Stretch injury is the commonest mechanism of neuronal injury. Mechanically, it results in sliding of the lipid bilayer of the cell membrane from the protein receptors and channels resulting in a phenomenon described as mechano-poration; this explains excitotoxicity as a mechanism (see below). Simultaneously, there is a breach in the blood–brain barrier and the release of intracellular adhesion molecules resulting in the ingress of leukocytes (Whalen *et al.* 1998). This leukocytic ingress triggers inflammatory cascades further poisoning the ionic pump. It has also been suggested that there is iron (hemorrhage) induced neuronal lipid peroxidation and excitotoxicity which explains the oxidative stress mechanism (Gennarelli *et al.* 1982) (see below).

Excitotoxicity as a mechanism

Both clinical and experimental studies have demonstrated an immediate and marked increase in the extracellular level of excitatory amino acids following brain injury (Katayama *et al.* 1990). There is a release of excitotoxic amino acids, causing further disturbance to the ionic pump mechanisms, resulting in escape of potassium into the extracellular space and ingress of calcium into the cell (Choi 1987). Increased extracellular potassium further increases neuronal excitability and may contribute to epileptogenesis (Nilsson *et al.* 1994). Intracellular calcium activates phospholipases causing free fatty acid release and the release of oxygen-free radicals which damage the blood–brain barrier and may induce DNA damage (Bramlett and Dietrich 2004). Intracellular calcium can also trigger cytoskeletal disruption.

Oxidative stress mechanism

It has been proposed that reactive oxygen species (ROS), especially hydroxyl radicals, are partially responsible for PTE (Gupta and Gupta 2006). Willmore (Willmore *et al.* 1978) suggested that after intracranial hemorrhage, red blood cells break down and release iron ions from hemoglobin, which then generate ROS. These free radicals react with the methylene group, adjacent to the double bond of polyunsaturated fatty acids and lipids, causing hydrogen abstractions and subsequent propagation of peroxidation reaction. Non-enzymatic initiation and propagation of lipid peroxidation causes disruption of membranes and subcellular organelles. Injury to

401

membranes impairs Na$^+$–K$^+$ ATPase activity (which maintains ionic gradients of neuron) and this decrease in activity lowers the convulsive threshold. Injury to the membrane also leads to neurotransmitter disorders. The release of aspartic acid, an excitatory neurotransmitter, increases and the release of γ-aminobutyric acid (GABA), which is an inhibitory neurotransmitter, decreases (Gupta and Gupta 2006). These findings suggest that oxidation by ROS, especially hydroxyl radicals, is involved in mechanisms leading to post-traumatic epilepsy.

Neuronal sprouting mechanism

Following trauma, induced neuronal loss and a neurorecovery process take place. These processes include axonal sprouting, neosynaptic genesis, and dentate gyrus region proliferation of progenitor cells (Dixon *et al.* 1987). Disorganization in this neosynaptogenesis process may result in epileptogenesis.

In summary, head trauma initiates a sequence of responses that includes altered blood flow and vasoregulation, disruption of the blood–brain barrier, an increase in intracranial pressure, focal or diffuse ischemic hemorrhage, inflammation, necrosis, disruption of fiber tract and blood vessels, and cerebral plasticity; all of these factors can contribute to post-traumatic epilepsy.

Risk factors for post-traumatic seizures

It is well established that TBI increases the risk of epilepsy; however, much less is known about the characteristics of TBI associated with that risk. Civilian patients who experience severe TBI may have up to a 30-fold increased incidence of epilepsy compared to the general population (Lowestein 2009). Overall the relative risks of epilepsy are raised twofold (relative risk 2.2) after a mild head injury and sevenfold (7.4) after severe head injury; risks are slightly greater in women than in men, and are increased with older age at time of injury (Shorvon and Neligan 2009). However, little is known about the magnitude and duration of increased risk and factors that modify risk.

Early seizures

The most consistent risk factor is the presence of intracranial blood, followed by higher injury severity (Frey 2003). Early seizures have been shown to occur 50–100% more frequently in children than in adults with comparable injuries (Annegers *et al.* 1998). Other risk factors influencing the occurrence of early PTS include diffuse cerebral edema, intracranial metal-fragment retention, residual focal neurologic deficits, and depressed or linear skull fractures (Frey 2003).

Late seizures

The presence of early seizures is the most consistently significant risk factor for the development of late PTS (Frey 2003). The relation between early PTS and the development of late PTS varies based on age and is more consistent in adults than in children. Intracerebral hemorrhage is also a risk factor for the occurrence of late PTS; subdural hematomas are likely responsible for most of this increased risk in both children and adults. Brain contusion was as strong a predictor of late seizure occurrence as subdural hematoma. Markers of increased injury severity have been shown to significantly increase the risk of late PTS. Age older than 65 years at the time of injury is a significant risk factor and premorbid chronic alcoholism likely increases that risk. Other risk factors for the development of late PTS include metal-fragment retention, skull fracture, residual cortical neurologic deficits, a single computed tomography (CT) lesion in the temporal or frontal regions, and persistent focal abnormalities on electroencephalogram (EEG) over 1 month after injury (Angeleri *et al.* 1999; Frey 2003).

There is a wide range of variability in individuals' responses to similar injuries. Some patients seize frequently after a head injury, whereas others may seize once or not at all, despite almost identical injury severity. There is speculation that much of this variability is due to genetic factors regulating response to cerebral injury (Caveness 1976). Multiple studies have attempted to demonstrate this genetic influence, with contradictory results. Some have found that family history of epilepsy is not a significant risk factor for the development of seizures after head injury whereas others have reported that the incidence of epilepsy was greater in head-injured people with a family history of epilepsy. Preliminary evidence indicates that the apoE-ε4 allele (Diaz-Arrastia *et al.* 2003) and haptoglobin Hp2-2 allele (Sadrzadeh *et al.* 2004) may be risk factors for PTE.

In summary, several patient and injury characteristics increase the likelihood for the development of late PTS. Some important patient characteristics include: increasing age, premorbid alcohol abuse, and family history. In terms of injury characteristics, markers of increasing injury severity such as penetrating injuries and depressed skull fracture increase the risk of late PTS. A seizure occurring immediately after injury substantially increases the risk of late PTS.

Natural history of post-traumatic seizures
Onset

In most cases of PTE, the risk of seizures is highest in the first year after trauma, and decreases progressively thereafter. One-half to two-thirds of patients who suffer PTS will experience seizure onset within the first 12 months, and 75–90% will have seizures by the end of the second year following the injury (Salazar *et al.* 1985; da Silva *et al.* 1990).

How long increased risk persists is a matter of controversy. After 5 years, adults with mild TBI no longer have a significantly increased risk relative to the general population (Annagers *et al.* 1998), whereas patients with moderate TBI remain at increased risk for more than 10 years post-injury and those with severe TBI have an increased risk for

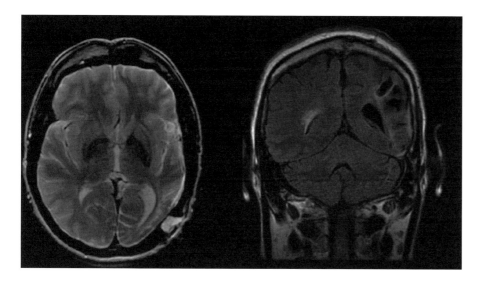

Fig. 58.1. Fifty-four-year-old right-handed man who sustained a severe closed head injury at the age of 10 and began having seizures a year later, whose MRI revealed left occipital, parietal, and temporal encephalomalacia. His seizures became refractory to AEDs, and he underwent presurgical evaluation. Seizure onset was found to be in the left mesial temporal region.

over 20 years after injury (Salazar *et al.* 1985; Annagers *et al.* 1998; Lowestein 2009).

Recurrence and remission

The total number of seizures over a lifetime in patients with PTS is not associated with any identifiable variables such as age or severity of injury, and often varies widely even within generally homogeneous populations (Frey 2003). Following early seizures post-TBI, only one-half of the patients experienced a single recurrence while another quarter experience a total of only two to three more seizures (Kollevold 1979). Most patients who will have a second unprovoked late PTS do so during the first 2 years after their first late PTS. Up to 86% of TBI survivors with a first PTS will also have a second within the following 2 years (Haltiner *et al.* 1997).

Remission rates among patients with PTS range from 25% to 40%, with higher overall remission rates reported in studies performed after the development of effective anti-epileptic drugs (AEDs) (Frey 2003). It is thought that no significant relation exists between the latency to first seizure and seizure duration or persistence, although patients with frequent seizures in the first year will often continue to have frequent seizures and have a smaller chance of seizure remission (Salazar *et al.* 1985).

Diagnosis of post-traumatic seizures

Investigation of seizures in patients who have sustained head injuries should focus on assessing whether the seizure was caused by a metabolic abnormality (e.g., hyponatremia) or an intracranial bleed. In a clinically stable patient whose serum electrolytes are within normal range and whose neurological examination appears to be similar to baseline, further laboratory studies are not indicated. If the patient presents with a seizure later after the head injury, standard

investigations including EEG, CT, and magnetic resonance imaging (MRI) are indicated.

Electroencephalography

Despite the important role that EEG plays in the evaluation of patients with epilepsy, particularly the diagnosis of seizures, it does not play a role in predicting the development of post-traumatic epilepsy (Jennet and van De 1975). Many patients who eventually develop post-traumatic epilepsy may have normal recordings early after injury. Risk factors in the EEG for late post-traumatic epilepsy may include delta slowing and focal epileptiform discharges, not uncommonly from the temporal lobes; however, these recordings may actually normalize in patients yet to evidence clinical seizures (Dalmady-Israel *et al.* 1993). Conversely, persistent focal disturbances are not necessarily related to future seizures.

Video-EEG long-term monitoring may be required if there is a need to record and analyze infrequent ictal and interictal EEG patterns as well as undefined nocturnal events. This test is always necessary when there is a suspicion that the events described by the patient may be non-epileptic in origin. Patients suffering severe closed head injury may develop post-traumatic stress disorder and may have non-epileptic attacks that can be confused with epileptic seizures. Furthermore, this test is indicated in patients who are candidates for epilepsy surgery when their seizures are therapy-resistant.

Neuroimaging

Magnetic resonance imaging of the brain is the investigation of choice (Fig. 58.1); however, when MRI is not available or in emergency situations, a CT scan of the head allows visualization of underlying pathology which may need urgent surgical intervention (e.g., intracranial hemorrhage, depressed fracture).

Structural imaging has shown promise for improving prediction of post-traumatic seizure risk. It has been demonstrated that the presence of focal hemorrhagic brain damage (with or without satellite extracerebral hematomas) on CT scans, performed within 48 hr following brain damage, is one of the most powerful predictive factors for early and late epilepsy (D´Alessandro et al. 1988). Magnetic resonance imaging is superior to CT scan in patients with late-onset post-traumatic epilepsy, particularly for demonstrating deposits of hemosiderin on T2-weighted sequences. The formation of gliotic scars around the hemosiderin is a significant predictive factor for the occurrence of seizures (Kumar et al. 2003). Furthermore, MRI is more sensitive for the detection of white-matter abnormalities, such as diffuse axonal injury.

Single photon emission computed tomography (SPECT) has limited value in the assessment of patients with closed head injury, although it has utility in the localization of an epileptogenic focus during presurgical evaluation of patients with therapy-resistant epilepsy, particularly in cases of dual pathology, where one of the lesions is post-traumatic (Chassagnon et al. 2006). Attempts to examine the relation between SPECT findings and specific post-concussive symptoms have yielded mixed and inconsistent results (Lewine et al. 2007). On the other hand, positron emission tomography (PET) is a technique for interictal study that has been extensively applied in presurgical evaluations of refractory seizures; however, due to its nature and the fact that epileptogenic areas as well as areas of encephalomalacia due to trauma would be hypometabolic, this test has a lesser value in cases of dual pathology.

Other tests

In general, the first seizure of late onset following closed head injury should be evaluated as with any new, unprovoked seizure, including consideration of other etiologies. If the patient becomes medically intractable, considerations for presurgical evaluation are warranted, including neuropsychology evaluation. This evaluation would also be recommended in those patients required to be on antiepileptic medication, in order to document the patient's baseline functioning (Agrawal et al. 2006).

Treatment of post-traumatic seizures

A seizure that occurs soon after a head injury may cause secondary brain damage, due to the increased metabolic demands of the brain soon after the injury, increased intracranial pressure, and excessive amounts of neurotransmitter release which may lead to additional brain injury (Agrawal et al. 2006). For this reason, the primary therapeutic objective in the use of anticonvulsant drugs has been the prevention of early seizures in an attempt to minimize the extent of brain damage following an injury (Agrawal et al. 2006). Recent pathophysiological studies have shown that some AEDs can also have neuroprotective effects (Agrawal et al. 2006). Animal models have indicated that phenytoin reduces neuronal damage in hypoxia, and that carbamazepine and valproate may also have neuroprotective effects (Watson and Lanthorn 1995; Bac et al. 1998); this suggests that AEDs have beneficial properties that are independent of their proposed anti-seizure activity. Conversely, AEDs have shown toxic effects even in stable patients, with impaired mental and motor function being the most common adverse effects, although serious adverse effects including deaths as a result of hematological reactions have also been reported (Schierhout and Roberts 2001).

Prophylactic anticonvulsant

Long-term prophylaxis after TBI is no longer warranted in the absence of a clinically definable seizure disorder (Temkin 2001; Beghi 2003). Prophylaxis during the first week after injury can suppress early seizures at a time when brain metabolism and blood flow may be compromised. After a week, prophylaxis should be discontinued (Agrawal et al. 2006). However, patients with early PTE, dural-penetrating injuries, multiple contusions, and/or subdural hematoma requiring evacuation may need continuation of anticonvulsant medication beyond the first week post-injury. Although AEDs appear to decrease the rate of early seizures, there is no evidence that the prevention of early seizures affects mortality, morbidity, or the development of late PTE (Beghi 2003).

Phenytoin has the most evidence to support its use to reduce early post-traumatic seizures. If treatment is limited to only 1 week, the risk of acute idiosyncratic reactions will be small.

Pharmacological treatment

Treatment of early-onset seizures is imperative, as there is evidence that they can result in secondary brain damage as a result of increased metabolic demands, raised intracranial pressure, and excess neurotransmitter release. As mentioned before, there is a lack of evidence regarding the prophylactic use of AEDs. On the other hand, antiepileptic drugs have had a significant impact on the treatment of psychiatric illnesses, especially in the role as mood stabilizers and for treatment of anxiety disorders, sometimes associated with post-traumatic stress disorder. Carbamazepine and valproate are well established (Temkin 2009), and accumulating data suggest that newer AEDs are also effective, including gabapentin, lamotrigine, and topiramate, although their efficacy needs to be established in placebo-controlled, randomized, clinical trials.

Surgical treatment

Head injuries frequently cause bilateral and multifocal injuries not amenable to surgical treatment. However, there are some cases in which surgery is a very effective treatment, particularly frontal-lobe epilepsy secondary to encephalomalacia. The results from surgical series are mixed. Marks and colleagues

(Marks *et al.* 1995) reviewed 25 patients with intractable post-traumatic complex partial seizures and found 17 with medial temporal seizure foci and 8 with neocortical (extra-hippocampal) foci. Of the mesial group, 14 underwent surgery, and 6 were found with hippocampal cell loss; in the remaining group there was non-specific gliosis with normal hippocampal cell count. Seizure-freedom or 90% reduction in seizures were seen in those with hippocampal cell loss, while only one patient without cell loss had more than a 50% reduction in seizure frequency.

References

Agrawal A, Timothy J, Pandit L, Manju M (2006) Post-traumatic epilepsy: an overview. *Clin Neurol Neurosurg* **108**:433–9.

Angeleri F, Majkowski J, Cacchio G, *et al.* (1999) Post-traumatic epilepsy risk factors: one-year prospective study after head injury. *Epilepsia* **40**:1222–30.

Annegers JF, Grabow JD, Groover RV, *et al.* (1980) Seizures after head trauma: a population study. *Neurology* **30**:683–9.

Annegers JF, Hauser WA, Coan SP, Rocca WA (1998) A population-based study of seizures after traumatic brain injuries. *N Engl J Med* **338**:20–4.

Armstrong KK, Sahgal V, Bloch R, Armstrong KJ, Heinemann A (1990) Rehabilitation outcomes in patients with post–traumatic epilepsy. *Arch Phys Med Rehabil* **71**:156–60.

Asikainen I, Kaste M, Sarna S (1999) Early and late post-traumatic seizures in traumatic brain injury rehabilitation patients: brain injury factors causing late seizures and influence of seizures on long-term outcome. *Epilepsia* **40**:584–9.

Bac P, Maurois P, Dupont C, *et al.* (1998). Magnesium deficiency-dependent audiogenic seizures (MDDASs) in adult mice: a nutritional model for discriminatory screening of anticonvulsant drugs and original assessment of neuroprotection properties. *J Neurosci* **18**:4363–73.

Beghi E (2003) Overview of studies to prevent post-traumatic epilepsy. *Epilepsia* **44**(Suppl 10):21–6.

Bramlett HM, Dietrich WD (2004) Pathophysiology of cerebral ischemia and brain trauma: similarities and differences. *J Cereb Blood Flow Metab* **24**:133–50.

Bruns J Jr., Hauser WA (2003) The epidemiology of traumatic brain injury: a review. *Epilepsia* **44**(Suppl 10):2–10.

Caveness WF (1976) Epilepsy, a product of trauma in our time. *Epilepsia* **17**:207–15.

Chassagnon S, Valenti MP, Sabourdy C, *et al.* (2006) Towards a definition of the "practical" epileptogenic zone: a case of epilepsy with dual pathology. *Epilept Disord* **8**(Suppl 2):S67–76.

Choi DW (1987) Ionic dependence of glutamate neurotoxicity. *J Neurosci* **7**:369–79.

Christensen J, Pedersen MG, Pedersen CB, *et al.* (2009). Long-term risk of epilepsy after traumatic brain injury in children and young adults: a population-based cohort study. *Lancet* **373**:1105–10.

D'Alessandro R, Ferrara R, Benassi G, Lenzi PL, Sabattini L (1988) Computed tomographic scans in post-traumatic epilepsy. *Arch Neurol* **45**:42–3.

da Silva AM, Vaz AR, Ribeiro I, *et al.* (1990) Controversies in post-traumatic epilepsy. *Acta Neurochir Suppl (Wien)* **50**:48–51.

Dalmady-Israel C, Zasler ND (1993) Post-traumatic seizures: a critical review. *Brain Inj* **7**:263–73.

Diaz-Arrastia R, Agostini MA, Frol AB, *et al.* (2000). TI: neurophysiologic and neuroradiologic features of intractable epilepsy after traumatic brain injury in adults. *Arch Neurol* **S7**:1611–16.

Diaz-Arrastia R, Gong Y, Fair S, *et al.* (2003) Increased risk of late post-traumatic seizures associated with inheritance of APOE epsilon4 allele. *Arch Neurol* **60**:818–22.

Dixon CE, Lyeth BG, Povlishock JT, *et al.* (1987) A fluid percussion model of experimental brain injury in the rat. *J Neurosurg* **67**:110–19.

Frey LC (2003) Epidemiology of post-traumatic epilepsy: a critical review. *Epilepsia* **44**(Suppl 10):11–17.

Gennarelli TA, Thibault LE, Adams JH, *et al.* (1982) Diffuse axonal injury and traumatic coma in the primate. *Ann Neurol* **12**:564–74.

Greenwald BD, Burnett DM, Miller MA (2003). Congenital and acquired brain injury. I. Brain injury: epidemiology and pathophysiology. *Arch Phys Med Rehabil* **84**:S3–7.

Gupta YK, Gupta M (2006) Post-traumatic epilepsy: a review of scientific evidence. *Indian J Physiol Pharmacol* **50**:7–16.

Haltiner AM, Temkin NR, Dikmen SS (1997) Risk of seizure recurrence after the first late posttraumatic seizure. *Arch Phys Med Rehabil* **78**:835–40.

Hauser WA, Annegers JF, Kurland LT (1991) Prevalence of epilepsy in Rochester, Minnesota: 1940–1980. *Epilepsia* **32**:429–45.

Jennett B, van De SJ (1975) EEG prediction of post-traumatic epilepsy. *Epilepsia* **16**:251–6.

Jensen FE (2009) Introduction: post-traumatic epilepsy – treatable epileptogenesis. *Epilepsia* **50**(Suppl 2):1–3.

Katayama Y, Becker DP, Tamura T, Hovda DA (1990) Massive increases in extracellular potassium and the indiscriminate release of glutamate following concussive brain injury. *J Neurosurg* **73**:889–900.

Kollevold T (1979) Immediate and early cerebral seizures after head injuries. IV. *J Oslo City Hosp* **29**:35–47.

Kumar R, Gupta RK, Husain M, *et al.* (2003). Magnetization transfer MR imaging in patients with posttraumatic epilepsy. *AJNR Am J Neuroradiol* **24**:218–24.

Lewine JD, Davis JT, Bigler ED, *et al.* (2007) Objective documentation of traumatic brain injury subsequent to mild head trauma: multimodal brain imaging with MEG, SPECT, and MRI. *J Head Trauma Rehab* **22**:141–55.

Lowenstein DH (2009) Epilepsy after head injury: an overview. *Epilepsia* **50**(Suppl 2):4–9.

Marks DA, Kim J, Spencer DD, Spencer SS (1995) Seizure localization and pathology following head injury in patients with uncontrolled epilepsy. *Neurology* **45**:2051–7.

Nilsson P, Ronne-Engstrom E, Flink R, *et al.* (1994). Epileptic seizure activity in the acute phase following cortical impact trauma in rat. *Brain Res* **637**:227–32.

Sadrzadeh SM, Saffari Y, Bozorgmehr J (2004) Haptoglobin phenotypes in epilepsy. *Clin Chem* **50**:1095–7.

Salazar AM, Jabbari B, Vance SC, *et al.* (1985). Epilepsy after penetrating head injury. I. Clinical correlates: a report of the Vietnam Head Injury Study. *Neurology* **35**:1406–14.

Schierhout G, Roberts I (2001). Anti-epileptic drugs for preventing seizures following acute traumatic brain injury. *Cochrane Database Syst Rev*:CD000173.

Shorvon S, Neligan A (2009) Risk of epilepsy after head trauma. *Lancet* **373**:1060–1.

Temkin NR (2001) Antiepileptogenesis and seizure prevention trials with antiepileptic drugs: meta-analysis of controlled trials. *Epilepsia* **42**:515–24.

Temkin NR (2009) Preventing and treating post-traumatic seizures: the human experience. *Epilepsia* **50**(Suppl 2):10–13.

Watson GB, Lanthorn TH (1995) Phenytoin delays ischemic depolarization, but cannot block its long-term consequences, in the rat hippocampal slice. *Neuropharmacology* **34**:553–8.

Whalen MJ, Carlos TM, Kochanek PM, *et al.* (1998) Soluble adhesion molecules in CSF are increased in children with severe head injury. *J Neurotrauma* **15**:777–87.

Willmore LJ, Sypert GW, Munson JB (1978) Recurrent seizures induced by cortical iron injection: a model of post-traumatic epilepsy. *Ann Neurol* **4**:329–36.

Chapter 59

De novo epilepsy after neurosurgery

Charles E. Polkey

Introduction

Epilepsy after neurosurgery is a complex subject. The literature regarding de novo seizures after neurosurgery is sparse, and much of it was published some years ago. It therefore deals with the use of older drugs and the distinction between early and late seizures is neglected. The incidence of seizures is influenced by factors including the underlying disease process, itself influenced by the nature and chronicity of the process and the neurosurgical procedure. Imposed upon these are the influences of other treatments ranging from immediate postoperative events to long-term effects such as radionecrosis which may present up to 15 years after therapeutic irradiation. There are very few clinical models that allow dissection of the provocative factors in de novo epilepsy after surgery. For some procedures, such as uncomplicated craniotomy, head injury may be considered a useful model but even here, in 20% of cases, epilepsy may present for the first time 4 years after injury. Another potential model is subarachnoid hemorrhage. Here the onset is relatively sudden in a previous normal brain and intervention often follows quickly. In addition, there are now good data comparing the outcome from interventional radiological treatment with microsurgical clipping of aneurysms. Similar comparisons can be made between the transsphenoidal and subfrontal approaches to a pituitary tumor, and cerebrospinal fluid (CSF) diversion or third ventriculostomy in treating the raised pressure associated with posterior fossa lesions.

It should also be recalled that anesthesia and in particular recovery from anesthesia can give conditions in which seizures may occur. Electrolyte imbalance, poor gaseous exchange, in particular hypercarbia, and certain anesthetic agents such as sevoflurane, can all produce seizures during recovery from anesthesia. Seizures in the first 48 hr after craniotomy require urgent assessment as their occurrence may indicate a significant postoperative complication. Fukamachi et al. (1985) noted seizures in 44 of 493 operations (8.9%) and in 12 of these patients there were significant lesions on computed tomography (CT) scans. However, other authors have not described significant intracranial complications such as hemorrhage with immediate postoperative seizures.

Frequency of epilepsy after neurosurgery

The frequency of epilepsy in certain conditions is well known, for example, de novo epilepsy after operative treatment of intracranial abscess is around 70% but this would probably occur independent of the surgical technique used. It is therefore difficult to assess the real influence of surgical technique and surgical intervention on de novo epilepsy in this condition. Studies of the incidence of epilepsy in patients with posterior fossa lesions shows that without a CSF diversion procedure such as a shunt or drain the incidence is 1.1% compared with 6.7% in shunted cases. In the shunted cases, in this series, epilepsy was associated with a blocked shunt or hematoma (Patir and Banerji 1990). Likewise the incidence of seizures after endoscopic ventriculostomy is low and usually associated with adverse events. Recent papers put it at 1% (Ersahin and Arslan 2008). Similar figures are quoted for epilepsy after operations involving the insertion of deep brain stimulating electrodes as in movement disorder treatment with lesioning or stimulators.

In a study of 716 patients undergoing posterior fossa surgery five patients had seizures within the first 24 hr (0.7%) and 13 within the first 2 weeks (1.8%). The causes of these seizures were mixed and included metabolic acidosis and hypernatremia in the first 24 hr and between 2 days and 14 days they were associated with shunting for hydrocephalus and remote supratentorial hemorrhage (Lee et al. 1990). In a study of early postoperative seizures (within 3 weeks of surgery) among 128 patients with chronic subdural hematomata, the incidence was 5.4%. In the subgroups analyzed according to CT lesion density, the incidences were 6.2% in the low-density group, 2.4% in the isodense group, and 13.7% in the mixed-density group (Chen et al. 2004). In the mixed density group, in which there was more active bleeding, epilepsy was most likely. In 118 craniotomies reported from Canada, performed for a miscellany of reasons, there were 87 patients who had not

The Causes of Epilepsy, eds. S. D. Shorvon, F. Andermann, and R. Guerrini. Published by Cambridge University Press. © Cambridge University Press 2011.

Table 59.1 Incidence of epilepsy in different methods of treatment in the International Subarachnoid Aneurysm Trial (ISAT)

	Endovascular treatment ($n = 1073$)		Neurosurgery ($n = 1070$)	
	Patients	Percent	Patients	Percent
Before first treatment	3 (3)	0.28	11 (6)	1.03
Procedure to discharge	16 (2)	1.49	33 (2)	3.08
Discharge to 1 year follow-up	27 (1)	2.52	44	4.11
After first year of follow-up	14 (1)	1.3	24	2.24
Total	**60**	**5.59**	**112**	**10.47**

Note:
Figures in brackets are numbers of patients rebleeding.
Source: After Molyneux *et al.* (2005).

experienced seizures before surgery and 11 of these had seizures within the first week after operation (12.6%), of whom six patients had seizures within the first 24 hr (Matthew *et al.* 1980).

A number of papers have reported the incidence of de novo epilepsy following craniotomy. Late-onset seizures were reported in 8% of patients undergoing craniotomy for astrocytic tumors (Hwang *et al.* 2001). In a series of 107 children undergoing craniotomy for a variety of causes, half of whom were receiving prophylactic anticonvulsants, 13 patients (12%) developed epilepsy within 12 months (Kombogiorgas *et al.* 2006). In another study involving 538 patients there was epilepsy after operation in 23 patients (4.3%) and de novo epilepsy in 18 of these (3.3%). Among 72 palliative craniotomies for glioblastoma multiforme there were 17 patients (23.6%) who had postoperative seizures and all except one of these seizures occurred after withdrawal of the prophylactic anticonvulsants (Telfeian *et al.* 2001).

It is interesting to compare the incidence of epilepsy in treatment modalities for the same condition which involve an intracranial approach with those which involve some other approach. Pituitary tumors are mostly treated by a transphenoidal approach now and the incidence of epilepsy in these patients is virtually zero, whereas when the transfrontal approach was used the incidence of epilepsy was 4–6%.

A slightly more complex situation is the treatment of aneurysmal subarachnoid hemorrhage. Here some patients are treated with a direct approach to the aneurysm involving craniotomy whereas others are treated using a closed endovascular approach. Of course, a certain liability to epilepsy will arise from the pathological consequences of the hemorrhage itself. A paper by Artiola Fortuny and colleagues in 1980 found that among 256 patients operated for aneurysmal subarachnoid hemorrhage who were followed up for between 18 months and 5 years there were nine who developed epilepsy, four in the first 24 hr and five later (Fabinyi and Artiola-Fortuny). Overall this is an incidence of 4.5% and according to these authors this is lower than other series at that time where the incidence varied between 8.4% and 15% (Fabinyi and Artiola-Fortuny 1980). A more modern series treated with

both clipping and coiling gives an incidence of symptomatic seizures 11.7% and unprovoked seizures 3.2%, giving an overall incidence of 15.3% in a group of 137 patients (Lin *et al.* 2008). When endovascular treatment of aneurysmal subarachnoid hemorrhage became practical, a trial, the International Subarachnoid Aneurysm Trial (ISAT), was set up to compare the results of endovascular coiling with direct surgery, usually clipping. Molyneux and colleagues (2005) compared the results in 1073 patients treated by endovascular coiling and 1070 patients treated by clipping. The results are shown in Table 59.1 at all stages of treatment and follow-up the incidence of epilepsy is lower in the coiled patients.

It seems that craniotomy probably increases the liability of de novo epilepsy by 5–10%. The complexity of the procedure also increases the incidence.

Pathophysiology

This is a broad and complex topic, bearing in mind the wide range of neurosurgical procedures both in terms of their underlying pathology, the severity of the intervention, and the region of the brain involved. There are few specific studies of these matters and some of these have already been alluded to.

The first point is a physiological one. A combination of the severity of the underlying disease and anesthetic conditions may produce a metabolic derangement such as hypoxia or electrolyte imbalance which could cause generalized convulsions. There may also be a secondary effect whereby acute cerebral edema is produced, itself significantly raising the threshold for seizures. These kinds of factors will produce seizures in the first 24–48 hr after surgery and if the edema is localized the seizures may be focal rather than generalized.

A second point is the effect of irritative substances on the brain, either directly or within the CSF. The commonest example of this is blood as in subarachnoid hemorrhage. This is mirrored by the well-known ability of certain chemicals, such as ferric chloride or penicillin, to produce an epileptic focus when applied to the cerebral cortex of experimental animals. An analogous clinical situation is the epileptogenic properties of the ring of hemoglobin breakdown products on the periphery of cavernomas.

A third point is the effect of gliosis, particularly in the cerebral cortex. Studies of post-traumatic epilepsy with modern imaging techniques have shown the relationship between cortical damage, in particular cortical contusions and post-traumatic epilepsy. There is a similar mechanism with cerebral abscesses which are surrounded by intense gliosis and have a 75% incidence of epilepsy. It is therefore clear that the underlying pathology will be one of the major factors that determine whether a patient will develop de novo epilepsy after neurosurgery.

Finally, it is evident from clinical experience that there are genetic and other factors that influence the development of epilepsy. For example the same or similar-sized meningiomas in the same location may cause raised pressure in one patient, neurological deficit in another, and seizures in a third. Again, series of patients operated upon for arteriovenous malformation show that the overall incidence of seizures before and after surgery is the same, some patients having lost their preoperative seizures and others having gained them after surgery. The influences of these factors are at present impossible to assess in any individual patient.

Surgical technique must play a part. The avoidance of conditions that provoke seizures such as hemorrhage and infection will reduce the incidence of epilepsy. Meticulous handling of tissue and retraction kept to a minimum will discourage gliosis and avoid damage to passing vessels which can produce distant lesions. Subpial dissection eliminates islands of gliotic tissue and also protects the adjacent underlying cortex and vessels from damage, and therefore should be used wherever possible.

Risk factors for epilepsy

As already suggested, there is some, as yet undefined, genetic factor that determines whether epilepsy develops in an individual patient. Outside of this, the location of the lesion and the nature of the lesion, particularly if it is destructive, will be potent factors in determining whether epilepsy develops. Although it might be thought that progressive lesions would be more likely to be associated with epilepsy than stationary ones, it must be remembered that even static lesions can slowly mature and produce epilepsy. The account above of the frequency of epilepsy illustrates how this varies with various conditions and increases with the complexity of the lesion.

Types of epilepsy

Accounts of this in the literature are sparse, but correspond to general principles and personal experience. The seizures that occur soon after the procedure, say within 48 hr, are likely to be generalized seizures because they are likely to relate to generalized brain dysfunction such as cerebral edema. Local cerebral edema at the site of intervention is less common but used to be seen after temporal lobectomy causing "neighborhood seizures" in the first week. By contrast, later seizures relating to localized brain dysfunction are likely to be complex partial seizures. The literature on cerebral tumors suggests that late postoperative seizures are more likely to be partial seizures and may be more difficult to control.

Principles of management

Management of the underlying condition is important and in some circumstances further surgery may be needed. One of the clearest predictors of success in surgery for drug-resistant epilepsy is the presence of a discrete, resectable lesion and this has also been noted in general surgery for gliomas where one author notes that complete resection is less likely to be followed by seizures. The majority of lesions encountered in this circumstance are, as it were, of natural origin such as cortical dysplasia or benign tumors, but even these are sometimes not completely removed when they could be. However, there are other conditions, such as cerebral abscess, where the primary treatment may not be surgical or the surgical management may not involve resection. In these circumstances serious consideration should be given to further surgery.

Drug treatment

This is a complex matter and individual advice about drug regimes is not appropriate to a review of this nature. Suffice it to say that most would agree that initially monotherapy is preferred to polytherapy. For generalized seizures the first choice is probably sodium valproate or if unsuccessful lamotrogine and for complex partial seizures carbamazepine or if unsuccessful valproate or phenytoin. More detailed advice can be found in Dulac et al. (2008) and an account of the clinical evidence for the use of various drugs is given by Glauser et al. (2006). Because of the many other considerations such as age, sex, coexistent disease, and so on, it is clearly essential for the non-specialist practitioner to seek advice in any individual case. Likewise the treatment of status epilepticus, which might arise in the immediate postoperative period, requires careful and expert management.

Prophylaxis

As with head injury, the prophylaxis of seizures by the use of anticonvulsant drugs remains a contentious issue with practice not governed by evidence. A survey by the American Association of Neurological Surgeons in 2005 showed that most still used prophylactic antiepileptic drugs (AEDs), and that the rate was higher amongst the neurosurgeons with the longer length of practice (Siomin et al. 2005). Michelucci in a review in 2006 concludes that AED prophylaxis is useful in the prevention of early seizures, those seizures that occur in the first week after surgery, but not otherwise (Michelucci 2006). This is in line with the recommendation of the Quality and Standards Committee of the American Academy of Neurology in 2000 that prophylactic AEDs were not useful in preventing first seizures, and should be discontinued after the seventh postoperative day (Glantz et al. 2000). In treating a group of 107 children subjected to supratentorial craniotomy for a variety of conditions, in whom the incidence of de novo seizures was 12%, Kombogiorgas and colleagues found that the use of prophylactic AEDs had no influence on the development of epilepsy (Kombogiorgas *et al.* 2006).

One of the important considerations in postoperative prophylaxis is the adequacy of treatment. Many of the early studies lack rigor, failing to distinguish between early and late seizures. Most of the studies relate to the use of older drugs; and, to use phenytoin as an example, it is clear, as suggested by Horwitz, that an adequate blood level is a prerequisite of successful prophylaxis (Horwitz 1989). This is of special importance in the immediate postoperative period when it seems that these drugs are most likely to be successful. Yeh and colleagues found that phenytoin levels could drop by as much as 26% as a result of craniotomy, mainly due to blood loss (Yeh *et al.* 2006). Lee and colleagues used intravenous phenytoin for prophylaxis in a group of 189 patients undergoing craniotomy and found that they could attain therapeutic levels in 59.8%. Compared with a control group given a placebo there were fewer seizures in the postoperative period. They also noted that in patients subjected to emergency surgery an appropriate loading dose should be administered 20 min before skin closure (Lee *et al.* 1989). One of the problems that arise with these drugs is the side effects; these will be dealt with later in discussing drug and treatment interactions. However, in a recent paper Milligan and colleagues compared levetiracetam with phenytoin, and noted that both prevented early seizures, and after adjusting for the proportion of patients with brain tumors, these drugs were equally effective but levetiracetam had fewer adverse effects and a higher retention rate at 1 year (Milligan *et al.* 2008).

The conclusion would seem to be that prophylactic AEDs are useful in reducing the likelihood of early postoperative seizures and that some thought should be given to using newer drugs. However, the ability to administer the drug parenterally and the means of identifying adequate treatment remain significant factors. Consideration also has to be given especially for continuing treatment of patients with established de novo epilepsy of the effects of other drugs and other treatments.

Antiepileptic drugs, especially the older drugs, are known to be metabolized along established pathways that they may share with other AEDs and also with non-anticonvulsant drugs. Of particular importance are the cytochrome P450 systems. When other drugs are given with the AEDs the pharmacokinetics of both are affected. For a detailed account consult Levy *et al.* (2008). Many recent papers emphasize the lower incidence of side effects and easier pharmacokinetics of the newer non-enzyme-inducing drugs such as levetiracetam.

In routine neurosurgery particular problems may occur with nimodipine, a calcium antagonist which is used very successfully to limit the effect of vasospasm after aneurysmal subarachnoid hemorrhage. Wong and colleagues note that nimodipine is metabolized via the cytochrome D450 3A4 system and that a number of AEDs (in particular phenytoin)

inhibit this system and therefore limit the availability of the nimodipine. They therefore suggest that valproate should be used instead (Wong and Poon 2005).

The same problem is seen with a number of antibiotics; for example, Michenfelder *et al.* (1990) examined retrospectively patients given penicillin after supratentorial procedures. The incidence of early seizures was 4.7% (20 cases) of the 427 patients given penicillins and only 1.8% (10 cases) of the 566 not given penicillins ($p < 0.01$). There are similar reports in regard to other antibiotics, especially those used in the intensive care setting.

Brain tumors present a special problem as discussed by van Breemen *et al.* (2007) For a number of reasons patients with brain tumors are more liable to develop side effects and adverse reactions to AEDs than the general population. Stevens–Johnson syndrome has been reported with several of these drugs. Nor should the cognitive effects of these drugs on patients whose intellectual capacity is already affected be ignored. Dexamethasone, which is commonly used to control peritumoral edema, has its half-life shortened by both phenytoin and phenobarbitone. Therefore phenytoin levels should be carefully monitored, especially when the steroid is being withdrawn, when phenytoin levels may easily go into the toxic range. The blood levels of chemotherapeutic agents may be lowered by concomitant administration of enzyme inducing AEDs. Conversely, valproate can inhibit the metabolism of some chemotherapeutic agents resulting in increased activity and possible toxic levels of these drugs. Other chemotherapeutic agents can lower the plasma levels of carbamazepine, valproate, and phenytoin. At present there are few reported problems with levetiracetam. Van Breemen *et al.* (2007) recommend the use of lamotrigine and valproate in localization-related epilepsy with levetiracetam and gabapentin as second-line drugs.

Adjuvant therapy

Aside from the complexities of drug interactions, adjuvant therapy of brain tumors, which chiefly relates to oncological diseases, can sometimes help to control seizures, including those that are produced or made worse by neurosurgical procedures.

The effect of radiotherapy on epilepsy arising from cerebral tumors is not well described. In treating arteriovenous malformations it is clear that epilepsy is only controlled when the lesion is totally obliterated whatever the means. On the other hand, it is well known that radiotherapy can cause cerebral damage, including damage from radionecrosis, which may cause epilepsy. Shuper *et al.* (2003) describing 219 children with cerebral tumors and epilepsy note that radiation damage is one cause of epilepsy and recommend that radiotherapy in these patients should be delayed as long as possible. There are two papers that describe the beneficial effects of radiotherapy, one in only nine patients with malignant gliomas and the other in five adults with low-grade astrocytomas (Rogers *et al.* 1993; Chalifoux and Elisevich 1996). Wick *et al.* (2005) noted that radiotherapy and chemotherapy made one-third of their patients seizure-free. Since radiotherapy is recommended in patients with brain tumors for survival rather than control of epilepsy, and a large number of patients are treated for this reason, it is clear that there is no consistent or striking effect of this treatment on seizures.

The effect of chemotherapy on epilepsy arising from cerebral tumors can be beneficial as summarized by Villaneuva *et al.* (2008). Pace and Brada both describe improvements in seizure control with temozolomide and Frenay with nitrosourea (Brada *et al.* 2003; Pace *et al.* 2003; Frenay *et al.* 2005).

Conclusions

(1) De novo seizures after neurosurgical procedures can be divided into early seizures in the first week and late seizures which have different origins.

(2) The incidence of the seizures depends upon the underlying pathology and the brain region. It also depends upon the complexity of the procedure, and the surgical technique. It can be reduced to some extent by surgical technique and by avoiding postoperative complications such as infection or hemorrhage.

(3) Treatment with AEDs should be used, conforming to the general principles for the use of these drugs.

(4) Prophylactic AEDs are not effective in preventing late seizures but may affect the occurrence of early seizures in the first postoperative week.

(5) Other treatments such as further surgery and adjuvant therapy for intracranial tumors may be useful in treating difficult de novo seizures.

References

Brada M, Viviers L, Abson C, et al. (2003) Phase II study of primary temozolomide chemotherapy in patients with WHO grade II gliomas. *Ann Oncol* **14**:1715–21.

Chalifoux R, Elisevich K (1996) Effect of ionizing radiation on partial seizures attributable to malignant cerebral tumors. *Stereotact Funct Neurosurg* **67**:169–82.

Chen CW, Kuo JR, Lin HJ, et al. (2004) Early post-operative seizures after burr-hole drainage for chronic subdural hematoma: correlation with brain CT findings. *J Clin Neurosci* **11**:706–9.

Dulac O, Leppik IE, Chadwick DW, Specchio L (2008) Starting and stopping treatment. In: Engel J, Pedley TA (eds.) *Epilepsy: A Comprehensive Textbook*, 2nd edn. Philadelphia, PA: Lippincott Williams and Wilkins, pp. 1301–25.

Ersahin Y, Arslan D (2008) Complications of endoscopic third ventriculostomy. *Childs Nerv Syst* **24**:943–8.

Fabinyi GC, Artiola-Fortuny L (1980) Epilepsy after craniotomy for intracranial aneurysm. *Lancet* **1**:1299–300.

Frenay MP, Fontaine D, Vandenbos F, Lebrun C (2005) First-line nitrosourea-based chemotherapy in symptomatic non-resectable supratentorial pure low-grade astrocytomas. *Eur J Neurol* **12**:685–90.

Fukamachi A, Koizumi H, Nukui H (1985) Immediate postoperative seizures: incidence and computed tomographic findings. *Surg Neurol* **24**:671–6.

Glantz MJ, Cole BF, Forsyth PA, et al. (2000) Practice parameter: anticonvulsant prophylaxis in patients with newly diagnosed brain tumors: Report of the Quality Standards Subcommittee of the American Academy of Neurology. *Neurology* **54**:1886–93.

Glauser T, Ben-Menachem E, Bourgeois B, (2006) ILAE treatment guidelines: evidence-based analysis of antiepileptic drug efficacy and effectiveness as initial monotherapy for epileptic seizures and syndromes. *Epilepsia* **47**:1094–120.

Horwitz NH (1989) Prophylactic anticonvulsants for prevention of immediate and early postcraniotomy seizures. *Surg Neurol* **32**:398.

Hwang SL, Lieu AS, Kuo TH, et al. (2001) Preoperative and postoperative seizures in patients with astrocytic tumors: analysis of incidence and influencing factors. *J Clin Neurosci* **8**:426–9.

Kombogiorgas D, Jatavallabhula NS, Sgouros S, et al. (2006) Risk factors for developing epilepsy after craniotomy in children. *Childs Nerv Syst* **22**:1441–5.

Lee ST, Lui TN, Chang CN, et al. (1989) Prophylactic anticonvulsants for prevention of immediate and early postcraniotomy seizures. *Surg Neurol* **31**:361–4.

Lee ST, Lui TN, Chang CN, Cheng WC (1990) Early postoperative seizures after posterior fossa surgery. *J Neurosurg* **73**:541–4.

Levy HR, Bourgeois BF, Hachad H (2008) Drug–drug interactions. In: Engel J, Pedley TA (eds.) *Epilepsy: A Comprehensive Textbook*, 2nd edn. Philadelphia, PA: Lippincott Williams and Wilkins, pp. 1235–48.

Lin YJ, Chang WN, Chang HW, et al. (2008) Risk factors and outcome of seizures after spontaneous aneurysmal subarachnoid hemorrhage. *Eur J Neurol* **15**:451–7.

Matthew E, Sherwin AL, Welner SA, Odusote K, Stratford JG (1980) Seizures following intracranial surgery: incidence in the first post-operative week. *Can J Neurol Sci* **7**:285–90.

Michelucci R (2006) Optimizing therapy of seizures in neurosurgery. *Neurology* **67**:(Suppl 4):S14–18.

Michenfelder JD, Cucchiara RF, Sundt TM Jr. (1990) Influence of intraoperative antibiotic choice on the incidence of early postcraniotomy seizures. *J Neurosurg* **72**:703–5.

Milligan TA, Hurwitz S, Bromfield EB (2008) Efficacy and tolerability of levetiracetam versus phenytoin after supratentorial neurosurgery. *Neurology* **71**:665–9.

Molyneux AJ, Kerr RS, Yu LM, et al. (2005) International subarachnoid aneurysm trial (ISAT) of neurosurgical clipping versus endovascular coiling in 2143 patients with ruptured intracranial aneurysms: a randomised comparison of effects on survival, dependency, seizures, rebleeding, subgroups, and aneurysm occlusion. *Lancet* **366**:809–17.

Pace A, Vidiri A, Galie E, et al. (2003) Temozolomide chemotherapy for progressive low-grade glioma: clinical benefits and radiological response. *Ann Oncol* **14**:1722–6.

Patir R, Banerji AK (1990) Complications related to pre-craniotomy shunts in posterior fossa tumors. *Br J Neurosurg* **4**:387–90.

Rogers LR, Morris HH, Lupica K (1993) Effect of cranial irradiation on seizure frequency in adults with low-grade astrocytoma and medically intractable epilepsy. *Neurology* **43**:1599–601.

Shuper A, Yaniv I, Michowitz S, *et al.* (2003) Epilepsy associated with pediatric brain tumors: the neuro-oncologic perspective. *Pediatr Neurol* **29**:232–5.

Siomin V, Angelov L, Li L, Vogelbaum MA (2005) Results of a survey of neurosurgical practice patterns regarding the prophylactic use of anti-epilepsy drugs in patients with brain tumors. *J Neurooncol* **74**:211–15.

Telfeian AE, Philips MF, Crino PB, Judy KD (2001) Postoperative epilepsy in patients undergoing craniotomy for glioblastoma multiforme. *J Exp Clin Cancer Res* **20**:5–10.

van Breemen MS, Wilms EB, Vecht CJ (2007) Epilepsy in patients with brain tumors: epidemiology, mechanisms, and management. *Lancet Neurol* **6**:421–30.

Villanueva V, Codina M, Elices E (2008) Management of epilepsy in oncological patients. *Neurologist* **14**:(Suppl 1):S44–54.

Wick W, Menn O, Meisner C, *et al.* (2005) Pharmacotherapy of epileptic seizures in glioma patients: who, when, why and how long? *Onkologie* **28**:391–6.

Wong GK, Poon WS (2005) Use of phenytoin and other anticonvulsant prophylaxis in patients with aneurysmal subarachnoid hemorrhage. *Stroke* **36**:2532.

Yeh JS, Dhir JS, Green AL, Bodiwala D, Brydon HL (2006) Changes in plasma phenytoin level following craniotomy. *Br J Neurosurg* **20**:403–6.

Chapter 60

Epilepsy after epilepsy surgery

Andre Palmini

Complete seizure control is the universal goal of treatment for persons with epilepsy. Fortunately, this goal is obtainable in the majority of patients with available antiepileptic drugs (AEDs) (Mattson *et al.* 1985, 1992; Kwan and Brodie 2000). However, because the worldwide prevalence of epilepsy is high, the percentage of patients with more severe epileptic syndromes defying complete medical control translates into millions of people with refractory seizures (Sander 2003; Noronha *et al.* 2007). This constitutes a challenging population, given the significant morbidity and pervasive negative impact on quality of life associated with recurrent, unexpected epileptic attacks (de Boer *et al.* 2008; Ngugi *et al.* 2010).

The challenge posed by refractory epileptic seizures has been the driving force behind a number of scientific efforts in epileptology, including a continuous justification for the development of new AEDs and also for the delineation of clinical trials to test the effectiveness of new and traditional AED regimens. This notwithstanding, the most pragmatic way to control medically refractory seizures is to evaluate patients for surgical candidacy. Multichannel video-electroencephalogram (EEG) recording capabilities and advances in structural and functional neuroimaging techniques have led to enormous progress in the field of epilepsy surgery in the past 25 years. The benefits of surgical treatment of surgically remediable epileptic syndromes are now beyond question and these procedures have improved the lives of thousands of children and adults in developed and developing countries (Engel 1996; Wiebe *et al.* 2001; Palmini 2009).

Understandably, the issues at stake are quite different when the neurologist discusses with a patient and his/her family the possibility to control seizures with AEDs or with surgery. To say the very least, potential failures with medications are more easily accepted than surgical failures, which is related to the different level of risks and expectations involved. Therefore, ideally, epilepsy surgery would be offered to and performed in patients with close to a 100% chance of complete seizure control for a very long time. Such a "hopeful" outcome scenario is inevitable in the minds of patients and relatives, but unfortunately is not realistic for many, in whom seizures recur following the surgical procedure.

The many aspects involved in the scenario of recurrent seizures following a surgical procedure for epilepsy are dealt with here. These vary according to a temporal dimension and also according to the reason for recurrence. There are acute or late postoperative seizures, as well as seizures related to the surgical procedure *itself* or surgical failures due to suboptimal localization and/or resection of the epileptogenic zone. The chapter is divided into five parts:

- an overview of biological and psychosocial issues that may be associated with seizure recurrence after epilepsy surgery
- an analysis of the dynamics of postoperative seizure recurrences
- considerations regarding seizure recurrence after temporal and extratemporal epilepsy surgery
- possible impact of modification or discontinuation of AED regimens on putative seizure recurrence
- de novo epilepsy after epilepsy surgery which includes postoperative seizures possibly related to surgically inflicted cortical damage and postoperative seizures possibly associated with disinhibition of potential (previously dormant) epileptogenic zones

Biological and psychosocial issues related to postoperative seizure recurrence

There are a number of reasons for the unwelcome scenario of epilepsy after epilepsy surgery, including the lack of reliable biological markers for the entire epileptogenic zone (EZ), the inevitable a posteriori verification of the correctness of the localization and resection of the EZ, the *dynamic* (as opposed to *static*, fixed) nature of the epileptogenic abnormalities, and the popular perception that epilepsy "cured" by surgery automatically means freedom from further treatment with AEDs.

The first issue concerns uncertainties related to the tissue to be excised. The ability to localize and resect the EZ varies according to the etiology and topography of the associated lesion and electrical abnormalities, *and there are no spatial*

The Causes of Epilepsy, eds. S. D. Shorvon, F. Andermann, and R. Guerrini. Published by Cambridge University Press. © Cambridge University Press 2011.

biological markers to delineate the EZ. Thus, such localization is always a matter of exploring targets and boundaries throughout the cerebral cortex. Owing to functional constraints, surgical procedures for electroclinical epilepsy syndromes in the temporal lobe often have a higher chance of fully resecting the EZ than procedures for extratemporal epilepsies. Furthermore, the strong impact of structural lesions upon epileptogenicity usually allow more pragmatic localization and extensive resections of the EZ in those epilepsies associated with a visible lesion in the magnetic resonance image (MRI), in contrast to MRI-negative scenarios. The identification of an epileptogenic lesion on MRI is, however, often related to the underlying etiology and a significant number of patients with refractory seizures – associated with milder forms of focal cortical dysplasia (FCD), for example (Palmini *et al.* 2004; Krsek *et al.* 2008) – have normal MRI.

It follows that the precise knowledge of the extent of tissue to be resected during epilepsy surgery is not fully available before the operation. The EZ – i.e., the amount of tissue to be resected to render a patient seizure-free – can only be confirmed retrospectively, and this confirmation cannot be separated from the surgical outcome itself. Thus, in many cases, recurring seizures indicate that the EZ was not completely resected.

In addition, epilepsy is highly dynamic and epileptogenic processes interact with brain circuits at different levels of development, generating complex anatomofunctional scenarios. Implicit in the idea of a surgical procedure to resect "the epileptic focus" is the expectation that such focus is an isolated, static, anatomical entity, with very little interference upon or from other brain regions. Such is not the case, as suggested by a number of findings, examples of which are discussed below.

The EZ associated with the most common etiology in patients with refractory partial seizures for which epilepsy surgery is performed – mesial temporal sclerosis (MTS) – has been apparently delineated (Engel 1996; Spencer *et al.* 2005; Paglioli *et al.* 2006). However, although the bulk of abnormalities is contained within a resectable part of the temporal lobe, even "complete" resections may not lead to lasting seizure freedom (Hennessy *et al.* 2000; McIntosh *et al.* 2004), suggesting that adjacent or interconnected regions, in the ipsilateral or contralateral hemisphere, may retain some epileptogenic potential. Upon closer scrutiny, different groups have shown that structural changes may be more widespread than previously thought in this entity, involving distant neocortical regions and also subcortical structures (de Santana *et al.* 2010; Labate *et al.* 2010). Possibly, this abnormal network interacts in a dynamic fashion leading either to a more spatially restricted or to a more diffuse "focus." A second example of a complex, dynamic, anatomofunctional scenario is the observation that distant cortical regions may be "disinhibited" by previous surgery in patients with FCD (Palmini 2010). The underlying mechanism of this is still to be understood, yet it is clear that following a resection of dysplastic cortex, some patients may present with recurrent seizures after months or even years of

seizure freedom. These seizures may arise from adjacent cortex (usually still harboring dysplastic tissue) or from more distant cortical regions, which were silent before operation and thus become independent, practically de novo, EZ in their own right. These observations revive the long-standing notion of a dormant "potential EZ" – a concept that itself has remained "dormant" for some time, although witnessing a rekindled interest recently (Penfield and Jasper 1954; Rosenow and Luders 2001). I will develop this aspect further in a later section. Finally, the *temporal dynamics* of "epileptic foci" associated with a number of etiologies can be confusing. The initial precipitating insult in patients with MTS may precede the onset of recurring complex partial seizures by decades. Similar observations are routinely seen in patients who suffered prenatal or perinatal vascular lesions or harbor certain types of malformative lesions such as polymicrogyria and nodular heterotopias, whose seizures may begin years or decades after the insult or the establishment of the malformation. The common denominator of these examples is that the dynamics of epileptogenesis challenges the "static" view of epilepsy. A significant challenge is to adapt epilepsy surgery procedures to this non-simplistic, dynamic view of focal epilepsy.

A final point concerns the management of AEDs following resective surgery and its potential impact on seizure recurrence postoperatively. Engaging in elective brain surgery is a major step for patients and families. Part of the psychological basis of agreeing to epilepsy surgery is not only having seizures controlled, but also being freed from AEDs. This very humane desire may lower the medical threshold for AED reduction or discontinuation, sometimes leading to seizure recurrence (see below).

The dynamics of postoperative seizure recurrences and its impact on outcome analysis

This section will review seizure recurrence without introducing the variable constituted by AED tapering or discontinuation. It may be difficult to differentiate seizure recurrence due to incomplete resection of the EZ from de novo epileptogenesis (to be discussed below); however, because the latter is probably less common (Hennessy *et al.* 2000), the discussion which follows assumes that seizures recurred because the EZ was not fully resected. As alluded to above, such incompleteness may even be related to the dynamics of epileptogenesis and does not necessarily mean a major failure of localization at the time of preoperative evaluation.

Clearly, studies in epilepsy surgery outcome vary significantly in methodology: this is a field plagued by a lack of studies providing clear-cut answers to the many questions posed by doctors, patients, and relatives. There are several reasons for this, including ethical, epileptological, and pragmatic aspects. It is debatable how ethically acceptable it is to deny or delay surgical treatment when candidacy is established, and only a few studies, employing creative protocols, have been able to circumvent these difficulties (Wiebe *et al.* 2001). Also, there are several interfering clinical, electrographic, imaging, and histological variables that make it difficult to focus strictly on homogeneous groups of patients, even when restricting the type of lesions and the topography. For instance, a hypothetical analysis of the outcome of the surgical treatment of low-grade tumors in the non-dominant temporal neocortex would still be affected by the fact that studied patients would have varying durations of epilepsy, some may have had a second insult, some may have presented with generalized seizures, the distribution of interictal spikes could be more or less extensive within and outside the temporal lobe, and the specific subtype of pathology could be more or less associated with microscopic extension beyond the visible lesion. All these factors may be relevant for the epileptogenicity of the lesion and ultimately impact on surgical outcome. Finally, there is the pragmatic aspect that epilepsy surgery centers tend to have particular (and at times peculiar) views on how to approach patients for presurgical evaluation and resective surgery, which often precludes comparison of results among centers.

Relevant to this discussion is the dynamic of surgical outcome which, in a sense, mirrors the dynamics of epileptogenicity in focal epilepsies. There are two extremes in the outcome continuum that would comply with a simplistic model of epileptogenesis and epilepsy surgery: patients who continue to have seizures some (short) time after operation (i.e., unquestionable failures) and patients who become and persist seizure-free for a really long time after the surgical procedure. These would be represented, respectively, by situations in which the EZ was not adequately localized/resected and by the opposite scenario, when the EZ was completely removed and no potential EZ re-emerged for a long time (see below). The latter would imply that the whole extent (macro- and microscopic) of the underlying pathology was identified by the available imaging techniques or inferred by EEG and that the epileptic focus did not impinge upon adjacent or synaptically connected cortical regions in the years preceding operation. However, this most favorable scenario is observed in only a limited number of patients undergoing presurgical evaluation and eventually taken to surgery. Many others have more dynamic evolutions.

When the surgical results of a group of patients are analyzed at a specific point in time, a number of possible outcomes may follow in the years to come. For instance, patients may be seizure-free for a number of months or years, including at the time of outcome analysis, and then relapse. These relapses may turn into recurrent attacks and constitute long-term failures ("running up") or seizure freedom may be possible again (McIntosh and Berkovic 2006), with or without modifications of the AED regimen. Conversely, patients may have had some postoperative seizures close to outcome analysis, but these may "run down" over the ensuing years (Salanova *et al.* 1996), and the patient may then become seizure-free, for a short or a very long time. Thus, the timing of outcome

analysis is crucial but the data are intrinsically fallible. The dynamic of outcome interferes even with survival analyses, because calculation of the probability of seizure recurrence takes into consideration the longest outcome of patients whose status may change in the future (Paglioli *et al.* 2004).

Furthermore, postoperative attacks may be identical, somewhat similar, or completely different from the refractory seizures that led to surgery. Such postoperative ictal semiology may suggest that the original EZ was at least partially missed or that some other factors may account for the seizures. Explaining semiologically distinct postoperative attacks is often difficult from a pathogenetic point of view, because it demands an understanding of epileptogenicity that challenges simplistic views. For instance, the appearance of different types of auras or the occurrence of motor seizures, including secondarily generalized seizures that were not present preoperatively in patients with temporal lobe epilepsy (TLE) (Hennessy *et al.* 2000; Henry *et al.* 2000) may suggest that potential, higher-threshold EZ were ignited (or "disinhibited") (Palmini 2006) and that "new" pathways of seizure propagation were created after operation. Not infrequently, however, postoperative attacks are less severe versions of those experienced preoperatively, particularly for the absence of secondary generalization, more focal involvement, occurrence only during sleep, or simply a reduced frequency overall. These suggest partial resection of a correctly localized EZ without disinhibition of a potential EZ.

Seizure recurrence after temporal and extratemporal epilepsy surgery

Unilateral mesial temporal lobe epilepsy due to hippocampal sclerosis (MTLE/HS) is the prototype of a surgically remediable epilepsy syndrome, in which the chances for medical control are reduced whereas the chances for surgical remediation are elevated. The proportion of patients with TLE/HS who *are* controlled by AED is somewhat variable, ranging from 10% to 60% according to patient referral source (Semah *et al.* 1998; Kobayashi *et al.* 2001; Yasuda *et al.* 2006). Patients recruited from the community or evaluated in studies of familial TLE tend to have higher rates of medical control, whereas these chances are very limited in patients who are seen in tertiary epilepsy outpatient clinics, because they have already proved refractory to medical management on community care. Focusing on those who did prove refractory and went to surgery, a number of studies have provided figures of recurrent postoperative seizures. In general, the longer the follow-up, the higher the probability of verifying recurrent seizures (Salanova *et al.* 1999; McIntosh *et al.* 2004; Schmidt *et al.* 2004a; Tellez-Zenteno *et al.* 2005). However, some studies report fairly stable seizure control over up to 10–12 years (Paglioli *et al.* 2004, 2006; Pimentel *et al.* 2010), suggesting that even unilateral TLE/HS may not be – as initially believed – an entirely homogenous syndrome, and also that other factors, including patient selection, might influence the chances of recurrent seizures in this entity.

Because TLE/HS has such a high relevance in the setting of epilepsy surgery, the issue of postoperative seizure recurrence needs to be approached in a way that helps counseling patients and families both before and after surgery. According to different series, around 50–80% of patients have lasting control of complex partial seizures following either temporal lobectomy or selective amygdalohippocampectomy for TLE/HS (Salanova *et al.* 1999; McIntosh *et al.* 2004; Paglioli *et al.* 2004, 2006). This prognosis has to accommodate, however, some variations which defy a simplistic view of resecting "the focus." The first is the persistence of auras in some patients. It has variably been shown that auras persist in 25–50% of patients after temporal lobe surgery (Bladin 1987; Fried *et al.* 1995; Binder *et al.* 2009). Why this happens is unclear but likely reflects a network view of the EZ – rather than a simplistic view of a single, isolated focus (Elliott *et al.* 2009a, b). Interestingly, persistence of aura has not been found to predict recurrence of complex partial or generalized seizures post-temporal lobectomy (McIntosh *et al.* 2004; Janszky *et al.* 2005; Tellez-Zenteno *et al.* 2005). Another important aspect of the surgical treatment of TLE/HS is that some patients may remain seizure-free for up to 8 years and then have one or more seizures. This late relapse is "almost" specific for this entity, at least in what concerns the many etiologies of temporal lobe epilepsy (McIntosh *et al.* 2004). Such delayed relapses raise obvious pathogenetic issues because the EZ was probably adequately resected, yet some part of the epileptic network gets somehow reactivated.

An elegant study from Melbourne (McIntosh and Berkovic 2006) analyzed the long-term outcome of 325 patients who underwent temporal lobectomy associated with different underlying etiologies during a 20-year period and who were followed for a median of 10 years. Of these patients 202 (62%) had at least one seizure after operation. The authors posed a practical question, namely, what happens after "the magic is broken" and a seizure occurs postoperatively. They showed that 80% of those who had a seizure ended up having a second attack and 70% a third seizure. The risk for further recurrence was related to the timing of the first postoperative seizure. When the latter occurred in the first 2 years after operation, the risk was four times greater than that in those patients in whom the first recurrence was after 2 years of postoperative seizure freedom. On average, however, half the patients who had one recurrent seizure had further attacks. Furthermore, the authors found that the probability of regaining seizure freedom diminishes progressively with each new relapse. For instance, of the 202 patients who had a first relapse, one-third achieved a minimum of 2 years of remission afterwards (median 4.4 years). On the other hand, when a second seizure ensued, the median time in "new" remission dropped to 2.8 years. The good news was that in those who did achieve a 2-year remission following seizure recurrence (that is, regained seizure freedom), the probability of being seizure-free 4 years later was 67%, and 7 years later 57%. How much, and through

which mechanisms, AEDs might interfere in this evolution is an open question.

Finally, as mentioned above, one has also to be prepared for the emergence of different types of seizures many months or years after surgery for TLE/HS (Hennessy *et al.* 2000; Henry *et al.* 2000). In a much-needed study, Hennessy and colleagues (2000) studied 44 patients with recurrent seizures following temporal lobe surgery. They showed that in 20 patients relapsing after surgery for unilateral TLE/HS, seizures variably originated from the ipsilateral frontal, contralateral frontal, ipsilateral temporal neocortex, contralateral temporal neocortex, ipsilateral hippocampal remnant, and contralateral hippocampus. In other words, months or years after an anterior temporal resection for what appeared to be clear-cut cases of TLE/HS, six different neurophysiological mechanisms of epileptogenicity were found to be associated with relapses.

Irrespective of this, pooling the results of different studies provides figures of around 65% of patients undergoing temporal lobe surgery as being seizure-free after 5 years (Wiebe *et al.* 2001; Tellez-Zenteno *et al.* 2005). Dissecting out these results shows that when the underlying etiology is HS or a low-grade tumor long-term results are better than when MRI is normal (McIntosh *et al.* 2004).

The prototype of refractory extratemporal epilepsy is FCD. Different from the subsyndromes associated with TLE, which are subdivided on the basis of the underlying pathology but have a common topographic denominator, FCD may occur in all cortical regions. However, most FCD lesions do impinge upon extratemporal regions. Seizure recurrence following surgical treatment of refractory partial epilepsies associated with FCD is more common than following temporal lobe surgery, particularly TLE/HS. Interestingly, however, although several features of recurrent seizures are clearly different in both entities, others are similar.

Two major aspects concerning surgery for FCD are that lesions often localize to the vicinity of eloquent cortical regions and that they may have a microscopic extension beyond the resolution of MRI. This poses significant challenges in terms of resection and often resections are incomplete. This is a major cause of seizure recurrence in these patients. In a recent study, two largely different patterns of postoperative seizures following incomplete resections for extratemporal FCD were found (Camargo *et al.* in preparation). The most common situation, observed in a significant proportion of patients, are semiologically similar yet milder seizures in that generalizations and/or attacks during wakefulness are controlled. Thus, semiology is similar but seizures are less frequent and the epilepsy less severe. In this new series of patients studied in Porto Alegre, we had difficulties similar to those reported two decades ago (Palmini *et al.* 1991) in classifying the surgical outcome, because the commonly used classification system fails to consider improvements in seizure severity when seizure frequency is not changed by the procedure. The other, opposite, scenario is represented by acutely worsened seizures, which are more severe and more frequent, and emerge in the first few days after operation. In many of these patients a second operation had to be performed acutely to control these worsening attacks, which suggest acute disinhibition within an epileptogenic network (Palmini 2010). Thus, major differences in comparison with temporal lobe surgery is that recurrences following FCD extratemporal operations are often more obviously driven by incomplete resections of the EZ, tend to occur early after operation and tend to either retain a similar semiology, although in a less severe degree or be associated with acute worsening of the epilepsy.

On the other hand, some other patients operated for FCD have an outcome dynamic which is smaller than that seen in those with TLE/HS. At times, there is a clear emergence of a different or previously dormant EZ, in the same or in the contralateral hemisphere (Palmini 2010), and this is associated with semiologically distinct seizures. A structural surrogate for these attacks originating from different cortical regions in patients with FCD was recently described (Fauser et al. 2009). Furthermore, in many patients recurrence may occur more than 2 years after operation. This delayed recurrence resembles that described after surgery for TLE/HS, in that no obvious explanation exists, besides emergence of a dormant, lower-threshold EZ that took time to mature. In contrast to delayed recurrences following TLE/HS surgery however, those related to FCD tend to be long-lasting and represent true "running up" phenomena. Whether these late recurrences may relate to de novo epileptogenesis around the surgical scar is unclear and expanded below.

De novo epilepsy after epilepsy surgery

The discussion that follows chiefly concerns what could be seen as de novo epilepsy after epilepsy surgery and is subdivided into two independent parts: postoperative seizures possibly related to surgically inflicted cortical damage; and postoperative seizures possibly associated with disinhibition of a potential (previously dormant) EZ.

For the first part, a circular argument could be made concerning resective surgery for epilepsy, in that the sheer act of resection is in itself an insult to the tissue, potentially leading to cortical disruption and reorganization conducive to the creation of "another" epileptic focus. This "resect-one-focus-create-another" scenario is not frequent (Hennessy et al. 2000) and thus resective epilepsy surgery is a widely used therapeutic procedure for refractory seizures. This discussion will start by sharing some views on why damage caused by the cortical resection usually does not create an independent epileptic focus. In doing so, evidence will be considered from general neurosurgery, particularly resective surgery for brain tumors, pointing to the high threshold for the production of an epileptic focus in or around the inevitable cortical scars. Next, clinical epileptological situations of seizure recurrence following epilepsy surgery will be discussed that are indeed possibly related to surgically inflicted tissue injury, including acute postoperative seizures and delayed partial seizures from more significant postresective scarring.

The second possibility is the long-standing notion of a dormant, "potential epileptogenic zone." Seizures following resection of a "primary" focus may arise either from adjacent or from more distant cortical regions, that were silent before operation and thus become independent, de novo epileptogenic zones in their own right. Cortical regions are highly interconnected and such connectivity carries both excitatory and inhibitory impulses. Thus, the possibility that resecting an epileptogenic region could "disinhibit" other, previously silent but potentially epileptogenic, areas should be considered.

Postoperative seizures possibly related to surgically inflicted damage

Recurrent unprovoked seizures, i.e., epilepsy, are a clinical common denominator following a number of different types of cortical insults. These molecular, dysplastic, gliotic (traumatic, vascular), neoplastic, and inflamatory insults, in themselves, have as a common denominator the fact that all disrupt the delicate balance of excitation and inhibition in more localized or more diffuse cortical networks. Therefore, it could be postulated that neurosurgical trauma to the cortex – inevitably incurred during resective epilepsy surgery and leading to variable degrees of reactive gliosis – could result in an "iatrogenic epileptic focus." However, because some of these neurosurgical procedures are performed exactly to resect previously existent epileptic regions, the scenario of epilepsy after epilepsy surgery would be a significant deterrent to surgical procedures for the treatment of epilepsy. Fortunately, the evidence accumulated so far suggests that the latter scenario is rare, and there may be a number of reasons for this.

It may be instructive to begin by analyzing the literature on the risk of single seizures or epilepsy in patients with brain tumors. This is an interesting point of departure because there has been an ongoing discussion on the need for prophylactic AEDs in these patients, i.e., after the diagnosis or resection of the tumor, irrespective of the occurence of seizures. The American Academy of Neurology (AAN) has issued a practice parameter (Glantz et al. 2000) based upon a careful review of the available literature (Glantz et al. 1996; Forsyth et al. 2003; Wen and Kesari 2008) which suggests that AEDs are not significantly better than placebo to prevent new-onset seizures in patients with recently diagnosed brain tumors. What is interesting in the context of the present chapter is that the findings from these studies and hence the AAN recommendations, are not modified by the performance of surgery in these patients. In other words, the "production" of a cortical scar by operating on the tumors did not increase the prevalence of seizures (between 25% and 35% of tumor patients) nor indicated that AED prophylaxis was warranted (Kuijlen et al. 1996; Glantz et al. 2000; De Santis et al. 2002; Forsyth et al. 2003). Another somewhat related aspect derived from the neurosurgical literature is that seizures occur in between 15% and 20% of patients after supratentorial neurosurgical procedures in general – i.e., including surgery for ruptured aneurysms, trauma, tumors, etc. (North *et al.* 1980, 1983). In this more varied pool of patients, the risk seems limited to between 2 and 3 months after operation and AED prophylaxis is apparently effective in reducing seizure occurrence during this period, although the issue is not settled (Kuijlen *et al.* 1996). No benefit is apparent after this period (North *et al.* 1980, 1983).

Combining the fact that cortical manipulation apparently does not increase the risk of seizures beyond that which already exists in patients with brain tumors and in other supratentorial pathologies, and that the risk for long-term seizures is small, it stands out that factors beyond the production of a cortical gliotic scar during a neurosurgical procedure must concur for the development of long-term epilepsy. Even though surgically inflicted, limited cortical damage during epilepsy surgery necessarily occurs in patients whose seizure threshold is, by definition, lower than that of the general population, the latter does not seem to represent a significant risk factor, given the low rates of epilepsy after epilepsy surgery (see below). Thus, it is likely that recurrent seizures following surgically inflicted cortical damage depend upon the interaction of a number of factors including, but not limited to, the cortical scar and genetic predisposition. This scenario may not be much different from that of post-traumatic epilepsies, which are related not only to the severity of the craniocerebral trauma but also to genetic aspects and to an imbalance in the impingement upon inhibitory and excitatory neuronal pools (Avramescu *et al.* 2009; Christensen *et al.* 2009; Stam *et al.* 2009).

The next aspect to be discussed when considering the possibility that surgically inflicted cortical damage may lead to epilepsy is that of acute postoperative seizures (APOS) in patients undergoing epilepsy surgery, which are variably defined as attacks occurring in the first 2 to 4 weeks after operation. Two aspects should be specifically reviewed: first, whether these seizures are semiologically similar or different from the habitual medically refractory seizures these patients had and which led to epilepsy surgery in the first place; second, the predictive value of APOS for long-term seizure recurrence. Perhaps most would agree that should APOS represent an iatrogenic effect of the operation (or a manifestation of some postoperative presumably precipitating factors such as reduced levels of AEDs, metabolic abnormalities) they would tend to be semiologically different from the habitual preoperative seizures and would tend to behave as "provoked seizures," i.e., not be associated with epilepsy and thus have a restricted impact on long-term seizure outcome. Indeed, traditionally, APOS have been regarded as "benign" (neighborhood) seizures without impact on the long-term outcome, and due to local cortical changes related to the surgical procedure (Penfield and Jasper 1954; Falconer and Serafetinides 1963; Ojeman and Bourgeois 1993); however, recent evidence

suggests that this may not be so (McIntosh *et al.* 2005; Mani *et al.* 2006; Jeha *et al.* 2007).

Acute postoperative seizures have been homogeneously reported in between 22% and 29% of patients, and these stable figures are somewhat surprising given the different types of epilepsy syndromes included in these reports (Tigaran *et al.* 2003; McIntosh *et al.* 2005; Mani *et al.* 2006; Jeha *et al.* 2007). From these and other studies it has become clear that the majority of APOS tend to be semiologically similar to the habitual preoperative attacks (Wingkun *et al.* 1991), do not seem related to postoperative precipitating factors (Tigaran *et al.* 2003), and have been interpreted as more likely representing active residual epileptogenic tissue (i.e., incomplete resection of the EZ) (Jeha *et al.* 2007). The latter is certainly supported by recent findings suggesting that APOS are not benign and constitute an important risk factor for seizure recurrence in the medium and long term (McIntosh *et al.* 2005; Mani *et al.* 2006). Should APOS be solely a manifestation of acute cortical damage from the epilepsy surgery procedures, they would more likely behave as cortical scars associated with tumor or other supratentorial resections and probably have no bearing on long-term seizure outcome (North *et al.* 1980, 1983; Forsyth *et al.* 2003).

Nevertheless, it should be acknowledged that some resections for epilepsy may cause more significant postresection scarring around the surgical area, and thus be more directly associated with postoperative seizures. Such scarring may be due to local ischemia or represent wallerian degeneration following partial resection of neuronal pools. It is also possible that patients vary in their vulnerability for significant scarring. The issue of cortical scars and epilepsy surgery has a long history, because for a long time in the past many or most epilepsy surgical procedures were performed to remove traumatic, inflammatory, or vascular cortical scars (Palmini 2006). A review of those resections showed that even when close to eloquent cortical areas in the central, parietal, or occipital regions, significant seizure control was achieved in more than 50% of patients (Rasmussen 1991). These results suggest that resecting scars does not carry a significant risk of creating new, potentially epileptogenic, scars.

Notwithstanding the considerations above, some operations for temporal or extratemporal epilepsies do result in significant tissue scarring (Fig. 60.1), and vascular involvement has been reported even during selective procedures such as selective amygdalohippocampectomies (Renowden *et al.* 1995; Schaller *et al.* 2002, 2004). When postoperative scars are extensive, they may lead to seizures. This, again, is not a settled issue (Renowden *et al.* 1995) but evidence recently obtained in Porto Alegre indirectly supports this (J. R. Hoefel *et al.* unpublished data). We evaluated postoperative MRIs of 60 fairly homogeneous patients who underwent transcortical selective amygdalohippocampectomy (Paglioli *et al.* 2004, 2006) for unilateral MTLE/HS and were followed for at least 2 years after operation. Twenty patients in whom seizures recurred were compared in a case–control study with 40 who had remained

A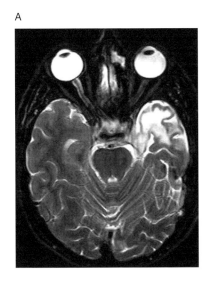

B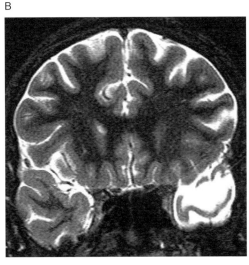

Fig. 60.1. Axial (A) and coronal (B) T2-weighted MRI sections from a patient who underwent a transcortical selective amygdalohippocampectomy which led to significant scarring involving temporal gyri and the temporal pole.

seizure-free for a number of clinical, neurophysiological, and imaging variables. The extent of resection of mesial temporal structures and the extent of the transcortical section on the second temporal gyrus did not differ between the groups. Furthermore, no demographic, epileptologic, or neurophysiological aspect correlated with outcome. The only variable that significantly correlated with postoperative seizure control was the extent of scarring in the temporal lobe. We devised a five-point quantitative scale to objectivate the severity of scarring on postoperative MRIs. One point was given for corticectomies on the second temporal gyrus larger than 2.5 cm and one point for the presence of scarring on T2 and fluid-attenuated inverse recovery (FLAIR) MR images on the white matter of each of the three temporal gyri and the temporal pole. The mean score for the patients who were seizure-free was 0.7 whereas it was 2.5 for those who had seizure recurrences ($p < 0.01$).

In summary, the available data suggest that the cortical and white matter manipulation during epilepsy surgery usually does not lead to independent, de novo epileptic foci, with the possible exception of those patients in whom the resultant scarring is extensive. Clearly, more research is needed in regard to this important aspect.

Seizures after epilepsy surgery: the putative role of disinhibition of "potential" epileptogenic zones

Disinhibition of synaptically interconnected neuronal pools is protean in disorders of all levels of the central nervous system. Here, the evidence for the possibility that following resection of an EZ, other, synaptically connected, adjacent or distant cortical regions may be disinhibited and develop into a de novo EZ will be considered.

This issue brings to the front an old concept, that of "dormant" epileptogenic regions (Penfield and Jasper 1954; Penfield 1958; Rasmussen 1983) that may become active

following resection of a "dominant" region that could have been keeping the former under some level of inhibition. In a sense, the currently used terminology "potential epileptogenic zones" may be relevant because these areas were probably already part of a more extensive epileptogenic zone, except that they did not manifest clinically before operation. Of course, a very important issue is how to anticipate the existence and the localization of these areas before resection. Probably, this kind of preoccupation was in Rasmussen's mind when he proposed the terminology "red versus green spikes" to differentiate those electrocorticographic discharges that might point to relevant epileptogenic cortex from those more clearly benign (Rasmussen 1983; Palmini 2006).

A recent publication drew attention to the fact that FCD can be multifocal, independently involving more than one non-adjacent region (at times in the contralateral hemisphere) (Fauser *et al.* 2009). This is an important finding because FCD is the most frequent cause of neocortical epilepsy and experience has shown that some of these dysplastic lesions may not be seen on MRI. The bona fide observation that FCD can be multifocal (Fauser *et al.* 2009) raises the possibility that in some patients the visible dysplastic lesion may be associated with other, non-visible lesions, at varying distances. Should that be true, it might explain some apparently puzzling findings of de novo epilepsy following resection of a dysplastic lesion.

We have described two young female patients with MRI-negative, medically refractory epilepsia partialis continua (EPC) histologically proven to be due to focal cortical dysplasia type II (Palmini *et al.* 2004) in the rolandic cortex. Even though continuous motor seizures were strictly unilateral for several months before operation, EPC re-emerged in the contralateral hemibody 48 hr after complete resection of the central cortex in one patient and one year later in the other. This led to the demise of one patient and a severe encephalopathy in the other (Silva *et al.* 1995). The fact that seizures emerged de novo from cortical tissue which had never produced seizures suggests that resection of dysplastic tissue in one rolandic area "disinhibited" a potential, secondary EZ, in these cases in the homologous region of the contralateral hemisphere. Should this reasoning prove correct, it follows that inhibitory mechanisms were probably operative within a network involving both rolandic regions. Such a network was disrupted by resection of the primary abnormality which interfered with an inhibitory equilibrium and led to seizures from the other side.

Another piece of evidence in the direction of de novo activation of a potential, previously dormant, EZ is the issue of seizure recurrence after a long seizure-free interval following complete resection of lesions for cortical dysplasia. We have just concluded an analysis of 63 patients – children and adults – operated for extratemporal FCD and followed for 5 or more years (A. Palmini *et al.* unpublished data). Half became seizure-free. The dynamics of seizure recurrence in the other half, however, suggested two different underlying mechanisms. Eighteen patients had seizure recurrence in the first 6 months, with a similar semiology and evidence of incomplete lesion resection on MRI. The other 12 patients, roughly one-fifth of the cohort, had a prolonged seizure-free interval after resection, which lasted for from 6 to 30 months, when seizures then recurrred. Seven of these 12 patients (around 10% of the total sample) had had complete lesion resection according to preoperative MRI and postexcision electrocorticography. In four of these patients a second evaluation showed that seizures originated from the contralateral hemisphere and three had seizure onset in another lobe in the operated hemisphere. Pathology in the three who were reoperated on showed the same underlying abnormalities. These cases show that the activation or disinhibition of potential epileptogenic zones may be protracted and involve an interconnected network probably related to microscopic, previously silent, FCD. Figure 60.2 illustrates an EEG counterpart of such disinhibition. This is a 50-year-old patient who had left-sided EPC following a peripheral injury to the left hand and underwent focal resection in the right rolandic region guided by acute electrocorticography (ECoG). Previous to the resection he had a few independent spikes in the right temporal lobe, related to a temporal lobe epilepsy he had had in the past and which had been cured for the last 10 years. The picture shows the striking activation (disinhibition) of this neocortical temporal focus which was virtually silent for a decade in the week following the ipsilateral rolandic resection of what proved to be a type I, MRI-negative, FCD. Indeed, he had postoperative recurrent electrographic seizures which his EEGs had never showed during preoperative evaluation.

In summary, there is evidence that at least in some pathologies epilepsy may be a release phenomenon following initial resection for epilepsy. Obviously, much more research is needed to untangle what differentiates patients in whom an initial resection will activate a dormant EZ, although some of the basic mechanisms have been recently advanced (Calcagnotto *et al.* 2005).

The possible impact of modification or discontinuation of antiepileptic drugs on seizure recurrence

A discussion of epilepsy after epilepsy surgery would not be complete without some considerations on the possible role of AED reduction or discontinuation on postoperative seizure recurrence. Stopping AEDs would be the closest construct for the "cure" of epilepsy. It is on the minds of patients and families and, more often than not, on the minds of doctors as well.

In a sense, the idea of a surgical cure stems from the idea of the epileptic focus as an isolated entity that could be clearly localized and resected. As discussed in the previous sections, such a model is not adequate for perhaps the majority of patients with refractory seizures undergoing epilepsy surgery. Nevertheless, when patients are seizure-free for a significant time after operation, the issue of AED tapering or discontinuation commonly arises. Below are summarized some reviews and original studies addressing this issue. Before reviewing these data, however, it is important to mention that no study has been delineated in a way to provide scientifically definitive answers to the many questions related to the issue of AED discontinuation after surgery. In fact, research to date provides only partial answers to questions such as: (1) how long to wait before initiating AED discontinuation in seizure-free patients; (2) which patients are ideal candidates for AED discontinuation; (3) what is the ideal rate of AED reduction; (4) what is the risk of seizure recurrence following planned AED discontinuation; (5) what is the timing of recurrence following discontinuation; (6) what are the chances of regaining seizure control when seizures recur following AED discontinuation; and (7) how patients in whom AEDs were discontinued compare with those who continued with medication in rates of seizure recurrence.

Schmidt and colleagues reviewed the literature and tried to collect data to inform these questions at least partially (Schmidt *et al.* 2004a, b). They found that around 48% of adults and 71% of children who were seizure-free after surgery eventually stopped medication. About one-third, however, had recurrent seizures during reduction or after dicontinuation. This figure compares with a recurrence rate of, respectively, 7% and 17% of recurrence after 1 and 5 years of operation in those who did not stop medication. They also showed that between 60% and 90% of patients regained seizure control when AEDs were reinstituted after recurrence.

A comprehensive review by Tellez-Zenteno and colleagues (2007), reports the dynamics of use of AEDs following epilepsy surgery. They showed that about 20% of patients operated for TLE were both seizure-free and off AEDs, 50% were on monotherapy, and 30% on polytherapy. This compares most favorably with control series in which no patient with TLE was off AEDs, only one-fourth were on monotherapy, and 76% were receiving two or more drugs. The figures for extratemporal

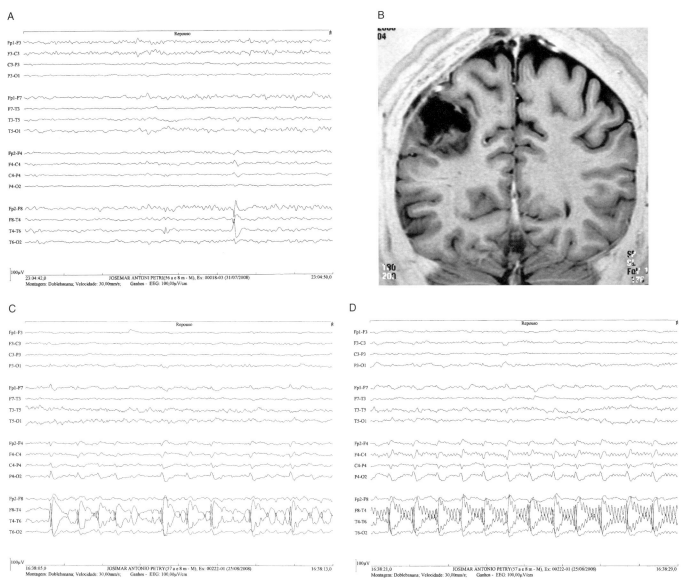

Fig. 60.2. (A) Pre-resection scalp EEG in the longitudinal montage showing isolated spike in the right temporal lobe. (B) Acute post-resection MRI indicating the right rolandic resection. (C, D) Post-resection EEGs showing that the right temporal focus, silent for years and which had displayed only rare spikes during preoperative evaluation, produced recurrent electrographic seizures following resection of an ipsilateral rolandic dysplastic lesion.

epilepsy surgery are, on the surface, even better, in that 36% of patients were seizure-free and off AEDs. However, these numbers are "contaminated" with infants and children who underwent large resections or hemispherectomies and also by patients operated for low-grade tumors. Both scenarios are associated with high grades of "surgical cure," facilitating discontinuation of AEDs. Pooling the data irrespective of type of surgery, about 25% of patients are seizure-free and off AEDs, 40% are on monotherapy, and 35% on polytherapy. Because most patients with refractory seizures considered for epilepsy surgery are on AED polytherapy at the time of referral, the fact that two-thirds are converted either to monotherapy or can stop medications is in itself a favorable result.

The Cleveland Clinic group reported on 97 children and adolescents with medically refractory partial epilepsies who had been seizure-free for at least 6 months after operation (Lachhwani *et al.* 2008). Ninety-seven percent of the 29 patients in whom AEDs were unchanged continued to be seizure-free for the last year before analysis. The other 68 patients had medications stopped after a median of 13 months after operation. Eighty-four percent of these continued to be seizure-free for a median of 5.5 years, whereas the other 16% (11 patients) had relapses.

In an interesting report coming from the Mayo Clinic including 210 patients who were seizure-free for longer than 1 year after epilepsy surgery, the authors studied the pattern of seizure recurrence according to different levels of manipulation of the AED regimen (Schiller *et al.* 2000). Seizure recurrence was documented in 7% of 30 patients whose AEDs were not changed, in 14% of the 96 in whom AEDs were reduced, and in 26% of the 84 in whom AEDs were stopped. There was a trend for seizure recurrence in those who had a structural pathology on MRI before operation, and apparently there was no relation between relapses and duration of seizure freedom before AED modification, particularly when comparing a "standard" period of 2 years to a "prolonged" period of 6 years.

In a prospective, non-randomized study of 291 patients who had attained at least 1-year remission at any time after surgery, Berg and colleagues (2006) evaluated the rate of seizure relapse in 129 patients who reduced or discontinued AEDs and in 162 who did not reduce AEDs. Overall, 39% of patients relapsed. Interestingly, relapses occurred in 45% of those patients who *did not* reduce AEDs and in 32% of those who reduced medication. Patients who reduced AEDs were more likely to have attained remission immediately after surgery (which encouraged reduction of AEDs after some time of seizure freedom). Of those who reduced, an increased rate of recurrence was (as expected) seen in those with "delayed remission," i.e., patients who had already demonstrated some tendency to epilepsy after epilepsy surgery.

Probably only prospective, randomized studies of homogeneous groups of patients will eventually provide more solid evidence to inform AED reduction or discontinuation after epilepsy surgery. For the time being, it is important to have a clear idea of the favorable and unfavorable prognostic factors reducing or increasing the risk of recurrence for the various epilepsy scenarios before attempting AED reduction and discontinuation in a given patient.

References

Avramescu S, Nita DA, Timofeev I (2009) Neocortical post-traumatic epileptogenesis is associated with loss of GABAergic neurons. *J Neurotrauma* **26**:799–812.

Berg AT, Vickrey BG, Langfitt JT, *et al.* (2006) Reduction of AEDs in postsurgical patients who attain remission *Epilepsia* **47**:64–71.

Binder DK, Garcia PA, Elangovan GK, Barbaro NM (2009) Characteristics of auras in patients undergoing temporal lobectomy. *J Neurosurg* **111**:1283–9.

Bladin PF (1987) Post-temporal lobectomy seizures. *Clin Exp Neurol* **24**:77–83.

Calcagnotto ME, Paredes MF, Tihan T, *et al.* (2005) Dysfunction of synaptic inhibition in epilepsy associated with focal cortical dysplasia. *J Neurosci* **25**:9649–57.

Christensen J, Pedersen MG, Pedersen CB, *et al.* (2009) Long-term risk of epilepsy after traumatic brain injury in children and young adults: a population-based cohort study. *Lancet* **373**:1105–10.

de Boer HM, Mula M, Sander JW (2008) The global burden and stigma of epilepsy. *Epilepsy Behav* **12**:540–6.

de Santana MT, Jackowski AP, da Silva HH, *et al.* (2010) Auras and clinical features in temporal lobe epilepsy: a new approach on the basis of voxel-based morphometry. *Epilepsy Res* **89**:327–38.

De Santis A, Villani R, Sinisi M, *et al.* (2002) Add-on phenytoin fails to prevent early seizures after surgery for supratentorial brain tumors: a randomized controlled study. *Epilepsia* **43**:175–82.

Elliott B, Joyce E, Shorvon S (2009a) Delusions, illusions and hallucinations in epilepsy. I. Elementary phenomena. *Epilepsy Res* **85**:162–71.

Elliott B, Joyce E, Shorvon S (2009b) Delusions, illusions and hallucinations in epilepsy. II. Complex phenomena and psychosis. *Epilepsy Res* **85**:172–86.

Engel J Jr. (1996) Surgery for seizures. *N Engl J Med* **334**:647–52.

Falconer MA, Serafetinides EA (1963) A follow-up study of surgery in temporal lobe epilepsy. *J Neurol Neurosurg Psychiatry* **26**:154–65.

Fauser S, Sisodiya SM, Martinian L, *et al.* (2009) Multi-focal occurrence of cortical dysplasia in epilepsy patients. *Brain* **132**:2079–90.

Forsyth PA, Weaver S, Fulton D, *et al.* (2003) Prophylactic anticonvulsants in patients with brain tumor. *Can J Neurol Sci* **30**:106–12.

Fried I, Spencer DD, Spencer SS (1995) The anatomy of epileptic auras: focal pathology and surgical outcome. *J Neurosurg* **83**:60–6.

Glantz MJ, Cole BF, Friedberg MH, *et al.* (1996) A randomized, blinded, placebo-controlled trial of divalproex sodium prophylaxis in adults with newly diagnosed brain tumors. *Neurology* **46**:985–91.

Glantz MJ, Cole BF, Forsyth PA, *et al.* (2000) Practice parameter: anticonvulsant prophylaxis in patients with newly diagnosed brain tumors. Report of the Quality Standards Subcommittee of the American Academy of Neurology. *Neurology* **54**:1886–93.

Hennessy MJ, Elwes RD, Binnie CD, Polkey CE (2000) Failed surgery for epilepsy: a study of persistence and recurrence of seizures following temporal resection. *Brain* **123**:2445–66.

Henry TR, Drury I, Schuh LA, Ross DA (2000) Increased secondary generalization of partial seizures after temporal lobectomy. *Neurology* **55**:1812–17.

Janszky J, Janszky I, Schulz R, *et al.* (2005) Temporal lobe epilepsy with hippocampal sclerosis: predictors for long-term surgical outcome. *Brain* **128**:395–404.

Jeha LE, Najm I, Bingaman W, *et al.* (2007) Surgical outcome and prognostic factors of frontal lobe epilepsy surgery. *Brain* **130**:574–84.

Kobayashi E, Lopes-Cendes I, Guerreiro CA, *et al.* (2001) Seizure outcome and hippocampal atrophy in familial mesial temporal lobe epilepsy. *Neurology* **56**:166–72.

Krsek P, Maton B, Korman B, *et al.* (2008) Different features of histopathological subtypes of pediatric focal cortical dysplasia. *Ann Neurol* **63**:758–69.

Kuijlen JM, Teernstra OP, Kessels AG, *et al.* (1996) Effectiveness of antiepileptic prophylaxis used with supratentorial craniotomies: a meta-analysis. *Seizure* **5**:291–8.

Kwan P, Brodie MJ (2000) Early identification of refractory epilepsy. *N Engl J Med* **342**:314–19.

Labate A, Cerasa A, Aguglia U, *et al.* (2010) Voxel-based morphometry of sporadic epileptic patients with mesiotemporal sclerosis. *Epilepsia* **51**:506–10.

Lachhwani DK, Loddenkemper T, Holland KD, et al. (2008) Discontinuation of medications after successful epilepsy surgery in children. Pediatr Neurol 38:340–4.

Mani J, Gupta A, Mascha E, et al. (2006) Postoperative seizures after extratemporal resections and hemispherectomy in pediatric epilepsy. Neurology 66:1038–43.

Mattson RH, Cramer JA, Collins JF, et al. (1985) Comparison of carbamazepine, phenobarbital, phenytoin, and primidone in partial and secondarily generalized tonic–clonic seizures. N Engl J Med 313:145–51.

Mattson RH, Cramer JA, Collins JF (1992) A comparison of valproate with carbamazepine for the treatment of complex partial seizures and secondarily generalized tonic-clonic seizures in adults. N Engl J Med 327:765–71.

McIntosh AM, Kalnins RM, Mitchell LA, et al. (2004) Temporal lobectomy: long-term seizure outcome, late recurrence and risks for seizure recurrence. Brain 127:2018–30.

McIntosh AM, Kalnins RM, Mitchell LA, Berkovic SF (2005) Early seizures after temporal lobectomy predict subsequent seizure recurrence. Ann Neurol 57:283–8.

McIntosh AM, Berkovic SF (2006) What happens now? Ongoing outcome after post-temporal lobectomy seizure recurrence. Neurology 67:1671–3.

Ngugi AK, Bottomley C, Kleinschmidt I, et al. (2010) Estimation of the burden of active and life-time epilepsy: a meta-analytic approach. Epilepsia 51:883–90.

Noronha AL, Borges MA, Marques LH, et al. (2007) Prevalence and pattern of epilepsy treatment in different socioeconomic classes in Brazil. Epilepsia 48:880–5.

North JB, Penhall RK, Hanieh A, et al. (1980) Postoperative epilepsy: a double-blind trial of phenytoin after craniotomy. Lancet 1:384–6.

North JB, Penhall RK, Hanieh A, et al. (1983) Phenytoin and postoperative epilepsy: a double-blind study. J Neurosurg 58:672–7.

Ojeman GA, Bourgeois BF (1993) Early post-operative management. In: Engel J Jr. (ed.) Surgical Treatment of the Epilepsies, 2nd edn. New York: Raven Press, pp. 539–40.

Paglioli E, Palmini A, da Costa JC, et al. (2004) Survival analysis of the surgical outcome of temporal lobe epilepsy due to hippocampal sclerosis. Epilepsia 45:1383–91.

Paglioli E, Palmini A, Portuguez M, et al. (2006) Seizure and memory outcome following temporal lobe surgery: selective compared with nonselective approaches for hippocampal sclerosis J Neurosurg 104:70–8.

Palmini A, Andermann F, Olivier A, et al. (1991) Focal neuronal migration disorders and intractable partial epilepsy: results of surgical treatment. Ann Neurol 30:750–7.

Palmini A, Najm I, Avanzini G, et al. (2004) Terminology and classification of the cortical dysplasias. Neurology 62:S2–8.

Palmini A (2006) The concept of the epileptogenic zone: a modern look at Penfield and Jasper's views on the role of interictal spikes. Epilept Disord 8(Suppl 2):S10–15.

Palmini A (2009) Epilepsy surgery in countries with limited resources. In: Shorvon S, Perucca E, Engel J Jr. (eds.) The Treatment of Epilepsy. Oxford, UK: Blackwell Publishing, pp. 1051–6.

Palmini A (2010) Electrophysiology of focal cortical dysplasias. Epilepsia 51:23–6.

Penfield W, Jasper HH (1954) Epilepsy and the Functional Anatomy of the Human Brain. London: Churchill.

Penfield W (1958) Pitfalls and success in surgical treatment of focal epilepsy. Br Med J 1:669–72.

Pimentel J, Bentes C, Campos A, et al. (2010) Long-term and late seizure outcome after surgery for temporal lobe epilepsy. Epilept Disord 12:54–8.

Rasmussen T (1983) Characteristics of a pure culture of frontal lobe epilepsy. Epilepsia 24:482–93.

Rasmussen T (1991) Surgery for central, parietal and occipital epilepsy. Can J Neurol Sci 18:611–16.

Renowden SA, Matkovic Z, Adams CB, et al. (1995) Selective amygdalohippocampectomy for hippocampal sclerosis: postoperative MR appearance. AJNR Am J Neuroradiol 16:1855–61.

Rosenow F, Luders H (2001) Presurgical evaluation of epilepsy. Brain 124:1683–700.

Salanova V, Andermann F, Rasmussen T, et al. (1996) The running down phenomenon in temporal lobe epilepsy. Brain 119:989–96.

Salanova V, Markand O, Worth R (1999) Longitudinal follow-up in 145 patients with medically refractory temporal lobe epilepsy treated surgically between 1984 and 1995. Epilepsia 40:1417–23.

Sander JW (2003) The epidemiology of epilepsy revisited. Curr Opin Neurol 16:165–70.

Schaller C, Klemm E, Haun D, et al. (2002) The transsylvian approach is "minimally invasive" but not "atraumatic". Neurosurgery 51:971–6; discussion 976–7.

Schaller C, Jung A, Clusmann H, et al. (2004) Rate of vasospasm following the transsylvian versus transcortical approach for selective amygdalohippocampectomy. Neurol Res 26:666–70.

Schiller Y, Cascino GD, So EL, Marsh WR (2000) Discontinuation of antiepileptic drugs after successful epilepsy surgery. Neurology 54:346–9.

Schmidt D, Baumgartner C, Loscher W (2004a) Seizure recurrence after planned discontinuation of antiepileptic drugs in seizure-free patients after epilepsy surgery: a review of current clinical experience. Epilepsia 45:179–86.

Schmidt D, Baumgartner C, Loscher W (2004b) The chance of cure following surgery for drug-resistant temporal lobe epilepsy: what do we know and do we need to revise our expectations? Epilepsy Res 60:187–201.

Semah F, Picot MC, Adam C, et al. (1998) Is the underlying cause of epilepsy a major prognostic factor for recurrence? Neurology 51:1256–62.

Silva LF, Palmini A, da Costa JC, et al. (1995) MRI-invisible rolandic cortical dysplasia presenting with intractable epilepsia partialis continua: the ominous question of unsuspected bilateral symmetrical lesions. Epilepsia 36:15.

Spencer SS, Berg AT, Vickrey BG, et al. (2005) Predicting long-term seizure outcome after resective epilepsy surgery: the multicenter study. Neurology 65:912–18.

Stam AH, Luijckx GJ, Poll-The BT, et al. (2009) Early seizures and cerebral edema after trivial head trauma associated with the CACNA1A S218L mutation. J Neurol Neurosurg Psychiatry 80:1125–9.

Tellez-Zenteno JF, Dhar R, Wiebe S (2005) Long-term seizure outcomes following epilepsy surgery: a systematic review and meta-analysis. Brain 128:1188–98.

423

Tellez-Zenteno JF, Dhar R, Hernandez-Ronquillo L, Wiebe S (2007) Long-term outcomes in epilepsy surgery: antiepileptic drugs, mortality, cognitive and psychosocial aspects. *Brain* **130**:334–45.

Tigaran S, Cascino GD, McClelland RL, *et al.* (2003) Acute postoperative seizures after frontal lobe cortical resection for intractable partial epilepsy. *Epilepsia* **44**:831–5.

Wen PY, Kesari S, (2008) Malignant gliomas in adults. *N Engl J Med* **359**:492–507.

Wingkun EC, Awad IA, Luders H, Awad CA (1991) Natural history of recurrent seizures after resective surgery for epilepsy. *Epilepsia* **32**:851–6.

Wiebe S, Blume WT, Girvin JP, Eliasziw M (2001) A randomized, controlled trial of surgery for temporal-lobe epilepsy. *N Engl J Med* **345**:311–18.

Yasuda CL, Tedeschi H, Oliveira EL, *et al.* (2006) Comparison of short-term outcome between surgical and clinical treatment in temporal lobe epilepsy: a prospective study. *Seizure* **15**:35–40.

Non-accidental brain injury

Renzo Guerrini and Alessio De Ciantis

Definitions and epidemiology

The definition non-accidental brain injury (NABI; also called *inflicted traumatic brain injury* [inflicted TBI] or *abusive head trauma* and *shaken baby syndrome* [SBS]) is used to describe the traumatic brain injury inflicted on an infant or young child (Case 2007; Minns *et al.* 2008). Non-accidental brain injury results from any external force that is severe enough to cause damage to the brain and represents a major cause of acquired brain injury in the pediatric population (Hawley *et al.* 2003; Bourgeois *et al.* 2008). In a population-based study in Scotland (Barlow and Minns 2000) SBS had an annual incidence of 24.6 per 100 000 children younger than age 1 year. The risk of a child suffering NABI by age 1 year was 1 in 4065 and injuries occurred almost exclusively in young infants (median age 2.2 months). Under age 2 years, 10% of all injuries of children are abusive. Between 40% and 50% of all abusive injuries are head injuries and about 80% of deaths related to head injuries are abusive (Case 2007). There is equal gender distribution with slight male predominance (Starling *et al.* 1995; Barlow and Minns 2000). According to Kinney and Armstrong (1997), in the USA, NABI was second only to sudden infant death syndrome (SIDS) as a cause of postneonatal death in infants under 12 months old, and according to Bechtel *et al.* (2004) NABI is the most common cause of traumatic death in the same age range. The estimated mortality rate ranges from 13% to 30% (Barlow *et al.* 2000).

Up to 50% of survivors suffer permanent cognitive or other neurological disability, and 30% have a chance for full recovery (Keenan *et al.* 2003; Bechtel *et al.* 2004; Case 2007; Gerber and Coffman 2007). Perpetrators, in descending order, include: fathers, mother's boyfriends, female babysitters, and mothers (Starling *et al.* 1995, 2004). Social and environmental risk factors include: young parents, a young or unmarried mother, maternal education level, low socioeconomic status, unstable family situations, single parents, multiple-birth pregnancy, extended family, a history of abuse toward the caregiver, and psychiatric illness and substance abuse histories (Keenan *et al.* 2003; Gerber and Coffman 2007; Ryan *et al.* 2008).

Clinical presentation and mechanisms of pathology

Infants and small children are especially vulnerable to head injuries because of the unique anatomical features of their head and brain: (1) relative to body size, the infant head is significantly larger than in adults; (2) the subarachnoid space is relatively large; (3) myelination is incomplete and the water content is high; (4) the neck musculature is weak, with consequent poor control of the weight of the head; (5) the skull is soft, with non-ossified bones and unfused sutures, open fontanelles, and extremely fragile blood vessels. The above components contribute to transmit impulse forces to deeper structures, producing subdural hemorrhage due to extravasated blood dissecting open the dura–arachnoid interface (Case 2007; Gerber and Coffman 2007).

Head injuries may result from impact (when the head strikes or is struck by an object) or shaking (cranial acceleration or deceleration) or a combination of these mechanisms, which act through translational or rotational forces. Translational forces occur when the brain's center of gravity moves in a straight line; rotational forces, which occur during shaking, cause the brain to turn about its center of gravity or at the attachment to the brainstem. These mechanisms submit the head of the child to acceleration–deceleration movements creating inertial movement of the brain within the skull and may result in subdural and subarachnoid hematoma, retinal hemorrhages, and diffuse axonal injury. With violent whiplash shaking starts the sequence of events in SBS. Cervical hyperextension causes neuraxis damage, which in turn produces breathing difficulty or apnea with subsequent brain hypoxia and cerebral edema. The consequent development of intracranial hypertension and hypoperfusion implies hypoxic ischemic cerebral injury and axonal injury (David 1999; Blumenthal 2002; Case 2007).

In autopsy series, the most common findings in infants with NABI are subdural hemorrhage (SDE), subarachnoid hemorrhage, retinal hemorrhages, hypoxic–ischemic axonal damage, axonal injury, and skull fractures (Geddes *et al.* 2001a; Oehmichen *et al.* 2008). The most usual cause of death

The Causes of Epilepsy, eds. S. D. Shorvon, F. Andermann, and R. Guerrini. Published by Cambridge University Press. © Cambridge University Press 2011.

A

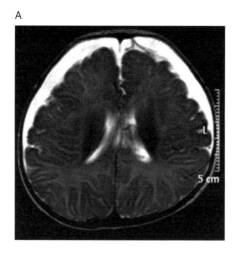

B

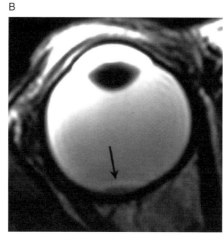

Fig. 61.1. Four-month-old infant with inconsolable crying, leftward eye and head version, and clonic movements. (A) Axial T2-weighted MR performed on the 3rd day after onset of symptoms. Bilateral subdural hemorrhages, especially in the frontal regions. (B) Right eye MRI performed on the 6th day after onset of symptoms. The retinal surface is uplifted at the posterior pole due to hemorrhage (arrow).

is raised intracranial pressure secondary to brain swelling (Geddes *et al.* 2001a).

Subdural hemorrhage, which occurs in up to 90% of cases (Case 2007), originates from stretching and tearing of the bridging veins which pass from the cortical surface to the dural venous sinuses. Blood is located along the interhemispheric fissure and over the convexities but also along the falx cerebri or focally within sulci along the hemispheres and can have unilateral or bilateral distribution (Ewing-Cobbs *et al.* 2000; Gerber and Coffman 2007). Occurrence of SDE is much less common following accidental head injury (Stoodley 2005).

Subarachnoid hemorrhage frequently co-occurs with subdural hemorrhage, which is often localized over the parasagittal cerebral convexities. Sometimes it is difficult to distinguish them because subarachnoid blood may be localized on the mesial surfaces and may be sparse (Case 2007).

Retinal hemorrhages are found in 70–85% of all shaken baby victims (Case 2007) and are one of the important elements in the diagnosis of NABI especially when other causes of inflicted head trauma are not apparent from history or clinical examination. They are usually bilateral and confluent but can be asymmetric and even occur unilaterally. There is correlation between their extension and severity and the severity of head trauma. The most common form is a flame-shaped hemorrhage that occurs in the superficial nerve fibers and ganglion cell layers. Less commonly, preretinal/subhyaloid, intraretinal, or vitreous hemorrhage occur (Chiesa and Duhaime 2009; Togioka *et al.* 2009). Unless they are very severe, retinal hemorrhages are not detectable by computed tomography (CT) or magnetic resonance imaging (MRI) (Sturm *et al.* 2008). Their absence does not exclude NABI (McCabe and Donahue 2000). The mechanism of injury resulting in retinal hemorrhages is not conclusively known but is probably linked to shaking of the globe and tearing of delicate retinal vessels.

Axonal damage is the best and most specific indicator of the acceleration–deceleration forces sustained by the brain (Case 2007; Gerber and Coffman 2007). It is consists of tears of axonal processes and small blood vessels. The shearing forces cause damage to the nerves because the young infant's brain has

not fully developed and the nerve fibers lack the myelin sheath. The most obvious lesions affect the corpus callosum, subcortical white matter, periventricular areas, and rostral brainstem (dorsolateral quadrants) (Sato 2009). Geddes *et al.* (2001b) found widespread axonal damage, interpreted as vascular, to be more frequent than traumatic axonal injury. Absence of axonal injury does not exclude SBS (Oehmichen *et al.* 2008).

Skull fractures give evidence of a significant impact injury (Stoodley 2005). In addition to skull fractures there may be other skeletal injuries. They occur in up to 50% of abused children, but their presence is not required for the diagnosis of SBS (Lancon *et al.* 1998).

The inflicted head injuries can take many forms. The classic presentation of NABI in infants is the SBS, which is characterized by widespread parenchymal damage, diffuse axonal injury, subdural and/or subarachnoid hemorrhages, and retinal hemorrhages (Fig. 61.1A, B). Most of the damage results from rotational acceleration–deceleration forces and there are usually limited or no signs of external trauma. This condition is often diagnosed based on finding retinal and subdural hemorrhage in infants referred for seemingly new-onset seizures (Bourgeois *et al.* 2008) or de novo status epilepticus and no history of trauma (Figs. 61.2, 61.3). In addition to loss of consciousness and seizures, other clinical presentations are observed, including, at times, subtle signs and symptoms such as reduced alertness, irritability, excessive salivation, episodes of vomiting, and impaired neck holding (Blumenthal 2002; Gerber and Coffman 2007). All of these signs can be difficult to assess if the child is having seizures. Children with NABI do not typically present with a lucid interval, they become symptomatic, most often losing consciousness, immediately after the abusive head trauma. Determining the timing of symptoms is crucial to identify the perpetrator (Starling *et al.* 1995, 2004; Case 2007). A summary list of the history or clinical elements that suggest or should raise the suspicion of NABI in the child presenting with new-onset seizures or de novo status epilepticus, as well as a list of procedures to follow if suspicion is confirmed, is presented in Table 61.1.

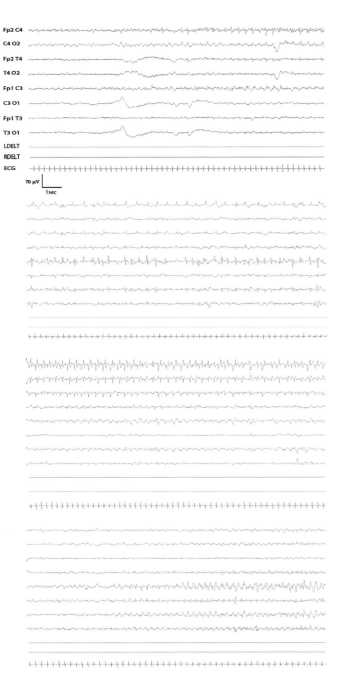

Fig. 61.2. Two-month-old boy with pallor, reduced reactivity, clonic eye jerking, and mild jerking of the upper limbs with alternating side. EEG recording, performed upon arrival, 3 days after the onset of symptoms captured continuous seizure activity, alternating in either hemisphere. Time lag between EEG traces is 1 min between the first and second trace, 2 min between the second and third, 17 min between the third and fourth.

Seizures and epilepsy following non-accidental brain injury

Seizures occur more frequently in children with inflicted (65–74%) versus non-inflicted traumatic brain injury (15–17%). They qualify as post-traumatic seizures (PTS) and are classified as immediate, early, or late seizures. Immediate seizures occur within 24 hr after the injury; early PTS occur between 24 hr and 1 week; late PTS occur after longer than 1 week following the trauma. In the series of Bourgeois *et al.* (2008) seizures were the presenting symptom in the acute phase of NABI in 296 of 404 children (73%). Occurrence of seizures is thought to betoken an unfavorable neurodevelopmental outcome (Barlow *et al.* 2000; Bourgeois *et al.* 2008). Status epilepticus is most often observed in children with severe injury and carries the greatest risk of adverse outcome (Yablon 1993). Subclinical status epilepticus was identified in 25% of children with NABI (Bourgeois *et al.* 2008). Deaths associated with status epilepticus are usually attributable to the lesion that precipitated it. Seizures following NABI, likewise seizures following head trauma of any type, are of different semiology, including generalized tonic–clonic, unilateral, or focal seizures (Hahn *et al.* 1988; Yablon 1993; Kumar *et al.* 2008). Multiple foci of cerebral injury may manifest with more than one seizure type (Hardman 1979).

Seizures, especially if prolonged, are likely to play an important role in the genesis of secondary brain damage since they raise metabolic requirements, intracranial pressure, cerebral hypoxia, and determine an excessive release of neurotransmitters (Schierhout and Roberts 1998; Duhaime and Durham 2007). Epileptogenesis in PTS is likely multifactorial. It may involve changes in the excitatory and inhibitory functions, altered calcium-mediated second-messenger activity mechanisms, changes in ionotropic receptor function and composition, altered endogenous neuroprotective activity, and generation of free radicals with brain parenchyma damage (Statler 2006).

Immediate and early PTS are thought to result from a direct reaction to the injury (direct neurologic or systemic effects of head trauma), while late seizures result from structural damage to the cerebral cortex (Gallagher 2002). Early seizures are more common than late seizures. Immediate seizures, which make up 50–80% of early seizures, are particularly frequent after severe traumatic brain injury but can also occur, occasionally, after mild or moderate injury (Hendrick and Harris 1968; Yablon 1993). In one retrospective series of children presenting at an average age of 5.9 months with an acute encephalopathy due to NABI, early seizures occurred in 32 (74%) of 44 patients (Barlow *et al.* 2000). Focal attacks were observed in 66% and status epilepticus in 41%. Seizures reached their peak frequency on the second day and ceased in all cases by day 10.

There are several accepted risk factors for early PTS. Severity of injury as expressed by Glasgow Coma Scale (GCS) score is a major indicator of early PTS. The risk of seizures after severe injury (GCS 3–8) is twofold that of children suffering moderate injury (GCS 9–12) and ten times greater than seen with mild injury (GCS 13–15). Early age also represents a definitive risk factor for early PTS. In one series, children ≤2 years of age were found to be two and half times more prone to

A

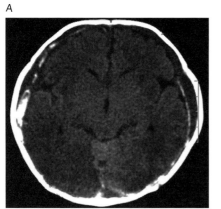

B

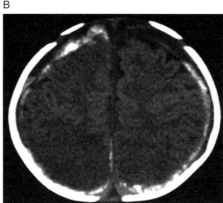

Fig. 61.3. (A, B) Same boy as in Fig 61.2. Axial brain CT scan showing bilateral frontotemporal, parieto-occipital, and interhemispheric subdural hematoma.

suffer convulsions after head injury than older children. Diffuse cerebral edema and intracranial hemorrhage, in particular subdural hematomas, carry the highest incidence of early PTS and of PTS in general. Depressed skull fractures represent an additional risk factor although less significant than edema and hemorrhage (Hahn *et al.* 1988; Ratan *et al.* 1999; Chiaretti *et al.* 2000).

Late PTS may occur weeks, months, or years after the injury and reflect permanent changes in the brain. Although it is expected that permanent changes are able to produce repeated unprovoked seizures, i.e., post-traumatic epilepsy, the operational definition of post-traumatic epilepsy is not always clear in follow-up studies of NABI. In the series of Barlow *et al.* (2000) and of Bourgeois *et al.* (2008) 22% and 20% of NABI survivors developed late post-traumatic epilepsy and the outcome in those with epilepsy was significantly worse than those without. The dynamics leading to late PTS are not completely understood. The main hypothesized risk factors include early seizures, depressed skull fracture, and intracranial hematoma (Asikainen *et al.* 1999). Prolonged unconsciousness, severity of brain injury, prolonged post-traumatic amnesia, and cortico/subcortical brain lesion have been variably associated with increased risk of late PTS (Hahn *et al.* 1988; Chadwick 2000). One putative mechanism of PTS, which is considered to be limited to the developing brain, is injury-related focal cortical dysplasia, resulting from dedifferentiation of the scarred area (Golden and Harding 2004). In a neuropathological study of the brain of two children who had survived several years after SBS, Marin-Padilla *et al.* (2002) observed post-injury reorganization including progressive cortical dysplasia with cytoarchitectural disorganization, laminar obliteration, synaptic reorganization, transformation of some neurons, preservation of layer 1 intrinsic fibers and Cajal-Retzius cells, and large hypertrophic neurons with intense neurofilament immunoreactivity. The authors proposed that this progressive dysplastic process might have played an important role in the pathogenesis of epilepsy. Additional reports of dysplastic cortical changes in children who had suffered early postnatal head injury and subsequent epilepsy are on record (Lombroso 2000).

Table 61.1 Checklist for suspected non-accidental brain injury in infants or children

(A) Elements that suggest or should raise the suspicion of, NABI in the child presenting with new onset seizures or de novo status epilepticus
Witnessed inflicted head injury
Confession by perpetrator to inflicting the head injury or shaking
Evidence of abusive injuries (e.g., pattern bruises, occult rib or limb fractures, old lesions without explanation)
History of traumatic event that is incompatible with neurological status
No history of traumatic event (fall, blow to head, motor vehicle crash) in the presence of traumatic injuries
Unlikely history
Changes in the history given by care-givers
Retinal hemorrhages
Presence of non-specific signs such as vomiting, irritability, lethargy
(B) Salient procedures if suspicion of NABI is confirmed
Whole body examination
Laboratory test (blood count, liver function, coagulation, cerebrospinal fluid)
CT scan (head: ask the neuroradiologist to check for subcutaneous hematomas)
X-ray skeletal screening
Abdominal CT
EEG or video-EEG monitoring
Ophthalmologic examination (funduscopy examination for detecting retinal hemorrhages)
MRI (head, eye)
Written description and photographs of the child's injuries
Inform social services and police if consistent evidence of NABI

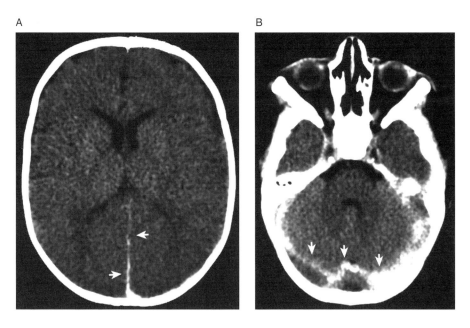

Fig. 61.4. Five-month-old boy. Axial brain CT scan, performed 48 hr after the onset of symptoms, shows acute hyperdense subdural hematomas along the posterior cerebral falx (A, arrows), in the posterior surfaces of the occipital lobes, and in the posterior fossa (B, arrows).

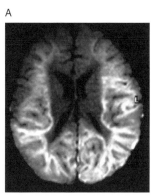
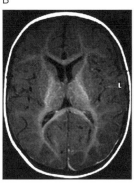
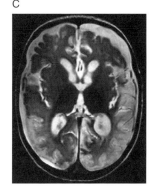

Fig. 61.5. Same boy as in Fig. 61.4. (A) Axial diffusion-weighted MRI performed on the fourth day after onset of symptoms. There is extensive bilateral hemispheric restricted diffusion corresponding to severe ischemia, with drop in the values of the apparent diffusion coefficient (ADC). (B) Axial T1-weighted MRI, performed at the same time as the above DWI, shows extensive hypointensity in the white matter. (C) Follow-up axial T2-weighted MRI performed 37 days after (B) and (C). There is diffuse brain atrophy with high-intensity abnormalities in the cerebral cortex and white matter, cortical thinning, and multiple subdural collections of different signal intensities and ages.

Diagnostic tests

Imaging

Radiological imaging plays a crucial role in investigating NABI, in order to assess intracranial complications, guide clinical management, and provide documentary evidence for forensic investigation (Jaspan *et al.* 2003). Imaging findings frequently include: traumatic diffuse axonal injury, severe brain swelling, subdural hemorrhage that can be diffuse, multifocal, or interhemispheric, exhibiting mixed density and associated with complex skull fractures (Sato 2009). The major imaging modalities used to investigate the sequelae of NABI include CT, MRI, skull radiography, and ultrasound. Computed tomography is the main imaging method in the evaluation of NABI. It is of rapid realization and can detect hemorrhage (Fig. 61.4A, B), edema, hypoxic–ischemic injury, bone fracture, and skin swelling with high sensitivity. Magnetic resonance imaging is more difficult to perform than CT in children, due to the length of time it takes, the sensitivity to patient motion, and the need for specialized monitoring equipment and general anesthesia in most cases. With respect to CT scan, MRI has a higher sensitivity in demonstrating parenchymal brain injury and detecting tiny volumes of subdural blood, especially in sites such as the posterior fossa and the anterior part of the middle cranial fossa (Jaspan *et al.* 2003; Stoodley 2005). Magnetic resonance imaging detects hemorrhage in the subacute stage (3–14 days) and demonstrates with high sensitivity early ischemic changes (especially with diffusion-weighted imaging) (Fig. 61.5 A–C) and diffuse axonal injury. This technique is also useful for characterizing retinal hemorrhages (Fig. 61.1B). Magnetic resonance spectroscopy (MRS) detects biochemical changes during the evolution of neuronal injury. Loss of integrity of the proton MR spectrum appears to announce irreversible neurological damage and occurs at a time when the clinical and neurological status gives no indication of long-term outcome (Haseler *et al.* 1997; Holshouser *et al.* 1997). Cranial ultrasound has a limited role. This technique provides information about parenchymal injury and extra-axial hemorrhage but has limited power in detecting subdural hemorrhage. Skull radiography is useful to diagnose fractures of the vault or base but does not give any direct information about intracranial injury (Jaspan *et al.* 2003).

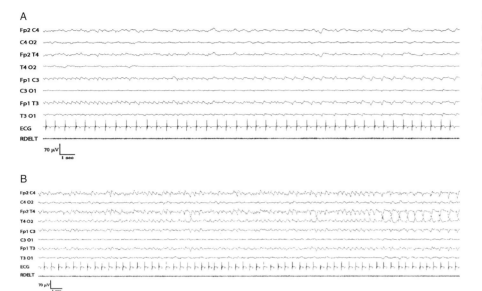

Fig. 61.6. Same boy as in Fig. 61.4 and 61.5. The EEG recording performed 6 days after onset of symptoms. At the time of recording the boy was drowsy and irritable but no clinically overt seizure activity was apparent. (A) Ictal activity originating from the left fronto-centro-temporal area. (B) A few minutes later, there is ictal electrographic activity over the centrolateral homologous regions.

Electroencephalography

In the series of Bourgeois *et al.* (2008) on admission, 11% of children with a diagnosis of NABI had a normal electro-encephalogram (EEG) while 25% exhibited subclinical status epilepticus. In our experience too, subclinical status epilepticus is a frequent and insidious manifestation of SBS (Fig. 61.6A, B). Early EEG was considered to be a good outcome predictor since a poor developmental outcome was observed in only 8% of children with normal EEG findings versus 71% of those with ictal abnormalities. Capturing electrographic seizures activity is of special diagnostic value when clinical manifestations are masked by the effects of the trauma or by iatrogenic intervention. Children tend to exhibit focal epileptiform discharges even after widespread brain damage. Additional features of interest that can be captured soon after the injury include voltage asymmetries, reactivity, depression of activity, localized or diffuse polymorphic delta activity, and coma patterns. The type of EEG activity soon after the injury is also helpful in predicting recovery from coma (Facco 1999).

Principles of treatment

Various drugs have been used with the purpose of preventing seizures and epilepsy in traumatic brain injury (TBI), although no study has specifically addressed NABI. Available evidence is insufficient to inform clinical practice in this area (Adelson *et al.* 2003) and antiepileptic drug (AED) prophylaxis of PTS with anticonvulsants is still a controversial issue. Some

authors suggest that prophylactic therapy with phenytoin, carbamazepine, or valproate can significantly reduce the incidence of PTS in pediatric head trauma (Langendorf *et al.* 1997; Gallagher, 2002). In particular, phenytoin has been considered the drug of choice for preventive treatment of early and late seizures while carbamazepine and valproate would be more suitable for the treatment of late seizures. However, while the role of prophylactic treatment with phenytoin during the first week after injury is substantiated by some original work (Temkin 2001), no positive effect on prevention of late seizures has been demonstrated. A systematic review of randomized controlled trials concluded that prophylactic treatment after acute traumatic head injury is likely to reduce early seizures but evidence was considered to be insufficient to support the view that prophylactic AEDs used at any time after head injury reduce death and overall disability (Schierhout and Roberts 1998). Prophylactic anticonvulsant therapy is not recommended to prevent late PTS in children; if a late PTS occurs, the patient should be managed in accordance with standard approaches to patients with new-onset seizures (Adelson *et al.* 2003). In general, it is recommended that post-traumatic epilepsy be treated the same as one would treat seizures of the same type of any etiology (Langendorf *et al.* 2008). The same rule applies to the medical treatment of status epilepticus occurring at any time after NABI. However, status epilepticus occurring as an early post-traumatic manifestation is often the expression of intracranial bleeding, especially subdural hematoma, and will therefore need accurate imaging monitoring for timely surgical treatment.

References

Adelson PD, Bratton SL, Carney NA, *et al.* (2003) Guidelines for the acute medical management of severe traumatic brain injury in infants, children, and adolescents. Chapter 19. The role of anti-seizure prophylaxis following severe pediatric traumatic brain injury. *Pediatr Crit Care Med* 4(3 Suppl):72–5.

Asikainen I, Kaste M, Sarna S (1999) Early and late posttraumatic seizures in traumatic brain injury rehabilitation patients: brain injury factors causing late seizures and influence of seizures on long-term outcome. *Epilepsia* **40**:584–9.

Barlow KM, Minns RA (2000) Annual incidence of shaken impact syndrome in young children. *Lancet* **356**:1571–2.

Barlow KM, Spowart JJ, Minns RA (2000) Early posttraumatic seizures in non-accidental head injury: relation to outcome. *Dev Med Child Neurol* **42**:591–4.

Bechtel K, Stoessel K, Leventhal JM, *et al.* (2004) Characteristics that distinguish accidental from abusive injury in hospitalized young children with head trauma. *Pediatrics* **114**:165–8.

Blumenthal I (2002) Shaken baby syndrome. *Postgrad Med J* **78**:732–5.

Bourgeois M, Di Rocco F, Garnett M, *et al.* (2008) Epilepsy associated with shaken baby syndrome. *Childs Nerv Syst* **24**:169–72.

Case ME (2007) Abusive head injuries in infants and young children. *Leg Med* **9**:83–7.

Chadwick D (2000) Seizures and epilepsy after traumatic brain injury. *Lancet* **355**:334–46.

Chiaretti A, De Benedictis R, Polidori G, *et al.* (2000) Early post-traumatic seizures in children with head injury. *Childs Nerv Syst* **16**:862–6.

Chiesa A, Duhaime AC (2009) Abusive head trauma. *Pediatr Clin N Am* **56**:317–31.

David TJ (1999) Shaken baby (shaken impact) syndrome: non-accidental head injury in infancy. *J R Soc Med* **92**:556–61.

Duhaime AC, Durham S (2007) Traumatic brain injury in infants: the phenomenon of subdural hemorrhage with hemispheric hypodensity ("Big Black Brain"). *Prog Brain Res* **161**:293–302.

Ewing-Cobbs L, Prasad M, Kramer L, *et al.* (2000) Acute neuroradiologic findings in young children with inflicted or noninflicted traumatic brain injury. *Childs Nerv Syst* **16**:25–33.

Facco E (1999) Current topics: the role of EEG in brain injury. *Intens Care Med* **25**:872–7.

Gallagher D (2002) Post traumatic epilepsy: an overview. *Einstein Q J Biol Med* **19**:5–9.

Geddes JF, Hackshaw AK, Vowles GH, Nickols CD, Whitwell HL (2001a). Neuropathology of inflicted head injury in children. I. Patterns of brain damage. *Brain* **124**:1290–8.

Geddes JF, Vowles GH, Hackshaw AK, *et al.* (2001b). Neuropathology of inflicted head injury in children. II. Microscopic brain injury in infants. *Brain* **124**:1299–306.

Gerber P, Coffman K (2007) Nonaccidental head trauma in infants. *Childs Nerv Syst* **23**:499–507.

Golden JA, Harding BN (2004). *Pathology and Genetics: Developmental Neuropathology*. Basel: ISN Neuropathology Press.

Hahn YS, Fuchs S, Flannery AM, Barthel MJ, McLone DG (1988) Factors influencing posttraumatic seizures in children. *Neurosurgery* **22**:864–7.

Hardman JM (1979) The pathology of traumatic brain injuries. *Adv Neurol* **22**:15–50.

Haseler LJ, Arcinue E, Danielsen ER, Bluml S, Ross BD (1997) Evidence from proton magnetic resonance spectroscopy for a metabolic cascade of neuronal damage in shaken baby syndrome. *Pediatrics* **99**:4–14.

Hawley CA, Ward AB, Long J, Owen DW, Magnay AR (2003) Prevalence of traumatic brain injury amongst children admitted to hospital in one health district: a population-based study. *Injury* **34**:256–60.

Hendrick EB, Harris L (1968) Post-traumatic epilepsy in children. *J Trauma* **8**:547–56.

Holshouser BA, Ashwal S, Luh GY, *et al.* (1997) Proton MR spectroscopy after acute central nervous system injury: outcome prediction in neonates, infants, and children. *Radiology* **202**:487–96.

Jaspan T, Griffiths PD, McConachie NS, Punt JA (2003) Neuroimaging for non-accidental head injury in childhood: a proposed protocol. *Clin Radiol* **58**:44–53.

Keenan HT, Runyan DK, Marshall SW, *et al.* (2003) A population-based study of inflicted traumatic brain injury in young children. *J Am Med Ass* **290**:621–6.

Kinney HC, Armstrong DD (1997). Perinatal neuropathology. In: Graham D, Lantos PL (eds.) *Greenfield's Neuropathology*, 6th edn. London: Arnold, pp. 535–99.

Kumar R, Singhal N, Mahapatra AK (2008) Traumatic subdural effusions in children following minor head injury. *Childs Nerv Syst* **24**:1391–6.

Lancon JA, Haines DE, Parent AD (1998) Anatomy of the shaken baby syndrome. *Anat Rec* **253**:13–18.

Langendorf FG, Pedley TA, Temkin NR (2008) Posttraumatic seizures. In: Engel J Jr.,

Pedley TA (eds.) *Epilepsy: A Comprehensive Textbook*. Philadelphia, PA: Lippincott Williams and Wilkins, pp. 2537–42.

Lombroso CT (2000). Can early postnatal closed head injury induce cortical dysplasia.? *Epilepsia* **41**:245–53.

Marín-Padilla M, Parisi JE, Armstrong DL, Sargent SK, Kaplan JA (2002) Shaken infant syndrome: developmental neuropathology, progressive cortical dysplasia, and epilepsy. *Acta Neuropathol* **103**:321–32.

McCabe CF, Donahue SP (2000) Prognostic indicators for vision and mortality in shaken baby syndrome. *Arch Ophthalmol* **118**:373–7.

Minns RA, Jones PA, Mok JY (2008) Incidence and demography of non-accidental head injury in southeast Scotland from a national database. *Am J Prev Med* **34**(4 Suppl):S126–33.

Oehmichen M, Schleiss D, Pedal I, *et al.* (2008) Shaken baby syndrome: re-examination of diffuse axonal injury as cause of death. *Acta Neuropathol* **116**:317–29.

Ratan SK, Kulshreshtha R, Pandey RM (1999) Predictors of posttraumatic convulsions in head-injured children. *Pediatr Neurosurg* **30**:127–31.

Ryan MA, Lloyd DW, Conlin AM, Gumbs GR, Keenan HT (2008) Evaluating the epidemiology of inflicted traumatic brain injury in infants of U.S. military families. *Am J Prev Med* **34**(4 Suppl):S143–7.

Sato Y (2009) Imaging of nonaccidental head injury. *Pediatr Radiol* **39**(Suppl 2):S230–5.

Schierhout G, Roberts I (1998) Prophylactic antiepileptic agents after head injury: a systematic review. *J Neurol Neurosurg Psychiatry* **64**:108–12.

Starling SP, Holden JR, Jenny C (1995) Abusive head trauma: the relationship of perpetrators to their victims. *Pediatrics* **95**:259–62.

Starling SP, Patel S, Burke BL, *et al.* (2004) Analysis of perpetrator admissions to inflicted traumatic brain injury in children. *Arch Pediatr Adolesc Med* **158**:454–8.

Statler KD (2006) Pediatric posttraumatic seizures: epidemiology, putative mechanisms of epileptogenesis and promising investigational progress. *Dev Neurosci* **28**:354–63.

Stoodley N (2005) Neuroimaging in non-accidental head injury: if, when, why and how. *Clin Radiol* **60**:22–30.

Sturm V, Landau K, Menke MN (2008) Optical coherence tomography findings in Shaken Baby Syndrome. *Am J Ophthalmol* **146**:363–8.

Temkin NR (2001) Antiepileptogenesis and seizure prevention trials with antiepileptic drugs: meta-analysis of controlled trials. *Epilepsia* **42**:515–24.

Temkin NR, Dikmen SS, Wilensky AJ, *et al.* (1990) A randomized, double-blind study of phenytoin for the prevention of post-traumatic seizures. *N Engl J Med* **323**:497–502.

Togioka BM, Arnold MA, Bathurst MA, *et al.* (2009) Retinal hemorrhages and shaken baby syndrome: an evidence-based review. *J Emerg Med* **37**:98–106.

Yablon SA (1993) Posttraumatic seizures. *Arch Phys Med Rehab* **74**:983–1001.

Chapter

62

Glioma

William P. Gray and Harry Bulstrode

Definitions and epidemiology

Gliomas are neoplasms derived from glial cell precursors. They comprise about 40% of primary central nervous system (CNS) tumors, with an incidence of 6 per 100 000 person–years (CBTRUS 2007). The only accepted risk factors are increasing age, radiation exposure, genetic predisposition, and male sex, which alone confers a 40% increase in incidence (Chandana *et al.* 2008). However, associations with environmental carcinogens, diet, and occupation have been reported, and the incidence is higher in developed industrialized countries (Ohgaki 2009).

Pathology

Classification is undertaken according to cell type, grade, and location. A simplified scheme based on the World Health Organization (WHO) classification (Louis *et al.* 2007) but concentrating on the gliomas of primary concern in epilepsy is provided (Fig. 62.1). The classification is primarily histological.

Astrocytomas are the commonest glioma subtype. Grade 1 is reserved for well-circumscribed lesions with benign behavior, found predominantly in children. Grade 2 astrocytomas, the typical "low-grade glioma," demonstrate cytological atypia, but are well differentiated and slow-growing, and usually demonstrate extensive diffuse infiltration at the time of diagnosis. Most will ultimately transform to high-grade tumors (WHO Grades 3 and 4). Grade 3 implies anaplasia, nuclear atypia, and brisk mitotic activity, while Grade 4 implies high mitotic rates and endothelial and microvascular proliferation, translating to rapid expansion and characteristic central necrosis. At a cellular level, there is disruption to cell-cycle control and

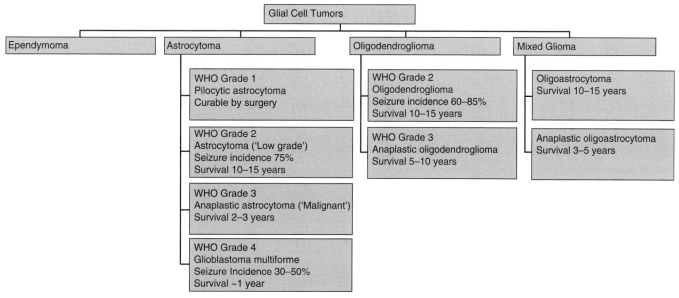

Fig. 62.1. Glioma classification, with seizure incidence and prognostic estimates (Louis *et al.* 2007).

The Causes of Epilepsy, eds. S. D. Shorvon, F. Andermann, and R. Guerrini. Published by Cambridge University Press. © Cambridge University Press 2011.

signal-transduction mechanisms, in two distinct patterns, corresponding to primary and secondary glioblastoma (Peiffer and Kleihues 1999; Ohgaki *et al.* 2004). The former is a de novo lesion manifesting at a mean age of 55 years with a clinical history usually of about 3 months' duration. The latter arises at a mean age of 40 in the context of a pre-existing Grade 2 or 3 lesion, and has distinct associated mutations including a 19q chromosomal deletion.

Oligodendrogliomas and ependymomas are relatively less common tumors arising respectively from oligodendrocytic and ependymal cell precursors. The same quintet of cellularity, mitotic rate, nuclear atypia, necrosis, and endothelial proliferation distinguish the high-grade examples of these lesions (Engelhard *et al.* 2002).

While not a feature of the WHO classification, distinctions in the genetic profile of gliomas are of increasing prognostic and even management importance. Chromosome 1p deletion is a positive prognostic marker in Grade 2 glioma (Iwamoto *et al.* 2008), and 1p/19q deletion is well established as an indicator of positive outcome and chemosensitivity in anaplastic oligodendroglioma (Kaloshi *et al.* 2007). O6-methylguanine DNA methyltransferase (MGMT) is a key enzyme involved in human DNA repair. Its inactivation is predictive of chemosensitivity in glioblastoma (Idbaih *et al.* 2007).

Clinical features

Gliomas may present with one or a combination of neurological deficits, symptoms of mass effect, and seizures, usually reflecting the anatomical location of the lesion. Most gliomas are supratentorial, 25% arising in frontal cortex, with 20% and 13% in temporal and parietal lobe locations respectively (CBTRUS 2007). These supratentorial tumors account almost exclusively for the burden of epilepsy in glioma. These lesions do not metastasize outside the CNS, although cerebrospinal fluid (CSF) dissemination to the spinal cord is well recognized.

Prognostic estimates for many of the different histological subtypes are provided in Fig. 62.1, with the proviso that outcomes are heavily influenced by clinical factors including age, neurological status, and tumor location. Other prognostic factors include contrast enhancement on imaging (typical of vascular high-grade lesions), extent of surgical resection, proliferation indices, and genetic profile.

Frequency and risk factors for epilepsy

Brain tumors represent the cause of epilepsy in about 6% of new cases presenting in general practice (Sander *et al.* 1990), but the figure is closer to 30% for adults aged 25–64. Historically 10–30% of cases of chronic intractable partial epilepsy were ultimately attributed to neoplasms (Spencer *et al.* 1984). Conversely, seizures are a feature in approximately one-third of gliomas (Hauser *et al.* 1993) and approximate figures for seizure incidence associated with some glioma subtypes are supplied in Fig. 62.1. Seizures occur with disproportionate frequency in low-grade gliomas. In a study group of patients who ultimately underwent surgical resection of low-grade glioma, 81% were symptomatic with seizures prior to surgery (Chang *et al.* 2008).

Seizures in the context of glioma appear to confer a significant prognostic benefit (Lote *et al.* 1998). Some of the benefit is likely to stem from early diagnosis, since seizures will often prompt referral for imaging well before symptoms of mass effect or neurological deficit appear and are acted upon. There is evidence, however, that glioma with epilepsy represents a distinct pathophysiological entity, characterized by specific immunohistochemistry (Piepmeier *et al.* 1993) as well as improved survival. Tumors identified as anaplastic gliomas histologically, arising in the context of intractable seizures, nevertheless seem to predominantly follow an indolent course (Fried *et al.* 1994; Piepmeier *et al.* 1996). Pooled 10-year survival rates of >90% have been reported for patients with intractable epilepsy in the context of Grade 2/3 astrocytomas (Luyken *et al.* 2003), compared to 21% in comparable cases without seizures as a presenting feature (Chandana *et al.* 2008).

Seizures are associated with cortical gray matter involvement, as recognized originally by Hughlings-Jackson in the nineteenth century. Temporal, parietal, and especially frontal lobe location predisposes to seizure, whilst seizures are rare in infratentorial tumors (Sirven *et al.* 2004), and tumors elsewhere rarely cause seizures unless there is cortical encroachment.

Of note, oligodendroglioma and oligoastrocytoma subtypes are significantly more likely to be associated with seizures than astrocytomas, probably a result of a tendency to gray matter spread as compared to the white matter predilection of astrocytomas (see "Mechanisms of epileptogenesis," below).

Characteristics of epilepsy in glioma

In a sample of 332 patients undergoing surgical resection of WHO Grade 2 gliomas (Chang *et al.* 2008), just over half of patients with seizures displayed generalized epilepsy, and about 60% had partial seizures, equally divided between simple and complex. Clearly in this context generalized epilepsy is likely to represent rapid secondary generalization of a focal event.

Where seizures were a feature preoperatively, about 25% of patients had a single ictus prior to resection, 25% had multiple seizures responsive to medication, and 50% had uncontrolled epilepsy, defined as seizure frequency greater than once per 3 months. These rates of response compare poorly to those achieved in other epilepsy syndromes, for reasons discussed in the "Principles of management" section below.

The nature of the seizures elicited by gliomas will generally correspond to tumor location. In up to one-third of cases, however, and especially in slow-growing temporal lobe tumors, the clinically apparent epileptic focus does not correspond to the tumor site. This indicates a process of secondary epileptogenesis, generally attributed to "dual pathology," such as hippocampal damage associated with an extrahippocampal lesion (Levesque *et al.* 1991).

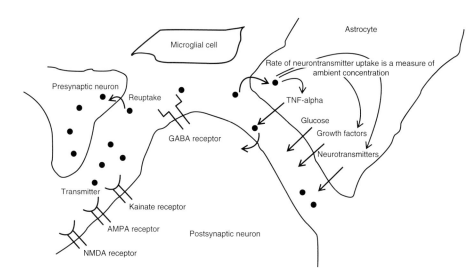

Fig. 62.2. The tripartite synapse. Glia modulate activity directly through uptake and release of neurotransmitters, including S100B, thought to be specific to gliotransmission. Additionally they act indirectly through release of growth factors and cytokines such as tumor necrosis factor (TNF)-α, which influence postsynaptic receptor expression and excitability. These processes are regulated in response to synaptic neurotransmitter concentrations.

Mechanisms of epileptogenesis

Epileptic foci are believed to develop within the cortex surrounding tumors, since the lesions themselves have no electroencephalographic (EEG) activity and are not electrically excitable (Hirsch *et al.* 1966). However, the mechanisms underlying glioma-induced epilepsy are poorly understood, and are likely to be multifactorial.

Structural mechanisms

The role of gross structural disruption in epileptogenesis is controversial. In the comparable situation of malformations of cortical development, structural disruption is associated with epilepsy. This is a more prominent feature in malformations with abnormalities of glioneuronal proliferation, so that the cellular substrate may be of primary importance (Wong 2008). The analogy is limited, however, since structural abnormality present during development is likely to differ in its potential for functional disruption. In gliomas, mechanical or vascular disruption of afferent pathways may render regions hyperexcitable (Wolf *et al.* 1996), but the lower seizure incidence in high-grade glioma and glioblastoma despite extensive disruption is difficult to reconcile with this explanation.

Intercellular mechanisms

At the intercellular level, increased excitability may result from synaptic and gap junction abnormalities, with altered expression of connexin gap junction proteins demonstrated in these tumors (Aronica *et al.* 2001).

There are speculative roles for abnormalities of oxygenation balance, electrolytes, pH, lactate, enzymes, and amino acids in the peritumoral milieu (Schaller and Ruegg 2003; Rajneesh and Binder 2009). Compromise of the blood–brain barrier in the laboratory setting produces seizures, with a mechanism related to elevated albumin levels implicated (Ivens *et al.* 2007). Again, the relatively low seizure incidence in high-grade tumors argues against a key role for edema, metabolic

dysfunction, or breakdown of the blood–brain barrier, which are associated most strongly with these lesions, but aspects of the microenvironment are clearly important predisposing factors (Schaller 2005).

Abnormalities in excitatory and inhibitory receptor expression are pertinent to seizure generation in certain gliomas. Highly epileptogenic glioneuronal tumors have shown strong expression of glutamate receptors on their neuronal component, as well as increased expression of metabotropic glutamate receptors in the astrocytes around these lesions (Aronica *et al.* 2001). The same group has demonstrated underexpression of γ-aminobutyric acid (GABA) receptors, following on from work demonstrating relative absence of neurons transmitting via GABA and somatostatin in peritumoral cortex as compared to non tumor-infiltrated cortex (Haglund *et al.* 1992).

Increased excitability may also result from changes in dedicated synaptic transmission mechanisms. Glial cells have not traditionally been accorded a central role in epileptogenesis, since the seizure ictus is a consequence of action potentials, which must originate in neurons. There is however growing evidence implicating glia, beyond their traditionally accepted structural and metabolic support roles. Glia may play an important role at this level as part of the "tripartite synapse" (Fig. 62.2). Astrocytes are involved in neurotransmitter reuptake, and synaptic modulation by means of growth factor secretion. Knock-out mice not expressing a glutamate reuptake (GLUT-1) transporter develop seizures (Tanaka *et al.* 1997). In the case of GABA transmission, synaptic release of the transmitter by neurons mediates phasic inhibitory postsynaptic currents, but excitability is dependent on a tonic GABA receptor-mediated conductance (Semyanov *et al.* 2003). The resting level of tonic inhibition depends heavily on glia and their neurotransmitter reuptake mechanisms, and disruption here may render neuronal networks hyperexcitable and predispose to seizure. Glial induced changes in number, size, and distribution of synaptic vesicles may also be of importance (Alger *et al.* 1990).

More novel is the suggestion that astrocytes may be directly involved in neural processing through active release of neurotransmitters including adenosine triphosphate (ATP) and glutamate (Newman 2003), a process upregulated in glioma cells as a means to promote invasion (Lyons *et al.* 2007). A calcium-binding protein, S100B, released by astrocytes is found at greater concentration in serum and CSF in epilepsy as well as other neuropathological conditions. Recently S100B has been shown to enhance kainate-induced gamma oscillations via activation of a specific receptor (Sakatani *et al.* 2008). Knock-out of either receptor or ligand is conversely associated with reduced excitability. This implies direct glial involvement in epileptogenesis, not only through modulation of traditional synaptic pathways, but also by separate dedicated mechanisms.

Glial cells have also been shown to express inflammatory cytokines at high levels in association with seizures in resected specimens. These cytokines, in particular interleukin-1 (IL-1), can be shown in turn to prolong seizures in rodent models (Vezzani *et al.* 2008), and tumor necrosis factor-α (TNF-α) among others is overexpressed in gliomas of all grades (Roessler *et al.* 1995). More generally, glia are seen to play a key role in the process of "synaptic scaling" (Stellwagen and Malenka 2006). The strength of excitatory synaptic inputs is modulated in response to activity levels, a process mediated by TNF-α released from glial cells. Chronic underexcitation, reproduced experimentally by receptor blockade, is detected in terms of reduced neurotransmitter reuptake by glial cells. Tumor necrosis factor-α is released in response, and stimulates increased neuronal glutamatergic receptor expression, as well as GABA receptor phagocytosis.

These mechanisms may explain the greater propensity of low-grade gliomas to induce epilepsy, since retention of some maladaptive astrocytic physiological properties by glioma cells in an invading edge of tumor in contact with functional glioneuronal synapses may alter the balance of excitability towards seizure generation.

Diagnostic tests

Imaging

Diagnosis of a space-occupying lesion as the cause of a seizure is made usually with the aid of cross-sectional imaging. Magnetic resonance imaging (MRI), with and without gadolinium contrast, is the investigation of choice, showing a higher sensitivity and specificity (greater than 90%) than computed tomography (CT) for detecting a glioma (especially WHO Grades 1–3, which may be isodense with surrounding tissue). Increased signal on T2-weighted and fluid-attenuated inversion recovery (FLAIR) imaging is characteristic of a glioma, but also of the swelling associated with seizures, especially status epilepticus. Persistence on follow-up imaging is therefore key to interpretation. An MRI scan may demonstrate characteristics of certain tumors and associated features of calvarial moulding or mass effect. Advances in MRI offer new insights into glioma. Diffusion-weighted sequences can establish the cellularity of lesions, useful for example in excluding abscess as a differential

for cystic tumors. Functional MRI can be used to plan resection by demonstrating the extent of eloquent cortex. Perfusion MR provides information on tumor vascularity and angiogenesis, predictive of grade, and MR spectroscopy (MRS) has been employed to differentiate tumor grade using algorithms to analyze the spectral signature of the lesions (Price 2007). Finally, MRI is necessary for the accurate assessment of tumor extent and for gaging whether total macroscopic resection has been achieved postoperatively (Luyken *et al.* 2003).

Biopsy

Definitive diagnosis is by surgical resection or biopsy. The oncological literature would suggest that all CT/MRI-identified mass lesions should be biopsied to identify curable conditions and predict prognosis, especially in light of the dependence of WHO criteria on histopathology. However, stereotactic biopsy is not without risk, and histopathological diagnosis may not alter management. If resective surgery is being contemplated for intractable epilepsy, against a background of stable appearances on surveillance imaging consistent with low-grade glioma, then pre-resection biopsy is not required.

Investigating epilepsy in known glioma

Strategies for identifying epileptic foci, including possibly secondary foci, are applied to a variable extent. The role of EEG in localizing foci has receded with the advent of cross-sectional imaging, but it remains a core diagnostic technique. Typical abnormalities include abnormal delta or theta wave activity which may be focal and therefore of assistance in localization, focal attenuation of activity over the tumor, and combinations of spike and wave discharges. Normal EEG is encountered in only 5% of tumors in the cerebral hemispheres, but in a higher proportion of tumors elsewhere (Fischgold *et al.* 1961).

The use of MRI and even positron emission tomography (PET) techniques allow increasingly confident preoperative identification of features such as hippocampal sclerosis suggestive of potential dual pathology. Novel techniques combining EEG and structural MRI to identify foci have shown promising early results (Ding *et al.* 2007).

The gold standard for establishing the location of epileptic foci prior to operation, however, remains the invasive placement of intracranial electrodes. The decision to proceed with this should be made through organized review of non-invasive data by a multidisciplinary team. This topic is covered in more detail in the "Principles of management" section.

Principles of management

Management of glioma

The mainstay of management of both newly diagnosed and recurrent glioma is usually surgical resection. Factors that may limit the extent of resection, or preclude it altogether, include the patient's functional status and tumor location. For example where there is involvement of eloquent cortex or other critical

Table 62.1 Low-grade glioma: to operate early, or watch and wait?

Favoring early resection	Favoring "watch and wait"
Patient preference	
Failure of pharmacological seizure control	Seizures as sole presenting feature
Developing neurological deficit	Eloquent/operatively challenging location
Progression on imaging	Diffuse infiltration on imaging
Need for histological verification	Poor functional status

Table 62.2 Postoperative outcomes for low-grade glioma patients presenting with seizures

Engel Class 1	Seizure-free	67%
Engel Class 2	Almost seizure-free	17%
Engel Class 3	Significant seizure reduction	7%
Engel Class 4	No significant seizure reduction	8%

Source: Chang *et al.* (2008).

structures, tissue diagnosis by open or stereotactic biopsy may be preferred. Initial treatment of ependymoma may be by radiotherapy or indeed by observation alone. Historically a "watch-and-wait" strategy has been advocated in preference to early surgery for patients with radiologically low-grade lesions who are able to achieve seizure control with anticonvulsants (Cairncross and Laperriere 1989). The intuitive belief that early and aggressive cytoreduction must slow progression has been challenged by retrospective data that demonstrate equivalent outcomes in this group (Recht *et al.* 1992). This seems at odds, however, with the improved outcome data associated with extensive rather than limited resection, replicated across multiple data series (Keles *et al.* 2001). Although retrospective analysis of survival rates in patients with low-grade glioma resections using intraoperative MR seemed to be significantly increased compared to Central Brain Tumor Registry of the United States (CBTRUS) results (Claus *et al.* 2005), there is only modest evidence that surgery leads to improved outcomes in low-grade glioma through a reduction in tumor burden (Pouratian *et al.* 2007). Faced with the natural history of continuous growth and ultimate transformation to higher grade (Mandonnet *et al.* 2003), early resection is usually favored by clinicians and patients. However the decision depends on a complex balance of conflicting concerns (Table 62.1).

Chemotherapy may be an appropriate adjuvant modality in low-grade gliomas, especially at relapse. A *Cochrane Review* in 2002 (Stewart 2002) established the role for chemotherapy in high-grade glioma, Grade 3 lesions demonstrating greater chemosensitivity to traditional agents when compared to glioblastomas. For these latter, systemic temozolomide confers significantly increased median and 2-year survival (Hart *et al.* 2008b), as does the local implantation of carmustine wafers inserted into the tumor cavity at the time of complete macroscopic excision (Hart *et al.* 2008a). Where near-complete resection is achieved, chemotherapeutic-impregnated polymer wafers (Gliadel®) can be inserted at the time of surgery, conferring an increase in median survival of about 2 months. Of note, the evidence suggests that these strategies do not prolong survival in recurrent disease.

Fractionated focal radiotherapy is a key component of adjuvant treatment, especially in high-grade lesions. In low-grade lesions, evidence points to a prolonged period before relapse in patients receiving radiotherapy immediately after surgery, but overall survival is not improved (van den Bent 2005). Therefore given the associated comorbidity, especially neurocognitive sequelae, observation alone may be judged appropriate.

Seizure control

Retrospective studies have demonstrated that macroscopic resection of gliomas provides seizure freedom in 60–80% of patients (Goldring *et al.* 1986; Boon *et al.* 1991; Cascino *et al.* 1992; Fried *et al.* 1994; Luyken *et al.* 2003). These reported series of lesional or glioma resections tend to be heterogeneous and have often focused on drug refractory epilepsy where low-grade astrocytomas and oligodendrogliomas were in the minority, or did not distinguish between glioma patients with easily controlled or drug-refractory epilepsy. A more recent retrospective evaluation of seizure outcomes in 332 cases of surgically treated low-grade glioma is detailed in Table 62.2 (Chang *et al.* 2008). Importantly, 39% of patients did not achieve seizure control on anticonvulsant drugs preoperatively, and their seizures were significantly more likely to be simple partial, to involve the temporal lobe, and to have been present for longer, prior to surgery. While the overall 12–month seizure-freedom rate after surgery was 69%, only 50% of patients who had uncontrolled seizures preoperatively were seizure-free at 6-month follow-up, compared to 80% in whom seizures had been controlled prior to surgery. Multivariate logistic regression analysis showed that gross total resection was a strong predictor of seizure control, whereas duration of seizures >1 year and simple partial seizures predicted failure to control seizures.

The additional value of preoperative electrocorticography (ECoG) using subdural grids to identify the seizure onset zone, and perhaps guide resection extension beyond the tumor mass, is limited in extratemporal gliomas which can be reasonably treated by macroscopic resection followed by a wait-and-see policy. This contrasts with the established role of preoperative ECoG in the treatment of dysembryoplastic neuroepithelial tumors, gangliogliomas, and other cortical lesions. Multivariate analysis in a recent prospective study of lesional surgery (where fewer than 5% were low-grade gliomas) has shown that removal of the seizure onset zone was the single independent predictor for achieving seizure freedom (Schwartz *et al.* 2000; Asano *et al.* 2009). Postresection ECoG can be misleading, as surgical trauma may produce postresection discharges where none existed preoperatively, and may lead to the removal of more functional brain tissue than necessary (Schwartz *et al.* 2000). Functionally critical eloquent cortex can be safely identified by cortical stimulation during awake surgery in adults, and intracranial grids for preoperative stimulation are often poorly tolerated in gliomas with mass effect.

A more established role for preoperative ECoG exists in temporal lobe lesional surgery as dual pathology in the mesial temporal lobe can be associated with neocortical lesions, including gliomas (Fried *et al.* 1992). One study (Berger *et al.* 1993) found a mesial temporal focus in 26 of the 29 low-grade temporal tumors studied. In general excision of both mesial temporal sclerosis and the extrahippocampal lesion generates the best seizure control (Li *et al.* 1999). In the presence of an atrophic hippocampus, resection of only the tumor achieves a seizure-free outcome in only 20% of patients (Li *et al.* 1997). If tumor exists in the lateral temporal lobe and non-concordant data suggest a mesial temporal onset with borderline verbal memory, intracranial monitoring is used to localize accurately the seizure onset zone. In either temporal lobe, if the hippocampal volume is reduced in the presence of a lateral tumor and borderline memory, then intracranial monitoring is used to identify dual pathology. If the tumor involves the dominant temporal mesial structures with normal verbal memory then resection is not indicated and a biopsy is obtained to guide treatment. Where a tumor is distinct from the dominant mesial structures with normal verbal memory a simple lesionectomy is performed, or if the verbal memory is severely impaired then the mesial structures are excised with the tumor.

Importantly, seizure recurrence after initial control is strongly predictive of tumor recurrence/progression, and is an important trigger for repeat imaging before further resective or adjuvant therapy.

It should also be recognized that surgical intervention may be a precipitant of seizures, either through local manipulation, edema, ischemia, and hemorrhage, or through associated systemic disturbance, such as electrolyte imbalance or omission of antiepileptic drugs (AEDs). Seizure incidence following craniotomy, regardless of indication, is quoted to be 5–10% (Gerstle de Paquet 1976).

Chemotherapy with temozolomide has been shown to be of seizure benefit in approximately 50% of Grade 2 gliomas (Brada *et al.* 2003). Chemotherapeutic agents, however, are also implicated in epileptogenesis through induction of encephalopathy (cyclosporin A, vincristine) and electrolyte disturbance (cisplatin). Acute hemorrhage in the tumor may trigger seizures, and is a recognized complication of chemotherapeutic agents including L-asparaginase.

Irradiation is an option to reduce seizure frequency in the context of biopsy-proven unresectable low-grade astrocytoma (Rogers *et al.* 1993). Stereotactic radiosurgery represents an alternative avenue for treatment of epileptic foci, reducing seizures when used in the context of arteriovenous malformations (Hoh *et al.* 2002), although recent results in patients treated for mesial temporal epilepsy have been disappointing (Vojtech *et al.* 2009). Applied to epilepsy in glioma, a retrospective series has reported significant improvement to Engel Class 1 or 2 in more than 50% of those treated (Schrottner *et al.* 2002). Complications of bleeding, edema, and tissue necrosis may lead to increases in seizure frequency after radiation treatment, as they may after surgery.

Antiepileptic drugs

For patients with gliomas presenting without seizures, there is no good evidence to suggest efficacy for AEDs as prophylaxis, confirmed by a recent *Cochrane Review* establishing no clear benefit, but a significant incidence of side effects (Tremont-Lukats *et al.* 2008).

Patients presenting with a single seizure in the context of a glioma have traditionally been treated with phenytoin first line, reflecting the lack of evidence for novel AEDs in this context to date. The enzyme-inducing effects of many traditional AEDs lead to decreased serum concentrations of corticosteroids and chemotherapeutic drugs (Yap *et al.* 2008), and this correlates with demonstrable reduced survival rates in glioblastoma patients receiving these agents alongside chemotherapy as compared to those receiving other AEDs (Oberndorfer *et al.* 2005). Novel non-enzyme-inducing AEDs therefore offer considerable potential benefits in this situation. Refractory seizures, those occurring with sufficient frequency and severity to limit daily life despite the use of AEDs at adequate serum concentrations, are common in glioma. This may reflect overexpression of transporter proteins, coded for by multidrug-resistance genes *MDR1* and *MRP*, which can limit intracellular concentrations of AEDs including carbamazepine, phenytoin, phenobarbital, lamotrigine, and felbamate (Loscher and Potschka 2002). Again, novel AEDs that are not substrates for these proteins, such as levetiracetam, may have an important role in intractable epilepsy (Maschio *et al.* 2006).

With these factors in mind, valproic acid and lamotrigine are considered good first-line drugs, and there is a case for addition of levetiracetam in refractory cases (van Breemen *et al.* 2007). Valproate's action as an inhibitor of histone deacetylases has incidentally recently been shown to lead to inhibition of cell proliferation and growth arrest in murine astrocytoma (Benitez *et al.* 2008), raising the interesting possibility of a secondary chemotherapeutic benefit.

References

Alger JR, Frank JA, Bizzi A, *et al.* (1990) Metabolism of human gliomas: assessment with H-1 MR spectroscopy and F-18 fluorodeoxyglucose PET. *Radiology* **177**:633–41.

Aronica E, Gorter JA, Jansen GH, *et al.* (2001) Expression of connexin 43 and connexin 32 gap-junction proteins in epilepsy-associated brain tumors and in the perilesional epileptic cortex. *Acta Neuropathol* **101**:449–59.

Aronica E, Yankaya B, Jansen GH, et al. (2001) Ionotropic and metabotropic glutamate receptor protein expression in glioneuronal tumors from patients with intractable epilepsy. Neuropathol Appl Neurobiol 27:223–37.

Asano E, Juhasz C, Shah A, et al. (2009). Role of subdural electrocorticography in prediction of long-term seizure outcome in epilepsy surgery. Brain 132:1038–47.

Benitez JA, Arregui L, Cabreva G, et al. (2008) Valproic acid induces polarization, neuronal-like differentiation of a subpopulation of C6 glioma cells and selectively regulates transgene expression. Neuroscience 156:911–20.

Berger MS, Ghatan S, Haglund MM, et al. (1993) Low-grade gliomas associated with intractable epilepsy: seizure outcome utilizing electrocorticography during tumor resection. J Neurosurg 79:62–9.

Boon PA, Williamson PD, Fried I, et al. (1991) Intracranial, intraaxial, space-occupying lesions in patients with intractable partial seizures: an anatomoclinical, neuropsychological, and surgical correlation. Epilepsia 32:467–76.

Brada M, Viviers L, Abson C, et al. (2003) Phase II study of primary temozolomide chemotherapy in patients with WHO grade II gliomas. Ann Oncol 14:1715–21.

Cairncross JG, Laperriere NJ (1989) Low-grade glioma: to treat or not to treat." Arch Neurol 46:1238–9.

Cascino GD, Kelly PJ, Hirschhorn KA, et al. (1992) Long-term follow-up of stereotactic lesionectomy in partial epilepsy: predictive factors and electroencephalographic results. Epilepsia 33:639–44.

CBTRUS (2007) Statistical Report: Primary Brain Tumors in the United States. Hinsdale, IL: Central Brain Tumor Registry of the United States.

Chandana SR, Movva S, Aora M, et al. (2008) Primary brain tumors in adults. Am Fam Physician 77:1423–30.

Chang EF, Potts MB, Keles GE, et al. (2008) Seizure characteristics and control following resection in 332 patients with low-grade gliomas. J Neurosurg 108:227–35.

Claus EB, Horlacher A, Hsu L, et al. (2005) Survival rates in patients with low-grade glioma after intraoperative magnetic resonance image guidance. Cancer 103:1227–33.

Ding L, Wilke C, Xu B, et al. (2007) EEG source imaging: correlating source locations and extents with electrocorticography and surgical resections in epilepsy patients. J Clin Neurophysiol 24:130–6.

Engelhard HH, Stelea A, Cochran EJ, (2002) Oligodendroglioma: pathology and molecular biology. Surg Neurol 58:111–17; discussion 117.

Fischgold HZ, Buisson B, Ferey J (1961) Electroencephalography and cerebral tumors: general comments on the use of EEG in the diagnosis and localization of cerebral tumors. EEG Clin Neurophysiol 19(Suppl):51–74.

Fried I, Kim JH, Spencer DD (1992) Hippocampal pathology in patients with intractable seizures and temporal lobe masses. J Neurosurg 76:735–40.

Fried I, Kim JH, Spencer DD (1994) Limbic and neocortical gliomas associated with intractable seizures: a distinct clinicopathological group. Neurosurgery 34:815–23; discussion 823–4.

Gerstle de Paquet EPM, Iniquez RA (1976) Epileptic seizures as an early complication of neurosurgery. Acta Neurol Latinoamericana 22:144–51.

Goldring S, Rich KM, Picker S (1986) Experience with gliomas in patients presenting with a chronic seizure disorder. Clin Neurosurg 33:15–42.

Haglund MB, Shamseldin M, Lettich E, Ojemann GA (1992) Changes in gamma-aminobutyric acid and somatostatin in epileptic cortex associated with low-grade gliomas. J Neurosurg 77:209–16.

Hart MG, Garside R, Rogers G, Somerville M, Stein K (2008a). Chemotherapeutic wafers for high grade glioma. Cochrane Database Syst Rev 3:CD007294.

Hart MG, Garside R, Rogers G, Somerville M, Stein K (2008b). Temozolomide for high grade glioma. Cochrane Database Syst Rev 4:CD007415.

Hauser WA, Annegers JF, Kurland LT (1993) Incidence of epilepsy and unprovoked seizures in Rochester, Minnesota: 1935–1984. Epilepsia 34:453–68.

Hirsch JB-F, Sachs M, Hirsch JC, Scherrer J (1966) Electrocorticogramme et activités unitaires lors de processus expansifs chez l'homme. EEG Clin Neurophysiol 21:417–28.

Hoh BL, Chapman PH, Loeffler JS, et al. (2002) Results of multimodality treatment for 141 patients with brain

arteriovenous malformations and seizures: factors associated with seizure incidence and seizure outcomes. Neurosurgery 51:303–9; discussion 309–11.

Idbaih A, Omuro A, Ducray F, Hoang-Xuan K (2007) Molecular genetic markers as predictors of response to chemotherapy in gliomas. Curr Opin Oncol 19:606–11.

Ivens S, Kaufer D, Flores LP, et al. (2007). TGF-beta receptor-mediated albumin uptake into astrocytes is involved in neocortical epileptogenesis. Brain 130:535–47.

Iwamoto FM, Nicolardi L, Demopoulos A, et al. (2008) Clinical relevance of 1p and 19q deletion for patients with WHO grade 2 and 3 gliomas. J Neurooncol 88:293–8.

Kaloshi G, Benouaich-Amiel A, Daikite F, et al. (2007) Temozolomide for low-grade gliomas: predictive impact of 1p/19q loss on response and outcome. Neurology 68:1831–6.

Keles GE, Lamborn KR, Berger S (2001) Low-grade hemispheric gliomas in adults: a critical review of extent of resection as a factor influencing outcome. J Neurosurg 95:735–45.

Levesque MN, Vinters HV, Babb TL (1991) Surgical treatment of limbic epilepsy associated with extrahippocampal lesions: the problem of dual pathology. J Neurosurg 75:364–70.

Li L, Cendes F, Watson C, et al. (1997) Surgical treatment of patients with single and dual pathology. Neurology 48:437–44.

Li L, Cendes F, Andermann F, et al. (1999) Surgical outcome in patients with epilepsy and dual pathology. Brain 122:799–805.

Loscher W, Potschka H (2002) Role of multidrug transporters in pharmacoresistance to antiepileptic drugs. J Pharmacol Exp Ther 301:7–14.

Lote K, Stenwig AE, Skullerud K, Hirschberg H (1998) Prevalence and prognostic significance of epilepsy in patients with gliomas. Eur J Cancer 34:98–102.

Louis DN, Ohgaki H, Wiestler OD, et al. (2007) The 2007 WHO classification of tumors of the central nervous system. Acta Neuropathol 114:97–109.

Luyken C, Blümcke I, Fimmers R, et al. (2003) The spectrum of long-term epilepsy-associated tumors: long-term seizure and tumor outcome and neurosurgical aspects. Epilepsia 44:822–30.

Lyons SA, Chung WJ, Weaver AK, *et al.* (2007) Autocrine glutamate signaling promotes glioma cell invasion. *Cancer Res* 67:9463–71.

Mandonnet E, Delattre JY, Tanguy ML, *et al.* (2003) Continuous growth of mean tumor diameter in a subset of grade II gliomas. *Ann Neurol* 53:524–8.

Maschio M, Dinapoli L, Zarabla A, Jandolo B (2006) Issues related to the pharmacological management of patients with brain tumors and epilepsy. *Funct Neurol* 21:15–19.

Newman EA (2003) New roles for astrocytes: regulation of synaptic transmission. *Trends Neurosci* 26:536–42.

Oberndorfer S, Piribauer M, Marosi C, *et al.* (2005) P450 enzyme inducing and non-enzyme inducing antiepileptics in glioblastoma patients treated with standard chemotherapy. *J Neurooncol* 72:255–60.

Ohgaki H (2009) Epidemiology of brain tumors. *Methods Mol Biol* 472:323–42.

Ohgaki H, Dessen P, Jourde B, *et al.* (2004) Genetic pathways to glioblastoma: a population-based study. *Cancer Res* 64:6892–9.

Peiffer J, Kleihues P (1999) Hans-Joachim Scherer (1906–1945), pioneer in glioma research. *Brain Pathol* 9:241–5.

Piepmeier J, Fried I, Makuch P (1993) Low-grade astrocytomas may arise from different astrocyte lineages. *Neurosurgery* 33:627–32.

Piepmeier J, Christopher S, Spencer D, *et al.* (1996) Variations in the natural history and survival of patients with supratentorial low-grade astrocytomas. *Neurosurgery* 38:872–8; discussion 878–9.

Pouratian N, Asthagiri A, Jagannathan J, *et al.* (2007) Surgery insight: the role of surgery in the management of low-grade gliomas. *Nat Clin Pract Neurol* 3:628–39.

Price SJ (2007) The role of advanced MR imaging in understanding brain tumor pathology. *Br J Neurosurg* 21:562–75.

Rajneesh KF, Binder DK (2009) Tumor-associated epilepsy. *Neurosurg Focus* 27:E4.

Recht LD, Lew R, Smith TW (1992) Suspected low-grade glioma: is deferring treatment safe? *Ann Neurol* 31:431–6.

Roessler K, Suchanek G, Breitschopf H, *et al.* (1995) Detection of tumor necrosis factor-alpha protein and messenger RNA in human glial brain tumors: comparison of immunohistochemistry with in situ hybridization using molecular probes. *J Neurosurg* 83:291–7.

Rogers LR, Morris HH, Lupica K (1993) Effect of cranial irradiation on seizure frequency in adults with low-grade astrocytoma and medically intractable epilepsy. *Neurology* 43:1599–601.

Sakatani S, Seto-Ohshima A, Shinohara Y, *et al.* (2008) Neural-activity-dependent release of S100B from astrocytes enhances kainate-induced gamma oscillations in vivo. *J Neurosci* 28:10 928–36.

Sander JW, Johnson AL, Shorvon SD (1990) National General Practice Study of Epilepsy: newly diagnosed epileptic seizures in a general population. *Lancet* 336:1267–71.

Schaller B (2005) Influences of brain tumor-associated pH changes and hypoxia on epileptogenesis. *Acta Neurol Scand* 111:75–83.

Schaller B, Ruegg SJ (2003) Brain tumor and seizures: pathophysiology and its implications for treatment revisited. *Epilepsia* 44:1223–32.

Schrottner O, Unger F, Eder HG, *et al.* (2002) Gamma-knife radiosurgery of mesiotemporal tumor epilepsy observations and long-term results. *Acta Neurochir* 84 (Suppl):49–55.

Schwartz TH, Bazil CW, Forgione M, *et al.* (2000) Do reactive post-resection "injury" spikes exist? *Epilepsia* 41:1463–8.

Semyanov A, Walker MC, Kullman DM (2003) GABA uptake regulates cortical excitability via cell type-specific tonic inhibition. *Nat Neurosci* 6:484–90.

Sirven JI, Wingerchuk DM, Drazkowski JF, *et al.* (2004) Seizure prophylaxis in patients with brain tumors: a meta-analysis. *Mayo Clin Proc* 79:1489–94.

Spencer DD, Spencer SS, Mattson RH, Williamson PD (1984) Intracerebral masses in patients with intractable partial epilepsy. *Neurology* 34:432–6.

Stellwagen D, Malenka RC (2006) Synaptic scaling mediated by glial TNF-alpha. *Nature* 440:1054–9.

Stewart L, Burdett S, Glioma Meta-Analysis Trialists Group (2002). Chemotherapy for high-grade glioma. *Cochrane Database Syst Rev* 3:CD003913.

Tanaka K, Watase K, Manabe T, *et al.* (1997) Epilepsy and exacerbation of brain injury in mice lacking the glutamate transporter GLT-1. *Science* 276:1699–702.

Tremont-Lukats IW, Ratilal BO, Armstrong T, *et al.* (2008) Antiepileptic drugs for preventing seizures in people with brain tumors. *Cochrane Database Syst Rev* (2):CD004424.

van Breemen MS, Wilms EB, Vecht CJ, *et al.* (2007) Epilepsy in patients with brain tumors: epidemiology, mechanisms, and management. *Lancet Neurol* 6:421–30.

van den Bent MJ, de Witte O, Ben Hassel M, *et al.* (2005). Long-term efficacy of early versus delayed radiotherapy for low-grade astrocytoma and oligodendroglioma in adults: the EORTC 22845 randomised trial. *Lancet* 366:985–90.

Vezzani A, Ravizza T, Balosso S, *et al.* (2008) Glia as a source of cytokines: implications for neuronal excitability and survival." *Epilepsia* 49(Suppl 2):24–32.

Vojtech Z, Vladyka V, Kalina M, *et al.* (2009) The use of radiosurgery for the treatment of mesial temporal lobe epilepsy and long-term results. *Epilepsia* 50:2061–71.

Wolf HK, Roos D, Blümcke I, *et al.* (1996) Perilesional neurochemical changes in focal epilepsies. *Acta Neuropathol* 91:376–84.

Wong M (2008) Mechanisms of epileptogenesis in tuberous sclerosis complex and related malformations of cortical development with abnormal glioneuronal proliferation. *Epilepsia* 49:8–21.

Yap KY, Chui WK, Chan A (2008) Drug interactions between chemotherapeutic regimens and antiepileptics. *Clin Ther* 30:1385–407.

Chapter 63

Ganglioglioma, dysembryoplastic neuroepithelial tumor, and related tumors

Thomas S. Jacques and William Harkness

Introduction

Tumors account for around 30% of cases of drug-resistant epilepsy in surgical series (reviewed in Thom *et al.* 2008). Most of these tumors are low-grade glioneuronal tumors; the two best described are dysembryoplastic neuroepithelial tumors (DNT) and ganglioglioma. Diagnosis of these tumors is important because they are potentially curable causes of drug-resistant epilepsy.

The majority of tumors that present with epilepsy comprise a group of tumors that include DNTs, ganglioglioma, gangliocytoma, and the more recently described angiocentric glioma. These tumors are the main focus of this chapter and their management is predominantly focused on seizure control rather than oncological concerns. However, as over 40% of patients with supratentorial tumors present with seizures, a much wider range of glial tumors may present with intractable epilepsy including pilocytic astrocytoma, diffuse and anaplastic astrocytoma, pleomorphic xanthoastrocytoma, and oligodendroglioma. Several of these tumors carry a much greater risk of tumor progression and so management involves not only seizure control but also the involvement of the multidisciplinary oncology team (Louis *et al.* 2007a).

Ganglioglioma and DNTs are the commonest tumors presenting with epilepsy, accounting for 40–50% and 10–20% of cases, respectively (Frater *et al.* 2000; Benifla *et al.* 2006; Bauer *et al.* 2007; Becker *et al.* 2007). However, there is variation in the reported figures and this is likely to be due to variations in diagnostic criteria, surgical practice, and local referral patterns. For example in our practice, DNT is more common than these figures suggest. We have avoided the term "hamartoma" in this context as it lacks specificity and has been used to describe a wide range of epilepsy-associated pathology including low-grade glioneuronal tumors, cortical tubers, and malformations.

In childhood, clinical presentation of epilepsy-associated tumors is often with drug-resistant partial seizures with or without secondary generalization. Patients should undergo a full presurgical evaluation but usually the magnetic resonance imaging (MRI) appearances of these lesions are characteristic. However, the true definitions of these tumors are histopathological (WHO Classification of tumors of the Central Nervous System) (Louis *et al.* 2007a).

Dysembryoplastic neuroepithelial tumor
Definition

Dysembryoplastic neuroepithelial tumor (DNT) is the archetype of epilepsy-associated tumors. It is a nodular cortical tumor presenting with intractable seizures in young patients. In its purest form it is defined by a characteristic histological feature, the "specific glioneuronal element." These tumors are considered Grade 1 in the WHO classification of central nervous system (CNS) tumors reflecting their benign clinical behavior (Daumas-Duport *et al.* 2007).

Epidemiology

An estimate for the age-specific incidence of DNT in children is 0.55 per million child–years and the tumor represents approximately 1% of brain tumors in childhood (O'Brien *et al.* 2007). Depending on definition, DNT can account for between 10% and 20% of tumors removed for control of seizures (Daumas-Duport *et al.* 2007).

Dysembryoplastic neuroepithelial tumor is predominantly a tumor of childhood and young adults. The first seizure is usually before the age of 20 years, although a diagnosis may not be made until later. Occasionally cases present with their first seizure as late as the fourth decade (Daumas-Duport *et al.* 2007).

Pathology

A typical DNT is cortical and has a nodular or multinodular architecture (Daumas-Duport *et al.* 2007; O'Brien *et al.* 2007). The main tumor cells resemble oligodendrocytes (uniform rounded cells with minimal cytoplasm) and are known as oligodendrocyte-like cells (OLCs) (Fig. 63.1A). The OLCs are

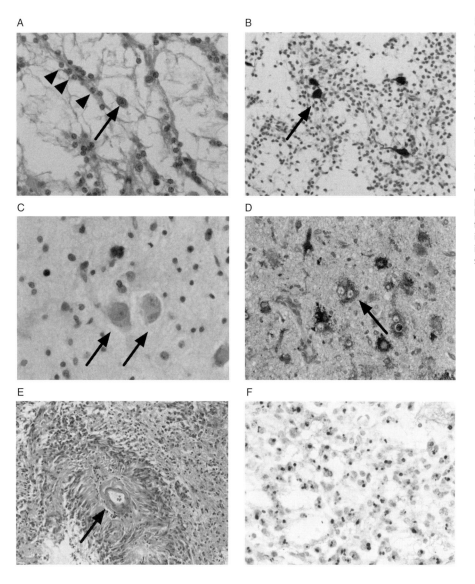

Fig. 63.1. Pathological features of dysembryoplastic neuroepithelial tumor (A and B), ganglioglioma (C and D), and angiocentric glioma (E and F). (A, B) The DNT consists of small round oligodendroglial-like cells arranged in columns separated by mucinous material (A: arrow heads). Scattered normally formed neurons are present in the tumor (A, B: arrows). (C, D) Dysplastic ganglion cells in a ganglioglioma (arrows), including some binucleate cells. The dysplastic cells show prominent staining for chromogranin (D). (E, F) Angiocentric glioma. The cells show a characteristic swirling pattern around blood vessels (E: arrow indicates the vessel lumen). They demonstrate evidence of ependymal differentiation, e.g., paranuclear dots of EMA staining (E). (A, C, E: hematoxylin and eosin; B: immunohistochemistry for the neuronal marker NeuN; DL: immunohistochemistry for chromogranin; F: immunohistochemistry for EMA.) See color plate section.

arranged in columns around axons. This columnar arrangement is the "specific glioneuronal element" that defines DNTs. The columns usually run perpendicular to the cortical surface and are separated by pools of matrix, which contains mature neurons. These neurons frequently sit within the pools of matrix without an apparent connection to the surrounding tissue and are therefore described as "floating neurons" (Fig. 63.1A, B).

The "simple form" of DNT consists entirely of this typical architectural pattern. However, other DNTs are more heterogeneous consisting of the typical nodules described above mixed with nodules of glial cells. These forms are called the "complex form" of DNT. The glial nodules may show a wide range of morphology containing astrocytic cells, oligodendroglial cells, or neuronal cells. Furthermore, the glial cells may show the changes typically associated with malignant tumors. Therefore small stereotactic biopsies can be particularly misleading.

Finally, some cortical tumors with a typical clinical picture of DNT lack the distinctive glioneuronal element or multinodular architecture. Some authors have suggested these tumors should be regarded as a "non-specific form" of DNT. This classification is controversial and clearly depends on a close correlation between the clinical and pathological findings.

The best chance to obtain a specific pathological diagnosis is with a complete resection with all the tissue sent to the pathologist. On a small resection sample or a stereotactic biopsy, the typical architectural features may be obscured and the differential diagnosis can be wide, including other tumors that contain uniform rounded cells (particularly oligondendroglioma but also pilocytic astrocytoma, neurocytoma, and ependymoma) and other glioneuronal tumors (ganglioglioma, papillary glioneuronal tumor) (Table 63.1).

Table 63.1. Comparison of the pathological features of DNT and ganglioglioma

Feature	DNT	Ganglioglioma
Macroscopy	Nodular or multinodular cortical tumor	Frequently cystic with mural nodule
Neuronal component	Floating neurons (normal appearing neurons floating in matrix)	Dysplastic neurons (neurons with abnormal cytoarchitectural features)
Glial component	Oligodendrocyte-like cells	Very variable but usually astrocytic
Calcification	Frequent	Frequent
Rosenthal fibers	Unusual	Frequent
Eosinophilic granular bodies	Unusual	Frequent
Perivascular lymphocytes	Unusual	Frequent

Associated pathology

Architectural changes in the cortex around a DNT are common and are often described as cortical dysplasia (Raymond *et al.* 1994; Sakuta *et al.* 2005; Takahashi *et al.*, 2005; Daumas-Duport *et al.* 2007). However, a distinction should be made between these architectural changes (often equivalent to type 1 focal cortical dysplasia [FCD] or mild cortical dysplasia [MCD]) and the more dramatic changes seen in type 2 FCD, which is rare in association with DNT. FCD associated with tumors been reclassified as FCD Type IIIb (Blümcke *et al.* 2010). In our experience, the architectural changes are usually rather subtle. Occasionally DNTs may also occur as a dual pathology with hippocampal sclerosis (Salanova *et al.* 2004).

Clinical features

Presentation is usually with seizures. Typically, the patients do not have focal neurological deficits. However, in rare cases, there may be a congenital, non-progressive deficit (Daumas-Duport *et al.* 2007; O'Brien *et al.* 2007). Most tumors do not show clinical or radiological features to suggest mass effect or peritumoral edema although in rare cases hemorrhage or ischemic change may occur which may be associated with mass effect (e.g., Thom *et al.* 1999). There are a very small number of case reports of malignant progression in DNT (Hammond *et al.* 2000; Nakatsuka *et al.* 2000; Rushing *et al.* 2003). However, some of these reported cases are not entirely straightforward and malignancy in DNT should be regarded as exceptional. As a general rule, tumor progression does not occur, even when surgical resection is incomplete.

In most cases, the tumors are sporadic but cases have been described in neurofibromatosis type 1 and XYY syndrome and in the latter, the tumor was multifocal (Lellouch-Tubiana *et al.* 1995; Krossnes *et al.* 2005).

Epilepsy

Usually DNTs present with partial seizures which may or may not show secondary generalization. The semiology of the seizures is dependent on the location of the lesion, the most common site being the mesial temporal cortex. Very rarely asymptomatic cases may be diagnosed as incidental findings or present due to hemorrhage (Thom *et al.* 1999). The epilepsy is usually resistant to antiepileptic drugs (AEDs). The pathological substrate for the seizures is not clear. Some studies based on ictal electrophysiological recordings and supported by ictal single photon emission computed tomography (SPECT) suggest that the source of seizures is the perilesional cortex, e.g., the surrounding cortical dysplasia (Kameyama *et al.* 2001).

Most studies of surgical resection for DNT report good control of seizures in the short term with many series reporting seizure freedom (Engel Class 1) in excess of 80% (Raymond *et al.* 1994; Kameyama *et al.* 2001; Nolan *et al.* 2004; Takahashi *et al.* 2005; Chan *et al.* 2006; Bilginer *et al.* 2009). However, this figure falls with time (Nolan *et al.* 2004; Chan *et al.* 2006), for example one study reported 85% Class 1 (Engel) at 1 year but this fell to 62% with prolonged follow-up (Nolan *et al.* 2004). Proposed risk factors for recurrent seizures after surgery include partial resection, long preoperative history of seizures, and adjacent cortical dysplasia (Daumas-Duport *et al.* 2007).

The tumors are diagnosed most frequently in the temporal lobe. However, their propensity for diagnosis in the temporal lobe may be due to likelihood of seizures arising from lesions in this area of the brain and the geographical association with the limbic system.

Diagnosis

The most important investigation in the preoperative diagnosis of DNT is a thin-slice MRI (Ostertun *et al.* 1996; Urbach 2008) (Fig. 63.2). These tumors are intracortical lesions that typically lack significant mass effect or peritumoral edema (but see comment under "Clinical features"). The tumors are hypointense on T1-weighted sequences and hyperintense on T2-weighted sequences. They may show multiple rings of enhancement. There may be a "soap bubble" texture on T2-weighted images and/or a "stripy" texture on T1-weighted images. On fluid-attenuated inversion recovery (FLAIR) sequences, there may be a ring of high signal around the periphery (FLAIR ring sign). Calcification of the tumor and scalloping of the overlying calvaric bone is common but may be seen in any slowly growing cortical lesion. The lesions usually encompass the thickness of the gyrus and can occasionally produce macrogyri. Evidence of tumor enlargement may occur in the presence of ischemic change or hemorrhage.

443

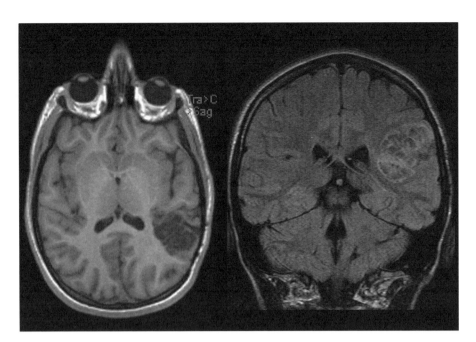

Fig. 63.2. A large left temporoparietal lobe DNT. The MR images show a lobulated peripherally based lesion with "soap bubble" internal structure and hyperintense rim on FLAIR images. (Images courtesy of Dr. Roxana Gunny, Great Ormond Street Hospital for Children, London.)

The differential diagnosis includes other low-grade epilepsy-associated tumors (e.g., ganglioglioma), cortical dysplasia, and diffuse gliomas. The most important differential diagnosis in terms of outcome is diffuse glioma. Features that favor DNT over glioma include lack of mass effect, lack of peritumoral edema, and cortical localization. The presence of the FLAIR ring sign or signal inhomogeneity are also useful indicators of a DNT. In practice, unequivocal differentiation from other low-grade epilepsy-associated tumors (especially ganglioglioma) is often not possible.

The diagnosis of DNT should be considered if there are the following features:

(1) Partial seizures (with or without generalization) beginning before the age of 20 years
(2) No progressive deficit
(3) A cortical lesion
(4) No significant mass effect and no peritumoral edema.

Management

The primary goal of management in DNT is seizure control and secondarily confirmation of the radiological diagnosis. Control of tumor growth and progression are minor considerations in most cases.

Surgical resection is the mainstay of treatment. Conservative treatment can be considered if seizure control, neurological development, and treatment side effects are acceptable. However, this should be weighed against the option of a potentially curative surgical option which also affords definitive diagnosis. There is also evidence to suggest that freedom from seizures following surgical resection is higher in those patients with a shorter history of seizures and this may be a further argument for early surgery (e.g., Aronica *et al.* 2001). As with all epilepsy

surgery, the decision to offer surgery or not to offer surgery should be made in the context of a multidisciplinary specialist referral service.

The main surgical options are resection with or without extension to include the adjacent dysplastic cortex. Biopsy is not recommended because, as discussed above, it presents significant diagnostic problems and offers little prospect of therapeutic benefit. On theoretical grounds, it is reasonable to suspect resection of adjacent dysplastic cortex would improve seizure freedom. Indeed, the evidence from SPECT and electrocorticography (ECoG) support a role for this dysplastic tissue in epileptogenesis (Kameyama *et al.* 2001). However, studies based on either tailored, local lesionectomy or wider excisions both produce good outcomes and direct comparisons are not available. Although in the UK, the Children's Cancer and Leukaemia Group have recommended extended resection for DNT, the arguments for this are rather theoretical, based on the epileptogenecity of the surrounding cortex (O'Brien *et al.* 2007). The evidence to support one or other approach is relatively weak. In one small series, the presence of cortical dysplasia predicted recurrent seizures (Sakuta *et al.* 2005) and in another, two recurrences were associated with incomplete resection, in one incomplete resection of the DNT and in one case of the cortical dysplasia (Chan *et al.* 2006). However, other studies have not shown a clear effect of surgical approach on outcome (Clusmann *et al.* 2002, 2004). It is notable, however, that many of these studies included a mix of pathology, not just DNTs. Given the good seizure outcome for DNT in all surgical series irrespective of surgical approach and the lack of clear evidence of an advantage of wide excision, the decision as to the extent of surgery may be more influenced by the effect of removing adjacent potentially eloquent cortex.

Ganglioglioma and gangliocytoma

Definition

Ganglioglioma and gangliocytoma are both tumors defined pathologically by the presence of dysplastic ganglion cells (Blümcke and Wiestler 2002; Becker *et al.* 2007; Louis *et al.* 2008). Dysplastic ganglion cells are mature neurons that are part of the lesion and show cytological or architecture abnormalities. In addition, ganglioglioma but not gangliocytoma contains neoplastic glial cells.

Gangliocytoma is always a low-grade tumor (WHO Grade 1) with a benign course. Most gangliogliomas are also Grade 1 tumors but a small percentage (<5%) show malignancy in the glial component and are designated anaplastic ganglioglioma (WHO Grade 3). A three-tier system with a Grade 2 tumor has been used but diagnostic criteria have not been agreed in the current WHO classification (Becker *et al.* 2007).

The lesions discussed here should be distinguished from the dysplastic gangliocytoma of the cerebellum (Lhermitte–Duclos syndrome) and desmoplastic infantile ganglioglioma.

Epidemiology

Ganglioglioma and gangliocytoma account for slightly more than 1% of all brain tumors (Becker *et al.* 2007). Ganglioglioma accounts for up to 50% of all tumors in patients undergoing surgery for control of epilepsy and is the commonest tumor associated with chronic epilepsy. Gangliocytoma is much less common in epilepsy practice. Both tumors can occur at any age but mostly present in late childhood, adolescence, or early adult life. Gangliocytoma tends to present later than ganglioglioma. There is no clear gender predisposition.

Pathology

The defining feature of both tumors is the presence of dysplastic ganglion cells (Blümcke and Wiestler 2002; Becker *et al.* 2007; Louis *et al.* 2008) (Fig. 63.1C, D; Table 63.1). These are mature neurons showing abnormal architectural or cytological differentiation. Features of dysplastic ganglion cells include increased cell size, abnormal neuronal clusters, abnormal neuronal architecture, and neurons containing more than one nucleus.

In ganglioglioma, in addition there is a neoplastic glial cell component, which commonly resembles a low-grade astrocytoma but can show a diverse range of morphology. It is this glial component that can proliferate and in the higher-grade tumors shows malignant transformation.

A number of additional histological features are very common in ganglioglioma including evidence of inflammation (perivascular cuffs of lymphocytes), glial inclusions (eosinophilic granular bodies [EGB] and Rosenthal fibers), and calcification.

The diagnosis of ganglioglioma depends on the identification of unequivocal dysplastic ganglion cells and this may be affected by sampling artifact. The presence of parenchymal staining for the endothelial marker CD34 has been suggested as a useful adjunct to diagnosis and is present in over 80% of gangliogliomas but is not entirely specific (Blümcke *et al.* 1999; Blümcke and Wiestler 2002). Immunostaining for neuronal markers may highlight the abnormal neuronal component. In particular, staining for chromogrannin may show dense granular staining around the cell bodies of dysplastic ganglion, a pattern not seen in normal cortical neurons (Hirose *et al.* 1997) (Fig. 63.1D).

Associated pathology

Architectural changes in the cortex around ganglioglioma can occur (cortical dysplasia) and the tumor may occur as a dual pathology with hippocampal sclerosis (Prayson and Frater 2003; Eriksson *et al.* 2005; Benifla *et al.* 2006).

Clinical features

Ganglioglioma and gangliocytoma may arise anywhere within the neuraxis. tumors in the cerebral cortex present most commonly with epilepsy and the temporal lobe is most commonly affected (Blümcke and Wiestler 2002). Presentation with features of a focal neurological deficit or mass effect is less common with cortical lesions than with lesions in the spinal cord or brainstem or with high-grade lesions.

Most gangliogliomas occur as sporadic isolated tumors. However, there is an association between ganglioglioma and a range of congenital malformations (e.g., partial agenesis of the corpus callosum, orofaciodigital synotosis). Ganglioglioma have been described in Down syndrome, Turcot syndrome, neurofibromatosis type 1 and type 2, fragile X syndrome, and Peutz–Jegher syndrome (reviewed in Louis *et al.* 2008).

Epilepsy

Ganglioglioma usually presents with partial seizures which may or may not show secondary generalization and are refractory to AEDs (Blümcke and Wiestler 2002). The semiology of the seizures is dependent on the location of the lesion. The most common site is the temporal cortex.

Most studies of surgical resection for ganglioglioma report good control of seizures (Morris *et al.* 1998; Aronica *et al.* 2001; Blümcke and Wiestler 2002; Benifla *et al.* 2006). In several studies, in excess of 80% of patients achieve seizure freedom (Engel Class 1), and many of the remainder show benefit from the surgery (Blümcke and Wiestler 2002; Benifla *et al.* 2006). There is reduction in seizure freedom with prolonged follow-up in some studies (Morris *et al.* 1998).

Diagnosis

The most important preoperative investigation is MRI (Urbach 2008) (Fig. 63.3). The tumor is usually a well-circumscribed mass, which is hypointense on T1-weighted images and hyperintense on T2-weighted images. There is frequently a cyst and an enhancing nodule. However, enhancement is not always present. Scalloping of the overlying calvaric bone and calcification of the tumor are common. The differential diagnosis includes FCD (when there is no enhancement or a cyst), DNT, and diffuse glioma.

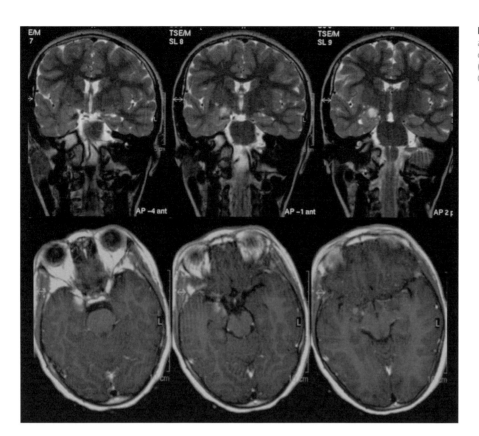

Fig. 63.3. A ganglioglioma in the right amygdala and inferior basal ganglia showing a cyst, calcifcation, and peripheral nodular enhancement. (Images courtesy of Dr. Roxana Gunny, Great Ormond Street Hospital for Children, London.)

Management

The goals of management are seizure control, confirmation of the radiological diagnosis, and control of tumor growth and progression. Optimal treatment of epilepsy-associated ganglioglioma involves complete surgical resection of the tumor. Complete resection, a long history of epilepsy, and low tumor grade are associated with the lowest recurrence rates (Lang *et al.* 1993; Luyken *et al.* 2004; Becker *et al.* 2007). Recurrence-free survival rates for ganglioglioma following surgical resection are in excess of 94% (Becker *et al.* 2007). Complete resection is not essential for seizure control but offers the best chance of achieving seizure freedom. While a conservative approach can be considered if the radiological diagnosis is certain, this decision must be taken in the context of a potential curative surgical approach that would prevent tumor progression. Limited biopsies (e.g., stereotactic biopsies) are sometimes undertaken but carry a significant risk of misdiagnosis or misgrading by the pathologist and do not offer tumor control or the best chance for seizure control. Adjuvant therapy has no established role for the treatment of low-grade ganglioglioma but is often offered to patients with anaplastic ganglioglioma. Due to the rarity of anaplastic ganglioglioma, there are few data to indicate the optimal management of these tumors.

Angiocentric glioma

Definition

Angiocentric glioma is a low-grade cortical tumor associated with epilepsy (Burger *et al.* 2007). It is defined on pathological grounds and is characterized by monomorphic bipolar glial cells with a distinctive arrangement around cortical blood vessels. Some of the features of the tumor indicate that the cells are undergoing ependymal differentiation. The alternative names angiocentric neuroepithelial tumor and monomorphous angiocentric glioma have been used in the past for this tumor. It is a low-grade tumor and designated Grade 1 in the WHO classification (Burger *et al.* 2007).

Epidemiology

The incidence of this tumor is unclear as fewer than 30 cases have been described (Lellouch-Tubiana *et al.* 2005; Wang *et al.* 2005; Louis *et al.* 2007b; Majores *et al.* 2007). Almost any age can be affected but it most commonly presents in adolescence or early adulthood. There is no gender predisposition.

Pathology (Figure 63.1D and 63.1E)

The tumors are composed of uniform spindled (bipolar) glial cells arranged in a rather distinctive pattern around blood vessels and aggregated under the pial surface in perpendicular structures (Burger *et al.* 2007) (Fig. 63.1E, F). There are regions of solid tumor and the tumor may trap host cortical neurons. Histological features of malignancy are unusual. Immunohistochemical studies and electron microscopy have shown evidence of ependymal differentiation, e.g., paranuclear dot staining with epithelial membrane antigen.

Clinical features and epilepsy

Presentation is typically with chronic seizures and like the other low-grade epilepsy-associated tumors are most likely to present with drug-resistant partial seizures, which may generalize. The tumors are most frequent in the frontal and temporal lobes. There is often a long history of seizures (mean 7.5 years). Within the limited literature, most patients achieve Engel Class 1 or 2 after surgical resection. The tumors usually behave in a benign manner with only one recurrent anaplastic tumor described (Wang *et al.* 2005).

Diagnosis

As with the other low-grade epilepsy-associated tumors, MRI is the key preoperative investigation. The tumor is intracortical and may extend to the white matter. It is typically well demarcated and solid. It is hyperintense on T2 weighted and FLAIR images and may show a stalk of hyperintensity running towards the ventricle. One case presenting as hippocampal atrophy has been described. Calcification is unusual. The differential diagnosis includes low-grade glioneuronal tumors (DNT and ganglioglioma), FCD, and diffuse glioma.

Management

There is a limited literature to inform the management of these tumors. Given the generally benign clinical course and good seizure control after surgery, complete surgical resection would usually be advocated. This has the advantage of good seizure control, tissue diagnosis, and prevention of recurrence.

References

Aronica E, Leenstra S, Van Veelen CW, *et al.* (2001) Glioneuronal tumors and medically intractable epilepsy: a clinical study with long-term follow-up of seizure outcome after surgery. *Epilepsy Res* **43**:179–91.

Bauer R, Dobesberger J, Unterhofer C, *et al.* (2007) Outcome of adult patients with temporal lobe tumors and medically refractory focal epilepsy. *Acta Neurochirurg* **149**:1211–16; discussion 1216–17.

Becker AJ, Wiestler OD, Figarella-Branger D, Blümcke I (2007) Ganglioglioma and gangliocytoma. In: Louis DN, Ohgaki H, Wiestler OD, Cavenee WK (eds.) *WHO Classification of Tumors of the Central Nervous System*. Lyon: International Agency for Reseach on Cancer (IARC).

Benifla M, Otsubo H, Ochi A, *et al.* (2006) Temporal lobe surgery for intractable epilepsy in children: an analysis of outcomes in 126 children. *Neurosurgery* **59**:1203–13; discussion 1213–14.

Bilginer B, Yalnizoglu D, Soylemezoglu F, *et al.* (2009) Surgery for epilepsy in children with dysembryoplastic neuroepithelial tumor: clinical spectrum, seizure outcome, neuroradiology, and pathology. *Childs Nerv Syst* **25**:485–91.

Blümcke I, Wiestler O (2002) Gangliogliomas: an intriguing tumor entity associated with focal epilepsies. *J Neuropathol Exp Neurol* **61**:575–84.

Blümcke I, Giencke K, Wardelmann E, *et al.* (1999) The CD34 epitope is expressed in neoplastic and malformative lesions associated with chronic, focal epilepsies. *Acta Neuropathol* **97**:481–90.

Blümcke I, Thom M, Aronica E, *et al.* (2010) The clinicopathologic spectrum of focal cortical dysplasias: a censusus classification proposed by an ad hoc Task Force of the ILAE Diagnostic Methods Commission. *Epilepsia* in press.

Burger PC, Jouvet A, Preusser M, *et al.* (2007) Angiocentric glioma. In: Louis DN, Ohgaki H, Wiestler OD, Cavenee WK (eds.) *WHO Classification of Tumors of the Central Nervous System*. Lyon: International Agency for Reseach on Cancer (IARC).

Chan CH, Bittar RG, Davis GA, *et al.* (2006) Long-term seizure outcome following surgery for dysembryoplastic neuroepithelial tumor. *J Neurosurg* **104**:62–9.

Clusmann H, Kral T, Fackeldey E, *et al.* (2004) Lesional mesial temporal lobe epilepsy and limited resections: prognostic factors and outcome. *J Neurol Neurosurg Psychiatry* **75**:1589–96.

Clusmann H, Schramm J, Kral T, *et al.* (2002) Prognostic factors and outcome after different types of resection for temporal lobe epilepsy. *J Neurosurg* **97**:1131–41.

Daumas-Duport C, Pietsch T, Hawkins C, Shankar SK (2007) Dysembryoplastic neuroepithelial tumor. In: Louis DN, Ohgaki H, Wiestler OD, Cavenee WK (eds.) *WHO Classification of Tumors of the Central Nervous System*. Lyon: International Agency for Reseach on Cancer (IARC).

Eriksson SH, Nordborg C, Rydenhag B, Malmgren K (2005) Parenchymal lesions in pharmacoresistant temporal lobe epilepsy: dual and multiple pathology. *Acta Neurol Scand* **112**:151–6.

Frater JL, Prayson RA, Morris HH, Bingaman WE (2000) Surgical pathologic findings of extratemporal-based intractable epilepsy: a study of 133 consecutive resections. *Arch Pathol Lab Med* **124**:545–9.

Hammond RR, Duggal N, Woulfe JM, Girvin JP (2000) Malignant transformation of a dysembryoplastic neuroepithelial tumor: case report. *J Neurosurg* **92**:722–5.

Hirose T, Scheithauer BW, Lopes MB, *et al.* (1997) Ganglioglioma: an ultrastructural and immunohistochemical study. *Cancer* **79**:989–1003.

Kameyama S, Fukuda M, Tomikawa M, *et al.* (2001) Surgical strategy and outcomes for epileptic patients with focal cortical dysplasia or dysembryoplastic neuroepithelial tumor. *Epilepsia* **42**(Suppl 6):37–41.

Krossnes BK, Wester K, Moen G, Mørk SJ (2005) Multifocal dysembryoplastic neuroepithelial tumor in a male with the XYY syndrome. *Neuropathol Appl Neurobiol* **31**:556–60.

Lang FF, Epstein FJ, Ransohoff J, *et al.* (1993) Central nervous system gangliogliomas. II. Clinical outcome. *J Neurosurg* **79**:867–73.

Lellouch-Tubiana A, Boddaert N, Bourgeois M, *et al.* (2005) Angiocentric neuroepithelial tumor (ANET): a new epilepsy-related clinicopathological entity with distinctive MRI. *Brain Pathol* **15**:281–6.

Lellouch-Tubiana A, Bourgeois M, Vekemans M, Robain O (1995)

Dysembryoplastic neuroepithelial tumors in two children with neurofibromatosis type 1. *Acta Neuropathol* **90**:319–22.

Louis DN, Ohgaki H, Wiestler OD, Cavenee WK (eds.) (2007a) *WHO Classification of Tumors of the Central Nervous System.* Lyon: International Agency for Research on Cancer (IARC).

Louis DN, Ohgaki H, Wiestler OD, *et al.* (2007b) The 2007 WHO classification of tumors of the central nervous system. *Acta Neuropathol* **114**:97–109.

Louis DN, Reifenberger G, Bart DJ, Ellison DW (2008) Tumors: Introduction and neuroepithelial tumors. In: Love S, Louis DN, Ellison DW (eds.) *Greenfield's Neuropathology*, 8th edn. London: Hodder Arnold.

Luyken C, Blümcke I, Fimmers R, *et al.* (2004) Supratentorial gangliogliomas: histopathologic grading and tumor recurrence in 184 patients with a median follow-up of 8 years. *Cancer* **101**:146–55.

Majores M, Niehusmann P, Von Lehe M, Blümcke I, Urbach H (2007) Angiocentric neuroepithelial tumor mimicking Ammon's horn sclerosis: case report. *Clin Neuropathol* **26**:311–16.

Morris HH, Matkovic Z, Estes ML, *et al.* (1998) Ganglioglioma and intractable epilepsy: clinical and neurophysiologic features and predictors of outcome after surgery. *Epilepsia* **39**:307–13.

Nakatsuka M, Mizuno S, Kimura T, Hara K (2000) A case of an unclassified tumor closely resembling dysembryoplastic neuroepithelial tumor with rapid growth. *Brain Tumor Pathol* **17**:41–5.

Nolan MA, Sakuta R, Chuang N, *et al.* (2004) Dysembryoplastic neuroepithelial tumors in childhood: long-term outcome and prognostic features. *Neurology* **62**:2270–6.

O'Brien DF, Farrell M, Delanty N, *et al.* (2007) The Children's Cancer and Leukaemia Group guidelines for the diagnosis and management of dysembryoplastic neuroepithelial tumors. *Br J Neurosurg*, **21**:539–49.

Ostertun B, Wolf HK, Campos MG, *et al.* (1996) Dysembryoplastic neuroepithelial tumors: MR and CT evaluation. *AJNR Am J Neuroradiol* **17**:419–30.

Prayson RA, Frater JL (2003) Cortical dysplasia in extratemporal lobe intractable epilepsy: a study of 52 cases. *Ann Diagn Pathol* **7**:139–46.

Raymond AA, Halpin SF, Alsanjari N, *et al.* (1994) Dysembryoplastic neuroepithelial tumor: features in 16 patients. *Brain* **117**:461–75.

Rushing E, Thompson LD, Mena H (2003) Malignant transformation of a dysembryoplastic neuroepithelial tumor after radiation and chemotherapy. *Ann Diagn Pathol* **7**:240–4.

Sakuta R, Otsubo H, Nolan MA, *et al.* (2005) Recurrent intractable seizures in children with cortical dysplasia adjacent to dysembryoplastic neuroepithelial tumor. *J Child Neurol* **20**:377–84.

Salanova V, Markand O, Worth R (2004) Temporal lobe epilepsy: analysis of patients with dual pathology. *Acta Neurol Scand* **109**:126–31.

Takahashi A, Hong SC, Seo DW, *et al.* (2005) Frequent association of cortical dysplasia in dysembryoplastic neuroepithelial tumor treated by epilepsy surgery. *Surg Neurol* **64**:419–27.

Thom M, Gomez-Anson B, Revesz, T, *et al.* (1999) Spontaneous intralesional hemorrhage in dysembryoplastic neuroepithelial tumors: a series of five cases. *J Neurol Neurosurg Psychiatry* **67**:97–101.

Thom M, Sisodiya S, Najm I (2008) Neuropathology of epilepsy. In: Love S, Louis DN, Ellison DW (eds.) *Greenfield's Neuropathology*, 8th edn. London: Hodder Arnold, pp. 833–88.

Urbach H (2008) MRI of long-term epilepsy-associated tumors. *Semin Ultrasound CT MR* **29**:40–6.

Wang M, Tihan T, Rojiani AM, *et al.* (2005) Monomorphous angiocentric glioma: a distinctive epileptogenic neoplasm with features of infiltrating astrocytoma and ependymoma. *J Neuropathol Exp Neurol* **64**:875–81.

Chapter 64

Hypothalamic hamartoma and gelastic epilepsy

John F. Kerrigan

The causal disease

Definition and epidemiology

Hypothalamic hamartomas (HH) are an uncommon human pathology resulting in a distinctive and often severe epilepsy syndrome, usually including gelastic (laughing) seizures. Two clinicoradiological subtypes are recognized. The first is the pedunculated or parahypothalamic HH subtype, associated with central precocious puberty (CPP), usually without neurological symptoms. The second is the sessile or intrahypothalamic subtype, which results in refractory epilepsy and associated neurobehavioral comorbidity. Brandberg and colleagues have reported that 1 in 200 000 children and adolescents in Sweden have been diagnosed with HH in association with epilepsy (Brandberg *et al.* 2004). It may be slightly more common in males. There are no recognized differences in incidence between different regions or ethnic groups. Unless otherwise indicated, this chapter will focus on HH associated with epilepsy.

Pathology, physiology, and clinical features of the disease

By definition, hamartomas consist of normal (non-neoplastic) appearing cells with disorganized three-dimensional relationships. Hypothalamic hamartomas are congenital mass lesions, and are sometimes referred to as tumors on this basis, but their size does not change relative to the brain, and they do not appear to undergo malignant transformation (Turjman *et al.* 1996).

Lesions in HH consist of intermixed well-differentiated neurons and glia. Most HH neurons are small (8–12 μm maximal diameter), comprising approximately 90% of the total neuronal population (Coons *et al.* 2007). Small HH neurons appear to have an interneuron phenotype, with relatively simple monopolar or bipolar morphology, and expression of the synthetic enzyme for γ-aminobutyric acid (GABA). These cells also show intrinsic pacemaker-like firing activity that is independent of synaptic input (Wu *et al.* 2005). Large HH neurons (>20 μm maximal diameter) make up approximately 10% of the neuronal population and are more likely to be excitatory projection-type neurons. Large HH neurons have the interesting property of depolarizing (firing) to $GABA_A$-receptor agonist administration (Kim *et al.* 2008; Wu *et al.* 2008). The microarchitecture of HH tissue is characterized by clusters or nodules of small HH neurons, with or without larger HH neurons. Although they are highly variable in size and abundance, these neuronal nodules are a universal feature of HH pathology, and may prove to be the "functional unit" responsible for the intrinsic epileptogenesis of HH tissue (Coons *et al.* 2007; Fenoglio *et al.* 2007).

The gross anatomy of HH lesions determines the nature of their clinical symptoms. Those HH lesions that are located more anteriorly within the hypothalamus, possessing a base of attachment to the tuber cinereum or infundibulum, are associated with CPP, while lesions attaching more posteriorly, typically in the region of the mammillary bodies, are more likely to be associated with epilepsy and comorbid neurological features. Larger lesions, with a broader base of attachment including both regions, are more likely to have both epilepsy and CPP (Freeman *et al.* 2004). Approximately 40% of HH patients with epilepsy have a history of CPP, although seizures are usually the presenting symptom. On the basis of physical proximity and limited indirect evidence, HH lesions associated with epilepsy may make their functional connection with the brain via the circuitry of the limbic system (locally, the columns of the fornix, mammillary bodies, and mammillothalamic tracts) but the specific nature of this connection remains unknown.

Epilepsy in the disease

Frequency of epilepsy

Completely asymptomatic HH lesions are uncommon. The onset of seizures is variable (as are all clinical features for HH), but in the majority of cases seizures begin during infancy or early childhood, with a progressively declining incidence of new cases during childhood, adolescence, and early adulthood. Given the often subtle or misleading nature of gelastic seizures,

The Causes of Epilepsy, eds. S. D. Shorvon, F. Andermann, and R. Guerrini. Published by Cambridge University Press. © Cambridge University Press 2011.

the correct clinical diagnosis of epilepsy associated with HH may be delayed months or even years from the onset of seizure activity. When questioned retrospectively, 85% of HH patients undergoing surgical treatment at our institution had a history of first seizure activity before 12 months of age, and 47% before 1 month of age. For over 90%, gelastic seizures are the first seizure type.

Types of epilepsy, specific characteristics, and natural history

Gelastic seizures

Gelastic seizures are brief, usually 5–20 s in duration, and frequent, typically with multiple events per day. Although characterized by laughter, they usually have a joyless character, and include a spectrum of behavioral features that can be suggestive of crying (in which case they are called dacrystic seizures). Most parents can readily identify the difference between gelastic seizures and true laughter in their children. Consciousness may be completely preserved, or may be impaired. However, this determination is difficult to make in young children. The frequency of gelastic seizures often decreases after the age of 10 years, and they may disappear entirely during adulthood. Gelastic seizures may be associated with pathology elsewhere in the brain, but are most strongly associated with HH.

Other seizure types

Unfortunately, most patients (80–100%) will acquire additional seizure types as they get older, commonly from 4 to 10 years of age (Berkovic et al. 1988; Mullati et al. 2003). Complex partial seizures that mimic temporal lobe epilepsy are most common, but seizures that suggest frontal lobe origin and secondarily generalized tonic–clonic seizures are also encountered. A gelastic component as the first ictal symptom may or may not be obvious.

The electroencephalogram (EEG) is usually normal or shows otherwise non-specific abnormalities during infancy. Interictal epileptiform abnormalities become more abundant as additional seizure types develop, most commonly revealing focal spike transients from the anterior to mid-temporal field, although focal spikes from any head region, including occipital, can be seen. For those HH lesions with unilateral attachment to the hypothalamus, interictal spikes are more commonly encountered ipsilateral to the lesion.

Ictal recordings with scalp electrodes during gelastic seizures may show *no change* in the EEG, or alternatively subtle and non-specific ictal changes such as a slight diffuse decrease in background amplitude, or a reduction in the frequency of interictal spikes. Complex partial seizures that mimic seizures of neocortical origin demonstrate simultaneous ictal patterns on scalp EEG, and may localize to temporal or frontal head regions. However, ictal recordings from scalp EEG electrodes must be interpreted with caution in HH patients, as these results are usually misleading with respect to localizing the site of seizure onset. False localization with video-EEG recordings from scalp electrodes has resulted in temporal or frontal lobe resection, with universally poor results (Cascino et al. 1993).

Generalized seizure types have also been widely reported in HH patients, including infantile spasms (Kerrigan et al. 2007). A review of published reports suggests that complex partial seizures occur in 50–60% of HH patients, tonic–clonic seizures in 40–60%, atypical absence in 40–50%, tonic seizures in 15–35%, and "drop attacks" in 30–50%. Freeman and colleagues have emphasized the occurrence of a generalized epilepsy phenotype in 12 of 20 patients undergoing HH resection, including patients with tonic seizures and generalized slow spike–wave abnormalities on EEG, consistent with Lennox–Gastaut syndrome (Freeman et al. 2003). Nevertheless, patients within this subgroup responded favorably to HH resection.

The EEG features in older children and adolescents with HH are diverse. A review by Tassinari and colleagues described interictal EEG findings for older children and adolescents with HH, with normal findings in 2%, generalized spike or spike–wave in 47%, multifocal independent spikes in 18%, and focal spikes (temporal > frontal) in 33% (Tassanari et al. 1997). (Our own experience with over 150 HH patients suggests that the true prevalence figures for generalized seizure types and generalized EEG abnormalities are somewhat lower.)

Secondary epileptogenesis

An additional issue contributing to the complexity of the natural history for patients with HH and epilepsy is the prospect of secondary epileptogenesis (SE), defined here as a process by which one seizure focus may cause the emergence of a second and perhaps ultimately independent seizure focus in a distant and previously normal brain region (Morrell 1985; Cibula and Gilmore 1997; Wilder 2001). Case reports of patients undergoing seizure recordings with intracranial EEG electrodes, including placement into the HH, have demonstrated that non-gelastic seizure types may arise from neocortical regions without involvement of the HH (Munari et al. 1995). Surgical treatment with HH resection may still be effective for these patients, however (Freeman et al. 2003). Up to 20% of HH patients undergoing surgical resection may experience the "running-down" phenomenon, in which seizures arising from neocortical regions may decrease in frequency and disappear over weeks or months following HH resection or disconnection (Freeman et al. 2003; Ng et al. 2006).

Regrettably, for some patients, the process of SE may have completely matured, so that the second, neocortical focus becomes completely independent of the HH, and seizures will persist even after successful HH removal. Clinical factors that differentiate patients with reversible SE from those with permanent SE have not yet been identified. This process occurs over time, so older patients are at higher risk for permanent SE, but the age at which this occurs appears to be highly variable. The basic cellular mechanisms responsible for SE are unknown (Dudek and Spitz 1997).

Principles of management

Treatment for epilepsy resulting from HH is based upon the following principles: (1) epilepsy associated with HH is a progressive disease for the majority of patients, with development of multiple seizure types, and coincident deterioration in cognition and behavior, (2) antiepilepsy drugs (AEDs) are unsuccessful in managing seizures associated with HH, (3) the HH is intrinsically epileptogenic, (4) eradication or complete disconnection of the HH is successful for controlling seizures, and may help ameliorate the comorbid problems with cognition and behavior, (5) on this basis, earlier surgical intervention is preferred, and (6) treatment choice is guided by the individual circumstances of the case, including the clinical course of the disease and an assessment of the size and attachment of the HH.

Classification and surgical anatomy

Several authors have proposed classification schemes for HH lesions, including Valdueza (Valdueza et al. 1994), Regis (Regis et al. 2004), and Delalande and Fohlen (Delalande and Fohlen 2003) (Fig. 64.1). Currently our preference is to use the Delalande and Fohlen classification, as the identified subtypes relate simply and directly to the surgical anatomy. The optimal surgical approach is determined primarily by the location of the base of attachment of the HH to the hypothalamus, as the following discussion will indicate (Polkey 2003; Feiz-Erfan et al. 2005).

Ventral surgical approach to hypothalamic hamartoma lesions

Type I lesions in the Delalande system are attached to the inferior (horizontal) surface of the hypothalamus. This type includes those HH lesions with a thin pedicle or stalk, often attached to the tuber cinereum, and associated with CPP only, but can also include HH lesions with a broader or more posterior base of attachment that are associated with epilepsy. These lesions are best resected or disconnected through a pterional approach or its modifications such as the orbitozygomatic or subfrontal approaches. Where total resection via a pterional approach is possible, seizure outcome is good (66% seizure-free with complete resection of the lesion) (Valdueza et al. 1994), but this approach is not suited to most HH cases, where a substantial component of

the HH has a vertical plane of attachment within the third ventricle (Delalande Types II–IV).

Dorsal surgical approach for hypothalamic hamartoma lesions

Delalande Type II lesions have a vertical plane of attachment within the third ventricle, and are best suited to a transcallosal interforniceal approach or transventricular endoscopic resection/disconnection. Delalande Types III and IV have both vertical and horizontal planes of attachment (both above and below the normal position of the floor of the third ventricle). The superior approaches noted above may be adequate, but management of some of these lesions may require a combined approach, with either simultaneous or staged resections from above and below.

Rosenfeld and colleagues in Melbourne, Australia were the first to utilize the transcallosal, anterior interforniceal (TAIF) approach to the third ventricle to resect HH lesions in patients with refractory epilepsy (Rosenfeld et al. 2004). This approach, utilizing microsurgical technique and intracranial guidance systems, creates excellent direct visualization of the HH and its attachment within the third ventricle. These authors have published a series of 29 consecutive patients undergoing HH resection via the TAIF approach (Harvey et al. 2003). Age at surgery ranged from 4 to 23 years (mean age 10 years). All patients had multiple seizure types, including gelastic seizures. Coexisting morbidities included a history of central precocious puberty in 13 (45%), intellectual disability in 21 (72%), and behavioral problems, most frequently rage and aggression, in 18 (62%).

Resection of at least 95% of the HH lesion was achieved in 18 patients (62%). Postoperative follow-up for a minimum of 12 months showed 15 patients (52%) that were completely seizure-free and seven patients (24%) with at least a 90% improvement in seizure frequency. Surgical resection was generally well tolerated. Small, unilateral ischemic strokes of the thalamus and internal capsule occurred in two cases (7%), both with complete recovery, and transient third cranial nerve injury was reported in one patient. The majority of patients (55%) developed mild, asymptomatic hypernatremia postoperatively, but there were no persistent disturbances in fluid or electrolyte homeostasis. Five patients (17%) required thyroid hormone replacement therapy following surgery. Impairment of short-term memory is a concern, as the TAIF procedure requires retraction of the columns of the fornix.

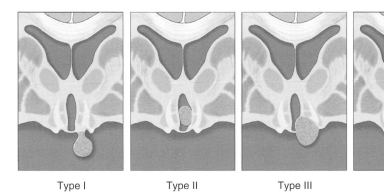

Type I   Type II   Type III   Type IV

© 2009, BNI

Fig. 64.1. Classification scheme of HH as proposed by Delalande and Fohlen (2003). Type I lesions are attached below the floor of the third ventricle, primarily in the horizontal plane, while Type II lesions attach to the wall of the hypothalamus with a vertical plane of attachment, above the floor of the third ventricle. Type III lesions attach both above and below the normal position of the floor of the third ventricle (either unilaterally or bilaterally), while Type IV lesions are defined as "giant" lesions. We have used a lesion volume of 10 cm^3 to demarcate Type IV lesions from Type III (Ng et al. 2006).

Transient memory disturbance was noted in 14 patients (48%) in the immediate postoperative period, but residual difficulties were reported by only four (14%). Attention and behavior were noted to improve in many of the patients in this series, but further details were not available (Harvey *et al.* 2003).

Similar results have been reported by Rekate and colleagues at the Barrow Neurological Institute in Phoenix (Ng *et al.* 2006). In this series of 26 consecutive patients undergoing TAIF, 54% were seizure-free following the procedure, which correlated with complete resection. The profile for surgical complications was also similar. Notably, transient short-term memory impairment was noted in 58% of the patients, but persisted in only two patients (8%). The impact of HH surgery on cognition and behavior requires further study.

Endoscopic resection and disconnection

Transcortical transventricular endoscopic resection and/or disconnection has also emerged as a treatment option for HH patients with refractory epilepsy (Akai *et al.* 2002). The Barrow group has reported a series of 37 consecutive HH patients treated with endoscopic resection/disconnection for treatment-resistant epilepsy (Ng *et al.* 2008). All patients had at least 1 year of follow-up. The mean age at the time of surgery was 11.8 years (range 0.7 to 55 years). All patients had a history of gelastic seizures at some point during their clinical course, and 29 (78%) had gelastic seizures at the time of surgery. Twenty-eight patients (76%) had Type II HH lesions by the Delalande classification.

Eighteen patients (49%) were completely seizure-free, while seizure frequency was reduced at least 90% in an additional eight patients (22%). Twelve patients were determined to have 100% of their HH lesions resected. Of these, eight (67%) were 100% seizure-free. As observed with the TAIF approach, most patients tolerated endoscopic resection well. However, the

endoscopic group had a significantly shorter postoperative hospital stay (mean 4.1 days) versus the previously noted transcallosal group (mean 7.7 days, $p < 0.001$). Only five patients (14%) experienced postoperative short-term memory loss, but this appeared to be a permanent residual problem in three (8%), comparable to the TAIF approach. Endocrine disturbance was not observed. However, 11 patients (30%) showed small unilateral thalamic infarcts on diffusion-weighted magnetic resonance imaging (MRI). These were asymptomatic in 9 of 11 cases, and the remaining two made a complete clinical recovery. These infarcts likely resulted from injury to small thalamic perforators.

Stereotactic radiosurgery

Gamma knife radiosurgery (GK) has also been investigated as an ablative or destructive therapy for HH lesions (Regis *et al.* 2000; Romanelli *et al.* 2008). This technique is non-invasive, and can deliver a "killing" dose to a small volume of tissue via a large number of independent trajectories, with little or no injury to surrounding brain. Limitations for its use in the hypothalamus include the need to avoid damage to the optic tracts, which are known to be relatively radiosensitive, and the large size and/or broad area of attachment of some HH lesions. There is also a significant time lag between treatment and therapeutic effect, up to 24 months, during which seizure frequency may temporarily increase for some patients.

Regis has described a series of 27 patients with intractable epilepsy and HH with at least 3 years of follow-up after GK therapy (Regis *et al.* 2006). The median radiosurgery dose to the 50% isodose margin was 17 Gy (range 13 to 26 Gy, mean 16.9 Gy). Of the 27 patients reported, 10 (37%) were completely seizure-free, and an additional six (22%) were substantially improved with only rare gelastic seizures. The GK technique has an excellent side-effect profile. Three patients

Table 64.1 Summary of HH treatment results by different techniques: transcallosal resection/disconnection (Harvey *et al.* 2003; Ng *et al.* 2006), endoscopic resection/disconnection (Ng *et al.* 2008), and gamma knife radiosurgery (Regis *et al.* 2006)

	Harvey *et al.* (2003)	Ng *et al.* (2006)	Ng *et al.* (2007)	Regis *et al.* (2006)
Treatment	Transcallosal	Transcallosal	Endoscopic	Gamma knife
Number of patients	29	26	37	27
Mean age at treatment	10.0 years	10.0 years	11.8 years	17.9 years
Mean lesion volume	NA	4.0 cm^3	1.0 cm^3	0.7 cm^3
Efficacy				
Percent seizure-free	52%	54%	49%	37%
Over 90% improvement	24%	35%	22%	22%
Cognitive function	"Majority improved"	65% "Better"	68% "Better"	33% "Dramatic improvement"
Short-term memory impairment				
Transient	48%	58%	14%	0%
Residual	14%	8%	8%	0%

Note:
NA, not available.

(11%) experienced transient poikilothermia, and none demonstrated evidence of residual complications following GK. The disadvantage of GK is the delayed onset of action for controlling seizures, and the more limited anatomical spectrum of HH lesions to which it is suited. Nevertheless, GK is a valuable treatment option for many patients with HH and epilepsy, and perhaps the preferred treatment modality for those with small lesions, who are clinically stable, and can tolerate the aforementioned delay in efficacy.

Table 64.1 compares HH treatment results following transcallosal and endoscopic resection and gamma knife radiosurgery. Differences in the patient population for each report are noted, however, such as HH lesion size, which limits direct comparison between techniques.

References

Akai T, Okamoto K, Iizuka H, Kakinuma H, Nojima T (2002) Treatments of hamartoma with neuroendoscopic surgery and stereotactic radiosurgery: a case report. *Minim Invas Neurosurg* **45**:235–9.

Berkovic SF, Andermann F, Melanson D, et al. (1988) Hypothalamic hamartomas and ictal laughter: evolution of a characteristic epileptic syndrome and diagnostic value of magnetic resonance imaging. *Ann Neurol* **23**:429–39.

Brandberg G, Raininko R, Eeg-Olofsson O (2004) Hypothalamic hamartoma with gelastic seizures in Swedish children and adolescents. *Eur J Pediatr Neurol* **6**:35–44.

Cascino GD, Andermann F, Berkovic S F, et al. (1993) Gelastic seizures and hypothalamic hamartomas: evaluation of patients undergoing chronic intracranial EEG monitoring and outcome of surgical treatment. *Neurology* **43**:747–50.

Cibula JE, Gilmore RL (1997) Secondary epileptogenesis in humans. *J Clin Neurophysiol* **14**:111–27.

Coons SW, Rekate HL, Prenger E C, et al. (2007) The histopathology of hypothalamic hamartomas: study of 57 cases. *J Neuropathol Exp Neurol* **66**:131–41.

Delalande O, Fohlen M (2003) Disconnecting surgical treatment of hypothalamic hamartoma in children and adults with refractory epilepsy and proposal of a new classification. *Neurol Med Chir (Tokyo)* **43**:61–8.

Dudek FE, Spitz M (1997) Hypothetical mechanisms for the cellular and neurophysiologic basis of secondary epileptogenesis: proposed role for synaptic reorganization. *J Clin Neurophysiol* **14**:90–101.

Feiz-Erfan I, Horn EM, Rekate IIL, et al. (2005) Surgical strategies to approach hypothalamic hamartomas causing gelastic seizures in the pediatric population: transventricular versus skull base approaches. *J Neurosurg (Pediatrics)* **103**:325–32.

Fenoglio KA, Wu J, Kim DY, et al. (2007) Hypothalamic hamartoma: basic mechanisms of intrinsic epileptogenesis. *Semin Ped Neurol* **14**:51–9.

Freeman JL, Harvey AS, Rosenfeld JV, et al. (2003) Generalized epilepsy in hypothalamic hamartoma: evolution and postoperative resolution. *Neurology* **60**:762–7.

Freeman JL, Coleman LT, Wellard RM, et al. (2004) MR imaging and spectroscopic study of epileptogenic hypothalamic hamartomas: analysis of 72 cases. *AJNR Am J Neuroradiol* **25**:450–62.

Harvey AS, Freeman JL, Berkovic SF, Rosenfeld JV (2003) Transcallosal resection of hypothalamic hamartomas in patients with intractable epilepsy. *Epilept Disord* **5**:257–65.

Kerrigan JF, Ng Y-T, Prenger E, et al. (2007) Hypothalamic hamartoma and infantile spasms. *Epilepsia* **48**:89–95.

Kim DY, Fenoglio KA, Simeone TA, et al. (2008) GABA$_A$ receptor-mediated activation of L-type calcium channels induces neuronal excitation in surgically resected human hypothalamic hamartomas. *Epilepsia* **49**:861–71.

Morrell F (1985) Secondary epileptogenesis in man. *Arch Neurol* **42**:318–35.

Mullati N, Selway R, Nashef L, et al. (2003) The clinical spectrum of epilepsy in children and adults with hypothalamic hamartoma. *Epilepsia* **44**:1310–19.

Munari C, Kahane P, Francione S, et al. (1995) Role of the hypothalamic hamartoma in the genesis of gelastic fits (a video-stereo-EEG study). *Electroencephalogr Clin Neurophysiol* **95**:154–60.

Ng Y-T, Rekate HL, Prenger EC, et al. (2006) Transcallosal resection of hypothalamic hamartoma for intractable epilepsy. *Epilepsia* **47**:1192–202.

Ng Y-T, Rekate HL, Prenger EC, et al. (2008) Endoscopic resection of hypothalamic hamartomas for refractory symptomatic epilepsy. *Neurology* **70**:1543–8.

Polkey CE (2003) Resective surgery for hypothalamic hamartoma. *Epilept Disord* **5**:281–6.

Regis J, Bartolomei F, de Toffol B, et al. (2000) Gamma knife surgery for epilepsy related to hypothalamic hamartomas. *Neurosurgery* **47**:1343–52.

Regis J, Hayashi M, Eupierre LP, et al. (2004) Gamma knife surgery for epilepsy related to hypothalamic hamartoma. *Acta Neurochir Suppl* **91**:33–50.

Regis J, Scavarda D, Tamura M, et al. (2006) Epilepsy related to hypothalamic hamartomas: surgical management with special reference to gamma knife surgery. *Childs Nerv Syst* **22**:881–95.

Romanelli P, Muacevic A, Striano S (2008) Radiosurgery for hypothalamic hamartomas. *Neurosurg Focus* **24**:e9 (1–7).

Rosenfeld JV, Freeman JL, Harvey AS (2004) Operative technique: the anterior transcallosal transeptal interforniceal approach to the third ventricle and resection of hypothalamic hamartomas. *J Clin Neurosci* **11**:738–44.

Turjman F, Xavier JL, Froment JC, et al. (1996) Late MR follow-up of hypothalamic hamartomas. *Childs Nerv Syst* **12**:63–8.

Valdueza JM, Cristante L, Dammann O, et al. (1994) Hypothalamic hamartomas: with special reference to gelastic epilepsy and surgery. *Neurosurgery* **34**:949–58.

Wilder BJ (2001) The mirror focus and secondary epileptogenesis. *Int Rev Neurobiol* **45**:435–46.

Wu J, Xu L, Kim DY, et al. (2005) Electrophysiological properties of human hypothalamic hamartomas. *Ann Neurol* **58**:371–82.

Wu J, DeChon J, Xue F, et al. (2008) GABA$_A$ receptor-mediated excitation in dissociated neurons from human hypothalamic hamartomas. *Exp Neurol* **213**:397–404.

453

Chapter

65

Meningioma

Sumeet Vadera and William Bingaman

Introduction

In adults, meningiomas are the second most frequent primary brain tumor after gliomas, with an incidence rate of 6 per 100 000. They are most commonly seen in the fourth to seventh decade of life and are four times more common in females than males (Claus *et al.* 2005).

The vast majority of meningiomas, at 90–95%, are slow-growing benign tumors that arise from the arachnoid cap cells of the arachnoid villi of the meninges; the remainder are classified as atypical or malignant. Meningiomas span the continuum from small, slow-growing, asymptomatic convexity lesions to large tumors that encase major blood vessels and other important structures along the skull base. Meningiomas can arise anywhere that dura is present, but are most commonly seen at the base of the skull, in parasellar regions, or along dural reflections such as the falx cerebri and tentorium cerebelli, and along venous sinuses. Patients commonly present with a solitary tumor except in certain genetic conditions such as neurofibromatosis type 2 in which there is a high incidence of multiple meningiomas (Claus *et al.* 2005).

Some evidence suggests that the development of meningiomas is a multifactorial process involving the upregulation and downregulation of various oncogenes and tumor suppressor genes (van Breemen *et al.* 2007). An increased risk has been noted with exposure to ionizing radiation, head trauma, or high doses of estrogen, such as during pregnancy or hormone replacement therapy, although this is very controversial (Claus *et al.* 2005).

This chapter will discuss the etiology, diagnosis, and principles of management of epilepsy in patients diagnosed with meningiomas. The authors will also present cases that demonstrate the broad spectrum of meningioma-related epileptogenesis and the challenges associated with their surgical management.

Epilepsy and meningiomas

As is the case with other intracranial tumors, seizures are often the presenting symptom associated with meningiomas (Lynam *et al.* 2007). The main predictive factor in the development of

epilepsy in the setting of a meningioma is the location of the tumor, with an increased incidence seen in patients with cortical lesions. Studies show an 80% increased seizure risk when in the parietal region, 74% in the temporal region, 62% in the frontal region, and no increased risk for seizures with meningiomas of the occipital region (Lynam *et al.* 2007). Sellar tumors rarely cause seizures unless they extend into the cerebral hemisphere.

There is a lack of information regarding the molecular, cellular, and pathophysiological mechanisms involved in tumor-related epilepsy (Gonzalez-Martinez and Najm 2008). Meningiomas and other slow-growing tumors are associated with epilepsy more often than rapidly growing tumors. The slow growth is thought to allow for local and remote changes required for epileptogenesis. There are a number of potential mechanisms that have been postulated to explain the association between intracranial tumors and seizures including peritumoral compression of the surrounding cortex causing local irritation, microscopic tumor invasion, and ischemic changes secondary to microvasculature occlusion (van Breemen *et al.* 2007).

Epilepsy can also occur after surgical resection of the meningioma. In this setting the tumor is no longer the primary concern, and the recurrent seizures that significantly impact the patient's life become the focus of care. When these seizures persist despite adequate trials of anticonvulsant therapy, surgery to localize and resect the epileptic cortex is often necessary. This cortex has usually been damaged by the tumor and/or its subsequent surgical removal. Successful treatment of the epilepsy revolves around identifying and removing the epileptogenic zone (EZ) while preserving function.

The diagnosis of epilepsy secondary to meningioma rests upon a detailed history and physical examination as well as radiographic evidence, most often magnetic resonance imaging (MRI) and computed tomographic (CT) imaging. On CT, these tumors are often well-demarcated, calcified, extra-axial lesions causing local mass effect. Bony erosion or invasion can be seen with skull-based meningiomas. Magnetic resonance imaging with and without gadolinium is the

The Causes of Epilepsy, eds. S. D. Shorvon, F. Andermann, and R. Guerrini. Published by Cambridge University Press. © Cambridge University Press 2011.

imaging study of choice because it allows an understanding of tumoral anatomy correlated to the underlying brain, usually shows the area of dural origin, and allows an understanding of the arterial and venous anatomy in relation to the tumor. A catheter angiogram or MR venogram (MRV) may be necessary for surgical planning to avoid injuring this surrounding vasculature (Kwan and Brodie 2000).

In the setting of medically resistant seizures, several other tests may be useful in helping to understand where the epilepsy is arising from in order to determine a surgical plan. Video-electroencephalography (video-EEG) will confirm the diagnosis of epilepsy and record the seizure semiology to help localize the cortical onset area. The EEG details will localize the seizure onset within a region of the brain, usually corresponding to the area involved with the tumor. When EEG information or semiology is obtained that is not in agreement (discordant) with the tumor location, further diagnostic testing should be performed including the use of invasive cortical EEG recordings to better define the EZ prior to removal. Additional testing can also be performed to better define the functional integrity of the cortical tissue involved. These include interictal positron emission tomography (PET), functional MRI (fMRI), intracarotid sodium amytal testing (Wada), single photon emission computed tomography (SPECT), and white matter tractography. Radionuclide PET scanning allows subjective quantification of the metabolism of the brain using a radioactively labeled glucose molecule. In regions of seizure onset, these areas appear as hypometabolic. Blood flow analysis by SPECT is done in both the interictal and ictal state and an area of regional blood flow increase during seizure onset corresponds to the site of seizure origin. Functional MRI and Wada testing are primarily used to identify eloquent cortical areas that may be involved in the planned cortical resection. After all these data are gathered, they are presented at a multidisciplinary conference and a hypothesis regarding the EZ and its relationship to the tumor or damaged cortex is formulated. The surgical aspects of removing the epileptogenic zone are then discussed and a final discussion with the patient takes place.

Principles of management

In terms of the medical management of epilepsy related to meningiomas, the choice of antiepileptic drugs (AED) depends on various factors including age, drug–drug interactions, and comorbid conditions. Lamotrigine, valproic acid, and topiramate are considered the first-line AEDs in these patients (van Breeman et al. 2007). Levetiracetam or gabapentin can be used as additional therapeutic agents as needed. Unfortunately even with double and triple agent therapy, pharmacoresistance is noted in a large number of cases. Medication related side effects also limit the overall efficacy of medical treatment alone (Lynam et al. 2007). Once medical intractability has been demonstrated or unacceptable side effects occur, surgical treatment should be considered and the patient referred to an experienced epilepsy center.

Meningiomas along the convexities are often readily accessible and so surgical resection is often indicated for treatment of the underlying neoplasm. In patients with preoperative seizures secondary to meningiomas, studies have shown postoperative seizure-free outcomes as high as 63.5% (Gonzalez-Martinez and Najm 2008). It was first noted by Wilder Penfield that surgical management of medically refractory epilepsy related to intracranial tumors had very good outcomes, and multiple subsequent studies have confirmed this finding (Penfield et al. 1940; Gonzalez-Martinez and Najm 2008). Other factors that effect postoperative seizure outcome include lesion location, preoperative EEG findings, and overall extent of tumor resection. Overall the majority of patients with seizures and a meningioma will become seizure-free with resection of the tumor. As the underlying cortex is typically not invaded or significantly affected by the tumor itself, cortical resection should be kept to a minimum during tumor removal to minimize the cortical damage postoperatively. When cortical tissue is involved and cortical resection is anticipated, intraoperative electrocorticography (ECoG) may be performed to define the interictal irritative zone (Engel and Pedley 2007). It remains controversial whether including this "irritated" tissue in the resection leads to better outcomes. Nonetheless, if the ECoG demonstrates continuous spiking, that tissue should be removed if possible.

It has been noted that approximately 20% of patients undergoing meningioma surgery will develop seizures after complete tumor resection even without a history of epilepsy prior to surgery. Factors noted to provoke new-onset postoperative epilepsy include extended amounts of intraoperative brain retraction, interruption of cortical arteries or veins, parietal meningiomas, and severe peritumoral edema (Gonzalez-Martinez and Najm 2008). Careful surgical technique during the initial tumor resection may help to prevent some of these cases, but when seizures occur or persist after surgery, and are not controlled by AEDs, the patient should be considered for further surgery to control the epilepsy.

The surgical decision-making process

Once the decision to perform surgery has been made, a hypothesis utilizing the information discussed earlier is completed and the risks and benefits are discussed with the patient. If the underlying meningioma is thought to be the cause of the epilepsy, the options are to remove the tumor with or without some surrounding cortical tissue as discussed in the preceding section. In patients who have had surgical resection of a meningioma previously and present with seizures, the main possibilities are that the surrounding damaged cortex is the cause of epilepsy or that there has been a recurrence of the tumor causing epilepsy. The preoperative imaging studies can likely differentiate between these two cases. If damaged cortex is believed to be the cause of epilepsy, then further cortical resection is required, but may be limited secondary to the location and functionality of surrounding cortex.

The following cases are useful to illustrate some of the points made earlier in this chapter.

Case 1

The patient is a 72-year-old right-handed male, who presents with a 6-month history of continuous jerking of the proximal right upper extremity. Symptoms began shortly after the patient underwent a craniotomy for the resection of a left parafalcine posterior frontal meningioma. This surgery was complicated by a postoperative sagittal sinus thrombosis and hemorrhagic venous infarct affecting the perirolandic cortex. Neurologic examination was consistent with this injury and the patient had hemiplegia initially that improved to a hemiparesis involving the arm and leg more than the face.

Approximately 1 week after the surgery, the patient was noted to develop intermittent focal motor seizures with mild jerking of the right hand, spreading to the forearm, arm, and shoulder. These progressed to more violent shaking episodes for approximately 1 min that would be followed by a gradual decline in intensity over 10 min. The patient initially noted one episode every 2 weeks, but this eventually increased to once every 3 days. Anticonvulsant therapy included phenytoin, valproate, and levetiracetam as well as rectal benzodiazepine on an as-needed basis, but eventually these became ineffective. These episodes progressed to continuous jerking of the right shoulder and upper extremity. Throughout these episodes, the patient denied loss of consciousness, incontinence, or tongue-biting, but did describe numbness in his right leg shortly after the "violent" jerking episodes began. There was no associated language impairment. The patient was diagnosed with epilepsia partialis continua – a syndrome of continuous focal jerking of a body part, usually localized to a distal limb, and referred to our institution for further evaluation.

The patient had a full preoperative work-up to confirm the diagnosis of epilepsy and establish the causal relationship between the previous area of surgery and the ictal onset zone. Examination revealed a right hemiparesis, necessitating the use of a wheelchair for ambulation, right partial homonymous hemianopsia, right central facial weakness, and decreased tone in the right upper limb. The patient had 2/5 strength in the proximal right upper extremity and no fine finger strength, and 4/5 strength in the right lower extremity proximally. The MRI of the brain showed evidence of a previous craniotomy and encephalomalacia involving the left perirolandic region and parietal lobe with increased fluid-attenuated inversion recovery (FLAIR) signal in both the pre- and postcentral gyri on the left. Video-EEG monitoring was performed that showed interictal spiking and seizure onset arising from the left parietocentral region.

The case was discussed in a multidisciplinary manner between the neurosurgeon, epileptologists, neuropsychologists, and neuroradiologists and the collective decision was made that the patient would benefit from further surgery. Discussion revolved around the question of using subdural electrodes to obtain extraoperative EEG recordings and functional information to guide the resection versus intraoperative recordings via ECoG and cortical stimulation. Because of the significant loss in motor function preoperatively and the stable spike focus on scalp EEG, it was decided to perform a second craniotomy with intraoperative ECoG to help define the seizure onset area. This was performed under general anesthesia with stereotactic guidance, somatosensory evoked potential identification of the central sulcus, and direct cortical stimulation to identify potential motor cortex (Fig. 65.1A). The patient underwent resection of the left perirolandic cortex guided by intraoperative ECoG and cortical stimulation. The EEG spiking corresponded directly to the hand and thumb motor cortex and because of the pre-existing weakness and desperate nature of the epilepsy, this area was resected (Fig. 65.1B). Postoperatively the epilepsia partialis continua disappeared, but he continues to have less severe and less frequent simple motor seizures affecting his leg. The family and patient have declined further surgical treatment.

This case is illustrative of the difficulties in treating epilepsy involving the perirolandic cortex which was damaged by surgical removal of a parafalcine meningioma. Surgical treatment is limited by eloquent cortex in this area and often removal of the entire damaged cortex is not possible. While we improved the quality of life of this patient, his daily activities are still impaired by the pre-existing hemiparesis and the occasional seizure activity. He will remain in anticonvulsant therapy for the remainder of his life.

Case 2

The patient is a 67-year-old right-handed woman who presented to the epilepsy monitoring unit with a 4-year history of intractable focal epilepsy. The seizures were described as a feeling that "something was wrong." This would occasionally be accompanied by a feeling of numbness in her right arm. After this, her husband stated that she would turn her head to the left and appear to "fumble with her hands." These spells lasted for several minutes, followed by a prolonged postictal state. There were no other lateralizing features. There were no reports of generalized motor seizures, status epilepticus, or other seizure types. Seizures occurred once every 3–4 months.

Evaluation of these events led to the identification of a right occipital meningioma. She underwent resection of the meningioma at an outside institution 1 year after seizures began. She was initially treated with phenytoin, then switched to levetiracetam, and finally to lamotrigine. Seizures continued despite levetiracetam (1500 mg twice a day).

The most recent MRI showed satisfactory postoperative changes from the right parasagittal meningioma resection (Fig. 65.2A). Video-EEG localized the seizure focus to the right parieto-occipital region, and PET scanning showed reduced activity in the right parasagittal region related to previous surgery, as well as hypometabolism in the right mesial temporal lobe (Fig. 65.2B).

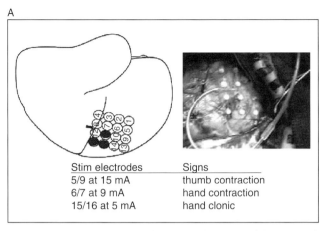
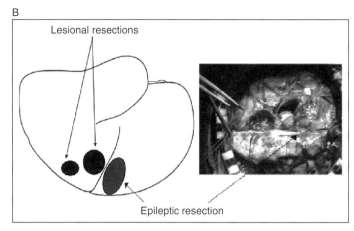

Fig. 65.1. (A) Somatosensory evoked potentials (SSEP) and direct cortical stimulation identify the central sulcus and specific motor functions. (B) Postoperative photograph depicting resection of the left perirolandic cortex.

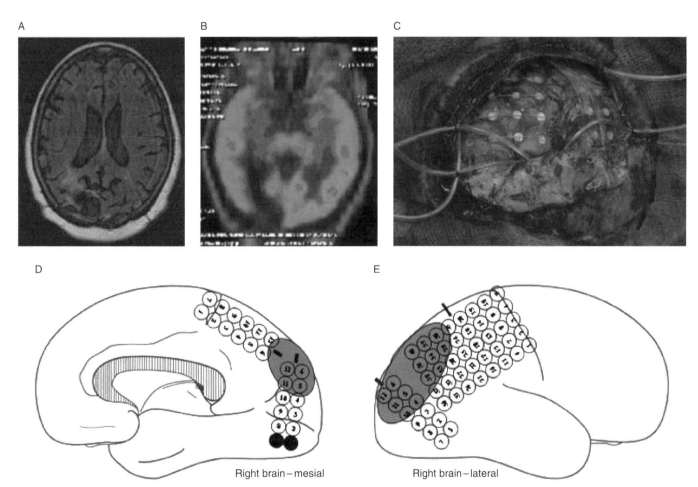

Fig. 65.2. (A) MRI showing previous parasagittal occipital meningioma resection. (B) PET scan demonstrating hypometabolism in the right mesial temporal lobe and reduced activity along the previous surgical cavity. (C) Intraoperative photograph depicting subdural grid placement. (D, E) Seizure focus localized to prior surgical resection bed.

After a thorough discussion involving neuroradiologists, epileptologists, neuropsychologists, and neurosurgeons, the decision was made to place subdural grids prior to resection in order to localize the focus of seizure onset and hopefully exclude temporal lobe involvement (Fig. 65.2C).

The patient underwent right parieto-occipital craniotomy with insertion of subdural grids for chronic epilepsy monitoring. After 2 weeks of invasive monitoring, the seizure focus was localized to the area of prior tumor resection with no definite involvement of her temporal lobe. She underwent resection of a portion of her parietal lobe and the entire occipital lobe (Fig. 65.2D, E). Postoperatively, the patient did well, and was discharged to an acute rehabilitation facility. Although follow-up is short, the patient was noted to have had only one seizure and continues on levetiracetam.

This patient presented with a long history of epilepsy and an underlying meningioma. Despite adequate removal of the tumor, the epilepsy persisted and she required more extensive removal of the underlying cortex. It remains unknown why some patients develop this type of epilepsy and how best to evaluate it. If one could predict the failure of her epilepsy to respond to tumor removal, an invasive cortical recording study prior to tumor resection would be indicated to help define extent of cortical resection. Perhaps the more aggressive use of intraoperative ECoG recordings would help to treat these types of patients more successfully.

Conclusion

Epilepsy is the presenting symptom of meningioma in 20–50% of cases, and so a complete work-up including imaging studies, EEG, and a therapeutic trial of medications is imperative in patients with new-onset seizures (Ramamurthi *et al.* 1980; Lynam *et al.* 2007).

In patients who have undergone a complete work-up and appropriate medication trial but still do not have good seizure control, surgical resection of the meningioma and related EZ can be very successful in the management of epilepsy. Depending upon the location of the meningioma and the EEG results, invasive monitoring, including subdural grids and depths may be required to accurately define the ictal onset zone and delineate it from structurally important regions of the brain that may be located in close proximity.

Studies comparing seizure-free postoperative outcomes after meningioma resection show equivalent or greater than average outcomes when compared with other epileptogenic lesions (Gonzalez-Martinez and Najm 2008). It is important to note that surgery for meningioma resection can in and of itself provoke postoperative seizures which may or may not be transient. A preoperative discussion is essential to ensure that the patient is aware of the risks and benefits of this surgery, especially when there is a particularly high risk for developing postoperative seizures such as with parietal lesions.

References

Claus EB, Bondy ML, Schildkraut JM, *et al.* (2005) Epidemiology of intracranial meningioma. *Neurosurgery* 57:1088–95.

Engel, J, Pedley TA (2007) *Epilepsy: A Comprehensive Textbook.* Philadelphia, PA: Lippincott Williams and Wilkins.

Gonzalez-Martinez JA, Najm IM (2008) Meningiomas and epilepsy. In Lee JH (ed.) *Meningiomas: Diagnosis, Treatment, and Outcome.* London: Springer-Verlag, pp. 243–6.

Kwan P, Brodie MJ (2000) Early identification of refractory epilepsy. *N Engl J Med* 342:464–8.

Lynam LM, Lyons MK, Drazkowski JF, *et al.* (2007) Frequency of seizures in patients with newly diagnosed brain tumors: a retrospective review. *Clin Neurol Neurosurg* 109:634–8.

Penfield W, Erickson TC, Tarlov I (1940) Relation of intracranial tumors and symptomatic epilepsy. *Arch Neurol Psychiatry* 44:300–15.

Ramamurthi B, Ravi R, Ramachandran V (1980) Convulsions with meningiomas: incidence and significance. *Surg Neurol* 14:415–16.

van Breemen MS, Wilms EB, Vecht C (2007) Epilepsy in patients with brain tumors: epidemiology, mechanisms, and management. *Lancet Neurol* 6:421–30.

Chapter

66

Metastatic disease

Rolando F. Del Maestro, Abdulrahman Sabbagh, Ahmed Lary, and Marie-Christine Guiot

Introduction

This chapter is the final of five that address the topic of brain tumors as causes of epilepsy. The first four chapters discussed a series of common primary intrinsic and extra-axial tumors of the central nervous system. This chapter will focus on secondary brain tumors, commonly referred to as solid metastatic brain tumors, and neoplastic meningitis.

Why brain metastasis is the focus of this chapter

There are three primary reasons to focus on brain metastatic disease related to epilepsy.

(1) The incidence of metastatic brain lesions is four to five times higher than primary brain tumors (Gavrilovic and Posner 2005). Approximately 1.4 million Americans were diagnosed with cancer in 2008 (American Cancer Society 2008) and up to 40% of these individuals, over half a million people annually in the United States, will develop one or more cerebral metastases during the course of their cancer. The treatment of metastatic disease involves a wide range of subspecialties and this, along with the public health impact of brain metastasis to the health profession and community, results in the need for a coordinated approach to this complex problem.

(2) Many of the medications needed to treat systemic cancer interact with antiepileptic medications and vice versa. Therefore knowledge of these interactions is crucial to the appropriate treatment of the patient with cerebral metastatic disease and epilepsy (Maschio et al. 2006).

(3) Evidence-based clinical practice guidelines have been developed concerning patients with solid metastatic brain tumors. Medical practitioners employing these guidelines will hopefully result in a significant impact on this area of neuro-oncology (Kalkanis and Linskey 2010).

Incidence proportions of brain metastasis

The estimate of the incidence of metastatic brain tumors has varied from 8.3 per 100 000 (Walker et al. 1985) to 11 per 100 000 (Percy et al. 1972) while the incidence rate for primary brain tumors is 6.6 per 100 000 (Ries et al. 2003). The number of metastatic brain tumors is felt to be increasing because of a number of factors. These include longer survival of cancer patients secondary to more effective treatments and earlier diagnosis along with the aging population in developed countries (van Breemen et al. 2007).

Depending on the type of data used, the incidence proportions of brain metastasis have varied from 20% to 50% (Bernholtz-Sloan et al. 2004). In a careful study of the incidence proportions of brain metastasis in patients diagnosed in the Metropolitan Detroit Surveillance System from 1973 to 2001 the total incidence percentage of brain metastases was 9.6% for all the primary sites studied. Lung (19.9%) had the highest number of brain metastases followed by melanoma (6.9%), renal (6.5%), breast (5.1%), and colorectal (1.8%) cancer. A number of factors such as race, age, sex, and type of cancer resulting in cerebral metastasis were important in this population-based study. A number of other population-based studies have looked at the issue of incidence proportion of brain metastasis in cancer patients with variable results. These have ranged from an Icelandic study (Guomundsson 1970) at less than 20%, a study from Finland (Fogelholm et al. 1984) at 18%, a Rochester, Minnesota study (Percy et al. 1972) at 41%, and a US National Survey at 51% (Walker et al. 1985). The studies including autopsy reports were consistently higher and may not reflect the number of individuals who are actively being treated for their metastatic disease (Mendez and Del Maestro 1988). In summary, the population-based observations suggest that between 10% and 20% of patients with a systemic cancer will present and need care for their cerebral metastasis and this will involve at least 20% of lung cancer patients.

The Causes of Epilepsy, eds. S. D. Shorvon, F. Andermann, and R. Guerrini. Published by Cambridge University Press. © Cambridge University Press 2011.

Incidence of epilepsy in metastatic brain disease

There is a paucity of data based on Class 1 evidence that addresses the issue of the incidence of epilepsy in patients who present with cerebral metastasis who have not experienced a seizure. There is only one underpowered randomized controlled trial that can be used to address this question. In this study, Forsyth et al. (2003) randomized 100 patients, 60 with metastatic disease and 40 with primary brain tumors to anticonvulsants versus no anticonvulsants. Twenty-six of the metastatic patients were treated with anticonvulsants (25 with phenytoin, one with phenobarbital). The primary end point was the incidence of seizures at 3 months post randomization. When the seizure rate was only 10% and the mortality rate was 30% the trial was terminated early since to reach a clinically relevant seizure occurrence rate was not going to be possible with the planned accrual. However, in this study, there was no significant difference in seizure incidence in patients receiving or not receiving prophylactic anticonvulsants. Based on this limited information the American Association of Neurological Surgeons and the Congress of Neurological Surgeons guidelines do not recommend the routine long-term prophylactic use of anticonvulsants in patients with cerebral metastatic disease who have never had a seizure (Mikkelsen et al. 2010). This is in keeping with two other published guidelines (Glantz et al. 2000; Perry et al. 2006).

The percentage of patients with cerebral metastasis who present with seizures varies widely depending on the type of patients being assessed. Cancer centers routinely employing investigations including cerebral computed tomography (CT), magnetic resonance imaging (MRI), and positron emission tomography (PET) scans would be expected to have lower incidence of epilepsy in their cancer patients as a presenting sign of cerebral metastatic disease in the range of 12% (Posner 1995). Neurosurgical series are generally higher; between 20% (Herman 2002) and 35% of patients with secondary tumors will develop epilepsy (Villemure and de Tribolet 1996). Careful prospective studies have not been carried out to determine which type of primary systemic cancer or specific brain location is more commonly associated with focal or generalized seizures although subcortical location is clearly felt to be important in epileptogenesis (van Breemen et al. 2007). Many factors such as the types of primary tumor, number of metastatic lesions, size of tumors, and their location all play a part in the type and number of seizures seen in individual patients. The supratentorial component of the brain is associated with about 85% of the solid cerebral metastasis. Location of the metastatic tumors in the frontal, parietal, and temporal lobes are associated with more tumors than the occipital lobes (Delattre et al. 1988) (Fig. 66.1A). Seizures also originate more frequently from the frontal, parietal, and temporal lobes than from metastatic lesions in the occipital lobes (Sirven et al. 2004). The expectation would be that seizures as a presenting sign of cerebral metastasis will decrease as more and more staging procedures are performed in cancer patients before definitive surgical or medical treatment. However, as patients live longer with their neoplastic disease as a consequence of both earlier diagnosis and more effective treatment, cerebral metastatic disease will continue to increase and more patients will develop epilepsy and require antiepileptic medication during their disease process (van Breemen et al. 2007).

Genetics of metastatic brain disease

The molecular basis of metastasis is a complex interplay involving the interaction of cancer cells and their microenvironment. This results in the ability of tumor cells to detach from a major tumor mass and invade the vascular system thereby allowing new cancer cell foci to exist and flourish in new environments resulting in death secondary to organ dysfunction. A number of random epigenetic and genetic events in tumor cells along with a conducive microenvironment allow the evolution of metastatic lesions. The genes involved in metastatic disease have been classified into initiation, progression, and virulence categories (see review Chiang and Massagué 2008). Based on the "seed versus soil" hypothesis proposed by Paget, certain circulating tumor cells such as those from lung tend to adhere to the endothelium of brain microvessels and then propagate in this "soil." This conducive "soil" in the supratentorial component of the central nervous system (CNS) appears to reside predominantly in the microvessels of the white-matter–gray-matter junction between the major arterial vessels, the watershed regions, and can involve single (Figs. 66.1B, D) and multiple sites (Fig. 66.1C). Since the brain receives 15–20% of the cardiac output, many circulating tumor cells may have the possibility of coming in contact with the conducive microvessels of watershed brain regions. The location of cerebral metastatic lesions in these regions has the ability to alter function of the overlying cerebral cortex and result in subsequent seizure activity.

Neoplastic meningitis

Neoplastic meningitis occurs when malignant tumor cells seed the leptomeninges of the brain. Between 1% and 5% of patients with solid cancer will develop neoplastic meningitis, a disorder which can affect all components of the neuroaxis, and in this situation it is called carcinomatous meningitis (Chamberlain 2008). Leukemia and lymphoma patients develop neoplastic meningitis in 5–15% of cases and primary brain tumor in about 1% of tumors (Chamberlain 1997). This disorder usually occurs in patients with progressive and widely disseminated cancer but occasionally can be the presenting feature of cancer. Seizures occur in 14% of patients and can be difficult to control (Kaplan et al. 1990). Since patient survival is very limited despite intrathecal therapy it would appear reasonable to continue antiepileptic medication in these patients who develop seizures during the course of their disease.

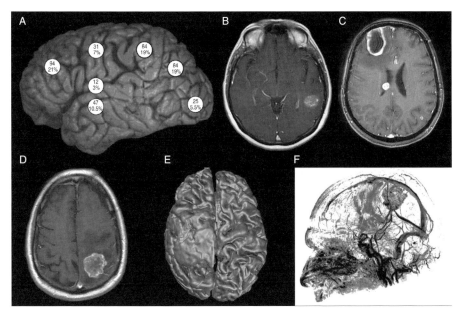

Fig. 66.1. Variability of metastatic lesions. Cerebral metastatic disease can present in a large number of ways. (A) Metastatic lesions are more frequently found in the frontal, parietal, and temporal regions and less frequently in the occipital area. (B) Non-symptomatic solitary left temporal lesion identified in a patient with a lung mass who underwent a PET scan for screening. (C) Patient presenting with headache and cognitive dysfunction. Multiple lesions were present on an enhanced MR scan. The right frontal lesion is associated with significant mass effect and peritumoral edema and the patient was started on anticonvulsant therapy and steroids before an operative procedure to resect the frontal lesion which was consistent with a large-cell carcinoma of the lung metastasis. (D) Patient with familial polyposis syndrome presenting with focal motor seizures of the right arm. MR demonstrates a single lesion in the left parietal region with peritumoral edema. (E) Three-dimensional reconstruction of the brain surface demonstrates the distortion of the cortex by the tumor (note left is on the left in this reconstruction). (F) Diffusion tensor imaging demonstrates the distortion of the white matter motor fibers by the tumor. (Part A adapted with permission from Delattre *et al. Arch Neurol* **45**:741–4, 1988. Copyright © (1988) American Medical Association. All rights reserved.)

Epileptogenesis of metastatic brain disease

The origin and nature of epileptogenesis involving metastatic lesions is poorly understood. Epileptic seizures in patients with cerebral metastatic disease are most likely multifactorial, however, a number of factors are considered to be contributing to the development and continuation of these seizures in a sub-group of individuals.

Metastatic tumors: cortical isolation and injury

Since metastatic deposits usually occur at the cortical gray–white matter junction this location must invariably alter the function of cortical efferents and afferents resulting in a shift to that of excitatory mechanisms (Fig. 66.1F). Metastatic lesions have the potential to produce chronic partial deafferentiated regions in the cortex adjacent or immediately above smaller metastatic deposits (Fig. 66.2A). Cannon (1939) suggested in his "law of denervation" that denervation and thus deafferentation of the cortex is a potent initiator of epileptogenesis. Both animal and human studies of resected epileptogenic lesions have supported these concepts (see review Fish 1999). Cannon noted that Hughlings Jackson had commented that "no-one could suppose that a tumor discharges, the tumor leads to instability of the gray matter and the discharge causing the convulsion of this unstable gray matter" (Fish 1999). Since metastatic lesions are not composed of nervous tissue, the cells within the tumor cannot be responsible for the epileptogenesis seen. However, these tumors can distort adjacent gray matter causing changes in mechanical forces resulting in microvascular alterations such as ischemia and direct tissue damage (Figs. 66.1E, 66.2B). The role played by chronic ischemia along with tumor necrosis and changes in the pH of the interstitial fluids in the microenvironment of the metastatic lesion is unknown. However, these conditions may predispose to the swelling of perilesional astrocytes and neurons resulting in changes in sodium flux and epileptogenesis (Fish 1999; van Breemen *et al.* 2007).

Metastatic tumors grow as distinct nodules with very little invasion of adjacent cortex (Fig. 66.2A, C). Therefore, unlike low-grade and malignant glioma in which invasive tumor cells may disrupt neural circuits, metastatic tumor cells would not be expected to result in epilepsy predominantly by this mechanism. Secondary epileptogenesis may not play a very significant role in the development of seizures in patients with metastatic disease because of the fast rate of growth of metastatic lesions and the short survival of many of these patients. Refractory seizures also do not seem to be as significant a problem in metastatic lesions as compared to low-grade tumors which also may be related to the failure of metastatic cells to directly invade brain tissue. Although very few data are available, surgery for intractable seizure disorders appears to be very infrequently carried out for patients with metastatic lesions (van Breemen *et al.* 2007).

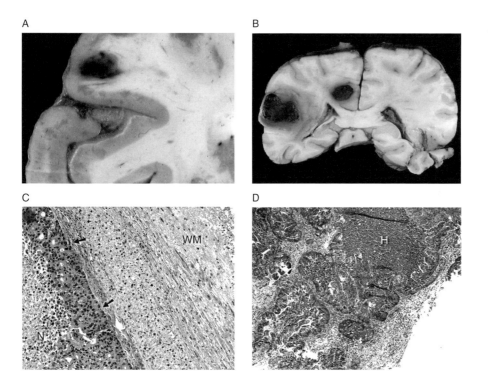

Fig. 66.2. Pathology of metastatic disease. The subcortical location and non-invasive characteristics of metastatic lesions. (A) A small metastatic lesion located just below the gray matter demonstrating how the position of even a small lesion could isolate and deafferent overlying cortex and result in seizures. (B) Multiple metastatic lesions associated with hemorrhage demonstrating how larger lesions can distort and damage overlying cortical tissue. (C) Photomicrograph showing the tumor–brain interface of a metastatic adenocarcinoma demonstrating the lack of invasion (arrows), necrosis (N) and alteration of the adjacent white matter (WM) (hematoxylin and eosin; original magnification ×200). (D) Photomicrograph demonstrating the disorganization of a metastatic adenocarcinoma from lung with hemorrhage (H) with distortion rather then invasion of white matter (WM) (hematoxylin and eosin; original magnification ×100).

The role played by changes in the white matter during metastatic tumor growth to epileptogenesis is poorly understood (Fig. 66.1C). No clear relationship between seizure frequency and the amount of peritumoral edema or tumor mass effect has been found (Fish 1999). Hoffman *et al.* (1994) carried out experiments in animals which demonstrated that both combined subcortical cutting and transcortical cutting resulted in significant epileptogenic changes. However, white matter undercutting did not result in significant changes suggesting that cortical gray matter circuits are more essential to epileptogenesis. Diffusion tensor imaging now allows the assessment of damage to white matter tracts going to and from specific cortical regions by metastatic tumors (Wong *et al.* 2009). This technique may allow a much more careful assessment of the role of white matter injury and cortical isolation in the generation of seizures originating from underlying metastatic deposits (Fig. 66.1F).

Hemorrhage into and around metastatic lesions can occur and there is evidence that the presence of hemosiderin deposits are associated with medically intractable seizures in primary brain tumors (see review in Willmore and Ueda, 2009) (Fig. 66.2B, D). The role of hemorrhage, the release of iron, and the subsequent alterations in membrane structure and function secondary to free-radical-induced membrane lipid peroxidation may play a role in the epileptogenesis in both traumatic cerebral injury and metastatic lesions associated with hemorrhage (Del Maestro 1980). The injection of ferric ions into rodent brain results in liberation of glutamate as has been seen in human epilepsy. The regulation of glutamate synaptic transporter proteins such as GLAST by glial cells is downregulated by free-radical injury and may be fundamental in the response of cerebral tissue to injury and associated hemorrhage (Willmore and Ueda 2009).

A growing metastatic cerebral lesion can be expected to deafferent the cortical tissue directly above and adjacent to this lesion and may further alter the immediate microenvironment by distortion, ischemia, or hemorrhage. All of these factors acting together result in the development of epileptogenesis in the adjacent cortical tissue and subsequent seizures in these patients.

Published guidelines for the treatment of patients with metastatic cerebral lesions

The American Association of Neurological Surgeons and Congress of Neurological Surgeons have defined a series of guidelines for the treatments of patients with single and multiple metastatic lesions (Kalkanis and Linskey 2010). Level 1 recommendations support the role of surgery followed by whole-brain radiation therapy (WBRT) in the treatment of patients with single metastatic lesions which can be safely resected since there is Class 1 evidence supporting this treatment (Kalkanis *et al.* 2010). In patients not presenting with seizures anticonvulsants are recommended preoperatively and if no seizures occur in the perioperative period the recommendation is that these medications be discontinued after 7 days (Mikkelsen *et al.* 2010). Once a seizure has occurred anticonvulsants should be used. No prospective long-term studies have been carried out to outline the response of the seizure disorder in these patients to specific medications or the operative procedure. Therefore no recommendations based on the type of anticonvulsant,

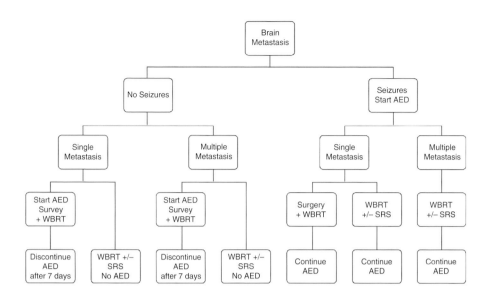

Fig. 66.3. Treatment algorithm of anticonvulsant treatment of patients with cerebral metastasis presenting with or without seizures. AED, antiepileptic drugs; SRS, stereotactic radiosurgery; WBRT, whole brain radiation therapy.

dose, or length of anticonvulsant treatment was recommended in the guidelines. The American Association of Neurological Surgeons and Congress of Neurological Surgeons guidelines have also attempted to assess the type of radiation treatment used to treat metastatic cerebral disease. A treatment algorithm can be developed based on the multiple radiation modalities assessed depending on whether the metastatic lesion is solitary or multiple (Fig. 66.3). A number of radiation options are available for treatment of specific cases and these appear to have equivalent results. Care must be employed in the treatment of lesions greater than 3 cm and careful follow-up is essential in patients treated with stereotactic radiosurgery (SRS) (Linskey *et al.* 2010). The routine use of chemotherapy following WBRT for brain metastases was not recommended since it has not been shown to increase survival (Mehta *et al.* 2010). A number of emerging and investigational therapies were considered reasonable including the use of temozolomide and WBRT for malignant melanoma brain metastasis and epidermal growth factor receptor inhibitors in the management of brain metastasis in selective cases of non-small-cell lung carcinoma (Olson *et al.* 2010). However, despite the advances in surgery, newer modalities of radiation therapy and experimental therapies, the prognosis of patients with cerebral metastases remains poor.

Issues related to the pharmacological management of a cancer patient who has cerebral metastases and epilepsy

Patients with metastatic cancer are commonly being treated with a wide variety of anticancer molecules many of which are known to interact with antiepileptic drugs (AEDs). Therefore knowledge of these interactions is critical to patient care. This topic is very extensive and only a brief overview of the important issues involved will be discussed.

When one drug modifies the activity of another, decreasing or increasing its efficacy, a pharmacological interaction is considered to have occurred. These interactions can occur between drugs that have similar or different mechanisms of action (pharmacodynamic interactions) or those that interface with the distribution of another drug altering its site of action or concentration (pharmacokinetic interactions).

Corticosteroids

The American Association of Neurological Surgeons and the Congress of Neurological Surgeons guidelines recommend that steroids only be used to treat patients with mild symptoms (4–8 mg/day dexamethasone) or severe symptoms secondary to increased intracranial pressure (16 mg/day or more) (Ryken *et al.* 2010). Phenobarbitol and phenytoin shorten the half-life of dexamethasone and both increased and decreased concentrations of phenytoin have been seen in patients taking dexamethasone (Maschio *et al.* 2006). Phenytoin concentrations need to be carefully monitored particularly postoperatively when dexamethasone is being decreased since this can result in toxic levels of phenytoin.

Chemotherapeutic drug interactions

Antiepileptic drugs are known to reduce the activity of chemotherapeutic drugs. Elimination of drugs by hepatic metabolism is associated with the most significant pharmacological interactions because of glucuronidation or induction of the P450 enzymes (Maschio *et al.* 2008). Phenytoin, carbamazepine, and phenobarbital are well-known enzyme inducers and decrease the activity of a large number of chemotherapeutic agents (Table 66.1A). A number of chemotherapeutic drugs result in a decreased activity of AEDs (Table 66.1B). The adverse effects of a number of antiepileptic drugs can be increased by the commonly used anticancer agents such as cisplatin and nitrosoureas (Table 66.1C). Cancer patients

Table 66.1 Drug interactions

(A) Antiepileptic medications that reduce the activity of chemotherapeutic drugs		
Phenytoin	**Carbamazepine**	**Phenobarbitol**
Busulfan	Methotrexate	Cyclophosphamide
Methotrexate	Vincristine	Ifosfamide
Vincristine	Paclitaxel	Thiotepa
Paclitaxel	9-Aminocamptothecin	Nitrosoureas
Irinotecan	Teniposide	Methotrexate
Topotecan		Vincristine
9-Aminocamptothecin		Paclitaxel
Teniposide		9-Aminocamptothecin
		Teniposide
		Doxorubicin
		Procarbazine
		Tamoxifen

(B) Chemotherapeutic drugs that reduce the activity of antiepileptic drugs		
Phenytoin	**Carbamazepine**	**Valproic acid**
Bleomycin	Cisplatin	Methotrexate
Nitrosoureas	Adriamycin	Cisplatin
Cisplatin		Adriamycin
Etoposide		
Dacarbazine		
Adriamycin		
Carboplatin		
Vinblastin		
Methotrexate		

(C) Chemotherapeutic drugs that increase the toxicity of antiepileptic drugs	
Phenytoin	**Valproic acid**
Fluorouracil	Cisplatin
Tegafur	Nitrosoureas
Tamoxifen	

Source: Modified with permission from Maschio *et al.* (2006); Copyright © (2006) CIC Edizioni Internazionale, Roma.

on phenytoin, carbamazepine, phenobarbital, and valproic acid have shown decreased cognitive performance when compared to individuals who were not on these drugs (Klein *et al.* 2003). This information suggests that the selection of AEDs to be used in cancer patients will not only have an influence on quality-of-life issues but may influence both the response of their cancer to chemotherapeutic treatment and AED toxicity and therefore must be carefully considered.

Practical guidelines for the antiepileptic drugs in patients with cerebral metastatic disease

There are very few Class 1 studies which can provide Level 1 recommendations to help with the treatment of these patients. Figure 66.3 presents a treatment algorithm that may be useful in the treatment of individual patients. The present guidelines are consistent in recommending that patients with cerebral metastatic disease who have not had a seizure should not be treated with antiepileptic medication. However, in patients who present without a seizure and evidence of cerebral metastatic disease amenable to and requiring urgent surgery, it is recommended to begin AEDs prior to surgery. One drug that is commonly used in this situation is phenytoin since it can be used both intravenously and by mouth in equivalent dosages. Careful monitoring of phenytoin levels is crucial since all these patients will also be on dexamethasone prior to surgery and on a decreasing dose after surgery. Phenytoin should be discontinued after 7 days if no postoperative seizures occur. In patients in whom phenytoin may alter the response of the patient's present chemotherapy and/or multiple liver metastatic lesions and hepatic failure is present then the use of levetiracetam should be considered.

Patients presenting with seizures secondary to an intracerebral metastasis and requiring urgent surgery can also be started on phenytoin and switched to another non-enzyme-inducing drug postoperatively such as levetiracetam or valproic acid (van Breemen et al. 2007). In countries where intravenous levetiracetam is available this medication would seem to be a reasonable alternative to phenytoin in the patient requiring urgent surgery.

One question that always comes up is when can these AEDs be withdrawn in patients who are seizure-free? Many patients with metastatic cerebral disease have very limited survival and therefore it seems reasonable to continue antiepileptic treatment in this subgroup of patients until carefully designed studies provide further guidelines on the prolonged treatment of these patients.

In patients with cerebral metastases presenting with seizures in whom urgent surgery is not felt to be applicable it may be reasonable to start these patients on a non-enzyme-inducing drug such as levetiracetam or valproic acid. Research related to the most appropriate drug to be used in patients with cerebral metastatic disease is needed and patients should be encouraged to participate in well-designed Phase III trials.

Conclusions

Cerebral metastatic disease is common and may become more frequent as the treatment options for patients with cancer prove more effective. The treatment of epilepsy in patients with secondary brain tumors should involve a multidisciplinary team that is knowledgeable about all the surgical, radiation, and therapeutic options in the management of these patients. Special consideration of the drug interactions between the medications utilized to treat seizures and drugs used in the treatment of each individual patient's cancer needs to be a priority. Seizures are common in these patients and their appropriate management not only influences the patients' quality of life but also may influence their response to treatment. A series of treatment guidelines have been developed by the American Association of Neurological Surgeons and the Congress of Neurological Surgeons which help guide surgical, radiotherapy, and therapeutic management. The reason for epileptogenesis in these patients is poorly understood and unfortunately not the focus of much of the research into lesion induced epilepsy. Research needs to be focused on the best AED or drug combination to use in these patients so that new practice guidelines can be developed to improve patient care.

Acknowledgments

This work is supported by the Franco Di Giovanni, the B-Foundation Strong, the Colannino Family, and Alex Pavanel Family along with the Raymonde and Tony Boeckh Funds for Brain Tumor Research. The authors also thank the Montreal English School Board and the Brainstorm and the Brain Tumor Foundation of Canada for their financial support. Dr. R. F. Del Maestro holds the William Feindel Chair in Neuro-Oncology at McGill University.

References

American Cancer Society (2008) Cancer facts and figures 2008. Available online at www.cancer.org/docroot/stt/content/stt_lx_cancer_.facts and_figures_2008.asp

Barnholtz-Sloan JS, Sloan JE, Davis FG, et al. (2004) Incidence proportions of brain metastases in patients diagnosed (1973 to 2001) in the Metropolitan Detroit Cancer Surveillance System. J Clin Oncol 22:2865–72.

Cannon WB (1939) A law of denervation. Am J Med Sci 198:737–50.

Chamberlain MC (1997) Carcinomatous meningitis. Arch Neurol 44:16–17.

Chamberlain MC (2008) Neoplastic meningitis. Curr Neurol Neurosci Rep 8:249–58.

Chiang AC, Massagué J (2008) Molecular basis of metastasis. N Engl J Med 359:2814–23.

Delattre J-Y, Krp G, Thaler HT, Posner JB (1988) Distribution of brain metastases. Arch Neurol 45:741–4.

Del Maestro RF (1980) An approach to free radicals in medicine and biology. Acta Physiol Scand (Suppl) 492:153–68.

Fish DR (1999) How do tumors cause epilepsy? In: Kotagal P Lüders HD (eds.) The Epilepsies: Etiologies and Prevention. L San Diego, CA: Academic Press, pp. 301–14.

Fogelholm R, Uutela T, Murros K (1984) Epidemiology of central nervous system neoplasms: a regional survey in Central Finland. Acta Neurol Scand 69:129–36.

Forsyth PA, Weaver S, Fulton D, et al. (2003) Prophylactic anticonvulsants in patients with brain tumor. Can J Neurol Sci 30:106–12.

Gavrilovic IT, Posner JB (2005) Brain metastases: epidemiology and pathophysiology. J Neurooncol 75:5–14.

Glantz MJ, Cole BF, Forsyth PA, et al. (2000) Practice parameters: anticonvulsant prophylaxis in patients with newly diagnosed brain tumors: report of the Quality Standards Subcommittee of the American Academy of Neurology. Neurology 54:1886–93.

Guomundsson KR (1970) A survey of tumors of the central nervous system in Iceland during the 10-year period 1954–1963. *Acta Neurol Scand* **46**:538–52.

Herman ST (2002) Epilepsy after brain insult. targeting epileptogenesis. *Neurology* **59**:S21–6.

Hoffman SN, Salin PA, Prince DA (1994) Chronic neocortical epileptogenesis in vitro. *J Neurophys* **71**:1762–73.

Kalkanis SN, Linskey ME (2010) Evidence-based clinical practice parameter guidelines for the treatment of patients with metastatic brain tumors: introduction. *J Neurooncol* **96**:7–10.

Kalkanis SN, Kondziolka D, Gaspar LE, *et al.* (2010) The role of surgical resection in the management of newly diagnosed brain metastases: a systematic review and evidence-based clinical practice guidelines. *J Neurooncol* **96**:33–43.

Kaplan JG, DeSouza TG, Farkash A, *et al.* (1990) Leptomeningeal metastases: comparison of clinical features and laboratory data of solid tumors, lymphomas and leukemias. *J Neurooncol* **9**:225–9.

Klein M, Engelberts NHJ, van der Ploeg S (2003) Epilepsy in low-grade gliomas: the impact on cognitive and quality of life. *Ann Neurol* **54**:514–20.

Linskey ME, Andrews DW, Asher AL, *et al.* (2010) The role of stereotactic radiosurgery in the management of patients with newly diagnosed brain metastasis: a systematic review and evidence-based clinical practice guidelines. *J Neurooncol* **96**:45–68.

Maschio M, Dinapoli L, Zarabla A, Jandolo B (2006) Issues related to the pharmacological management of patients with brain tumors and epilepsy. *Funct Neurol* **21**:15–19.

Mehta MP, Paleologos NA, Mikkelsen T, *et al.* (2010) The role of chemotherapy in the management of newly diagnosed brain metastases: a systematic review and evidence-based clinical practice guideline. *J Neurooncol* **96**:71–83.

Mendez IM, Del Maestro RF (1988) Cerebral metastases from malignant melanoma. *Can J Neurol Sci* **15**:119–23.

Mikkelsen T, Paleologos NA, Robinson PD, *et al.* (2010) The role of prophylactic anticonvulsants in the management of brain metastases: a systemic review and evidence-based clinical practice guideline. *J Neurooncol* **96**:97–102.

Olson JJ, Paleologos NA, Gaspar LE, *et al.* (2010) The role of emerging and investigational therapies for metastatic brain tumors: a systematic review and evidence-based clinical practice guideline of selected topics. *J Neurooncol* **96**:115–42.

Percy AK, Elveback LR, Okazaki H, Kurland LT (1972) Neoplasms of the central nervous system: epidemiologic considerations. *Neurology* **22**:40–8.

Perry J, Zinman L, Chambers A, *et al.* (2006) The use of prophylactic anticonvusants in patients with brain tumors: a systematic review. *Curr Oncol* **13**:222–9.

Posner JB (1995) Brain metastases. *J Neurooncol* **27**:287–93.

Ries LAG, Eisner MP, Kosary CL (eds.) (2003) *SEER Cancer Statistics Review, 1975–2000* Bethesda, MD: National Cancer Institute. Available online at http://seer.cancer.gov/csr/

Ryken TC, McDermott M, Robinson PD, *et al.* (2010) The role of steroids in the management of brain metastases: a systematic review and evidence-based clinical practice guideline. *J Neurooncol* **96**:103–4.

Sirven JI, Wingerchuk DM, Drazkowski JF, Lyons MK, Zimmerman RS (2004) Seizure prophylaxis in patients with brain tumors: a metanalysis. *Mayo Clin Proc* **79**:1489–94.

Walker RA, Robins M, Weinfeld FD (1985) Epidemiology of brain tumors: the national survey of intracranial neoplasms. *Neurology* **35**:219–26.

Van Breeman MSM, Wilms EB, Vecht CJ (2007) Epilepsy in patients with brain tumors: epidemiology, mechanisms and management. *Lancet Neurol* **6**:421–30.

Willmore LJ, Ueda Y (2009) Posttraumatic epilepsy: hemorrhage, free radicals and the molecular regulation of glutamate. *Neurochem Res* **34**:688–97.

Wong W, Stewart CE, Desmond PM (2009) Diffusion tensor imaging in glioblastoma multiforme and brain metastases: the role of q, p, L, and fractional anisotropy. *AJNR Am J Neuroradiol* **30**:203–8.

Villemure JG, De Tribolet N (1996) Epilepsy in patients with central nervous system tumors. *Curr Opin Neurol* **9**:424–8.

Viral encephalitis

Jane E. Adcock

Overview

Viral encephalitis is an uncommon complication of otherwise common viral infections. Viral encephalitides include acute viral encephalitis, postinfectious encephalomyelitis, slow viral infections of the central nervous system (CNS), and chronic degenerative diseases of the CNS of presumed viral origin. All of these disorders may result in seizures. This chapter presents the diagnostic and clinical challenges that accompany the management of seizures following CNS infection by the herpes viruses, RNA viruses, enteroviruses, and arenaviruses. The HIV-related encephalitides and infections are discussed in Chapter 74. Emerging and less common viral infections are discussed in Chapter 75.

Epidemiology

The incidence of acute viral encephalitis is geographically diverse. In Westernized industrial countries an incidence of 10.5 per 100 000 cases in children and 2.2 per 100 000 in the adult population has been calculated from a systematic review of the epidemiological literature (Jmor *et al.* 2008). Incidence is generally higher in tropical regions, and hotspots have developed in communities with high levels of HIV infection, or with inadequate vaccination programs.

Community-based studies suggest that infections account for just 2% of etiological diagnoses in cases with newly diagnosed epileptic seizures in the UK (Sander *et al.* 1990). Of these, half may be caused by viral infections, although the virus is unidentified in many cases (Jmor *et al.* 2008). Mild viral meningitis is common and may go unnoticed, but acute viral encephalitis has a fatality ratio of up to 70% in untreated cases. Infants, elderly people, and patients who are immunocompromised are most at risk of serious complications. There are many forms of viral encephalitis, and all are associated to varying degrees with subsequent epilepsy. The risk of developing epilepsy following viral encephalitis is increased seven- to tenfold over premorbid levels. This risk increases to 22 times the premorbid risk if the patient experiences early seizures during the acute infection. Most seizures occur within 5 years of the acute illness although the risk of unprovoked seizures remains elevated for 15 years (Annegers *et al.* 1988; Duncan *et al.* 1995). It carries a significantly higher risk of ongoing seizures compared to bacterial meningitis (Annegers *et al.* 1988; Duncan *et al.* 1995). Chronic epilepsy may develop in up to 25% of survivors (Duncan *et al.* 1995). Viral meningitis is not associated with an increased risk of epilepsy (Annegers *et al.* 1988).

Sporadic forms of viral encephalitis include the herpes viruses (herpes simplex 1 and 2, herpes varicella–zoster, human herpesvirus 6, Epstein–Barr virus, and cytomegalovirus), the RNA viruses (measles, mumps, and influenza), and enteroviruses (coxsackie viruses and echoviruses). It is herpes simplex encephalitis that remains the most common sporadic fatal encephalitis with high mortality rates and significant morbidity in survivors.

Clinical features of disease

Viral encephalitis is characterized by acute onset of a febrile illness. Fever, headache, lethargy, nausea, and non-specific flu-like symptoms are often the first clinical signs of infection, with subsequent symptoms of leptomeningeal irritation becoming prominent. Advancing viral infection of the brain parenchyma produces edema, neuronal and glial cell degeneration, inflammatory infiltration, and eventual tissue necrosis. Early neurological signs may include behavioral disturbance including agitation, irritability, or confusion, and speech disturbance or dysphasia. Hemiparesis may occur in up to one-third of cases. It is often only when a patient develops seizures, stupor, or coma that the severity of the condition is recognized. Early recognition, diagnosis, and treatment are therefore key, and should always be considered in the differential diagnosis in any patient who presents with the above features.

A detailed history will give clues to the viral etiology. Essential to elicit is a detailed travel history, particularly to

The Causes of Epilepsy, eds. S. D. Shorvon, F. Andermann, and R. Guerrini. Published by Cambridge University Press. © Cambridge University Press 2011.

endemic areas (Japanese encephalitis, malaria, West Nile), a history of a rash in the patient or close contacts (measles, varicella–zoster, human herpesvirus 6, meningococcus), any interaction with animals (e.g., rodents and lymphocytic choreomeningitis virus), any bites or scratches from animals or insects, and risk factors for HIV. A history to suggest simple or complex partial seizures of temporal lobe type should be specifically explored (herpes simplex virus 1). Physical examination should include assessment of conscious level and orientation, inspection of skin for any lesions/rashes/bites/scratches, and specific examination for oral candidiasis (HIV), oral or genital ulcers (herpes simplex 1 and 2, syphilis), parotid swelling and deafness (mumps), meningism, focal neurological signs including cranial nerve palsies (enterovirus, listeria), hemiparesis (cerebral abscess), movement disorders (West Nile virus), and evidence of radiculopathy (Epstein–Barr virus, cytomegalovirus).

Investigations

Initial investigations should include a full blood count (which may show abnormal lymphocytes of Epstein–Barr virus, leukocytosis, or leukopenia), electrolytes (syndrome of inappropriate antidiuretic hormone [SIADH] is common in encephalitis), blood cultures, and a chest X-ray (atypical pneumonias can present with encephalitic-like illness). Brain imaging should be performed to exclude space-occupying pathology or hemorrhage, and to assess for edema or focal abnormalities. A lumbar puncture should be performed as soon as possible once imaging has excluded a space occupying lesion, marked cerebral edema, or midline shift. Cerebrospinal fluid (CSF) examination is critical to establish the diagnosis. A typical viral CSF picture may include a mildly raised opening pressure, a mild to moderate lymphocytic pleocytosis (5–1000 cells/mm), and mild to moderately elevated protein (0.6–1.0 g/L) with a normal or mildly reduced glucose. This typical viral picture helps to differentiate from an acute bacterial infection which is usually associated with the CSF showing high neutrophil count, high protein, and low glucose. However, early in severe viral encephalitis polymorphs may predominate, giving a confusing picture. In some instances, the red cell count can be significantly raised (HSV-1 can be associated with an acute necrotizing hemorrhagic encephalitis).

Specific viruses can now be detected in the CSF using polymerase chain reaction (PCR) where previously specific viral diagnoses could only be made by brain biopsy. Herpes simplex virus (HSV-1 and HSV-2), cytomegalovirus (CMV), varicella-zoster virus (VZV), Epstein–Barr virus (EBV), and human herpesvirus 6 (HHV-6) can all now be reliably diagnosed via PCR.

If there is to be a significant delay in obtaining CSF in a very ill patient in whom there is a high suspicion of viral encephalitis, treatment for both viral encephalitis and possible bacterial meningitis should be commenced with the antiviral agent acyclovir as well as with broad-spectrum antibiotics, until more CSF results can be obtained.

Up to 5–10% of patients subsequently proven to have HSV-1 encephalitis may initially have normal CSF, i.e., normal protein, glucose, and cell count, particularly if the CSF has been tested less than 3 days after the onset of symptoms (Davies et al. 2005; Mook-Kanamori et al. 2009). Such patients should therefore be treated with acyclovir if the clinical suspicion is high pending final HSV-1 PCR results, and repeat CSF testing should be considered.

Herpes viruses

Herpes simplex virus (HSV-1 and HSV-2)

Infection from the herpes simplex virus (HSV) is the most common form of sporadic encephalitis, and it remains a serious disease with a high mortality and morbidity. HSV-1 encephalitis is the most common form, affecting children older than 3 months and adults, affecting predominantly the temporal and frontoparietal areas. It accounts for up to 20% of all viral encephalitis cases. HSV-2 affects predominantly neonates. HSV is transmitted from the infected mother via fetal intrapartum contact with genital HSV-2 infection in 85% of such cases. Skin lesions typically signal infection within the first week of life, but isolated HSV-2 encephalitis may present 2 weeks after birth. Brain involvement is generalized (Whitley 1997, 2006). HSV-2 encephalitis also occurs in immunosuppressed adults, e.g., HIV/AIDS. Both viruses can also cause meningitis which does not have long-term sequelae. Discussion of HSV in this chapter will focus on HSV-1 encephalitis.

In the majority of cases, HSV-1 encephalitis results from a reactivation of latent infection of the virus, usually in older patients, with only one-third of cases a primary infection, which tends to occur in younger patients under the age of 20. Primary infection with HSV-1 occurs in the oral mucosa, and may cause oral herpes or may be completely asymptomatic. The viral route into the CNS is predominantly via the trigeminal nerve to cause latent infection in the trigeminal ganglion. Other case studies have suggested routes via the olfactory bulb, consistent with the temporal and orbitofrontal localization of the virus evident on magnetic resonance imaging (MRI) and in autopsy studies. Animal studies suggest that the potency of the virus is linked to its ability to replicate within specific areas of the brain (Stroop and Schaefer 1989). Why reactivation of latent infection occurs in immunocompetent patients is unknown.

Diagnosis

Abnormalities in the CSF are typical of viral encephalitis, with a lymphocytic pleocytosis (5–100 cells/mL), a moderately elevated protein (0.6–1.0g/L) and a normal or only mildly reduced glucose. Very early in the course of the illness, CSF white cells may be only mildly elevated, or show a preponderance of neutrophils. The CSF red cell count is usually normal,

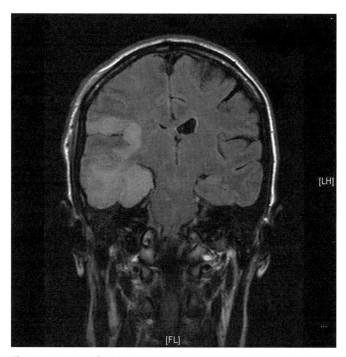

Fig. 67.1. Coronal fluid-attenuated inversion recovery (FLAIR) MRI brain scan demonstrating extensive T2-weighted high signal in the right temporal lobe and insula in a 45-year-old man with HSV-1 encephalitis. (Image courtesy of Dr. Philip Anslow).

but may be markedly elevated as HSV-1 can occasionally be hemorrhagic (Solomon *et al.* 2007). As described previously, amplification of viral nucleic acids from CSF, via PCR, is the non-invasive diagnostic test of choice. PCR has a >95% sensitivity and specificity for HSV-1, but it may be negative in the first few days of the illness. Therefore, if the clinical suspicion is high, treatment should continue, and PCR of the CSF should be repeated after a few days. The CSF PCR can also be negative late in the illness, i.e., after 10 days. In this circumstance, should there be strong clinical suspicion; the CSF can be tested for immunoglobulin (IgG and IgM) antibodies against HSV-1 (Solomon *et al.* 2007).

Imaging

Computed tomography (CT) is often normal in the first week of illness, but may show subtle swelling or low density in the frontotemporal region(s). The neuroradiological investigation of choice is MRI, and typical findings include high signal intensities, edema, hemorrhage, and localized loss of gray/white matter differentiation in temporal lobes, insula cortex, and cingulated cortex (Fig. 67.1). However, even MRI can be normal if performed very early. Diffusion-weighted MRI may be particularly useful in demonstrating early changes (Solomon *et al.* 2007).

Electroencephalography

Although the electroencephalogram (EEG) is abnormal in most patients with HSV-encephalitis, only 40% present with seizures during the acute infection (Labar 1997). The EEG patterns change over the course of the illness. The most common finding is that of diffuse high-amplitude slowing over the temporal regions. However, early EEG changes may include focal temporal or lateralized polymorphic delta activity with paroxysmal lateralizing epileptiform discharges (PLEDS) repeating at intervals of 1–5 s over the temporal regions, usually within 4 weeks of disease onset. These complexes may be unilateral or bilateral, synchronous or asynchronous, and are usually concordant with the extent of the pathology on the affected side (Whitley 1997). These discharges were once thought to be diagnostic of HSV-encephalitis, but are now known to be present in other conditions including stroke, tumor, traumatic brain injury, and dysplasia.

Treatment

The nucleoside analog acyclovir 10 mg/kg every 8 hr for 14 days is the antiviral treatment of choice. Some advocate treatment for up to 21 days in severe cases as relapses have been reported after cessation of treatment (Yamada *et al.* 2003). Hydration should be maintained and renal function monitored because of the small risk of renal failure.

The management of seizures during the acute infection may be a critical factor in the long-term prognosis of the patient. Animal studies have demonstrated that highly epileptogenic strains of HSV are associated with high mortality rates in rats. However, the mortality rates were halved in rats who were administered phenobarbital, following infection with the same strain (Schlitt 1988). Clinical studies also suggest that patients with a greater extent of parenchymal damage are more vulnerable to acute symptomatic seizures (Kim *et al.* 2008). These studies emphasize the poor prognosis associated with uncontrolled comorbid seizures during the acute infection, as well as emphasizing the need for aggressive anticonvulsant therapy.

Prognosis

Untreated HSV-1 encephalitis carries a mortality rate of up to 70%. Mortality rates remain high at 20% in treated patients, but these rates vary by region and are associated with the duration of illness prior to commencement of treatment. However, even following appropriate early treatment mortality rates still approach 10% (Labar 1997). Morbidity rates are high and over 60% of surviving patients will continue to have significant neurological and neuropsychological problems following resolution of the acute infection. Younger patients and those who present within 4 days of the onset of the infection, with minimal neurological disturbance at the commencement of treatment, tend to have the best prognosis.

Neuropsychological sequelae are a significant concern for many patients. A profound anterograde amnesic syndrome is a rare but catastrophic complication associated with bilateral destruction of the mesial temporal lobe structures (Baxendale 1998). More commonly, the disruption of memory functions associated with the mesial temporal lobe structures, and executive functions associated with damage to frontal regions, leave many without any realistic prospects of returning to their premorbid roles. Personality changes associated with frontal lobe disturbance can also be marked. Neurorehabilitation efforts should focus on helping the family and patient adjust to their new circumstances. The transition from intensive medical input to very long-term outpatient rehabilitation can be difficult for many patients and their families to manage, leading to frustration and confusion regarding recovery. Having been very ill and often close to death, patients and their families can associate survival with anticipated full recovery. It is important for the clinician to manage these expectations appropriately.

Chronic epilepsy may develop due to irreparable damage, particularly if the mesial temporal lobe structures are involved. Seizures may be partial seizures with frequent secondary generalization. If the damage is discrete, surgical resection may be a suitable option for some patients, but on the whole encephalitis is associated with poorer postoperative outcomes in surgical cases compared to other etiologies.

A small number of case studies in the literature have raised the possibility that ongoing chronic herpes simplex encephalitis infection may underlie subsequent medically intractable epilepsy in some patients. Whilst immunohistochemical and ultrastructural studies were negative for viral pathogens in these cases, PCR analysis revealed HSV-1 genome demonstrating the persistence of viral genome in brain parenchyma long after the initial episode of treated herpes encephalitis (Jay 1995, 1998).

Epstein–Barr virus

Epstein–Barr virus (EBV) is one of the most common human viruses. The majority of the world's population will have been infected at sometime prior to the age of 40. Infections with EBV are common in the pediatric population and rarely cause significant illness. When EBV is contracted in adolescence it results in infectious mononucleosis in one-third to one-half of all cases.

Involvement of the CNS in EBV infection is unusual but can result in encephalitis, aseptic meningitis, meningoencephalitis, and cerebellitis. The virus may be the cause in up to 5% of patients with acute encephalitis. It is seen more commonly in children, but should be particularly considered in immunocompromised adults. Interestingly, patients with EBV encephalitis do not typically show the classic symptoms of infectious mononucleosis, but tend to present with a non-specific prodrome or with seizures (Doja et al. 2006). Seizures have been reported acutely in 36–48% in pediatric series (Hung et al. 2000; Doja et al. 2006). Status epilepticus is a rare complication (Ross 1997). Although usually considered a self-limiting illness with few sequelae, death may occur, and ongoing epilepsy has been reported in some series in up to one-third of children (Domachowske et al. 1996).

Human herpesvirus 6

Like EBV, human herpesvirus 6 (HHV-6) is extremely prevalent in the population worldwide. Primary infection with HHV-6B is a common disease of childhood causing fever, irritability, cough, and the classic rash known as roseola infantum. Symptoms usually settle spontaneously. However, HHV-6 has been associated with febrile convulsions in children under the age of 5, occurring in up to 10% of infected children. A prospective study of children presenting to a hospital emergency department found that HHV-6 infection was associated with one-third of all febrile seizures in children up to 2 years old (Hall 1994). Approximately one-third of children who have a febrile seizure have another seizure during a subsequent febrile illness, but only 2% of children whose first seizure is associated with fever will go on to develop epilepsy (Fenichel 1997). In a follow-up study spanning 2–4 years, Rantala et al. (1990) found that children with a history of febrile convulsions in the context of a proven viral infection had no more recurrences than those without any proven infection. Occasionally HHV-6 encephalitis occurs in non-immunocompromised children. However, as with CMV and VZV, immunocompromised patients are much more susceptible to developing encephalitis, either as an acute infection (usually seen in transplant patients), as well as reactivation of latent infection (seen more often in patients with HIV) (Dockrell et al. 1999). Seizures occur commonly as part of the encephalitic illness. Recommended treatment is with ganciclovir and foscarnet. Mortality is high in these immunocompromised patient groups, over 50%, but there are few published data on long-term morbidity and the incidence of long-term epilepsy.

Cytomegalovirus

Cytomegalovirus (CMV) encephalitis is a significant opportunistic infection in HIV-infected patients, second only to HIV encephalitis in prevalence in this patient group. It is rarely seen in immunocompetent groups, although a study by Studahl et al. (1994) suggests that CMV encephalitis in the normal host may be more common than previously suspected. Transmission can occur via blood transfusion or donor organs. In otherwise healthy individuals, the infection manifests itself with a febrile illness and headache, followed by confusion, dysphasia, seizures, cranial nerve palsies, and eventual coma. Cytomegalovirus radiculitis may also occur, which may give a clue to the diagnosis. During the acute phase MRI may show periventricular enhancement (ventriculitis) and increased signal in the subcortical areas of the frontal and parietal regions on a T2-weighted image.

Cytomegalovirus encephalitis can be prolonged and complicated by seizures during the acute infection. Neuropsychological deficits are common, with language and memory problems the most common complaints. Whilst immunocompetent patients usually recover well and ongoing seizures are uncommon, immunocompromised patients surviving an acute episode can be left with complex long-term neurological problems, including epilepsy (Griffiths 1997). Chronic epilepsy occurs in 20–25% of children with symptomatic congenital CMV, and may be associated with hearing loss, microcephaly, and learning disability (Stagno 1996).

Nucleosides are the only true antiviral agents active against CMV. The antiviral therapy of choice for CMV encephalitis remains ganciclovir and the pyrophosphate analogue foscarnet. Cidofovir could also be considered.

Varicella–zoster virus

Varicella–zoster virus (VZV) is second only to HSV as a common cause of viral encephalitis, and has an incidence of 1 in 2000 infected persons, most commonly infants and adults. Encephalitis can occur as part of the acute varicella (commonly known as chickenpox) infection in non-immunocompromised patients, with encephalitic symptoms of fever, headache, altered mental state, etc. occurring a week after the onset of the vesicular rash. Herpes varicella–Zoster encephalitis can also occur as a reactivation of latent infection (commonly known as shingles, usually reactivating years after the initial varicella infection), particularly in immunocompromised patients, when the typical skin rash may not necessarily occur. Focal neurological signs may occur, and seizures occur acutely in 29–52% of cases. Cerebellitis and viral meningitis may also occur. Direct viral invasion and autoimmune-mediated vasculitis are the two major mechanisms leading to VZV encephalitis (Hausler et al. 2002). Accordingly MRI may show vasculitic ischemic lesions, with discrete non-enhancing subcortical areas of high signal which subsequently may enhance and then coalesce. The diagnosis should therefore be considered in the presence of subcortical lesions, even in the absence of typical skin lesions. Temporal lobe abnormalities may also occur.

Treatment is with intravenous acyclovir using the same regime as with herpes simplex encephalitis. Corticosteroids are also recommended because of the significant vasculitic component of the disease (Hausler et al. 2002; Solomon et al. 2007). In immunodeficient patients with VZV reactivation, acyclovir can prevent the skin rash but may not prevent the neurologic complications of VZV encephalitis.

Encephalitis due to VZV has a reported mortality rate of up to 15% in immunocompetent patients and is significantly higher in immunosuppressed patients (Hausler et al. 2002).

RNA viruses

Measles

Measles is still endemic in countries where immunisation is limited. Involvement of the CNS, even in uncomplicated measles, is common. Measles encephalitis and the late complications of measles, subacute sclerosing panencephalitis, still occur in relatively high numbers in school-age children.

Measles encephalitis occurs in 1 in 1000 cases of measles. Encephalitis usually develops within 1 week after the onset of measles although encephalitis may occasionally occur during

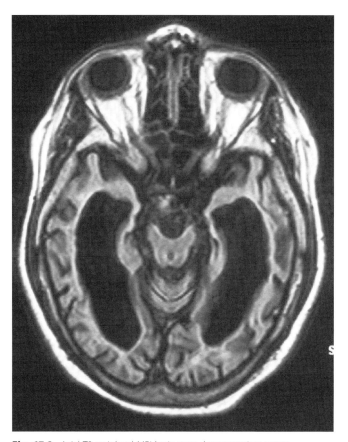

Fig. 67.2. Axial T2-weighted MRI brain scan demonstrating severe global cerebral atrophy in a 10-year-old child with SSPE. (Image courtesy of Dr. Philip Anslow).

the prodromal stage and has been reported up to 3 weeks after the onset of the characteristic measles rash. The mortality rate is approximately 15%. Approximately one in three survivors are left with residual neurological sequelae including epilepsy and cognitive difficulties (Cherry 2004; Moss et al. 2004; Perry and Halsey 2004).

The CSF findings in measles encephalitis include mild pleocytosis. Measles antibodies are absent.

Subacute sclerosing panencephalitis (SSPE) is a rare, progressive degenerative condition that occurs in 1 in 100 000 cases of measles. It affects children and young adults approximately 7 years after the primary infection. Disease progression can be highly variable but usually results in death 1–3 years following onset. The syndrome is characterized by severe myoclonic epilepsy, progressive dementia, and motor deficits. The CSF has high levels of antibodies against measles virus. The MRI findings include high-signal changes in the deep white matter and severe cerebral atrophy (Tuncay et al. 1996) (Fig. 67.2).

A vaccination program with high participation rates is the most effective protection against the measles virus. Recent media scares surrounding the measles–mumps–rubella (MMR) vaccine in the UK have led to decreased participation in the childhood vaccination program leading to an increase in incidence in UK, although levels remain low at present. People exposed to the virus can be protected by the administration of human anti-measles γ-globulin within 72 hr of exposure. This is particularly important in the immunocompromised and children with other chronic debilitating diseases, who are most at risk of developing encephalitis. However, once infected, the treatment of acute measles encephalitis is focused on symptom relief. Treatment with ribavirin is recommended (Solomon et al. 2007). Effective treatments for SSPE remain elusive, although ribavirin and intraventricular interferon A have been used in some cases (Boos and Esiri 2003).

Mumps

Infection of the CNS is the most common extrasalivary gland manifestation of mumps but the severity of parotiditis does not predict CNS involvement. Mumps meningitis is relatively common, occurring in up to 10% of cases, and is usually a benign illness with no significant risk of mortality or long-term sequelae. Pleocytosis in CSF is present in approximately half of all mumps infections even in the absence of any neurological symptoms. Mumps encephalitis is rare, occurring in 0.1% of cases, and is signaled by the presence of seizures, pronounced changes in the level of consciousness, or focal neurological symptoms. Mortality associated with mumps encephalitis is low (about 1.5%), and long-term morbidity is rare although occasionally hydrocephalus due to ependymal cell involvement can occur. Sensorineural deafness is a well-known complication, but occurs in less than 1 per 20 000 cases. Epilepsy and cognitive problems have been reported infrequently. Unfavorable outcomes are more common in adults than in children and in men than women (Hviid et al. 2008).

Influenza

Both influenza A and B are associated with febrile convulsions and a risk of encephalitis, although influenza A more predominantly so. The influenza A virus is associated with febrile convulsions in approximately 20% of children hospitalized with influenza A. The risk of febrile convulsion in influenza A appears higher than parainfluenza or adenovirus infection. Risks of multiple recurrent seizures within the illness also appear to be increased in influenza A infection, but the long-term risks of epilepsy associated with complex febrile convulsions in the context of influenza A infection are unknown (Chiu 2001).

Encephalitis is relatively uncommon, but when it occurs it usually affects children under the age of 5, although young adults may also be affected. It has usually been described during epidemics or outbreaks of influenza. Rates of mortality (up to 31%) and morbidity (27–50%) are high.

No discussion of RNA viruses and seizure risk would be complete without a word on vaccines. Whilst the MMR vaccination increases the risk of febrile seizures for 2 weeks following the inoculation, the absolute risk remains small, even in children with other predisposing factors. Whilst febrile seizures are associated with an increased risk of epilepsy that reaches well into adulthood, febrile seizures are common and are associated with a benign outcome for the vast majority of children (Vestergaard and Christensen).

Enteroviruses

Human enteroviruses include the polioviruses, coxsackieviruses, echoviruses, and enterovirus 71. These viruses are transmitted by the fecal–oral route and CNS spread is through the hematogenous route. The viruses normally replicate in the gastrointestinal (GI) tract, where the infection results in mild GI disorder. Following the viremic phase the virus may target specific organs such as the spinal cord, brain, meninges, myocardium, or skin. Incubation periods are varied and range from 2 to 40 days, with children and young adults most at risk. All human enteroviruses are associated with aseptic meningitis. Coxsackievirus meningitis is seen most frequently in preschool children. Fortunately, complete recovery is the norm, in contrast to polioviruses. Enterovirus 71 is associated with severe CNS involvement with paralyses similar to those seen in poliovirus and is discussed in detail in Chapter 75. Febrile seizures and status epilepticus are associated with the acute febrile illness in a substantial number of patients following CNS invasion by enteroviruses. The enterovirus is usually detectable by PCR of CSF of infected patients (Hosoya 1997). Treatment with intravenous administration of specific immunoglobulin has limited value in eradicating the virus from the CSF, but is used in the treatment of severely affected children, although there is limited evidence for its efficacy (Steiner et al. 2005).

Although recovery rates are generally good, damage to the hypothalamic–pituitary axis can result in long-term endocrine disturbance. Neurological sequelae including cognitive disturbance and recurrent seizures, largely depend on the extent and site of cerebral damage associated with the encephalitis.

Arenaviruses

Arenaviruses are associated with rodents, their natural hosts. Numerous arenaviuses have been isolated from various rodents without any evidence of transmission to humans. Arenaviruses that can cause human infection include lymphocytic choriomeningitis virus (LCMV) and Lassa virus. They are transmitted to humans by contact with feces/urine from infected rodents or via dust containing infective particles. Human-to-human transmission has been documented in transplant cases, and occasional outbreaks from laboratories handling the viruses have been reported in the past (Peter 2005).

Lymphocytic choriomeningitis virus occurs in North and South America and Europe, with seroprevalence of 2–4%. Its natural host is the common house mouse. Whilst approximately one-third of infections are subclinical, half may have some neurological involvement. The course of the disease is biphasic. In the first 3–5 days the patient may present with a non-specific flu-like illness with fever, a headache, lymphadenopathy, and a maculopapular rash. After 1 week, symptoms may progress to a more severe headache, photophobia, neck stiffness, and vomiting consistent with meningitis. More overt encephalitis with seizures and confusion may occur during this stage. Overall mortality rates are less than 1%, but higher in those who develop LCMV encephalitis (Peters 2005, 2006). Patients with severe disease tend to be immunocompromised patients. Studies of CSF demonstrate lymphocytic pleocytosis with elevated protein, and the virus can be cultured from the CSF or blood. Using IgM enzyme-linked immunosorbent assay (ELISA) and PCR methods LCMV may also be detected in CSF. The virus is highly teratogenic and results in fetal loss in one-third of cases of maternal transmission. Over 80% of surviving infants have neurodevelopmental disorders, including cerebral palsy, seizures, blindness, learning difficulties, and progressive hydrocephalus. Neuroimaging reveals hydrocephalus or intracranial periventricular calcifications in the majority of surviving infants. Cortical dysplasia may be present in infants who were exposed to the virus in the first trimester of in utero development (Peters 2005). Treatment is supportive, with no antiviral agents specifically recommended, although there is some evidence of efficacy with ribavirin.

The Lassa virus is prevalent in *Mastomys natalensis*, a rodent that has a wide distribution in sub-Saharan and West Africa. The reported incidence of human Lassa fever cases in West African countries is increased during the dry season. Like LCMV, Lassa fever usually presents with non-specific flu-like symptoms. In some cases facial edema occurs with hemorrhagic conjunctivitis, and bleeding from the nose, gums, and vagina. Neurological signs include impaired consciousness and seizures, which may progress to coma and death. Deafness also occurs, which may be permanent. A poor prognosis is associated with a high viremia and the development of encephalitis and edema. Case fatality rates range from 15% to 20% for hospitalized cases, although the overall death rate is approximately 1%. As with LCMV, the risk of fetal death is high, particularly if the infection occurs during the final trimester of pregnancy. The diagnostic tests of choice are ELISA methods on blood and CSF although the virus can be cultured. Ribavirin treatment may be an effective treatment in Lassa fever. Efficacy is increased if treatment is commenced within the first 6 days of illness. It is contraindicated in pregnancy, but may be warranted if the mother's life is at risk.

Conclusions

Viral encephalitis is associated with seizures during the acute stage of the infection (early seizures) and leads to an increased risk of the development of epilepsy (late seizures) following resolution of the illness. The mechanisms that underlie early and late seizures differ. Early seizures vary in their prognostic significance dependent on the underlying process associated with the modus operandi of specific viruses. With the exception of herpes simplex encephalitis, where risks of developing epilepsy have been documented to be as high as 60%, the incidence of late unprovoked seizures in different viral encephalitides has not been systematically evaluated, partly due to the historical difficulties in identifying and reporting viral agents (Misra *et al.* 2008).

The risk of late seizures is partly dependent on the extent and site of damage left by the virus, together with any ongoing "slow" infections. Wider applications of PCR may help to determine individual risks for some of the more common viral agents. In the meantime, it is clear that active management of early seizures during the acute phase of the infection may help to reduce the risk of developing late seizures following viral encephalitis.

References

Annegers JF, Hauser WA, Beghi E, Nicolosi A, Kurland LT (1988) The risk of unprovoked seizures after encephalitis and meningitis. *Neurology* **38**:1407–10.

Baxendale S (1998) Amnesia in temporal lobectomy patients: historical perspective and review. *Seizure* **7**:15–24.

Boos J, Esiri MM (2003) *Viral Encephalitis in Humans*. Washington, DC: ASM Press.

Cherry JD (2004) Measles virus. In: Feigin RD, Cherry JD (eds.) *Texbook of Pediatric Infectious Diseases,* 5th edn. Philadelphia, PA: WB Saunders, pp. 2283–99.

Chiu S (2001) Influenza A infection is an important cause of febrile seizures. *Pediatrics* **108**:e63.

Davies NW, Brown LJ, Gonde J, *et al.* (2005) Factors influencing PCR detection of viruses in cerebrospinal fluid of patients with suspected CNS infections. *J Neurol Neurosurg Psychiatry* **76**:82–7.

Dockrell DH, Smith TF, Paya CV (1999) Human herpesvirus-6. *Mayo Clin Proc* **74**:163–70.

Doja A, Bitnun A, Jones EL, *et al.* (2006) Pediatric Epstein–Barr virus-associated encephalitis: 10-year review. *J Child Neurol* **21**:385–91.

Domachowske JB, Cunningham CK, Cummings DL, *et al.* (1996) Acute manifestations and neurological sequelae of Epstein–Barr virus encephalitis in children. *Paediatr Infect Dis J* **15**:871–5.

Duncan JS, Shorvon S, Fish DR (1995) *Clinical Epilepsy*. London: Churchill Livingstone.

Fenichel GM (1997) *Clinical Pediatric Neurology*. Philadelphia, PA: WB Saunders.

Griffiths PD (1997) Cytomegalovirus. In: Scheld WM (ed.) *Infections of the Central Nervous System*. Philadelphia, PA: Lippincott-Raven, pp. 107–15.

Hall S (1994) Human herpesvirus 6 infection in children: a prospective study of complications and reactivation. *N Engl J Med* **331**:432–8.

Hausler M, Schaade L, Kemeny S, *et al.* (2002) Encephalitis related to primary varicella–zoster virus infection in immunocompetent children. *J Neurol Sci* **195**:111–16.

Hosoya M (1997) Detection of enterovirus by PCR and culture in CSF of children with transient neurologic complications associated with acute febrile illness. *J Infect Dis* **175**:700–3.

Hung KL, Liao HT, Tsai ML (2000) Epstein–Barr virus encephalitis in children. *Acta Paediatr Taiwan* **41**:140–6.

Hviid A, Rubin S, Muhlemann K (2008) Mumps. *Lancet* **371**:932–44.

Jay V (1995) Pathology of chronic herpes infection associated with seizure disorder: a report of HSV-1 detection by PCR. *Pediatr Pathol Lab Med* **15**:146.

Jay V (1998) Intractable seizure disorder associated with chronic herpes infection. *Childs Nerv Syst* **14**:20.

Jmor F, Emsley HC, Fischer M, Solomon T, Lewthwaite P (2008) The incidence of acute encephalitis syndrome in Western industrialised and tropical countries. *Virol J* **5**:134.

Kim MA, Park KM, Kim SE, Oh MK (2008) Acute symptomatic seizures in CNS infection. *Eur J Neurol* **15**:38–41.

Labar D (1997) Infection and inflammatory diseases. In: J Engel Jr. (ed.) *Epilepsy: A Comprehensive Textbook*. Philadelphia, PA: Lippincott-Raven, pp. 2587–96.

Misra UK, Tan CT, Kalita J (2008) Viral encephalitis and epilepsy. *Epilepsia* **49**(Suppl 6):13–18.

Mook-Kanamori B, van de Beek D, Wijdicks EF (2009) Herpes simplex encephalitis with normal initial cerebrospinal fluid examination. *J Am Geriatr Soc* **57**:1514–15.

Moss WJ, Ota MO, Griffin DE (2004) Measles: immune suppression and immune responses. *Int J Biochem Cell Biol* **26**:1380–5.

Perry RT, Halsey NA (2004) The clinical significance of measles: a review. *J Infect Dis* **189**(Suppl 1):S4–16.

Peter CJ (2005) Lymphocytic choriomeningitis, Lassa virus, and the South American hemorrhagic fever. In: Mandell GL, Bennett JE, Dolin R (eds.) *Principles and Practice of Infectious Diseases*, 6th edn. New York: Churchill Livingstone, pp. 2090–6.

Peters CJ (2006) Lymphocytic choriomeningitis virus: an old enemy up to new tricks. *N Engl J Med* **354**:2208–11.

Rantala H, Uhari M, Tuokko H (1990) Viral infections and recurrences of febrile convulsions. *J Pediatr* **116**:195–9.

Ross JP (1997) Epstein–Barr virus. In: Scheld WM (ed.) *Infections of the Central Nervous System*. Philadelphia, PA: Lippincott-Raven, pp. 117–27.

Sander JW, Hart YM, Johnson AL, Shorvon SD (1990) National General Practice Study of Epilepsy: newly diagnosed epileptic seizures in a general population. *Lancet* **336**:1267–71.

Schlitt M (1988) Neurovirulence in an experimental focal encephalitis: relationship to observed seizures. *Brain Res* **440**:298.

Solomon T, Hart IJ, Beeching NJ (2007) Viral encephalitis: a clinician's guide. *Pract Neurol* **7**:288–305.

Stagno S (1996) Cytomegalovirus. In: Weatherall DJ, Ledingham J, Warrell DA (eds.) *Oxford Textbook of Medicine*, 3rd edn, vol. 1. Oxford, UK: Oxford University Press, pp. 359–70.

Steiner I, Budka H, Chaudhuri A, et al. (2005) Viral encephalitis: a review of diagnostic methods and guidelines for management. *Eur J Neurol* **12**:331–43.

Stroop WG, Schaefer DC (1989) Neurovirulence of two clonally related HSV-1 strains in a rabbit seizure model. *J Neuropathol Exp Neurol* **48**:171–83.

Studahl M, Ricksten A, Sandberg T, et al. (1994) Cytomegalovirus infection of the CNS in non-compromised patients. *Acta Neurol Scand* **89**:451–7.

Tuncay R, Akman-Demir G, Gokvigit A, et al. (1996) MRI in subacute sclerosing panencephalitis. *Neuroradiology* **38**:636–40.

Vestergaard M, Christensen J (2009) Register-based studies on febrile seizures in Denmark. *Brain Dev* **31**:372–7.

Whitley RJ (1997) Herpes simplex virus. In: Scheld WM (ed.) *Infections of the Central Nervous System*. Philadelphia, PA: Lippincott-Raven, pp. 73–89.

Whitley RJ (2006) Herpes simplex encephalitis: adolescents and adults. *Antiviral Res* **71**:141–8.

Yamada S, Kameyama T, Nagaya S, Hashizume Y, Yoshida M (2003) Relapsing herpes simplex encephalitis: pathological confirmation of viral reactivation. *J Neurol Neurosurg Psychiatry* **74**:262–4.

Chapter

68

Bacterial meningitis and focal suppurative intracranial infections in children

Suresh S. Pujar and Richard F. M. Chin

Epilepsy is one of the most common neurological disorders of the brain. It is estimated that globally there are over 50 million people with epilepsy, 85% of whom live in developing countries, and 2.4 million new cases occur each year (World Health Organization 2005). A significant proportion of these individuals have neuropsychiatric comorbidities that can have an impact not only on their quality of life, but also on that of their family members. At least half the cases of epilepsy begin in childhood or adolescence as a result of congenital or acquired brain disorders. Of the acquired causes, central nervous system (CNS) infections are common in childhood and include bacterial meningitis, viral encephalitis, and intracranial suppurative infections such as brain abscess, subdural empyema, and cranial epidural abscess.

A true picture of the contribution of CNS infections to the incidence of epilepsy is best provided by well-designed population-based studies, but there are few such studies. In the Rochester Epidemiology project, CNS infections contributed to 3% of newly diagnosed epilepsies, a proportion roughly similar to that caused by traumatic brain injury (Annegers et al. 1996). In a systematic review of studies from sub-Saharan Africa, CNS infections were the cause of epilepsy in up to 26% of patients, suggesting that the burden of epilepsy from CNS infections is much higher in developing countries (Preux and Druet-Cabanac 2005). In addition to bacterial and viral CNS infections, high prevalence of parasitic infections such as malaria and cysticercosis account for the higher proportions in the African, Asian, and Latin American regions.

In this chapter, we will discuss the burden and the changing epidemiology of acute bacterial meningitis (ABM) and the incidence of epilepsy following ABM and intracranial abscesses in children, and identify the predictive factors, therapeutic implications, and prevention of ABM and consequent epilepsy in these conditions.

Acute bacterial meningitis
Epidemiology

There have been dramatic changes in the epidemiology of ABM in recent decades which will consequently result in changes in the epidemiology of epilepsy associated with ABM. The introduction of a vaccine against *Haemophilus influenzae* type B (HiB), which was the major pathogen causing ABM in children, has virtually eradicated this infection in the developed world. As a result, *Streptococcus pneumoniae* has become the most common pathogen beyond the neonatal period and the median age of patients with ABM has increased from 15 months to 25 years (Yogev and Guzman-Cottrill 2005). Similarly, introduction of a seven-valent pneumococcal conjugate vaccine (PCV7) has resulted in substantial reduction in invasive pneumococcal disease in the developed countries. However, an increase in infections caused by non-PCV7 serotypes of pneumococci and the emergence of penicillin and cephalosporin-resistant pneumococci are a growing concern.

The estimated incidence of ABM in children is 1.5 in 100 000 per year in developed countries and 20 in 100 000 per year in developing countries (Murthy and Prabhakar 2008). In addition, the African "meningitis belt" has frequent epidemics of meningococcal meningitis. Recent studies suggest that in the developed countries, *S. pneumoniae* and *Neisseria meningitidis* are the leading pathogens causing ABM in children. However, in the developing countries with no universal immunization against HiB, it continues to be a major pathogen causing ABM in children.

The incidence of bacterial meningitis in neonates is 0.25–1 in 1000 live births (Pong and Bradley 1999). The risk factors for developing meningitis include perinatal/intrauterine maternal infections (chorioamnionitis, endometritis, urinary tract infection), prolonged rupture of membranes, prematurity, and low birth weight. The major pathogens causing neonatal meningitis are Group B streptococci, *Escherichia coli*, *Listeria*, and other Gram-negative bacteria (Pong and Bradley 1999).

Incidence of epilepsy following acute bacterial meningitis in children

The incidence of long-term neurological sequelae following ABM is mostly determined by the presence or absence of

---

complications such as brain abscess, or infarction from raised intracranial pressure (ICP) or venous thrombosis. Most children who suffer from an episode of uncomplicated ABM have a favorable outcome, but a small proportion have long-term neurological sequelae that include epilepsy.

During the acute phase of ABM, 20–30% of children and about 40% of neonates have seizures before admission or within 2 days of hospitalization (Feigin *et al.* 1992). Case series of ABM in children from developing countries however report much higher seizure occurrence (as high as 80%) during the acute phase (Rosman *et al.* 1985). The figures for occurrence of convulsive status epilepticus (CSE) during the acute phase of ABM are not clearly reported. The risk of ABM in CSE with fever was 15–18% in a pediatric population-based study (Chin *et al.* 2005).

The 20-year risk of developing unprovoked seizures in a population-based cohort of 714 survivors of encephalitis or meningitis from Olmsted County, Minnesota, was 6.8%, of which almost all developed epilepsy (Annegers *et al.* 1988). Therefore, the incidence of unprovoked seizures and epilepsy can be regarded as similar in this population. Six out of 199 surviving patients who had bacterial meningitis (3%) developed epilepsy. The occurrence of epilepsy was 4.2 times higher than expected in this population. The corresponding observed : expected (O : E) ratios were 16.2 for encephalitis and 2.3 for aseptic meningitis. In a prospective study from England and Wales, 116 out of 1584 (7.3%) children suffering meningitis in infancy had developed epilepsy by 5 years (relative risk 2.7, 95% confidence interval [CI] 1.9 to 3.9) (Bedford *et al.* 2001). A higher proportion of children (8/47, 17%) developed epilepsy following bacterial meningitis in a 1966 birth cohort from northern Finland (Rantakallio *et al.* 1986). In a meta-analysis of 45 studies (22 prospective with prospective evaluation of outcomes, 18 retrospective with prospective evaluation of outcomes, and 5 retrospective with retrospective evaluation of outcomes) examining the outcome of bacterial meningitis in 4418 children, the mean incidence of epilepsy was 4.2% (95% CI 2.1 to 7.0) in prospective studies from developed countries and 5.0% (95% CI 3.6 to 6.8) in non-prospective cohorts or studies from developing countries (Baraff *et al.* 1993). In a recent systematic review which included 29 studies on bacterial meningitis in children, 0.9–20.6% of survivors of bacterial meningitis developed epilepsy (Carter *et al.* 2003).

The incidence of epilepsy following neonatal meningitis is reported to be 5.4–12% in prospective studies with at least 5 years' follow-up (Bedford *et al.* 2001; Stevens *et al.* 2003).

Time of development of epilepsy following acute bacterial meningitis in childhood

The majority of children who develop unprovoked seizures/epilepsy following an episode of bacterial meningitis will have their first unprovoked seizure within 5 years of the episode (Annegers *et al.* 1988; Pomeroy *et al.* 1990). In the Minnesota study, the incidence of epilepsy was 10.8 times higher than

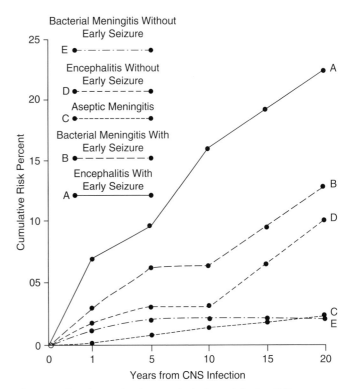

Fig. 68.1. Cumulative risks of unprovoked seizures following CNS infection. (Reproduced from Annegers *et al.* [1988] with permission.)

expected for 0–4 years follow-up, 3.8 times expected for 5–9 years follow-up, and 5.4 times expected for 10 or more years of follow-up. Assuming the association of CNS infections and epilepsy is causal, 80% of cases 10 years or more following the CNS infection were ascribable to the prior CNS infection in that study.

Predictive factors for development of epilepsy following acute bacterial meningitis in childhood

Most studies have investigated predictive factors for major neurological sequelae following ABM rather than examining predictive factors for subsequent epilepsy.

From the published studies, there is a strong association between occurrence of seizures during acute meningitis, younger age (less than 5 years), presence of persistent neurological deficits and the etiologic agent, and development of late unprovoked seizures (Annegers *et al.* 1988; Pomeroy *et al.* 1990; Baraff *et al.* 1993; Grimwood *et al.* 1996; Arditi *et al.* 1998; Akpede *et al.* 1999; Saez-Llorens and McCracken 2003; Chang *et al.* 2004). In the study from Minnesota, the risk of developing late unprovoked seizures was 11.5 times higher than expected in children with bacterial meningitis who had early seizures, compared to 2.6 in those who did not have early seizures (Annegers *et al.* 1988) (Fig. 68.1). The type of seizures during acute phase (focal or generalized) do not seem to have any influence on development of late seizures (Pomeroy *et al.* 1990; Chang *et al.* 2004). A meta-analysis examining the outcomes of bacterial meningitis in children revealed that survivors of *S. pneumoniae* meningitis had the highest incidence of long-term neurological sequelae and that of *N. meningitidis* meningitis, the lowest (Baraff *et al.* 1993). Other predictive factors for development of late seizures/neurological sequelae following ABM observed by some authors include duration of illness before diagnosis/treatment (Akpede *et al.* 1999), presence of electroencephalographic (EEG) abnormalities (Pomeroy *et al.* 1990), abnormal neuroimaging (Chang *et al.* 2004), low cerebrospinal fluid (CSF) glucose concentration (Pomeroy *et al.* 1990; Chang *et al.* 2004), high CSF protein concentration (Edwards *et al.* 1985; Chang *et al.* 2004), abnormalities in CSF leukocyte count (Edwards *et al.* 1985), altered state of consciousness, and poor perfusion during acute illness (Edwards *et al.* 1985; Chang *et al.* 2004).

Nature and prognosis of unprovoked seizures/epilepsy following acute bacterial meningitis in children

In the majority of children who develop late unprovoked seizures following ABM, the seizures are recurrent, i.e., they develop epilepsy (Annegers *et al.* 1988; Pomeroy *et al.* 1990; Chang *et al.* 2004). The seizures are commonly of a focal nature, with or without secondary generalization, though other seizure types such as generalized or myoclonic seizures may occur (Annegers *et al.* 1988; Pomeroy *et al.* 1990; Chang *et al.* 2004). The incidence of partial-onset seizures was increased 12-fold and that of generalized-onset threefold after CNS infections in the Minnesota study (Annegers *et al.* 1988).

Limited available data on the course of epilepsy after ABM from hospital-based studies suggests that about one-third of patients achieve good seizure control (fewer than two seizures per year) with one or two antiepileptic drugs (AEDs) (Pomeroy *et al.* 1990; Chang *et al.* 2004). The remainder, however, continue to have two or more seizures per year despite treatment with multiple AEDs. The prognosis of epilepsy following ABM may be comparable to that of patients with epilepsies of remote symptomatic etiology (Berg *et al.* 2001).

In a community-based cohort of 63 children with new-onset temporal lobe epilepsy from Australia, four (6%) had a history of ABM (Harvey *et al.* 1997). Of these, three had evidence of hippocampal sclerosis on magnetic resonance imaging (MRI). In a surgical series from China, 6% of patients undergoing surgery for temporal lobe lesion and 4.7% for extratemporal lobe lesion had suffered an episode of meningitis. The corresponding figures for febrile seizure were 11.4 and 0.7 (Xiao *et al.* 2004). Studies on patients undergoing surgery for refractory partial epilepsy suggest that unilateral mesial temporal sclerosis (MTS) is more frequent in children suffering from an episode of CNS infection at a younger age (<4 years) (Lancman and Morris 1996; O'Brien *et al.* 2002). There is also a suggestion that the postsurgical outcome may be favorable in a group of patients who had epilepsy following

meningitis compared to encephalitis (Marks *et al.* 1992; O'Brien *et al.* 2002).

Pathogenesis of seizure disorder following acute bacterial meningitis

Experimental work suggests that the brain injury and neuronal death due to ABM is not mediated simply by the presence of viable bacteria but occurs as a consequence of the host reaction to bacterial components (Scheld *et al.* 2002; Saez-Llorens and McCracken 2003). The host inflammatory reactions, if not modulated effectively, eventually cause alteration of CSF dynamics (brain edema, intracranial hypertension), of brain metabolism, and of cerebrovascular autoregulation (reduced cerebral blood flow). Whether or not a person suffering an episode of ABM develops neurological sequelae such as epilepsy probably depends on the maturity of the brain at the time of the insult, the severity of the brain injury, and the part of the brain affected.

There is some suggestion that children who suffer an episode of CNS infection (meningitis or encephalitis) at an early age (<4 years) have a higher frequency of MTS than children who suffer prolonged febrile convulsions (Marks *et al.* 1992; Lancman and Morris 1996; Harvey *et al.* 1997; O'Brien *et al.* 2002; Xiao *et al.* 2004). It is not clear whether MTS developing in children suffering CNS infection at an early age is the result of having status epilepticus during the acute illness, a direct effect of the etiologic agent on the hippocampi, or an immune-mediated injury due to host immune reaction to the infection. Further studies are required to understand this association and the pathogenesis.

Therapeutic implications

The changing epidemiology of bacterial meningitis and the emergence of antibiotic resistant strains of pneumococcal meningitis demand regional guidelines for initial empirical treatment of ABM based on the knowledge of regional epidemiologic factors.

Initial empirical antibiotic treatment should be administered without delay in all suspected cases of ABM. Even in cases in whom a computed tomography (CT) scan of the head is considered to exclude focal pathology in the brain, blood cultures should be collected and initial empirical antibiotics administered prior to the CT scan (Tunkel *et al.* 2004). Lumbar puncture could be performed after ruling out a focal pathology. The antibiotic treatment could be changed to target specific organisms after obtaining polymerase chain reaction (PCR) or culture and sensitivity results.

The effectiveness of administration of dexamethasone before the first effective parenteral antibiotic dose in reducing neurologic and/or audiologic sequelae in children with HiB meningitis has been demonstrated in several studies. There is however no convincing evidence on the beneficial effects of adjuvant dexamethasone in non-HiB meningitis or in children from low-income countries (Saez-Llorens and McCracken 2007). A recent study confirmed the benefit of corticosteroid therapy in adults with pneumococcal meningitis, but such evidence is lacking in children. A recent *Cochrane Review* of 20 randomized controlled trials (six from low-income and 14 from high-income countries) concluded that overall the use of adjuvant dexamethasone in ABM significantly reduced the rates of mortality, severe hearing loss, and neurological sequelae (van de Beek *et al.* 2007). Subanalysis for children in high-income countries showed a protective effect of corticosteroids on severe hearing loss overall (mostly in the HiB group), and for short-term neurological sequelae. For children in low-income countries, however, the use of corticosteroids was associated neither with benefit nor with harmful effects. The possible factors responsible for this difference in efficacy are delay in presentation, clinical severity, underlying anemia, malnutrition, the antibiotics used, and the higher incidence of positive HIV status. The conclusions of the *Cochrane Review* would suggest the use of corticosteroids in high-income countries. However, *S. pneumoniae* is now the most common pathogen in high-income countries and at present there is insufficient evidence for the benefit of corticosteroids in ABM caused by this pathogen in children. Corticosteroids on the other hand may inhibit the absorption of antibiotics (especially vancomycin) into the CSF across the blood–brain barrier (Tunkel *et al.* 2004). Therefore, a risk–benefit assessment should be weighed carefully for use of corticosteroids in ABM in children and will vary according to the geographical location and available resources.

A recent prospective, randomized, double-blind, placebo-controlled study from Latin American nations on the beneficial effects of adjuvant oral glycerol on the outcome of childhood ABM presents some encouraging results (Peltola *et al.* 2007). There is a suggestion that glycerol acts by increasing the serum osmolality resulting in reduced CSF secretion and reduced CSF volume as a consequence, enhanced water movement back to plasma by osmosis, increased cerebral blood flow, and thus improved brain oxygenation (Singhi *et al.* 2008). The most common pathogen in the Latin American study was HiB followed by *S. pneumoniae* and *N. meningitidis*. The incidence of severe neurological sequelae was significantly reduced among patients who received glycerol alone and patients who received dexamethasone–glycerol combination, whereas in the dexamethasone-alone group, no more than a tendency towards a reduction in severe neurological sequelae was observed. Also, receipt or non-receipt of pretreatment antimicrobials and the timing of their administration with respect to the initiation of an adjuvant medication did not alter the findings. The beneficial effects were best seen in the HiB meningitis group. This study assumes importance as the study population and the clinical situations represent those in low-income countries where the burden of ABM is highest. Also, glycerol can be given orally, is inexpensive and easily available, has no special storage requirements, and has no major side effects,

and therefore would be very beneficial in low-income countries. If further studies confirm that glycerol improves the prognosis of children with ABM, this would immensely influence the management of ABM in resource-poor countries and have profound effects on the long-term sequelae.

Prevention of acute bacterial meningitis
Vaccines

The most effective strategy for prevention of ABM and its sequelae is by implementing large-scale immunization against the common meningeal pathogens. Meningitis due to HiB has been virtually eradicated in countries where universal immunization is implemented. Introduction of pediatric heptavalent pneumococcal conjugate vaccine (PCV7) has resulted in substantial reduction in the rates of pneumococcal meningitis in the USA. There has however been a recent increase in meningitis caused by non-PCV7 serotypes, and the advent of new conjugated vaccines that include larger number of serotypes could help reduce this. The tetravalent (A,C,Y,W-135) meningococcal conjugate vaccine provides protection against the majority of cases of meningitis in adolescents. The majority of cases of meningococcal meningitis in infants however are caused by serotype B, for which there is no licensed vaccine available yet, but candidate vaccines are undergoing trials and should be available for use soon. Use of conjugated Group B streptococcal (GBS) vaccines could be effective in prevention of neonatal meningitis due to this organism. There is pressing need for a collaborative effort from the vaccine manufacturers, governmental and non-governmental organizations, charities, and global health organizations to ensure availability of the vaccines and effective implementation of vaccine programs in the resource-poor countries where the burden of ABM is greatest.

Chemoprophylaxis

Secondary prevention of HiB and meningococcal meningitis could be achieved by chemoprophylaxis among contacts. Intrapartum antibiotic prophylaxis given to women with prenatal vaginal or rectal GBS colonization has been associated with a significant reduction in rates of GBS meningitis in the newborns.

Brain abscess

Pyogenic intracranial abscesses are rare in children. Brain (parenchymal) abscesses are the most common followed by subdural and epidural abscesses. The overall incidence of brain abscess in a prospective population-based study from Olmsted County, Minnesota, was 1.3 in 100 000 person–years (Nicolosi *et al.* 1991). The incidence rate in children 5–9 years old was slightly higher (2.4 in 100 000 person–years). About 25% of all brain abscesses occur in children less than 15 years of age, but abscesses are rare in children between 1 month and 2 years of age (Woods 1995). Abscesses are two to three times more common in boys. Congenital cyanotic heart disease is the most common condition predisposing to brain abscess in children in developed countries, followed by sinusitis, ear infection, head trauma, and neurosurgery. In the developing countries, however, congenital cyanotic heart disease and ear infection are the commonest predisposing conditions, followed by bacterial meningitis and sinusitis. Unlike in the developing countries, brain abscess can occur as a rare complication of bacterial meningitis in the developed countries. The site of the abscess and the causative organism depend on the predisposing condition, and isolation of mixed aerobic and anaerobic organisms is not uncommon.

Brain abscesses in neonates are commonly associated with Gram-negative bacillary meningitis and multiple abscesses are often present. Group B streptococcus is the most common cause of neonatal bacterial meningitis, and E. coli and Klebsiella pneumoniae rarely cause brain abscess in neonates.

The occurrence of seizures during the acute phase of brain abscess depends on the location of the abscess. In general, 30–45% of children present with seizures (Saez-Llorens, 2003).

The incidence of epilepsy following brain abscess is difficult to assess and depends mainly on the type of study and the duration of follow-up. The reported rate of epilepsy following brain abscess ranges from as low as 3% to as high as 95%, but in most studies, including the population-based study from Minnesota, it is about 30–35% (Nicolosi et al. 1991; Kilpatrick 1997). Various predictive factors for later development of epilepsy, such as age (higher incidence in children), causative organism, and size and site of the abscess have been reported by some but not by others (Legg et al. 1973; Nielsen et al. 1983; Buonaguro et al. 1989; Kilpatrick 1997). Epilepsy is very unlikely following infratentorial abscess. Children who manifest with seizures during the acute illness are more likely to develop later epilepsy (Kilpatrick 1997). Also, those with persistent changes on CT scan following the acute episode, suggesting tissue damage, and those with more spikes and sharp waves on EEG seem to have a higher likelihood of developing epilepsy (Legg et al. 1973; Wispelwey and Scheld 1987; Aebi et al. 1991). The relationship between the nature of treatment of brain abscess and development of subsequent epilepsy is unclear. Some authors report higher incidence following treatment by excision of the abscess compared to antibiotics alone and/or aspiration, as a result of tissue damage and subsequent gliosis; however, others have not seen any difference in the two groups (Legg et al. 1973; Hirsch et al. 1983; Buonaguro et al. 1989; Aebi et al. 1991; Kilpatrick 1997).

The majority of patients develop seizures within 12–18 months following the episode of brain abscess. However, this interval can be longer especially in younger children (mean of 4.2 years in one of the studies) (Legg et al. 1973; Buonaguro et al. 1989). There is also a suggestion that the latent interval is shorter for temporal lobe abscess and longer for frontal lobe abscess (Legg et al. 1973). The seizures can be generalized, focal with or without secondary generalization, or mixed. In a study with mean follow-up of 26 years, the incidence and the severity of epilepsy was highest in the fourth and fifth years following brain abscess (Legg et al. 1973). The prognosis of epilepsy in children following brain abscess is likely to be poor as a result of brain parenchymal damage sustained during the acute phase (symptomatic epilepsy). Treatment with epilepsy surgery could be considered if a focal epileptogenic lesion is identified upon neuroimaging. These children are also more likely to have other neurologic sequelae such as hemiparesis, cranial nerve palsy, hydrocephalus, and behavioral and intellectual disorders (especially children younger than 5 years of age).

Subdural empyema

Subdural empyema, the collection of pus in the potential space between the dura and the arachnoid, is the second most common intracranial suppurative infection in children. In children, it occurs predominantly in those under 3 years or over 12 years of age. The peak incidence is in the second decade of life and the condition is more common in males. In younger children, subdural empyema usually occurs as a complication of ABM; and it develops in about 2% of infants with ABM (Woods 1995). In older children and adults, it results from contiguous spread of infection from chronic sinusitis or mastoiditis. It can rarely occur as a complication of neurosurgery. Formerly HiB was the predominant pathogen causing subdural empyema associated with ABM in the pre-HiB vaccine era, but it has now probably been replaced by S. pneumoniae.

The incidence of epilepsy and other neurological sequelae following a subdural empyema depends on the degree of parenchymal injury resulting from an associated brain abscess or infarction or from raised ICP or venous thrombosis. The morbidity and mortality is increased in those who develop complications such as venous sinus thrombosis. Epilepsy develops in about one-third of people following subdural empyema and the majority develop unprovoked seizures within a couple of years following the episode (Cowie and Williams 1983; Yogev 2003). The prognosis of epilepsy following subdural empyema is likely to be similar to that of any epilepsy of remote symptomatic etiology.

Epidural abscess

Isolated intracranial epidural abscess, the collection of pus in the potential space between the dura and the inner aspect of the cranium, is rare. It occurs almost exclusively in older children and adults. As the dura adheres tightly to the cranium, especially at the suture lines, epidural abscess rarely becomes large enough to exert pressure on the underlying brain or cause parenchymal injury. It may however serve as a focus for subdural spread of infection and is frequently associated with subdural empyema, meningitis, and/or brain abscess. Osteomyelitis of the overlying diploic bone is often present. Common predisposing conditions include sinusitis, otitis media, trauma, neurosurgical procedures, orbital cellulitis, and fetal scalp monitoring (Woods 1995).

The prognosis of uncomplicated cranial epidural abscess is excellent. The long-term neurological sequelae such as epilepsy would primarily depend on the presence of coexisting lesions such as brain abscess and subdural empyema (Yogev 2003).

Conclusion

Intracranial infections in children still make a significant contribution to the development of epilepsy, especially in resource-poor countries. This contribution can however be reduced by implementing universal immunization programmes. Bacterial meningitis, which is the commonest of CNS infections in children, is generally associated with a good long-term prognosis. Focal intracranial suppurative infections such as brain abscess and subdural empyema are uncommon in children but are associated with a higher incidence of subsequent epilepsy. There are limited data in the literature on the incidence of epilepsy following subdural empyema and

Table 68.1 Risk of developing epilepsy following acute bacterial meningitis in children and focal intracranial suppurative infections

Etiology	Risk of epilepsy
Bacterial meningitis	0.9–20.6%
Brain abscess	30–35%[a]
Subdural empyema	15–40%
Epidural abscess	Very low

Note:
[a]Best estimate as derived from population-based study, but the range may be as high as 3–95%.

hardly any following epidural abscess, possibly due to the rarity of these conditions in childhood. Most available data on the nature and clinical features of epilepsy after bacterial infection are based on hospital-based reports, and prospective, community-based studies would provide a true picture of the clinical features and extent of the long-term burden of epilepsy in these conditions.

References

Aebi C, Kaufmann F, Schaad UB (1991) Brain abscess in childhood: long-term experiences. *Eur J Pediatr* **150**:282–6.

Akpede GO, Akuhwa RT, Ogiji EO, Ambe JP (1999) Risk factors for an adverse outcome in bacterial meningitis in the tropics: a reappraisal with focus on the significance and risk of seizures. *Ann Trop Paediatr* **19**:151–9.

Annegers JF, Hauser WA, Beghi E, Nicolosi A, Kurland LT (1988) The risk of unprovoked seizures after encephalitis and meningitis. *Neurology* **38**:1407–10.

Annegers JF, Rocca WA, Hauser WA (1996) Causes of epilepsy: contributions of the Rochester epidemiology project. *Mayo Clin Proc* **71**:570–5.

Arditi M, Mason EO Jr., Bradley JS, et al. (1998) Three-year multicenter surveillance of pneumococcal meningitis in children: clinical characteristics, and outcome related to penicillin susceptibility and dexamethasone use. *Pediatrics* **102**:1087–97.

Baraff LJ, Lee SI, Schriger DL (1993) Outcomes of bacterial meningitis in children: a meta-analysis. *Pediatr Infect Dis J* **12**:389–94.

Bedford H, De LJ, Halket S, et al. (2001) Meningitis in infancy in England and Wales: follow up at age 5 years. *Br Med J* **323**:533–6.

Berg AT, Shinnar S, Levy SR, et al. (2001) Two-year remission and subsequent relapse in children with newly diagnosed epilepsy. *Epilepsia* **42**:1553–62.

Buonaguro A, Colangelo M, Daniele B, Cantone G, Ambrosio A (1989) Neurological and behavioral sequelae in children operated on for brain abscess. *Childs Nerv Syst* **5**:153–5.

Carter JA, Neville BG, Newton CR (2003) Neuro-cognitive impairment following acquired central nervous system infections in childhood: a systematic review. *Brain Res Brain Res Rev* **43**:57–69.

Chang CJ, Chang HW, Chang WN, et al. (2004) Seizures complicating infantile and childhood bacterial meningitis. *Pediatr Neurol* **31**:165–71.

Chin RFM, Neville BGR, Scott RC (2005) Meningitis is a common cause of convulsive status epilepticus with fever. *Arch Dis Childh* **90**:66–9.

Cowie R, Williams B (1983) Late seizures and morbidity after subdural empyema. *J Neurosurg* **58**:569–73.

Edwards MS, Rench MA, Haffar AA, et al. (1985) Long-term sequelae of group B streptococcal meningitis in infants. *J Pediatr* **106**:717–22.

Feigin RD, McCracken GH Jr., Klein JO (1992) Diagnosis and management of meningitis. *Pediatr Infect Dis J* **11**:785–814.

Grimwood K, Nolan TM, Bond L, et al. (1996) Risk factors for adverse outcomes of bacterial meningitis. *J Paediatr Child Health* **32**:457–62.

Harvey AS, Berkovic SF, Wrennall JA, Hopkins IJ (1997) Temporal lobe epilepsy in childhood: clinical, EEG, and neuroimaging findings and syndrome classification in a cohort with new-onset seizures. *Neurology* **49**:960–8.

Hirsch JF, Roux FX, Sainte-Rose C, Renier D, Pierre-Kahn A (1983) Brain abscess in childhood: a study of 34 cases treated by puncture and antibiotics. *Childs Brain* **10**:251–65.

Kilpatrick C (1997) Epilepsy and brain abscess. *J Clin Neurosci* **4**:26–8.

Lancman ME Morris HH III (1996) Epilepsy after central nervous system infection: clinical characteristics and outcome after epilepsy surgery. *Epilepsy Res* **25**:285–90.

Legg NJ, Gupta PC, Scott DF (1973) Epilepsy following cerebral abscess: a clinical and EEG study of 70 patients. *Brain* **96**:259–68.

Marks DA, Kim J, Spencer DD, Spencer SS (1992) Characteristics of intractable seizures following meningitis and encephalitis. *Neurology* **42**:1513–18.

Murthy JM, Prabhakar S (2008) Bacterial meningitis and epilepsy. *Epilepsia* **49**(Suppl 6):8–12.

Nicolosi A, Hauser WA, Musicco M, Kurland LT (1991) Incidence and prognosis of brain abscess in a defined population: Olmsted County, Minnesota, 1935–1981. *Neuroepidemiology* **10**:122–31.

Nielsen H, Harmsen A, Gyldensted C (1983) Cerebral abscess: a long-term follow-up. *Acta Neurol Scand* **67**:330–7.

O'Brien TJ, Moses H, Cambier D, Cascino GD (2002) Age of meningitis or encephalitis is independently predictive of outcome from anterior temporal lobectomy. *Neurology* **58**:104–9.

Peltola H, Roine I, Fernandez J, *et al.* (2007) Adjuvant glycerol and/or dexamethasone to improve the outcomes of childhood bacterial meningitis: a prospective, randomized, double-blind, placebo-controlled trial. *Clin Infect Dis* **45**:1277–86.

Pomeroy SL, Holmes SJ, Dodge PR, Feigin RD (1990) Seizures and other neurologic sequelae of bacterial meningitis in children. *N Engl J Med* **323**:1651–7.

Pong A, Bradley JS (1999) Bacterial meningitis and the newborn infant. *Infect Dis Clin N Am* **13**:711–33.

Preux PM, Druet-Cabanac M (2005) Epidemiology and etiology of epilepsy in sub-Saharan Africa. *Lancet Neurol* **4**:21–31.

Rantakallio P, Leskinen M, von Wendt L (1986) Incidence and prognosis of central nervous system infections in a birth cohort of 12 000 children. *Scand J Infect Dis* **18**:287–94.

Rosman NP, Peterson DB, Kaye EM, Colton T (1985) Seizures in bacterial meningitis: prevalence, patterns, pathogenesis, and prognosis. *Pediat Neurol* **1**:278–85.

Saez-Llorens X (2003) Brain abscess in children. *Semin Pediatr Infect Dis* **14**:108–14.

Saez-Llorens X, McCracken GH Jr. (2003) Bacterial meningitis in children. *Lancet* **361**:2139–48.

Saez-Llorens X, McCracken GH Jr. (2007) Glycerol and bacterial meningitis. *Clin Infect Dis* **45**:1287–9.

Scheld WM, Koedel U, Nathan B, Pfister HW (2002) Pathophysiology of bacterial meningitis: mechanism(s) of neuronal injury. *J Infect Dis* **186**(Suppl 2):S225–33.

Singhi S, Jarvinen A, Peltola H (2008) Increase in serum osmolality is possible mechanism for the beneficial effects of glycerol in childhood bacterial meningitis. *Pediatr Infect Dis J* **27**:892–6.

Stevens JP, Eames M, Kent A, *et al.* (2003) Long term outcome of neonatal meningitis. *Arch Dis Child Fetal Neonatal Ed* **88**:F179–84.

Tunkel AR, Hartman BJ, Kaplan SL, *et al.* (2004) Practice guidelines for the management of bacterial meningitis. *Clin Infect Dis* **39**:1267–84.

Van de Beek D, GJ, McIntyre P, Prasad K (2007) Corticosteroids for acute bacterial meningitis. *Cochrane Database Syst Rev* Jan 24:CD004405.

Wispelwey B, Scheld WM (1987) Brain abscess. *Clin Neuropharmacol* **10**:483–510.

Woods CR Jr. (1995) Brain abscess and other intracranial suppurative complications. *Adv Pediatr Infect Dis* **10**:41–79.

World Health Organization (2005) *Epilepsy Care in the World 2005*. Available online at www.who.int/mental_health/neurology/Epilepsy_atlas/

Xiao B, Huang ZL, Zhang H, *et al.* (2004) Etiology of epilepsy in surgically treated patients in China. *Seizure* **13**:322–7.

Yogev R (2003) Focal suppurative infections of the central nervous system. In: Long S, Pickering L, Prober C (eds.) *Principles and Practice of Pediatric Infectious Diseases*, 2nd edn. Philadelphia, PA: Churchill Livingstone, pp. 302–11.

Yogev R, Guzman-Cottrill J (2005) Bacterial meningitis in children: critical review of current concepts. *Drugs* **65**:1097–112.

Chapter

69

Bacterial meningitis and pyogenic abscess in adults

Lina Nashef and Fahmida A. Chowdhury

Definitions and epidemiology

Bacterial meningitis

Bacterial meningitis is infection of the nervous system confined to the meninges and subarachnoid space. It is nowadays in the Western world most commonly caused by *Neisseria meningitidis* and *Streptococcus pneumoniae* (Schut *et al.* 2008).

The estimated incidence of bacterial meningitis in adults in developed countries ranges from 0.6 to 6 per 100 000 adults per year, possibly up to ten times higher in the developing world (Weisfelt *et al.* 2006; Fitch and Van der Beek 2007). Worldwide, it is estimated that at least 890 000 cases of bacterial meningitis occur annually (500 000 in Africa, 210 000 in Asia, 100 000 in Europe, and 80 000 in the Americas) (Tikhomirov *et al.* 1997).

Pyogenic abscess (cerebral, epidural, and subdural)

Cranial suppurative disorders include (1) intracranial abscesses (which constitute the majority of these disorders in the developed world) and (2) subdural empyemas (commonly seen where otorhinological infections are neglected) and, less commonly, epidural (extradural) empyemas. These disorders occur with contiguous purulent spread, hematogenous/metastatic spread, head trauma, neurosurgical procedures, and immunosuppression (Ersin and Cansever 2008). Most series report mainly on brain abscesses. These occur at any age, with males more often affected. Incidence is higher in developing countries. In the classic Mayo Clinic study of residents of Olmsted County, Minnesota, from 1935 to 1981, based on 38 cases, nine diagnosed at autopsy, the overall incidence of brain abscess was 1.3 per 100 000 person–years (1.9 in males, 0.6 females). The incidence was higher in children and in those over 60 years old and decreased over the period of the study. Mortality was 38%. Of 18 survivors, five had epilepsy (Nicolosi *et al.* 1991). The demography, case mix, and outcome (see below) have changed since this landmark study. There is a reported decrease in incidence in developed countries (Nicolosi *et al.* 1991; Sharma *et al.* 2009). Older series reported brain abscess to be particularly common in children with otitis media. While sinus disease is still a cause, particularly amongst teenagers and young adults, in more recent series, the incidence of brain abscess secondary to congenital heart disease and otitis media is lower, while that related to immunosuppression, trauma, or neurosurgery is higher. Series from South Africa focus on empyemas seen between 1983 and 1997 (Nathoo *et al.* 1999a, b, 2001), with subdural (699) and epidural empyemas (82) accounting respectively for 15% and 2% of all admissions for intracranial sepsis.

Pathology, physiology, and clinical features of disease

Bacterial meningitis

Neisseria meningitidis and *Streptococcus pneumoniae* cause 80% of all cases in the Western world (Van de Beek 2006). Less common causes in adults include *Listeria monocytogenes*, *Staphylococcus aureus*, Enterobacteriaceae, and *Mycobacterium tuberculosis* (Stoll 1997; Tikhomirov *et al.* 1997). Mycobacterial infections are discussed in Chapter 73.

Bacteria reach the meninges through direct contact between the meninges and the nasal cavity or skin or by hematogenous spread. Bacteria colonize the mucosal surfaces, cross the epithelium, and spread via the bloodstream to the choroid plexus, where they cross the blood–brain barrier into the subarachnoid space. Direct contamination of the cerebrospinal fluid (CSF) may also occur from indwelling devices and skull fractures. The majority of pathogens are capsulated bacteria which resist phagocytosis and complement mediated bactericidal activity in the bloodstream. Bacterial products in the subarachnoid space cause an inflammatory response within hours by triggering the release of proinflammatory cytokines that upregulate adhesion molecules on endothelial cells and promote granulocyte penetration into the CSF, leading to further release of inflammatory mediators. Increased vascular permeability causes vasogenic cerebral edema. Toxins released from bacteria and granulocytes result in loss of cellular homeostasis and further cerebral edema. This

The Causes of Epilepsy, eds. S. D. Shorvon, F. Andermann, and R. Guerrini. Published by Cambridge University Press. © Cambridge University Press 2011.

together with systemic hypotension and reduced perfusion leads to apoptosis of cerebral neurons and glia. Purulent exudates can also obstruct the normal flow of the CSF and cause hydrocephalus.

The most common symptoms of meningitis are headache, photophobia, phonophobia, nausea, and vomiting (Schut *et al.* 2008). The main signs are fever, reduced conscious level, and signs of meningism, such as nuchal rigidity, Brudzinski's sign (flexion of the neck causing involuntary flexion of the knee and hip), and Kernig's sign (pain provoked by attempting to extend the knee with the hip flexed). Signs of meningism have poor sensitivity (5%) but high specificity (95%). In a large study, only two-thirds of patients had the classic triad of fever, meningism, and change in mental status, but all had at least one of these findings (Durand *et al.* 1993). Meningitis caused by meningococci may be accompanied by a characteristic rash. Symptoms can develop over several hours or 2 to 3 days. Severe bacterial meningitis may also be associated with cerebral edema, raised intracranial pressure and seizures. In some patients, notably neonates and infants (see Chapter 68), immunocompromised patients and the very old, signs are often more subtle. Complications of bacterial meningitis include hearing loss, mental retardation, paralysis, and seizures.

Suppurative intracranial disorders

Pyogenic bacterial abscesses can be single or multiple. Most are supratentorial. The frontal lobe is most commonly affected followed by temporal or parietal lobes. Local pathology includes sinusitis, mastoiditis, orbital or dental sepsis, trauma with dural tear, or neurosurgery. Spread occurs from contiguous local infection; for example, frontal sinusitis leads to frontal empyema or abscess formation, mastoiditis to temporal or cerebellar infection, while infection in the sphenoid sinus can spread to the cavernous sinus. With hematogenous or metastatic spread, more common in recent years, abscesses can be multiple, often involve middle cerebral artery territory, and are associated with a higher mortality. Predisposing conditions include intravenous drug use, septicemia, heart disease (e.g., cyanotic congenital heart disease and/or bacterial endocarditis), diabetes, alcoholism, bronchiectasis, pulmonary arteriovenous shunts, gastrointestinal sepsis, and immune suppression such as in oncology, HIV, and organ transplantation. With immunosuppression, atypical abscesses are more common. In a significant minority of abscesses, no cause is identified. With empyemas, which may coexist with brain abscess, young male patients in the second or third decade of life are the most commonly affected and local infections are usually the cause. Which bacterial pathogens are implicated depends on the origin of the sepsis with two or three species of bacteria often isolated, most commonly: *Streptococcus anginosus* group (formerly *Streptococcus milleris*); anaerobes especially *Bacteroides* spp.; Enterobacteriaceae (that is coliforms such as *Escherichia coli*, *Klebsiella* spp.); *Staphylococcus aureus*; and various species of *Haemophilus*. With postneurosurgical

implants, very commonly coagulase-negative staphylococci such as *Staphylococcus epidermidis* are isolated as are *Staphylococcus aureus* and Enterobacteriaceae. Microbiology is discussed further in the section on treatment.

Untreated brain abscess was often fatal. Outcome improved with surgical drainage and antibiotic treatment. Cranial imaging, leading to earlier detection, reduced mortality from 40–60%, prior to the era of computed tomography (CT) scanning, to 10%. However, it has risen again since 2000 to between 17% and 32% with changes in demographics and case mix (Ersin and Cansever 2008). Poor prognostic factors include immunocompromise, comorbidities, lower Glasgow Coma Scale (GCS) scores at presentation, pretreatment neurological status, and intraventricular rupture. Residual neurological deficit, cognitive dysfunction, and epilepsy are long-term consequences. Subdural empyema is also potentially fatal with 12% mortality in one series (Nathoo *et al.* 1999a). Mortality was around 1% with epidural empyemas (Nathoo *et al.* 1999b).

With intracranial abscess, a localized area of cerebritis develops into a collection of pus with a well-vascularized capsule and surrounding gliosis, immune reaction, and swelling. Recognized stages include: early and late cerebritis, and early and late capsule formation. Intracranial sepsis predisposes to venous sinus thrombosis. Cranial suppurative disorders present commonly with headache, altered mental state, nausea and vomiting, pyrexia, or seizures with neurological symptoms and signs depending on the site of the lesion. Signs of systemic infection may be absent, with fever of more than 38.5°C reported in 20–55% of patients. The classical triad in brain abscess of headache, fever, and neurological deficit is seen in some 15–30% of cases. In those without evidence of sepsis, more rapid deterioration favors abscess over tumor. Intraventricular rupture, a risk with deep-seated lesions, is a devastating complication. Other clinical features, often seen with empyemas, include neck stiffness, periorbital edema or cellulitis, purulent nasal/aural discharge or "Pott's puffy tumor" (subgaleal abscess, an abscess in the potential space between the skull periosteum and the scalp galea aponeurosis) (Nathoo *et al.* 1999a, b).

Epilepsy in the disease

A distinction is made between acute (provoked) and remote symptomatic seizures/epilepsy. In general, acute symptomatic seizures due to neurological insults increase the risk for unprovoked seizures/epilepsy, this risk being less than the risk of a second seizure following an unprovoked seizure. The risk of later seizures/epilepsy is much higher with status epilepticus (Singh and Prabhakar 2008a, b).

Bacterial meningitis
Frequency of epilepsy
Acute seizures

In developed countries, the risk of provoked seizures (acute symptomatic) in adults ranges from 7% to 27% (Durand *et al.*

483

1993; Wang *et al.* 2005; Weisfelt *et al.* 2006; Zoons *et al.* 2008). In developing countries, the high incidence of seizures/epilepsy is thought to be partly attributable to central nervous system (CNS) infections (ILAE 1994), but there are very few prospective community based studies. In one study in Swaziland, 19% of patients with bacterial meningitis had provoked seizures (Ford and Wright 1994). These early seizures are a sign of severe disease, and a poorer prognosis, with a significant association between seizures and mortality as well as neurological sequelae.

Chronic epilepsy

In developed countries, the risk of unprovoked seizures/epilepsy was 6.8% in a population-based adult cohort of survivors of meningitis (Annegers *et al.* 1988). In the Rochester study, 3% of newly diagnosed epilepsies were attributed to prior CNS infection compared to 11% and 4% to cerebrovascular disease and traumatic brain injury respectively (Hauser and Kurland 1975). Retrospective studies in developing countries reported that CNS infections are responsible for between 5.2% and 26% of epilepsies; 5.2% in a hospital-based study in Equador (Carpio *et al.* 2001), 10.6% in a Chilean study (Lavados *et al.* 1992), 24.5% in a hospital-based study in South India (Murthy and Yangala 1998), and 26% in sub-Saharan Africa (Preux and Druet-Cabanac 2005).

Risk factors for seizures/epilepsy in the disease

Acute seizures

Reported associated factors, some not consistent across studies, include the following.

1. Increased age (Zoons *et al.* 2008).
2. Reduced consciousness on admission (Wang *et al.* 2005; Zoons *et al.* 2008).
3. Abnormal investigations. Abnormal neuroimaging and CSF findings (low glucose and high protein) and increased erythrocyte sedimentation rate (ESR) were associated with acute seizures (Zoons *et al.* 2008). Evidence of electroencephalogram (EEG) abnormalities was also associated with early seizures in another study which, conversely, reported no relationship between seizures and neuroimaging abnormalities (Wang *et al.* 2005).
4. Etiological agent. Two studies reported *Streptococcus pneumoniae* as the causal agent in a higher percentage of patients with seizures than without (58% vs. 30%: Durand *et al.* 1993; and 79% vs. 46%: Zoons *et al.* 2008). However, another study found no significant relation between causative pathogens and seizures (Wang *et al.* 2005).

Chronic epilepsy

The probability of developing epilepsy following meningitis has been associated with the following.

1. Acute provoked seizures during the acute illness. The 20-year risk of developing unprovoked seizures/epilepsy after bacterial meningitis was found to be 13% for those

with early seizures, and 2.4% for those without (Annegers *et al.* 1988). In another retrospective study, 31 of 117 patients with culture-proven bacterial meningitis had seizures. No adult without seizures in the acute phase of bacterial meningitis developed late seizures (Wang *et al.* 2005).
2. Etiological agent. The incidence of epilepsy was highest after *S. pneumoniae* (14.8%) compared to *Haemophilus influenzae* (6.1%) and *N. meningitidis* (1.4%) (Annegers *et al.* 1988).
3. In a pediatric study, EEG abnormalities, an initial CSF glucose concentration <1.1 mmol\L (20 mg/dL), and persistent neurological deficits were found to be associated with late unprovoked seizures (Pomeroy *et al.* 1990).

Types of seizures/epilepsy, specific characteristics, treatment, and prognosis

Acute seizures

Following bacterial meningitis, these are usually generalized but may be of focal onset, 13% vs. 7% (Durand *et al.* 1993), 22% vs. 4% (Wang *et al.* 2005), and 10% vs. 6% (Zoons *et al.* 2008). In one study, EEG during the acute stages in those with seizures showed unilateral abnormality in 6% and diffuse abnormality in 94% (Wang *et al.* 2005). In another study, EEG showed focal changes in 38%, generalized discharges in 16%, and status epilepticus in 14% (Zoons *et al.* 2008). Acute seizures tend to occur early. In one study, 80% (25/31) of the episodes occurred within 24 hr of presentation (Wang *et al.* 2005). In another, two-thirds of the cases occurred within 24 hr of admission, but more than one-third of patients with such early-onset seizures in this study had a history of alcoholism (Durand *et al.* 2008).

Studies suggest that mortality is higher in those with acute seizures. In a retrospective study of 117 patients with culture-proven bacterial meningitis, 31 had early provoked seizures, of whom 10 progressed to status epilepticus (6/10 died, 4 completely recovered and were seizure-free). Overall, 19/31 died of meningitis during the acute stage. At follow-up after completing treatment 10 of 12 survivors completely recovered and were seizure-free, the other 2 progressed to chronic epilepsy. Mortality rates for those patients with and without seizures during acute bacterial meningitis were 39% (12/31) and 34% (29/86), respectively (Wang *et al.* 2005). Durand *et al.* (2008) reported that patients who had seizures within 24 hr of admission had a higher mortality rate (72% vs. 18%). In another study, mortality in those with seizures was 41% compared with 16% in those without, and those with seizures were more likely to have long-term neurological sequelae such as hearing loss or hemiparesis at discharge (24% vs. 6%) (Zoons *et al.* 2008).

Chronic epilepsy

Following meningitis, epilepsy is usually focal, with partial onset seizures in 23/31 cases (Annegers *et al.* 1988). Although, the majority of unprovoked seizures following bacterial meningitis occur within 5 years, the risk remains elevated for 15 years (Annegers *et al.* 1988). There is little literature regarding prognosis and remission rates of seizures following CNS infections. In general, seizure prognosis in the aftermath of bacterial meningitis is likely to correspond to outcome in other symptomatic epilepsies. The average recurrence risk after a first unprovoked seizure due to any cause is estimated to be about 50%. When the first unprovoked seizure is due to a remote symptomatic etiology, the estimated rate of recurrence over 2 years is 57% (Berg and Shinnar 1994). Remission rates following antiepileptic drug (AED) therapy are thought to be similar to other epilepsies with remote symptomatic etiology, i.e., ~50% (Pomeroy *et al.* 1990). The average risk estimate of relapse of seizure(s) 1 year after AED withdrawal following a period of remission for all types of epilepsies is 25% at 1 year (Berg and Shinnar 1994). Remote symptomatic epilepsy of any etiology increases this risk by 1.5 times.

Suppurative intracranial disorders

Acute symptomatic seizures

Intracranial suppurative disorders can present with seizures, partial or generalized, reportedly in 7–19% of cases of brain abscess (Carpenter *et al.* 2007; Sharma *et al.* 2009). Seizures were observed during the acute illness in 7% (Roche *et al.* 2003), 13.4% (Tseng and Tseng 2006), and 26% (Carpenter *et al.* 2007). In the largest series of subdural empyemas, along with fever, neck stiffness, and headache, the occurrence of focal seizures was a common initial presenting feature with almost 40% of patients experiencing seizures, usually focal. Status epilepticus has also been reported. In epidural abscess, seizures can occur in the acute phase with 9/82 patients presenting with seizures in one study (Nathoo *et al.* 1999b).

Late seizures/epilepsy

There is a significantly increased risk of long-term epilepsy following brain abscess, which in older series ranges from very low to 72% or higher (Legg *et al.* 1973; Koszewski 1991). The epilepsy can occur early or after many years. Lower reported rates of later epilepsy may reflect shorter duration of follow-up in some series. The epilepsy is usually focal with partial seizures and secondary generalization. Results of studies are not consistent in relation to incidence or reported risk factors for the development of later epilepsy (Adcock and Oxbury 2000). This may in part be due to differences in follow-up and use of prophylactic AEDs. Factors that need to be considered in this regard include age (longer latency in children), sex, the occurrence of acute symptomatic seizures or status epilepticus, site of abscess (temporal), associated meningitis, whether the abscess is single or multiple, abscess size, stage at detection, treatment modalities and surgical procedures, focal neurological deficit, imaging changes, causative organisms, and the presence of immunocompromise.

Examples of some earlier series

An old series from the London Hospital in the United Kingdom was based on 186 patients treated between 1939 and 1966. Eighty-six of 160 cases with supratentorial abscess survived beyond 1 month, of whom 70 (age range 18 months to 62 years, mean 26 years, 52 male) were followed up for 3 to 30 years (mean 11) (Legg *et al.* 1973). Treatment with phenobarbital or phenytoin was only given in the event of seizures. Epilepsy developed in 51 of 70 patients (72%), including all 12 with preoperative seizures. In this study, the incidence was not influenced by the site of the abscess ("intracerebral or extracerebral"), anatomical site, the introduction of penicillin, the use of thorotrast (a carcinogenic radioactive contrast medium with a half-life of years), the final method of surgical treatment (burr hole aspiration alone or with craniotomy/total excision), age, nor the presence of residual neurological deficit in 34% of cases. The interval to the development of epilepsy ranged from 1 month to 15 years (mean 3.3 years) and was shorter in adults than children. Of those aged 20 to 40 years who developed epilepsy, 50% had their initial seizure during the first year, compared with only 20% of those aged 20 years or less. Given a broadly similar percentage of cases developing epilepsy in the first year to other series (30% in their series), the authors argued that earlier studies quoted had underestimated the incidence of epilepsy (42–63%) because of limited follow-up. They observed a shorter latent interval for temporal lobe than frontal lobe abscess. They noted that epileptic activity was highest 4 to 5 years after operation and concluded that this supported a continuing pathological process progressive over a number of years.

A later study from Poland (Koszewski 1991) retrospectively reported on 108 survivors following treatment for brain abscess (single: 91 supratentorial, 10 infratentorial; multiple: 7 supratentorial including 1 with cerebellar abscesses) in the years 1948–88 with follow-up between 3 to 21 years (average 11 years). All patients were treated prophylactically with AEDs (mostly phenobarbital) for at least 1 year after discharge. The incidence of epilepsy reported was 37% in supratentorial abscesses. The one case of epilepsy with cerebellar abscess also had meningitis, this being the more likely cause of the epilepsy. In 32 of 37 patients (86%), seizures occurred within 1 year after discharge. It is surprising that the proportion with late seizures is so much less than in Legg's study, raising the possibility that later seizures were underestimated. This study found the following risk factors for developing epilepsy to be significant: gender (male sex), age 15–45 years, site of supratentorial abscess (temporal a little more common than frontal or parietal, with no cases observed amongst 11 occipital abscesses), and abscess size greater than 4 cm. Koszewski states that:

> The incidence of epilepsy following brain abscess ranged widely in various reports from the very low figures such as: 0%, 3% or 15% to 72%, and even up to 95%, but in most papers it oscillated at the level of about 40%. The incidence of seizures in our series is rather "average" being 34%, in spite of a

Table 69.1 Lumbar puncture findings in different meningitides

	Normal	Acute bacterial meningitis	Viral meningitis	TB meningitis
Appearance	Clear	Turbid/purulent	Clear/opalescent	Clear/opalescent
Pressure	$<20\,cm\,H_2O$	$>20\,cm\,H_2O$	$<20\,cm\,H_2O$	Usually $>20\,cm\,H_2O$
Cells	$0\text{–}5/mm^3$	$5\text{–}2000/mm^3$	$5\text{–}500/mm^3$	$5\text{–}1000/mm^3$
Polymorphs	0	$>50\%$	$<50\%$	$<50\%$
Glucose	2.2–3.3 mmol/L (40–60 mg/dL) (always look at ratio to blood; CSF glucose is normally more than half of blood glucose)	Low ($<40\%$ blood)	Normal	Low ($<40\%$ blood)
Protein	$<400\,mg/L$	Often $>900\,mg/L$	400–900 mg/L	Often $>1\,g/L$
Other		Bacterial Gram stain/DNA PCR	Viral nucleic acid by PCR	Zn/auramine fluorescent stain

Source: Schut *et al.* (2008).

relatively long follow-up period. It is remarkable that the reports, presenting an extraordinary low seizures rate are usually the ones dealing with prolonged anticonvulsant treatment.

More recent series

Extrapolation with regard to incidence and risk factors from older series may not be valid. Diagnosis is now earlier with better imaging. Surgical treatment has evolved. Furthermore, the case mix is different. An additional factor that could affect the incidence of epilepsy is the increased number of cases with immunocompromise, where the local immune reaction, which in itself is thought to contribute to brain damage, is altered.

Of recent series, many do not report on long-term epilepsy (Tseng and Tseng 2006; Carpenter *et al.* 2007) and clearly more large-scale studies are needed with longer-term follow-up. In a series from South Africa, of 121 patients who underwent a neurosurgical procedure for the treatment of a brain abscess (44% frontal), 16 died and 13 were known to have developed epilepsy (Sichizya *et al.* 2005). In the Dublin series of cases operated on for suppurative intracranial disorders (mainly abscesses but including empyema), of 163 patients, 10% died before discharge or transfer and 18 (11%) developed epilepsy. The authors, however, acknowledged that follow-up was incomplete (Roche *et al.* 2003). These figures are lower than expected from older series and are very likely to be underestimates with incomplete follow-up. In their review article, Ersin and Cansever (2008), quoting Cansever, report that after surgical removal of abscesses compared with stereotactic aspiration, more focal neurological deficits (5.2% compared with 0%) and seizures (47.7% compared with 31.2%) were seen. They concluded that the type of surgical intervention chosen for the management of the abscess is one of the most important factors both in seizure and neurological outcome, noting larger hypodense areas in surgically treated patients, reflecting damaged brain parenchyma leading to neurological deficits and epileptic

activities. Without knowing what influenced the choice of procedure, interpretation is difficult.

In the largest subdural empyema series, 103 of 509 patients (14.7%) who were followed-up experienced postoperative seizures (Nathoo *et al.* 1999a). No information is provided on duration of follow-up. In the 82 cases with epidural empyemas, only four patients required long-term treatment with antiepileptic medication but follow-up was not possible in 29 cases (35%). Mean follow-up was 250 ± 651.54 days.

Diagnostic tests for the disease
Bacterial meningitis

Initial immediate investigations include lumbar puncture in the absence of evidence of raised intracranial pressure, blood cultures, and routine blood tests including inflammatory markers, before prompt empirical therapy (Schut *et al.* 2008). The CSF is examined for protein, glucose, and red and white blood cells (Table 69.1).

Papilledema and focal neurological signs are found in $<1\%$ of cases and should prompt urgent imaging to exclude a significant space occupying lesion by CT or magnetic resonance imaging (MRI), where lumbar puncture is contraindicated. In addition to focal signs and raised intracranial pressure, other indications for brain imaging before considering lumbar puncture include seizures, reduced GCS, and severe immunocompromise. In other cases, the lumbar puncture should not be delayed by imaging. If it does not cause delay then imaging may be carried out prior to lumbar puncture but this is not required in many cases. Antibiotic treatment should be started urgently in any case (see below).

In bacterial meningitis, CSF Gram stain may demonstrate bacteria in up to 60% of cases, but this figure is reduced by 20% where antibiotics have already been administered. Culture is more sensitive and identifies the organism in 70–85% of

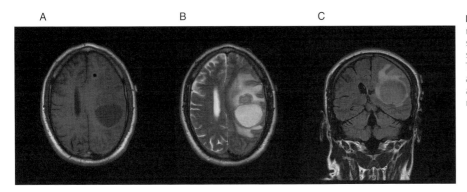

Fig. 69.1. MR images from a patient with confirmed mature cerebral abscess. (A) Axial T1-weighted image showing the abscess as a hypodense area with surrounding edema and mass effect. (B) Axial T2-weighted image demonstrating a hyperdense abscess and surrounding edema with hypodense abscess capsule. (C) Coronal fluid-attenuated inversion recovery (FLAIR) image with hypodense abscess.

untreated cases but can take up to 48 hr. Various more specialized tests may be used to distinguish between various types of meningitis. For example, the latex agglutination test may be positive in meningitis due to *S. pneumoniae*, *N. meningitidis*, *H. influenzae*, *E. coli* and Group B streptococci (*Streptococcus agalactiae*). Many laboratories, however, while carrying out latex agglutination on blood for pneumococcus, do not carry this out on CSF, preferring polymerase chain reaction (PCR), which has better sensitivity and specificity. Limulus lysate test may be positive in meningitis caused by Gram-negative bacteria, although this is not done routinely. The PCR may assist in identifying various causes of meningitis. Routine tests must include blood and CSF for culture and meningococcal and pneumococcal PCR as well as CSF Gram stain. Additional tests are performed as indicated, particularly in the immunocompromised, including for non-bacterial causes (see Chapter 75) such as India ink stain of CSF and cryptococcal antigen. Partial treatment with antibiotics, for example in the community, may affect CSF findings. Viral meningitis may present with polymorphs in the first few hours.

Suppurative intracranial disorders

Imaging

Brain imaging has greatly facilitated diagnosis in suppurative cranial disorders; MRI is more sensitive than CT in early changes and multiple lesions, especially if small, and is the investigation of choice in suspected abscesses, subdural, or epidural collections. In early cerebritis, T1-weighted MR images, show an ill-defined area of iso- or hypointensity with hyperintensity on T2-weighted MR images. There is subtle mass effect with minimal or no contrast enhancement. A mature abscess is seen as an intracerebral space-occupying lesion, often with mass effect and, usually, surrounding edema. A thin ring around a central area of necrosis with peripheral edema is typical. There may be ring enhancement, depending on the stage of abscess development. The abscess capsule may demonstrate hypointensity on T2-weighted imaging. The rim of enhancement is usually thinnest on its central aspect with potential satellite lesions. On MRI, mature pyogenic brain abscesses are centrally hypointense on T1- and hyperintense on T2-weighted images with restricted diffusion (Fig. 69.1). Although malignant lesions are more likely to have thick irregular ring enhancement, distinction between pyogenic brain abscess and necrotic brain tumor can be difficult on conventional MR imaging. Diffusion and perfusion imaging, and possibly spectroscopy, may help in the differential diagnosis. Other investigations needed to identify the cause of the abscess are guided by the individual case. The differential diagnosis includes other non-pyogenic infective causes, malignancy, and inflammatory processes. Subdural and epidural empyemas are characterized by extra-axial intensely rim-enhancing fluid collection. There may be associated parenchymal sepsis or venous infarction.

Blood tests

Raised ESR, C-reactive protein (CRP), and white count are frequently but not always observed. Although the yield is not high, blood cultures are indicated.

Microbiology

Brain abscesses are commonly caused by bacteria. These can be identified from the surgical specimen in the majority (73% in one study: Roche *et al.* 2003). Although the yield is lower, even if the patient is already on antibiotics, organisms can still be identified from surgical specimens, thus emphasizing the diagnostic value of surgical drainage. Polymicrobial infection may be present, both aerobic and anaerobic, the latter reportedly present in some 30–50% of abscesses, sometimes more often. The underlying etiology influences the organisms found. Members of the *S. anginosus* group are commonly isolated, as are staphylococci, which can predominate in cases following neurosurgical procedures. Methicillin (Meticillin) resistance is common among the coagulase-negative staphylococci, and methicillin-resistant *S. aureus* may also cause postneurosurgical infection. Other relatively common organisms include *Bacteroides* spp., Enterobacteriaceae (e.g., *E. coli* or *Proteus* spp.), *Pseudomonas* spp., and *Haemophilus* spp. Anaerobic bacteria other than *Bacteroides* may also be cultured, including *Clostridium* (rarely) and *Actinomyces* spp., the latter occurring in immunocompromised patients. Other less common infective agents include *Propionibacterium acnes*, *Listeria*, and *Nocardia*. *Propionibacterium acnes* is a Gram-positive bacillus, part of cutaneous flora and sometimes a contaminant. It is an infrequent but recognized cause of often indolent infections complicating neurosurgery, particularly where there is foreign tissue. *Listeria* causes both meningioencephalitis and brain abscesses, frequently infratentorial, often in the immunocompromised. *Nocardia* are environmental aerobic acid-fast Gram-positive branching rods, fastidious in culture, which uncommonly cause cerebral infection, including abscesses in both immunocompetent and immunocompromised subjects.

Positive identification of causative organisms, essential for selection of the most appropriate treatment, depends on meticulous processing of surgical specimens. This relies on conventional stains and specimen cultures, conventional biochemical identification methods, PCR–restriction fragment length polymorphism (RFLP) analysis, and, more recently, multiple sequenced 16S ribosomal DNA PCR amplifications. The latter technique, although rarely available, reportedly identifies significantly more strains, some new.

Lumbar puncture

This is contraindicated in the majority in view of the presence of mass lesions and raised intracranial pressure (Garfield 1960). It may be justified in a few selected patients with very small abscess lesions and associated meningitis *in the absence* of increased intracranial pressure. Reported yield in relation to positive culture is 10–30%, often compatible with abscess culture. (Tseng and Tseng 2006).

Principles of management
Meningitis
Antimicrobial treatment in adults

Effective and timely antibiotic treatment is essential. Delay in treatment is associated with a poorer outcome. Thus, treatment with broad-spectrum antibiotics should not await confirmatory tests. A third-generation cephalosporin in adequate dosage (e.g., parenteral ceftriaxone or cefotaxime) is suitable empirical therapy for previously well non-immunosuppressed adults with pneumococcal, meningococcal, *H. influenzae*, and *E. coli* meningitis (Chaudhuria *et al.* 2008). In countries with a high level of cephalosporin resistance, vancomycin is added. If *Listeria* is suspected, such as in patients above 50 years of age or those who are immunocompromised, then amoxicillin or ampicillin is also added. Once the bacterial pathogen is isolated and sensitivities confirmed, antimicrobial therapy is modified accordingly. At all stages advice should be sought from an expert in infection. If a neurosurgical implant is present, and/or there is severe ventriculitis, intrathecal or intraventicular antibiotics may be appropriate in some patients.

Corticosteroid treatment

Significant morbidity and mortality, despite effective antibiotic therapy, is partly attributed to the intense inflammatory response to bacterial infection. Thus, corticosteroids constitute an adjuvant therapeutic strategy. A systematic review in adults with community-acquired acute bacterial meningitis showed that adjunctive corticosteroid treatment reduced mortality and neurological sequelae, including deafness, specifically when the causative agent is *S. pneumoniae* (van de Beek *et al.* 2007). This is recommended 15–20 min before or with the first dose of antibiotic and given for 4 days (De Gans and van de Beek 2002). No study has specifically examined the effect of adjuvant corticosteroid therapy on subsequent epilepsy. Nevertheless, since persistent neurological deficits have been reported as risk factors for late unprovoked seizures following bacterial meningitis, it is possible that corticosteroids may influence the incidence of late unprovoked seizures/epilepsy.

Supportive measures

These are essential and include fluid replacement, antiemetics, AEDs (see section "Management of acute symptomatic seizures" below), and treatment of raised intracranial pressure.

Bacterial meningitis

The burden of epilepsy due to bacterial meningitis can be reduced by (1) early diagnosis and effective therapy of the meningitis, and (2) reduction in rates of bacterial meningitis and thereby associated epilepsy though vaccinations, disease surveillance, and treatment of close contacts.

Vaccination

Vaccination programs against common meningeal pathogens have resulted in a decline in incidence of meningitis in both the developed and developing world (Dery and Hasbun 2007). There are vaccines against *H. influenzae* type B, some strains of *N. meningitidis*, and many types of *S. pneumoniae*. However, there are still large parts of Africa and other parts of the developing world where little progress has been made in this regard.

Disease reporting and surveillance

This is also important to allow health authorities to trace contacts and recognize outbreaks. Close contacts of a person with meningitis caused by *N. meningitidis* are given prophylactic antibiotics such as rifampicin, ciprofloxacin, or ceftriaxone (in pregnancy).

Suppurative intracranial disorders

Combined medical and surgical treatment is usual. Medical treatment alone can be successful in those with small lesions and in the early cerebritis stage.

Surgical treatment

Brain abscess

In general, urgent surgical drainage is recommended and surgical intervention indicated for most cases with brain abscess, except those with early cerebritis or in those with small lesions and a known organism. Current practice favors burr hole aspiration usually using stereotaxy or image guidance. Aspiration removes pus, decompresses, and provides material for analysis and culture. Repeated aspiration is sometimes needed. Routine craniotomy with resection is now out of favor because of the risk of hemorrhage. Because of the risk of recurrence, weekly imaging is recommended followed by monthly scans until resolution, with continuing surveillance over the next year. Inflammatory markers such as CRP and white cell counts should also be monitored.

Subdural and epidural empyema

Craniotomy is associated with a better outcome (Nathoo *et al.* 1999b, 2001) as it allows for adequate decompression of the brain and complete evacuation of pus. In the early stages of the disease process, or when collections complicate meningitis, the pus may be thin. However, subdural and extradural collections can be loculated, tenacious, and extensive, and brain swelling is usually present which may lead to secondary complications. Thus, burr holes are not considered as effective.

Antimicrobial treatment

In a stable non-immunocompromised patient, prompt investigations (blood or other cultures) to identify the organisms are carried out before empirical treatment is started. Antibiotics therapy should not, however, be delayed by urgent transfer of the patients to a neurosurgical unit for surgery. Initial antimicrobial treatment should take into account the clinical setting and site of abscess and cover Gram-positive and Gram-negative organisms as well as anaerobes, until culture and sensitivity data are available to guide treatment. A third-generation cephalosporin, such as cefotaxime or ceftriaxone, together with metronidazole is a reasonable combination, with vancomycin, where infection follows neurosurgery. Additional empirical treatment with gentamicin, or high doses of benzyl penicillin, flucloxacillin (nafcillin), or rifampicin (rifampin) have also been used depending on the case (Carpenter *et al.* 2007). If *Listeria* is suspected, high-dose ampicillin or amoxycillin is indicated. Treatment is later adjusted depending on culture and sensitivity. Antibiotics are given intravenously then followed by oral therapy for a variable but prolonged period. It should be noted that certain antibiotics can be neurotoxic and cause seizures and encephalopathy

Corticosteroids

These have been used to reduce vasogenic edema and they are thought to possibly retard capsule formation. However, appropriate and adequate antimicrobial cover is essential if corticosteroids are given, and steroids should only be commenced under the guidance of the neurosurgeons.

Management of acute symptomatic seizures

Antiepileptic drug treatment

In bacterial meningitis the advice is to treat acute symptomatic seizures. In cases of suppurative intracranial disorders, the literature advocates routine prophylactic cover with AEDs as acute symptomatic seizures occur frequently. Gradual withdrawal, in the absence of evidence for epilepsy, is later carried out when the patient is stable. The choice of AED depends on urgency and available route of administration. Those that can be given intravenously and orally (with loading where appropriate for early efficacy) include phenytoin, phenobarbital, valproate, and levetiracetam. The latter two have a better profile in relation to interactions, but are not as well established. If there is no evidence of seizures, it is appropriate to gradually withdraw antiepileptic medication at the end of the acute phase of the illness and restart if late seizures occur. For those with acute symptomatic seizures, gradual withdrawal over weeks to months, depending on the case, is also usually advised after recovery. As appropriate, patients should be counseled not to drive for a period dependent on assessment of individual risk and advised of local driving regulations. If there are continuing seizures, long-term AED treatment is indicated as per focal/generalized seizures of any cause.

Drug interactions

Several antibiotics can affect the metabolism of AEDs (Patsalos and Perucca 2003; Patsalos 2005) and AEDs can also affect the metabolism of antibiotics and steroids. Enzyme-inducing medication such as rifampicin (rifampin) and a number of AEDs, such as phenytoin, phenobarbital, and carbamazepine, can reduce levels and efficacy of some metabolized drugs, although it should be noted that enzyme induction does not occur instantly. The effect of enzyme inhibition on the half-life of the other drug on the other hand (e.g., with valproate) is immediate. Conversely, carbapenem antibiotics, in particular meropenem, can significantly reduce plasma levels of valproate by increasing clearance of valproate (Haroutiunian *et al.* 1999). There are other mechanisms for drug interaction other than enzyme inhibition and induction. Caution is required with co-medication in any clinical setting and potential interactions always considered.

Epilepsy surgery

Epilepsy surgery may also be considered in any focal epilepsy associated with a focal lesion if the lesion is shown to be the source of seizures and is resectable without significant risk of deficit. Epilepsy surgery can be successful in cases with intractable epilepsy secondary to previous intracranial sepsis. A subset of intractable postmeningitic epilepsy comprises mesial temporal lobe epilepsy, often with unilateral mesial temporal sclerosis (MTS), amenable to surgical treatment. Patients with temporal lobe epilepsy may have a previous history of meningitis or encephalitis leading to concern whether more diffuse damage precludes epilepsy surgery. This need not be the case, although a history of a CNS infection, particularly encephalitis, carries some adverse prognostic significance for outcome after epilepsy surgery (O'Brien *et al.* 2002) and can be associated with bilateral memory loss (Donaire *et al.* 2007). In a series from the Mayo Clinic (O'Brien *et al.* 2002), 39 of 383 patients who underwent anterior temporal lobectomy for temporal lobe epilepsy had a remote history of meningitis or encephalitis. There was a non-significant trend for worse outcome in the meningitis/

encephalitis group compared to those without (Class 1 outcomes 61.5% vs. 73.1%). This study also confirmed previous reports (Berg and Shinnar 1994) demonstrating better outcome within this group if the infection occurred under the age of 4 years and with MTS seen on MRI.

Acknowledgments

The authors would like to acknowledge Dr. John Philpott-Howard, Consultant and Senior Lecturer in Medical Microbiology, Mr. Keyoumars Ashkan, and Mr. Daniel Walsh, Consultant Neurosurgeons, King's College Hospital, for their helpful comments on the manuscript.

References

Adcock JE, Oxbury JM (2000) Brain infections. In: Oxbury JM, Polkey CE, Duchowny M (eds.) *Intractable Focal Epilepsy*. Philadelphia, PA: W.B. Saunders.

Al-Rajeh S, Abomelha A, Awada A, *et al.* (1990) Epilepsy and other convulsive disorders in Saudi Arabia: a prospective study of 1000 consecutive cases. *Acta Neurol Scand* **82**:341–5.

Annegers JF, Hauser WA, Beghi E, Nicolosi A, Kurland LT (1988) The risk of unprovoked seizures after encephalitis and meningitis. *Neurology* **38**:1407–10.

Annegers JF, Rocca WA, Hauser WA, (1996). Causes of epilepsy: contributions of the Rochester epidemiology project. *Mayo Clin Proc* **71**:570–5.

Berg AT, Shinnar S (1994) Relapse following discontinuation of antiepileptic drugs: a meta-analysis. *Neurology* **44**:601–8.

Carpenter J, Stapleton S, Holliman R (2007) Retrospective analysis of 49 cases of brain abscess and review of the literature. *Eur J Clin Microbiol Infect Dis* **26**:1–11.

Carpio A, Hauser WA, Lisanti N, *et al.* (2001) Etiology of epilepsy in Ecuador. *Epilepsia* **42**(Suppl 2):122.

Chang CJ, Chang HW, Chang WN, *et al.* (2004) Seizures complicating infantile and childhood bacterial meningitis. *Paediatr Neurol* **31**:165–71.

Chaudhuria A, Martin PM, Kennedy PGE, *et al.* (2008) EFNS guideline on the management of community-acquired bacterial meningitis: report of an EFNS Task Force on acute bacterial meningitis in older children and adults. *Eur J Neurol* **15**:649–59.

De Gans J, van de Beek D (2002) Dexamethasone in adults with bacterial meningitis. *N Engl J Med* **347**:1549–56.

Dery M, Hasbun R (2007) Changing epidemiology of bacterial meningitis. *Curr Infect Dis Rep* **9**:301–7.

Desai J (2008) Perspectives on interactions between antiepileptic drugs (AEDs) and antimicrobial agents. *Epilepsia* **49**Suppl(6):47–9.

Donaire A, Carreno M, Agudo R, *et al.* (2007) Presurgical evaluation in refractory epilepsy secondary to meningitis or encephalitis: bilateral memory deficits often preclude surgery. *Epilept Disord* **9**:127–33.

Durand ML, Calderwood SB, Weber DJ, *et al.* (1993) Acute bacterial meningitis in adults – a review of 493 episodes. *N Engl J Med* **328**:21–8.

Ersin E, Cansever T (2008) Pyogenic brain abscess. *Neurosurg Focus* **24**:E2.

Fitch M, Van der Beek D (2007) Emergency diagnosis and treatment of adult meningitis. *Lancet Infec Dis* **7**:191–200.

Ford H, Wright J (1994) Bacterial meningitis in Swaziland: an 18-month prospective study of its impact. *J Epidemiol Commun Health* **48**:276–80.

Garfield J (1960) Management of supratentorial intracranial abscess: a review of 200 cases. *Br Med J* **2**:7–11.

Grondahl TO, Langmoen IA (1983) Epileptogenic effect of antibiotic drugs. *J Neurosurg* **78**:938–43.

Hantson P, Léonard F, Maloteaux JM, Mahieu P (1999) How epileptogenic are the recent antibiotics? *Acta Clin Belg* **54**:80–7.

Haroutiunian S, Ratz Y, Rabinovich B, *et al.* (1999) Valproic acid plasma concentration decreases in a dose-independent manner following administration of meropenem: a

retrospective study. *J Clin Pharmacol* **49**:1363–9.

Hauser WA, Kurland LT (1975) The epidemiology of epilepsy in Rochester, Minnesota, 1935 through 1967. *Epilepsia* **16**:1–66.

ILAE (1994) Commission on Tropical Diseases: relationships between epilepsy and tropical diseases. *Epilepsia* **35**:89–93.

Koszewski W (1991) Epilepsy following brain abscess: the evaluation of possible risk factors with emphasis on new concept of epileptic focus formation. *Acta Neurochir (Wien)* **113**:110–17.

Lavados J, Germain L, Morales A, *et al.* (1992) A descriptive study of epilepsy in the district of El Salvador, Chile, 1984–1988. *Acta Neurol Scand* **85**:249–56.

Legg NJ, Gupta PC, Scott DF (1973) Epilepsy following cerebral abscess, a clinical and EEG study of 70 patients. *Brain* **96**:259–68.

Murthy JMK, Yangala R (1998) Aetiological spectrum of symptomatic localization related epilepsies: a study from South India. *J Neurol Sci* **158**:65–70.

Nathoo N, Nadvi SS, van Dellen JR, *et al.* (1999a) Intracranial subdural empyemas in the era of computed tomography: a review of 699 cases. *Neurosurgery* **44**:529–35.

Nathoo N, Nadvi SS, Gouws E, *et al.* (2001) Craniotomy improves outcomes for cranial subdural empyemas: computed tomography-era experience with 699 patients. *Neurosurgery* **49**:872–7.

Nathoo N, Nadvi SS, van Dellen JR (1999b). Cranial extradural empyema in the era of computed tomography: a review of 82 cases. *Neurosurgery* **44**:748–53.

Nicolosi A, Hauser WA, Musicco M, *et al.* (1991) Incidence and prognosis of brain abscess in a defined population: Olmsted County, Minnesota, 1935–1981. *Neuroepidemiology* **10**:122–31.

O'Brien TJ, Moses H, Cambier D, Cascino GD (2002). Age of meningitis or encephalitis is independently predictive of outcome from anterior temporal lobectomy. *Neurology* **58**:104–9.

Patsalos PN, Perucca E (2003) Clinically important drug interactions in epilepsy: interactions between antiepileptic drugs and other drugs. *Lancet Neurol* **2**:473–81.

Patsalos PN (2005) *Antiepileptic Drug Interactions: A Clinical Guide*. Guildford, UK: Clarius Press.

Pomeroy SL, Holmes SJ, Dodge PR, Feigin RD (1990) Seizures and other neurological sequelae of bacterial meningitis in children. *N Engl J Med* **323**:1651–7.

Preux P, Druet-Cabanac M (2005) Epidemiology and etiology of epilepsy on sub-Saharan Africa. *Lancet Neurol* **4**:25–31.

Rantakallio P, Leskinen M, von Wendt L (1986) Incidence and prognosis of central nervous system infections in a birth cohort of 12 000 children. *Scand J Infect Dis* **18**:287–94.

Roche M, Humphreys H, Smyth E, *et al.* (2003) A twelve-year review of central nervous system bacterial abscesses: presentation and etiology. *Clin Microbiol Infect* **9**:803–9.

Sander JW, Perucca E (2003) Epilepsy and comorbidity: infections and antimicrobials usage in relation to epilepsy management. *Acta Neurol Scand* **108**(Suppl 180):16–22.

Schut ES, de Gans J, van de Beek D (2008) Community acquired bacterial meningitis in adults. *Pract Neurol* **8**:8–23.

Sharma R, Mohandas K, Cooke RPD (2009) Intracranial abscesses: changes in epidemiology and management over five decades in Merseyside. *Infection* **37**:39–43.

Sichizya K, Fieggen G, Taylor A, *et al.* (2005) Brain abscesses: the Groote Schuur experience, 1993–2003. *S Afr J Surg* **43**:79–82.

Singh G, Prabhakar S (2008a) The association between central nervous system (CNS) infections and epilepsy: epidemiological approaches and microbiological and epileptological perspectives. *Epilepsia* **49**(Suppl 6):2–7.

Singh G, Prabhakar S (2008b) The effects of antimicrobial and antiepileptic treatment on the outcome of epilepsy associated with central nervous system (CNS) infections. *Epilepsia* **49**(Suppl 6):42–6.

Stoll BJ (1997) The global impact of neonatal infection. *Clin Perinatol* **24**:1–21.

Tikhomirov E, Santamaria M, Esteves K (1997) Meningococcal disease: public health burden and control. *World Health Status Q* **50**:170–7.

Tseng J-H, Tseng M-Y (2006) Brain abscess in 142 patients: factors influencing outcome and mortality. *Surg Neurol* **65**:557–62.

Van de Beek D, de Gans J, Tunkel AR, *et al.* (2006) Community acquired bacterial meningitis in adults. *N Engl J Med* **354**:44–53.

Van de Beek D, de Gans J, McIntyre P, Prasad K (2007) Corticosteroids in acute bacterial meningitis. *Cochrane Database Syst Rev.* Jan 24:CD004405.

Wallace KL (1997) Antibiotic-induced convulsions. *Crit Care Clin* **13**:741–62.

Wang KW, Chang WN, Chang HW, *et al.* (2005) The significance of seizures and other predictive factors during the acute illness for the long-term outcome after bacterial meningitis. *Seizure* **14**:586–92.

Weisfelt M, van de Beek D, Spanjaard L, *et al.* (2006) Clinical features, complications, and outcome in adults with pneumococcal meningitis: a prospective case series. *Lancet Neurol* **5**:123–9.

Zoons E, Weisfelt M, de Gans J, *et al.* (2008) Seizures in adults with bacterial meningitis. *Neurology* **70**:2109–15.

491

Chapter 70

Malaria

Charles R. J. C. Newton

Introduction

There are four species of *Plasmodium* that naturally infect humans, but only *P. falciparum* is associated with epilepsy, although seizures are reported during acute *P. vivax* infections. *Plasmodium falciparum* is the most severe form of malaria and is responsible for most of the neurological complications. It accounts for almost all the mortality and neurological sequelae following malaria infections.

Epidemiology of malaria

It is estimated that *P. falciparum* infects over 2 billion people in the world, causing 500 million clinical episodes of malaria, with more than 1 million deaths per year (Snow *et al.* 2005). Over 70% of the infections occur in young children living in sub-Saharan Africa, most of whom live in endemic areas where they can receive up to 300 bites from infected mosquitoes per year. There are differences in the clinical presentation between African children and non-immune individuals. In particular, seizures during acute infections and neurological sequelae following severe malaria are more common in African children than non-immune individuals (Newton and Warrell 1998).

Pathogenesis of malaria

The erythrocyte stages of *P. falciparum* are responsible for the acute symptoms and probably the development of epilepsy. One of the unique features of *P. falciparum* is that the late stages of the erythrocytic cycle, i.e., schizonts, sequester within the vascular beds of the internal organs, particularly the brain. The infected erythrocytes adhere to the postcapillary venules via parasite-derived proteins exported to the erythrocyte surface which attach to ligands upregulated in the endothelium. The sequestration of the infected erythrocytes is thought to be responsible for many of the neurological complications of *P. falciparum* malaria, through stimulation of mediators such as cytokines and nitric oxide, and microvascular obstruction leading to a reduction in the perfusion of brain tissue. However, frank ischemia is rarely documented in *P. falciparum* malaria, since most patients recover without any evident sequelae.

Manifestations of *P. falciparum* malaria

The manifestations of severe *P. falciparum* malaria include coma, seizures, severe anemia, metabolic acidosis, and, in non-immune individuals, renal impairment and pulmonary edema.

Cerebral malaria is the most severe neurological complication. It is a diffuse encephalopathy, characterized by coma, decorticate or decerebrate posturing, and occasionally brainstem signs. Malaria retinopathy is a pathognomic feature in African children (Lewallen *et al.* 2008), but its significance in non-immune individuals is less clear. Pathologically, the brains of people dying with cerebral malaria are often swollen (particularly African children), gray (from hemozoin, the pigment produced by the breakdown of hemoglobin by the parasite), and the cut surfaces reveal petechial hemorrhages throughout the brain. Microscopically the pathological hallmark is sequestration of the infected erythrocytes within the venules of the brain (Fig. 70.1). There are two types of hemorrhages, petechial and ring hemorrhages. The petechial hemorrhages consist of normal erythrocytes surrounding a ruptured cerebral vessel, appear more common in the white matter, and are associated with sequestration. The ring hemorrhage is unique to malaria, since it consists of a ring of infected erythrocytes, pigment, and monocytes surrounding a layer of uninfected erythrocytes and gliosis, with a central thrombosed vessel. Durck's granulomata are seen in patients (particularly adults) who have died following a prolonged illness. These are circumscribed cellular reactions scattered throughout the brain, and may represent the residue of ring hemorrhages.

Seizures are common during the acute infection in children, and can occur in association with cerebral malaria or in non-comatose patients. They are less common in adults. Over 80% of African children with cerebral malaria present with a history of seizures, and about 60% have seizures during the admission. Status epilepticus occurs in about 28% of children with cerebral malaria and this is associated with neurological sequelae (Crawley *et al.* 2001). The cause of acute seizures in *P. falciparum*

The Causes of Epilepsy, eds. S. D. Shorvon, F. Andermann, and R. Guerrini. Published by Cambridge University Press. © Cambridge University Press 2011.

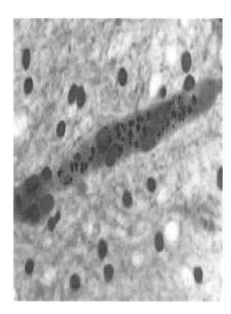

Fig. 70.1. Histological section of the brain of a patient who died of cerebral malaria, showing sequestration of the parasitized erythrocytes in a cerebral venule.

malaria is unclear. Since this type of malaria is the most common cause of fever in children aged between 6 months and 6 years in endemic areas, the seizures are often classified as febrile seizures. However, in contrast to febrile seizures not associated with malaria, the seizures associated with malaria tend to be repetitive, focal, and often prolonged (Idro *et al.* 2007).

Epilepsy and malaria

Although an association between malaria and epilepsy was first suggested in the 1940s (Talbot *et al.* 1949), only recently have epidemiological studies demonstrated the association between *P. falciparum* malaria and the development of epilepsy. The first study that reported an association was conducted in Kenyan children who had had cerebral malaria or malaria and complicated seizures (Carter *et al.* 2004). Of the children exposed to cerebral malaria or who had complicated seizures during their acute illness, 9% and 12% had developed epilepsy 2–9 years later. Thus the risk of developing epilepsy was in the order of four and six times that of the general population respectively. In a similar study of children in Mali, the incidence of epilepsy was 17.0 per 1000 person–years following cerebral malaria, with a relative risk 14.3 (95% confidence interval [CI] 1.6–132.0), after adjusting for age and duration of follow-up (Ngoungou *et al.* 2006a). In a case–control study of Gabonese children with epilepsy, the odds ratio for exposure to cerebral malaria was 3.9 (95% CI 1.7–8.9) (Ngoungou *et al.* 2006b).

The epilepsy documented in these epidemiological studies and from case series are characterized by generalized and focal seizures. In the seizures that occur following recovery from cerebral malaria, 40–66% are generalized seizures, with a remainder of focal or partial becoming generalized seizures. Complex partial seizures are infrequently reported from the African children, but this may be caused by difficulties in describing the semiology in this patient group. Complex partial seizures have been reported in case reports of epilepsy following cerebral malaria in travelers (Schijns *et al.* 2008).

Epilepsy is reported to start from 1 month after the episode of cerebral malaria, but the range of time interval is wide (Carter *et al.* 2004; Ngoungou *et al.* 2006a, b) and the cumulative incidence is likely to increase with longer follow-up. The frequency of seizures in the African studies varied considerably from one per week to less than one in the last 2 years. Most of the children with epilepsy in these studies were not on treatment at the time of assessment (Carter *et al.* 2004; Ngoungou *et al.* 2006a, b). There are no comparable studies following adults exposed to cerebral malaria.

Electroencephalographic (EEG) abnormalities occur in about one-third of the African children with epilepsy following cerebral malaria (Carter *et al.* 2004; Ngoungou *et al.* 2006a, b). Focal features, e.g., slowing, are the most common feature, with only one-fourth having epileptiform abnormalities (Carter *et al.* 2004). Discharges over the temporal lobe are recorded in only a few patients.

In most of the patients in the African studies neuroimaging was not available. Computed tomography (CT) identified cerebral atrophy in some patients (Newton *et al.* 1994). Magnetic resonance imaging (MRI) demonstrated hippocampal sclerosis in one adult (Schijns *et al.* 2008), but studies in patients with epilepsy have not been reported.

The epilepsy in Kenyan children, particularly the active epilepsy, was associated with other neurological deficits such as hemiparesis and quadriparesis. Behavioral problems, e.g., attention deficit disorder and cognitive impairment, appear to be more common in children with active epilepsy.

Epileptogenesis of *P. falciparum* malaria

The cause of epilepsy following *P. falciparum* malaria is unknown. Since complicated seizures during the acute episode have similar features to complex febrile seizures, the mechanisms by which these cause epilepsy may be similar.

Several interacting mechanisms could be responsible. The most likely are vascular or ischemic damage, secondary to microvascular obstruction (Newton and Krishna 1998), since ischemic lesions are detected in a few adults with severe malaria (Looareesuwan *et al.* 1995; Cordoliani *et al.* 1998). Family history of seizure disorders is more common in children who develop seizures during acute malaria than those who do not have seizures, suggesting that genetic predisposition may contribute to the epilepsy (Versteeg *et al.* 2003). An increase in excitotoxins, particularly quinolinic acid and glutamate, have been measured in the cerebrospinal fluid of patients during the acute illness (Dobbie *et al.* 2000; Medana *et al.* 2002). Antibodies against voltage-gated channels are increased during the acute infection and this may lead on to epilepsy (Lang *et al.* 2005).

Management of epilepsy

Most patients who develop epilepsy following severe malaria respond to first-line antiepileptic drugs (AEDs), such as phenobarbital, phenytoin, and carbamazepine, used in resource-poor countries. During the acute illness, the control of seizures appears to be relatively resistant to benzodiazepines, perhaps because falciparum malaria downregulates the γ-aminobutyric acid (GABA) receptors (Ikumi *et al.* 2008). However, this latter finding is unlikely to affect the control of seizures in patients with epilepsy following severe malaria. The epilepsy following malaria is often associated with considerable comorbidity, particularly behavioral and neurocognitive impairment in children. The epilepsy appears relatively easy to treat with standard AEDs, although a few patients may require more aggressive treatment, including surgery. In an adult who developed mesial temporal lobe epilepsy following cerebral malaria, anteromedial temporal lobe resection with amygdalo-hippocampectomy stopped the seizures for at least 3 years after the treatment (Schijns *et al.* 2008).

Antimalarial drugs and epilepsy

Antimalarial drugs are used to prevent and treat malaria. There are many case reports and case series that have suggested that antimalarial drugs are associated with increasing seizure frequency in patients with epilepsy or precipitating seizures (Richens and Andrews 2002). However, there are not any carefully conducted studies reported to establish the association.

The aminoquinolones, such as chloroquine and mefloquine, are contraindicated in patients with epilepsy, based upon a number of case reports. Mefloquine is used as chemoprophylaxis but has been reported to increase seizure frequency in people with epilepsy as well as to precipitate seizures in people without epilepsy or predisposing neurological conditions (Bem *et al.* 1992; Richens and Andrews 2002).

The safest and most effective chemoprophylaxis for people with epilepsy is the atovaquone/proguanil combination (Richens and Andrews 2002), although the suitability of this combination for the area of travel should be checked with an authorative source. Doxycycline (100 mg daily) is often prescribed as an alternative chemoprophylactic agent; however, it is less effacious than atovaquone/proguanil. Furthermore since AEDs such as carbamazepine, phenytoin, and phenobarbital may increase the metabolism of doxycycline, the dose should be doubled (100 mg twice daily). Other drugs such as proguanil alone or pyrimethamine/dapsone are less effective in preventing malaria, but may be useful in some areas. Prevention against being bitten by infected mosquitoes, with bed nets and suitable clothing in the evening, reduces the risk considerably.

References

Bem JL, Kerr L, Stuerchler D (1992) Mefloquine prophylaxis: an overview of spontaneous reports of severe psychiatric reactions and convulsions. *J Trop Med Hyg* **95**:167–79.

Carter JA, Neville BG, White S, *et al.* (2004) Increased prevalence of epilepsy associated with severe falciparum malaria in children. *Epilepsia* **45**:978–81.

Cordoliani YS, Sarrazin JL, Felten D, *et al.* (1998) MR of cerebral malaria. *AJNR Am J Neuroradiol* **19**:871–4.

Crawley J, Smith S, Muthinji P, Marsh K, Kirkham F (2001) Electroencephalographic and clinical features of cerebral malaria. *Arch Dis Childh* **84**:247–53.

Dobbie M, Crawley J, Waruiru C, Marsh K, Surtees R (2000) Cerebrospinal fluid studies in children with cerebral malaria: an excitotoxic mechanism? *Am J Trop Med Hyg* **62**:284–90.

Idro R, Ndiritu M, Ogutu B, *et al.* (2007) Burden, features, and outcome of neurological involvement in acute falciparum malaria in Kenyan children. *J Am Med Ass* **297**:2232–40.

Ikumi ML, Muchohi SN, Ohuma EO, Kokwaro GO, Newton CR (2008) Response to diazepam in children with malaria induced seizures. *Epilepsy Res* **85**:215–18.

Lang B, Newbold CI, Williams G, *et al.* (2005) Antibodies to voltage-gated calcium channels in children with falciparum malaria. *J Infect Dis* **191**:117–21.

Lewallen S, Bronzan RN, Beare NA, *et al.* (2008) Using malarial retinopathy to improve the classification of children with cerebral malaria. *Trans R Soc Trop Med Hyg* **102**:1089–94.

Looareesuwan S, Wilairatana P, Krishna S, *et al.* (1995) Magnetic resonance imaging of the brain in patients with cerebral malaria. *Clin Infect Dis* **21**:300–9.

Medana IM, Hien TT, Day NP, *et al.* (2002) The clinical significance of cerebrospinal fluid levels of kynurenine pathway metabolites and lactate in severe malaria. *J Infect Dis* **185**:650–6.

Newton CR, Krishna S (1998) Severe falciparum malaria in children: current understanding of pathophysiology and supportive treatment. *Pharmacol Ther* **79**:1–53.

Newton CR, Warrell DA (1998) Neurological manifestations of falciparum malaria. *Ann Neurol* **43**:695–702.

Newton CR, Peshu N, Kendall B (1994) Brain swelling and ischaemia in Kenyans with cerebral malaria. *Arch Dis Childh* **70**:281–7.

Ngoungou EB, Dulac O, Poudiougou B, *et al.* (2006a) Epilepsy as a consequence of cerebral malaria in area in which malaria is endemic in Mali, West Africa. *Epilepsia* **47**:873–9.

Ngoungou EB, Koko J, Druet-Cabanac M, *et al.* (2006b) Cerebral malaria and sequelar epilepsy: first matched case-control study in Gabon. *Epilepsia* **47**:2147–53.

Richens A, Andrews C (2002) Clinical practice: antimalarial prophylaxis in patients with epilepsy [corrected]. *Epilepsy Res* **51**:1–4.

Schijns OE, Visser-Vandewalle V, Lemmens EM, Janssen A, Hoogland G (2008) Surgery for temporal lobe epilepsy after cerebral malaria. *Seizure* **17**:731–4.

Snow RW, Guerra CA, Noor AM, Myint HY, Hay SI (2005) The global distribution of clinical episodes of *Plasmodium falciparum* malaria. *Nature* **434**:214–17.

Talbot DR, Elerding AC, Westwater JO (1949) Epilepsy as a sequela of recurrent malaria. *J Am Med Ass* **141**:1130–2.

Versteeg AC, Carter JA, Dzombo J, Neville BG, Newton CR (2003) Seizure disorders among relatives of Kenyan children with severe falciparum malaria. *Trop Med Int Health* **8**:12–16.

Neurocysticercosis

Hector H. Garcia

Neurocysticercosis is a major contributor to the burden of seizures in the world, and is also one of the few preventable causes of seizures and epilepsy (Garcia and Del Brutto 2005). The pig is the usual host of the larval stage of the pork tapeworm *Taenia solium,* a condition called porcine cysticercosis. However, the larvae or cysticerci can also infect the human host. Cysticercosis lesions in the human nervous system (neurocysticercosis: NCC) are a common cause of neurological morbidity in most developing countries, particularly seizures and intracranial hypertension. Highly endemic areas include Latin America, India, parts of China and Africa, Indonesia, and parts of the Asian Southeast. In these areas, cysticercosis is responsible for approximately one-third of all epilepsy cases. Serological evidence of exposure to the parasite can be found in 10–25% of the general population, and residual brain calcifications can also be found in 10% or more of the general population (Del Brutto *et al.* 2005; Medina *et al.* 2005; Montano *et al.* 2005). Because of increased immigration and travel patterns, NCC is now seen with some frequency in non-endemic, industrialized countries (Schantz *et al.* 1998). Mortality in NCC is associated with the presence of hydrocephalus or intracranial hypertension (associated with extraparenchymal NCC), and also with increased mortality in individuals with seizures. Extraparenchymal NCC carries a poor prognosis with a mortality that may reach 20%.

Infection is caused by ingestion of the eggs of the tapeworm, excreted with the feces of an infected human tapeworm carrier. Pigs acquire cysticercosis due to their coprophagic habits, and humans get infected by fecal–oral contamination. Current evidence implicates a tapeworm carrier as the direct source of human cysticercosis infection (probably through contaminated hands, food, or fomites), rather than common source infections from contaminated water or short-stem vegetables. Once ingested by a suitable host, the egg is exposed to the gastric acid and intestinal juices and liberates an embryo the size of a red blood cell, which actively crosses the mucosa of the small intestine until reaching the circulatory system. From there, embryos are distributed into the tissues but apparently most of the invading parasites are destroyed by the immune system of the host. Cysts survive mostly in the brain and the eye, by using active immune evasion mechanisms and probably helped by the blood–brain barrier or the hemato-ocular barrier (Flisser 1994).

The disease follows different courses depending on whether the cysts locate in the brain parenchyma (intraparenchymal NCC) or in the ventricles or subarachnoid space (extraparenchymal NCC). Seizures are the main clinical presentation of intraparenchymal disease. Larvae in the brain parenchyma initially form as cysts with clear liquid content and, thanks to several active mechanisms of immune evasion, elicit a minimal inflammatory reaction. After a period of time, estimated to be about 3 to 5 years on the basis of seizure cases in English soldiers deployed to India in the early twentieth century (Dixon and Lipscomb 1961) the cysts begin to degenerate. This period of degeneration is associated with severe local inflammation around the degenerating cyst(s). Finally, the cyst is collapsed and becomes an inflammatory nodule (enhancing lesion or cysticercal granuloma) (Rajshekhar and Chandy 2000). The cellular clearance process continues, inflammation decreases, and finally a calcified scar replaces the larval material (Fig. 71.1). Seizures may appear at any stage, but are more common in the degenerative phase.

Conversely, extraparenchymal NCC usually follows a progressive course. It is frequently associated with obstructive hydrocephalus which requires the placement of a ventricular shunt. Intraventricular cysts may grow and block the circulation of cerebrospinal fluid (CSF). Cysts located into the sylvian fissure and surrounded by parenchyma commonly continue to grow, slowly, until reaching several centimeters in diameter and producing a mass effect (giant cysts) (Fig. 71.2). Cysts in the basal subarachnoid space tend to grow and infiltrate the neighboring cisterns, also leading to intracranial hypertension and hydrocephalus. A thick cellular and protein-rich CSF response is characteristic which is many times the consistency of normal CSF. This can result in the formation of membranes which can block a ventricular shunt, causing a relapse of hydrocephalus

The Causes of Epilepsy, eds. S. D. Shorvon, F. Andermann, and R. Guerrini. Published by Cambridge University Press. © Cambridge University Press 2011.

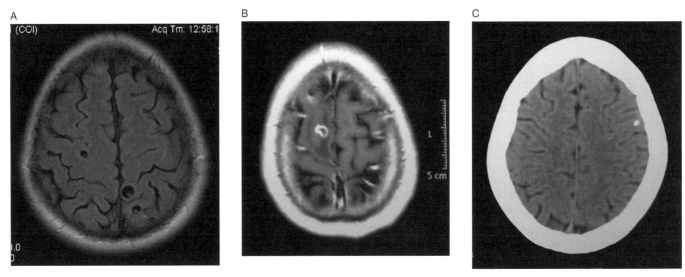

Fig. 71.1. Intraparenchymal brain cysticercosis. (A) Live, viable cysts. (B) Degenerating cyst (single cysticercal granuloma). (C) Residual calcifications.

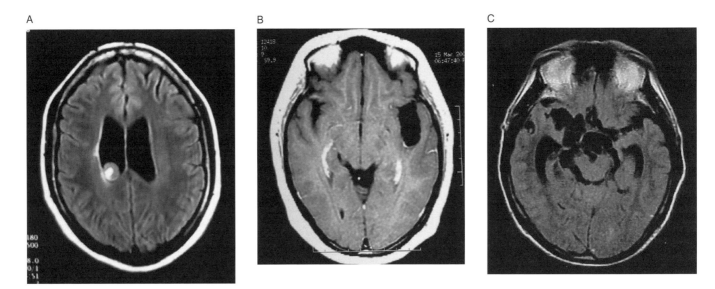

Fig. 71.2. Extraparenchymal neurocysticercosis. (A) Intraventricular cyst. (B) Giant cyst in the sylvian fissure. (C) Basal subarachnoid cysticercosis.

and intracranial hypertension which again requires surgical management. Seizures are not a primary nor a frequent manifestation of subarachnoid NCC (Bandres *et al.* 1992).

In the Indian subcontinent, the majority of cysticercosis cases are in older children and young adults, presenting as a single degenerating intraparenchymal lesion (single cysticercal granuloma). This clinical presentation is frequently seronegative and follows a very benign course: it leaves a residual calcification in less than 30% of cases, and with seizure activity continuing also in a minority of cases (~20%) (Rajshekhar and Jeyaseelan 2004). This clinical profile differs strikingly from that in Latin America where multiple cystic lesions or multiple calcifications probably account for more than 50% of clinical cases, and are commonly associated with chronic seizure disorders. Since helminth infections are overaggregated (meaning

that most infected individuals carry few parasites, and only a few are infected with heavy burdens), we have hypothesized that the typical human cysticercosis infection is very mild, with infestation with small numbers of parasites and resolves as part of its natural history (Garcia *et al.* 2003a). In this case, established cystic infections like those seen in Latin America or China would represent a subset of infections, probably those challenged with a heavier load of parasites, or resulting from a particular immune status of the host.

Epilepsy in neurocysticercosis

Seizures and epilepsy are a frequent presentation of intraparenchymal NCC. Most series find seizures in 70–95% of cases of symptomatic intraparenchymal NCC (Del Brutto *et al.* 1992).

Neurology services in endemic areas find NCC in a significant proportion (30–50%) of epilepsy cases.

Seizures are usually of focal onset, commonly with secondary generalization. Complex partial seizures are also common. While seizures in patients with multiple cysts or calcifications tend to recur, most patients with a single cysticercal granuloma experience a short period of seizure activity and then enter in remission. Patients who have a single granuloma seizure relapse in about 30% of cases, and relapse is associated with the presence of residual calcification or breakthrough seizures at presentation (Del Brutto et al. 1994; Singh et al. 2000; Nash et al. 2004).

In endemic regions, high backgrounds of exposure and asymptomatic infection are the rule. Seroprevalence of specific antibodies in the general population may easily reach 15–20% of all villagers, and when community studies based on computed tomography (CT) scans became available, 10–20% of all these villagers were found to have intraparenchymal brain calcifications, in most cases without apparent neurological symptoms. These high background levels of infection led to significant confusion in regard to the causative role of cysticercosis for seizures and epilepsy. Appropriate comparisons, however, demonstrate that in the same areas, epilepsy is two to three times more frequent in people with cerebral NCC lesions, and two to three times more frequent in seropositive individuals, and evidence of NCC is found in 30–50% of all epilepsy cases in endemic regions (Garcia et al. 2003b). Factors associated with epilepsy are the number and localization of the lesions, inflammation around at least one of the brain parasites, and edema around at least one calcified lesion. Factors associated with seizure relapse are the presence of residual calcification after cyst death (which occurs in most cysts but only in a minority of individuals presenting with single granuloma), numbers and location of residual calcifications, time with seizures before appropriate antiepileptic drug (AED) regimen, and AED compliance (Singh et al. 2000; Del Brutto et al. 2005; Nash et al. 2008).

Another particular clinical setting associated with seizures is the occurrence of perilesional edema around a dead, calcified parasite. This is responsible for approximately 50% of episodes of seizures in patients with only calcified brain lesions despite the fact that parasites are already dead. The presence of edema around dead tissue is on the face of it surprising, but the likely causative mechanism is exposure to antigenic epitopes trapped in the calcium matrix, which then trigger an inflammatory response with associated edema and seizures. The role of seizures as the primary cause of this perilesional edema has not been ruled out. Episodes of perilesional edema tend to decrease in frequency over the years (Nash and Patronas 1999; Nash et al. 2001, 2008).

Since NCC is thought to be one of a few eradicable diseases, one of the particularities of epilepsy associated with NCC is its potential to be eliminated. There have been attempts to control transmission of T. solium in endemic regions, usually restricted to one or a few small villages, using human chemotherapy to eliminate the tapeworm, health education, pig immunotherapy, or other measures. Currently a massive elimination program is being performed in Tumbes, northern coastal Peru, funded by the Bill and Melinda Gates Foundation. After two primary rounds of controlled testing of several possible interventions, a final strategy using human and pig chemotherapy plus a porcine vaccine (TSOL18, developed by Prof. M. Lightowlers at the University of Melbourne) (Gonzales et al. 2005) is being applied in a population of approximately 100 000 inhabitants. If successful, this program would provide a base model for elimination which should be expanded to other endemic areas. Baseline seizure prevalence and incidence were estimated and found to be extremely high (Montano et al. 2005; Villaran et al. 2009). The effect of NCC elimination should theoretically decrease these rates over the following years.

Diagnostic tests
Clinical settings

The primary diagnostic approach when neurocysticercosis is suspected is the use of brain imaging. A good-quality brain CT scan should uncover 90% or more cases, while older-generation scanners are usually of too limited sensitivity for this purpose. In most endemic regions, cost is a major factor in access to care. For those patients who can afford it, the more expensive magnetic resonance imaging (MRI) examinations will provide better assessment and detection of smaller lesions, better definition of those close to the skull, and images in diverse planes. As a drawback, MRI is not good for the detection of small calcifications, although new imaging protocols seem to have improved the pick-up rate (Garcia and Del Brutto 2003; Garcia et al. 2005). Serology is quite helpful in confirming the diagnosis, particularly if the brain lesions are not pathognomic. Immunoblot (Western blot) using purified antigens is the assay of choice (Tsang et al. 1989). Newly developed monoclonal-based antigen detection enzyme-linked immunosorbent assay (ELISA) technologies can confirm the presence of live parasites but their sensitivity for diagnosing patients with few intraparenchymal cysts seems to be much lower. A promising use for antigen detection is the follow-up of patients of subarachnoid NCC (Dorny et al. 2004; Zamora et al. 2005).

The differential diagnosis of a single brain enhancing lesion is problematic. Biopsy-based evidence from India suggests that a vast majority of these lesions, at least in the Indian subcontinent, are cysticercal granulomas (Chandy et al. 1991). However, tuberculosis, brain abscess, toxoplasmosis, fungal infections, and neoplasia are among many other potential causes. Ruling out progressive disease (neoplasia, tuberculosis) should be a primary objective in this setting. A set of criteria to distinguish cysticercosis from tuberculosis, developed by Rajshekhar et al. (Rajshekhar and Chandy 2000) is useful. Lesions bigger than 2 cm in maximal diameter without a shift of the midline structures due to the surrounding edema, in patients presenting with seizures with no evidence of persistent raised intracranial pressure, progressive neurological deficit, or an active systemic disease, are highly suggestive of tuberculosis rather than cysticercosis. Magnetic resonance spectroscopy (MRS) could differentiate malignant processes (decrease in N-acetylaspartate (NAA) with increased choline and some lactate, with moderate reduction in creatine) and in some cases tuberculosis (a high peak of lipids), although large series have not been reported to confirm these assumptions (Tripathi et al. 2000; Pretell et al. 2005). A full work-up for tuberculosis should be carried out, in spite of the fact that extra-SNC tuberculosis is an uncommon finding in patients with a single enhancing brain lesion. A positive immunoblot supports the diagnosis of NCC but its sensitivity in this type of lesion seems to be of only approximately 70%. Follow-up with frequent imaging is mandatory whenever a definitive diagnosis has not been reached.

Histopathology is only available in the rare cases where a lesion biopsy is indicated, or a big cyst is excised. Intraventricular cysts can be taken out by neuroendoscopy. Ruling out taeniasis in the patient or his or her household members is frequently neglected despite the fact that it can be positive in 10% or more of cases, particularly in young children or individuals with many viable brain lesions (Gilman et al. 2000). Finding a T. solium tapeworm carrier in the household very strongly supports NCC as the etiology of brain lesions. Diagnosis of taeniasis is normally made by microscopy, which has poor sensitivity despite the use of concentration methods or multiple samples. Coproantigen ELISA detection greatly increases the sensitivity of the screening but it is of very limited availability.

Field settings

In endemic villages only a small proportion of the population harbors viable brain cysts. Most individuals infected with NCC have brain calcifications only, and the vast majority is neurologically asymptomatic. Calcifications represent dead parasites, thus they do not necessarily occur with detectable antibodies. Results of antibody or even antigen serology in these settings are quite difficult to interpret. Cross-reactions are common for assays using non-purified antigens. Even if we assume absolute specificity, circulating specific antibodies may also represent past exposure, aborted infections, or established infections outside the nervous system. The specificity of antigen detection tests has not been extensively studied. When tested in the field, a substantial proportion of antigen-positive cases do not have brain parasites.

Similarly, the few studies using CT in the general population in endemic areas have consistently shown a very high background of intraparenchymal brain calcifications, present in 10–20% of all villagers (usually over 10% even in seronegative villagers) (Cruz et al. 1999; Garcia-Noval et al. 1996). At a community level, viable cysts have a low prevalence, usually below 1–2%, calcifications are frequent, and most infected patients are apparently asymptomatic. There is no evidence that "preventative" killing of viable cysts with antiparasitic therapy could benefit asymptomatic individuals and avoid the appearance of seizures. It follows that diagnostic screening for cysticercosis in field conditions should focus on individuals with defined neurological symptoms, especially those with epilepsy (particularly late onset epilepsy) or intracranial hypertension.

Principles of management

Treatment of epilepsy secondary to NCC follows standard guidelines for the management of any other secondary epilepsies. Neurocysticercosis is rarely associated with refractory seizures, and first-line AEDs usually achieve good seizure control. The most commonly used, for reasons of cost and availability, are phenytoin and carbamazepine. The overall prognosis of epilepsy secondary to NCC is good. Appropriate seizure control is the rule, and 50% or more of patients will not relapse following discontinuation of AEDs (Del Brutto et al. 1992). Since seizures in NCC are mostly sparse, patients do not feel the need to resume antiepileptic treatment after an interruption, and late relapses following self-withdrawal are frequent. Seizures may relapse after several years (Del Brutto et al. 1992; Singh et al. 2000; Rajshekhar and Jeyaseelan 2004).

Management of NCC involves symptomatic treatment (including AEDs) and antiparasitic agents. Antiparasitic treatment of NCC should only be applied after the neurological symptoms, in particular the intracranial hypertension, have been adequately investigated and stabilized. The need for antiparasitic therapy will depend on the type (stage), location, and numbers of parasitic cysts, and may be contraindicated in some disease types where abrupt inflammation could endanger the patient's life. Both albendazole and praziquantel kill between 60% and 70% of brain parasites after an initial course of treatment, with a slightly better efficacy for albendazole (Sotelo et al. 1990). The usual regime of albendazole is 15 mg/kg per day divided into two doses per day, for 7 to 15 days. Longer regimens seem required for extraparenchymal NCC. The usual regimen of praziquantel is 15 mg/kg per day, for 15 days. A short course of three doses of 25 mg/kg per day of praziquantel at 2-hourly intervals in the same morning, followed by steroids on demand if symptoms appear, was reported in Mexico (Corona et al. 1996), and seems effective for patients with a single cyst. Antiparasitic treatment is normally given with concomitant steroid therapy to modulate the inflammation caused by the death of the parasites. Most of these patients are also taking AEDs. There are a series of pharmacological interactions between these drugs. Phenytoin, carbamazepine, and dexamethasone may affect bioavailability of praziquantel. Dexamethasone does not significantly affect albendazole levels; it is not clear whether phenytoin or carbamazepine affect bioavailability of albendazole. A summary of the currently most accepted treatment approaches are presented in Table 71.1.

Table 71.1 Usual treatment approaches in neurocysticercosis (in addition to appropriate symptomatic therapy)

Location	Stage	Treatment
Parenchymal	Viable or degeneration	Antiparasitic treatment, with steroids (excepting individuals with massive infection)
	Calcified	No need for antiparasitic treatment
Extraparenchymal	Intraventricular	Neuroendoscopical removal, when available
	Subarachnoid	Antiparasitic treatment with steroids; ventricular shunt if there is hydrocephalus

Antiparasitic treatment aims to destroy living parasites on the assumption that once inactive they will cause fewer seizures. Assessment needs to account for the stage of the parasitic infection, and in particular whether they were viable cysts or already degenerating parasites. In Latin America, patients presenting with multiple viable intraparenchymal cysts are a sizeable proportion of NCC cases, while a single cysticercal granuloma occurs in ~15% of all cases. Conversely, in India (and apparently also in travelers), a single enhancing lesion is by far the commonest manifestation. This difference in clinical presentation affects the need for, and the perception of the effects of, antiparasitic treatment. Radiologically, the use of albendazole or praziquantel is clearly associated with parasite destruction of viable cysts, but only faster resolution of degenerating granulomas (Del Brutto *et al.* 2006).

The assessment of the effect of parasite destruction in improving seizure prognosis should also take into account the baseline characteristics of the patient population. Antiparasitic drugs and in some cases steroids have been associated with better prognosis of the seizure disorder which again clearly varies according to the type of NCC. Unfortunately, a sizable portion of the literature provides mixed estimates which are thus difficult to interpret. There are also other factors affecting seizure relapses, which include the number and location of lesions, presence of residual calcifications, and compliance with AED therapy. An overall analysis of the scarce available evidence suggests that fewer seizures occur in patients who are treated with antiparasitic drugs, and that this improvement is most marked in patients with viable cysts, but is not conclusive in patients who had a single cysticercal granuloma (Garcia *et al.* 2004; Del Brutto *et al.* 2006).

References

Bandres JC, White AC Jr., Samo T, Murphy EC, Harris RL (1992) Extraparenchymal neurocysticercosis: report of five cases and review of management. *Clin Infect Dis* 15:799–811.

Chandy MJ, Rajshekhar V, Ghosh S, *et al.* (1991) Single small enhancing CT lesions in Indian patients with epilepsy: clinical, radiological and pathological considerations. *J Neurol Neurosurg Psychiatry* 54:702–5.

Corona T, Lugo R, Medina R, Sotelo J (1996) Single-day praziquantel therapy for neurocysticercosis. *N Engl J Med* 334:125.

Cruz ME, Schantz PM, Cruz I, *et al.* (1999) Epilepsy and neurocysticercosis in an Andean community. *Int J Epidemiol* 28:799–803.

Dixon HB, Lipscomb FM (1961) *Cysticercosis: An Analysis and Follow-Up of 450 Cases.* London: Medical Research Council.

Del Brutto OH (1994) Prognostic factors for seizure recurrence after withdrawal of antiepileptic drugs in patients with neurocysticercosis. *Neurology* 44:1706–9.

Del Brutto OH, Santibanez R, Noboa CA, *et al.* (1992) Epilepsy due to neurocysticercosis: analysis of 203 patients. *Neurology* 42:389–92.

Del Brutto OH, Santibanez R, Idrovo L, *et al.* (2005) Epilepsy and neurocysticercosis in Atahualpa: a door-to-door survey in rural coastal Ecuador. *Epilepsia* 46:583–7.

Del Brutto OH, Roos KL, Coffey CS, Garcia HH (2006) Meta-analysis: cysticidal drugs for neurocysticercosis: albendazole and praziquantel. *Ann Intern Med* 145:4351.

Dorny P, Brandt J, Geerts S (2004) Immunodiagnostic approaches for detecting *Taenia solium*. *Trends Parasitol* 20:259–60; author reply 60–1.

Flisser A (1994) Taeniasis and cysticercosis due to *Taenia solium*. *Prog Clin Parasitol* 4:77–116.

Garcia HH, Del Brutto OH (2003) Imaging findings in neurocysticercosis. *Acta Tropica* 87:71–8.

Garcia HH, Del Brutto OH (2005) Neurocysticercosis: updated concepts about an old disease. *Lancet Neurol* 4:653–61.

Garcia HH, Gilman RH, Gonzalez AE, *et al.* (2003a) Hyperendemic human and porcine *Taenia solium* infection in Peru. *Am J Trop Med Hygiene* 68:268–75.

Garcia HH, Gonzalez AE, Gilman RH for The Cysticercosis Working Group in Peru (2003b) Diagnosis, treatment and control of Taenia solium cysticercosis. *Curr Opin Inf Dis* 16:411–19.

Garcia HH, Pretell EJ, Gilman RH, *et al.* (2004) A trial of antiparasitic treatment to reduce the rate of seizures due to cerebral cysticercosis. *N Engl J Med* 350:249–58.

Garcia-Noval J, Allan JC, Fletes C, *et al.* (1996) Epidemiology of *Taenia solium* taeniasis and cysticercosis in two rural Guatemalan communities. *Am J Trop Med Hygiene* 55:282–9.

Gilman RH, Del Brutto OH, Garcia HH, Martinez M (2000) Prevalence of taeniosis among patients with neurocysticercosis is related to severity of infection. *Neurology* 55:1062.

Gonzalez AE, Gauci CG, Barber D, *et al.* (2005) Vaccination of pigs to control human neurocysticercosis. *Am J Trop Med Hygiene.* 72:837–9.

Medina MT, Duron RM, Martinez L, *et al.* (2005) Prevalence, incidence, and etiology of epilepsies in rural Honduras: the Salama Study. *Epilepsia* 46:124–31.

Montano SM, Villaran MV, Ylquimiche L, *et al.* (2005) Neurocysticercosis: association between seizures, serology, and brain CT in rural Peru. *Neurology* **65**:229–33.

Nash TE, Del Brutto OH, Butman JA, *et al.* (2004) Calcific neurocysticercosis and epileptogenesis. *Neurology* **62**:1934–8.

Nash TE, Patronas NJ (1999) Edema associated with calcified lesions in neurocysticercosis. *Neurology* **53**:777–81.

Nash TE, Pretell J, Garcia HH (2001) Calcified cysticerci provoke perilesional edema and seizures. *Clin Infect Dis* **33**:1649–53.

Nash TE, Pretell EJ, Lescano AG, *et al.* (2008) Perilesional brain edema and seizure activity in patients with calcified neurocysticercosis: a prospective cohort and nested case-control study. *Lancet Neurol* **7**:1099–105.

Pretell EJ, Martinot C Jr., Garcia HH, *et al.* (2005) Differential diagnosis between cerebral tuberculosis and neurocysticercosis by magnetic resonance spectroscopy. *J Comput Assist Tomogr* **29**:112–14.

Rajshekhar V, Chandy MJ (2000) *Solitary Cysticercus Granuloma: The Disappearing Lesion.* Chennai: Orient Longman.

Rajshekhar V, Jeyaseelan L (2004) Seizure outcome in patients with a solitary cerebral cysticercus granuloma. *Neurology* **62**:2236–40.

Schantz PM, Wilkins PP, Tsang VCW (1998) Immigrants, imaging and immunoblots: the emergence of neurocysticercosis as a significant public health problem. In: Scheld WM, Craig WA, Hughes JM (eds.) *Emerging Infections*, 2nd edn. Washington, DC: ASM Press, pp. 213–41.

Singh G, Sachdev MS, Tirath A, Gupta AK, Avasthi G (2000) Focal cortical–subcortical calcifications (FCSCs) and epilepsy in the Indian subcontinent. *Epilepsia* **41**:718–26.

Sotelo J, del Brutto OH, Penagos P, *et al.* (1990) Comparison of therapeutic regimen of anticysticercal drugs for parenchymal brain cysticercosis. *J Neurol* **237**:69–72.

Tripathi RP, Gupta A, Gupta S, *et al.* (2000) Co-existence of dual intracranial pathology clinical relevance of proton MRS. *Neurol India* **48**:365–9.

Tsang VC, Brand JA, Boyer AE (1989) An enzyme-linked immunoelectrotransfer blot assay and glycoprotein antigens for diagnosing human cysticercosis (*Taenia solium*). *J Infect Dis* **159**:50–9.

Villaran MV, Montano SM, Gonzalvez G, *et al.* (2009) Epilepsy and neurocysticercosis: an incidence study in a Peruvian rural population. *Neuroepidemiology* **33**:25–31.

Zamora H, Castillo Y, Garcia HH, *et al.* (2005) Drop in antigen levels following successful treatment of subarachnoid neurocysticercosis. *Am J Trop Med Hygiene* **73**:S41.

Chapter 72

Other parasitic diseases

Manish Modi and Gagandeep Singh

Introduction

Parasitic infections and human infirmity have been known to be closely related since time immemorial. A number of parasites (about 300 species of helminth worms and over 70 species of protozoa) are known to infest humans (Cox 2002). Fortunately, the majority of the parasites are rare; and only about 90 or so parasitic species cause familiar human diseases. Most parasites have complex life cycles, often involving multiple hosts. Human beings may figure in the parasite life cycles as definite, intermediate, or accidental hosts.

Helminths are eukaryotic, multicellular organisms with well-developed organs. The relationship between helminths and epilepsy has been known for quite some time. The causative role of helminths in the so-called *epilepsia verminosa* has been in the past variously attributed to competition for nutrition between the host and parasite or to the irritation of peripheral nerves leading to seizures (Snyder and Cohen 2001). Table 72.1 enumerates specific helminthic organisms that are known to produce infestation of the human central nervous system (CNS). Here we review some of the parasitic disorders other than *Taenia solium* cysticercosis (which is covered in Chapter 71), which may involve the CNS and for which an association with seizures and epilepsy has been described. Nearly all the parasitic disorders discussed below are of local importance in certain selected geographic regions of the world. Nevertheless, the scale of modern travel across the world both from and to endemic regions has led to the sporadic recognition of the rare parasitic disorders in regions far away and distinct from their usual geographic boundaries. Hence, it is important that neurologists across the globe are aware of the epidemiology, clinical manifestations, and treatment of the parasitic disorders.

Sparganosis

Sparganosis is a tapeworm infection caused by sparganum, the migratory larva of genus *Spirometra*. The infestation typically involves subcutaneous tissue, skeletal tissue, and visceral organs; involvement of the nervous system is exceedingly rare.

Epidemiology

Sparganosis occurs mainly in the Far East and Southeast Asia (including China, Japan, Korea, and Taiwan). However, cases have been documented from other regions too, in particular, the United States and India, where freshwater fish is a common food item (Murata *et al.* 2007). Three species are responsible for infestation in Asia: *S. ranarum*, *S. mansoni*, and *S. erinaei*. In the western hemisphere, however, the most common species responsible for human infestation is *S. mansonoides*.

Life cycle

Domestic and wild carnivores (cats and dogs) harbor the adult worm in the small intestines and are hence the definitive hosts. Eggs from the adult worm in this location are shed in feces into fresh water. The eggs grow into coracidia in fresh water and are ingested by cyclops, the first intermediate host, in which they develop into procercoid larvae. When infested cyclops are subsequently ingested by the second intermediate hosts, i.e., frogs, snakes, and freshwater fish, the larvae penetrate the intestinal wall in order to settle eventually in the subdermal tissue and muscles as plerocercoid larvae, i.e., sparganum. When the second intermediate hosts are ingested by cats or dogs (the definitive hosts), the spargana settle in intestines and grow into adult worms (Fig. 72.1).

Humans are accidental hosts and get infested by drinking fresh water containing cyclops; ingesting raw or inadequately cooked flesh of infected fish, frogs, or snakes; or by direct application of infected tissues to the eye or open wounds in the practice of traditional medicine in endemic regions (Kim *et al.* 1996). In humans, the larvae are mainly located in the subcutaneous tissue of the abdominal wall and inguinal region, orbit and urinary organs, etc., where they produce nodules and abscesses. The parasite rarely infests the brain parenchyma, ventricles, or spinal cord (Murata *et al.* 2007).

Clinical manifestations

Brain involvement is perhaps seen in fewer than 3% of cases of sparganosis. Neurological involvement can be acute, subacute,

The Causes of Epilepsy, eds. S. D. Shorvon, F. Andermann, and R. Guerrini. Published by Cambridge University Press. © Cambridge University Press 2011.

Table 72.1 Parasitic diseases affecting the central nervous system (CNS)

Parasite family	Organisms	Disease	Clinical features	CNS involvement
Cestodes (tapeworms)	*Taenia solium*	Cysticercosis	Subcutaneous nodules	Seizures, stroke, hydrocephalus, myelopathy
	Spirometra	Sparganosis	Subcutaneous nodules, abscesses	Space-occupying lesion, seizures, meningioencephalitis
	Echinococcus	Hyadatid disease	Large cystic masses in lungs, liver	Focal signs, raised intracranial pressure
Nematodes (roundworms)	*Trichinella*	Trichinosis	Intestinal symptom, larval migration	Myositis
	Angiostrongyloides	Angiostrongyliasis	Migrating lesions	Meningioencephalitis
	Strongyloides	Strongyloidiasis	Skin lesions, lung and intestinal lesions	Encephalitis
	Toxocara canis	Larva migrans	Visceral larva migrans, ocular larva migrans, covert toxocariasis	Vasculitis, myelitis, meningoencephalitis, seizures
	Onchocerca volvulus	Onchocerciasis	Blindness, skin changes, Nakalanga syndrome	Musculoskeletal pains, seizures
Trematodes (flukes)	*Schistosoma*	Schistosomiasis	Swimmer's itch, Katayama fever, granulomas in intestine, liver, urinary bladder	Mass lesions, raised intracranial pressure, myelopathy, seizures
	Paragonimus	Paragonimiasis	Pulmonary symptoms, diarrhea, hepatosplenomegaly	Seizures, meningitis, tumor-like, subacute, and chronic encephalopathy, infarction, intracranial bleed

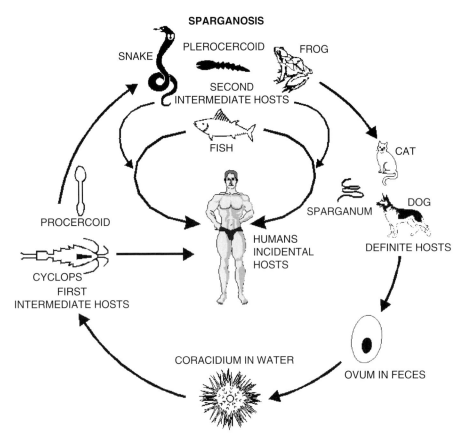

Fig. 72.1. Life cycle of *Spirometra*. (Modified from Garcia and Modi 2008.)

or chronic. The most frequent manifestations of cerebral sparganosis are headache, seizures, and focal neurological deficits (Youn *et al.* 1994; Murata *et al.* 2007). Furthermore, memory disturbances, dysphasia, dysarthria, dizziness, or hemianopia may occur depending on the site of infestation in the brain. The clinical manifestations resemble that of any other focal space-occupying lesion and may be protracted over months to years. An acute presentation may mimic encephalitis or subarachnoid hemorrhage. When the migratory worms penetrate the ventricular system, intraventricular hemorrhage and obstructive hydrocephalus may occur (Okamura *et al.* 1995; Nobayashi *et al.* 2006).

Diagnosis and treatment

A diagnosis of cerebral sparganosis may be suspected in individuals from endemic areas with a history of ingestion of frogs, fish, or snakes. Imaging (computed tomography [CT] or magnetic resonance imaging [MRI]) studies reveal granulomas that may be associated with small hemorrhages and surrounding edema in the acute stage and fibrosis and calcification in the chronic stage. Trivial shift in the location of the worm as demonstrated on serial imaging is another characteristic, albeit rare feature (Chang *et al.* 1987; Okamura *et al.* 1995). Immunological studies using enzyme-linked immunosorbent assay (ELISA) are in use in centers in endemic regions, and when performed on the cerebrospinal fluid (CSF), have been found to be highly specific and sensitive (Chang *et al.* 1987; Murata *et al.* 2007). Peripheral blood eosinophilia is another supporting laboratory feature.

Surgical excision of the granuloma and worm is the standard way of treating cerebral sparganosis (Nobayashi *et al.* 2006; Murata *et al.* 2007). Medical treatment (with praziquantel 50 mg/kg per day for 14 days) may be of use in surgically inaccessible lesions (Munckhof *et al.* 1994).

Toxocariasis

Human toxocariasis is a parasitic zoonosis caused by larval stages of *Toxocara canis* and *T. catis*, the common roundworms of dogs and cats, respectively. Toxocariasis occurs in the setting where the human–soil–dog relationship is particularly close (Nicoletti *et al.* 2007).

Epidemiology

Toxocariasis appears to be widely prevalent throughout the world. Whereas serological studies suggest prevalence rates of 3–6% in developed countries, the estimated seroprevalence is much higher in the resource-poor less-developed countries (e.g., 63.2% in Bali and 86% in Saint Lucia, West Indies) (Chomel *et al.* 1993; Magnaval *et al.* 2001). It has been suggested that the humid climates favor the survival of *Toxocara* eggs in soil while poor hygiene of hosts increases the probability of being infested in less-developed countries (Lynch *et al.* 1988).

Life cycle

Human toxocariasis is primarily a soil-transmitted zoonosis. The adult forms of *T. canis* inhabit the upper digestive tracts of their definitive hosts, dogs. The worms produce up to 200 000 eggs daily and these are passed into feces. Humans are infected when they ingest toxocara eggs or infective stage larvae in contaminated soil (geophagia, pica). The larvae penetrate the human small intestine and migrate to various tissues such as liver, heart, lungs, muscles, eyes, and CNS (Fig. 72.2). The larvae release an array of enzymes, waste products, and cuticular components that mediate tissue damage, necrosis, and inflammatory reaction (Xinou *et al.* 2003). Neurological involvement is related to the number of larvae entering the brain and to the severity of the host inflammatory response within the brain.

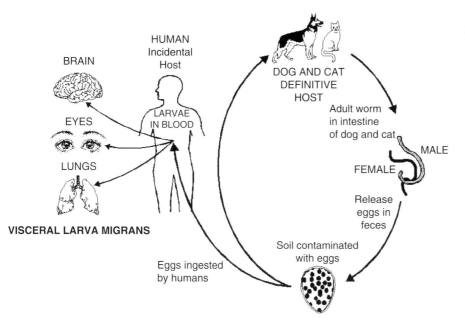

Fig. 72.2. Life cycle of *Toxocara*. (Modified from Garcia and Modi 2008.)

Clinical manifestations

Human toxocariasis commonly presents in the form of one of the three clinical syndromes: visceral larva migrans (VLM), ocular larva migrans, and covert toxocariasis (Magnaval *et al.* 2001). Toxocariasis is the most common cause of VLM worldwide especially in children. Features of VLM include fever, lethargy, sore throat, cough, wheezing, lymphadenopathy, abdominal pain, anorexia, vomiting, and hepatomegaly. Ocular larva migrans produces visual loss and eye pain due to endophthalmitis with retinal detachment, retinochoroiditis, and optic papillitis. Covert toxocariasis presents with non-specific symptoms.

Neurological involvement occurs in up to 28% of infected patients. Neurological manifestations include eosinophilic meningoencephalitis, vasculitis, seizures, myelitis, behavioral disturbances, and, rarely, acute disseminated encephalomyelitis (Despommier 2003; Marx *et al.* 2007). In one community-based association study, seropositive status for *Toxocara* was found to be associated with both partial and generalized seizures, though the association with partial seizures was stronger (Nicoletti *et al.* 2002). The association of toxocariasis and epilepsy is discussed further below.

Diagnosis and treatment

The laboratory features of toxocariasis are non-specific. Peripheral blood eosinophilia is a common feature. Immunological tests, including ELISA and Western blot may be of use. Descriptions of neuroimaging findings are sparse and somewhat inconsistent. Enhancing subcortical lesions, focal meningeal enhancement, and granulomatous lesions have been described (Xinou *et al.* 2003; Marx *et al.* 2007). Once diagnosis is confirmed, the anthelminthic drug albendazole (15mg/kg

per day orally for 5–15 days) is the treatment of choice. Other drugs like mebendazole, diethylcarbamazine, and thiabendazole may be useful (Magnaval *et al.* 2001). Systemic corticosteroids may be given for 4–6 weeks in case of ocular, pulmonary, myocardial, or neurological involvement.

Onchocerciasis

Onchocerciasis, also known as river blindness, is caused by the roundworm *Onchocercus volvulus*. It is a chronic systemic infestation manifesting with skin, musculoskeletal, and immunological disturbances, growth arrest (Nakalanga dwarfism), and, possibly, seizures and epilepsy (Burnham 1998).

Epidemiology

Onchocerciasis occurs in over 30 countries in Africa (including Nigeria, Cameroon, Ethiopia, Uganda, and the Congo), Latin America, and the Arabian Peninsula. An estimated 17.7 million persons are infected with this parasite, the majority being from Central Africa (Burnham 1998).

Life cycle

Larvae of the *O. volvulus* enter the human body during the blood-meal of an infected female *Simulium* fly. The larvae develop into bisexual adult worms, the females of which reside in skin nodules and release microfilariae, which invade the skin, eyes, and possibly other human organs. The life cycle is completed when the *Simulium* fly ingests blood from an infected person (Burnham 1998; Marin *et al.* 2006) (Fig. 72.3).

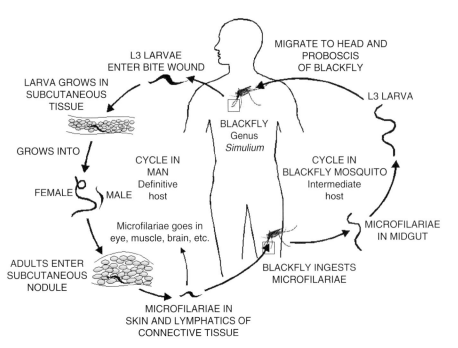

Fig. 72.3. Life cycle of *Onchocerca*. (Modified from Garcia and Modi 2008.)

Clinical manifestations

Onchocerciasis presents predominantly with blindness and skin changes. However, weight loss, musculoskeletal pain, and growth arrest (affecting children, known as Nakalanga syndrome) are other features that may be attributed to infestation. Visual impairment is predominantly due to sclerosing keratitis and iridocyclitis. Posterior segment lesions, optic neuritis, and optic atrophy have also been reported (Burnham 1998). Skin lesions vary from localized maculopapular rash with itching to generalized papular lesions with severe itching. Widespread lichenified, hyperkeratotic lesions are intensely itchy and distressing (Burnham 1998; Marin *et al.* 2006).

Diagnosis and treatment

Excision skin biopsy is a convenient means of confirming diagnosis, though ELISA tests are also available. The parasiticidal drug ivermectin is the mainstay of treatment (Burnham 1998; Newell *et al.* 1997). The drug has been systematically distributed for mass treatment in endemic regions through several agencies (Marin *et al.* 2006). The association of epilepsy and onchocerciasis is discussed further below.

Schistosomiasis

Schistosomiasis occurs due to infestation with blood flukes residing in abdominal veins of certain vertebrate definite hosts. Five species of *Schistosoma* are known to infect humans: *S. mansoni*, *S. japonicum*, *S. mekongi*, *S. intercalatum*, and *S. haematobium*. The infestation is most often characterized by chronic inflammation of the intestines and urinary bladder. Neurological manifestations, albeit rare, occur in *S. japonicum* infestation (Ross *et al.* 2002; Betting *et al.* 2005).

Epidemiology

Worldwide, more than 200 million people are currently infected and more than 600 million are at risk of infestation. Of these, approximately 120 million people have symptoms and 20 million have severe illness. The majority of *S. haematobium*, *S. mansoni*, and *S. intercalatum* infections are found in sub-Saharan Africa. *Schistosoma mansoni* infestation remains endemic in parts of Brazil, Venezuela, and the Caribbean. *Schistosoma japonicum* infestation occurs in East and Southeast Asia. *Schistosoma haematobium* infestation has been reported from Africa, the Middle East, and southwest Asia, and *S. mekongi* infestation from Cambodia and Laos (Ross *et al.* 2002).

Life cycle

Humans are the definitive hosts. Schistosome eggs are passed through urine and feces in to fresh water. Here, they transform to ciliated miracidia, which in turn penetrate freshwater snails. Within the snail hosts, the parasites mature into sporocysts and then cercariae, which are again released into water. From here, they infest humans by cutaneous penetration. Once the cercariae penetrate human skin, they shed their bifurcated tails and the resulting schistosomulae enter capillaries and lymphatic venules en route to the lungs and liver. These organisms then mature into mating pairs of male and female worms that migrate through the portal vein into venules draining the pelvic viscera. Each worm lays several hundreds of ova that eventually penetrate the wall of the urinary bladder (*S. haematobium*) or rectum (*S. mansoni* and *S. japonicum*) and are excreted in urine or feces (Betting *et al.* 2005) (Fig. 72.4).

Various mechanisms have been proposed for invasion of the brain: the eggs may reach the brain through the valveless

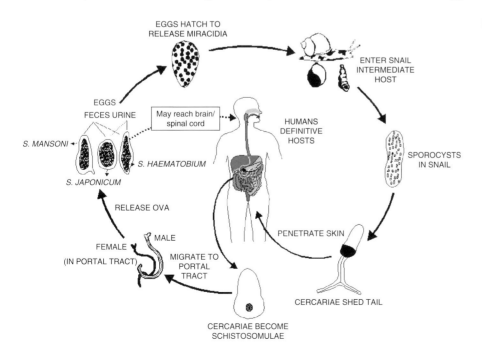

Fig. 72.4. Life cycle of *Schistosoma*. (Modified from Garcia and Modi 2008.)

venous plexus of Batson, which joins the deep iliac veins and inferior vena cava with veins of spinal cord and brain or they may migrate to the brain via pulmonary arteriovenous shunts or portal pulmonary arteriovenous shunts. The worms themselves may enter the cerebral veins and deposit their eggs in the cerebrum, cerebellum, brainstem, choroid plexus, and leptomeninges (Preidler *et al.* 1996).

Clinical features

Three stages of schistosomiasis are recognized. The first stage comprises of cercarial dermatitis (swimmer's itch), while the second stage is known as Katayama fever and is characterized by fever, myalgias, headaches, hepatosplenomegaly, bloody diarrhea, and respiratory embarrassment beginning 2–8 weeks following initial infection. Finally, chronic schistosomiasis is the result of granulomatous and fibrotic reactions to the parasite antigens. The intestines and liver are more severely affected in *S. mansoni* and *S. japonicum* infestation, while the genitourinary tract is commonly afflicted in *S. haematobium* infestation. However, infestation is also observed in other organs such as skin, lungs, adrenal glands, skeletal muscle, brain, and spinal cord (Betting *et al.* 2005). In autopsy studies, cerebral involvement is common; however, most cases have remained asymptomatic during life. Clinical manifestations related to cerebral involvement occur in only 1–2% of cases. The cerebral manifestations include seizures with raised intracranial pressure and focal signs, depending on the site of the granulomas (Betting *et al.* 2005).

Diagnosis and treatment

In the case of systemic schistosomiasis, diagnosis is established by the demonstration of ova in the urine or feces. Immunological tests are in use. Cerebral involvement has been demonstrated upon imaging studies in the form of large granulomas, tumor-like enhancement, or even intracerebral hematomas (Preidler *et al.* 1996; Artal *et al.* 2006). The treatment comprises mainly the administration of praziquantel (60mg/kg orally in three divided doses) (Scrimgeour and Gajdusek 1985). Corticosteroids and surgical resection are adjuncts to anthelminthic treatment (Fowler *et al.* 1999).

Paragonimiasis

Paragonimiasis is a benign lung disease caused by the trematode *Paragonimus*. Of the 20 species described, *P. westermani* (also known as Oriental lung fluke) is the best known (Cha *et al.* 1994). Cerebral infestation occurs in 2–27% of cases in clinic-based populations and in fewer than 1% in community-based populations (Oh *et al.* 1969).

Epidemiology

Paragonimiasis is endemic in Southeast Asia, Korea, Japan, and China. Other endemic foci include Africa (Cameroon and Nigeria) and the west coasts of Central and South America.

Life cycle

Adult worms reside in the lungs of cats, dogs, wild carnivores, and human beings, and produce eggs which are coughed out in sputum or eventually excreted through feces. When these eggs reach fresh water, they become embryonated and release miracidia. These miracidia penetrate their first intermediate hosts, i.e., snails and develop into cercariae. The cercariae, after being released into water, are ingested by the second intermediate hosts, crayfish or crabs, and develop into metacercariae. Human beings are infested by ingesting un(der)cooked crayfish and crabs containing metacercariae. The metacercariae excyst in the human small intestine, penetrate the intestinal wall, migrate into the peritoneum, and invade the pleural cavity and lung parenchyma in 2–8 weeks, during which period, they mature into adults (Robertson *et al.* 2006) (Fig. 72.5).

Infection of brain occurs when the worm strays into the intracranial cavity. The worm reaches the cranium through the jugular foramen, penetrates meninges, or invades brain parenchyma directly. Lesions are most common in temporal and occipital lobes. The initial lesions of cerebral paragonimiasis include exudative aseptic inflammation, cerebral hemorrhage, or infarction. The wandering adult *Paragonimus* makes tunnels along its track of migration. Toxic substances like proteases released by the worm may be responsible for aseptic inflammation within the brain tissue (Cha *et al.* 1994).

Clinical manifestations

Paragonimiasis usually presents with pulmonary symptoms (Chen *et al.* 2008). Cerebral involvement is heralded by seizures, headache, hemiparesis, hypesthesia, blurred vision, diplopia, homonymous hemianopia, and meningitic symptoms. Neurological presentations are pleomorphic and at least seven different presentations have been described: (1) seizures, (2) meningitis, (3) tumor-like syndrome, (4) subacute progressive encephalopathy, (5) infarction, (6) chronic brain syndrome, and (7) intracranial hemorrhage (intracerebral, subdural, or subarachnoid). Seizures have been reported in up to 80% of those with neurological involvement (Kusner and King 1993; Choo *et al.* 2003; Chen *et al.* 2008).

Diagnosis and treatment

The geographic origin of patients, ingestion of un(der)cooked crustaceans, pulmonary symptoms, abnormal chest roentgenograms, and peripheral blood eosinophilia, are clues to the diagnosis of cerebral paragonimiasis. Antibody tests by complement fixation in CSF are sensitive and specific in diagnosis. Definitive diagnosis is only possible by biopsy of brain lesions in order to demonstrate eggs (Kusner and King 1993; Cha *et al.* 1994). Imaging studies may reveal meningitis, cerebral hemorrhage, or infarction and granulomatous lesions (often appearing as conglomerate enhancing lesions or grape-like clusters) (Cha *et al.* 1994; Zhang *et al.* 2006; Chen *et al.* 2008). Treatment comprises administration of praziquantel (25 mg/kg thrice daily for 2–3

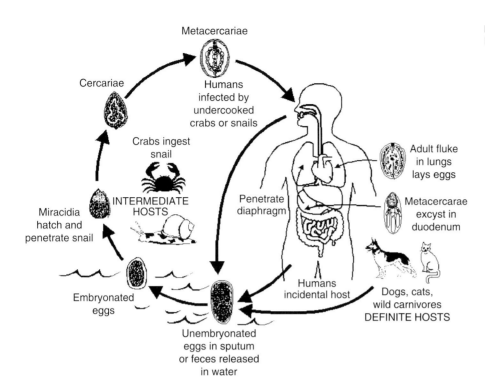

Fig. 72.5. Life cycle of *Paragonimus*. Miracidia hatch and Penetrate Snail.

Metacercariae

Cercariae

Humans infected by undercooked crabs or snails

Crabs ingest snail

INTERMEDIATE HOSTS

Miracidia hatch and penetrate snail

Embryonated eggs

Unembryonated eggs in sputum or feces released in water

Humans incidental host

Penetrate diaphragm

Adult fluke in lungs lays eggs

Metacercarae excyst in duodenum

Dogs, cats, wild carnivores DEFINITE HOSTS

days), which is highly effective for pulmonary disease and in the early stages of neurological disease. Corticosteroids may be added to reduce inflammation. Hydrocephalus may require surgical intervention (Cha *et al.* 1994; Chen *et al.* 2008).

Association of parasitic diseases with epilepsy

Although the association between epilepsy and parasitic diseases has been generally recognized, most research and literature concerning the association is related to infection with *Taenia solium* cysticercosis. For several other helminthic parasites, the association has neither been adequately studied, nor even proven in geographically diverse regions of the world. The other parasitic diseases have restricted geographical distributions as described above, and do not attract global attention. In these regions, reports of series or sometimes individual cases alone of seizures (or epilepsy) occurring in verified cases of the parasitic disorder form the basis of the literature.

When brain lesions are demonstrated on imaging studies of individuals presenting with seizures (or epilepsy), histological examination of these lesions through biopsy provides proof of the causal association between the parasitic disorder and seizures. Histological evidence may be sought from parasitic lesions that are located outside the nervous system and hence are easily approachable, e.g., biopsy of subcutaneous nodules due to cysticercosis or onchocerciasis. In other situations, evidence of parasitic infection is provided by immunological tests performed on serum or CSF.

Population-based studies to explore the association of parasitic disorders with epilepsy have been undertaken in only few instances. These studies have either a cross-sectional or case–control design. Odds ratios (or risk ratios) are then calculated for the exposed (to parasite) and unexposed populations. An odds ratio of above 5 is implicit with a certain causal association. Population-based studies have explored the association between exposure to *Toxocara*, *Onchocerca*, and *Spirometra* and epilepsy in selected geographical regions.

In the case of *Toxocara* infection, association studies were fueled by early anecdotal reports and uncontrolled studies of *Toxocara* exposure in highly selected populations of people with epilepsy (Glickman *et al.* 1979; Arpino *et al.* 1990). More recently, three case–control studies performed in Bolivia (South America), Burundi (Africa), and Catania (Italy) found age-adjusted odds ratios of 2–5 for exposure to *Toxocara* as measured by antibody responses in the serum in community-based samples of people with epilepsy (Nicoletti *et al.* 2002, 2007, 2008). Together, these studies, with more or less similar design provide evidence of a modest to strong association between *Toxocara* exposure and epilepsy. The association appeared to be even stronger for partial epilepsy in the Bolivian and Catanian studies but not in the Burundian study.

The interpretation of the association between *Toxocara* exposure and epilepsy is however not straightforward and caution is needed on several accounts. First, evidence of exposure to *Toxocara* (the outcome variable) is presumed on the basis of antibody tests performed on the serum or plasma. These tests at best detect exposure to the organism but do not necessarily indicate active infestation. Second, the symptoms and signs of human toxocariasis are relatively non-specific. Hence, it is often difficult to suspect a diagnosis of toxocariasis in the clinical setting. Third, so far, the neuropathological correlates or the structural basis of the presumed cerebral infestation in people with epilepsy remains elusive. Imaging studies in those infested people with epilepsy have not been performed largely due to economic reasons and the lack of access to imaging studies in resource-poor regions, where *Toxocara* infestation is common. In the few confirmed cases of brain infestation with *Toxocara*, the reports of imaging abnormalities are not consistent. Hence, although there appears to be a modest association of *Toxocara* infestation with epilepsy in selected geographic locations, it still remains to be determined if this association is causal. It is possible that exposure to *Toxocara* in people with epilepsy is related to poor socioeconomic status, overcrowding, and illiteracy. It may also be surmised that the people with epilepsy are more likely to keep dogs as domestic pets in order to give a warning of seizures and hence may be exposed to *Toxocara*. Or else they may fall down to the ground during seizures and get exposed to *Toxocara* eggs contaminating the soil. In order to confirm a causal association, studies of the association need to be undertaken in incident samples of epilepsy. Besides, the association needs to be biologically plausible; hence it is desirable to demonstrate the brain lesions in toxocariasis that might be responsible for seizures.

A modest number of studies, mostly from Central Africa, have explored the association between another helminthic infestation, *Onchocerciasis*, and epilepsy (Kilian 1994; Kipp *et al.* 1994; Kabore *et al.* 1996; Kaiser *et al.* 1996, 1998, 2007, 2008; Newell *et al.* 1997; Duke 1998; Druet-Cabanac *et al.* 1999, 2004; Farnarier *et al.* 2000; Boussinesq *et al.* 2002; Dozie *et al.* 2006). Many of the studies have had a cross-sectional design and another three studies were matched case–control studies (Druet-Cabanac *et al.* 1999; Farnarier *et al.* 2000; Boussinesq *et al.* 2002). Nine published studies from Africa reviewed recently lacked consistency with relative risks varying from 0.84 to 6.80 and pooled crude relative risk of 1.21 (95% confidence interval [CI]: 0.99–1.47) (Druet-Cabanac *et al.* 2004). The relative risks in most African studies have not been controlled for age and levels of endemicity of onchocerciasis in the general population. In sub-Saharan Africa, where onchocerciasis is common, prevalence rates vary between 13% and 89% (Ovuga *et al.* 1992; Kabore *et al.* 1996). Moreover, the published studies have not made adjustments for confounding factors. It has been suggested that *T. solium* cysticercosis is also widely prevalent in much of sub-Saharan Africa. Seizures are the most common presentation of cysticercosis and subcutaneous nodules quite similar to those encountered in onchocerciasis are not uncommon. In a biopsy study from Togo, onchocerci were found in

68% of subcutaneous nodules and cysticerci in 28% (Dumas *et al.* 1989). Hence, it is possible that a proportion of cases of epilepsy among those exposed to *Onchocerca* have neurocysticercosis-related seizures (Kaiser *et al.* 2008).

As in the case of toxocariasis, imaging and pathological descriptions of brain involvement by *Onchocerca* are either limited or unavailable. Various mechanisms have been proposed for the occurrence of seizures in onchocerciasis and hence the association between infestation and epilepsy. Direct brain invasion, though not adequately demonstrated, is the most likely mechanism. Immunological mechanisms, specifically the involvement of cytokines, have also been surmised to play a role in the generation of seizures (Marin *et al.* 2006). Indeed, it has been suggested that the variations in the association between the parasitic infestation and epilepsy in different geographic regions within Africa may be related to different strains of *O. volvulus* and differences in their pathogenicity to the brain (Druet-Cabanac *et al.* 2004; Marin *et al.* 2006). In one study, the occurrence of seizures correlated with the parasitemic load as determined on dermal biopsies (Boussinesq *et al.* 2002). Finally, a cause–effect relationship between *Onchocerca* infestation and epilepsy can only be established in studies of samples of incident seizure and to the best of our knowledge such studies have not been undertaken.

In the case of sparganosis, a clinic-based, case–control serological study using an anti-*Spirometra* antibody (IgG) assay in Korea found seropositivity rates among 2667 randomly selected epileptic patients to be 2.5% in comparison to 1.9% in unmatched healthy controls, yielding an odds ratio of 1.32 (Kong *et al.* 1994). Population-based studies of the association of epilepsy with other parasitic disorders such as schistosomiasis and paragonimiasis are not available.

Conclusions

The causal association between CNS infestation and epilepsy is predictable, but poorly documented due to constraints in epidemiological, epileptological, and microbiologic methods. Further studies of association between various parasitic infestations of the brain and epilepsy and the natural history of seizures following these infestations with documentation of their structural correlates on imaging are desirable. In addition the effects of anthelminthic drugs and the role of antiepileptic drugs on the seizure outcome also need to be considered. The ultimate aim is to eradicate these disorders through scientifically established and properly legislated preventive measures.

References

Arpino C, Gattinara GC, Piergili D, Curatolo P (1990) Toxocara infection and epilepsy in children: a case control study. *Epilepsia* **31**:33–6.

Artal FJ, Mesquita HM, Gepp Rde A, Antunes JS, Kolil RK (2006) Brain involvement in a *Schistosoma mansoni* myelopathy patient. *J Neurol Neurosurg Psychiatry* **77**:512.

Betting LE, Pirani C Jr., de Souja Queiroz LS, Damasceno BP, Cendes F (2005) Seizures and cerebral schistosomiasis. *Arch Neurol* **62**:1008–10.

Boussinesq M, Pion SD, Demanga-Ngangue, Kamgno J (2002) Relationship between onchocerciasis and epilepsy: a matched case–control study in the Mbam Valley, Republic of Cameroon. *Trans R Soc Trop Med Hyg* **96**:537–41.

Burnham G (1998) Onchocerciasis. *Lancet* **351**:1341–6.

Cha SH, Chang KH, Cho SY, et al. (1994) Cerebral paragonimiasis in early active stage: CT and MR features. Am J Roentgenol 162:141–5.

Chang KH, Cho SY, Chi JG, et al. (1987) Cerebral sparganosis: CT characteristics. Radiology 165:505–10.

Chen Z, Zhu G, Lin J, Wu N, Feng H (2008) Acute cerebral paragonimiasis presenting as hemorrhagic stroke in a child. Pediatr Neurol 39:133–6.

Chomel BB, Kasten R, Adams C, et al. (1993) Serosurvey of some major zoonotic infections in children and teenagers in Bali, Indonesia. Southeast Asian J Trop Med Health 24:321–6.

Choo JD, Suh BS, Lee HS, et al. (2003) Chronic cerebral paragonimiasis combined with aneurysmal subarachnoid hemorrhage. Am J Trop Med Hyg 69:466–9.

Cox FEG (2002) History of human parasitology. Clin Microbiol Rev 15:595–612.

Despommier D (2003) Toxicariasis: clinical aspects, epidemiology, medical ecology, and molecular aspects. Clin Microbiol Rev 16:265–72.

Dozie IN, Onwuliri CO, Nwoke BE, et al. (2006) Onchocerciasis and epilepsy in parts of the Imo river basin, Nigeria: a preliminary report. Publ Health 120:448–50.

Druet-Cabanac M, Boussinesq M, Dongmo L, et al. (2004) Review of epidemiological studies searching for a relationship between onchocerciasis and epilepsy. Neuroepidemiology 23:144–9.

Druet-Cabanac M, Preux PM, Bouteille B, et al. (1999) Onchocerciasis and epilepsy: a matched case–control study in the Central African Republic. Am J Epidemiol 149:565–70.

Duke BO (1998) Onchocerciasis, epilepsy and hyposexual dwarfism. Trans R Soc Trop Med Hyg 92:236.

Dumas M, Grunitzky E, Deniau M, et al. (1989) Epidemiological study of neuro-cysticercosis in northern Togo (West Africa). Acta Leiden 57:191–6.

Farnarier G, Diop S, Coulibaly B, et al. (2000) Onchocerciasis and epilepsy: epidemiological survey in Mali. Med Trop 60:151–5.

Fowler R, Lee C, Keystone JS (1999) The role of corticosteroids in the treatment of cerebral schistosomiasis caused by Schistosoma mansoni: case report and discussion. Am J Trop Med Hyg 61:47–50.

Garcia HH, Modi M (2008). Helminthic parasite and seizures. Epilepsia 49(Suppl 6):25–32.

Glickman LT, Cypess RH, Crumrine PK, Gitlin DA (1979) Toxocara infection and epilepsy in children. J Pediatr 94:75–8.

Kabore JK, Cabore JW, Melaku Z, Druet-Cabanac M, Preux PM (1996) Epilepsy in a focus of onchocerciasis in Burkina Faso. Lancet 347:836.

Kaiser C, Kipp W, Asaba G, et al. (1996) The prevalence of epilepsy follows the distribution of onchocerciasis in a west Ugandan focus. Bull World Health Org 74:361–7.

Kaiser C, Asaba G, Leichsenring M, Kabagambe G (1998) High incidence of epilepsy related to onchocerciasis in West Uganda. Epilepsy Res 30:247–51.

Kaiser C, Asaba G, Kasoro S, et al. (2007) Mortality from epilepsy in an onchocerciasis endemic area in West Uganda. Trans R Soc Trop Med Hyg 101:48–55.

Kaiser C, Pion S, Preux PM, et al. (2008) Onchocerciasis, cysticercosis, and epilepsy. Am J Trop Med Hyg 79:643–4.

Kilian AH (1994) Onchocerciasis and epilepsy. Lancet 343:983.

Kim DG, Paek SH, Chang KH, et al. (1996) Cerebral sparganosis: clinical manifestations, treatment, and outcome. J Neurosurg 85:1066–71.

Kipp W, Kasoro S, Burnham G (1994) Onchocerciasis and epilepsy in Uganda. Lancet 343:183–4.

Kong Y, Cho SY, Kang WS (1994) Sparganum infections in normal adult population and epileptic patients in Korea: a seroepidemiologic observation. Kisaengchunghak Chapchi 32:85–92.

Kusner DJ, King CH (1993) Cerebral paragonimiasis. Semin Neurol 13:201–8.

Lee KJ, Bae YT, Kim DH, Deung YK, Ryang YS (2002) A seroepidemiologic survey for human sparganosis in Gangweon-do. Korean J Parasitol 40:177–80.

Lynch NR, Eddy K, Hodgen AN, Lopez RI, Turner KJ (1988) Seroprevalence of toxocara canis infection in tropical Venezuela. Trans R Soc Trop Med Hyg 82:275–81.

Magnaval JF, Glickman LT, Dorchies P, Morassin B (2001) Highlights of human toxicariasis. Korean J Parasitol 39:1–11.

Marin B, Boussinesq M, Druet-Cabanac M, et al. (2006) Onchocerciasis related epilepsy? Prospects at a time of uncertainty. Trends Parasitol 22:17–20.

Marx C, Lin J, Masruha MR, et al. (2007) Toxocariasis of the CNS simulating acute disseminated encephalomyelitis. Neurology 69:806–7.

Munckhof WJ, Grayson ML, Susil BJ, Pullar MJ, Turnidge J (1994). Cerebral sparganosis in an East Timorese refugee. Med J Austral 161:263–64.

Murata K, Abe T, Gohda M, et al. (2007) Difficulty in diagnosing a case with apparent sequel cerebral sparganosis. Surg Neurol 67:409–12.

Newell ED, Vyungimana F, Bradley JE (1997) Epilepsy, retarded growth and onchocerciasis, in two areas of different endemicity of onchocerciasis in Burundi. Trans R Soc Trop Med Hyg 91:525–7.

Nicoletti A, Bartoloni A, Reggio A, et al. (2002) Epilepsy, cysticercosis, and toxocariasis: a population-based case control study in rural Bolivia. Neurology 58:1256–61.

Nicoletti A, Bartoloni A, Sofia V, et al. (2007) Epilepsy and toxicariasis: a case-control study in Burundi. Epilepsia 48:894–9.

Nicoletti A, Sofia V, Mantella A, et al. (2008) Epilepsy and toxocariasis: a case-control study in Italy. Epilepsia 49:594–9.

Nobayashi M, Hirabayashi H, Sakaki T, et al. (2006) Surgical removal of a live worm by stereotactic targeting in cerebral sparganosis: case report. Neurol Med Chir (Tokyo) 46:164–7.

Oh SJ (1969) The rate of cerebral involvement in paragonimiasis: an epidemiologic study. Jpn J Parasitol 18:211–14.

Okamura T, Yamamoto M, Ohta K, Matsuoka T, Uozumi T (1995) Cerebral sparganosis mansoni: case report. Neurol Med Chir (Tokyo) 35:909–13.

Ovuga E, Kipp W, Mungherera M, Kasoro S (1992) Epilepsy and retarded growth in a hyperendemic focus of onchocerciasis in rural western Uganda. East Afr Med J 69:554–6.

Preidler KW, Riepl T, Szolar D, Ranner G (1996) Cerebral schistosomiasis: MR and CT appearance. AJNR Am J Neuroradiol 17:1598–600.

Ross AG, Bartley PB, Sleigh AC, *et al.* (2002) Schistosomiasis. *N Engl J Med* **346**:1212–20.

Scrimgeour EM, Gajdusek DC (1985) Involvement of the central nervous system in *Schistosoma mansoni* and *S. hematobium* infection: a review. *Brain* **108**:1023–38.

Snyder PJ, Cohen H (2001) Epilepsia verminosa. *J Hist Neurosci* **10**:163–72.

Xinou E, Lefkopoulos A, Gelagoti M, *et al.* (2003) CT and MR imaging findings in cerebral toxocaral disease. *AJNR Am J Neuroradiol* **24**:714–18.

Youn SH, Hu C, Pyen JS, *et al.* (1994) Clinical analysis of cerebral sparganosis. *Korean Neurosurg Soc* **23**:299–304.

Zhang JS, Huan Y, Sun LJ, *et al.* (2006) MRI features of pediatric cerebral paragonimiasis in the active stage. *J Magn Reson Imag* **23**:569–73.

Chapter

73

Tuberculosis

Nadir E. Bharucha, Roberta H. Raven, and Vivek Nambiar

The organism

Tuberculosis (TB) is a disease now commonest in developing countries and caused by the species *Mycobacterium tuberculosis* complex. The important organism in that complex is *M. tuberculosis*. Two-thirds of all TB patients have pulmonary disease and one-third are affected in all other sites, including the central nervous system (CNS) (Zuger and Lowy 1997; Raviglione and O'Brien 2008).

Mycobacterium tuberculosis is Gram-positive, and aerobic; it divides slowly and hence produces chronic disease. It has in its cell wall complex lipids linked to glycolipids and sugars. The cell wall prevents penetration of antibiotics, is acid-fast, and is responsible for interacting with the host defense system and even for surviving inside macrophages. Its genome has a sequence of about 4000 genes, one of the largest among bacteria. It is relatively stable, producing all requirements for its own successful replication.

Different strains of the organism have distinctive insertion sequences (IS) which can be identified by restriction fragment length polymorphism (RFLP) analysis, thus permitting genotyping (Barnes and Cave 2003). The most widely analyzed is IS6110. Therefore, it is possible to ascertain strain virulence, or to identity whether the infection in a patient is a reactivation of old TB or a new infection, as well as to find drug-resistant strains. Using this technology, it is now known that, even in developed countries, new infection is responsible for 20–25% of urban cases.

Epidemiology

Though the disease is known to be underreported, no reliable incidence or prevalence data for TB are available. The incidence of TB of the CNS tracks TB in general. The prevalence of TB is greatest in developing countries. The World Health Organization (WHO) in 2005 reported 8.8×10^6 new cases worldwide, of which 95% were in developing countries with 1.6×10^6 deaths overall. Of the new cases 80% were pulmonary. With associated HIV infection, extrapulmonary TB rose to

about 70%. Although the incidence of all TB in developed countries fell from 1900 till the late 1980s, it has subsequently begun to increase due to immigration from areas with a high prevalence, poor socioeconomic circumstances, and healthcare, and most importantly also to the arrival of human immunodeficiency virus (HIV). From 1990 to 2005 in countries in which HIV prevalence $\geq 5\%$, the incidence of TB rose by 7% per year, whereas in those with lower HIV prevalence, it rose by only 1.3% per year (Reid *et al.* 2006). The chance of infection by the TB bacillus depends on the presence of "open" TB cases, patients with sputum positive for *M. tuberculosis* who usually have pulmonary cavitation. Even a single droplet of infected sputum can contain up to 3000 organisms and can float for hours in an aerosol remaining infectious. Whether a person infected by the *M. tuberculosis* bacillus actually develops the disease depends on endogenous host susceptibility. After inhalation, only about 10% of organisms reach the pulmonary alveoli, where they are phagocytosed by alveolar macrophages as "phagosomes." Sometimes the glycolipid in the wall of the organism inhibits the calcium calmodulin pathway, preventing fusion of the phagosome with lysosomes and permitting bacterial proliferation. This results in macrophage rupture and hematogenous spread to other organs, including the CNS. After 2–4 weeks of infection, cell-mediated immunity and delayed-type hypersensitivity occur, resulting in tubercle formation.

A tubercle is an accumulation of activated macrophages, lymphocytes, and giant cells with a caseous, necrotic center. The significance of the granuloma is currently under debate. Generally granulomas are believed to contain infections but another view suggests that macrophages may promote infection by sheltering *M. tuberculosis* intracellularly (Rubin 2009).

Tubercles may rupture either into the subarachnoid space, releasing tubercular protein and producing meningoencephalitis, arteritis, and hydrocephalus, or they may rupture into the brain parenchyma, resulting in a tuberculoma or rarely an abscess. In children with neurotuberculosis, rupture of the primary tubercle leading to CNS infection occurs soon after

The Causes of Epilepsy, eds. S. D. Shorvon, F. Andermann, and R. Guerrini. Published by Cambridge University Press. © Cambridge University Press 2011.

initial exposure, whereas in adults the two events are often separated by years. Formation of tuberculomas involving cell-mediated immunity releases proinflammatory cytokines which lower the seizure threshold. (Vezzani and Granata 2005). The presence of status epilepticus also leads to production of proinflammatory cytokines with macrophage migration and hence cerebral inflammation (Vezzani et al. 2009). Thus in tuberculosis, the occurrence both of seizures and inflammation converge (via macrophages) to increase the likelihood of further seizures.

Clinical features
Tuberculous meningitis

Tuberculous meningitis is usually heralded by a non-specific prodrome of 2–6 weeks' duration (generally 2 weeks) (British Medical Research Council Stage I) which is then followed by the subacute onset of symptoms and signs of meningitis for 1–2 weeks with mildly impaired sensorium and/or cranial nerve palsies, involving particularly cranial nerves III, IV, and VI but also II, VII, and VIII (British Medical Research Council Stage II). This phase is followed by deepening unconsciousness and limb paralysis 3–8 weeks into the illness (British Medical Research Council Stage III). Seizures are common, particularly in children and the elderly (Karstaedt et al. 1998; Thwaites et al. 2000).

There may or may not be signs of systemic infection. History of contact with and the presence of pulmonary tuberculosis on chest X-ray are more often found in children than in adults. Children less often complain of headache and more often have hydrocephalus.

Clinical features of tuberculous meningitis are largely unaltered by HIV, but there is more tuberculosis in other systems and tuberculomas are more common.

Tuberculoma

Tuberculoma presents as an intracranial space-occupying lesion with any or all of the following symptoms: seizures, focal progressive neurological deficit, raised intracranial pressure. The history and systemic findings are similar to those of tuberculous meningitis. Tuberculomas often occur in patients with tuberculous meningitis, but patients with a granuloma presenting as an intracranial space-occupying lesion do not usually have meningitis. In India in the era before computed tomography (CT), 21.5% of all intracranial space-occupying lesions at pathology were tuberculomas (Dastur et al. 1968). In children, the proportion of tuberculomas was even higher, at 46.4%. The clinical issue of differentiating tuberculoma and neurocysticercosis on CT scanning is discussed below.

Tuberculous abscesses

Tuberculous abscesses are rare. They may result from liquefaction of the caseous necrotic core of a pre-existing granuloma, or more rarely, appear de novo. Clinical presentation is similar to tuberculoma, but duration of the illness is briefer

and patients appear more febrile and toxic. Such patients usually require neurosurgical attention for stereotactic aspiration of pus or excision biopsy.

Tuberculous encephalitis

Border zone encephalitis is almost invariably associated with meningitis and is responsible for the meningoencephalitic presentation of tuberculous meningitis. Isolated encephalitis does not occur in TB. An entity known as tuberculous encephalopathy was reported in the earlier literature by Dastur and Udani (1966) and has been reviewed more recently (Lammie et al. 2007). In the original paper, patients were children who presented with seizures and altered sensorium, and considerable brain swelling was found at autopsy. There was little or no meningitis. The changes in brain were thought to resemble allergic encephalomyelitis. This condition as originally described must be exceedingly rare and we have not encountered it.

Investigations
Cerebrospinal fluid

Examination of the cerebrospinal fluid (CSF) in tuberculous meningitis reveals a lymphocytic pleocytosis with raised proteins and low glucose. In about 25% of patients, there may be an initial predominance of neutrophils in the CSF, which, within days converts to the usual lymphocytic pattern. Neutrophil predominance may persist in immunocompromised patients. After commencing antituberculous treatment, the lymphocytic response may be converted to a neutrophilic response, the so-called "therapeutic paradox," which is the earliest manifestation of the immune reconstitution syndrome. Simultaneously, the patient declines clinically. In Turkey, in one reported series (Sutlas et al. 2003) this therapeutic paradox occurred in 32% of patients in the first weeks of treatment and resolved in the following weeks. Half these patients deteriorated clinically and four died. The CSF is sometimes relatively acellular in those with HIV, but also in non-HIV infected patients (Karstaedt et al. 1998). The acid-fast stain reveals the organism in only a very small percentage of patients, 25% in the literature and much less in our experience. Usually too few bacilli are present to be detected by the laboratory. Culture of the CSF is positive in up to 50% patients, if adequate volumes are examined. Culture requires 4–8 weeks. Although not useful for initial therapy, it may confirm the diagnosis and is useful to test drug sensitivity. Fully automated liquid culture systems have reduced culture time to 1–3 weeks. As bacteriology has limitations, biochemical, immunological, and molecular diagnostic methods have evolved. A biochemical marker is CSF adenosine deaminase activity (ADA), which is elevated in CSF in tuberculous meningitis (ADA results from lymphocyte and monocyte activity in CSF) (Thwaites et al. 2000). Although said to have high sensitivity and specificity, raised ADA also occurs in the CSF of patients with pyogenic meningitis, neurobrucellosis, lymphoma, and sarcoid. It can help discriminate

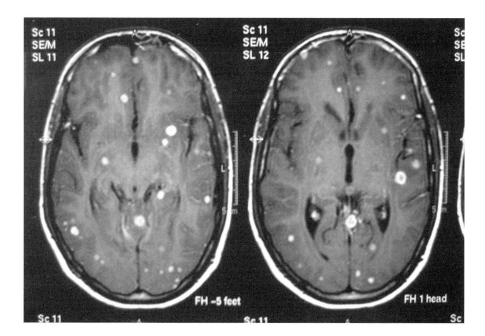

Fig. 73.1. Brain scan of 21-year-old man, presenting with headache and complex partial seizures. Gadolinium-enhanced MRI brain shows multiple tuberculomas. Fundi showed choroids and tubercles; and chest X-ray showed miliary tuberculosis.

aseptic meningitis. Serological tests can detect mycobacterial antibodies and antigens in CSF. However, the choice of antibodies and antigens in test kits determines the reliability of the test and antibody detection does not necessarily imply current infection and may be negative if the patient is immunocompromised. The future may lie in refinement of nucleic acid amplification (NAA) tests such as polymerase chain reaction (PCR) (Pai *et al.* 2003). They are rapid, but have not yet been found to have adequate sensitivity and specificity. Low sensitivity may be due to small sample size and low bacillary level, and false positives may occur due to cross-contamination with an outside source of *M. tuberculosis* DNA in the laboratory. At present, NAA assays are not practical in resource-poor countries (Nahid *et al.* 2006). Indeed, even in a major centre in the USA, only 24% patients with CSF culture-positive CNS TB had a positive PCR and none had a CSF smear positive for acid-fast bacilli (AFB) (Christie *et al.* 2008). The CSF examination is usually not performed in patients with granuloma for the following reasons: (1) if granulomas are large, there may be risk of herniation, (2) if the granulomas are small, CSF examination is usually normal, particularly if lesions are largely intraparenchymal or few in number.

Tuberculin skin test and interferon-γ releasing assays

The tuberculin skin test and its immunological equivalent with blood, the interferon-γ releasing assay (IGRA) which measures interferon-γ release by T cells, both measure development of cell-mediated immunity after exposure to *M. tuberculosis*. The IGRA has the advantage of a rapid result and being unaffected by previous Bacille Calmette–Guérin (BCG) vaccine (Richeldi 2006). However, both tests fail to distinguish latent from active

tuberculosis and would therefore be useful only in children in non-endemic areas when suspecting active TB (Davies and Pai 2008).

Neuroimaging

Neuroimaging, both CT and magnetic resonance imaging (MRI), with and without intravenous (IV) contrast, is able to identify most of the pathology of CNS TB, unless it is in the very early stages. It shows basal exudates, early hydrocephalus, granulomas, infarcts, and cerebritis (Fig. 73.1). Magnetic resonance angiography may help in identifying arteritis, but often does not as the arteries involved are too small to be visualized. The granuloma in TB is hyperintense in T1-weighted images and often hypointense in T2-weighted images.

Differentiation of tuberculoma and neurocysticercosis

If there are isolated granulomas, then neurocysticercosis is a major diagnostic consideration. Indeed, in India, in the early CT scan era, small (<10 mm), single, CT-enhancing lesions were found often in patients presenting with acute symptomatic seizures and they often resolved after 3 months without treatment, so-called "disappearing lesions." As anti-TB treatment had been started empirically in some of these patients, the lesions were thought to be tuberculomas. It was only after excision biopsy on some patients they were found to be cysticercal granulomas (Chandy *et al.* 1991). On MRI, neurocysticercosis in its cystic form is T1-weighted hypointense and T2-weighted hyperintense, the opposite of tuberculous granulomas. In general, large (>2 cm) irregular granulomas with midline shift on CT or MRI and producing a raised intracranial pressure and a progressive focal neurological deficit are more likely to be tuberculomas rather than cysticercal in origin (Rajshekhar and Chandy 1996). Neurocysticercosis is a commoner cause of acute symptomatic seizures than tuberculosis in several parts of India (Murthy and Yangala 1999). In addition to tuberculomas and neurocysticercosis, if the patient has HIV, it is necessary to rule out toxoplasma, lymphoma, and progressive multifocal leukoencephalopathy.

Diagnosis

To diagnose neurotuberculosis, several factors need consideration.

(1) History: exposure to a person with the disease, birth in or travel to an endemic area, past history of tuberculosis, immunosuppression, lifestyle factors, and socioeconomic circumstances.

(2) Clinical history of present illness and findings. A longer duration of illness favors tuberculous meningitis rather than bacterial meningitis.

(3) Laboratory findings: CSF pleocytosis with predominantly lymphocytes and blood white cell counts <15 000/mm^3. The AFB smear is usually negative and hence negative Gram stain, cryptococcal antigen test, and cytology for malignant cells are essential. Diagnostic algorithms using some of the above data have been developed for resource-poor countries (Torok et al. 2007). They have been found to be reasonably sensitive and specific and indeed superior to bacteriology in a routine laboratory.

(4) Neuroimaging findings consistent with tuberculosis are helpful in tuberculous meningitis and the only means of diagnosing a tuberculoma.

(5) Evidence of tuberculosis elsewhere: high-resolution CT scan of chest and ultrasound of abdomen and pelvis are useful. Routine chest X-ray is often negative.

(6) Response to anti-TB treatment should be monitored constantly, clinically, and with periodic CSF examination and imaging.

A high index of suspicion is essential. Most delays occur because the condition is not suspected. Delay in diagnosis and consequently treatment is the most important cause of a bad prognosis in tuberculosis (Storla et al. 2008).

Epilepsy in neurotuberculosis
Acute stage

In 10% of cases, tuberculous meningitis can present with acute symptomatic seizures (Kennedy and Fallon 1979). Seizures also occur during the course of the illness. One study found a varying frequency of about 7–10% in adults and 10–55% in children (Garcia-Monco 1999). A more recent survey of 61 adult patients from a neurological center in Turkey reported a higher frequency of seizures (16.3%) of which 50% were focal and 50% generalized (Sutlas et al. 2003). In a prospective study from a neurological center in India, which included 54 patients of all ages, the frequency of seizures was found to be 31.5%,

the majority being partial with secondary generalization (Misra et al. 2000). Occasionally neurotuberculosis presents with status epilepticus. It accounted for 9 of 93 patients (9.7%) with status epilepticus in Lucknow, India (Misra et al. 2008), 6 out of 85 (7%) patients in Hyderabad, India (Murthy et al. 2007), and 8 of 119 (6.7%) patients in Addis Ababa, Ethiopia (Amare et al. 2008). In neurotuberculosis, seizures can result from encephalitis, tuberculomas, vasculitis, hydrocephalus, hyponatremia, and isoniazid. Factors increasing the risk of seizures in neurotuberculosis are the same as for acute symptomatic seizures following any bacterial meningitis (Tyler 2008; Zoons et al. 2008). These include altered consciousness, a clinical focal deficit, systemic illness, a focal brain lesion on imaging (cortical granuloma, infarction, cerebritis) or hydrocephalus in children or associated chronic diseases like diabetes or alcoholism.

At the Bombay Hospital, a large well-equipped general hospital, averaging 25 000 admissions annually, we looked for records of neurotuberculosis for the years 2007–2008 (Bharucha et al. 2009). There were 166 admissions with this diagnosis. Case papers of 100 of these were studied. Thirty-seven patients had acute symptomatic seizures, of whom 31 had seizures related to the present admission and six had had seizures in the past. The current admission was for symptoms associated with tuberculosis or its treatment. Twenty-eight patients had generalized tonic–clonic seizures, six being secondarily generalized. Nine patients had partial seizures, four complex partial, and five simple partial. In all, 15/37 patients had partial seizures. Generalized convulsive status epilepticus occurred in seven of 37 patients (18.9%), with a partial onset in four.

Neuroimaging was carried out in all 37 patients (MRI = 28, CT = 7). Reports for two of these were unavailable. One or more granulomas were found in the majority, 27/35 patients. In 12 of these, granulomas were associated with tuberculous meningitis, in 11 granulomas occurred alone; in two, granulomas were associated with hyponatremia and in two with an infarct. Six patients had only tuberculous meningitis.

Seven of the 37 patients who had been on antituberculous treatment and were responding, developed new granulomas and presented with seizures – paradoxical worsening of tuberculosis. This phenomenon is more often seen after commencement of antiretroviral treatment (ART) in patients with HIV infection, and is known as immune reconstition inflammatory syndrome or IRIS. The recovery of the immune system results in increased inflammation in pre-existing lesions due to tuberculosis producing tuberculosis-associated IRIS (TB-IRIS) (Meintjes et al. 2008). In one study, cited by Meintjes et al. (2008), paradoxical reactions following antituberculous treatment occurred in 36% of patients with HIV who were receiving concurrent ART, 70% of HIV patients not on ART, and 2% of patients without HIV. Whether to start ART and antituberculous treatment simultaneously, or whether to start ART 3 months after antituberculous treatment is contentious. Although delaying ART may prevent the paradoxical reaction,

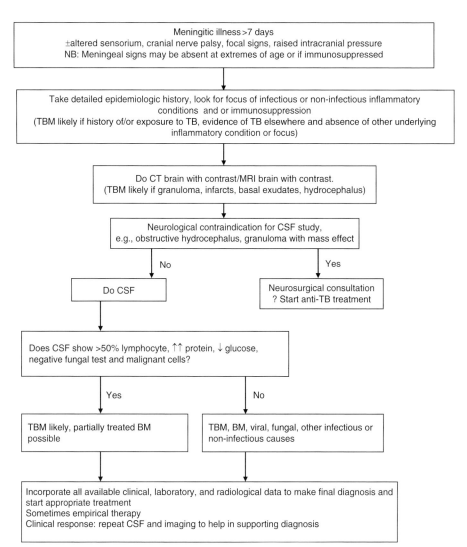

Fig. 73.2. Management of suspected tuberculous meningitis (TBM) in developing countries where bacteriological tests are usually negative.

if the patient is severely immunocompromised, he or she may succumb to the complications of acquired immune deficiency syndrome (AIDS). Indeed, a recent clinical trial to test this very hypothesis had to be modified because the mortality rate in the sequential treatment group (ART started after antituberculous treatment completed) was twice as high as in the integrated treatment group (ART started simultaneously with antituberculous treatment or 2 months after antituberculous treatment had begun) (Ryan 2008).

Chronic stage

Neurotuberculosis is associated with an increased risk of epilepsy. Quantifying this risk is difficult because of the multiple CNS pathologies involved. No modern prospective, community-based data are available for neurotuberculosis. In the pre-HIV era, community-based data from Rochester, Minnesota showed an increased risk of subsequent epilepsy after CNS infection, but there was no neurotuberculosis in this group. Risk of epilepsy was higher if there were early seizures and particularly status

epilepticus. It was greatest during the first 5 years, but persists for the subsequent 15 years (Annegers *et al.* 1988; Hesdorffer *et al.* 1998).

In a retrospective chart review of 147 patients with CNS infection from a neurology department in South Korea, among whom there were 63 patients with tuberculous meningitis, those without seizures at the time of the acute illness had no later epilepsy. Of those with CNS infection of all causes, 34/147 had acute symptomatic seizures and 14 of these patients later developed remote symptomatic epilepsy. Ten of the 34 with acute asymptomatic seizures had status epilepticus, the presence of which correlated with both later epilepsy and antiepileptic drug (AED) resistance. Most seizures in this study were due to viral encephalitis, not meningitis (Kim *et al.* 2008).

Principles of management

There are two different settings in which neurotuberculosis can present with seizures and epilepsy (Fig. 73.2). The first is in the context of the meningitic illness, together with a range of associated pathologies, involving the brain parenchyma and including granulomas, encephalitis, arteritis, and hydrocephalus. The epilepsy can present as acute symptomatic seizures, and/or status epilepticus. The differential diagnosis includes all other causes of CNS infection, bacterial meningitis, viral meningoencephalitis, cerebral malaria, fungal meningitis, and even non-infective causes. Once tuberculous meningitis is suspected and other conditions have been excluded, and the clinical findings and CSF picture are compatible, treatment should be started as quickly as possible without waiting for bacteriological confirmation

The second setting is the patient with one or more granulomas presenting with seizures, with or without symptoms and signs of an intracranial space-occupying lesion. Here the differential diagnosis is that of any space-occupying lesion and the key is where the patient has come from or traveled to and whether that place is endemic for infections such as tuberculosis or cysticercosis (Case Records of the Massachusetts General Hospital 2000), and whether there is evidence of infection in other organs. Knowledge of the presence of immunosuppression, especially HIV, is important in both situations.

Antiepileptic drugs

Initiation of treatment

Treatment with AEDs should not begin before a seizure occurs, unless there is a granuloma in the cortex or considerable cerebritis or large cortical infarcts or considerable hydrocephalus. Antiepileptic drugs should be initiated, however, if there is a history of seizures or a seizure occurs. Subtle seizures may be difficult to ascertain in a patient with altered consciousness and electroencephalography (EEG) is warranted. Status epilepticus should be treated promptly using established protocols.

Choice of drug

The choice of drug is limited by what is both affordable and locally available. The first-line AEDs, phenytoin, carbamazepine, valproate, and phenobarbitone, are most widely used in developing countries. However, there are problems due to interactions with antituberculous drugs and antiretroviral drugs, and with comorbidities. The hepatic side effects of antituberculous drugs are an important consideration.

Interaction with antituberculous drugs

Whereas isoniazid raises serum levels of phenytoin, valproate, carbamazepine, and ethosuximide by slowing their metabolism, rifampicin lowers their levels by accelerating their metabolism and that of lamotrigine.

Presence of coexisting diseases

Human immunodeficiency virus

The half-life of antiretroviral drugs, such as nevirapine, is reduced by enzyme-inducing AEDs, resulting in the failure

of ART. Levels of AEDs can also be altered by antiretroviral therapy. In the Bombay Hospital study, four of the 37 patients with seizures had HIV co-infection. All had granulomas and were being treated with phenytoin, ART, and antituberculous treatment. In addition, empirical antitoxoplasmosis treatment was given to three patients. The seizures in three out of these four patients were related to subtherapeutic phenytoin levels because of non-compliance or drug interaction, so phenytoin was switched to levetiracetam.

Phenytoin may produce a hypersensitivity reaction in patients with HIV, 14% in one study (Holtzman *et al.* 1989).

The use of valproate is controversial. It has been variously reported to induce viral replication or inhibit the virus (Jennings and Romanelli 1999; Ylisastigui *et al.* 2004).

Chronic liver disease

In general, the newer AEDs are safer, particularly levetiracetam, which is easy to use and the metabolism of which is unaffected by hepatic disorders.

Chronic renal failure

The dosage of those drugs such as levetiracetam, which are mostly excreted unchanged, needs to be modified according to glomerular filtration rate. In severe renal failure, it may need to be halved.

Stopping treatment

All the usual considerations for discontinuing AED treatment apply. In addition, the high risk of epilepsy for at least the first 5 years following neurotuberculosis, together with the nature of the initial illness and the presence of residual pathology should be borne in mind when deciding whether to continue treatment or stop it.

Managing the CNS inflammatory response

Corticosteroids are thought probably to reduce morbidity and mortality in tuberculous meningitis by altering the inflammatory cascade (Girgis *et al.* 1998). A controlled clinical trial of dexamethasone (Thwaites *et al.* 2004) showed that it decreased mortality but not severe disability. In this study, there were also significantly fewer side effects in the group receiving dexamethasone, particularly hepatic side effects. Antituberculous drugs therefore did not need to be changed or stopped. A beneficial effect of dexamethasone in patients with tuberculosis and HIV was not seen, probably because of their small proportion (18%). This subgroup had a higher fatality rate, possibly because antiretroviral drugs were not used or they may have had undiagnosed opportunistic infection.

In general the use of intravenous dexamethasone is warranted in all moderately and severely affected patients, particularly those with seizures, altered sensorium, and focal deficits, even if the patient is co-infected with HIV. Steroids are also used if the patient has one or more tuberculomas and presents with acute symptomatic seizures but has no tuberculous meningitis. Although steroids may not prevent the paradoxical enlargement of tuberculomas, they are useful in their treatment. In the Turkish study (Sutlas *et al.* 2003), all patients were given corticosteroids from the onset of treatment, but 23% developed tuberculomas, in keeping with what might be expected without steroids. Before using steroids in this situation, it is important to exclude antituberculous drug resistance, non-compliance with treatment, or the possibility of another infection altogether. Steroid usage should always be carefully considered in case the meningitis or granuloma is not tuberculous or is due to a resistant strain of tuberculosis. In a study from South Africa, rifampicin-resistant tuberculosis was discovered in 10.1% of patients with tuberculosis IRIS (Meintjes *et al.* 2009). Steroids could worsen cryptococcal meningitis.

Treating the underlying tuberculosis

Those drugs to be used in first-line antituberculous treatment are well established: rifampicin, isoniazid, pyrazinamide, ethambutol, and optional streptomycin. The first three are bacteriocidal. Pyrazinamide and isonazid have the best penetration of the CSF. Their side effects are well known. In the context of seizures, isoniazid may lower the seizure threshold particularly in newborns and in older patients with pyridoxine deficiency (McKenzie *et al.* 1976). The combination and duration of treatment of first-line drugs is debated. Minimal treatment consists of the first four drugs for 2 months, followed by rifampicin and isoniazid for 10 months (NICE 2006). Another common protocol recommends the continuation of four drugs for the full 12 months, possibly even 18 months as granulomas take time to resolve. Two important considerations are the severity of the illness and possible drug resistance. If drug sensitivity is not known and the patient lives in an endemic area, it is safer to use more drugs and to err on the side of longer duration, while constantly monitoring clinical, CSF, and imaging responses, in addition to drug toxicity, particularly hepatotoxicity.

Drug resistance in tuberculosis occurs at different levels: single drug resistance to any first-line drug, usually isoniazid, multi-drug resistance (MDR-TB) to isoniazid and rifampicin, extensive drug resistance (XDR-TB), resistance to isoniazid, rifampicin, fluoroquinolone, and a second-line injectable agent (Mitnick *et al.* 2008). Drug-resistant strains should be suspected in patients with HIV or with a history of antituberculous treatment. The WHO Report (2008), suggests that 2.9% of new cases of tuberculosis and 15.3% of previously treated tuberculosis are due to MDR-TB (Grant *et al.* 2008). The size of the problem is unknown, since facilities for identifying drug sensitivity are largely non-existent in most developing countries (Donald and van Helden 2009). Treatment is complicated, uses second-line drugs that are less effective and may be toxic, and must continue for a long time with good compliance.

Prevention of tuberculosis

The role of BCG vaccination in preventing pulmonary tuberculosis is uncertain. Its role in preventing miliary tuberculosis and tuberculous meningitis is better established and it should be given to newborn children living in endemic areas (Trunz 2006). It should not be given if the child is known to have HIV. Isoniazid prophylaxis is used to prevent activation of latent tuberculosis in immunosuppressed patients.

Symptomatic treatment

The presence and cause of concomitant hyponatremia should be ascertained and treated since low serum sodium exacerbates seizures. Raised intracranial pressure and hydrocephalus should be managed medically and with early surgical intervention, if required.

HIV-associated tuberculosis

(1) Rifampicin interferes with antiretroviral drugs. Rifabutin is often substituted. There are specific recommendations for concomitant treatment of HIV and tuberculosis (CDC 2007).

(2) IRIS in association with tuberculosis is more common in the presence of HIV, particularly in those in whom ART has been recently started and who have low CD4 counts. Management has been discussed earlier.

Acknowledgments

We gratefully acknowledge the help of Dr. Neeta J. Kulkarni and her staff in the Medical Records Department, Mrs. Apoline Fernandes for her help in preparing the manuscript, and Mrs. Aksha Endigeri for data analysis.

References

Amare A, Zenebe G, Hammack J, Davey G (2008) Status epilepticus: clinical presentation, cause, outcome, and predictors of death in 119 Ethiopian patients. *Epilepsia* **49**:600–7.

Annegers JF, Hauser WA, Beghi E, Nicolosi A, Kurland LT (1988) The risk of unprovoked seizures after encephalitis and meningitis. *Neurology* **38**:1407–10.

Barnes PF, Cave MD (2003) Molecular epidemiology of tuberculosis. *N Engl J Med* **349**:1149–56.

Bharucha NE, Raven RH, Nambiar V (2009) Review of status epilepticus (SE) in HIV and tuberculosis with preliminary view of Bombay Hospital experience. The Innsbruck Colloquium on Status Epilepticus, April 2–4, 2009. International League Against Epilepsy: Commission on European Affairs, Abstract IL24, 66.

Case Records of the Massachusetts General Hospital (2000) Weekly clinicopathological exercises. Case 24–2000: a 23-year-old man with seizures and a lesion in the left temporal lobe. *N Engl J Med* **343**:420–7.

Centers for Disease Control (2007) *Managing Drug Interactions in the Treatment of HIV-Related Tuberculosis.* Available online at www.cdc.gov/tb/TB_HIV_Drugs/default.htm

Chandy MJ, Rajshekhar V, Ghosh S, *et al.* (1991) Single small enhancing CT lesions in Indian patients with epilepsy: clinical, radiological and pathological considerations. *J Neurol Neurosurg Pscyhiatry* **54**:702–5.

Christie LJ, Loeffler AM, Honarmand S, *et al.* (2008) Diagnostic challenges of central nervous system tuberculosis. *Emerg Infect Dis* **14**:1473–5.

Dastur DK, Lalitha VS, Prabhakar V (1968) Pathological analysis of intracranial space-occupying lesions in 1000 cases including children. I. Age, sex and pattern; and the tuberculomas. *J Neurol Sci* **6**:575–92.

Dastur DK, Udani PM (1966) Pathology and pathogenesis of tuberculous encephalopathy. *Acta Neuropatholigica (Berlin)* **6**:311–26.

Davies PDO, Pai M (2008) The diagnosis and misdiagnosis of tuberculosis. *Int J Tuberc Lung Dis* **12**:1226–34.

Donald PR, van Helden PD (2009) The global burden of tuberculosis: combating drug resistance in difficult times. *N Engl J Med* **360**:2393–5.

Garcia-Monco JC (1999) Central nervous system tuberculosis. *Neurol Clin* **17**:737–59.

Girgis NI, Sultan Y, Farid Z, *et al.* (1998) Tuberculous meningitis, Abbasia Fever Hospital, Naval Medical Research Unit No. 3, Cairo, Egypt, from 1976 to 1996. *Am J Trop Med Hyg* **58**:28–34.

Grant A, Gothard P, Thwaites G (2008) Managing drug resistant tuberculosis. *Br Med J* **337**:a1110.

Hesdorffer DC, Logroscino G, Cascino G, Annegers JF, Hauser WA (1998) Risk of unprovoked seizure after acute symptomatic seizure: effect of status epilepticus. *Ann Neurol* **44**:908–12.

Holtzman DM, Kaku DA, So YT (1989) New-onset seizures associated with human immunodeficiency virus infection: causation and clinical features in 100 cases. *Am J Med* **87**:173–7.

Jennings HR, Romanelli F (1999) The use of valproic acid in HIV-positive patients. *Ann Pharmacother* **33**:1113–16.

Karstaedt AS, Valtchanova S, Barriere R, Crewe-Brown HH (1998) Tuberculous meningitis in south African urban adults. *Q J Med* **91**:743–7.

Kennedy DH, Fallon RJ (1979) Tuberculous meningitis. *J Am Med Ass* **241**:264–8.

Kim MA, Park KM, Kim SE, Oh MK (2008) Acute symptomatic seizures in CNS infection. *J Neurol* **15**:38–41.

Lammie GA, Hewlett RH, Schoeman JF, Donald PR (2007) Tuberculous encephalopathy: a reappraisal. *Tuberculous Neuropathology* **113**:227–34.

McKenzie SA, Macnab AJ, Katz G (1976) Neonatal Pyridoxine-responsive convulsions due to isoniazid therapy. *Arch Dis Child* **51**:567–8.

Meintjes G, Lawn SD, Scano F, *et al.* (2008) Tuberculosis-associated immune reconstitution inflammatory syndrome: case definitions for use in resource-limited settings. *Lancet Infect Dis* **8**:516–23.

Meintjes G, Rangaka MX, Maartens G, *et al.* (2009) Novel relationship between tuberculosis immune reconstitution inflammatory syndrome and antitubercular drug resistance. *Clin Infect Dis* **48**:667–76.

Misra UK, Kalita J, Roy AK, Mandal SK, Srivastava M (2000) Role of clinical, radiological, and neurophysiological changes in predicting the outcome of tuberculous meningitis: a multivariable analysis. *J Neurol Neurosurg Psychiatry* **68**:300–3.

Misra UK, Kalita J, Nair PP (2008) Status epilepticus in central nervous system infections: an experience from a developing country. *Am J Med* **121**:618–23.

Mitnick CD, Shin SS, Seung KJ, *et al.* (2008) Comprehensive treatment of extensively drug-resistant tuberculosis. *N Engl J Med* **359**:563–74.

Murthy JMK, Yangala R (1999) Acute symptomatic seizures: incidence and etiological spectrum – a hospital-based study from south India. *Seizure* **8**:162–5.

Murthy JMK, Jayalaxmi SS, Kanikannan MA (2007) Convulsive status epilepticus: clinical profile in a developing country. *Epilepsia* **48**:2217–23.

Nahid P, Pai M, Hopewell PC (2006) Advances in the diagnosis and treatment of tuberculosis. *Proc Am Thorac Soc* **3**:103–10.

NICE (2006) *Clinical Guideline 33: Tuberculosis – Clinical Diagnosis and Management of Tuberculosis, and Measures for Its Prevention and Control.* London: National Institute for Health and Clinical Excellence.

Pai M, Flores LL, Pai N, *et al.* (2003) Diagnostic accuracy of nucleic acid amplification tests of tuberculous meningitis: a systematic review and meta-analysis. *Lancet Infect Dis* **3**:633–43.

Rajshekhar V, Chandy MJ (1996) Comparative study of contrast computerised tomography and magnetic resonance imaging in patients with solitary cysticercus granulomas and seizures. *Neuroradiology* **38**:542–6.

Raviglione MC, O'Brien RJ (2008) Tuberculosis. In: Fauci AS, Braunwald E, Kasper DL, Hauser SL, Longo DL, Jameson JL, Loscalzo J (eds.) *Harrison's Principles of Internal Medicine.* New York: McGraw Hill Medical, pp. 1006–21.

Reid A, Scano F, Getahun H, *et al.* (2006) Towards universal access to HIV prevention, treatment, care, and support: the role of tuberculosis/HIV collaboration. *Lancet Infect Dis* **6**:483–95.

Richeldi L (2006) An update on the diagnosis of tuberculosis infection. *J Respir Crit Care Med* **174**:736–42.

Rubin EJ (2009) Granuloma in tuberculosis: friend or foe? *N Engl J Med* **360**:2471–3.

Ryan CT (2008) Concurrent ART/TB treatment finally proven to be beneficial. *AIDS Clin Care* **20**:89.

Storla DG, Yimer S, Bjune GA (2008) A systematic review of delay in the diagnosis and treatment of tuberculosis. *BMC Publ Health* **8**:15.

Sutlas PN, Unal A, Forta H, Senol S, Kirbas D (2003) Tuberculous meningitis in adults: review of 61 cases. *Infection* **31**:387–91.

Thwaites G, Chau TTH, Mai NTH, *et al.* (2000) Tuberculous meningitis. *J Neurol Neurosurg Psychiatry* **68**:289–99.

Thwaites GE, Bang ND, Dung NH, *et al.* (2004) Dexamethasone for the treatment of tuberculous meningitis in adolescents and adults. *N Engl J Med* **351**:1741–51.

Török ME, Nghia HD, Chau TT, *et al.* (2007) Validation of a diagnostic algorithm for adult tuberculous meningitis. *Am J Trop Med Hyg* **77**:555–9.

Trunz BB, Fine P, Dye C (2006) Effect of BCG vaccination on childhood tuberculous meningitis and miliary tuberculosis worldwide: a meta-analysis and assessment of cost-effectiveness. *Lancet* **367**:1173–80.

Tyler KL (2008) Bacterial meningitis: an urgent need for further progress to reduce mortality and morbidity. *Neurology* **70**:2095–6.

Vezzani A, Granata T (2005) Brain inflammation in epilepsy: experimental and clinical evidence. *Epilepsia* **46**:1724–43.

Vezzani A, Balosso S, Aronica E, Ravizza T (2009) Basic mechanisms of SE due to infection and inflammation. The Innsbruck Colloquium on Status Epilepticus, April 2–4, 2009. International League Against Epilepsy: Commission on European Affairs, Abstract IL21, 60.

WHO (2008) *Global Tuberculosis Control 2008: Surveillance, Planning, Financing*. Geneva: World Health Organization.

Ylisastigui L, Archin N, Lehrman G, Bosch RJ, Margolis DM (2004) Coaxing human immunodeficiency virus type 1 from resting $CD4^+$ T cells: can the reservoir of HIV be purged? *AIDS* **18**:1101–8.

Zoons E, Weisflet M, de Gans J, *et al.* (2008) Seizures in adults with bacterial meningitis. *Neurology* **70**: 2109–15.

Zuger A, Lowy FD (1997) Tuberculosis. In: Scheld WM, Whitley RJ, Durack DT (eds.) *Infections of the Central Nervous System*, 2nd edn. Philadelphia, PA: Lippincott-Raven Publishers, pp. 417–43.

Chapter 74

HIV infection

P. Satishchandra and S. Sinha

Introduction

Involvement of the nervous system at autopsy is noted in about 90% of HIV-seropositive patients. There are reports of neurological disorders as the presenting manifestation in 5–10% of patients with HIV infection (Rachlis 1988). Although seizures can be due to HIV infection per se, they are more commonly observed to be due to underlying opportunistic infections, systemic illness, drug or alcohol abuse, and even antiretroviral usage (Dal Pan et al. 1997; Satishchandra and Sinha 2008). The treatment of these seizures, includes the administration of antiepileptic drugs (AEDs) as well as the specific treatment of the underlying conditions and antiretroviral drugs where indicated (Romanelli et al. 2000; Romanelli and Ryan 2002).

Epidemiology

The majority of the data related to occurrence of seizures among HIV-seropositive patients are hospital-based. Seizures occur in 2–20% of HIV-seropositive individuals (Levy et al. 1985). The variation in the prevalence in different reports is probably due to the different inclusion criteria (Table 74.1). In developing countries, the increasing occurrence of HIV infection and therefore of opportunistic brain infections are likely to be an increasingly important cause of acute symptomatic seizures in future (Rachlis 1988; Garg 1999). Kellinghaus et al. (2008) in a recent series of 831 HIV-infected patients reported that 51 patients (6.1%) had seizures, and that only three among them (6%) were diagnosed with epilepsy before the onset of the HIV infection. Over the last 18 years (1989–2007), there were 1457 patients of HIV-seropositive subjects with associated neurological manifestations at our tertiary referral centre: opportunistic infections – 1213 (83.2%) and non-infective disorders – 243 (16.7%) (Fig. 74.1a–c). Analysis of a cohort of 500 patients from this group revealed new-onset acute symptomatic seizures in about one-fifth of patients (Sinha et al. 2005). The majority were young (mean: 32.1 ± 7.5 years) males ($M:F = 11.4:1$) and in their most productive period of life (although the male predominance might be due to the

selection bias of admissions to the National Institute of Mental Health and Neurosciences [NIMHANS]) (Sinha et al. 2005) (Fig. 74.1a). Dal Pan et al. (1997) reported seizures in 15 out of 268 (5.6%) patients of AIDS dementia complex. Similar frequencies of 3% to 8% were reported by others (Pascual-Sedano et al. 1999; Chadha et al., 2000).

The higher frequency of seizure (approx 20%) in our cohort of patients is due to the fact that all patients had neurological illness (referred as they were to a neurological unit) and predominantly neuro-HIV with underlying brain lesions. Because of the upsurge in the number of HIV-infected cases in India, with the increasing number of neuro-AIDS cases, seizures among HIV infected patients are an important and common cause of acute symptomatic seizures.

Type of seizures

In our cohort of 99 HIV-seropositive patients with new-onset acute symptomatic seizures, 20 patients presented with seizure as the initial presenting symptom (Sinha et al. 2005). The types of seizures in our cohort were: generalized ($n = 62$), partial ($n = 37$) including status epilepticus ($n = 8$). The mean duration of symptoms of underlying neurological illness was 23.7 ± 52.1 days. A total of 25/99 patients (25.3%) with seizures died, mainly due to underlying opportunistic illnesses during the course of illness. Seizure was difficult to control in 6.1% cases in this cohort (Sinha et al. 2005). Both simple and complex partial seizures had been noted in such patients with diffuse brain disease, e.g., HIV encephalopathy and meningoencephalitis, but the seizure type does not necessarily imply the presence of focal mass lesions (Holtzman et al. 1989; Garg 1999). As in our study, other authors also had reported generalized seizures to be more common than partial seizures (Pesola and Westfal 1998; Chadha et al. 2000), which might be because of rapid secondary generalization or the lack of a detailed. The documented incidence of convulsive status epilepticus ranges between 8% and 18% in different studies and is often associated with poor prognosis (Holtzman et al. 1989; Wong et al. 1990; Van Paesschen et al. 1995; Sinha et al.

The Causes of Epilepsy, eds. S. D. Shorvon, F. Andermann, and R. Guerrini. Published by Cambridge University Press. © Cambridge University Press 2011.

Table 74.1 Seizures in HIV-seropositive individuals: comparison of various studies in the literature

Sample size (of HIV-positive patients)	No. of individuals with seizures	No. of individuals with seizure as the first symptom (n or %)	No. of individuals with status epilepticus (SE or recurrence)	Common etiologies	Reference
—	100	18	SE: 12	Toxoplasmosis HIV encephalopathy Meningitis	Holtzman et al. (1989)
630	70 (11.1%)	80%	SE: 10	Toxoplasmosis Lymphoma Metabolic mass lesion	Wong et al. (1990)
—	68	—	SE: 12	Meningoencephalitis	Wong et al. (1990)
—	26	—	—	Idiopathic HIV encephalopathy CNS toxoplasmosis	Pesola and Westfal (1998)
550	17 (3.1%)	—	—	Drug toxicity Intracranial lesions	Pascual-Sedano et al. (1999)
455	23 (5.05%)	—	Recurrence: 16	Opportunistic infections	Chadha et al. (2000)
—	60	—	—	Space-occupying lesion Meningitis	Modi et al. (2000)
500	99 (19.8%)	4.0%	SE: 8	Opportunistic infections	Sinha et al. (2005)
831	51 (6.1%)	17	—	PML, neuroinfection Toxoplasmosis	Kellinghaus et al. (2008)

2005). Pascual-Sedano et al. (1999) reported a rate of 3% new-onset seizures in their series and 70.6% of this group had generalized seizure; three out of the 17 patients had recurrent uncontrolled seizures, and eight patients (47%) died during follow-up, within 4 months of their first reported seizure. This suggests that seizures are an indicator of poor prognosis in HIV-seropositive subjects (Holtzman et al. 1989). The majority of seizures in HIV-seropositive patients occur during the later part of the disease as the disease progresses, as indicated by available viral load and CD4+ cell count information. Seizures are also often associated with mass lesions secondary to opportunistic infections.

Etiology of seizures

In our cohort of 500 patients evaluated at NIMHANS from 1989 to 2000, opportunistic infections were detected as the primary cause of seizures in 93% of patients: monomicrobial 77% and polymicrobial 16%. Non-infective neurological illness of the brain was evident in only 3% patients (Sinha et al. 2005) (Fig. 74.1b, c). Very often, more than one cause could be responsible for the seizures. Similarly, electrolyte and metabolic disturbances, such as hyponatremia, hypomagnesemia, and

renal failure, are associated with an increased risk of seizure recurrence and increased occurrence of convulsive status epilepticus. The annual incidence and its underlying causes of all HIV-seropositive patients with neurological involvement ($n = 1457$) evaluated at our center from 1989 to 2007 are described in Fig. 74.1 a–c. In other series, Wong et al. (1990) also found that opportunistic infections were the commonest cause: herpes simplex encephalitis (HSV) 46%, toxoplasmosis 28%, and bacterial meningitis 10%. Similar findings were reported by Holtzman et al. (1989): HSV 45.7%, toxoplasmosis 15.7%, and bacterial meningitis 10%. Modi et al. (2000) found in their 60 HIV-infected patients with new-onset seizures, 55% had space-occupying lesions, 22% had meningitis, and in the remaining (23%) no specific etiology was evident. However, Pesola and Westfal (1998) reported idiopathic seizures in 30.7%, herpes simplex encephalitis in 30%, and unclear diagnosis in the remainder. Various electrolyte and metabolic disturbances, such as hyponatremia, hypomagnesemia, and renal failure, are associated with an increased risk of seizure recurrence and increased occurrence of convulsive status epilepticus (Holtzman et al. 1989; Van Paesschen et al. 1995). Kellinghaus et al. (2008) reported 51 seizures in their series of 831 HIV patients, and three of them had previous history of epilepsy.

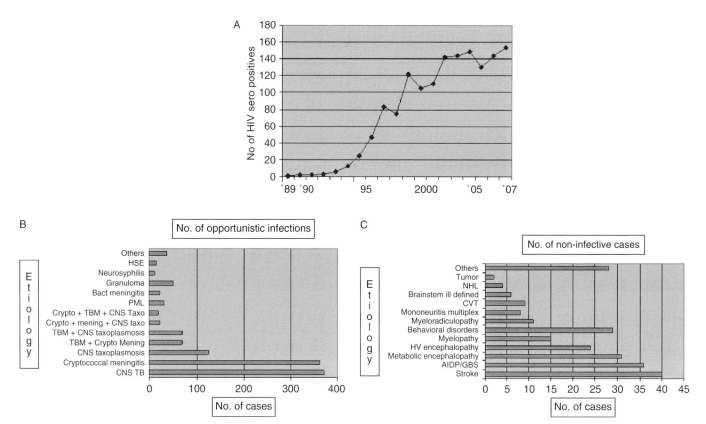

Fig. 74.1. Neurological disorders associated with HIV/AIDS at NIMHANS, Bangalore (1989–2007). (A) Line diagram showing increasing trend in the number of cases over 18 years. (B) Opportunistic infections (OIs) associated with HIV infection at NIMHANS, Bangalore. (C) Non-opportunistic infections associated with HIV infection.

Fourteen patients only had single or few provoked seizures in the setting of acute cerebral disorders ($n = 8$), drug withdrawal or sleep withdrawal ($n = 2$), or of unknown cause ($n = 4$), while 34 patients (67%) developed epilepsy in the course of their HIV infection: central nervous system (CNS) toxoplasmosis ($n = 7$), progressive multifocal leukencephalopathy ($n = 7$), and other acute or subacute cerebral infections ($n = 5$) were the most frequent causes of seizures.

Intracranial focal lesions account for nearly half the neurological disorders in neuro-AIDS patients. The nature of these focal cerebral lesions can be broadly divided into two distinct groups: opportunistic infections and non-infective lesions. Seizures are the dominant manifestations of most of these disorders. In patients without mass lesions, meningoencephalitis caused by some opportunistic infection is a frequent source of seizures. The incidence of meningitis and encephalitis in HIV-infected patients with new onset seizures varies from 12% to 16% (Garg 1999).

HIV and cerebral toxoplasmosis

In a retrospective analysis of all neurological opportunistic infections (OI) associated with HIV at NIMHANS, Bangalore from 1993 to 2005, there were 72 patients with CNS toxoplasmosis among 1005 patients (7.2%). Of these, 25, i.e., one-third (34.7%; age range: 5–60 years; M : F = 16 : 9) had manifested with seizures. Interestingly, eight patients had seizures as the sole neurological manifestations. The patterns of seizures were: simple partial ($n = 14$) and generalized ($n = 11$). The abnormal neuroimaging findings (21 with computed tomography [CT] and four with magnetic resonance imaging [MRI]) were: enhancing ring/disk lesions predominantly in basal ganglia, thalamus or in frontal cortex along with hydrocephalus, and meningeal enhancement with cortical atrophy (Fig. 74.2). Diagnosis was confirmed in 10 patients at autopsy, while in the remaining 15 diagnosis was made on the basis of a positive cerebrospinal fluid (CSF) anti-*Toxoplasma* antibody. Thirteen patients (54%) expired during the course of their illness (Shobha *et al.* 2006).

In other series, central nervous system (CNS) toxoplasmosis has also been found to be the most common cause of intracranial mass lesions in AIDS and occurs in 3–50% of patients (American Academy of Neurology 1998). Seizures have been reported as an early manifestation in 15–40% of these patients (Aronow *et al.* 1989; Wong *et al.* 1990).

The diagnosis is established by demonstrating the presence of characteristics neuroimaging findings, positive toxoplasma antibody titers in CSF, and clinical improvement and radiological resolution with anti-*Toxoplasma* treatment (Provenzale and Jinkins 1997). A variable frequency (12–28%) of toxoplasmosis in patients with new-onset seizures among HIV-infected persons has been described in the literature (Holtzman *et al.* 1989; Wong

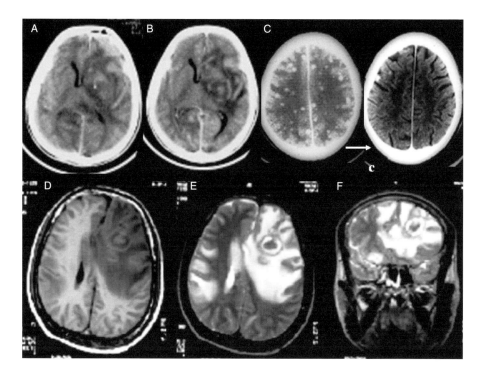

Fig. 74.2. Axial computed tomography (CT) scan (A, B) showing mixed-density lesion with mild enhancement and mass effect; (C) multiple small disk-like enhancing lesion (starry sky) resembling neurocysticercosis appearance but responding remarkably to anti-*Toxoplasma* treatment; D (T1-weighted axial), E (T2-weighted axial), F (T2-weighted coronal): magnetic resonance imaging (MRI) showing mixed-intensity toxoplasma granuloma.

et al. 1990; Dore *et al.* 1996). A high index of suspicion of CNS toxoplasmosis needs to be kept whenever a known HIV-seropositive individual presents with focal seizures of recent onset. Early, rapid, and correct diagnosis and management of CNS toxoplasmosis is extremely important because of the availability of effective treatment and with appropriate treatment a good prognosis.

HIV and cryptococcal meningitis

In a retrospective analysis of case records of all neurological disease associated with HIV at NIMHANS, Bangalore from 1989 to 2005, a large series of 335/1005 patients with CSF-culture-proven cryptococcal meningitis has been reported (Satishchandra *et al.* 2007). Mean age was 33.8 ± 8.3 years and M : F ratio = 7.3 : 1; among these 84 patients (25%) had acute symptomatic seizures. Seizures were most commonly generalized. Cranial CT scan was normal in 45%, showed diffuse atrophy in 25%, diffuse edema in 6%, focal hypodensity in 9%, hydrocephalus in 5%, granuloma in 5%, and basal exudates in 4%. Autopsy in 57 of these patients confirmed the diagnosis of cryptococcal meningitis. Additional coexistent opportunistic infections were toxoplasmosis (7), tuberculous meningitis (2), and cytomegalovirus encephalitis (1) (Satishchandra *et al.* 2007). Millogo *et al.* (2004) had reported that in their series, cryptococcal meningitis accounted for 16% of all patients with seizures.

HIV and neurotuberculosis

Neurotuberculosis, and especially tuberculoma, is a common cause of seizures in HIV-seropositive patients. Among 99 patients, 44 (45%) of those with neurotuberculosis had manifested with seizures in our earlier cohort (Sinha *et al.* 2005). Millogo *et al.* (2004) had reported that CNS tuberculosis formed about 7% of total patients causing seizures. Daikos *et al.* (2003) presented eight patients with multidrug-resistant tuberculous meningitis and AIDS. All developed meningitis as a terminal complication and among them only one had seizures.

HIV and progressive multifocal leukoencephalopathy

A total of 26 patients of progressive multifocal leukoencephalopathy (PML) associated with HIV-seropositivity were reviewed at our center over the last 10-year period. There were 19 males and 7 females with mean age being 39.3 ± 9.9 years. Five (19.2%) manifested with seizures, generalized in two patients and partial in form in three. Sixteen patients had characteristic MR imaging abnormalities suggestive of PML (Fig. 74.3). Seven patients died in the hospital and three died after discharge from the hospital. Five patients are being followed up at 6–30 months and are on first-line highly activ antiretroviral therapy (HAART) regimen (Shobha *et al.* 2005). Moulignier *et al.* (1995) had reported 10 HIV-infected patients with PML in whom partial or generalized seizures were the presenting neurological manifestations. They suggested that demyelinating lesions adjacent to the cerebral cortex act as an irritative focus. Axonal conduction abnormalities or disturbance of the neuron–glia balance are other possible mechanisms for a pure white-matter disorder producing seizures (Millogo *et al.* 2004). The advent of HAART has significantly improved life span of patients with PML associated with HIV infection, and hence the importance of making early diagnosis.

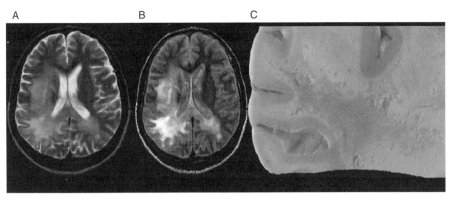

Fig. 74.3. (A,B) Axial MRI T2-weighted and fluid-attenuated inversion recovery (FLAIR) sequences revealing white-matter signal intensity changes in the parietal and frontal (right) and occipital (both sides) lobes without any mass effect; (C) demyelination of the white matter; (D,E) Luxol fast blue stain showing demyelination – these features are consistent with PML. See color plate section.

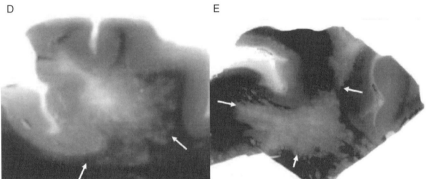

HIV and CNS lymphoma

Primary CNS lymphoma, the second most common cause of intracranial mass lesions, occurs in about 2% of patients with AIDS (American Academy of Neurology 1998). It is also the second most common mass lesion producing seizures in HIV-infected persons in Western countries. However, CNS lymphoma is extremely uncommon in India where HIV is primarily due to clade C virus (Satishchandra *et al.* 2000). A number of imaging features are helpful in distinguishing this condition from cerebral toxoplasmosis. Involvement of, and extension across, the corpus callosum is frequent in primary CNS lymphoma. Exclusive involvement of white matter, a periventricular location, and subependymal spread (seen as contrast enhancement along the ventricular surface) are also common in lymphoma (Provenzale and Jinkins 1997). Single-photon emission computed tomography (SPECT) scan is being increasingly used to differentiate CNS lymphoma from toxoplasmosis – with the latter showing decreased uptake. In our series of 99 patients with acute symptomatic seizures and HIV, only one patient had a primary CNS lymphoma (Sinha *et al.* 2005).

HIV and drugs and alcohol

Dal Pan *et al.* (1997) had reported that among the drug abusers with HIV infection, intravenous cocaine use was an important cause of acute symptomatic seizures. In our series, the HIV infection was acquired predominantly by heterosexual transmission, and no case was related to intravenous drug use.

Electroencephalography among HIV-seropositive patients with seizures

Kellinghaus *et al.* (2008) discussed the electroencephalographic (EEG) data in their series and found 38/51 (74.5%) of patients showed regional slowing, 14 generalized diffuse slowing and 9 regional slowing, and epileptiform discharges in 1. Ozakaya *et al.* (2006) described an HIV-infected, bilingual patient presenting with Wernicke aphasia due to partial status epilepticus with EEG revealing periodic lateralized epileptiform discharges (PLEDs), as the first sign of AIDS–toxoplasmosis complex. Similar reports of PLEDs have been documented by Cury *et al.* (2004). We had earlier reported non-specific EEG changes even among asymptomatic HIV-seropositive individuals (Sinha and Satishchandra 2003). Enzenberger *et al.* (1985) found that 50% of the 26 asymptomatic HIV-positive subjects had non-specific EEG abnormalities, and that five of them developed subacute encephalopathy subsequently. Whether EEG changes predict the future development of clinical seizures or encephalopathy is uncertain and requires further systematic study.

Magnitude and mechanisms of seizures

In various series, approximately half of HIV-seropositive patients with seizures have no definite identifiable disease of the brain, and direct cerebral HIV infection seems to be the most likely cause of the seizures (Holtzman *et al.* 1989; Wong *et al.* 1990; Garg 1999). Udgirkar *et al.* (2003) reported seizures in 75% of eight children with HIV encephalopathy. Navia *et al.* (1986) reported nine patients with AIDS–dementia complex who had new-onset seizures and in whom autopsies did not reveal any secondary infections or neoplastic processes. The authors considered direct HIV infection of the brain to be the cause of these seizures. Holtzman *et al.* (1989) reported HIV encephalopathy as the cause for seizures in 24% of the patients. The diagnosis was established with the help of characteristic clinical features and histopathology of brain tissues. Later, in a series by Wong *et al.* (1990), 6/17 patients following autopsy had diagnosis suggestive of HIV infection as a primary cause of seizures. In a series by Van Paesschen *et al.* (1995), 41% of patients had cerebral atrophy on CT scan without meningitis or other demonstrable CT lesions, and autopsy of two patients who died after seizure-onset revealed subacute HIV-associated encephalitis in one patient and cytomegalovirus encephalitis in the other. In a more recent study, Dore *et al.* (1996) observed that 42% of cases had no identifiable cause of seizures, although 18% of patients were receiving foscarnet therapy. They suggested that foscarnet therapy and subclinical HIV-1 involvement of the brain might be factors responsible for seizure activity in their series. In our previous study, one patient had epilepsia partialis continua, probably due to primary HIV infection, since this individual had no other underlying opportunistic infections (Sinha *et al.* 2005). Epilepsia partialis continua secondary to HIV encephalitis and PML had been reported (Pesola and Westfal 1998). Thus, available data strongly suggest that epilepsy is one of the neurological manifestations of HIV/AIDS. In our cohort, about 93% of the seizures occurred in patients with underlying opportunistic infections.

There is strong evidence for the existence of HIV- or immune-related toxins that produce injury or death of neurons via a potentially complex interaction between macrophages, microglia, or monocytes, especially after interacting with astrocytes. Interactions between macrophages (microglia), astrocytes, and neurons produce neurotoxic substances which include eicosanoids, platelet-activating factor, quinolinate, cysteine, cytokines, and free radicals. Macrophages activated by HIV-1 envelope protein gp120 release similar toxins and the final common pathway is through increased glutamate activity, activation of voltage-dependent calcium channel and *N*-methyl-D-aspartate (NMDA) receptor-operated channels and influx of calcium into the cells ultimately leading to neuronal death. The resultant relative imbalance of excitatory and inhibitory neurotransmitters and neurotoxicity of other substances in brain may predispose to seizures or decreased glutamate reuptake. The same mechanisms, which have been proposed for the pathogenesis of the AIDS–dementia complex, are considered responsible for early and late occurrences of seizures in these patients. The frequent occurrence of generalized seizures and status epilepticus suggests that the HIV-infected brain has a low cortical excitability and impaired mechanisms for terminating seizure activity. Concentrations of CSF β2-microglobulin and neopterin (markers that have been associated with HIV-1 involvement within the CNS) were found in 100% of patients with no identifiable cause of seizure activity (Lipton 1994).

Antiepileptic drug use in HIV-seropositives

Seizure recurrence after a single acute symptomatic seizure is likely to be as high as 70% among HIV-seropositive patients, and hence long-term antiepileptic therapy needs to be considered, even in those presented with single seizure, except when reversible metabolic derangements are detected. There are no definite guidelines regarding this. Clinicians faced with the task of controlling seizures in HIV-seropositive patients must consider a number of potential drug–disease and drug–drug interactions when selecting AED therapy in the face of limited data (Romanelli *et al.* 2000). We have proposed a therapeutic approach for such patients (Fig. 74.4). Phenytoin has been the most widely prescribed AED for these patients, but a significant number of patients are likely to experience undesirable side effects, including skin rashes, leukopenia, thrombocytopenia, and hepatic dysfunction; and phenytoin has a significant interaction with AZT.

In our previous series of 99 patients (Sinha and Satishchandra 2003), the commonest AEDs used in our setting in India were phenytoin (50.5%) and phenobarbitone (27.3%). Sometimes a combination of two (14.8%) and even rarely, three (1.9%) AEDs were required in managing acute symptomatic seizures. Seizures were poorly controlled in six cases. Staging of our cases could not be done because of scarcity of CD4 counts and viral load data. However, all our patients were HIV-1 clade C and drug naive with regard to antiretroviral therapy. Dal Pan *et al.* (1997) reported skin rashes and leukopenia with phenytoin and carbamazepine in HIV-seropositive patients. However, Chadha *et al.* (2000) did not find any serious adverse effects with phenytoin among their 23 cases. Romanelli *et al.* (2000) opined that, when AEDs are used with antiretroviral therapy, drug interactions are more frequent than when used without antiretrovirals.

Drug interactions

The concurrent use of anticonvulsants and antiretrovirals is a poorly researched field that poses a therapeutic dilemma for the clinician caring for HIV-seropositive individuals requiring both classes of medications. HIV-seropositive patients are likely to be receiving multiple medications both for HIV and for prophylaxis against various opportunistic infections, and sometimes for the treatment of opportunistic infections. The selection of AEDs in these situations must be made with careful consideration of the risk of drug interactions. Current HIV treatment guidelines include consideration of the risk of drug interactions. Current guidelines (HAART) advocate the use of a minimum of three antiretroviral medications most often including two nucleoside reverse transcriptase inhibitors and one protease inhibitor (Panel on Clinical Practice for Treatment of HIV Infection 2004). Antiepileptic and antiretroviral drugs have the potential for interacting through multiple mechanisms including competition for protein binding, enhanced or reduced liver metabolism, and increased viral

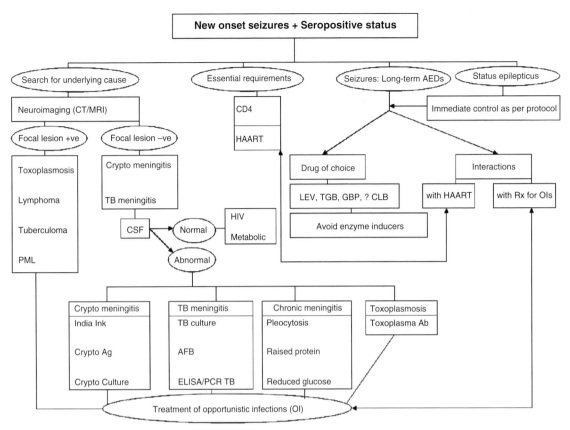

Fig. 74.4. Suggested approach to new-onset seizures in HIV-infected individuals. AEDs, antiepileptic drugs; AFB, acid-fast bacilli; Ag, antigen; Ab, antibody; CLB, clobazam; CSF, cerebrospinal fluid; GBP, gabapentin; HAART, highly active antiretroviral therapy; Lev, levetiracetam; OI, opportunistic infection; PML, progressive multifocal leucoencephalopathy; TB, tuberculosis; TBG, tiagabine; RX, treatment.

replication. Each of these factors must be considered when selecting appropriate therapy.

Some AEDs have strong protein binding and AIDS-associated hypoalbuminemia often causes an increase in free AED levels and hence the toxic effects. It is also true for most of the antiretroviral drugs (Romanelli *et al.* 2000). HIV-induced alterations of blood–brain integrity that are most commonly seen in the late stages of the disease may result in increased CNS penetration of anticonvulsants, but this is a poorly studied area and the clinical significance is not well characterized.

A number of anticonvulsants including primarily first-line AEDs: phenytoin, phenobarbitone, and carbamazepine have been shown to induce CYP3A activity. Therefore, the concurrent use of these AEDs with protease inhibitors may result in insufficient serum Pi protein concentrations, leading to increased viral replication and the emergence of resistance (Romanelli *et al.* 2000). Decrease in indinavir levels in patients while on carbamazepine and conversely elevation of carbamazepine levels in patients that were on ritonavir have been reported. Both protease inhibitors and AEDs such as phenytoin and phenobarbital have been associated with new-onset osteoporosis. Clinicians should be cautious when concurrently prescribing these two classes of drugs, particularly in patients who may be osteopenic, and should consider aggressive monitoring with calcium and vitamin D supplementation.

Effects on viral replication

Valproic acid has been shown in vitro to stimulate replication of HIV (Moog *et al.* 1996). The mechanism by which this happens is poorly understood, but may relate to the effects of the drug on intracellular levels of glutathione, a known regulator of HIV transcription. Until well-controlled in vivo studies are available, it may be advisable to use valproic acid cautiously or better to avoid its use in HIV-seropositive patients (Romanelli *et al.* 2000).

Recommendations

Seizure activity in HIV-seropositive patients is a relatively common occurrence that poses a real therapeutic dilemma for clinicians faced with caring for these patients. Few evidence-based data to guide drug selection and decision-making exist. Therefore, clinicians must rely upon their best judgment. Caution is needed when AEDs and antiretrovirals are co-administered. Antiepileptic drugs such as levetiracetam or gabapentin, which are minimally metabolized by the CYP system, may be the better alternatives for avoiding interactions involving enzyme inhibition or induction (Liedtke *et al.* 2004). In our experience, we find clobazam is a useful drug in these situations, as it has minimal drug interactions with antiretroviral drugs (used at a dose of 10–20 mg/day for an adult and 5 mg/day in a child).

References

American Academy of Neurology (1998) Report of the Quality Standards Subcommittee. Evaluation and management of intracranial mass lesions in AIDS. *Neurology* **50**:21–6.

Aronow HA, Feraru ER, Lipton RB (1989) New-onset seizures in AIDS patients: etiology, prognosis, and treatment. *Neurology* **39**(suppl 1):428.

Chadha DS, Handa A, Sharma SK, Varadarajulu, Singh AP (2000) Seizures in patients with HIV infection. *J Ass Physicians India* **48**:573–6.

Cury RF, Wichert-Ana L, Sakamoto AC, Fernandes RM (2004) Focal non-convulsive status epilepticus associated to PLEDs and intense focal hyperemia in an AIDS patient. *Seizure* **13**:358–61.

Daikos GL, Cleary T, Rodriguez A, Fischl MA (2003) Multidrug-resistant tuberculous meningitis in patients with AIDS. *Int J Tuberc Lung Dis* **7**:394–8

Dal Pan GJ, McArther JC, Harrison MJG (1997) Neurological symptoms in HIV infection. In: Berger JR, Levy RM (eds.) *AIDS and Nervous System*, 2nd edn. Philadelphia, PA: Lippincott-Raven, pp. 141–72.

Dore GJ, Law MG, Brew BJ (1996) Prospective analysis of seizures occurring in human immunodeficiency virus type-1 infection. *J Neuro AIDS* **1**:59–69.

Enzenberger W, Fischer PA, Helm EB, Stille W (1985) Value of EEG in AIDS. *Epilepsia* **36**:146–50.

Garg RK (1999) HIV medicine: HIV infection and seizures. *Postgrad Med J* **75**:387–90.

Holtzman DM, Kaku DA, So YT (1989) New-onset seizures associated with human immunodeficiency virus infection: causation and clinical features in 100 cases. *Am J Med* **87**:173–7.

Kellinghaus C, Engbring C, Kovac S, *et al.* (2008) Frequency of seizures and epilepsy in neurological HIV-infected patients. *Seizure* **17**:23–33.

Levy RM, Bredesen DE, Rosenblum ML (1985) Neurological manifestations of acquired immunodeficiency syndrome (AIDS): experience at UCSF and review of the literature. *J Neurosurg* **65**:475–96.

Liedtke MD, Lockhart SM, Rathbun RC (2004) Anticonvulsant and antiretroviral interactions. *Ann Pharmacother* **38**:482–9.

Millogo A, Lankoande D, Yameogo I, *et al.* (2004) New-onset seizures in patients with immunodeficiency virus infection in Bobo-Dioulasso Hospital. *Bull Soc Pathol Exot* **97**:268–70.

Modi G, Modi M, Martinus I, Saffer D (2000) New-onset seizures associated with HIV infection. *Neurology* **55**:1558–61.

Moog C, Kuntz-SimonG, Caussin-Schwemling C, *et al.* (1996) Sodium valproate, an anticonvulsant drug, stimulates human immunodeficiency virus type 1 replication independently of glutathione levels. *J Gen Virol* **196**:496–505.

Moulignier A, Mikol J, Pialoux G, *et al.* (1995) AIDS-associated progressive multifocal leukoencephalopathy revealed by new-onset seizures. *Am J Med* **99**:64–8.

Ozkaya G, Kurne A, Unal S, *et al.* (2006) Aphasic status epilepticus with periodic lateralized epileptiform discharges in a bilingual patient as a presenting sign of "AIDS-toxoplasmosis complex." *Epilepsy Behav* **9**:193–6.

Navia B, Jordan B, Price R (1986) The AIDS dementia complex. I. Clinical features. *Ann Neurol* **19**:517–24.

Panel on Clinical Practice for Treatment of HIV Infection (2004) Panel convened by the Department of Health and Human Services (DHHS) and the Henry J. Kaiser Family Foundation. Guidelines for the use of antiretroviral agents in HIV-infected adults and adolescents. Available online at www.hivatis.org/www.hivatis.org.

Pascual-Sedano B, Iranzo A, Marti-Fabregas J, *et al.* (1999) Prospective study of new onset seizures in patients with HIV infection: etiologic and clinical aspects. *Arch Neurol* **56**:609–12.

Pesola GR, Westfal RE (1998) New-onset generalized seizures with AIDS presenting at an emergency department. *Acad Emerg Med* **5**:905–11.

Provenzale JM, Jinkins JR (1997) Brain and spine imaging findings in AIDS patients. *Radiol Clin N Am* **35**:1127–66.

Rachlis AR (1988) Neurologic manifestations of HIV infection. *Postgrad Med J* **103**:1–11.

Romanelli F, Ryan M (2002) Seizures in HIV seropositive individuals: epidemiology and treatment. *CNS drugs* **16**:91–98.

Romanelli F, Jennings HR, Nath A, Ryan M, Berger J (2000) Therapeutic dilemma: the use of anticonvulsants in HIV positive individuals. *Neurology* **54**:1404–7.

Satishchandra P, Nalini A, Gourie-Devi M, *et al.* (2000) Profile of neurologic disorders associated with HIV/AIDS from Bangalore, south India (1989–96). *Indian J Med Res* **111**:14–23.

Satishchandra P, Sinha S (2008) Seizures in HIV seropositive individuals: NIMHANS experience and review. *Epilepsia* **49**:33–41.

Satishchandra P, Mathew P, Gadre G, *et al.* (2007) Cryptococcal meningitis: clinical, diagnostic and therapeutic overviews. *Neurol India* **55**:226–32.

Shobha N, Satishchandra P, Mahadevan A, *et al.* (2005) Clinical, radiological and pathological features of progressive multifocal leukoencephalopathy (PML) associated HIV clade C infection. Presented at International Conference on CNS Opportunistic Infections Associated with HIV, Frascati, Italy, 2005.

Shobha N, Satishchandra P, Desai A, *et al.* (2006) Seizure as the initial manifestation of cerebral toxoplasmosis in HIV clade C infected patients. Presented at an International Continued Medical Education conference, at Chennai, February 2006.

Sinha S, Satishchandra P (2003) Nervous system involvement in asymptomatic HIV seropositive individuals: a cognitive and electrophysiological study. *Neurology (India)* **51**:466–9.

Sinha S, Satishchandra P, Nalini A, *et al.* (2005) New-onset seizures among HIV infected drug naïve patients from south India. *Neurology Asia* **10**:29–33.

Udgirkar VS, Tullu MS, Bavdekar SB, *et al.* (2003) Neurological manifestations of HIV infection. *Ind Pediatr* **40**:230–4.

Van Paesschen W, Bodian C, Maker H (1995) Metabolic abnormalities and new-onset seizures in human immunodeficiency virus-seropositive patients. *Epilepsia* **36**:146–50.

Wong MC, Suite NDA, Labar DR (1990) Seizures in human immunodeficiency virus infection. *Arch Neurol* **47**:640–2.

Chapter

75

Emerging and less common central nervous system viral encephalitides

H. T. Chong and C. T. Tan

Introduction

Seizures are a common manifestation of encephalitis and the commonest cause of encephalitis is viral infection. There are hundreds of viruses that affect human beings, and many can cause encephalitis (Taylor *et al.* 2001). The overall incidence of viral encephalitides is approximately 3.5–7.4 in 100 000 per year. The incidence is higher among children; in children under 1 year of age, the incidence is 22.5 in 100 000 per year, and that in children 1 to 5 years of age, 15.2 in 100 000 per year (Koskiniemi *et al.* 1991). Viruses that cause human central nervous system infections can be divided into three broad categories – the primary human viruses, the arthropod-borne viruses or arboviruses, and the zoonotic viruses. The primary human viruses are important causes of encephalitis worldwide, and the arboviruses affect large geographical areas often across continents. The zoonotic viruses, apart from rabies, tend to be more localized (Fig. 75.1). Some of these viruses are important because of the size of population involved, others because they are emerging. The common causes of viral encephalitides with seizure are discussed elsewhere (see Chapter 67). This chapter focuses on the emerging and less common viruses that cause encephalitis and seizures.

Overview

In principle, any virus that causes encephalitis could potentially cause seizures. Clinically, however, certain viral agents are more likely to cause seizures while others only do so rarely. This is probably due to the differences in the underlying pathological process of infection, the anatomic sites involved, the immune and reparative responses elicited by the infection, and other host factors. Most viral infections of the central nervous system cause acute brain parenchymal inflammation with perivascular lymphocytic and mononuclear cell cuffing and infiltration, ballooning and death of neurons leading to subsequent gliosis. There are, however, significant differences among different infections in terms of histopathological appearance and the specific anatomic sites involved. In herpes simplex encephalitis, for example, the inflammation may progress to necrosis and hemorrhage; and homogenous eosinophilic intranuclear inclusion bodies (Cowdry type A) are seen in about half of the patients. Herpes simplex virus has a predilection to affect the temporal and frontal lobes, the cingulate gyrus, and the insular cortex. In rabies, intracytoplasmic inclusions, or Negri bodies, are seen in 80% of patients, and the virus tends to affect the spinal cord, brainstem, hypothalamus, cerebellum, and the hippocampus. Japanese encephalitis virus causes a non-specific parenchymal inflammation and has a propensity to affect the various deep brain nuclei, such as the thalamus, besides the brainstem and the cerebellum. Tick-borne encephalitis virus first infects the Langerhans cells before invading the lymphoid and reticuloendothelial system, and finally causes inflammation not just in the brain, but also in the spinal cord and the leptomeninges. Other viruses result in different pathological changes. The Venezuelan and Eastern equine viruses, Nipah and Hendra viruses cause widespread vasculitic changes and microvascular infarcts. Rarely, some viruses, such as the human herpesvirus 6, cause the unusual picture of a demyelinating encephalitis.

The occurrence of seizures and epilepsy are generally not well studied in viral encephalitides. Most infections cause focal with or without secondary generalized tonic–clonic seizures or myoclonic seizures. Little is known about the predictive factors of seizures in most infections. In some instances, for instance in Japanese B encephalitis, seizures carry a poor prognosis in terms of immediate outcome, but in most infections, the presence of seizures does not influence the prognosis.

Emerging encephalitides
Japanese encephalitis virus

Japanese encephalitis virus is a flavivirus transmitted by mosquitoes from birds and pigs to humans. It is found in East, South, and South-East Asia from eastern Russia to the northern tip of Australia, and from India to the Guam Islands. It causes 20 000–50 000 infections and 15 000 deaths annually, and thus is

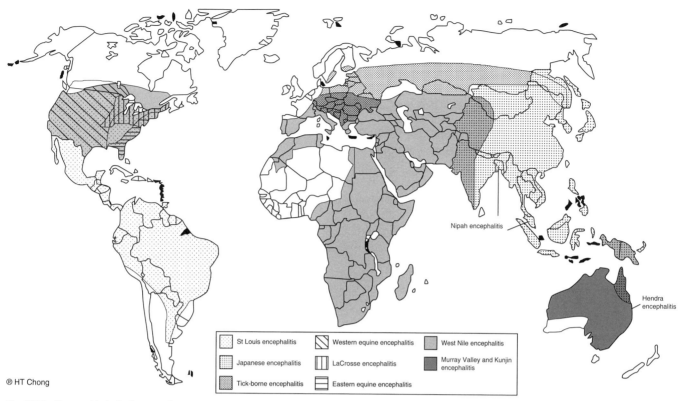

Nipah encephalitis

Hendra encephalitis

® HT Chong

	St Louis encephalitis		Western equine encephalitis		West Nile encephalitis
	Japanese encephalitis		LaCrosse encephalitis		Murray Valley and Kunjin encephalitis
	Tick-borne encephalitis		Eastern equine encephalitis		

Fig. 75.1. Geographical distribution of emerging and some less common viral encephalitides.

the most important viral encephalitis globally. The virus causes diffuse encephalitis, affecting the midbrain, thalamus, and basal ganglia more severely (Mackenzie 1999; Solomon et al. 2000).

Only 1 in 250 to 1000 patients infected with the virus becomes symptomatic. The infection ranges from mild, flu-like illness, to fatal meningoencephalitis. In endemic areas, it is mainly a childhood disease, though visiting naive adults are at particular risk of developing severe illness. After an incubation period of 5 to 15 days, symptomatic patients present first with fever, headache, vomiting, seizure, and impaired consciousness. Extrapyramidal signs such as mask-like face, tremor, rigidity, choreoathetosis, dystonia, dyskinesia, and generalized hypertonia are common, so are brainstem signs. Brain magnetic resonance imaging (MRI) is sensitive and shows hyperintensities in brainstem, cerebellum, basal ganglia, and even the cerebral region. Diagnosis is mainly by serology or polymerase chain reaction (PCR) in the acute stage. Effective vaccines are available, though treatment is mainly supportive (Solomon et al. 2000).

Seizures occur in approximately 40–60% of patients, though the rate is as high as 80% in children. Of these patients 45–57% have generalized clonic or tonic–clonic seizures, 18–43% have focal motor seizures, and up to 25% may have status epilepticus. The seizure manifestations can be subtle, especially in children, and include minimal clonic movements of the eyes, eyebrows, eyelids, mouth, or digits, with or without tonic eye movements, nystagmus, salivation, and irregular breathing. Seizures are associated with focal weakness and

abnormalities on the electroencephalogram (EEG) and brain computed tomography (CT) scan. Seizures also herald a poorer prognosis, and are associated with higher mortality, and poorer conscious state. This is especially the case in multiple or prolonged seizures or status epilepticus, probably because the seizures lead to raised intracranial pressure and a higher risk of herniation syndrome (Solomon et al. 2002).

Acutely, the EEG is abnormal in the vast majority of patients though in a non-specific manner. More than 60% of patients exhibit slow waves, usually of high amplitudes, often with reactivity to external stimuli. Other EEG changes included focal discharges, electrical status epilepticus, periodic lateralized epileptiform discharges (about 10% of patients), burst suppression, generalized attenuation, and alpha coma in about 10% of patients. An EEG tracing that is non-reactive to external stimuli carries a poorer prognosis (Kalita and Misra 1998; Solomon et al. 2002; Misra et al. 2008a).

During convalescence, more than a third of patients have normal EEG and over half have only mild abnormalities, signifying good recovery in the survivors. By 3 to 12 months after the onset of illness, three-quarters of the patients have a normal EEG recording. However, in patients with more severe infection, especially in situations where adequate medical facilities are not accessible, mortality may be as high as 30% in those admitted, and half of the survivors have severe neurological sequelae, which include motor deficit, fixed flexion deformities of the limbs, cognitive deficits, and in up to 20%, remote symptomatic epilepsy (Solomon et al. 2002).

West Nile virus

West Nile virus is a flavivirus closely related to the Kunjin virus and, somewhat less closely, to the Japanese encephalitis virus. First identified in Uganda in 1939, the reservoirs of West Nile virus are birds and the vector *Culex* mosquitoes. Human and other mammals are dead-end hosts. West Nile viral infection is endemic in Africa, the Mediterranean, and the Middle East. Migratory birds are believed to be important in the long-distance spread of the virus. The first outbreaks outside the endemic area occurred in Romania in 1996 and in the Volgograd and Krasnodar regions of Russia in 1999, which coincided with a major change in neurovirulence. In August the same year, the virus affected 62 patients in New York, and by 2002, it had spread throughout the United States and reached the Pacific coast.

In endemic areas, the infection is often asymptomatic. After an incubation period of 3 to 15 days, the patients present with flu-like illness, with a non-pruritic roseolar or maculo-papular rash that lasts for about a week. Only about 15% of patients, usually the elderly, develop central nervous system involvement, which could present as optic neuritis, myelitis, acute flaccid paralysis presumably from anterior horn cell involvement, aseptic meningitis, and encephalitis.

About 20% of patients infected with the virus develop a mild febrile illness and about 1 in 150 develops central nervous system infection. In non-endemic areas, as well as among the elderly, neurological involvement is more common and more severe. Fever, headache, neck pain, myalgia, back pain, nausea, chills, and rigors are the commonest symptoms, while altered mental state, neck stiffness, parkinsonism, including tremor, rigidity, and bradykinesia, were common signs. Other clinical features include signs of brainstem involvement and acute flaccid paralysis. Cerebrospinal fluid (CSF) analysis shows pleocytosis, often lymphocytic, with raised protein and normal sugar levels. Magnetic resonance imaging of the brain shows bilateral hyperintense lesions in the basal ganglia, thalamus and pons on T2-weighted images. Diagnosis is based on serologic testing of serum or CSF, or PCR analysis of CSF during the early part of the illness. There is no specific antiviral therapy for West Nile infection. Treatment is mainly supportive. Long-term outcomes are often good, though persistent fatigue, myalgia, and cognitive deficits have been reported.

Seizures occur in 5–30% of patients with West Nile encephalitis, and often present during the later part of the illness. Rarely, non-convulsive status epilepticus may occur. Electroencephalographic changes are often non-specific, such as diffuse irregular slow waves, and even in patients with non-convulsive status epilepticus the EEG may show only polymorphic delta slow waves. Focal sharp waves are seen occasionally (Sejvar *et al.* 2003; Gea-Banacloche *et al.* 2004).

Nipah virus

Nipah virus is a paramyxovirus endemic among the giant fruit bats (*Pteropus* species) in South and South-East Asia and in east African coastal regions. In 1998 it caused a fatal outbreak of encephalitis among pig farmers in Malaysia, when pigs contracted the virus by consuming fruits partially eaten by fruit bats. The disease continues to cause small annual outbreaks in Bangladesh and north-east India, probably related to the local practice of consuming raw, contaminated, date palm juice.

After an incubation period of about 2 weeks (range 1–32 days), Nipah infection causes a severe encephalitis characterized by sudden onset of fever, headache, giddiness, drowsiness, nausea, anorexia, vomiting, abdominal pain, cough, focal neurological deficits, and seizures. Over the ensuing 1 to 2 weeks, the patient's consciousness continues to deteriorate. In the Malaysian outbreak, more than 60% of patients required mechanical ventilatory support and mortality was about 40%. Terminal events were often heralded by severe hypertension, tachycardia, and hyperthermia, and then irreversible shock. A previous history of diabetes mellitus, brainstem signs, and positive CSF viral cultures were poor prognostic factors. Analysis of CSF shows features typical of viral encephalitis in 50–60% of patients with raised lymphocytes and protein levels, but normal sugar values. Computed tomography scan of the brain is almost invariably normal, while almost all patients would have abnormal MRI, showing widespread, focal, vasculitic-like lesions in the subcortical and deep white matter. Nipah immunoglobulin M (IgM) serology is positive in almost all patients by day 12 of illness, and that of immunoglobulin G (IgG) by day 26. In a non-randomized historical controlled trial, ribavirin was found to reduce mortality by about 30%, though supportive treatment is equally, if not more, important. (Chong *et al.* 2000; Goh *et al.* 2000).

Seizures are common in patients with acute Nipah encephalitis; about a quarter of the patients have generalized tonic–clonic seizures and one-third to half of the patients have segmental myoclonus, involving the diaphragmatic, limbs, and facial muscles. The myoclonus may be persistent over hours. Interestingly, myoclonus was absent in the reports of Nipah encephalitis in Bangladesh, though this could be due to reporting bias.

During the acute phase of infection, more than 96% of patients have abnormal EEG and 88% of patients have continuous diffuse slow waves with or without focal discharges. Focal discharges are seen in about half of the patients and bitemporal periodic complexes in a quarter of the patients. The periodic complexes are stereotypical with single spike or sharp wave followed by a slow wave of 200–250 ms. This is repeated irregularly every 1–2 s (Fig. 75.2). Almost all patients with periodic complexes were comatose in the initial Malaysian outbreak and none survived (Chew *et al.* 1999; Goh *et al.* 2000).

During the acute illness, the focal discharges and the periodic complexes seen in EEG do not correlate with focal neurological deficits, clinical seizure, or segmental myoclonus, though the degree of slowing correlates with the severity of illness (Chew *et al.* 1999).

A

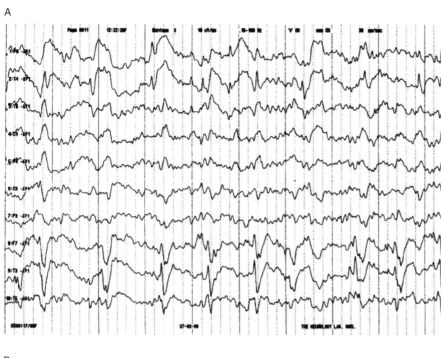

B

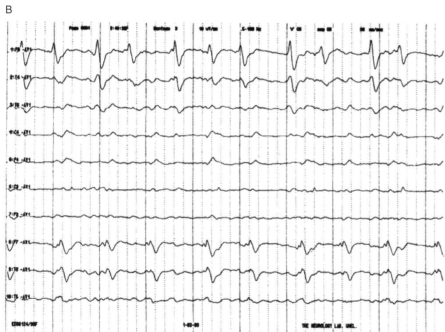

Fig. 75.2. (A) Bitemporal periodic complexes in Nipah encephalitis; (B) the same patient 2 days later, who died on the same day. (Reproduced from Chew *et al.* [1999] with kind permission.)

The mortality rates were 32–41% in the Malaysian outbreaks, and on average, as high as 73% in the Bangladesh outbreaks. About half of the Malaysian patients recovered totally and of the rest 15–30% or so recovered with residual neurological deficits. The incidence of late unprovoked seizure was 2.2% in an 8-year study of 137 patients in Malaysia – higher among the relapsed (4.0%) than the patients who had only acute Nipah encephalitis (1.8%) (Misra *et al.* 2008b). During convalescence and recovery, more than half of the patients had normal EEG. About 24% had intermittent diffuse slow waves, 18% intermittent focal slow waves, and 6% showed focal slow waves and focal discharges (Chew *et al.* 1999).

Relapsed Nipah encephalitis

In up to 10% of symptomatic and 3.4% of patients with asymptomatic infection, Nipah virus infection may cause a relapse of encephalitis 4 years or more after the initial acute infection. These patients present with recurrence of fever, headache, focal neurological deficits, and seizure. Brain MRI showed diffuse gray matter involvement suggesting neuronal invasion by the virus. Mortality is as high as 18%, and half have residual neurological deficits. There is no treatment of proven value of the relapse.

Seizures are seen in approximately half of the patients with a relapse, taking the form of mainly focal motor or generalized tonic–clonic seizures. Segmental myoclonus, prominent during acute infection, was not seen in any of the patients with the relapse disease.

The EEG shows continuous diffuse slow waves with focal preponderance and frontal or temporal discharges. The ominous bitemporal periodic complexes in acute infection are not seen in relapse patients. The EEG is abnormal in almost all patients with clinical cerebral involvement, and the laterality of EEG changes corresponds with MRI changes. Focal discharges on EEG do not predict mortality or the occurrence of clinical seizures (Tan *et al.* 2002). Late unprovoked seizures were documented in about 4.0% of patients in relapse in the Malaysian series. (Misra *et al.* 2008b).

Hendra virus

Hendra virus is a paramyxovirus closely related to the Nipah. Like Nipah virus, its natural reservoirs and hosts are the pteropid bats. It was first discovered in Queensland, Australia, in 1994, when it caused infection in horses and encephalitis in horse-handlers. Sporadic cases of human infections are still reported, though the transmissions from bats to horses and from horses to humans are not efficient. In symptomatic patients, after a short incubation period of 6 to 12 days, the patients presented with fever, flu-like symptoms, myalgia, headache, and vertigo. Mortality is approximately 50%. In a report of four patients, two recovered with no residual neurological deficit; one had relapse Hendra encephalitis 13 months after the initial acute infection and she presented with focal neurological deficits, altered conscious state, seizures, and ultimately died (Wong *et al.* 2009).

Enterovirus 71

Enteroviruses are small, single RNA stranded, non-enveloped, viruses that belong to the family of *Picornaviridae*. There are more than 60 different serotypes of enteroviruses, and humans are the only host. They are mostly transmitted by fecal–oral route or by respiratory droplets. Transmission is facilitated during warm weather; therefore, the incidence of infection is high in warm countries all year round. A few serotypes predominate in a particular locality, and these cause cyclical outbreaks depending on a variety of factors, including the availability of new, susceptible hosts; usually young children. Some serotypes are more likely to cause central nervous system infection, and among these, enterovirus 71 is probably the most important as it has caused large, multiple outbreaks in the United States, Europe, Australia, and East and South-East Asia since its discovery in California in 1969. The largest outbreak occurred in Taiwan in 1998 when the virus caused a massive epidemic affecting over a million people.

Clinically, enterovirus 71 affects mainly children, and those under 5 years of age are more severely affected. Enterovirus 71 infections may be asymptomatic, or there may be diarrhea, hand–foot–and–mouth disease, herpangina, myocarditis, acute flaccid paralysis, Guillian–Barré syndrome, aseptic meningitis, acute cerebellar ataxia, encephalitis, and rhombencephalitis, the last of which is associated with fatal pulmonary edema and hemorrhage. Analysis of CSF shows increased protein and normal sugar levels, and pleocytosis, often lymphocytic, though in up to 40% it may be neutrophilic. Magnetic resonance imaging of the brain shows hyperintense lesions in the brainstem and spinal cord on T2-weighted images, which can enhance in the acute illness. Diagnosis is by viral isolation or PCR. There is no proven antiviral therapy for enterovirus 71, though various agents had been tried, such as steroid and intravenous immunoglobulin. Supportive care remains the most important aspect of care.

Among children with rhombencephalitis, 68–86% are reported to exhibit myoclonic jerks, which could range from mild and intermittent jerks during sleep, or persistent jerks during both sleeping and waking, and may continue after the patient recovers from the acute encephalitis. Other seizures and opsomyoclonus have been documented, though there are few details in the current literature. The EEG shows bilateral central and parietal slow waves or sporadic sharp or spindle waves.

The overall outlook is good; in children without pulmonary edema or hemorrhage, mortality is close to zero. The outlook for children with pulmonary edema and/or hemorrhage is poor, however, with a mortality rate of about 80%. Among the survivors, 5% or fewer have residual neurological deficits which include poor motor skills and lower IQ. Remote symptomatic epilepsy is not documented in survivors of enterovirus 71 infection (Huang *et al.* 1999).

Dengue

Dengue virus, a flavivirus, causes one of the most important viral infections in human, affecting over 50 million individuals yearly, with half a million of hospital admissions. The virus is pandemic in South and South-East Asia and South America, as well as affecting northern Australia and sub-Saharan Africa. In recent years, outbreaks have been recorded in Hawaii, Cuba and Singapore.

The incubation period of dengue infection ranges from 3 to 14 days. The infection is asymptomatic in the majority of patients, especially among children. In symptomatic patients, it often causes sudden rise of high fever, headache, retro-ocular pain, myalgia, arthralgia, backache, nausea, anorexia, vomiting, and a non-pruritic macular or petechial rash. The rash may be florid, or may even become confluent, with associated flushing around the face, neck, and chest and islands of pale, normal skin. Leukopenia and thrombocytopenia are common, and so are bruises on the skin and subcutaneous bleeding after venepuncture. The febrile period lasts a week or less. However, thrombocytopenia and vascular leakage may worsen suddenly, and hemorrhagic complications and shock arise rapidly. There is a tendency for the disease to deteriorate within 48 to 72 hr after defervescence. Vascular leakage is evident by hemoconcentration, severe thrombocytopenia (platelet count $\leq 10^5/\mu l$), ascites, pleural effusion, hypoalbuminemia, or hypoproteinemia. This is termed dengue hemorrhagic fever, and it is an indication of impending shock. Therefore, intensive observation and prophylactic replenishment of loss intravascular fluid are indicated. If not treated, the patient may progress into dengue shock syndrome, which may be heralded by intense abdominal pain, persistent vomiting, restlessness, lethargy, or hypothermia with sweating. Other uncommon, but often severe manifestations of dengue infection include severe hemorrhage, hepatic damage, cardiomyopathy, and encephalopathy/encephalitis. Diagnosis is by serologic testing. Since dengue virus is closely related to other flaviviruses, the serologic test may be falsely positive in Japanese encephalitis, West Nile fever, or St. Louis encephalitis. Treatment is supportive, with particular attention to adequate fluid replacement titrated against clinical findings and the patient's hematocrit.

Neurological involvement in dengue infection is well documented, though whether the virus causes an encephalopathy or encephalitis is still debated. The incidence is low, and is seen especially among pediatric patients. Patients with neurological involvement present with confusion, altered conscious state, limb weakness, and seizures. Approximately 10–15% of those with neurological involvement have seizures; commonly generalized tonic–clonic seizures, but occasionally myoclonic jerks as well. The EEG often shows non-specific theta slow waves (Rigau-Perez et al. 1998; Misra et al. 2006, 2008a; Halstead 2007).

The overall mortality of dengue infection is low; however, if shock sets in, the mortality rate can rise to 12–44%. Among the patients with central nervous system involvement, mortality is approximately 30%; and another 20–30% have long-term neurological deficits.

Human herpesvirus 6

Human herpesvirus 6 is a beta-herpes virus, a DNA virus closely related to the cytomegalovirus and human herpesvirus 7. Humans are the primary and perhaps the only host. The mode of transmission is not clear, though the virus is secreted in saliva and urine. About 77% to 90% of children become seropositive by age 2 years and it has been reported to cause outbreaks in daycare centers in Brazil. The primary infection is symptomatic in 93% of children, and the symptoms include fever, irritability, rhinorrhea, cough, diarrhea, and rash. The typical roseolar rash (roseola infantum, exanthema subitum, or sixth disease) is seen in only 23% of children. About 10% of patients with a primary infection may suffer from febrile seizures. Uncommonly, focal demyelinating encephalitis may occur in young children. Primary infection in immunocompetent adults or older children is rare,

and may result in infectious mononucleosis-like illness, and the patients may have fever, lymphadenopathy, hepatitis, or encephalitis. Generally, the outcome of uncomplicated primary infection is excellent.

Immunocompromised hosts are more susceptible to human herpesvirus 6 infections, either from primary or reactivation of latent infection. The rate of infection in transplant patients varies from 24% to 66%, and symptomatic disease is more likely to result from primary infection than reactivation of latent infection. Clinical features include fever, leukopenia, rash, interstitial pneumonitis, and encephalitis, and in bone marrow transplant patients, bone marrow suppression. In patients with reactivation of latent infection, including patients with human immunodeficiency virus infection, human herpesvirus 6 infections often manifest as fever, though encephalitis, including limbic encephalitis, and interstitial pneumonitis have been documented.

In immunocompromised patients with human herpesvirus 6 encephalitis common clinical features include confusion, altered conscious states, headache, focal neurological deficits, and seizures, which occur in about 25% of patients. Scan findings with CT and MRI are non-specific and the EEG may show focal discharges. The gold standard of diagnosis is viral culture of peripheral mononuclear cells, while anti-complement immunofluorescence assay is an alternative. Serologic tests are not specific in detecting recent infection, as IgM may be produced in both primary and reactivation of latent infection. Treatment is largely supportive, though ganciclovir and foscarnet have been tried. In transplant patients with human herpesvirus 6 encephalitis mortality is in excess of 50%, though residual neurological deficits are not common among the survivors (Dockrell et al. 1999; Singh and Paterson 2000).

Chandipura virus

Chandipura virus is a rhabdovirus transmitted to humans by sandflies. Although the virus is found in both India and Africa, so far only two possible outbreaks of human infections have been reported, and both in India – the first in Andhra Pradesh in 2003 with 329 patients, and the second in Gujarat state in 2004 with 26 patients. Children, especially boys under 16 years of age in rural areas, are more at risk of acquiring Chandipura infections. Typically, the patients present with sudden onset of fever, follow by vomiting, altered conscious state, diarrhea, focal neurological deficits, and meningism. Seizures occur in over 80% of patients. Although the mortality ranges from 55.6% to 78.3%, and most deaths occur within 24 hr of onset of disease, residual neurological deficits are rare in children who recover. Diagnosis is made by viral culture or PCR of throat swab, brain aspirate, or peripheral blood mononuclear cell co-culture. Serologic tests are not helpful; in the two outbreaks in India, only 4.5–13% of patients had positive IgM and 65.3–97.7% had positive neutralizing antibodies. Serologic tests are less sensitive among children. Because of this, the role of Chandipura virus in these outbreaks is still debated, and Chandipura viral infection was proven in only 8.5–45% of patients in these two outbreaks. In all of the affected patients,

CSF pleocytosis was not observed, and in the autopsy cases, brain parenchymal inflammation was not observed (Rao *et al.* 2003; Chadha *et al.* 2005).

Monkeypox virus

Monkeypox virus is an orthomyxovirus closely related to variola or smallpox virus. The virus causes outbreaks in central and western Africa and was brought into the United States in 2003 through the importation of infected Gambian rats for the pet trade. Clinically it causes fever and acute pustular rash. Among the 34 patients infected in the Midwestern United States outbreak, a 6-year-old girl developed acute encephalitis and seizures (Sejvar 2006).

Other uncommon encephalitides

Rabies

Rabies, a rhabdovirus which is spread by the bites of infected animals, is an important health problem worldwide. Although only 15% of the bite victims develop rabies, worldwide there are more than 35 000 reported human cases annually, the majority of which occur in India. Dogs are the primary vectors in developing countries, while small terrestrial mammals and bats are the primary vectors in developed countries. After an incubation period of 3 weeks to 2 months, the patient develops fever, flu-like symptoms, mood changes, and local pruritus, pain, and paresthesiae at the sites of bite. If the brainstem, limbic system, hypothalamus, and the autonomic center are involved, the patient develop furious or agitated rabies, characterized by hydrophobia, aerophobia, and episodes of generalized arousal associated with confusion, agitation, and hyperesthesia punctuated by periods of lucidity. Death often ensues within a week. If the spinal cord is primarily involved, the patient may develop weakness, paresthesiae, pain, and muscle fasciculation, starting from the affected limb spreading to the rest of the body, and eventually involving all the other limbs as well as the bulbar and respiratory muscles. Uncommonly, patients may present with subtle or focal seizures, which are easily missed. Vaccines are available for pre- and post-exposure prophylaxis and treatment. Treatment involves thorough washing of the wounds with soap, water, and if available, virucidal agents. The standard vaccine is given intramuscularly in five doses on days 0, 3, 7, 14, and 28 into deltoid or the anterolateral aspect of thigh, and passive immunization with human rabies immunoglobulin infiltrated around the wounds. The mortality of rabies in unvaccinated individuals is 100% (Warrell and Warrell 2004).

Tick-borne encephalitis

The three subtypes of tick-borne encephalitis virus (Far Eastern, Siberian [previously known as Russian spring–summer encephalitis], and Western European) are the commonest causes of encephalitis in Europe, accounting for 29–54% of encephalitis with a diagnosis and 10 000 to 20 000 cases annually. The flavivirus is transmitted by the *Ixodes* and *Haemaphysalis* ticks, with rodents and wolves acting as reservoirs and amplifying hosts. Shrews, hedgehogs, moles, and other insectivores are additional hosts. The risk of acquiring the infection is, therefore, higher among men, especially among farmers, hunters, forest workers, and those participating in outdoor leisure activities. The virus is found in a large geographical area stretching from Scandinavia to Jilin in northern China and Hokkaido, Japan.

Humans are the dead-end host of the virus, and 70–95% of infections are subclinical. In symptomatic patients, the virus causes a biphasic illness after an incubation period of 4 to 28 days. The first, viremic, phase lasts 4 to 18 days, and the patients complain of fever, myalgias, nausea, fatigue, and headache. After an interval of 8 to 133 days, 74–87% of patients suffer from central nervous system involvement; half of these develop meningoencephalitis, the other half meningitis, radiculitis, or myelitis. Patients with meningoencephalitis have recurrence of fever, headache, altered consciousness, confusion, tremor, ataxia, weakness, dysphasia, cranial nerve palsies, and, uncommonly, seizures which are seen in 0.3–3.3% of patients. The EEG is abnormal in 77% of patients, but the changes of diffuse and/or intermittent focal slow waves are non-specific. Magnetic resonance imaging of the brain shows abnormalities in the thalamus, cerebellum, brainstem, and caudate nucleus in 18% of patients. Mortality is low at 0.1–1.4%, though 26–46% of patients have residual symptoms, and up to 30% have significant neurological deficits. Approximately 4–5% of patients develop focal motor status epilepticus partialis continua, known as Kozhevnikov epilepsy among Russian neurologists (Gritsun *et al.* 2003). The disease is more severe among the elderly, and mortality is reportedly higher in far-eastern Russia, though it is not known whether this is due to the strain of the virus or underreporting of milder cases. Diagnosis at the first stage is by PCR, and the second stage by serology. There is no definitive treatment though effective vaccines are available (Lindquist and Vapalathi 2008).

LaCrosse encephalitis

The commonest cause of encephalitis in the United States is caused by the Californian serogroup of bunyaviruses; and among this group of viruses, LaCrosse virus is responsible for almost all infections. LaCrosse virus is transmitted by *Aedes triseriatus* mosquito with chipmunks and squirrels as the natural reservoirs and amplifying hosts. Occurring mainly in the upper Midwestern states during summer months, the incidence of LaCrosse infection has been stable over the years with 70–100 cases annually. More than 90% of the cases occur in young people under 15 years of age, with males being twice as likely to contract the virus compared with females. In endemic areas, up to 18% of residents are seropositive.

Probably only 1 in 1000 person infected with the virus becomes symptomatic, and in the symptomatic, fever is near universal, and three-quarters have headache and half have meningism. Other common features are seizures, an altered consciousness state, focal neurological deficits, abdominal pain, cough, and sore throat. About 12% of patients become comatose though the outcome is usually good.

LaCrosse encephalitis is highly epileptogenic. About 40–49% of patients with symptomatic infection develop acute symptomatic seizures and up to 20% of patients develop remote symptomatic epilepsy even after recovery from the infection. Abnormal EEG findings were reported in up to 75% of children 3 to 4 years after the infection. Apart from epilepsy, the overall outcomes remain good; the mortality rate is only 0.3–0.5%, and residual neurological deficits, such as weakness, learning disabilities, cognitive deficits, and behavioral changes, are seen in about 2% of the patients with central nervous system infection.

St. Louis encephalitis

St. Louis encephalitis, caused by a flavivirus, is the second commonest cause of viral encephalitis in the United States. It occurs primarily in the Ohio–Mississippi valley, but human infections have been documented in other regions from southern Canada to Argentina. The virus is transmitted by the *Culex* mosquito, the amplifying hosts are birds, and the virus spills out of the zoonotic cycle when there is a sufficient number of mosquitoes. This causes periodic outbreaks of human disease once every decade or so. Only 1 in 800 to 100 000 human infection results in clinical illness and the elderly are most at risk; while 40% of symptomatic young patients suffer from mild aseptic meningitis only, 90% of the symptomatic elderly develop encephalitis. The onset of encephalitis can be abrupt or slow, and the clinical features include fever, headache, dizziness, nausea, malaise, meningism, seizures, confusion, tremor, ataxia, apathy, cranial nerve palsies, and urinary frequency, urgency, or retention. The patients often recover from the acute infection after a week or so, though 30–50% continue to have prolonged asthenia, insomnia, irritability, depression, poor memory, headache, tremor, and even gait and speech disturbance which can last up to 2 years. The mortality rate is 5–20% though it can be as high as 70% in those who age 75 years and above. Analysis of CSF shows raised protein and pleocytosis, and MRI T2-weighted images show substantia nigra edema in about 20% of patients. Diagnosis is by serologic test and treatment is supportive. A mosquito control program has proven effective in breaking the cycle of transmission.

In patients with acute St. Louis encephalitis, generalized tonic–clonic seizure occur in 30% of patients, myoclonic jerks in about 10%, and status epilepticus in another 10%. The EEG shows diffuse background slow waves in 70% of patients, bilateral periodic lateralized epileptiform discharges in 10%, and status epilepticus in another 10%.

Western equine encephalitis

Western equine encephalitis virus is an alphavirus, from the *Togaviridae* family. It is mainly transmitted by *Culex tarsalis* mosquito and its natural reservoirs are birds. In summer, the mosquito switches its feeding pattern from birds to mammals, causing outbreaks in horses, mules, and humans. Western equine encephalitis is limited to North America and the last human outbreak was reported in Colorado in 1988. Since then, fewer than five sporadic cases have been reported annually.

Only 1 in 100–2000 infections results in clinical disease, which ranges from mild fever to aseptic meningitis and encephalitis. Infants are more likely to develop central nervous system infection and neurological sequelae. After an incubation period of 5 to 10 days, those with encephalitis present with sudden onset of fever, headache, nausea, vomiting, and respiratory symptoms. After a few days, the patients develop lethargy, an altered consciousness, meningism, and vertigo. In infants less than 1 year of age, irritability, tremor, weakness, and focal or generalized seizures are common features. Long-term sequelae of Western equine encephalitis are mild and include fatigue, headache, and tremor, and the mortality rate is 3–4%. In children, severe neurological deficits are common and are seen in 56% of infants younger than 1 month of age and 10% in older infants. A quarter to a third of children with acute symptomatic seizures will develop remote symptomatic epilepsy, sometimes up to 2 years after the acute illness. Diagnosis is by viral isolation or serologic test. Treatment is mainly supportive as there is no specific antiviral agent available (Lowry 1997).

Eastern equine encephalitis

Eastern equine virus causes the most lethal arboviral encephalitis in the United States. It is an alphavirus from the family *Togaviridae*, and it is found almost exclusively along the Atlantic and Gulf coasts of the United States, extending as far inland as Wisconsin, Indiana, and Michigan. The chief vector is *Culiseta melanura*, a fastidious mosquito that breeds in a specific microenvironment of dark, organic-rich water in peat soil and is strictly ornithophilic. Human infections occur when other less fastidious mosquitoes venture into this environment. There are about five reported cases of Eastern equine encephalitis a year in the United States.

Almost all infections are symptomatic, which could manifest as either systemic infection or encephalitis. Young children are more susceptible to develop encephalitis with its subsequent serious neurological deficits. Systemic infection begins abruptly with high fever, followed by myalgia, arthralgia, and malaise, and lasts 1 to 2 weeks, and recovery is mostly complete. In patients with encephalitis, headache, irritability, restlessness, drowsiness, anorexia, vomiting, diarrhea, seizure, and coma occur a few days after the onset of systemic infection. Children may develop generalized or facial edema, weakness, tremor, muscular twitching, or dysautonomia. In fatal cases, death often occurs as a result of either severe encephalitis or dysautonomia causing myocardial insufficiency and respiratory failure, and usually occurs 2 to 10 days after the onset of symptoms. Diagnosis is by serologic testing and treatment is largely supportive. A vaccine for Eastern equine encephalitis has been developed and used successfully in humans, but it is not available for general use.

Eastern equine encephalitis is the most lethal arboviral encephalitis in North America; the mortality rate ranges between 30% and 75% and the majority of the survivors are left with severe, disabling, and often progressive intellectual and physical disabilities, which include personality disorders, cranial nerve palsies, weakness, and remote symptomatic seizures. The long-term outcome is even poorer; 9 years after infection, up to 90% of patients eventually died because of associated neurological deficits, and only 3% recovered (Calisher 1994; Sejvar 2006).

Murray Valley encephalitis

Murray Valley encephalitis virus is a flavivirus found only in Australia, Papua New Guinea, and perhaps the eastern islands of Indonesia. *Culex* mosquito, especially *C. annulirostris*, is the vector, and wading birds its natural reservoir and host. Horses, feral pigs, and cattle may act as additional reservoir or amplifying hosts. Outbreaks of Murray Valley encephalitis have been reported throughout Australia, and sporadic cases occur annually, mainly in the Kimberly region of northern Western Australia and in the Northern Territory. Only 1 in 500 to 5000 infections is symptomatic though infection is more common and severe in children and infants. Clinically the patients present with sudden onset of fever, headache, vomiting, dizziness, weakness, brainstem signs, seizures, and myoclonus. Mortality ranges from 15% to 31% and half of the survivors have significant residual neurological deficits. There is no specific antiviral therapy for Murray Valley encephalitis (Russell and Dwyer 2000).

References

Calisher CH (1994) Medically important arboviruses of the United States and Canada. *Clin Microbiol Review* 7:89–116.

Chadha MS, Arankalle VA, Jadi RS, *et al.* (2005) An outbreak of Chandipura virus encephalitis in the eastern districts of Gujarat state, India. *Am J Trop Med Hyg* 73:566–70.

Chew NK, Goh KJ, Tan CT, Ahmad Sarji S, Wong KT (1999) Electroencephalography in acute Nipah encephalitis. *Neurol J Southeast Asia* 4:45–51.

Chong HT, Kunjapan SR, Thayaparan T, *et al.* (2000) Nipah encephalitis outbreak in Malaysia, clinical features in patients from Seremban. *Neurol J Southeast Asia* 5:61–7.

Dockrell DH, Smith TF, Paya CV (1999) Human herpesvirus 6. *Mayo Clin Proc* 74:163–70.

Gea-Banacloche J, Johnson RT, Bagic A, *et al.* (2004) West Nile virus: pathogenesis and therapeutic options. *Ann Intern Med* 140:545–53.

Goh KJ, Tan CT, Chew NK, *et al.* (2000) Clinical features of Nipah virus encephalitis among pig farmers in Malaysia. *N Engl J Med* 342:1229–35.

Gritsun TS, Lashkevich VA, Gould EA (2003) Tick-borne encephalitis. *Antivir Res* 57:129–46.

Halstead SB (2007) Dengue. *Lancet* 370:1644–52.

Huang CC, Liu CC, Chang YC, *et al.* (1999) Neurologic complications in children with enterovirus 71 infection. *N Engl J Med* 341:936–42.

Kalita J, Misra UK (1998) EEG in Japanese encephalitis: a clinicoradiological correlation. *Electroencephalogr Clin Neurophysiol* 106:238–43.

Koskiniemi M, Rautonen J, Lehtokoski-Lehtiniemi E, Vaheri A (1991) Epidemiology of encephalitis in children: a 20-year survey. *Ann Neurol* 29:492–7.

Lindquist L, Vapalathi O (2008) Tick-borne encephalitis. (Seminar.) *Lancet* 371:1861–71.

Lowry PW (1997) Arbovirus encephalitis in the United States and Asia. (Seminar of the University of Minnesota.) *J Lab Clin Med* 129:405–11.

Mackenzie JS (1999) Emerging viral diseases: an Australian perspective. *Emerg Infect Dis* 5:1–8.

Misra UK, Kalita J, Syam UK, Dhole TN (2006) Neurological manifestations of dengue virus infection. *J Neurol Sci* 244:117–22.

Misra UK, Tan CT, Kalita J (2008a) Seizures in encephalitis. *Neurology Asia* 13:1–13.

Misra UK, Tan CT, Kalita J (2008b) Viral encephalitis and epilepsy. *Epilepsia* 49:13–18.

Rao BL, Basu A, Wairagkar NS, *et al.* (2003) A large outbreak of acute encephalitis with high fatality rate in children in Andhra Pradesh, India, in 2003, associated with Chandipura virus. *Lancet* 364:869–74.

Rigau-Perez JG, Clark GG, Gubler DJ, *et al.* (1998) Dengue and dengue hemorrhagic fever. *Lancet* 352:971–9.

Russell RC, Dwyer DE (2000) Arboviruses associated with human diseases in Australia. *Microbes Infect* 2:1693–704.

Sejvar JJ (2006) The evolving epidemiology of viral encephalitis. *Curr Opin Neurol* 19:350–7.

Sejvar JJ, Haddad MB, Tierney BC, *et al.* (2003) Neurologic manifestations and outcome of West Nile virus infection. *J Am Med Ass* 290:511–15.

Singh N, Paterson D (2000) Encephalitis caused by human herpesvirus-6 in transplant recipients: relevance of a novel neurotropic virus. (Overview.) *Transplantation* 69:2474–9.

Solomon T, Dung NM, Kneen R, *et al.* (2000) Japanese encephalitis. *J Neurol Neurosurg Psychiatry* 68:405–15.

Solomon T, Dung NM, Kneen R, *et al.* (2002) Seizures and raised intracranial pressure in Vietnamese patients with Japanese encephalitis. *Brain* 125:1084–93.

Tan CT, Goh KJ, Wong KT, *et al.* (2002) Relapsed and late-onset Nipah encephalitis. *Ann Neurol* 51:703–8.

Taylor LH, Latham SM, Woolhouse ME (2001) Risk factors for human disease emergence. *Phil Trans R Soc Lond B* 356:983–9.

Warrell MJ, Warrell DA (2004) Rabies and other lyssavirus diseases. (Seminar.) *Lancet* 363:959–69.

Wong KT, Robertson T, Ong BB, *et al.* (2009) Human Hendra virus infection causes acute and relapsing encephalitis. *Neuropathol Appl Neurobiol* 35:296–305.

Chapter

76

Cerebral hemorrhage

Henry B. Dinsdale

Intracerebral hemorrhage

Intracerebral hemorrhage (ICH) accounts for 5–10% of all patients with stroke (Wolfe and D'Agostino 1998). It is twice as common as subarachnoid hemorrhage (SAH) and more likely to result in death or major disability. Hypertension and advancing age are important risk factors.

Half the deaths from ICH occur in the first 3 days and up to 52% of patients with a diagnosis of primary ICH are dead at 1 month (Broderick et al. 2007). Only 20% of patients are functionally independent at 6 months (Counsell et al. 1995). Hematoma volume and growth are determinants of mortality and functional outcome. Imaging studies record active bleeding and hematoma growth for several hours in 20–40% of patients, especially those with initially large hematomas. Other factors influencing survival are age, mean arterial pressure, blood glucose, lateral shift of midline structures, intraventricular and subarachnoid spread of blood, infratentorial location, and hydrocephalus (Fogelholm et al. 2005).

Usually ICH is a consequence of a long-term process. In spite of important advances in the diagnosis and care of patients with ICH, most reduction in death and disability will come from the more mundane task of dealing with its precursors, especially adequate treatment of hypertension and careful monitoring of anticoagulants.

Rupture of microaneurysms in small and medium-sized penetrating cerebral arteries is a frequent cause of ICH (Ross Russell 1963; Dinsdale 1964). Common locations are the basal ganglia, thalamus, cerebellum, and pons. A finding of ICH in normotensive patients and at uncommon sites, such as the head of the caudate nucleus, suggests a mechanism other than hypertension. Other causes include anticoagulants, amyloid angiopathy, primary and secondary tumors, drug abuse, thrombolytic agents such as tissue-type plasminogen activator, vascular malformations, granulomatous angiitis, and antiplatelet agents. Leukoariosis may be a risk factor for warfarin-related ICH. Cocaine, amphetamines, and other sympathomimetic drugs may cause ICH in younger patients.

Cerebral amyloid angiopathy (CAA), characterized by deposits of amyloid in the adventitia and media of medium-sized cortical arteries, accounts for 10–20% of ICH. Anticoagulant, thrombolytic, or antiplatelet agents promote CAA-related ICH (Rosand et al. 2000), which is most frequent in the occipital lobe and rare in deep hemisphere or brainstem structures. Pathologic examination is required to determine CAA-related ICH but the diagnosis is suggested when imaging studies demonstrate multiple, strictly lobar hemorrhages. In CAA-related ICH there is a 3-month mortality rate of 25%.

Lobar hematomas due to CAA may be multifocal and recurrent. Increased recurrence is associated with the E-2 and E-4 alleles of apolipoprotein E. A mutation in the amyloid precursor protein (APP) gene is present in a number of families with hereditary cerebral amyloid angiopathy (HCAA) (Zhang-Nunes et al. 2006). Although dementia is often present in patients with CAA, the location of the APP mutation in families with HCAA differs from that in familial Alzheimer disease.

Initial symptoms of ICH are due to increased intracranial pressure and depend on the location of bleeding. Severe headache and vomiting are frequent but not universal. Gradual increase in symptoms is common but some patients present with sudden deterioration and loss of consciousness. Hypertension is present in 90% of patients. Putamenal ICH produces hemiplegia, sensory abnormalities, speech defects, and hemisensory inattention. Thalamic ICH causes decreased consciousness, hemiparesis, gaze palsies, and pupillary abnormalities due to compression or hemorrhage into the midbrain tegmentum. With cerebellar hemorrhage, bleeding occurs in or near the dentate nucleus causing ataxia, vomiting, headache, ipsilateral cerebellar signs, nystagmus, and a variety of gaze problems. Primary pontine hemorrhage causes coma, miosis, slow irregular breathing, conjugate deviation of eyes, hyperthermia, and usually early death. Patients may survive a small, lateral pontine hemorrhage.

Epilepsy in intracerebral hemorrhage

Cerebrovascular disease (CVD) is the most commonly identified antecedent of epilepsy in adults, accounting for 11% of

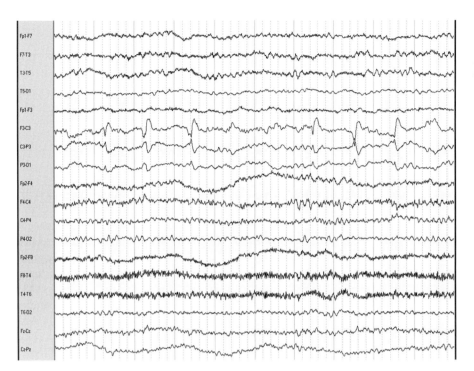

Fig. 76.1. Electroencephalogram in 79-year-old patient with tonic–clonic and focal seizures resulting from cerebral hemorrhage due to cerebral amyloid angiopathy. The EEG shows slow waves and repetitive discharges from C3.

cases (Hauser *et al.* 1996). Post-ICH seizures are defined as single or multiple convulsive episodes resulting from reversible or irreversible cerebral damage, regardless of the time of onset following the stroke (Myint *et al.* 2006). Intracerebral hemorrhage is less frequent than ischemic CVD, but carries twice the risk for seizures compared to patients with ischemic stroke; ICH patients have an incidence of seizures ranging from 4% to 15.4% (Kammersgaard and Olsen 2005). Of those experiencing seizures, 45% have seizures within 24 hr of ICH, often accompanied by clinical worsening and increasing midline shift. Seizures are usually partial, predominantly motor and more frequent with frontal lobe hematomas (De Rueck *et al.* 2007). Complex partial and primary generalized seizures are uncommon. A small minority develops recurring seizures.

Post-ICH seizures may be partial, generalized, or secondary generalized, convulsive (CSE) or non-convulsive status epilepticus (NCSE) (Fig. 76.1). About one-third of patients present with generalized seizures and most of the remainder with partial seizures, especially with lobar ICH. Early-onset seizures are usually partial; late-onset seizures tend to be generalized. Convulsive status epilepticus is more frequent in patients with a history of alcoholism and carries a higher mortality rate. It occurs in 9% of patients experiencing post-stroke seizures (Rumbach *et al.* 2000).

Seizures may be non-convulsive and contribute to coma in up to 10% of patients. Electrographic seizures, usually focal with secondary generalization, were found in 28% of patients with ICH, compared with 6% with ischemic stroke (Vespa *et al.* 2003). Atypical seizures, acute confusional states, behavioral change, syncope of unknown origin, and Todd's paralysis may cause diagnostic problems. Non-convulsive status epilepticus is more common than is generally appreciated. It causes decreased levels of consciousness, confusion, and coma. Twitching or occasional blinking may be present.

Products of blood metabolism, excitotoxic neurotransmitter release and global hypoperfusion are considered factors causing early post-ICH seizures. Gliosis, meningocerebral cicatrix, and hemosiderin deposits may be sources of continuing irritability. Seizures occur most frequently with lobar hematomas, especially frontal or parietal. Seizures are more frequent with cortical lesions on computed tomography (CT) scan, persisting paresis and in the elderly. Electroencephalogram (EEG) abnormalities and partial seizures carry a higher recurrence rate. There is no correlation between post-ICH seizures and hemorrhage size, cerebrospinal fluid (CSF) blood, the presence of hydrocephalus, intracranial shift, Glasgow Coma Scale score, level of consciousness or neurological deficit (Bladin *et al.* 2000).

Early seizures are associated with an increased risk of seizure recurrence but almost half of those with ischemic stroke or ICH experience only one seizure (Burn *et al.* 1997). Stroke survivors functionally independent 1 to 6 months following stroke have a low risk of seizures.

Diagnostic tests

Intracerebral hemorrhage is the most lethal form of stroke and is a medical emergency. Prompt imaging studies are required because clinical presentation alone is insufficient to differentiate ICH from stroke due to other causes. Scanning with CT and magnetic resonance imaging (MRI) are first-choice options (Fig. 76.2). They have equal and excellent ability to identify an acute hematoma, its size, location, enlargement, and ventricular extension (Fiebach *et al.* 2004). Catheter angiography may be

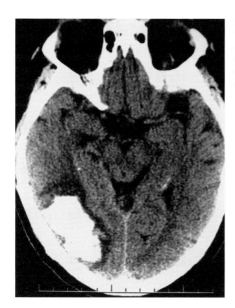

Fig. 76.2. Computed tomography scan demonstrating posterior cerebral hemorrhage due to ruptured arteriovenous malformations.

indicated when there is SAH, blood in unusual locations, obvious vascular abnormalities, or unusual calcifications. Hemosiderin deposits from earlier bleeds may be present with CAA-related ICH. Cortical damage on imaging studies is more predictive of epilepsy than any single EEG finding.

The degree of post-ICH abnormality in the EEG depends on the site, size, and speed of development of the hematoma. Polymorphic high-amplitude delta is usually present over all or part of the affected hemisphere; it may be prominent in the temporal region in slowly evolving hematomas. Delta activity tends to be intermittent and rhythmic when present at a distance from the hematoma. Focal or diffuse slowing is associated with a low risk of seizures whereas focal spikes or periodic lateralized epileptiform discharges (PLEDs) carry a higher risk. Sharp transients are more frequent with ICH than with ischemic stroke. Moderate depression of alpha activity often accompanies capsular and thalamic hemorrhage. Widespread poorly reactive alpha may be the only finding with brainstem hemorrhage. Cerebellar hemorrhage is associated with little EEG change, unless there is tonsillar herniation causing diffuse slowing.

Continuous electroencephalographic monitoring (cEEG) in ICH patients revealed seizures in one-third (Classen et al. 2007). One-half of the purely electrographic seizures were detected within the first hour in 56% of patients and within 48 hr in 94%. Electrographic seizures are more common with an increase in ICH volume of 30% or more during the first 24 hr. Periodic lateralized epileptiform discharges are associated with poor outcome.

Principles of management

Although the effect of post-ICH seizure on outcome remains unclear, the high mortality and morbidity of ICH make it advisable to avoid, if possible, the presumptive neuronal injury or destabilization that may occur with early seizures. Longer-term management must recognize that few post-ICH seizures recur.

The optimal timing and type of treatment of post-ICH seizures have yet to be determined. Stroke Council Guidelines of the American Heart Association recommend prompt treatment of onset seizures with intravenous diazepam, followed by loading doses of phenytoin (Broderick et al. 2007). Prophylactic treatment from the outset with phenytoin is recommended for all ICH patients, to be tapered and discontinued if no seizure activity occurs after 1 month. Others suggest a more nuanced approach with the decision to initiate antiepileptic drugs (AEDs) after a first or second post-stroke seizure individualized, based on the functional impact of the first seizure and the patient's preference (Ryvlin et al. 2006). They note the lack of level A evidence supporting the use of first-generation AEDs and prefer low-dose extended-release carbamazepine, lamotrigine, or gabapentin. The National Institute for Health and Clinical Excellence (NICE) in the UK recommends carbamazepine, lamotrigine, sodium valproate, or topiramate if focal or generalized seizures recur. A brief period of prophylactic antiepileptic therapy soon after lobar ICH may reduce the risk of early seizures (National Institute for Clinical Excellence 2004). For all AEDs, the chief limiting adverse effect is sedation.

First-line treatment for CSE is a benzodiazepan (lorazepam or diazepam) followed by phenytoin. Close monitoring of respiratory and cardiovascular function is required. Refractory CSE requires anesthesia induced by barbiturate or non-barbiturate drugs such as thiopentone, pentobarbitone, propofol, or midazolam.

Prompt clinical evaluation is required followed by transfer of patients with supratentorial ICH to a stroke unit. Objectives of acute treatment include stopping or slowing initial bleeding, controlling intracranial pressure (ICP), and providing general supportive measures. Early intensive blood-pressure-lowering treatment may reduce hematoma growth in ICH but rapid decline in blood pressure that compromises brain perfusion is associated with an increased death rate. Hemostatic therapy with recombinant activated factor VIII reduces growth of the hematoma but remains investigational concerning its effect on survival or functional outcome (Broderick et al. 2007). Persistent hyperglycemia following ICH may require insulin and is associated with poor outcome. Therapeutic cooling lowers ICP but carries a high rate of complications. More aggressive therapies, such as osmotic diuretics and drainage via ventricular catheter, require ICP monitoring with the goal to maintain cerebral perfusion pressure >70 mm Hg. A clinical grading scale that enables risk stratification can provide guidance for treatment decisions (Hemphill et al. 2001).

Intermittent pneumatic compression decreases the incidence of deep-vein thrombosis and pulmonary embolism. Low-dose subcutaneous low-molecular-weight heparin may be required for patients with hemiplegia. The coagulation defect in warfarin-related ICH requires prompt reversal with vitamin K1. Reinstitution of warfarin in patients with prosthetic heart valves or chronic non-valvular atrial fibrillation is considered safe after a period of 10 days (Claassen et al. 2008).

Protamine sulfate should be used for heparin-related ICH. Acute ischemic stroke is followed by symptomatic ICH in 3–9% of patients treated with tissue-type plasminogen activator. Treatment by infusion of platelets and factor VIII are recommended (Grotta *et al.* 2001).

Decisions about surgery remain controversial. Craniotomy produced insignificant benefit in patients with supratentorial ICH randomized to surgery or medical treatment (Mendelow *et al.* 2005). Surgery was not helpful for supratentorial ICH and harmful for those in coma. Surgery may benefit those with lobar hemorrhages within 1 cm of the cortex. Non-randomized patients with cerebellar hemorrhage >3 cm are helped by surgery when there is compression of the brainstem or obstruction of the fourth ventricle (van Loon *et al.* 1993). There is no evidence supporting either early or delayed evacuation. Catheter-directed or minimally invasive endoscopic surgery for clot evacuation using tissue-type plasminogen activator may hold promise in selected patients.

Subdural hematoma

Subdural hematomas (SDH) usually arise from venous bleeding in the potential space between the dural and arachnoid membranes. Low-pressure bleeding is caused by trauma that tears small bridging veins between the brain surface and dural sinuses. Cerebral atrophy in older patients increases the length that bridging veins traverse between the meningeal layers and the likelihood of bleeding. Head injury may be trivial or absent, particularly in patients on anticoagulants. Subdural hematomas are located usually over the lateral convexities but blood may collect along the medial surface of the hemisphere, below the temporal lobe or in the posterior fossa. After 1 week, fibroblasts in the inner surface of the dura form a thick outer membrane. An inner membrane forms later and encapsulates the clot, which begins to liquefy. Recurrent bleeding or osmotic effects can cause further enlargement. Chronic subdural hematomas (CSH) may become symptomatic weeks following trauma. An altered mental status, sometimes mistaken for dementia, may be the only clinical feature. Alcoholism and pre-existing epilepsy are common. Arachnoid cysts are a risk factor for SDH following trauma in the young.

Acute subdural hematoma (ASDH) is a medical emergency with a high mortality rate. Half of the patients lose consciousness at the time of injury and 25% are in coma when they arrive at the emergency room. Half of those who awaken lose consciousness again after an interval. Ipsilateral pupillary dilation and contralateral hemiparesis are common clinical findings. Acute subdural hematoma is found along the posterior interhemispheric fissure and the tentorium in shaken baby syndrome.

Epilepsy

Brain contusion with SDH is a risk factor for later seizures, so there is a strong relation between the severity of head injury and the risk of subsequent unprovoked seizures (Annegers

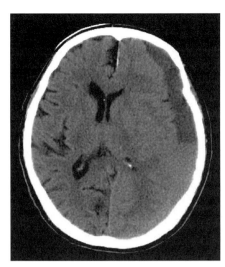

Fig. 76.3. Computed tomography scan demonstrating left anterolateral subdural hematoma with compression of lateral ventricle and shift of midline structures.

et al. 1998). New seizures occurred in 18.5% of patients requiring surgery for CSH (Sabo *et al.* 1995). Periodic lateralized epileptiform discharges may be associated with focal seizures and altered consciousness both before and after surgical evacuation, usually of large hematomas. Ethanol withdrawal is often a factor in these patients.

Diagnostic tests

Acute SDH presents as a hyperdense, crescent-shaped mass overlying and deforming the surface of the brain (Fig. 76.3). It becomes isodense after 1 week and hypodense thereafter. Membranes may enhance with intravenous contrast. Longstanding CSH may liquefy and form a hygroma, occasionally with membrane calcification. Scanning by MRI is preferred in the non-acute setting because of its high sensitivity and specificity. Multiplanar capabilities of MRI make it the study of choice for detecting small SDH, especially in the middle cranial and posterior fossa. Small SDH may be missed with CT.

The EEG may be normal in patients with CSH. Background activity is usually reduced in amplitude or abolished over the affected hemisphere. Focal, ipsilateral slow activity may be the most prominent feature. The EEG may not localize the lesion or reliably distinguish CSH from other space-occupying lesions. Non-convulsive seizures after brain injury will be detected by cEEG (Vespa 2005). Periodic lateralized epileptiform discharges have been recorded over the side of the hematoma, usually before but also after surgical evacuation (Westmoreland 2001).

Management

Acute and chronic subdural hematomas with mass effect should be evacuated. Depending on the clinical condition of the patient, small lesions need not be treated surgically. Prophylactic AED is recommended for patients treated surgically for CSH (Sabo *et al.* 1995). Periodic lateralized epileptiform discharges and seizures usually resolve after a few days treatment with anticonvulsant drugs.

Extradural hemorrhage

Most extradural hemorrhage (EDH) is due to blunt trauma, occurs in the potential space between the dura and the skull, and is present in 1–3% of head injuries. It often results from blows to the pterion region with laceration of the underlying middle meningeal artery. Bleeding is usually arterial and rapid, causing shift of midline structures and brainstem compression. Bleeding can also be due to disruption of venous sinuses and diploic veins. Rarely, EDH is contrecoup. It is a common traumatic lesion in the posterior fossa, especially in children. Between 12% and 20% of patients with EDH die. Some patients regain consciousness only to descend later into coma, the so-called "lucid interval." Associated brain injury and best motor responses are important prognostic indicators. Dura mater also covers the spine, so EDH can occur in the spinal column, spontaneously during childbirth or as a complication of epidural anesthesia or laminectomy.

Epilepsy

As with other forms of cerebral trauma, the extent of the brain injury and local tissue destruction are factors predicting the appearance of early and late epilepsy (Annegers *et al.* 2000). Focal brain damage on CT is a powerful predictor of increased risk for post-traumatic epilepsy (PTE) (D'Alessandro *et al.* 1982). Non-contusional, extradural hematoma not requiring evacuation appears not to put patients at additional risk for PTE (Englander *et al.* 2003). Gliotic scarring around hemosiderin deposits on T2-weighted imaging is a risk factor for seizure recurrence. Abnormal EEG records, which are more common in patients who develop late PTE, appear to reflect the extent of brain damage rather than the likelihood of developing epilepsy (Jennett and van de Sand 1975).

Diagnostic tests

The expanding hematoma strips the dura from the skull producing on CT or MRI a characteristic, high-attenuation, biconvex (lentiform) hematoma with a well-defined margin (Fig. 76.4). Hypodense areas may reflect active bleeding. There is often significant mass effect with compression of the ipsilateral ventricle, occasionally with dilatation of the opposite ventricle due to obstruction of the foramen of Munro. As with SDH, dural attachment at skull sutures limits expansion of the hematoma.

Management

Because these lesions can enlarge rapidly, the threshold for operative removal of the hematoma is low. Small EDH may be managed conservatively if the neurological examination is normal. Seizure management is described elsewhere (see Chapter 58).

Subarachnoid hemorrhage

Subarachnoid hemorrhage (SAH) arises from rupture of a cerebral aneurysm in 85% of patients and accounts for 20% of all nontraumatic, fatal intracranial hemorrhages (Whisnant *et al.* 1993). The incidence increases with age, smoking, hypertension, and

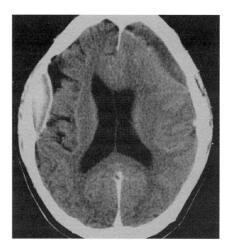

Fig. 76.4. Computed tomography scan of left anterior subdural hematoma and right extradural hemorrhage due to trauma.

excessive alcohol, and SAH is more common in women (Ingall *et al.* 1989). Familial and heritable disorders such as polycystic kidneys and Marfan syndrome are risk factors. It is also caused by trauma, arteriovenous malformations, and bleeding disorders. The prevalence of unruptured aneurysms in the American population is between 0.5% and 1.0% with an annual 1–2% risk of bleeding for aneurysms greater than 3 mm in diameter (Mayberg *et al.* 1994). There is a post-SAH risk of re-bleeding of 1–2% a day during the first 4 weeks. Subarachnoid hemorrhage has a mortality rate of 25% with significant morbidity in 50% of survivors. Delayed cerebral vasospasm (DCV) is common, more frequent with large amounts of subarachnoid blood, and accounts for 30% of death or dependence (Kassell *et al.* 1990).

The usual onset is sudden intense headache, often with brief loss of consciousness, vomiting, and later neck stiffness. There may be oculomotor nerve abnormalities and intraocular hemorrhage. Misdiagnosis is common, especially with smaller hemorrhages. A low Glasgow Coma scale score, older age, and loss of consciousness at the outset predict poor outcome (Brouwers *et al.* 1993).

Epilepsy

Seizures at the time of hemorrhage (onset seizures) occur in 8.5–17.9% of patients with SAH (Silverman *et al.* 2002). Most seizures are partial, secondary generalized or generalized tonic–clonic. Seizure-like episodes after SAH are not all epileptic, and include transient decerebrate posturing due to elevated intracranial pressure. Non-convulsive status epilepticus may account for unexplained coma or neurological deterioration in 8% of patients. The prevalence of seizures months and years following SAH ranges from 12% to 15% (Olaffson *et al.* 2000). Independent predictors of epilepsy 12 months after SAH include middle cerebral artery location, intraparenchymal hematoma, cerebral infarction, hypertension, and thickness of the cisternal clot.

Diagnostic tests

Computed tomography demonstrates a high-density clot in the subarachnoid space within 24 hr in the majority of patients. Aneurysm is not detected in initial imaging studies in 15–20%. Conventional catheter angiography, which can be repeated, may be required to demonstrate an aneurysm. Multiple aneurysms occur in 1% of patients.

The EEG may be normal or show bilateral variations in background activity reflecting varying degrees of consciousness. Local delta or sharp wave activity is associated with vasospasm. Hematomas may produce focal abnormalities. Morphological criteria and response to stimulation are helpful in distinguishing triphasic waves from NCSE (Boulanger *et al.* 2006). Patients suspected to have NCSE may require cEEG.

Management

Urgent evaluation is necessary because of the risk of rebleeding. Measures to stabilize the patient include intubation and ventilation, analgesia, and transfer to an intensive care unit. The calcium channel blocker nimodipine reduces secondary ischemia and cerebral infarction, and improves outcome after SAH. Aneurysms are treated by clipping or endovascular coiling, the latter the desired method for basilar artery aneurysms. Sound evidence on the timing of surgery is lacking; however, early aneurysm ablation is the policy in most centers (de Gans *et al.* 2002). Avoidance of hypovolemia, hypotension, and hyponatremia help minimize neurological and systemic complications

Retrospective studies of small numbers of patients conclude that the routine use of prophylactic anticonvulsants is of no benefit after clipping or coil embolization (Byrne *et al.* 2004).

References

Annegers JF, Hauser WA, Coan SP, Rocca WA (1998) A population-based study of seizures after traumatic brain injuries. *N Engl J Med* **338**:20–4.

Bladin CF, Alexandrov AV, Bellavance A, et al. (2000) Seizures after stroke: a prospective multicenter study. *Arch Neurol* **57**:1617–22.

Boulanger J-M, Deacon C, Lecuyer D, Gosselin S, Reiher J (2006) Triphasic waves versus nonconvulsive status epilepticus: EEG distinction. *Can J Neurol Sci* **33**:175–80.

Broderick J, Connolly S, Feldman E, et al. (2007) American Heart Association/ American Stroke Association Stroke Council, High Blood Pressure Council, and the Quality Care Outcomes in Research Interdisciplinary Working Group. Guidelines for the management of spontaneous intracerebral hemorrhage in adults: 2007 update. *Circulation* **116**:e391–e413.

Brouwers PJ, Dippel DW, Vermeulen M, et al. (1993) Amount of blood on computed tomography as an independent predictor after aneurysm rupture. *Stroke* **24**:809–14.

Burn J, Dennis M, Bamford J, et al. (1997) Epileptic seizures after a first stroke: the Oxfordshire community stroke project. *Br Med J* **315**:1582–7.

Byrne JV, Boardman P, Ioannidis I, Adcock J, Traill Z (2004) Seizures after aneurysmal subarachnoid hemorrhage treated with coil embolization. *Neurosurgery* **52**:542–52.

Claassen DO, Kazemi N, Zubkov AY, Wijdicks EFM, Rabinstein AA (2008) Restarting anticoagulation therapy after warfarin-associated intracerebral hemorrhage. *Arch Neurol* **65**:1313–18.

Claassen J, Jette N, Chum F, et al. (2007) Electrographic seizures and periodic discharges after intracererbal hemorrhage. *Neurology* **69**:1356–65.

Counsell C, Boonyakarnkul S, Dennis M, et al. (1995) Primary intracerebral hemorrhage in the Oxfordshire Community Stroke Project. II. Prognosis. *Cerebrovasc Dis* **5**:26–34.

D'Alessandro R, Tinuper P, Ferrara R, et al. (1982) CT scan prediction of post-traumatic epilepsy. *J Neurol Neurosurg Psychiatry* **45**:1153–5.

De Gans K, Nieuwkamp D, Rinkel GJE, Algra A (2002) Timing of aneurysm surgery in subarachnoid hemorrhage: a systematic review of the literature *Neurosurgery* **50**:336–42.

De Rueck J, Hemelsoet D, Van Maele G (2007) Seizures and epilepsy in patients with a spontaneous intracerebral hematoma. *Clin Neurol Neurosurg* **109**:501–4.

Dinsdale HB (1964) Spontaneous hemorrhage in the posterior fossa: a study of primary pontine and cerebellar hemorrhage with observations on the pathogenesis *Arch Neurol* **10**:200–17.

Englander T, Bushnik T, Duong TT, et al. (2003) Analyzing risk factors for late posttraumatic seizure. *Arch Phys Med Rehab* **84**:365–73.

Fiebach JB, Schellinger PD, Gass A, et al. (2004) Stroke magnetic resonance imaging is accurate in hyperacute intracerebral hemorrhage. *Stroke* **35**:502–6.

Fogelholm R, Murros K, Rissanen A, Avikainen S (2005) Admission blood glucose level and short term survival in primary intracerebral hemorrhage: a population based study. *J Neurol Neurosurg Psychiatry* **76**:349–53.

Grotta JC, Burgin WS, El-Mitwalli A, et al. (2001) Intravenous tissue-type plasminogen activator therapy for ischemic stroke: houston experience 1996 to 2000. *Arch Neurol* **58**:2009–13.

Hauser A, Annegers JF, Rocca WA (1996) Descriptive epidemiology of epilepsy: contributions of population-based studies from Rochester, Minnesota. *Mayo Clin Proc* **71**:576–86.

Hemphill JC, Bonovich DC, Besmertis L, Manley GT, Johnston SC (2001) The ICH score: a simple, reliable grading scale for intracerebral hemorrhage *Stroke* **32**:891–7.

Ingall TJ, Whisnant JP, Wiebers DO, O'Fallon WM (1989) Has there been a decline in subarachnoid hemorrhage mortality? *Stroke* **20**:718–24.

Jennett B, van de Sande J (1975) EEG prediction of post-traumatic surgery. *Epilepsia* **16**:251–6.

Kammersgaard LP, Olsen TS (2005) Poststroke epilepsy in the Copenhagen stroke study: incidence and predictors. *J Stroke Cerebrovasc Dis* **14**:210–14.

Kassell NF, Torner JC, Haley EC Jr., et al. (1990) The International Cooperative Study on the timing of aneurysmal surgery. I. Overall management and results. *J Neurosurg* **73**:18–36.

Mayberg MR, Batjer HH, Dacey R, et al. (1994) Guidelines for the management of aneurysmal subarachnoid hemorrhage: a statement for healthcare professionals from a special writing group of the Stroke

Council, American Heart Association. *Circulation* **90**:2592–605.

Mendelow AD, Gregson BA, Fernandes HM, *et al.* (2005) Early surgery versus initial conservative treatment in patients with spontaneous supratentorial intracerebral hematomas in the International Surgical Trial in Intracerebral Hemorrhage (STICH): a randomized trial. *Lancet* **365**:387–97.

Myint PK, Staufenberg EFA, Sabanathan K (2006) Post-stroke seizure and post-stroke epilepsy. *Postgrad Med J* **82**:568–72.

National Institute for Clinical Excellence (2004) *The Epilepsies: The Diagnosis and Management of the Epilepsies in Adults and Children in Primary and Secondary Care.* London: NICE.

Olafsson E, Gudmundsson G, Hauser WA (2000) Risk of epilepsy in long-term survivors of surgery for aneurysmal subarachnoid hemorrhage: a population-based study in Iceland. *Epilepsia* **41**:1201–5.

Rosand J, Hylek EM, O'Donnell HC, Greenberg SM (2000) Warfarin-associated hemorrhage and cerebral amyloid angiopathy: a genetic and pathologic study. *Neurology* **55**:947–51.

Ross Russell RW (1963) Observations on intracerebral aneurysms. *Brain* **86**:425–42.

Rumbach L, Sablot D, Berger E, *et al.* (2000) Status epilepticus in stroke. *Neurology* **54**:350–3.

Ryvlin P, Montavant A, Noghoghossian N (2006) Optimizing therapy of seizures in stroke patients. *Neurology* **67**:S3–9.

Sabo RA, Hanigan WC, Aldag JC (1995) Chronic subdural hematomas and seizures: the role of prophylactic anticonvulsive medication. *Surg Neurol* **43**:579–82.

Silverman IE, Restrepo L, Mathews GC (2002) Poststroke seizures. *Arch Neurol* **59**:195–201.

Van Loon J, Van Calenbergh F, Goffin J, Plets C (1993) Controversies in the management of spontaneous cerebellar hemorrhage: a consecutive series of 49 cases and review of the literature. *Acta Neurochir (Wien)* **122**:187–93.

Vespa P (2005) Continuous EEG monitoring for the detection of seizures in traumatic brain injury, infarction, and intracerebral hemorrhage: "to detect and protect". *J Clin Neurophysiol* **22**:99–106.

Vespa PM, O'Phelan K, Shah M, *et al.* (2003) Acute seizures after intracerebral hemorrhage: a factor in progressive midline shift and outcome. *Neurology* **60**:1441–6.

Westmoreland BF (2001) Periodic lateralized epileptiform discharges after evacuation of subdural hematomas. *J Clin Neurophysiol* **18**:20–4.

Whisnant JP, Sacco SE, O'Fallon WM, Fode NC, Sundt TM (1993) Referral bias in aneurysmal subarachnoid hemorrhage. *J Neurosurg* **78**:726–32.

Wolfe PA, D'Agostino RB (1998) Epidemiology of stroke. In: Barnett H, Mohr J, Stein B, Yatsu F (eds.) *Stroke: Pathophysiology, Diagnosis and Management.* New York: Churchill Livingstone, pp. 3–28.

Zhang-Nunes SX, Maat-Scheiman ML, van Duinen SG, *et al.* (2006) The cerebral beta-amyloid angiopathies: hereditary and sporadic. *Brain Pathol* **16**:30–9.

Chapter 77

Cerebral infarction and occult degenerative cerebrovascular disease

Ruth E. Nemire and R. Eugene Ramsay

Introduction

Stroke is among the most frequent causes of death and disability worldwide. Evidence for the relationship between cerebrovascular disease and epilepsy is based on data from studies that ask the questions: what are the risks for developing epilepsy; what diagnostic tests might be used; and what treatments are appropriate? There are few studies, they have different methodologies and patient numbers, and they are often based on retrospective chart reviews and case histories. Based on the neurobiology and pathophysiology of cerebrovascular disease, little evidence exists to support the use of any particular one of the currently available antiepileptic medications when stroke is the cause of seizures; however, in specific populations there may be good reasons to use one drug rather than another because of issues of patient tolerance or the absence of adverse impacts on comorbid diseases. The best approach is prevention, and, in lieu of that, design of future treatments should be aimed at reducing cell death and the cascade of events which may lead to development of epilepsy.

Cerebrovascular disease

The World Health Organization (2004, 2009a, b) defines cerebrovascular disease (stroke) as an interruption of blood supply by hemorrhage or clot which causes a reduction in oxygen and nutrient supply resulting in damage to the brain. Risk factors include age, hypertension, and hypercholesterolemia. Hematologic disorders such as sickle-cell disease and coagulopathies also put patients at risk for stroke (Gordon 2008). About 10% of children with sickle-cell disease have at least one stroke. (American Stroke Association 2009) Males (adult and children) are reported to have a higher occurrence of stroke than women. (Hart and Kantor 1990; Gordon 2008; World Health Organization 2009a).

Stroke is a leading cause of death and disability across the globe. The prevalence of stroke is estimated to be approximately 5–10 per 1000 persons. Worldwide, stroke is the second highest cause of death after cardiovascular disease. The World Health Organization (2009a) estimates that approximately 5.5 million persons die annually from stroke worldwide, accounting for approximately 10% of all deaths. People living in low- and middle-income countries account for more than 85% of those dying from stroke. Stroke is one of the top 10 causes of death in children (Pappachan and Kirkham 2008). The incidence of stroke in the pediatric population is estimated to be 2–8 cases per 100 000 children per year in North America (Chung and Wong 2004; Bernard and Goldenberg 2008). The population of people over 70 years of age account for two-thirds of those affected. Stroke is the leading cause of disability in adults. More than 50% of patients who have a stroke will be left with some type of impairment (World Health Organization 2004).

Brief overview of cerebrovascular (stroke) pathophysiology

The initiating event for ischemic stroke is one of three pathophysiologic occurrences resulting in the interruption of oxygen and glucose delivery to brain cells (Smith Wade *et al.* 2006) (Fig. 77.1):

- occlusion of a vessel by an embolus that develops at a distant site
- thrombosis of an intracranial vessel
- hypoperfusion of intracranial or extracranial arteries causing limited blood flow (Osuga *et al.* 2000; Rashidian *et al.* 2005; Rami *et al.* 2008; Wang *et al.* 2009).

Patients with hypercoagulable disorders are at risk for thrombosis leading to ischemic stroke and the risk may be unknown until the first presentation (Hart and Kantor 1990; Smith Wade *et al.* 2006) (Table 77.1).

Once one of these initial events occurs, a cascade of actions occurs along two major pathways: the first pathway leads to cell death owing to the energy failure of the cell; the second pathway consists of apoptosis or programmed cell death. Cell death can occur within 4 min if a total lack of oxygen exists

The Causes of Epilepsy, eds. S. D. Shorvon, F. Andermann, and R. Guerrini. Published by Cambridge University Press. © Cambridge University Press 2011.

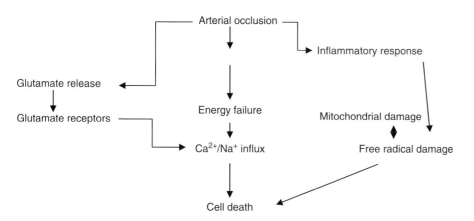

Fig. 77.1. Probable events leading to cell death. (Adapted from: Smith Wade *et al.* [2006].)

Table 77.1 Cerebrovascular and primary hematologic pathophysiology of disease

Etiology	Pathophysiology
Cerebrovascular	Ischemic
	Hypoperfusion
	Embolic
	Thrombolic
Hematologic	Elevated concentrations of coagulation factors
	Factor V
	Factor VIII
	Reduced concentration or function of anticoagulant factors
	Protein S
	Protein C
	Erythrocyte disorders
	Sickle-cell disease
	Thrombotic angiopathies
Homocysteinemia	Thrombocytopenia
	Hemolytic uremic syndrome

and there is no collateral blood flow to the area of the infarction. Cell death occurs when cells are deprived of glucose and mitochondrial cells cannot produce ATP or energy. This causes depolarization of neurons and a rise in intracellular calcium. Glutamate is also released upon depolarization and causes a rise in neuronal calcium influx. Free radicals are formed and released, causing general destruction and cell death (Wilmore and Rubin 1981; Osuga *et al.* 2000; Rashidian *et al.* 2005; Hailer 2008; Rami *et al.* 2008; Wang *et al.* 2009).

Clinical features of cerebrovascular disease

Stroke is a major international public health problem, despite the fact that much of the cause is recognizable and preventable.

The incidence, prevalence, and high financial impact make cerebrovascular disease a matter of public health concern for developed as well as underdeveloped populations (World Health Organization 2009a). Risk factors are divided into those that are preventable risks and those that are not. Preventable risks include obesity, smoking, alcoholism, lack of exercise, hypertension, and hypercholesterolemia. Those risks that are not preventable include heredity, ethnicity, male sex, and increasing age. Education and support for the reduction of risk factors among the public is at the forefront of reducing the morbidity and high cost of stroke.

Presenting symptoms in both adult and pediatric populations may not immediately be recognized by patients or providers until progression and/or diagnostic testing by a physician to rule out other disease. Presenting symptoms in adults may include any of the following depending on affected area and size of the ensuing area of damage: visual disturbance, hemiparesis, dysarthria, persistent numbness and mild sensory loss, weakness, and incoordination or epilepsy. The exception is cortical stroke which may occur without presenting clinical symptoms (Ramsay *et al.* 2004).

The vascular and nervous system in neonates, infants, and children is different from adults and clinical presentation are often not the same (Pappachan and Kirkham 2008). Presenting symptoms in children may include nausea, vomiting, headache, and seizures instead of, or in addition to, those described for adults.

Epilepsy and cerebrovascular disease

Risk factors for epilepsy and what are the features of the disease that influence epilepsy?

The prevalence of epilepsy worldwide is estimated at 0.4–1%, with the numbers reported from studies in developing countries slightly higher at 0.6–1% (World Health Organization 2009a). Wright *et al.* (2000) observed a 4.5 in 1000 prevalence rate of epilepsy in the United Kingdom which is similar to worldwide data. North American data on incidence and prevalence is reported to be similar to that estimated worldwide for developed countries. (Theodore *et al.* 2006).

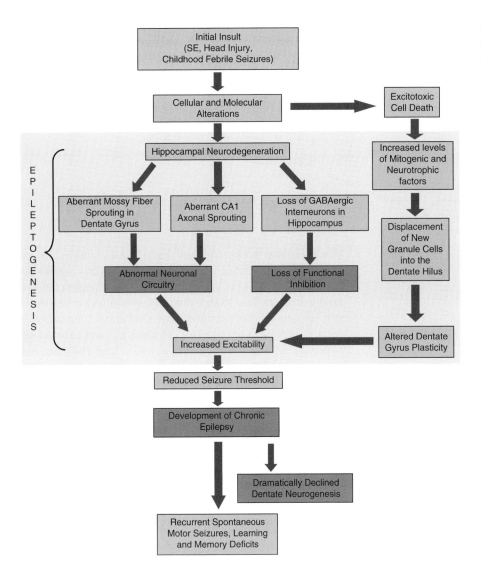

Fig. 77.2. Potential mechanisms leading to the development of seizures. (Reprinted with permission from Acharya et al. [2008].)

The number of patients and the relative risk for those who will proceed clinically to develop post-stroke epilepsy (PSE) is difficult to establish, particularly since seizures may be secondary to a subclinical cortical stroke. The incidence of PSE is reported to be as great as 50% within 5 years from the initial event (Burn et al. 1997). Lack of homogeneity in methodology limits the understanding of the actual prevalence of PSE. Studies are most often retrospective, and the history, diagnosis, and the classification of epilepsy is often not noted. Despite the lack of homogeneity and methodological approach, stroke and brain injuries or trauma in adults are found high on the list among common causes of seizures (Granieri et al. 1983; Bladin et al. 2000; Silverman et al. 2002; Lossius et al. 2005; Szaflarski et al. 2008). Underlying genetic hematologic disorders (Smith Wade et al. 2006) (Table 77.1), such as sickle-cell disease, or coagulopathies that cause thrombosis or hypoperfusion may lead to stroke and finally epilepsy (Prengler et al. 2005). Among the pediatric population those with sickle-cell disease and recurrent stroke are at risk of developing epilepsy (Wright et al. 2000; Prengler et al. 2005; Matta et al. 2006; Gordon 2008).

The mechanisms that cause cerebrovascular disease to lead to seizures or the development of epilepsy are not well defined by animal models or clinical research. Animal studies indicate various mechanisms (Acharya et al. 2008) (Fig. 77.2), including cell injury, programmed cell death, inflammation, and immune responses (Acharya et al. 2008; Hailer 2008; Wang et al. 2009). In animal models of epilepsy, pretreatment with antioxidants significantly reduces the development of epileptiform activity (Wilmore and Rubin 1981).

The Seizures After Stroke Study (SASS) is one of the few prospective, multicenter trials conducted to determine the risk and frequency of seizures after stroke, mortality, neurological and functional outcome, and the relationship to underlying cerebral pathologic lesions (Bladin et al. 2000; Silverman et al. 2002). A total of 1897 patients were enrolled. Seizures occurred in 8.9% of patients (ischemic and hemorrhagic). Post-stroke epilepsy developed in 2.5% of patients overall.

Observations by others provide a glimpse into the relationship between cerebrovascular disease and PSE in diverse populations. In a retrospective study, Lossius and colleagues (2005) investigated patients diagnosed with PSE to identify predictors and outcome of treatment in a stroke unit. They estimated a 3% prevalence of PSE. In a study by Wright and colleagues (2000) an underlying etiology was identified in 29% of patients presenting with seizures or epilepsy. Cerebrovascular disease and head injuries were among the most common causes of PSE (Wright *et al.* 2000). In a community-based epidemiologic study of a population in northern Italy, perinatal brain injuries were found to be the most frequent event causing seizures (Granieri *et al.* 1983). In a study of Tanzanian communities, Matuja (1989) found that in adults the onset of seizures or epilepsy was due to head injury or cerebrovascular disease in 74% of the cases.

Types of epilepsy and other characteristics

Authors of multiple studies (So *et al.* 1996; Bladin *et al.* 2000; De Reuck *et al.* 2005; Lossius *et al.* 2005; Menon and Shorvon 2009) offer various views and provide conflicting evidence of the significance of the anatomic location of the stroke, the severity of patient neurological scores, and incidence of early or late seizures, on the patient risk for development of PSE. DeReuck and colleagues (2005) retrospectively reviewed records for 110 patients with either a single seizure or epilepsy and added 367 patients admitted to the hospital from the years 2000 to 2002, with stroke as a matched control group. A diagnosis of anterior circulation stroke was the most common among all patients with or without seizures. This group of patients with anterior circulation stroke represented the group with the most potential to develop seizures among all patients. The severity of neurological deficit was similar across groups and it did not make a difference whether the patient developed late-onset seizures. The results of this retrospective review indicate that anterior circulation stroke was the only risk factor for seizure development among those patients with cerebrovascular disease (De Reuck *et al.* 2005). Alternatively, the outcome of the Akershus Stroke Study completed by Lossius and colleagues (2005), did not identify a specific location as an indicator for the development of PSE. Lossius found patients with a Scandanavian Stroke Scale score of less than 30 to be at risk. In another population-based study to identify seizures in Rochester, Minnesota, researchers defined early seizures as those occurring within the first week after stroke. Thirty-five patients (6%) developed early seizures. The type of stroke and location in these 35 patients tended to be embolic and anterior. The percentage of patients with an anterior hemisphere stroke that developed PSE approached 90% by year 5 (So *et al.* 1996). The outcome of the SASS trial (Bladin *et al.* 2000) indicates that 40% of seizures occurred within the first 24 hr after ischemic stroke. Five percent of patients had an early seizure and 4% had a late-onset seizure defined as more than 2 weeks after the event. Post-stroke epilepsy developed in half of the patients with late-onset seizures. Patients with seizures had worse neurological scores during the hospital stay (Bladin *et al.* 2000).

Diagnostic tests: electroencephalogram and imaging

Electroencephalogram (EEG) and imaging studies are standard diagnostic tools for both cerebrovascular disease and epilepsy. Exponential advances in medical technology have changed how physicians review the findings, and what abnormalities can be detected since the earliest PSE studies were conducted. However, clinical decisions in patient care and treatment are based on judgment and experience because imaging tests often do not yield information that changes decisions or improves outcome (Yu *et al.* 2009). There are few observations and no conclusive evidence regarding the use of diagnostic testing – either EEG or imaging – to predict whether a patient will develop seizures (Shorvon *et al.* 1984; Gupta *et al.* 1988). In a retrospective review of 90 patients with PSE, there were 61 EEGs and computed tomography (CT) scans completed. Focal slowing was the most common EEG abnormality and was present in 60% of cases (Gupta *et al.* 1988). Patients with a CT scan indicating a larger infarction were reported to have a larger number of seizures than those patients with a smaller area of damage. In another study looking at the utility of CT in patients with late-onset epilepsy, 74 patients were compared with age-matched controls for evidence of cerebrovascular disease. Patients with epilepsy had an excess of ischemic lesions, and low attenuation of the periventricular white matter. These changes were present in 13 of the patients with epilepsy and only two of the control group. In six of the 13 cases a clinical examination was normal (Shorvon *et al.* 1984). Ramsay and colleagues (2004) looked at a population of veterans ($n = 594$) to determine prospectively what treatments were most efficacious, given the special needs of the elderly population. A subset of patients ($n = 23$) were reviewed after initial EEG. Fourteen patients exhibited abnormal slowing, and nine had a normal EEG. Extended EEG recordings were then completed and 12 of the patients had epileptiform activity noted when the routine EEG was not diagnostic. The diagnosis of epilepsy was confirmed in these patients based on 24-hr monitoring.

Special populations

Late-onset epilepsies: risk of stroke

Stroke may follow late-onset epilepsy. Cleary and colleagues (2004) collected retrospective data on 4709 individuals 60 years and older with new-onset seizures and an equal number without a history of seizures matched for age, sex, and lifestyle. The relative hazard of stroke at any point for people developing late-onset seizures compared with the control group was 2.89 (95% confidence interval [CI] 2.45–3.41). The occurrence of late-onset epilepsy was a stronger predictor of stroke than either smoking or high cholesterol.

Patient population over 55 years of age

There is consensus that the incidence and prevalence of stroke and epilepsy increases with age (Lesser *et al.* 1985; Fish *et al.*

1989; Hauser *et al.* 1993; Schreiner *et al.* 1995; Annegers *et al.* 1996; So *et al.* 1996; Li *et al.* 1997; Wright *et al.* 2000; Timmons *et al.* 2002; Cleary *et al.* 2004; World Health Organization 2009c, 46). The studies specific to determining the epidemiology of epilepsy associated with stroke in the older population bear the same methodological problems as those completed in the general population, in addition to limited numbers. Li and colleagues (1997) investigated the relationship between what they considered vascular determinants of epilepsy in an older population. Their data are part of the Rotterdam study which was designed to investigate the risk factors for chronic disease in the elderly. Patients were screened to determine a diagnosis of epilepsy and to determine the type of seizure. Sixty-five out of 4944 subjects over age 55 had a diagnosis of epilepsy. The outcome of the study confirmed an association of epilepsy and vascular factors of stroke or myocardial infarction, peripheral vascular disease, hypertension, serum total cholesterol, and left ventricular hypertrophy. The number of patients studied by Shreiner and colleagues (1995) is small but the outcome may provide guidance for future studies to determine risks for developing PSE. A total of 18 patients with subcortical vascular encephalopathy (SVE) were followed prospectively after their first hospital admission for a seizure and compared to a group matched for sex, age, risk factors, and neurological deficits and SVE without epilepsy. The group which developed epilepsy ($n = 10$) had a statistically higher rate of lacunar infarctions in subcortical white matter when compared to the group without. In 10 patients with epilepsy, a constant theta or delta EEG focus was present on EEG but only present in one of the patients without epilepsy ($p < 0.005$). The authors conclude that "the association of SVE, multiple subcortical lacunas and temporal EEG abnormalities are suggestive for an increased risk for epileptic seizures" (Schreiner *et al.* 1995). In a study of 130 cases of patients over age 50 (average age 65 years) diagnosed with epilepsy, the most common type of seizure was partial (66%) followed by secondary generalized tonic–clonic (34%). In this cohort of cases epilepsy was determined to have been caused by cerebrovascular disease 50% of the time and more often in patients who were over 74 years of age (Paradowski and Zagrajek 2005). Timmons and colleagues (2002) retrospectively reviewed the charts of patients 65 years or older with a diagnosis of epilepsy to determine the underlying etiology of the seizures, prescribing practices, and long-term follow up. Sixty-eight cases are included in the review and subsequent analysis. Five of the patients presented in status epilepticus as the first seizure. Approximately 40% of the patients with seizures ($n = 28$) presented clinically with partial seizures. Approximately half of those patients presenting with partial seizures had an EEG performed. The rest of the patients presented with seizures that were generalized or described as absence. Approximately 40% of this group had an EEG completed. In addition to the stroke, patients were identified who were taking medications known to lower seizure threshold (20%) and 2% of patients had been withdrawn from benzodiazepines within days prior to the event. Approximately 13% of

patients had a metabolic disturbance that could provoke seizures. Finally, at least 9% were reported to have recently imbibed in too much alcohol intake. Forty-one percent of the total number of patients had a diagnosis of hypertension and 40% had been diagnosed with ischemic heart disease. Seizures in the patient with stroke, while categorized as complex partial, may not present with the same features as those of a younger individual (Ramsay *et al.* 2004). The older patient may present with signs and symptoms subsequently diagnosed by the primary care physician as altered mental status, confusion, or loss of memory rather than a seizure. In the Veterans Administration Cooperative #428 trial 25% of patients who were diagnosed with epilepsy were not even considered to have had seizures by primary care physicians or internists (Ramsay *et al.* 2004).

Patient population under 18 years of age

There is a paucity of large or prospective studies in pediatric patients to determine the incidence or prevalence of seizures or epilepsy following stroke, largely because of the low incidence. However, in two studies with relatively small numbers the association with epilepsy and pediatric stroke was clear. In a study of 76 pediatric patients with sickle-cell disease Prengler and colleagues (2005) "collected data on the prevalence of cerebral vasculopathy in patients with sickle-cell disease with and without seizures and of magnetic resonance (MR) perfusion abnormality in those with recent seizures ($n = 6$)." All six patients with epilepsy exhibited decreased cerebral perfusion on magnetic resonance imaging (MRI) and four of the six had abnormal angiography and abnormal transcranial Doppler. Five of the patients had an abnormal EEG. In a retrospective review of children admitted under the Hospital Authority in Hong Kong, Chung and Wong (2004) determined that the prevalence of stroke was slightly lower than reported in other countries at two cases per 100 000 children–years. There was no sickle-cell disease or thrombophilia reported in this population. The long-term neurologic deficits reported include development delay, epilepsy, and hemiplegia (Chung and Wong 2004). Matta *et al.* (2006) describe a series of pediatric cases with cerebrovascular disorders. Twenty-three patients were identified with a diagnosis of stroke sequelae. The most frequent etiology was heart disease and sickle-cell anemia. Nine of these patients experienced seizures.

Principles of management

A prospective chart review to assess the incidence, etiology, medication use, and quality of life in patients who had their first seizure after 50 was completed by Ruggles and colleagues (2001). All patients in the Marshfield Epidemiology Study Area (MESA) of the United States between July 1996 and June 1998 who were over 50 and had a first seizure were identified by the diagnostic coding system records. There were 48 patients identified. Vascular etiology accounted for seizures in 21 patients (44%). Twelve patients were diagnosed with epilepsy. In the first year of monitoring another six patients experienced a second seizure and were diagnosed with epilepsy. Patients were treated with phenytoin, carbamazepine, or valproate and 75% of patients were reported to have seizures controlled, although that is not defined by the authors as seizure-free. One-fourth of the patients reported adverse events (Ruggles *et al.* 2001).

The VA Coop #428 trial (Rowan *et al.* 2005) involved 18 study centers and researchers enrolled 593 patients. The purpose of the study was to determine efficacy and long-term tolerability of one of three antiepileptic medications: carbamazepine, gabapentin, or lamotrigine. The most common etiology for seizures was stroke in 50% of patients; however, an additional 30% had significant vascular disease risk factors (e.g., hypertension, hypercholesterolemia, and/or diabetes). Patients taking lamotrigine tolerated the drug better than either carbamazepine or gabapentin. The seizure-free rate for patients achieving 12 months' participation in the study was 53%, with lamotrigine eliciting the highest seizure-free rate. Twenty percent of patients withdrew from the study prior to 12 months owing to adverse events.

Summary

Stroke is a killer and causes long-term disability. It is among the most frequent causes of death in adults and children across the globe. Prevention and reduction of risk behaviors will improve the prevalence and the incidence. However, not all stroke is preventable, nor will all patients do what is necessary to reduce their risk, even with improved health literacy and wellness incentives. Thus, PSE will continue to be a focus for research, and necessitate advances in treatment for the practitioner.

Case reports, retrospective chart reviews, and a few prospective trials are reported by researchers around the world. The problem with these multiple studies and case reports is that they use varying methodologies, the number of patients is often small, technology has improved for diagnosis, and different outcomes are measured. It does seem apparent, despite the weakness of the research, that as patients age their risk for stroke and resultant seizures increases due to vascular disease. Patients both adult and pediatric with hematologic disorders that cause thrombosis or hypoperfusion are also at risk for stroke and resultant seizures. There are three important issues that continue to be unclear relating to cerebrovascular causes of epilepsy which impact current and future trends for treatment, and potential for outcome. These issues include the need for further definition of the mechanisms for vascular damage during and after stroke that lead to seizures and epilepsy, determination of the risk of epilepsy with early or late seizures, and best treatment options for PSE.

References

Acharya MM, Hattiangady B, Shetty AK (2008) Progress in neuroprotective strategies for preventing epilepsy. *Prog Neurobiol* **84**:363–404.

American Stroke Association (2009) *Pediatric Stroke.* Available online at www.strokeassociation.org/presenter.jhtml?identifier=3030392

Annegers JF, Rocca WA, Hauser WA (1996) Causes of epilepsy: contributions of the Rochester epidemiology project. *Mayo Clin Proc* **71**:570–5.

Bernard TJ, Goldenberg NA (2008) Pediatric arterial ischemic stroke. *Pediatr Clin N Am* **55**:323–38.

Bladin C, Alexandrov A, Bellavance A, *et al.* (2000) Seizures after stroke: a prospective multicenter study. *Arch Neurol* **57**:1617–22.

Boggs JB (2001) Elderly patients with systemic disease. *Epilepsia* **42**(suppl 8):18–23.

Burn J, Dennis M, Bamford J, *et al.* (1997) Epileptic seizures after a first stroke: the Oxfordshire community stroke project. *Br Med J* **315**:1582–7.

Chung B, Wong V (2004) Pediatric stroke among Hong Kong Chinese subjects. *Pediatrics* **114**:e206–12.

Cleary P, Shorvon S, Tallis R (2004) Late onset seizures as a predictor of subsequent stroke. *Lancet* **363**:1184–6.

De Reuck J, Goethals M, Vonck K, Van Maele G (2005) Clinical predictors of late-onset seizures and epilepsy in patients with cerebrovascular disease. *Eur Neurol* **54**:68–72.

Fish DR, Miller DH, Roberts RC, Blackie JD, Gilliatt RW (1989) The natural history of late-onset epilepsy secondary to vascular disease. *Acta Neurol Scand* **80**:524–6.

Gordon N (2008) Childhood strokes. *J Pediatr Neurol* **6**:197–201.

Granieri E, Rosati G, Tola R, *et al.* (1983) A descriptive study of epilepsy in the district of Copparo, Italy, 1964–1978. *Epilepsia* **24**:502–14.

Gupta SR, Naheedy MH, Elias D, Rubino FA (1988) Postinfarction seizures: a clinical study. *Stroke* **19**:1477–81.

Hailer NP (2008) Immunosuppression after traumatic or ischemic CNS damage: it is neuroprotective and illuminates the role of microglial cells. *Prog Neurobiol* **84**:211–33.

Hart RG, Kantor MC (1990) Hematologic disorders and ischemic stroke: a selective review. *Stroke* **21**:1111–21.

Hauser WA, Annegers JF, Kurland LT (1993) Incidence of epilepsy and unprovoked seizures in Rochester, Minnesota: 1935–1984. *Epilepsia* **34**:453–68.

Lesser RP, Lüders H, Dinner DS, Morris HH (1985) Epileptic seizures due to thrombotic and embolic cerebrovascular disease in older patients. *Epilepsia* **6**:622–30.

Li X, Breteler MM, de Bruyne MC, *et al.* (1997) Vascular determinants of epilepsy: the Rotterdam Study. *Epilepsia* **38**:1216–20.

Lossius MI, Rønning OM, Slapø GD, Mowinckel P, Gjerstad L (2005) Poststroke epilepsy: occurrence and predictors – a long-term prospective controlled study (Akershus Stroke Study). *Epilepsia* **46**:1246–51.

Matta AP, Galvão KR, Oliveira BS (2006) Cerebrovascular disorders in childhood: etiology, clinical presentation, and neuroimaging findings in a case series study. *Arq Neuropsiquiatr* **64**(2A):181–5.

Matuja WB (1989) Aetiological factors in Tanzanian epileptics. *E Afr Med J* **66**:343–8.

Menon B, Shorvon SD (2009) Ischaemic stroke in adults and epilepsy. *Epilepsy Res* doi:10.1016/j.eplepsyres.2009.08.007.

Osuga H, Osuga S, Wang F, *et al.* (2000) Cyclin-dependent kinases as a therapeutic target for stroke. *Proc Natl Acad Sci USA* **97**:10 254–9.

Pappachan J, Kirkham FJ (2008) Cerebrovascular disease and stroke. *Arch Dis Childh* **93**:890–8.

Paradowski B, Zagrajek MM (2005) Epilepsy in middle-aged and elderly people: a three-year observation. *Epileptic Disord* **7**:91–5.

Prengler M, Pavlakis SG, Boyd S, *et al.* (2005) Sickle cell disease: ischemia and seizures. *Ann Neurol* **58**:290–302.

Rami A, Bechmann I, Stehle JH (2008) Exploiting endogenous anti-apoptotic proteins for novel therapeutic strategies in cerebral ischemia. *Prog Neurobiol* **85**:273–96.

Ramsay RE, Rowan AJ, Pryor FM (2004) Special considerations in treating the elderly patient with epilepsy. *Neurology* **62**(Suppl 2):S24–9.

Rashidian J, Iyirhiaro G, Aleyasin H, *et al.* (2005) Multiple cyclin-dependent kinases signals are critical mediators of ischemia/hypoxic neuronal death in vitro and in vivo. *Proc Natl Acad Sci USA* **102**:14 080–5.

Ribacoba-Montero R, Pujols-Castillo Y, Vallina-García MI, *et al.* (2007) Clinical epidemiological study of vascular epilepsy. *Rev Neurol* **45**:719–24.

Rowan AJ, Ramsay RE, Collins JF, *et al.* (2005) New onset geriatric epilepsy: a randomized study of gabapentin, lamotrigine, and carbamazepine. *Neurology* **64**:1868–73.

Ruggles KH, Haessly SM, Berg RL (2001) Prospective study of seizures in the elderly in the Marshfield Epidemiologic Study Area (MESA). *Epilepsia* **42**:1594–9.

Schreiner A, Pohlmann-Eden B, Schwartz A, Hennerici M (1995) Epileptic seizures in subcortical vascular encephalopathy. *J Neurol Sci* **130**:171–7.

Shorvon SD, Gilliatt RW, Cox TC, Yu YL (1984) Evidence of vascular disease from CT scanning in late onset epilepsy. *J Neurol Neurosurg Psychiatry* **47**:225–30.

Silverman IE, Restrepo L, Mathews GC (2002) Poststroke seizures. (Review). *Arch Neurol* **59**:195–201.

Smith Wade S, English JD, Johnston SC (2006) Cerebrovascular diseases. In: Fauci AS, Braunwald E, Kasper DL, *et al.* (eds.) *Harrison's Manual of Medicine*, 17th edn. New York: McGraw-Hill, pp. 79–87.

So EL, Anneger JF, Hauser WA, O'Brien PC, Whisnant JP (1996) Population-based study of seizure disorders after cerebral infarction. *Neurology* **46**:350–5.

Szaflarski JP, Rackley AY, Kleindorfer DO, *et al.* (2008) Incidence of seizures in the acute phase of stroke: a population-based study. *Epilepsia* **49**:974–81.

Theodore WH, Spencer SS, Wiebe S, *et al.* (2006) Epilepsy in North America: a report prepared under the auspices of the Global Campaign against Epilepsy, the International Bureau for Epilepsy, the International League Against Epilepsy, and the World Health Organization. *Epilepsia* **47**:1700–22.

Timmons S, Sweeney B, Hyland M, O'Mahony D, Twomey C (2002) New onset seizures in the elderly: etiology and prognosis. *Ir Med J* **95**:47–9.

Wang W, Bu B, Xie M, *et al.* (2009) Neural cell cycle dysregulation and central nervous system diseases. *Prog Neurobiol* **89**:1–17.

Wilmore LJ, Rubin JJ (1981) Antiperoxidnat treatment and iron-induced epileptiform discharges in the rat: EEG and histopathologic studies. *Neurology* **31**:63–9.

World Health Organization (2004) *Neurology Atlas*. Available online at www.who.int/mental_health/neurology/neurogy_atlas_review_references.pdf

World Health Organization (2009a) *Stroke: Cerebrovascular Accident*. Available online at www.who.int/topics/cerebrovascular_accident/en/

World Health Organization (2009b) STEPwise approach to surveillance. Available online at www.who.int/chp/steps/en/

World Health Organization (2009c) *Epilepsy*. Available online at www.who.int/topics/epilepsy/en/

Wright J, Pickard N, Whitfield A, Hakin N (2000) A population-based study of the prevalence, clinical characteristics and effect of ethnicity in epilepsy. *Seizure* **9**:309–13.

Yu EH, Codrin L, Kanner RM, Libman RB (2009) The use of diagnostic tests in patients with acute ischemic stroke. *J Stroke Cerebrovasc Dis* **18**:178–84.

Chapter

78

Arteriovenous malformations

Suzanne A. Tharin, Autumn Marie Klein, and Robert M. Friedlander

Definition and epidemiology

Arteriovenous malformations (AVMs) are vascular malformations in which one or more high-flow fistulous connections, without intervening capillary beds, exist between arterioles and veins. The AVM nidus comprises a tangle of abnormal fistulous connections, which are often compact, but at times more diffuse. A hallmark of AVMs compared with some other cerebral vascular malformations is the absence of intervening brain parenchyma within the lesion. Some AVMs are associated with feeding artery aneurysms and intranidal aneurysms. Venous drainage from the AVM may be superficial or deep. The weakened vessel walls in AVMs are susceptible to rupture with consequent intracerebral hemorrhage. The overall risk of hemorrhage from AVMs is approximately 3% per year (Friedlander 2007). Deep location, deep venous drainage, previous history of hemorrhage, and presence of aneurysms have been described as high-risk features for hemorrhage (Perret and Nishioka 1966; Stapf et al. 2006).

The prevalence of AVMs in the general population is estimated at 0.01% (0.001–0.52%). They are widely accepted to be congenital, but a recent report by Gonzalez et al. (2005) of a case of de novo AVM (Du et al. 2007), has raised the possibility that AVMs may exist on a spectrum from congenital to acquired, with the majority being congenital. The great majority of AVMs arise in the absence of family history and are not heritable. However, a small proportion of AVMs are seen in patients with Osler–Weber–Rendu syndrome, also known as hereditary hemorrhagic telangiectasia (HHT). Rare families with a preponderance of AVMs in the absence of this syndrome have been reported (Herzig et al. 2000), some in association with RASA1 mutations (Eerola et al. 2003; Revencu et al. 2008).

Pathology, physiology, and clinical features

Arteriovenous malformations are high-flow lesions as there is a direct connection between the arteries and veins without a capillary bed. As a result, pathologic vascular changes occur including arterialization of veins, development of aneurysms of nidal and feeding arteries, and vascular recruitment. Surrounding and intervening brain may also undergo pathologic gliosis.

Secondary pathologies then produce several clinical features of AVMs. Venous outflow restriction or obstruction, aneurysm rupture, and rupture of nidal vessels result in hemorrhage. Cortical pathology, vascular steal, and hemosiderin deposition can result in epilepsy. Mass effect and steal can result in focal neurologic deficits.

Hemorrhage is the most frequent presenting symptom in AVMs. The risk of hemorrhage of an unruptured AVM is approximately 3% per year. Following AVM rupture, the risk of re-rupture increases to approximately 6% during the first year following rupture, then declines back to the baseline 3% per year after 1 year (Friedlander 2007). The consequences of AVM hemorrhage are clinically significant. Hemorrhage in AVM carries a 30–50% risk of permanent neurologic deficit and a 5–10% risk of death. The primary goal of AVM management is to assess the overall risk of the patient, and then develop a management plan that minimizes risks, i.e., deciding whether obliteration or observation is safest. The primary goal of obliterative AVM treatment by any modality is the prevention of hemorrhage.

Seizures are the second most frequent presenting symptom in patients with AVMs. Approximately one-third of patients with symptomatic AVMs present with seizures (Hofmeister et al. 2000; Hoh et al. 2002; Stapf et al. 2003). Other presenting symptoms include headache and focal neurologic deficits.

Epilepsy in the setting of arteriovenous malformations

Risk factors for seizure

In establishing the cause of epilepsy in the presence of an AVM, one must consider the AVM itself, hemorrhage from the AVM, and AVM treatment all as potential causes of

The Causes of Epilepsy, eds. S. D. Shorvon, F. Andermann, and R. Guerrini. Published by Cambridge University Press. © Cambridge University Press 2011.

Table 78.1 Anatomic and clinical characteristics of AVMs associated with a presentation of epilepsy: summary of the literature

Characteristic	Association with epilepsy[a]	Reference
AVM characteristic		
AVM size >3 cm	+	Piepgras *et al.* (1993), Hoh *et al.* (2002)
AVM in "epileptogenic" location[b]	+	Crawford *et al.* (1986), Piepgras *et al.* (1993), Hoh *et al.* (2002)
Middle cerebral artery feeders	+	Turjman *et al.* (1995)
Presence of varices	+	Turjman *et al.* (1995)
Hemorrhage	0	Thorpe *et al.* (2000), Hoh *et al.* (2002)
Deep/posterior fossa location	−	Hoh *et al.* (2002)
Patient characteristic		
Male sex	+	Hoh *et al.* (2002)
Age <65	+	Hoh *et al.* (2002)

Notes:
[a]+, positive association; −, negative association; 0, no association.
[b]Includes temporal lobe, frontal lobe.

epilepsy. The literature is not extensive on these points with only a few studies devoted to the topic of epilepsy and AVMs, all of them retrospective.

Anatomic characteristics of AVMs associated with a presentation of epilepsy include superficial location, location in an "epileptogenic" region (Crawford *et al.* 1986; Piepgras *et al.* 1993), including the temporal lobe (Hoh *et al.* 2002), size greater than 3 cm (Piepgras *et al.* 1993; Hoh *et al.* 2002), middle cerebral artery feeders, and the presence of varices (Turjman *et al.* 1995). Additional clinical characteristics associated with AVMs presenting with epilepsy include age older than 65 and male sex (Crawford *et al.* 1986; Heikkinen *et al.* 1989; Piepgras *et al.* 1993; Turjman *et al.* 1995; Eisenschenk *et al.* 1998; Hoh *et al.* 2002) (Table 78.1).

The epileptogenicity resulting from a hemorrhage and from hemosiderin deposition has been documented (Moriwaki *et al.* 1990). Curiously, AVM hemorrhage has not been found to be associated with a presentation of epilepsy (Thorpe *et al.* 2000; Hoh *et al.* 2002). In fact, in terms of treatment outcome, one study surprisingly found a positive association between hemorrhage-associated pretreatment seizures and favorable seizure outcome following treatment (Hoh *et al.* 2002). Risk factors for seizures (superficial/epileptogenic location, large size, MCA feeders) appear to be distinct from risk factors for hemorrhage (deep location, deep venous drainage, previous history of hemorrhage, and presence of aneurysms).

Treatment of AVMs, with surgery, radiation, embolization, or a combination of these, can cause new seizures in some patients with AVMs, albeit with a risk which is much smaller than the risk of the AVM itself causing seizures. For instance, the risk of AVM surgery causing new seizures is less than 10% in several series (Yeh *et al.* 1990, 1993; Piepgras *et al.* 1993; Dodick *et al.* 1994), comparable to the reported rates of new-onset seizures with embolization (Fournier *et al.* 1991). Radiosurgery appears to carry an even lower risk of new-onset seizures (0–6% in several retrospective series) (Kjellberg *et al.* 1983; Heikkinen *et al.* 1989; Lunsford *et al.* 1991; Steiner *et al.* 1992; Sutcliffe *et al.* 1992; Gerszten *et al.* 1996; Huang *et al.* 1996; Falkson *et al.* 1997; Eisenschenk *et al.* 1998; Kurita *et al.* 1998; Kida *et al.* 2000).

Etiology of seizures

Three pathologic mechanisms have been proposed to explain the epileptogenicity of AVMs: (1) steal phenomenon, whereby arteriovenous shunting in the AVM nidus causes focal ischemia in surrounding cortex, provoking seizures; (2) irritative effect, whereby hemosiderin deposits from subclinical hemorrhage and subsequent gliosis produce a seizure focus surrounding the AVM; and (3) kindling phenomenon, or secondary epileptogenesis, whereby epileptic discharges from a distant ipsi- or contralateral seizure focus are enhanced by excitatory connections to neurons at the AVM (Morrell 1981; Morrell *et al.* 1987; Yeh and Privitera 1991; Yeh *et al.* 1993).

Seizure frequency and characteristics

Partial and complex partial seizures, with and without secondary generalization, as well as generalized tonic–clonic (GTC) seizures have been described in patients with AVMs. Seizure frequency and severity also appear to vary significantly. Not surprisingly, seizure characteristics in AVM appear to have as much to do with the location and size of the AVM as with the inherent nature of the lesion.

Histopathologic case series from the 1960s revealed that although AVMs occur throughout the brain, brainstem, and spinal cord, large AVMs occur more frequently in the territory of the middle cerebral artery (McCormick 1966), and that smaller (<3 cm) AVMs are found more frequently in the frontal and temporal lobes than in the parietal and occipital lobes (McCormick and Nofzinger 1966). Clinical seizures from the frontal lobes classically begin with forced eye deviation away from the side of the seizure focus (Fig. 78.1). Mesial frontal seizures often occur from sleep with odd, at times arrhythmic, movements (e.g., pelvic thrusting, bicycling) with quick generalization and little postictal period. Temporal lobe seizures are typically preceded by a déjà vu, autonomic changes (e.g., heart rate changes), odd smells, staring, lip-smacking, automatisms, and, at times, amnesia for the event. Parietal lobe seizures are usually sensory alterations in the contralateral hemibody and occipital lobe seizures can be characterized by a wide range of unusual contralateral visual changes.

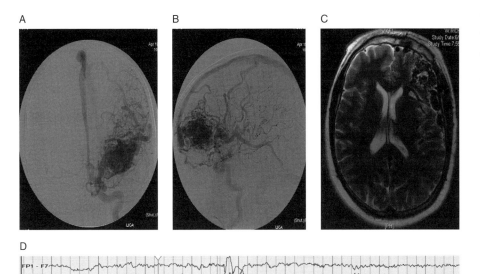

Fig. 78.1. Example of left frontal AVM and EEG showing left frontal discharges. Posteroanterior (A) and lateral (B) views of an angiogram demonstrating left frontal AVM. T2-weighted magnetic resonance (MRi) image from the same patient (C) with left frontal AVM. Electroencephalograph (EEG) tracing (D) showing left frontal spike.

Treatment and prognosis of epilepsy in arteriovenous malformations

The two treatment strategies for epilepsy in AVMs are treatment of the lesion itself and medical management of the seizures. There are no randomized controlled trials comparing seizure outcome in treated and untreated AVMs. While the primary goal of AVM treatment is the prevention of hemorrhage, several retrospective series have also demonstrated a benefit in seizure outcome with AVM treatment with surgery, radiation, embolization, or multimodality treatment (Hoh *et al.* 2002). There are no randomized controlled trials comparing seizure outcome by treatment modality. One retrospective study, however, suggests that if the AVM is completely obliterated, then surgery, radiation, embolization, and multimodality treatment are all equally effective in improving seizure outcome in treated AVM patients who presented with epilepsy (Hoh *et al.* 2002).

Epilepsy may be managed medically in patients with untreated AVMs, as well as pre- and postoperatively in patients undergoing AVM treatment. There are no randomized studies looking at medical treatment of epilepsy in AVMs. Epilepsy treatment is largely similar to that in other focal epilepsies. Medication choice should be directed toward an antiepileptic drug regimen that best treats focal lesions and that considers medical comorbidities. There is no data or clear guideline on the best medication for treatment of AVMs, although antiepileptic drugs such as carbamazepine and lamotrigine are typically used as first-line treatment for focal epilepsies. Levetiracetam, given its ease of administration and intravenous formulation, has gained favor in surgical patients, especially if they are an in acute situation. Follow-up electroencephalograms (EEGs) and medication serum levels should be performed if breakthrough seizures or other suspicious neurological events occur.

Interestingly, among patients with untreated lesions and localization-related (partial) epilepsy, those with untreated AVMs as the cause of their epilepsy have better outcomes with medical treatment than those with untreated mesial temporal sclerosis as the cause (Stephen *et al.* 2001).

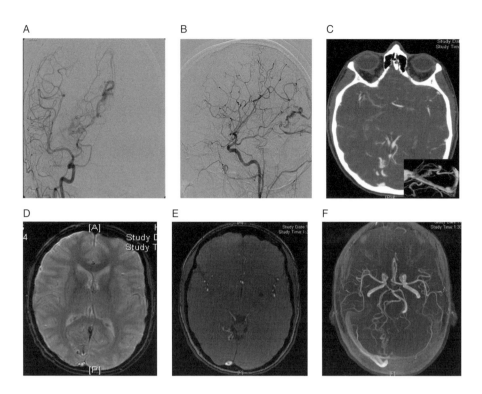

Fig. 78.2. Angiography, MRI angiography, (MRA), and CTa angiography (CTA) may be used to image AVMs: example of different imaging modalities from the same patient with right occipital AVM. Posteroanterior (A) and lateral (B) angiogram; (C) CTA, inset: three-dimensional reconstruction of lesion from CTA; (D) gradient echo MRI; (E) MRA; (F) three-dimensional reconstruction of MRA.

Diagnosis

Imaging arteriovenous malformations

Imaging is the key diagnostic tool for evaluating patients with AVMs. The gold standard imaging modality for AVMs is cerebral angiography, which delineates critical features of the lesion required to develop a rational approach for management. Cerebral angiography identifies feeding arteries, the AVM nidus, drainage pattern, as well as the presence of feeding artery and intranidal aneurysms (Fig. 78.2A, B). Computed tomography (CT) and magnetic resonance imaging (MRI) are less invasive and offer additional complementary information regarding specific anatomic localization. Location of the AVM provides information pertaining to determining both seizure risk and therapeutic options. Computed tomography is the best method of revealing acute hemorrhage as well as calcifications; CT angiography (CTA) provides considerable vascular detail and is less invasive than conventional angiography (Fig. 78.2C). Magnetic resonance imaging provides the most detailed cerebral anatomy (Fig. 78.2D) and can also demonstrate both acute hemorrhage and hemosiderin deposits. Magnetic resonance angiography (MRA) will demonstrate vascular anatomy but at present with less resolution than either CTA or conventional angiography (Fig. 78.2E, F). Preoperative CT and/or MRI can also assist in image-guided operative approaches.

There may be a role for functional imaging in the workup of AVMs. Functional MRI (fMRI) can be used to identify eloquent cortex adjacent to an AVM as well as along a potential surgical approach. Diffusion tensor imaging (DTI) can be used to visualize the location and displacement of surrounding white matter tracts.

Evaluation of epilepsy in the setting of arteriovenous malformations

While there are no clear guidelines on evaluation of epilepsy in the setting of an AVM or other vascular malformations, given the epileptogenic nature of AVMs, EEG should be considered even in asymptomatic patients identified with an AVM, particularly if the lesion has high seizure risk features as described in Table 78.1. In conjunction with imaging, the electrographic evaluation of AVMs is similar to that performed in other brain mass lesions such as tumors. An EEG prior to surgery, embolization, or radiation as well as after surgical treatment is suggested. Surgical interventions with a resulting skull defect or subsequent microhemorrhage can cause a breach rhythm on EEG or additional cortical irritative foci. In the absence of overt clinical seizure activity, if there is suggestion of cortical irritability or rhythmic activity on the EEG, a prophylactic antiepileptic drug should be considered. If seizures are not well controlled or if there is suspicion of repeated hemorrhage of the AVM, further EEG is recommended.

Principles of management

Treatment of arteriovenous malformations

Because AVM hemorrhage is associated with significant morbidity and mortality, the primary goal of AVM treatment is the prevention of hemorrhage or of repeated hemorrhage.

An important secondary goal of treatment in patients with AVM-associated epilepsy is the improvement of seizure outcome. Arteriovenous malformations may be treated with resective surgery, with radiation (stereotactic radiosurgery), with embolization, or with a combination of these. Incomplete obliteration of AVMs has been associated with an even greater risk of hemorrhage than untreated AVMs, although this is controversial; a recent report suggests a reduction in hemorrhage rate with partial treatment (Maruyama et al. 2005). The anatomic goal of treatment by any modality is the complete obliteration of the AVM.

The advantage of surgical resection is that it results in immediate AVM obliteration, thereby eliminating the risk of hemorrhage. The suitability of an AVM for surgery is assessed, in part, according to the Spetzler–Martin grading system (Spetzler and Martin 1986). (Table 78.2). In general terms, patients with grades I–III AVMs are good candidates for surgical resection. In contrast, patients with grade IV and V AVMs are generally poor surgical candidates, as attempts at resection of these lesions are associated with much higher rates of serious complications or death. Compactness of the AVM and absence of deep perforating arterial supply are also associated with favorable surgical outcome (Du et al. 2007). Postoperatively, particularly in patients with large AVMs, there is an approximately 5% risk of brain swelling and intracerebral hemorrhage, termed normal perfusion pressure breakthrough, which is thought to be caused by a failure of autoregulation and which is managed with aggressive maintenance of normotension and euvolemia in an intensive care unit setting during the immediate postoperative period (Staph et al. 2006).

In Spetzler and Martin's original series, resection of grade I AVMs resulted in 100% no deficit, grade II in 95% no deficit and 5% minor deficit, grade III 84% no deficit, 12% minor deficit, and 4% major deficit (Spetzler and Martin 1986). Subsequent series revealed that resection of grade IV resulted in 65% deficit, 4% disabling deficit, and of grade V resulted in 33% major deficit, (Steiner et al. 1992).

Embolization is frequently used in conjunction with surgery or radiation in the treatment of AVMs, although it may be used on its own. Use of newer agents, such as ONYX, have in some centers resulted in increased cure rates with embolization alone, especially for smaller AVMs (van Rooij et al. 2007; Panagiotopoulos et al. 2009).

Stereotactic radiosurgery is most appropriate for the treatment of deep and some large AVMs that are not candidates for surgery. One disadvantage of radiation is that it can take up to 5 years for an AVM to become obliterated following radiation treatment, during which time the patient remains at risk for hemorrhage (Maruyama et al. 2005). The radiosurgery-based AVM score (RBAS) was developed to predict patient outcomes following radiosurgery, in a manner analogous to the Spetzler–Martin system for open surgery. It is based on the identification of five factors affecting radiosurgery outcome: AVM volume, patient age,

Table 78.2 The Spetzler–Martin grading system is used to predict AVM surgical outcome

Feature		Points
Maximum diameter	<3 cm	1
	3–6 cm	2
	>6 cm	3
Eloquence of adjacent brain	noneloquent	0
	eloquent	1
Venous drainage	superficial	0
	deep	1
AVM grade		Sum of points: I–V

AVM location, history of previous embolization, and number of draining systems (Pollock and Flickinger 2002; Raffa et al. 2009). Curiously, it seems that improvement in seizure outcome from radiation is seen prior to AVM obliteration, suggesting that radiation may provide a treatment effect for seizure independent of AVM obliteration (Heikkinen et al. 1989).

Multimodality treatment, e.g., preoperative embolization followed by resective surgery, is increasingly common in the treatment of AVMs. Surgical resection can also be performed following subtotal obliteration of the AVM with radiosurgery, and vice versa. Controversy exists regarding the safety and efficacy of embolization performed prior to radiosurgery.

Finally, conservative management of AVMs is an option, depending on the perceived natural history of the particular lesion, the treatment risk, and the patient's age and preference. In 2001, a special writing group of the American Stroke Association published management recommendations for cerebral AVMs. The authors point out that there are no data available from randomized controlled trials on which to base these recommendations, which must be interpreted accordingly. In general, surgical resection is recommended for Spetzler–Martin grade I and II AVMs, embolization followed by surgical resection for grade III AVMs, radiosurgery for AVMs in eloquent brain or with vascular anatomy thought to present a high surgical risk, and expectant management for grade IV and V lesions, as for many of these the risks of treatment outweigh those associated with the natural history (Ogilvy et al. 2001).

Seizure outcome following treatment

There are no randomized controlled prospective trials comparing seizure outcome in treated vs. untreated AVMs. Nor are there any such trials comparing seizure outcomes by treatment modality. A number of retrospective (and one prospective) series describe relationships between AVM treatment and seizure

Table 78.3 Seizure outcome following AVM treatment: summary of the literature

Treatment	Percent of patients with seizures who improved	Percent of patients with seizures made seizure-free	Percent of patients with new-onset seizures post-resection	Reference
Surgery	4–100%	4–100%	8–26%	Parkinson and Bachers (1980), Wharen *et al.* (1982), Heros *et al.* (1990), Yeh *et al.* (1990, 1993), Piepgras *et al.* (1993)
Radiation	19–85%	19–85%	0–7%	Heikkinen *et al.* (1989), Falkson *et al.* (1997), Elsenschenk *et al.* (1998), Schauble *et al.* (2009)
Embolization	24%	Not available	8%	Fournier *et al.* (1991)
Multimodality	77%	66%[a]	6%	Hoh *et al.* (2002)

Note:
[a]Free from disabling seizures.

outcome in patients with epilepsy as a consequence of their AVM (summarized in Table 78.3). Factors associated with favorable seizure outcome following treatment include short pretreatment seizure history, association of pretreatment seizures with hemorrhage, GTC seizures, deep or posterior fossa AVM location, surgical resection (vs. other treatment modalities), and complete AVM obliteration (Hoh *et al.* 2002). Of note, among those patients with completely obliterated AVMs, no differences in seizure outcome between surgery, radiation, and embolization have been reported (Hoh *et al.* 2002), although it is possible that some subclinical seizures were missed.

Medical management of seizures in patients with arteriovenous malformations

Most outcome studies regarding epilepsy in AVM do not name the antiepileptic drugs the patients are taking; and some provide the number of antiepileptic drugs and others do not.

The medical management of seizures associated with AVMs is challenging. The epilepsy is often refractory to treatment, perhaps because of the hemorrhagic nature of these lesions. In addition, repeated microhemorrhage can lead to recurrent irritability that prevents optimal seizure control. The location of the lesion is also likely to be a factor, but there have been no studies relating seizure outcome in AVMs to location or the type of antiepileptic drug used to treat AVM-related seizures.

There are various possible causes of recurrent seizures in postprocedural AVM patients on seizure medication. The AVM may have re-bled. Medication compliance, interfering medications, other new medical illnesses, or fever are all other possible causes of seizure breakthrough. If none of these factors are present, then the antiepileptic drug dosage can be insufficient. Antiepileptic drug levels can be helpful, and the dosage adjusted or increased. If the patient is not tolerating medication, or if the level is inadequate, then alternatives should be considered. If the seizure is atypical for the patient, then reimaging may be needed to confirm AVM stability.

Another issue is the question of discontinuation of prophylactic antiepileptic drugs in a patient who has had a resection and has never had a seizure. A routine or prolonged ambulatory EEG is strongly recommended prior to weaning medications to determine if there is any epileptiform activity. If discharges or seizures are present, then it is unwise to wean antiepileptic drugs. If there is no epileptiform activity, no concern for clinical seizure, and postsurgical imaging shows no blood products in the region of the AVM, then weaning antiepileptic drugs cautiously is reasonable. Warning the patient to limit activities (e.g., driving) while weaning medication and afterwards for a short period of time is advisable given the chance that seizures could occur.

References

Awad IA, Magdinec M, Schubert A (1984) Intracranial hypertension after resection of cerebral arteriovenous malformations: predisposing factors and management strategy. *Stroke* 25:611–20.

Crawford PM, West CR, Shaw MDM (1986) Cerebral arteriovenous malformations and epilepsy: factors in the development of epilepsy. *Epilepsia* 27:270–5.

Dodick DW, Cascino GD, Meyer FB (1994) Vascular malformations and intractable epilepsy: outcome after surgical treatment. *Mayo Clin Proc* 69:741–5.

Du R, Keyoung HM, Dowd CF, Young WL, Lawton MT (2007) The effects of diffuseness and deep perforating artery supply on outcomes after microsurgical resection of brain arteriovenous malformations. *Neurosurgery* 60:638–48.

Eerola I, Boon LM, Mulliken JB, *et al.* (2003) Capillary malformation–arteriovenous malformation: a new clinical and genetic disorder caused by *RASA1* mutations. *Am J Hum Genet* 73:1240–9.

Eisenschenk S, Gilmore RL, Friedman WA, Henchey RA (1998) The effect of LINAC stereotactic radiosurgery on epilepsy associated with arteriovenous malformations. *Stereotact Funct Neurosurg* **71**:51–61.

Falkson CB, Chakrabarti KB, Doughty D, Plowman PN (1997) Stereotactic multiple arc radiotherapy. III. Influence of treatment of arteriovenous malformations on associated epilepsy. *Br J Neurosurg* **11**:12–15.

Fournier D, TerBrugge KG, Willinsky R, Lasjaunias P, Montanera W (1991) Endovascular treatment of intracerebral arteriovenous malformations: experience in 49 cases. *J Neurosurg* **75**:228–33.

Friedlander RM (2007) Clinical practice: arteriovenous malformations of the brain. *N Engl J Med* **356**:2704–12.

Gerszten PC, Adelson PD, Kondziolka D, Flickinger JC, Lunsford LD (1996) Seizure outcome in children treated for arteriovenous malformations using gamma knife radiosurgery. *Pediatr Neurosurg* **24**:139–44.

Gonzalez LF, Bristol RE, Porter RW, Spetzler RF (2005) De novo presentation of an arteriovenous malformation: case report and review of the literature. *J Neurosurg* **102**:726–9.

Hartmann A, Stapf C, Hofmeister C, et al. (2000) Determinants of neurological outcome after surgery for brain arteriovenous malformation. *Stroke* **31**:2361–4.

Heikkinen ER, Konnov B, Melnikov L, et al. (1989) Relief of epilepsy by radiosurgery of cerebral arteriovenous malformations. *Stereotact Funct Neurosurg* **53**:157–66.

Heros RC, Korosue K, Diebold PM (1990) Surgical excision of cerebral arteriovenous malformations: late results. *Neurosurgery* **26**:570–8.

Herzig R, Burval S, Vladyka V, et al. (2000) Familial occurrence of cerebral arteriovenous malformation in sisters: case report and review of the literature. *Eur J Neurol* **7**:95–100.

Hofmeister C, Stapf C, Hartmann A (2000) Demographic, morphological, and clinical characteristics of 1289 patients with brain arteriovenous malformation. *Stroke* **31**:1307–10.

Hoh BL, Chapman PH, Loeffler JS, et al. (2002) Results of multimodality treatment for 141 patients with brain arteriovenous malformations and seizures: factors associated with seizure incidence and seizure outcomes. *Neurosurgery* **51**:303–11.

Huang CF, Somaza S, Lunsford L, Kondziolka D, Flickinger JC (1996) Radiosurgery in the management of epilepsy associated with arteriovenous malformations. In: Kondziolka D (ed.) *Radiosurgery 1995*, vol. **1**. Basel: Karger, pp. 195–200.

Kida Y, Kobayashi T, Tanaka T, et al. (2000) Seizure control after radiosurgery on cerebral arteriovenous malformations. *J Clin Neurosci* **7**(Suppl 1):6–9.

Kjellberg RN, Hanamura T, Davis KR, Lyons SL, Adams RD (1983) Bragg–Peak proton-beam therapy for arteriovenous malformations of the brain. *N Engl J Med* **309**:269–74.

Kurita H, Kawamota S, Suzuki I, et al. (1998) Control of epilepsy associated with cerebral arteriovenous malformations after radiosurgery. *J Neurol Neurosurg Psychiatry* **65**:648–55.

Lunsford LD, Kondziolka D, Flickinger JC, et al. (1991) Stereotactic radiosurgery for arteriovenous malformations of the brain. *J Neurosurg* **75**:512–24.

Maruyama K, Kawahara N, Shin M, et al. (2005) The risk of hemorrhage after radiosurgery for cerebral arteriovenous malformations. *N Engl J Med* **352**:146–53.

McCormick WF (1966) The pathology of vascular ("arteriovenous") malformations. *J Neurosurg* **24**:807–16.

McCormick WF, Nofzinger JD (1966) "Cryptic" vascular malformations of the central nervous system. *J Neurosurg* **24**:865–75.

Moriwaki A, Hattori Y, Nishida N, Hori Y (1990) Electrocorticographic characterization of chronic iron-induced epilepsy in rats. *Neurosci Lett* **110**:72–6.

Morrell F (1985) Secondary epileptogenesis in man. *Arch Neurol* **42**:318–35.

Morrell F, Wada JA, Engel J Jr. (1987) Potential relevance of kindling and secondary epileptogenesis to the consideration of surgical treatment of epilepsy. In: Engel J Jr. (ed) *Surgical Treatment of Epilepsies*. New York: Raven Press, pp. 699–707.

Ogilvy CS, Stieg PE, Awad I, et al. (2001) Recommendations for the management of intracranial arteriovenous malformations: a statement for healthcare professionals from a Special Writing Group of the Stroke Council, American Stroke Association. *Stroke* **32**:1458–71.

Panagiotopoulos V, Gizewski E, Asgari S, et al. (2009) Embolization of intracranial arteriovenous malformations with ethylene-vinyl alcohol copolymer (onyx). *AJNR Am J Neuroradiol* **30**:99–106.

Parkinson D, Bachers G (1980) Arteriovenous malformations: summary of 100 consecutive supratentorial cases. *J Neurosurg* **57**:520–6.

Perret G, Nishioka H (2005) Arteriovenous malformations: an analysis of 545 cases of cranio-cerebral arteriovenous malformations and fistulae reported to the Cooperative Study. *J Neurosurg* **102**:726–9.

Piepgras DG, Sundt TM Jr., Ragoonwansi AT, Stevens L (1993) Seizure outcome in patients with surgically treated cerebral arteriovenous malformations. *J Neurosurg* **78**:5–11.

Pollock BE, Flickinger JC (2002) A proposed radiosurgery-based grading system for arteriovenous malformations. *J Neurosurg* **96**:79–85.

Raffa SJ, Chi YY, Bova FJ, Friedman WA (2009) Validation of the radiosurgery-based arteriovenous malformation score in a large linear accelerator radiosurgery experience. *J Neurosurg* **111**:832–9.

Revencu N, Boon LM, Mulliken JB, et al. (2008) Parkes Weber syndrome, vein of Galen aneurysmal malformation, and other fast-flow vascular anomalies are caused by *RASA1* mutations. *Hum Mutat* **29**:959–65.

Schäuble B, Cascino GD, Pollock BE, et al. (2004) Seizure outcomes after stereotactic radiosurgery for cerebral arteriovenous malformations. *Neurology* **63**:683–7.

Spetzler RF, Martin NA (1986) A proposed grading system for arteriovenous malformations. *J Neurosurg* **65**:476–83.

Stapf C, Khaw AV, Sciacca RR, et al. (2003) Effect of age on clinical and morphological characteristics in patients with brain arteriovenous malformation. *Stroke* **34**:2664.

Staph C, Mast H, Mohr JP, et al. (2006) Predictors of hemorrhage in patients with untreated brain arteriovenous malformation. *Neurology* **66**:1350–5.

Steiner L, Lindquist C, Adler JR, et al. (1992) Clinical outcome of radiosurgery for cerebral arteriovenous malformations. *J Neurosurg* **77**:1–8.

Stephen LJ, Kwan P, Brodie MJ (2001) Does the cause of localization-related epilepsy influence the response to antiepileptic drug treatment? *Epilepsia* **42**:357–62.

Sutcliffe JC, Forster DMC, Walton L, Dias PS, Kemeny AA (1992) Untoward clinical effects after stereotactic radiosurgery for intracranial arteriovenous malformations. *Br J Neurosurg* **6**:177–85.

Turjman F, Massoud TF, Sayre JW, Vinuela F, *et al.* (1995) Epilepsy associated with cerebral arteriovenous malformations: a multivariate analysis of angioarchitectural characteristics. *AJNR Am J Neuroradiol* **16**:345–50.

Thorpe ML, Cordato DJ, Morgan MK, Herkes GK (2000) Postoperative seizure outcome in a series of 114 patients with supratentorial arteriovenous malformations. *J Clin Neurosci* **7**:107–11.

van Rooij WJ, Sluzewski M, Beute GN (2007) Brain AVM embolization with onyx. *AJNR Am J Neuroradiol* **28**:172–7.

Wharen RE Jr., Scheithauer BW, Laws ER Jr. (1982) Thrombosed arteriovenous malformations of the brain: an important entity in the differential diagnosis of intractable focal seizure disorders. *J Neurosurg* **57**:520–6.

Yeh HS, Kashiwagi S, Tew JM Jr., Berger TS (1990) Surgical management of epilepsy associated with cerebral arteriovenous malformations. *J Neurosurg* **72**:216–23.

Yeh HS, Privitera MD (1991) Secondary epileptogenesis in cerebral arteriovenous malformations. *Arch Neurol* **48**:1122–4.

Yeh SH, Tew JM Jr., Gartner M (1993) Seizure control after surgery on cerebral arteriovenous malformations. *J Neurosurg* **78**:12–18.

Cavernous malformations

79

Adrian M. Siegel

Cavernous malformations (CMs) were first described postmortem by Hubert von Luschka in 1854 (Luschka 1854). He found a tumorous malformation ("Geschwulst") of cerebral vessels in a man who committed suicide. Initially, CMs were considered to be tumors as shown by the classification of tumors by Rudolf Virchow in 1863. In their monumental book *Tumors Arising from the Blood Vessels of the Brain* (1928) Cushing and Bailey also classified CMs as a solid subtype of hemangioblastomas. It is for this reason that the term "cavernoma" containing the Greek suffix "oma" meaning "neoplasm" has been used for a long time. Today, however, CMs are classified pathologically as true vascular malformations. Interestingly, despite of this reclassification recent insights into the pathophysiological mechanisms of CMs have shown a tumor-like nature.

Demographic data

In autopsy and radiological series, CMs have a prevalence of 0.1 to 0.5% (Otten *et al.* 1989; Robinson *et al.* 1991). Among the four vascular malformations (CMs, artierovenous malformations, venous malformations, and capillary telangiectases) CMs account for 8% to 15% (McCormick *et al.* 1968; Sarvar and McCormick 1978). The prevalence in males and females is similar. Solitary lesions are more common than multiple CMs. The latter may be found up to 15% and are frequently associated with familial cases. The exact prevalence of the inherited form of CMs is still unknown, but selected radiological and genetic series have shown a familial form in up to 20% of individuals harboring CMs. Cavernous malformations may be found throughout the central nervous system. Several studies have shown predilections for certain brain sites, but in our own compilation of 512 patients, we did not find any marked differences. Of the cerebral CMs, about 75% were supratentorial and 25% infratentorial, a proportion which reflects respective brain volumes. Spinal CMs were found in about 3% of our cases. Cavernous malformations clinically manifest in all age groups but usually CMs become symptomatic between the second and fourth decade (Simard *et al.* 1986). However, CMs may also manifest at birth or in the elderly.

Pathological characteristics

Cavernous malformations are lobulated, well-circumscribed, mulberry-like non-encapsulated lesions. They can vary greatly in size from one millimeter to several centimeters (McCormick *et al.* 1968; Simard *et al.* 1986; Russell and Rubenstein 1989). The size may also change over time, and expression of vascular endothelial growth factor within CM has been demonstrated (Bertalanffy *et al.* 2002). Cavernous malformations are characterized by low-flow sinusoidal vessels lined by thin endothelial walls with no obvious feeding arteries or venous drainage. The lack of intervening brain parenchyma is a *conditio sine qua non* for the diagnosis (Russell and Rubenstein 1989). Usually, there are no smooth muscles or elastic fibers. Calcification, however, may be present, and such cases have been described as hemangioma calcificans. Perilesional hemosiderin deposits due to chronic microhemorrhages are a common finding (Del Curling *et al.* 1991).

Although CMs are most likely congenital lesions, there is clear evidence of de novo development. Such de novo CMs have often been found both in children treated with radiation and in familial cases (Zabramski *et al.* 1994; Detwiler *et al.* 1997). Moreover, there is clear evidence for the concept that capillary telangiectases may evolve into CMs.

Pathophysiological mechanisms of epilepsy in cavernous malformations

For an optimal therapeutic approach it is mandatory to understand the epilepsy inducing mechanisms associated with CMs. In contrast to tumors such as ganglioglioma, CMs are not epileptogenic per se. There are several underlying mechanisms for epilepsy in CMs. The changes are related to increased concentration of iron and free radicals, neurotransmitter alterations, neuronal cell loss and gliosis, dysfunctions of astrocytes, and ischemia (Kraemer and Awad 1994). The key factor underlying epileptogenicity, however, is the pathological changes in the surrounding tissue due to the ubiquitous hemosiderin deposits. Hemosiderin is a multivalent ironhydroxid

The Causes of Epilepsy, eds. S. D. Shorvon, F. Andermann, and R. Guerrini. Published by Cambridge University Press. © Cambridge University Press 2011.

complex that likely represents a degradation product of ferritin. In addition, destruction of red blood cells leads to the oxidation of oxyhemoglobin with dissociation of heme iron from the globin component. Iron may exist in a number of valence states. Thus, it is an exellent electron donor for the production of free radicals and lipid peroxides as well as an exellent electron acceptor for oxidation/reduction reactions. The increased concentration of free iron and radicals may cause various pathophysiological intracellular processes which could all generate epileptogenic changes in the brain tissue surrounding CMs. Free radicals can also cause peroxidation of membrane lipids and proteins which affect cell membrane fluidity and protein function with subsequent malfunction of receptors, ion channels, and transport proteins. One of the most important ions affected is calcium, which increases in intracellular concentration due to iron-induced free radical generation and lipid peroxidation. In addition, iron in the surrounding tissue may interfere with excitatory mechanisms. First, iron retards two major mechanisms that are important in excitatory amino acid uptake and regulation: (1) it decreases glutamate reuptake in synaptosomes; and (2) it inhibits glutamine synthetase. Second, loss of inhibitory interneurons which have been demonstrated on immunhistochemical findings including (1) a decrease in the staining of GABAergic and somatostain immunoreactive neurons, and (2) a decrease in glutamic acid decarboxylase (GAD) from the cortex adjacent to tumors. Other factors considered in the pathogenesis of epilepsy associated with vascular malformations are gliosis, dysfunction of astrocytes, and neuronal cell loss. Gliosis may be induced by iron in the tissue adjacent to the lesion. Moreover, the imbalance of iron and calcium ions may lead to the dysfunction of astrocytes which play an active role in modulating neurotransmitters and extracellular ion physiology. Whether neuronal cell loss occurs on cortex adjacent to vascular malformations remains controversial. Secondary epileptogenesis at a distant site attributable to a "kindling" phenomenon, in which epileptic discharges are enhanced by excitatory synaptic connections from the vascular malformation, may also result in seizures.

Genetic aspects of cavernous malformations

Familial CMs of the central nervous system were first described in 1928. Hugo Friedrich Kufs reported a family in which he assumed a common pathological basis in two members (Kufs 1928). The index case was an 81-year-old man in whom multiple cerebral and hepatic cavernomas had been found in an autopsy. His daughter presented with an apoplexia pontis with a right-sided hemiparesis and hemihyperesthesia at the age of 17 years. Although CMs have not been pathologically confirmed in the daughter, Kufs has to be given the credit for the first description of this entity. By the use of magnetic resonance imaging further families have increasingly reported. Thus, since the first description almost 1000 families have been reported all over the world.

Genetic analysis identified three loci for familial CMs: *CCM1* on chromosome 7q21–q22 accounting for 40% of all familial cases, *CCM2* on 7p13–p15 accounting for 13–20%, and *CCM3* on 3q25.2–q27 for up to 40%. The gene *CCM1* encodes for a 736 amino acids protein called the Krev Interaction Trapped 1 (KRIT1) protein (Laberge-le Couteulx *et al.* 1999). KRIT1 contains three ankyrin repeats, a FERM (Band 4.1, ezrin, radixin, moesin) domain, and a NPXY (Asn-Pro-X-Tyr) motif. Molecular studies have shown that the NPXY motif seems to modulate a strong interaction with the integrin cytoplasmic domain-associated protein 1 (ICAP1), suggesting that this protein might be involved in bidirectional signaling between the integrin and the cytoskeleton in *CCM1* pathogenesis. In addition, KRIT1 has been shown to be a microtubule-associated protein that may help determine endothelial cell shape and function in response to cell–cell and cell–matrix interactions by guiding cytoskeletal structure. The *CCM2* gene found at locus 7p13–p15 encodes for the Malcavernin protein (Liquori *et al.* 2003). Malcavernin is a similar protein as the KRIT 1 binding partner ICAP1, a protein with a phosphotyrosin binding (PTB) domain. Recently, the PDCD10 (Programmed Cell Death 10) gene also called TFAR15 has been identified as the *CCM3* gene (Bergametti *et al.* 2005). Although the product and function of PDCD10 is still not known it is thought to interact with angiogenesis.

Although accurate prevalence data are still not available the familial occurrence of CMs seems to be underestimated. It is therefore important to obtain detailed family histories from all patients. The identification of other affected family members will be facilitated by the use of genetic testing. Currently, genetic studies are also focusing on the search for additional genes causing familial CMs.

Clinical features

Cavernous malformations may remain asymptomatic throughout life in up to 20% of cases (Del Curling *et al.* 1991; Bertalanffy *et al.* 2002). However, CMs often present with clinically significant (major) hemorrhages, focal neurological deficits, headache, or seizures. Hemorrhages occur in 20–40%. The annual bleeding risk is reported between 0.7% to 1.2% per lesion, with a higher risk of hemorrhage after an initial bleed and in cases localized to deep structures or the brainstem (Kondziolka *et al.* 1995; Porter *et al.* 1997). Thus, the annual risk of a repeat hemorrhage is about 25% in the first 28 months and subsequently decreases to 9% per year. Interestingly, patients with CMs and major hemorrhages rarely present with chronic epilepsy. Focal neurological deficits were reported at 10% to 25%. Whether headache is a "real" symptom due to CMs is controversial. Since headache has been reported only at 10% and 20% it cannot be ruled out that headache in a patient with CMs reflects sporadic headache of tension type, for instance.

The fact that CMs cause epilepsy has been known for a long time (Bremer and Carson 1890; Ohlmacher 1899). Epileptic seizures are the presenting symptom in about half of the patients with all types of seizures occurring (Maraire and Awad 1995; Moran *et al.* 1999). Some studies analyzed the risk for new onset seizures in asymptomatic CMs and found a rate between 1.5% and 2.4% per patient–year. It is known, that seizures are more common in lesions in the frontal and temporal lobe (Simard *et al.* 1986; Yaşargil 1987). In an own series of 206 patients surgically treated by Gazi Yaşargil at Zurich, 91 (44%) had epileptic seizures due to a CM. Of these, 80% had at least three seizures and in 75% the seizures were medically refractory. Detailed information regarding the type of seizures was available in 86 patients: 42 (49%) had complex partial seizures, 31 (36%) simple partial seizures, 12 (14%) tonic-clonic, and 1 status epilepticus. Seizures were medically refractory in 74% of the patients. In another series of 47 patients with epileptic seizures 44.7% had a seizure history of more than 10 years and 90% were refractory to therapy (Casazza *et al.* 1996). In general, the mean age of onset of symptoms is between the second and fourth decade. In our series of 206 surgically treated patients, the age of symptom onset was 21 years for epilepsy and focal neurological deficits, 24 years for headache, and 29 years for major hemorrhages.

Diagnostic tools

Scalp electroencephalography

The findings of scalp electroencephalography (scalp EEG) in CMs are similar to those in other lesions. In many cases, the main findings are focal slowing above the site of the lesion but the EEG may also be completely normal. Thus, in an own surgically oriented series, 135 out of 151 patients (89%) had an epileptic focus with topographic relationship corresponding to the site of the CMs whereas 11% revealed a normal interictal EEG.

Magnetoencephalography

Numerous studies of magnetoencephalography (MEG) in medically intractable epilepsy have shown that MEG can detect interictal and ictal epileptiform activity. In vascular malformations, however, MEG does not play an important role in the presurgical evaluation due to its limitations as a tool for localization and its high costs.

Imaging

The role in diagnosis and the history of imaging techniques such as cerebral angiography, computed tomography (CT), and magnetic resonance imaging (MRI) as well as the radiological characteristics of CM have been extensively reviewed in recent literature (Bertalanffy *et al.* 2002). Magnetic resonance imaging as the gold standard for the diagnosis does not only localize the lesion but also gives important information about the tissue adjacent to the vascular malformations. Based on the different signal characteristics in T1-weighted, T2-weighted, and particularly in gradient-echo MRI, CMs can be classified into four types (Zabramski *et al.* 1994) (Table 79.1). This classification is of help in the characterization of lesions with

Table 79.1 The four types of cavernous malformations

Type of CM	MRI signal characteristics	Pathologic characteristics
Type IA	T1: hyperintense focus of hemorrhage	"Overt" subacute focus of hemorrhage extending outside the lesion capsule of hemosiderin-stained gliotic brain
	T2: hyper- or hypointense focus of hemorrhage extending through at least one wall of the hypointense rim that surrounds the lesion. Focal edema may be present	
Type IB	T1: hyperintense focus of hemorrhage	Subacute focus of hemorrhage surrounded by a rim of hemosiderin-stained macrophages and gliotic brain
	T2: hyper- or hypointense focus of hemorrhage surrounded by a hypointense rim	
Type II	T1: reticulated mixed signal core	Loculated areas of hemorrhage and thrombosis of varying age surrounded by gliotic, hemosiderin-stained brain; in large lesions areas of calcification may be seen; chronic resolved hemorrhage
	T2: reticulated mixed signal core surrounded by a hypointense rim	
Type III	T1: iso- or hypointense	With hemosiderin-staining within and around the lesion
	T2: hypointense with a hypointense rim that magnifies size of lesion	
Type IV	T1: poorly seen or not visualized at all	Has been pathologically documented to be telangiectases
	T2: poorly seen or not visualized at all	
	Gradient-echo sequences: punctuate hypointense lesions	

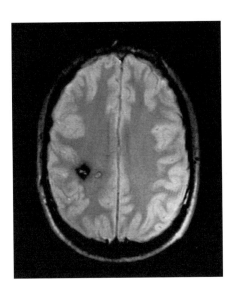

Fig. 79.1. Magnetic resonance image of multiple CMs of type II.

a history of bleeding. Thus, lesions at risk for hemorrhages and epilepsy are type I and, in particular, type II (Fig. 79.1). In modern neurosurgery, intraoperative MRI can be useful for the localization of the lesion.

Single photon emission computed tomography and positron emission tomography

Aside from structural imaging for the detection of vascular malformations, functional imaging constitutes a helpful extension of the presurgical diagnostic work-up. In the presurgical evaluation, interictal and ictal single photon emission computed tomography (SPECT) as well as interictal positron emission tomography (PET) are performed. Ictal SPECT has a maximal sensitivity of 80–90% for localizing the epileptogenic zone. Although less sensitive interictal SPECT has its value in the presurgical work-up, in particular for co-registered interictal–ictal SPECT studies. Positron emission tomography shows the highest sensitivity (60–90%) in temporal epilepsy. Although neither SPECT nor PET provides additional information about the location of a lesion, both tests are helpful tools in defining the epileptogenic zone in the tissue surrounding vascular malformations. Moreover, SPECT and PET may be pivotal in determining the epileptogenic lesion in patients with multiple CM.

Therapeutic options
Antiepileptic treatment

The optimal management of CMs presenting with epileptic seizures is still a matter of debate. In many patients, it is not clear whether CMs should be treated conservatively with antiepileptic drugs (AEDs) or whether resective brain surgery is mandatory. Only a few studies have carefully addressed this question, but usually only in small series. The risks of seizures in medically refractory epilepsy and the risks of hemorrhage have to be balanced against the risks of surgery. Of the AEDs, valproic acid should be avoided in the treatment of CMs due to

its high incidence of valproate-induced coagulation disorders, potentially resulting not only in a higher risk of a minor or gross hemorrhage but also a potential intraoperative coagulation problem in any subsequent surgery.

Surgical treatment

The first surgical treatment was carried out in 1890 by Bremer and Carson, in a patient with epilepsy due to a CM in the central region (Bremer and Carson 1890). Subsequently, more cases have been published with review of the literature by Walter Dandy, later by Hugo Krayenbühl, and Gazi Yaşargil.

There are many studies analyzing the epileptological outcome following removal of CMs. For example, Stefan and Hammen (2004) found complete seizure-freedom in 53% of 30 patients and in another series 31% of the patients became seizure-free (Folkersma and Mooij 2001). In an own multicenter study (Baumann *et al.* 2007) comprising 168 patients with an epileptogenic CM surgically treated, 1 year after surgery 70% of patients were seizure-free (48% of these 168 patients were in Engel class Ia), and in 25% of patients only rare seizures or a worthwhile improvement (Engel classes II – III) was observed. No improvement or deterioration (Engel class IV) was found in 5%. Of our patients, 68% remained seizure-free after 2 years, and 66% after 3 years. The seizure outcome 1 year following the surgery classified according to the localization of the CM is depicted in Fig. 79.2. In this series, significant predictors of good outcome were (1) age at operation >30 years, (2) age at epilepsy onset in later life, (3) mesiotemporal CMs, (4) size of CMs <1.5 cm, (5) seizure type consisting of simple partial, complex partial, and primarily generalized type and, (6) EEG reveals only a focus attributable to the CM, i.e., no additional seizure focus. In our series of 168 surgically treated patients, there was no mortality and persistent mild postoperative focal neurological deficits were found in 8% of patients. Postoperatively, AEDs were still taken by 95% and 85% of patients 1 and 2 years after surgery, respectively, and by 76% after 3 years.

Our own results have been confirmed by a recent study of 164 epileptic patients operated on for a CM (Chang *et al.* 2009). In this study, 72.7% were rendered completely seizure-free (Engel class I), 11.4% had rare seizures (Engel class II), 4.5% had a worthwhile improvement (Engel class III), and 11.4% had no improvement (Engel class IV). Predictors of complete seizure-freedom were gross total resection, smaller CMs, and the absence of secondary generalized seizures (94% of patients were seizure-free with all three predictors).

It is still unclear whether surgical treatment of CM should also include resection of the perilesional tissue. A few mainly anecdotal studies reported a better seizure outcome following resection of CM with the removal of the hemosiderin-stained surrounding brain tissue, whereas others found no correlation with better outcome. In an own study of 31 patients (Baumann *et al.* 2006), there was a more favorable outcome 3 years after operation in patients in whom hemosiderin had been removed completely, when compared to patients in whom postoperative

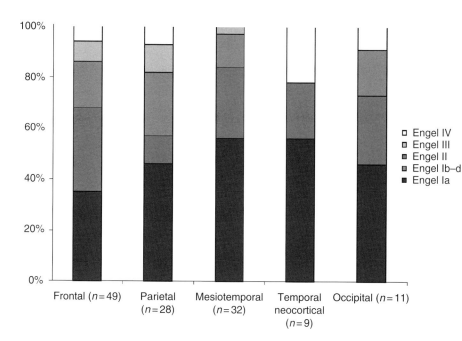

Fig. 79.2. Seizure outcome 1 year after resective surgery, classified according to localization of CMs.

- □ Engel IV
- □ Engel III
- ■ Engel II
- ■ Engel Ib–d
- ■ Engel Ia

hemosiderin still was detected by MRI. However, in the two first postoperative years, we did not find significant differences in seizure outcome between patients with and without complete removal of hemosiderin. The finding of a better long-term outcome in patients with complete resection of hemosiderin was not clearly affected by the localization or multiplicity of cavernoma, epilepsy classification, or demographic data such as gender or age.

Another controversial issue is the optimal therapeutic strategy in children with symptomatic CMs. Although one-fourth of all CMs affect the pediatric age group, the current literature mainly focuses on adult patients. In an own multicenter study we have analyzed this subgroup of patients. We studied 41 children with epilepsy due to a CM. The mean age at epilepsy onset was 9.7 years and the mean age at surgery was 11.3 years (range, 10 months to 17.8 years). In this series, there was no mortality due to the surgical procedures performed. Of the 41 children, in five no sufficient follow-up was available. Of the remaining children, 26 (72%) were rendered seizure-free (Engel class 1) following resection of the CM and the surrounding hemosiderin rim. Four patients (11%) had rare seizures (Engel class II), three patients (8%) showed a worthwhile improvement (Engel class III), and three patients (8%) had no worthwhile improvement (Engel class IV). Thus, most of the patients (91%) with preoperative seizures showed an improvement after surgical intervention (Engel classes I to III). There was no significant difference in the seizure outcome between children harboring a temporal lesion compared to those with CMs in other locations. However, there was a significant correlation between the preoperative duration of epilepsy and the postoperative outcome, i.e., the longer the epilepsy lasts the worse is the outcome. Based on these data, the surgical approach seems to be the favorable therapy of CMs causing epilepsy not only in adults but also in the pediatric age group.

In the context of surgical treatment, there are further particular aspects to be considered. For example, in patients with multiple CMs a question still unanswered is whether more than the symptomatic malformation should be removed. Moreover, in such cases it is still an open-ended question whether multiple CMs should be removed during the same surgical procedure or in a subsequent operation. In my own experience, there was no additional morbidity due to removal of a second symptomatic or asymptomatic CM during the same surgery, if this could be technically acheived.

Another important issue is the management of asymptomatic affected individuals. Here, the annual risk of hemorrhages or seizures has to be weighed in contrast to the risk of an operation. Even so, each case has to be considered individually and there are no clear guidelines applicable to all, so any decision to operate should be taken rather cautiously.

References

Baumann CR, Schuknecht B, Lo Russo G, *et al.* (2006) Seizure outcome following resection of cavernous malformations is better when surrounding hemosiderin-stained brain is also removed. *Epilepsia* **47**:563–6.

Baumann CR, Acciarri N, Bertalanffy H, *et al.* (2007) Seizure outcome after resection of supratentorial cavernous malformations: a study of 168 patients. *Epilepsia* **48**:559–63.

Bergametti F, Denier C, Labauge P, *et al.* (2005) Mutations within the programmed cell death 10 gene cause cerebral cavernous malformations. *Am J Hum Genet* **76**:42–51.

Bertalanffy H, Benes L, Miyazawa T, *et al.* (2002) Cerebral cavernomas in the adult: review of the literature and analysis of 72 surgically treated patients. *Neurosurg Rev* **25**:1–53.

Bremer L, Carson NB (1890) A case of brain tumor (*angioma cavernosum*), causing spastic paralysis and attacks of tonic spasms: operation. *Am J Med Sci* **100**:219–42.

Casazza M, Broggi G, Franzini A, *et al.* (1996) Supratentorial cavernous angiomas and epileptic seizures: preoperative course and postoperative outcome. *Neurosurgery* **39**:26–32.

Chang EF, Gabriel RA, Potts MB, *et al.* (2009) Seizure characteristics and control after microsurgical resection of supratentorial cerebral cavernous malformations. *Neurosurgery* **65**:31–7.

Del Curling O Jr., Kelly DL, Elster AD, Craven TE (1991) An analysis of the natural history of cavernous angiomas. *J Neurosurg* **75**:702–8.

Detwiler PW, Porter RW, Zabramski JM, Spetzler RF (1997) De novo formation of a central nervous system cavernous malformation: implications for predicting risk of hemorrhage – case report and review of the literature. *J Neurosurg* **87**:629–32.

Folkersma H, Mooij JJ (2001) Follow-up of 13 patients with surgical treatment of cerebral cavernous malformations: effect on epilepsy and patient disability. *Clin Neurol Neurosurg* **103**:67–71.

Kondziolka D, Lunsford LD, Kestle JR (1995) The natural history of cerebral cavernous malformations. *J Neurosurg* **83**:820–4.

Kraemer DL, Awad IA (1994) Vascular malformations and epilepsy: clinical considerations and basic mechanisms. *Epilepsia* **35**:S30–43.

Kufs H (1928) Über die heredofamiläre Angiomatose des Gehirns und der Retina, ihre Beziehungen zueinander und zur Angiomatose der Haut. *Z Neurol Psychiatrie* **113**:651–86.

Laberge-le Couteulx S, Jung HH, Labauge P, *et al.* (1999) Truncating mutations in *CCM1*, encoding KRIT1, cause hereditary cavernous angiomas. *Nat Genet* **23**:189–93.

Liquori CL, Berg MJ, Siegel AM, *et al.* (2003) Mutations in a gene encoding a novel protein containing a phosphotyrosine-binding domain cause type 2 cerebral cavernous malformations. *Am J Hum Genet* **73**:1459–64.

Luschka H (1854) Cavernöse Blutgeschwulst des Gehirnes. *Virchows Archiv pathol Anat* **6**:458–70.

Maraire JN, Awad IA (1995) Intracranial cavernous malformations: lesion behavior and management strategies. *Neurosurgery* **37**:591–605.

McCormick WF, Hardman JM, Boulter TR (1968) Vascular malformations (angiomas) of the brain, with special reference to those occurring in the posterior fossa. *J Neurosurg* **28**:241–51.

Moran NF, Fish DR, Kitchen N, *et al.* (1999) Supratentorial cavernous haemangiomas and epilepsy: a review of the literature and case series. *J Neurol Neurosurg Psychiatry* **66**:561–8.

Ohlmacher AP (1899) Multiple cavernous angioma, fibroendothelioma, osteoma and hematomyelia of the central nervous system in a case of secondary epilepsy. *J Nerv Ment Dis* **26**:395–412.

Otten P, Pizzolato GP, Rilliet B, Berney J (1989) A propos de 131 cas d'angiomas caverneux (cavernomas) du S.N.C, repérés par l'analyse retrospective de 24535 autopsies. *Neurochirurgie (Paris)* **35**:82–3.

Porter PJ, Willinsky RA, Harper W, Wallace MC (1997) Cerebral cavernous malformations: natural history and prognosis after clinical deterioration with or without hemorrhage. *J Neurosurg* **87**:190–7.

Robinson JR, Awad IA, Little JR (1991) Natural history of the cavernous angioma. *J Neurosurg* **75**:709–14.

Russel DS, Rubinstein LJ (1989) *Pathology of Tumors of the Nervous System*, 5th edn. Baltimore, MD: Williams and Wilkins, pp.727–90.

Sarwar M, McCormick WF (1978) Intracerebral venous angioma: case report and review. *Arch Neurol* **35**:323–5.

Simard JM, Garcia-Bengochea F, Ballinger WE, Jr., Mickle JP, Quisling RG (1986) Cavernous angioma: a review of 126 collected and 12 new clinical cases. *Neurosurgery* **18**:162–72.

Stefan H, Hammen T (2004) Cavernous haemangiomas, epilepsy and treatment strategies. *Acta Neurol Scand* **110**:393–7.

Yaşargil MG (1987) *Microneurosurgery*, vols. IIIA and B. Stuttgart, Germany: Thieme.

Zabramski JM, Wascher TM, Spetzler RF, *et al.* (1994) The natural history of familial cavernous malformations: results of an ongoing study. *J Neurosurg* **80**:422–32.

Chapter

80

Other vascular disorders

Leif Gjerstad and Erik Taubøll

Introduction

Most systemic vascular disorders may affect the brain, either primarily or secondarily, and cause acute and/or chronic ischemic lesions or hemorrhages. Ischemic lesions and hemorrhages may develop into an epileptogenic focus. The frequency of this depends upon such factors as the location and size of the lesion and the elapsed time from the insult. In ischemic stroke, epileptogenesis takes often months or years to develop and occurs with a relatively low frequency of 3–4% after 5 years (Lossius *et al.* 2005). The rate is somewhat higher after hemorrhagic stroke. The other less common vascular diseases have pathogenetic mechanisms that may increase the frequency of seizures and epilepsy, such as the presence of inflammation and/or immunological mechanisms.

In addition to being secondary to vascular lesions, epilepsy may be caused by other aspects of the disease, such as the genetic influences on brain development and function in the case in Ehlers–Danlos syndrome. Another problem in addressing rare diseases and syndromes is the possibility that an association between epilepsy, itself relatively common, and the disease is not a causal one. Many reports of epilepsy apparently associated with rare diseases should be critically reviewed in this light.

The present chapter is a brief description of some uncommon vascular disorders that can characteristically cause epilepsy and/or seizures. A more extensive and complete description of the many uncommon vascular disorders that may affect the brain has recently been published (Caplan 2008).

Moyamoya syndrome

Moyamoya syndrome and disease are both angiopathies that present with a range of neurological symptoms, including seizures, mostly in young people. The pathognomonic abnormality is the characteristic angiographic pattern of a mesh of vessels in the anterior cerebral circulation. This moyamoya, or "puff of smoke," is a progressive condition that may be caused by the idiopathic moyamoya disease, or be part of the syndrome

that is secondary to other causes. The idiopathic disease is genetic and almost exclusively associated with genetic factors commonly from North-East Asia, while the secondary syndrome may be caused by different vascular etiologies. The prevalence is highest in Japan where a recent study (Ikeda *et al.* 2006) found a prevalence of 50 per 100 000 people. The prevalence is much lower in other ethnic groups and probably represents the syndrome. A female predominance of about 2 : 1 has been reported from both Asia and the United States.

The high prevalence in the Japanese population supports a genetic basis for the disease, and different genetic associations have been suggested. The lack of atherosclerotic and inflammatory changes makes it likely that a metabolic disturbance influences the development of the arteries. The angiographic changes develop from the early narrowing of the anterior and median cerebral arteries. Second, the ischemic changes may facilitate the growth of small new vessels, resulting in the characteristic appearance. The presence of changes extracranially also suggests that moyamoya in some patients may be a more generalized vasculopathy. The narrowing of the arteries finally leads to infarction in the distribution of the anterior circulation.

Clinically different neurological signs and symptoms occur. Seizures, headaches, and focal motor impairment are common presentations in children and young adults. Intracerebral hemorrhage may be the initial sign in adults.

In a study of 334 Korean patients, the occurrence of seizures was the presenting symptom in 23.1% of children 16 years or younger and in 3.8% of adults (Han *et al.* 2000). The seizures have been reported to be generalized, but in all likelihood are secondarily generalized. In a report of 35 patients at a university hospital in Houston, USA none had seizures as their presenting symptom (Chiu *et al.* 1995). Treatment is with conventional antiepileptic drugs, and there are no reports of any systematic studies of specific individual antiepileptics. In one case report, a 6-year-old girl with a small infarction in her left frontal lobe had apparently typical absence seizures which ceased after extraintracranial bypass surgery (Kikuta *et al.* 2006).

The Causes of Epilepsy, eds. S. D. Shorvon, F. Andermann, and R. Guerrini. Published by Cambridge University Press. © Cambridge University Press 2011.

Cerebral angiography shows the characteristic changes in the vessels. Today, this can be performed non-invasively by magnetic resonance angiography. A classification system describing six stages is useful for grading the disease (Houkin *et al.* 2005). Positron emission tomography (PET), single photon emission computed tomography (SPECT), and perfusion magnetic resonance imaging (MRI) demonstrate the associated changes in cerebral hemodynamics in relation to reduced perfusion pressure (Kuroda and Houkin 2008). In children there is a characteristic electroencephalogram (EEG) finding with high amplitude slow waves occurring *after* hyperventilation ("re-build-up"). This phenomenon is probably triggered by hypoxia and is related to cerebral ischemia (Kuroda 1995).

The epilepsy is usually not the main clinical problem. In cases with moyamoya syndrome, the prognosis depends upon identification and treatment of the underlying cause of the condition. In the specific moyamoya disease, arterial bypass surgery is possible either from the superficial temporal artery to the medial cerebral artery, or directly by the use of donor tissue like muscle or dura mater (Kuroda and Houkin 2008). Surgery seems to improve the cerebral hemodynamics and protect against infarction. There are currently no medical treatments, but gene therapies may become a future option. Untreated, there is progression of symptoms in many patients.

Eclampsia

Pre-eclampsia, the combination of hypertension, edema, and proteinuria, is estimated to complicate 5–10% of all gestations in Caucasians, and even more in other ethnic groups. Hypertension is the most common initial feature but any one of the three signs may not occur. A seizure, which results in recategorization as eclampsia, may occur before, during, and after delivery (Sibai 2005). It also may occur before hypertension and proteinuria. A recent Scandinavian study found an incidence of 5 per 10 000 (Andersgaard *et al.* 2006) which is very similar to that of an earlier study from UK. Before the seizure, 86% had pre-eclampsia, and 33% had one or more major complications to the eclampsia.

Pre-eclampsia occurs more frequently in women with a predisposition towards vascular diseases, e.g., hypertension and diabetes. New data suggest that placental renin–angiotensin system activation and release of antiangiogenic factors are essential pathophysiological mechanisms (Shah 2007). The cerebral vascular changes most commonly occur in the posterior circulation and have features such as hypertensive encephalopathy, including cerebral edema. Magnetic resonance imaging (MRI) shows hyperintense signals on T2-weighted images, similar to those seen in reversible posterior leukoencephalopathy. Women with early pre-eclampsia usually have no clinical symptoms. Headaches, visual problems, and mental slowing indicate a progression to severe pre-eclampsia. In eclampsia, seizures occur and may be accompanied by stroke, cortical blindness, and coma. Intracerebral hemorrhage,

pulmonary edema, liver and kidney failure, and the HELLP syndrome (hemolysis, elevated liver function tests, and low platelets) are other complications. The seizures are generalized tonic–clonic in form.

In a pregnant woman blood pressure measurements and testing for proteinuria can identify those that may progress to severe pre-eclampsia/eclampsia. Cerebral MRI shows characteristic findings in eclampsia (see above), and is essential for excluding sinus thrombosis. Elevation of uric acid, thrombocytopenia, decreased levels of antithrombin III, disseminated intravascular coagulation (DIC), and HELLP may support the diagnosis.

Eclamptic seizures are usually treated with magnesium sulfate, which has also been shown in a randomized controlled trial to be superior to phenytoin and diazepam in preventing the occurrence of seizures (Lucas *et al.* 1995). In this study of 1049 patients with hypertension before labor who were treated with magnesium sulfate, none suffered seizures, as compared with 10 of 1089 that were treated with phenytoin. The therapeutic effect of magnesium sulfate is most likely multifactorial, including both an action on *N*-methyl-D-aspartate (NMDA) receptors as well as reversal of vasoconstriction and edema (Euser and Cipolla 2009). Some patients do not respond to magnesium sulfate, and may require more intense anticonvulsive treatment, including anesthesia. Prophylactic treatment with new antiepileptic drugs has not been systematically investigated. Hypertension does not respond to magnesium sulfate and needs separate treatment. Permanent treatment of the eclamptic condition is by termination of pregnancy.

Cerebral autosomal dominant arteriopathy with subcortical infarcts and leukoencephalopathy (CADASIL)

This disease is an inherited angiopathy caused by mutations of the NOCTCH3 gene and characterized by subcortical ischemic lesions. In western Scotland, the prevalence of genetically proven CADASIL was 1.98 per 100 000 with a mutation prevalence of 4.14 per 100 000 (Razvi *et al.* 2005).

The mutations in the gene cause changes in the encoded NOTCH3 protein, which is essential for normal development and function of vascular muscle cells. The vascular abnormality predominates in subcortical white matter, but also occurs in other parts of the brain and in other organs. The characteristic finding is thickening of arteriolar walls with granular material within the media, sparing the endothelium. In an analysis of 105 published cases with a mean age of symptom onset of 36.7 years, stroke and transient ischemic attacks were the initial symptoms in 45 patients, and migraine in 42 patients (Desmond *et al.* 1999). Occurrence of seizures was the initial symptom in three patients, and a total of six patients had subsequent seizures. Mood disturbance and cognitive impairment can occur in both early and late phases of the disease, and dementia associated with apathy is found in one-third of patients (Buffon *et al.* 2006).

Seizures may be the initial symptom or occur in the course of the condition, with a frequency of 5–10% of all cases. The seizures can be generalized or focal.

Cerebral MRI may show characteristic bilateral changes in subcortical areas. Skin biopsy and immunostaining with a NOTCH3 antibody and genetic testing for mutations are more specific tests.

No studies have specifically investigated the treatment of epilepsy caused by the CADASIL ischemic lesions, and the principles of treatment are no different from those of other post-strokes epilepsies. There is no specific treatment for the CADASIL to date, and the use of antiplatelet drugs and anti-coagulants may increase the risk of intracerebral hemorrhage. This may influence the choice of antiepileptic therapy.

Cerebral venous thrombosis

Thrombosis of the cerebral venous system is less common than in the arterial system. The incidence ranges from 3–4 cases per million in adults, and up to 7 cases per million in children (Stam 2005). It is more common in women due to the association with pregnancy and oral contraceptives, and the incidence is particularly high peri- and postpartum.

Hypercoagulability, dehydration, inflammation, hematologic conditions, compression by tumors, and low cerebrospinal fluid pressure are other predisposing factors. The thrombosis may occur in various cerebral veins and venous sinuses. The obstruction is usually not complete initially and collateral flow may also help to reduce the initial consequences. This probably explains why the onset of symptoms is often gradual, and in some cases progresses over months. When the obstruction becomes more developed, the venous pressure, and, consequentially the intracerebral pressure, increases, causing edema, venous infarction, and hemorrhage.

Headache is the most common symptom, and may be the only early symptom, and has been reported in about 90% of patients. Focal neurological symptoms and altered consciousness are also common and are related to the part of the brain that is most affected.

Seizures are common, and in the largest follow-up study of 624 patients they occurred before the diagnosis was made in 40% (Ferro et al. 2008). These seizures were focal in 9% of patients, generalized in 20%, and of both types in 10%. Seizures as a presenting symptom were strongly associated with supratentorial lesions. In 7% of patients, seizures occurred within 2 weeks of diagnosis. These findings support the prophylactic use of antiepileptic drugs in patients with cerebral venous thrombosis supratentorial lesions.

Cerebral computed tomography (CT) may show edema and venous infarcts, which can be hemorrhagic. The CT venogram may demonstrate contrast surrounding the thrombus (the delta sign). Cerebral MRI will show the thrombotic part of the vein on T2-weighted images, and MR venography (MRV) may demonstrate the disturbance of circulation. With the advent of reliable MRV, conventional angiography is now used less commonly, but can also demonstrate the obstruction in circulation.

As soon as the diagnosis has been established, anticoagulation should be considered. Heparin is accepted as the first choice (Bousser and Ferro 2007), but cerebral hemorrhage may be a contraindication. After the initial treatment, warfarin should be continued for at least 3 months, or lifelong, depending upon the underlying cause of the condition. There have been case reports of successful treatment with thrombolysis and mechanical removal of the thrombus. The seizures should be treated in a standard way, considering the necessity for intravenous infusion, and possible interactions with other drugs being used should also be considered.

The antiphospholipid syndrome

This autoimmune state, characterized by the presence of antiphospholipid antibodies, may cause thrombosis both in arteries and in veins. The syndrome is classified as primary when it occurs alone and secondary when it is associated with other diseases, most commonly systemic lupus erythematosus. The international classification criteria include thrombosis or fetal losses, together with the presence of lupus anticoagulant, anti-cardiolipin, and anti-beta-2-glycoprotein antibodies on two occasions 12 weeks apart (Miyakis et al. 2006). The incidence of primary antiphospholipid syndrome is unknown.

The antibodies of the antiphospholipid syndrome are heterogeneous and probably exert their prothrombotic effects through different mechanisms. Infections and immunization may trigger the syndrome by inducing the production of antibodies (Gharavi and Pierangeli 1998). Antibodies from patients produced a dose-dependent effect on aggregation of human platelets when investigated in vitro (Campbell et al. 1995). To explain the localized thrombosis, the possibility exists that this occurs when a second factor, such as infection or injury, triggers the clotting.

Thrombotic stroke may occur in any cerebral artery. Young age, female gender, a history of fetal loss, and the presence of an immunological disorder are associated with the antiphospholipid syndrome. Stroke may also be secondary to cardiac valvular lesions. Cerebral venous thrombosis also occurs. Transient global amnesia has been reported. Ischemia occurs in ocular arteries causing visual manifestations, and hearing loss is probably also related to vascular occlusions. An association between antiphospholipid antibodies and cognitive deficits has also been reported (Jacobsen et al. 1999).

Epilepsy is associated with the presence of stroke, and there is probably also a primary effect of antibodies on brain cells. Sneddon syndrome, which is a combination of livedo reticularis and cerebral ischemic lesions, has been associated with antiphospholipid syndrome (Frances et al. 1999). Epilepsy is more common in this syndrome than in other conditions with cerebral infarction.

The presence of the antibodies included in the definition (see above) is the most important diagnostic test. This laboratory finding, together with the occurrence of recurrent thrombotic episodes and fetal losses, strongly support the diagnosis. Cerebral MRI may show hyperintensities and infarction but these changes, as with other neurological symptoms and signs, are non-specific.

Anticoagulation or antiplatelet aggregation both seem to be effective in protection against new thrombotic episodes. In addition, the underlying disorder, if identified, may be treated. Catastrophic antiphospholipid syndrome must be treated with intravenous immunoglobulin (IGG) or plasma exchange.

Cerebral amyloid angiopathy

The common feature of the amyloid angiopathies is deposition of amyloid in cerebral arteries and veins. Beta-amyloid and cystatin C are the two most common amyloids. Both sporadic and hereditary cases occur. The frequency of sporadic cerebral amyloid angiopathy increases with age, and is a cause of lobar hemorrhage, with an estimated incidence of about 10 per 100 000 in persons older than 70 years (Schütz et al. 1990). Dementia is frequent. The prevalence of amyloid deposits is even higher in Alzheimer disease, but the type of amyloid found in vessels differs from that in senile plaques. The relationship between the angiopathy and Alzheimer disease is currently unresolved.

The beta-amyloid is a part and product of the larger amyloid precursor protein that has several isoforms. Some forms of beta-amyloid tend to accumulate in vessels (Hendricks et al. 1992). Cystatin C may colocalize. The deposit gradually changes the wall of the vessels and occlusion may occur. Hereditary amyloid angiopathies are autosomal dominant diseases caused by specific mutations in the amyloid precursor protein (APP) gene on chromosome 21. (The hereditary cystatin amyloid angiopathy is related to changes in the cystatin gene on chromosome 20.) The amyloid angiopathy is associated with inflammation.

The common clinical presentation of both sporadic and hereditary amyloid angiopathy is recurrent intracranial hemorrhages in the temporal and occipital regions. In addition, the cerebral ischemia probably contributes to the leukoencephalopathy. Small infarcts are frequent and may be responsible for the dementia, but this may also be caused by changes similar to those seen in Alzheimer disease.

Seizures related to the lobar hemorrhages are common. As bleeding often occurs in temporal lobes, many seizures are typical for those arising in this part of the brain. In familial oculoleptomeningeal amyloidosis, seizures are common, probably due to involvement of superficial cortical areas (Goren et al. 1980).

There are no specific tests in sporadic cases, although rectal biopsy may be helpful. The demonstration of small hemorrhages and leukoencephalopathy support the diagnosis. In hereditary cases, genetic testing may help in diagnosing the disease.

There is currently no specific treatment of the amyloid deposition. Anticoagulation and antiplatelet aggregation drugs may increase the tendency for bleeding. The hypertension should be treated and surgery for the lobar hematomas should be avoided.

Reversible posterior leukoencephalopathy syndrome/reversible cerebral vasoconstriction syndrome/hypertensive encephalopathy

A reversible vasoconstriction probably represents the common pathophysiology of these conditions, known by different names but characterized by bilateral hypoperfusion in medium-sized cerebral arteries, most often in the posterior circulation (Calabrese et al. 2007). Pregnancy/puerperium, legal and illegal drugs, head trauma, and migraine are included among those features that have been associated with these conditions. Hypertension seems to be a common factor in many cases (Pavlakis et al. 1999).

Reversible posterior leukoencephalopathy

In reversible posterior leukoencephalopathy, the most common symptoms are headache, seizures, and visual loss, in addition to mental abnormalities (Hinchey et al. 1996). Edema in the parieto-occipital regions is the characteristic finding on MRI. In addition to antihypertensives, immunosuppressive drugs may be useful and have a particular effect on the blood–brain barrier. Complications occur, and reversibility is normal; however, some patients may experience permanent deficits (Stott et al. 2005). The generalized seizures are probably caused by the edema and have a good prognosis. Post-stroke seizures may occur.

Reversible cerebral vasoconstriction

Reversible cerebral vasoconstriction, also called "thunderclap headache associated vasospasm," "benign angiopathy," and "reversible angiitis," is diagnosed by the demonstration by angiography of a reversible constriction of arteries. The exact mechanism for the vasoconstriction is unknown, but vasospasm induced by chemical or neurogenic effects may be crucial. It seems less likely that inflammation is involved, but a hormonal influence is probable in women.

A severe and subacute headache, often occipital, nausea, and photophobia are common at the onset. Generalized seizures and symptoms caused by local ischemia may occur. An emotional factor often seems to be an initiating factor. The symptoms usually resolve within a few days. In a recent study, the syndrome was secondary to one risk factor in 63% of patients, and idiopathic in 37% (Ducros et al. 2007). Women are affected more often than men. The condition usually has a benign prognosis, but brain infarcts and hemorrhages and brain edema may occur.

The demonstration of a reversible cerebral vasoconstriction and/or edema proves the diagnosis of these syndromes. Most important is the exclusion of other conditions which may also start abruptly with headache and neurological symptoms. Cerebral CT/MRI, followed by a non-invasive angiography and examination of cerebrospinal fluid, are essential investigations. These overlapping syndromes are probably caused by a variety of risk factors that have one, or a few, common effect(s) on cerebral vessels.

There is no specific treatment, but it is important to discontinue all drugs that may have been involved in the development of the syndrome, treat hypertension, and, if necessary, give anticonvulsants. It is important to optimize the cerebral circulation, but avoid both hypertension and hypotension. If an angiitis cannot be excluded, steroids can be given. Some patients need a more intensive treatment and permanent deficits can occur.

Ehler–Danlos syndrome

Ehler–Danlos syndrome is the name for a group of connective tissue disorders with different genetic and clinical features. The common features are hyperelastic skin and hyperextensible joints. Type IV of the syndrome has a defect in type III procollagen, resulting in an abnormal structure of vessel tissue. Type IV occurs in 1 in 50 000–500 000 individuals and is associated with cerebrovascular events (Byers 1995). Other types of the syndrome have been associated with brain abnormalities, including heterotopias, polymicrogyria, and epilepsy (Cupo et al. 1981; Jacome 1999; Echaniz-Laguna et al. 2000).

The fragile tissue of cerebral vessels in type IV can explain the association with intracranial aneurysm, carotid–cavernous fistula, and arterial dissection. Strokes (or local pressure effects) related to these complications can cause epilepsy. The failure in normal synthesis of collagen and/or tenascin also has implications for neuronal growth and differentiation, which may explain the associated heterotopias and polymicrogyria which can also cause epilepsy (Echaniz-Laguna et al. 2000) (see Chapters 48 and 49). In these syndromes, the clinical neurological features are therefore sometimes due to the underlying genetic defect in addition to the secondary cerebrovascular complications. The abnormal neuronal development is probably the cause of the neurological symptoms and signs, and the epilepsy, which occurs in early infancy.

The seizures reported have been both partial and generalized. The EEG may interictally be normal and prolonged EEG recording may be necessary to explore episodic events in patients (Jacome 1999).

The diagnosis can be made from the characteristic skin and joint features, and the history of vascular lesions. In type IV, the demonstration of defect collagen III proves the diagnosis. The vascular complications are diagnosed by MRI and MRI angiography. The MRI images also demonstrate cortical dysplasia.

The fragility of vessels makes ordinary surgery difficult and dangerous, and invasive angiography may also lead to dissections of the artery. Endovascular embolization has been performed for cavernous fistulas.

Marfan syndrome

This heritable connective tissue disorder, with a prevalence of 1 in 5000–10 000, is caused by mutations in the *FBN1* gene which codes for fibrillin. The characteristic features of the span exceeding the height and of the high arched palate are only part of the multiple organ defects including cardiovascular abnormalities.

The abnormal fibrillin, and also defects induced by other mutations (Mizuguchi et al. 2004), are probably the basis for the disturbed organ development. Skeletal malformations including long limbs, scoliosis, and atlantoaxial translation, lens dislocation, dissection of aorta, cardiac valve lesions and abnormal rhythmicity, cerebral aneurysms, mental retardation, lumbosacral dural ectasia, high arched palate, and skin changes are manifestations occurring in many patients. Embolism from cardiovascular abnormalities and cerebral aneurysms are probably the cause of the epilepsy reported in some patients (Chu 1983), but the basic protein defects may also play a role in causing neuronal dysfunction.

Both focal and generalized seizures have been reported but no data exist on their incidence. There have been case reports of recurrent complex partial status and myoclonus (Ambrosetto et al. 1988) and petit mal absence seizures (Goenka and Metha 1999).

A single diagnostic test has not yet been developed. The clinical features and demonstration of the characteristic organ abnormalities in a patient with a family history are crucial. Phenotypic variation and absence of heredity in many cases adds further to the diagnostic difficulties.

Prognosis and survival rate can be improved by careful follow-up and protective treatments. Cardiovascular surgery may be necessary, and beta-blockers can reduce vascular stress.

Isolated cerebral angiitis

Different names have been used to describe isolated angiitis, illustrating the difficulty in identifying this rare disorder that has an estimated incidence of 1 per 2 000 000 (Moore 1999). One of the names of this disorder, giant cell granulomatous angiitis, reflects the characteristic finding of granulomas in samples from many patients, but this may be a late phenomenon in the inflammatory process (Hankey 1991). The angiitis is probably an inflammatory reaction caused by a variety of disorders, such as infections, but also cerebral amyloid angiopathy (Calabrese et al. 1997).

The inflammatory reaction involves small arteries, and sometimes veins, in the leptomeningeal area, in all parts of the central nervous system. The narrowing of the arterial wall can be very restricted. Headaches, strokes, hemorrhages, seizures, and cranial neuropathies occur and disturbed consciousness and cognition have also been reported.

Epileptic seizures, which may be partial or generalized, occur in 30% of patients.

Angiography may show the characteristic multifocal stenoses, but normal findings have been reported in 50%

of patients due to the involvement of small-sized arteries (Zuber *et al.* 1999). Conventional angiography is still superior to MRI angiography in demonstrating the changes. Hyperintense vessels and leptomeningeal contrast enhancement may be seen by MRI. Slight inflammatory abnormalities can be found in the cerebrospinal fluid (Calabrese *et al.* 1997). The definitive diagnosis can often only be made by brain biopsy.

Combination of intravenous cyclophosphamide and corticosteroids is the most favorable therapy.

Takayasu arteritis

Takayasu disease/arteritis is a chronic arteritis of the aortic arch, with narrowing of the proximal part of the major branches. It is much more common in Asian populations and in women. In North America the incidence has been suggested to be 2.6 per 1 000 000 (Hall *et al.* 1985).

The chronic inflammation of unknown etiology gradually affects the major branches from the aorta and narrows the vessels, which finally become rigid tubes sometimes with aneurysms. The early generalized symptoms are usually related to the inflammation and the reduced circulation in extremities. Hypertension and embolism may cause intracerebral hemorrhages and infarctions.

As with other diseases with cerebrovascular complications, epilepsy can occur, but is probably not common. A recent case report illustrates the possible association between seizures and changes in the left common carotid artery in a 40-year-old man (Ioannides *et al.* 2009).

The main diagnostic features are MRI angiography of the aortic arch with the main branches, and inflammatory findings in blood samples.

Treatment of the arteritis includes corticosteroids, often in combination with other immunosupressive drugs. Vascular surgery may become necessary.

References

Ambrosetto G, Tinuper P, Tassinari CA (1988) Marfan's syndrome, recurrent complex partial status epilepticus and myoclonus: a case report. *Clin Electroencephalogr* **19**:33–6.

Andersgaard AB, Herbst A, Johansen M, *et al.* (2006) Eclampsia in Scandinavia: incidence, substandard care, and potentially preventable cases. *Acta Obstet Gynecol Scand* **85**:929–36.

Bousser MG, Ferro JM (2007) Cerebral venous thrombosis: an update. *Lancet Neurol* **6**:162–70.

Buffon F, Porcher R, Hernandez K, *et al.* (2006) Cognitive profile in CADASIL. *J Neurol Neurosurg Psychiatry* **77**:175–80.

Byers PH (1995) Ehlers–Danlos syndrome type IV: a genetic disorder in many guises. *J Invest Dermatol* **105**:311–13.

Calabrese LH, Dodick DW, Schwedt TJ, Singhal AB (2007) Narrative review: reversible cerebral vasoconstriction syndromes. *Ann Intern Med* **146**:34–44.

Calabrese LH, Duna GF, Lie JT (1997) Vasculitis in the central nervous system. *Arthritis Rheum* **40**:1189–201.

Campbell AL, Pierangeli SS, Wellhausen S, Harris EN (1995) Comparison of the effects of anticardiolipin antibodies from patients with the antiphospholipid syndrome and with syphilis on platelet activation and aggregation. *Thromb Haemost* **73**:529–34.

Caplan LP (ed.) (2008) *Uncommon Causes of Strokes* 2nd edn. Cambridge, UK: Cambridge University Press.

Chiu D, Sheddon P, Bratine P, Grotta JC (1998) Clinical features of moyamoya in the United States. *Stroke* **29**:1347–51.

Chu N-S (1983) Marfan's syndrome and epilepsy: report of two cases and review of the literature. *Epilepsia* **24**:49–55.

Cupo LN, Pyeritz RE, Olson JL, *et al.* (1981) Ehlers–Danlos syndrome with abnormal collagen fibrils, sinus of Valsalva aneurysms, myocardial infarction, panacinar emphysema and cerebral heterotopias. *Am J Med* **71**:1051–8.

Desmond DW, Moroney JT, Lynch T, *et al.* (1999) The natural history of CADASIL: a pooled analysis of previously published cases. *Stroke* **30**:1230–3.

Ducros A, Boukobza M, Porcher R, *et al.* (2007) The clinical and radiological spectrum of reversible cerebral vasoconstriction syndrome. *Brain* **130**:3091–101.

Echaniz-Laguna A, de Saint-Martin A, Lafontaine AL, *et al.* (2000) Bilateral focal polymicrogyria in Ehlers–Danlos syndrome. *Arch Neurol* **57**:123–7.

Euser AG, Cipolla MJ (2009) Magnesium sulfate for the treatment of eclampsia: a brief review. *Stroke* **40**:1169–75.

Ferro JM, Canhão P, Bousser MG, *et al.* (2008) Early seizures in cerebral vein and dural sinus thrombosis: risk factors and role of antiepileptics. *Stroke* **39**:1152–8.

Frances C, Papo T, Wechsler B, *et al.* (1999) Sneddon syndrome with or without antiphospholipid antibodies: a comparative study of 46 patients *Medicine (Baltimore)* **78**:209–19.

Gharavi AE, Pierangeli SS (1998) Origin of antiphospholipid antibodies: induction of aPL by viral peptides. *Lupus* **7**(Suppl2):52–4.

Goenka S, Mehta AV (1999) Petit mal seizure in a child with Marfan's syndrome. *Tenn Med* **92**:53–4.

Goren H, Steinberg MC, Farboody GH (1980) Familial oculoleptomeningeal amyloidosis. *Brain* **103**:473–95.

Hall S, Barr W, Lie JT, *et al.* (1985) Takayasu arteritis. *Medicine* **94**:89–99.

Han DW, Kwon OK, Byun BJ, *et al.* (2000) The Korean Society for Cerebrovascular Disease. A co-operative study: clinical characteristics of 334 Korean patients with moyamoya disease treated at neurosurgical institutes (1976–1994) *Acta Neurochirurg (Wien)* **142**:1263–73.

Hankey GJ (1991) Isolated angiitis/ angiopathy of the central nervous system. *Cerebrovasc Dis* **1**:2–15.

Hendriks L, van Duijn CM, Cras P, *et al.* (1992) Presenile dementia and cerebral hemorrhage linked to a mutation at codon 692 of the beta-amyloid precursor protein gene. *Nat Genet* **1**:218–21.

Hinchey J, Chaves C, Appignani B, *et al.* (1996) A reversible posterior leukoencephalopathy syndrome. *N Engl J Med* **334**:494–500.

Houkin K, Nakayama N, Kuroda S, *et al.* (2005) Novel magnetic resonance angiography stage grading for moyamoya disease. *Cerebrovasc Dis* **20**:347–54.

Ikeda K, Iwasaki Y, Kashihara H, *et al.* (2006) Adult moyamoya disease in the asymptomatic Japanese population. *J Clin Neurosci* **13**:334–8.

Ioannides MA, Eftychiou C, Georgiou GM, Nicolaides E (2009) Takayasus arteritis presenting as epileptic seizures: a case report and brief review of the literature. *Rheumatol Int* **29**:703–5.

Jacobson MW, Rapport LJ, Keenan PA, Coleman RD, Tietjen GE (1999) Neuropsychological deficits associated with antiphospholipid antibodies. *J Clin Exp Neuropsychol* **21**:252–64.

Jacome DE (1999) Epilepsy in Ehlers–Danlos syndrome. *Epilepsia* **40**:467–73.

Kikuta K, Takagi Y, Arakaa Y, Miyamoto S, Hashimoto N (2006) Absence epilepsy associated with moyamoya disease: case report. *J Neurosurg* **104**(Suppl 4):265–8.

Kuroda S (1995) Near-infrared monitoring of cerebral oxygenation during cerebral ischemia. *Hokkaido Igaku Zasshi* **70**:401–11. (In Japanese.)

Kuroda S, Houkin K (2008) Moyamoya disease: current concepts and future perspectives. *Lancet Neurol* **7**:1056–66.

Lossius MI, Rønning OM, Slapø GD, Mowinckel P, Gjerstad L (2005) Poststroke epilepsy: occurrence and predictors: a long-term prospective controlled study (Akershus Stroke Study). *Epilepsia* **46**:1246–51.

Lucas MJ, Leveno KJ, Cunningham FG (1995) A comparison of magnesium sulfate with phenytoin for the prevention of eclampsia. *N Engl J Med* **333**:201–5.

Miyakis S, Lockshin MD, Atsumi T, *et al.* (2006) International consensus statement on an update of the classification criteria for definite antiphospholipid syndrome (APS). *J Thromb Haemost* **4**:295–306.

Mizuguchi T, Collod-Beroud G, Akyiama T, *et al.* (2004) Heterozygous TGFBR2 mutations in Marfan syndrome. *Nat Genet* **36**:855–60.

Moore PM (1999) The vasculitides. *Curr Opin Neurol* **12**:383–8.

Pavlakis SG, Frank Y, Chusid R (1999) Hypertensive encephalopathy, reversible occipitoparietal encephalopathy, or reversible posterior leukoencephalopathy: three names for an old syndrome. *J Child Neurol* **14**:277–81.

Razvi SS, Davidson R, Bone I, Muir KW (2005) The prevalence of cerebral autosomal dominant arteriopathy with subcortical infarcts and leucoencephalopathy (CADASIL) in west of Scotland. *J Neurol Neurosurg Psychiatry* **76**:739–41.

Schütz H, Bödeker RH, Damian M, Krack P, Dorndorf W (1990) Age-related spontaneous intracerebral hematoma in a German community. *Stroke* **21**:1412–18.

Shah DM (2007) Preeclampsia: new insights. *Curr Opin Nephrol Hypertens* **16**:213–20.

Sibai BM (2005) Diagnosis, prevention, and management of eclampsia. *Obstet Gynecol* **105**:402–10.

Stam J (2005) Thrombosis of the cerebral veins and sinuses. *N Engl J Med* **28**:1791–8.

Stott VL, Hurrell MA, Anderson TJ (2005) Reversible posterior leukoencephalopathy syndrome: a misnomer reviewed. *Intern Med J* **35**:83–90.

Zuber M, Blustajn J, Arquizan C, *et al.* (1999) Angiitis of the central nervous system. *J Neuroradiol* **26**:101–17.

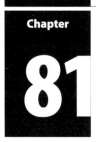

Chapter

Rasmussen encephalitis and related conditions

Antonio Gambardella and Frederick Andermann

Rasmussen encephalitis

Definition and epidemiology of Rasmussen encephalitis

In 1958, Theodore Rasmussen and co-workers at the Montreal Neurological Institute reported three patients suffering from severe focal seizures, accompanied by progressive hemiparesis and cognitive decline, in association with pathologic features of chronic encephalitis (Rasmussen *et al.* 1958). In the following years, most researchers and clinicians have adopted the term Rasmussen encephalitis (RE) for this condition characterized by chronic encephalitis and epilepsy (Andermann 1991). More recently, important new insights have added to our understanding of the pathophysiology, the diagnosis, and the management of this condition.

Rasmussen encephalitis is a rare, sporadic disease with no evidence for a genetic component (Andermann 1991). So far, no geographic, seasonal, or clustering effect has been detected; moreover there is no apparent increase in pre-existent febrile convulsions or immediately preceding viral illnesses (Antel and Rasmussen 1996).

Pathology

The histopathological properties of RE are non-specific and are suggestive of chronic multifocal encephalitis (Robitaille 1991). The affected hemisphere shows microglial nodules with or without neuronophagia, perivascular cuffs of small lymphocytes and monocytes, and gliosis, with destructive changes appearing first as laminar necrosis and later spongy degeneration. Four stages of the condition have been delineated that correspond to disease duration (Robitaille 1991). In the more active cases, there are numerous microglial nodules, with or without neuronophagia, accompanied by perivascular round cells and glial scarring. In later stages (groups 2 and 3), the smaller foci of inflammation tend to coalesce into larger areas of structural collapse, and there is associated neuronal loss and spongiosis in the inflamed cortex. Finally, latest cases showed no or few microglial nodules, neuronal loss and mild

perivascular inflammation, combined with various degrees of gliosis and glial scarring (Robitaille 1991). The round cell infiltrates in RE brains consist almost exclusively of T lymphocytes (Farrell *et al.* 1995). About 10% of children with RE have histologic evidence of a dual pathology that includes cortical dysplasia, low-grade tumor, tuberous sclerosis, vascular abnormalities, or old ischemic lesions in addition to typical findings (Hart *et al.* 1998).

Physiology

There has been much debate about the pathophysiology of RE, which still remains elusive. Rasmussen hypothesized a viral etiology, based on the constituents of the immune reaction in the brain such as lymphocyte infiltration and microglial nodules (Rasmussen *et al.* 1958). The viral hypothesis was further strengthened by the similarities that RE shares with Russian spring–summer meningoencephalitis, which is caused by a flavivirus (Asher and Gajdusek 1991) (see Chapter 75). Nonetheless, so far all attempts to identify a pathogenic viral agent have been contradictory and inconclusive, and a direct role of viruses in causing RE remains a matter of speculation.

Available data continue to suggest an immune basis to the pathogenesis of RE, with a role of both autoantibodies as well as cytotoxic T cells. A primary role for pathogenic antibodies in the etiology of RE was suggested by Rogers *et al.* (1994), who described seizure activity in rabbits that developed high titers of specific antibodies against subunit 3 of the ionotropic glutamate receptor (GluR3). Of greater interest, neuropathologic examinations in GRIA3-immunized rabbits revealed lesions similar to those seen in RE in humans. Subsequent studies in RE patients showed GluR3 antibodies, of whom one improved transiently after plasma exchange (Rogers *et al.* 1994). Other reports of temporary or longer-lasting improvement of the symptoms of RE by removal of antibodies from the circulation have subsequently been published (Andrews *et al.* 1996; Granata *et al.* 2003). Nonetheless, additional studies have illustrated that GluR antibodies are not present in all RE patients, and they are also found in patients with

The Causes of Epilepsy, eds. S. D. Shorvon, F. Andermann, and R. Guerrini. Published by Cambridge University Press. © Cambridge University Press 2011.

severe intractable epilepsy who do not have the clinical features of RE (Wiendl *et al.* 2001). Overall, the pathogenic role of elevated GluR3 autoantibodies in RE remains unclear, even though a humoral or complement-dependent pathogenesis (not necessarily mediated by GluR3 antibodies) probably contributes to the pathogenesis of RE.

In recent years, the focus of attention has shifted towards the role for autoimmune cytotoxic T lymphocytes early in the pathogenesis of RE (Farrell *et al.* 1995), by initiating an inflammatory process that progresses with the activation of astroglial and microglial cell populations and ultimately produces neuronal and cortical injury (Li *et al.* 1997; Bien *et al.* 2002a). Taken altogether, these data suggest that a cascade of events may occur in RE, with cytotoxic T cells playing a role at the onset of the disease by damaging neurons, and so realizing autoantigenic peptides which in turn generate an antibody response. What remains unknown, however, is the initiating event in this hypothetical cascade.

Since the brain involvement in RE is mainly unilateral, some other factors must contribute to the pathogenesis in order to cause unilaterality. One factor could be focal seizures per se, which might functionally damage both neurons and the blood–brain barrier and thus allow the access of antibodies, as well as the migration of immune cells mediating cellular and humeral immune responses back to the site of the initial injury. In analogy to other epileptic encephalopathies of childhood, it is also possible that the epileptic activity itself may contribute to the functional decline (Nabbout and Dulac 2003).

Clinical features

Rasmussen encephalitis usually starts in childhood, and its diagnosis is facilitated by the characteristic clinical picture of intractable focal epilepsy, epilepsia partialis continua (EPC), and other forms of status epilepticus, accompanied by progressive hemiparesis and cognitive decline that develops in association with obvious progressive loss of tissue involving one hemisphere (Rasmussen *et al.* 1958). The neurologic deficits can appear at any time between 3 months to a few years after the onset of seizures. The initial course of RE is one of relentless progression, but at a stage when moderate to severe neurologic deficits and cognitive decline have occurred, the disease eventually burns itself out (Bien *et al.* 2002b). The patient is left with significant neurologic morbidity. Death is rare. There is also a much more rare, early-onset variant of RE with an increased risk of bilateral disease. In these patients, there is no evidence of dual pathology; the course is malignant with a high risk of death (Andermann and Farrell 2006).

Although the onset of RE characteristically occurs in childhood, adolescent and adult patients have been increasingly recognized, and they account for about 10% of all cases of RE (Oguni *et al.* 1991; Hart *et al.* 1997; Villani *et al.* 2001). This adolescent/adult form of RE shares similar histopathological as well as clinical, electrophysiological, and neuroimaging findings with childhood RE (Hart *et al.* 1997; Bien *et al.* 2002b), even though it is usually less severe and tends to respond better to immunological treatment (Leach *et al.* 1999; Villani *et al.* 2001). Occipital onset to the seizures appears to be more common than in the childhood form, and bilateral disease may also occur (Hart *et al.* 1997).

More recently, a limited and relatively non-progressive form of RE has been emphasized (Gambardella *et al.* 2008), confirming Rasmussen's insightful suspicion of the existence of a more limited and less malignant form of the disorder. In such patients, the disease starts during early adolescence or adult life and may remain circumscribed, without the development of a marked fixed neurological deficit (although mild signs may be present) nor episodes of EPC or convulsive status epilepticus. A remarkable finding in some of these patients was the appearance of involuntary choreoathetotic movements, which could precede or follow the appearance of seizures. The presence of movement disorder in RE was also addressed by other authors and seems to correlate with atrophy of the caudate nucleus (Frucht 2002). Awareness of the possibility of movement disorder as a presenting symptom of RE is important because it may lead to some confusion in the diagnosis, especially in the less common adolescent or adult patients. The early atrophy of the caudate nuclei is an important marker of this diagnosis although not specific (Leach *et al.* 1999; Frucht 2002). In particular, the combination of movement disorder and focal epilepsy should arouse suspicion of RE.

Related conditions and differential diagnosis

The diagnosis of RE can usually be made clinically, although other conditions such as cortical dysplasia, tumor, cerebral vasculitis, and mitochondrial encephalopathy with lactic acidosis and stroke-like episodes (MELAS) need to be considered (for review see Bien *et al.* 2005). Moreover, clinical and laboratory features observed in RE, especially in those patients with a limited chronic focal form of RE, must be differentiated from those reported in VGKC-Ab-associated limbic encephalitis (Vincent *et al.* 2004). In the latter, the mean age at diagnosis is old age, and the typical presentation is with subacute onset of confusion, behavioral changes and psychosis, short-term memory loss, and seizures. The difference is also reflected by the normal level of VGKC antibodies in antibodies in RE patients (Gambardella *et al.* 2008).

Epilepsy in Rasmussen encephalitis

Although seen in adulthood, RE typically starts in childhood, between the ages of 14 months and 14 years, with an average age at disease manifestation of 6 years (Oguni *et al.* 1991). A European consensus has recently proposed three disease stages (Bien *et al.* 2005). At the onset, there may be a *prodromal phase* characterized by a relatively low seizure frequency and rarely mild hemiparesis with a median duration of 7.1 months (range: 0 months to 8.1 years). Following this, all patients enter an *acute stage* of the disease, although for one-third of cases, this appears to be the initial clinical disease manifestation. It is characterized by frequent seizures, with approximately one-fifth of patients presenting with generalized or focal status epilepticus. Focal motor seizures occur in the vast majority of patients during the course of the illness, frequently in the form of EPC. Todd paresis is common prior to the development of a fixed neurological deficit. In each patient, there may be a great heterogeneity of seizure semiologies, which is best explained as a march (of the epileptic focus) across the hemisphere (Oguni *et al.* 1991). The neurological deterioration becomes manifest by progressive hemiparesis, hemianopia, cognitive deterioration, and, if the language dominant hemisphere is affected, aphasia (Oguni *et al.* 1991). Exceptionally, progressive hemiparesis may precede seizures of several months (Korn-Lubetzki *et al.* 2004). It has been found that the mean duration of this acute stage is 8 months (range 4–8 months). The Montreal group (Rasmussen and Andermann 1991), however, suggested that the median duration of progressive neurological deterioration is about 3 years, ranging from a few months to several years. After that, the patients pass into the *residual stage* with permanent and stable neurological deficits and still many seizures, although less frequent than in the acute stage. Any significant improvement in the seizure disorder usually only occurs after the development of major neurological deficit, when the disease eventually burns itself out.

Treatment of the seizures themselves with standard antiepileptic medications, singly or in various combinations, has proved disappointing. No anticonvulsive mono-or combination-therapy has been described to be superior to other regimens (Andermann 1991). The mainstay of treatment of RE is functional hemispherectomy, which produces a remarkable decline in seizure burden and improves cognitive outcome, at the cost of postoperative hemiparesis with or without aphasia and visual field deficits (Bien *et al.* 2005).

Diagnostic tests

The diagnosis of RE can usually be made clinically, although the particular challenge is the early recognition of the disease. Ten years ago, formal diagnostic criteria for RE were proposed, which are still adequate in cases with EPC (Hart *et al.* 1994). More recently the European consortium (Bien *et al.* 2005) integrated such criteria and proposed a two-step approach to allow the diagnosis of RE at all stages (see Table 81.1). In these diagnostic criteria, at least two sequential clinical examinations or magnetic resonance imaging (MRI) studies are required to meet the criteria of progression of a neurological deficit, or the hematrophy over time on MRI (Bien *et al.* 2005). It was also addressed that, when brain biopsy is not performed, MRI with administration of gadolinium and cranial computed

Table 81.1 *Diagnostic criteria for Rasmussen encephalitis.* Rasmussen encephalitis can be diagnosed if either all three criteria of Part A or two out of three criteria of Part B are present. Check first for the features of Part A; then, if these are not fulfilled, check Part B

Part A		
(1) Clinical	Focal seizures (with or without epilepsia partialis continua) and unilateral cortical deficit(s)	
(2) EEG	Unihemispheric slowing with or without epileptiform activity and unilateral seizure onset	
(3) MRI	Unihemispheric focal cortical atrophy and at least one of the following:	
	Gray or white matter T2-weighted/FLAIR hyperintense signal	
	Hyperintense signal or atrophy of the ipsilateral caudate head	
Part B		
(1) Clinical	Epilepsia partialis continua or progressive unilateral cortical deficit(s)	
(2) MRI	Progressive unihemispheric focal cortical atrophy	
(3) Histopathology	T-cell-dominated encephalitis with activated microglial cells (typically, but not necessarily forming nodules) and reactive astrogliosis	
	Numerous parenchymal macrophages, B cells or plasma cells or viral inclusion bodies exclude the diagnosis of RE	

Source: From the European Consortium (Bien *et al.* 2005).

tomography (CT) needs to be performed to document the absence of gadolinium enhancement and calcifications to rule out a unihemispheric vasculitis (Bien *et al.* 2005).

Electroencephalography

In the vast majority of patients, very early after disease onset, the electroencephalogram (EEG) shows an impairment of background activity and sleep spindles, which predominates over the affected hemisphere, although it is usually bilateral (So and Gloor 1991). Interictal epileptiform discharges occur in most patients, most commonly multiple independent foci lateralized over one hemisphere. Ictal patterns are almost always strictly ipsilateral to the affected hemisphere (So and Gloor 1991). In cases with the secure diagnosis of RE, the documentation of an independent contralateral seizure onset may raise the suspicion of bilateral disease.

Neuroimaging

Magnetic resonance imaging of the brain shows progressive hematrophy of variable degree in the involved cerebral

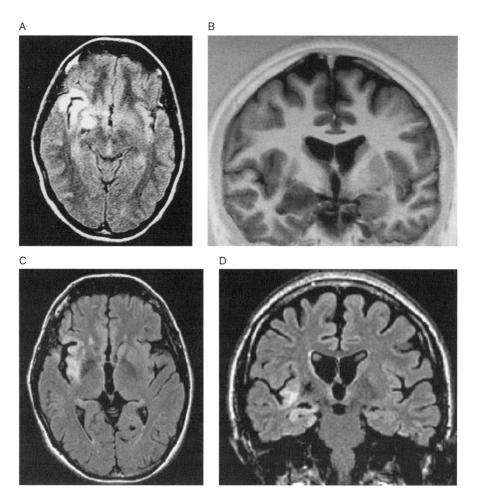

Fig. 81.1. Brain magnetic resonance imaging (MRI) scan of a 36-year-old woman with Rasmussen encephalitis. (A) Axial fluid-attenuated inversion recovery (FLAIR) images showed an increased signal without swelling of the right temporal insular structures and of the right caudate nucleus. (B) Coronal inversion recovery images revealed a moderate atrophy of the head of the right caudate nucleus and the corpus striatum with a mild dilatation of the horn of the right lateral ventricle. (C, D) After 5 months, there was a similar increased signal of the right temporal insular structures on axial and coronal FLAIR images. In comparison with the previous MRI, it was evident a marked dilatation of the sylvian fissure and temporal horn, and a much increased atrophy of the head of the right caudate nucleus and the corpus striatum with dilatation of the horn of the right lateral ventricle. There was also a hypointense signal within the head of the right caudate nucleus.

hemisphere (Fig. 81.1). In the early stages of RE, cerebral atrophy may be apparent only in the temporoinsular area, with enlargement of the temporal horn and sylvian fissure, and subsequent spread to involve the rest of the hemisphere. In addition to these changes, there is an abnormal cortical or subcortical (or both) hyperintense signal in the T2-weighted and fluid-attenuated inversion recovery (FLAIR) images (Fig. 81.1C, D). A transient focal cortical swelling on early scans with subsequent spread of signal changes and atrophy within the affected hemispheres may occasionally occur. Totally normal findings on very early scans have been reported, but are rare (Geller *et al.* 1998; Lee *et al.* 2001). Gadolinium enhancement is very rare in RE (Bien *et al.* 2005).

Fluorodeoxyglucose positron emission tomography (PET) studies showed large areas of hypometabolism which were confined to the affected hemisphere. In early stages these abnormalities were confined to frontotemporal areas, while in later stages, they extended to posterior cortical regions (Lee *et al.* 2001). Similar changes were seen using single photon emission computed tomography (SPECT) (Leach *et al.* 1999). Magnetic resonance spectroscopy studies consistently showed decreased N-acetyl-aspartate (NAA) levels and increased (or normal) choline (cho) peaks resulting in a decreased NAA/cho ratio suggestive of neuronal loss or dysfunction (Matthews *et al.* 1990). Partly observed increased lactate peaks seemed to be associated with the presence of EPC (Matthews *et al.* 1990).

Laboratory tests

No laboratory test is available to positively support the diagnosis of RE (Fig. 81.2). In about half of the cerebrospinal fluid (CSF) examinations that were carried out in a group of 51 patients with RE, cell counts and protein levels were in the normal range. In the remainder, elevated cell counts (16–70 cells/mL, predominantly lymphocytes), an increased protein content (50–100 mg/dL) or a first or midzone elevation of the colloidal gold curve were observed. In only 15% of the abnormal CSF tests, all three parameters were abnormal (Andermann 1991). Oligoclonal bands seem to be an inconsistent finding (Andermann 1991). Overall, either a normal or abnormal CSF examination does not enable one to exclude or confirm the diagnosis of RE. Serological CSF tests are usually applied to rule out a CNS infection by known neurotropic agents.

Brain biopsy is usually not required in RE because there are valuable criteria that may allow the correct diagnosis of the condition (see Table 81.1). In uncertain cases, brain biopsy can contribute considerably to diagnostic certainty. Since

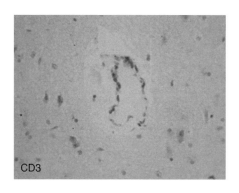
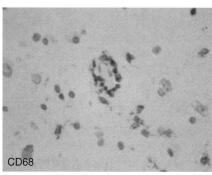

Fig. 81.2. Immunohistochemical study in a 31-year-old right-handed woman with RE. Immunohistochemistry showing sparse perivascular collection T cells (CD3 immunohistochemistry) and macrophages/microglia (CD68), which were also seen away from the blood wall. These changes are suggestive of RE. See color plate section.

abnormal and normal tissue elements may be located in very close apposition (Robitaille 1991), to avoid false-negative results an open biopsy comprising meninges and gray and white matter is preferable. There is evidence, indeed, that more limited surgical tissue collection, especially stereotactic procedures, increases the risk of false-negative results in an unacceptable manner (Bien *et al.* 2005).

Principles of management

No known treatment has been shown to have a long-term effect sufficient to obviate the need for surgery, and the difficult decision of whether to delay hemispherectomy until hemiparesis has already developed (Andermann 1991), perhaps allowing more time for trials of medical treatment, or to operate early in the hope of preventing intellectual decline, is still matter of a great debate. An early surgery seems to be favored in view of the progressive neurologic devastation and dementia that may directly result from the catastrophic epilepsy. Early surgery in young children may also improve chances of the transfer of neurologic function to the good hemisphere, especially when speech is at stake because of involvement of the dominant hemisphere.

Hemispherectomy and its modern variants (HE) (Villemure *et al.* 1997) controls seizures in most RE patients, with a seizure freedom rate ranging between 62.5% and 85% (Bien *et al.* 2005). The late complications of the early surgical techniques, including superficial hemosiderosis and hydrocephalus, have been largely overcome by the introduction of disconnective procedures such as functional hemispherectomy and hemispherotomy (Villemure 1997). After HE, patients will have a spastic hemiplegia of the contralateral side with loss of the (functionally highly relevant) fine

motor hand movements. However, only a minority of patients are unable to walk without the use of assistive devices. On the other hand, the improvement in seizure control is usually accompanied by improvement in behavior and sometimes in cognitive performances. Another inevitable consequence of HE is a homonymous hemianopia to the contralateral side, but even this consequence is tolerable because it does not interfere with the patient's overall functioning (Villemure *et al.* 1997). Although concern remains about left hemispherectomy in patients developing seizures after early childhood, there is good evidence that language recovery may occur after left hemispherectomy in children with late-onset seizures.

Immunosuppressive, immunomodulatory, and antiviral treatment approaches against the proposed mechanisms of RE have been applied, and the following regimens have been recently recommended (Bien *et al.* 2005): (1) corticosteroids; (2) intravenous immunoglobulins (IVIG); (3) corticosteroids plus IVIG; (4) plasmapheresis or protein A IgG immunoadsorption (PAI); and (5) tacrolimus. Overall these medical treatments of RE have remained unsatisfactory. It seems fairly clear that immune modulating agents such as IVIG, or plasmapheresis, as well as steroids tend to modify the course. This results in much less tissue loss, which at times is difficult to demonstrate. There is also no or considerably less hemiparesis and there are fewer other focal clinical features. The paucity of these changes renders a surgical decision much more difficult. The endpoint of the disease does not appear to be modified by current treatments. Further trials of immune modification should hopefully result in a better prognosis of this dreadful disease, as Theodore Rasmussen described it.

References

Andermann F (ed.) (1991). *Chronic Encephalitis and Epilepsy: Rasmussen's Syndrome*. Boston, MA: Butterworth-Heinemann.

Andermann F, Farrell K (2006) Early onset Rasmussen's syndrome: a malignant often bilateral form of the disorder. *Epilepsy Res* 70(Suppl): S259–62.

Andrews PI, Dichter MA, Berkovic SF, Newton MR, McNamara JO (1996) Plasmaphcrcsis in Rasmussen's encephalitis. *Neurology* 46:242–6.

Antel JP, Rasmussen T (1996) Rasmussen's encephalitis and the new hat. *Neurology* 46:9–11.

Asher DM, Gajdusek DC (1991) Virologic studies in chronic encephalitis. In:

Andermann F (ed.) *Chronic Encephalitis and Epilepsy: Rasmussen's Syndrome*. Boston, MA: Butterworth-Heineman pp. 147–58.

Bien CG, Bauer J, Deckwerth TL, *et al.* (2002a) Destruction of neurons by cytotoxic T cells: a new pathogenic mechanism in Rasmussen's encephalitis. *Ann Neurol* 51:311–18.

Bien CG, Widman G, Urbach H, *et al.* (2002b) The natural history of Rasmussen's encephalitis. *Brain* 125:1751–9.

Bien CG, Granata T, Antozzi C, *et al.* (2005) Pathogenesis, diagnosis and treatment of Rasmussen encephalitis: a European consensus statement. *Brain* 128:454–71.

Farrell MA, Droogan O, Secor DL, *et al.* (1995) Chronic encephalitis associated with epilepsy: immunohistochemical and ultrastructural studies. *Acta Neuropathol Berl* 89:313–21.

Frucht S (2002) Dystonia, athetosis, and epilepsia partialis continua in a patient with late-onset Rasmussen's encephalitis. *Mov Disord* 17:609–12.

Gambardella A, Andermann F, Shorvon S, Le Piane E, Aguglia U (2008) Limited chronic focal encephalitis: another variant of Rasmussen syndrome? *Neurology* 70:374–7.

Geller E, Faerber EN, Legido A, *et al.* (1998) Rasmussen encephalitis: complementary role of multitechnique neuroimaging. *AJNR Am J Neuroradiol* 19:445–9.

Granata T, Fusco L, Gobbi G, *et al.* (2003) Experience with immunomodulatory treatments in Rasmussen's encephalitis. *Neurology* 61:1807–10.

Hart YM, Cortez M, Andermann F, *et al.* (1994) Medical treatment of Rasmussen's syndrome (chronic encephalitis and epilepsy): effect of high-dose steroids or immunoglobulins in 19 patients. *Neurology* 44:1030–6.

Hart YM, Andermann F, Fish DR, *et al.* (1997) Chronic encephalitis and epilepsy in adults and adolescents: a variant of Rasmussen's syndrome? *Neurology* 48:418–24.

Hart YM, Andermann F, Robitaille Y, *et al.* (1998) Double pathology in Rasmussen's syndrome: a window on the etiology? *Neurology* 50:731–5.

Korn-Lubetzki I, Bien CG, Bauer J, *et al.* (2004) Rasmussen encephalitis with active inflammation and delayed seizure onset. *Neurology* 62:984–6.

Leach JP, Chadwick DW, Miles JB, Hart IK (1999) Improvement in adult-onset Rasmussen's encephalitis with long-term immunomodulatory therapy. *Neurology* 52:738–42.

Lee JS, Juhasz C, Kaddurah AK, Chugani HT (2001) Patterns of cerebral glucose metabolism in early and late stages of Rasmussen's syndrome. *J Child Neurol* 16:798–805.

Li Y, Uccelli A, Laxer KD, *et al.* (1997) Local-clonal expansion of infiltrating T lymphocytes in chronic encephalitis of Rasmussen. *J Immunol* 158:1428–37.

Matthews PM, Andermann F, Arnold DL (1990) A proton magnetic resonance spectroscopy study of focal epilepsy in humans. *Neurology* 40:985–9.

Nabbout R, Dulac O (2003) Epileptic encephalopathies: a brief overview. *J Clin Neurophysiol* 20:393–7.

Oguni H, Andermann F, Rasmussen TB (1991) The natural history of the syndrome of chronic encephalitis and epilepsy: a study of the MNI series of fortyeight cases. In: Andermann F (ed.) *Chronic Encephalitis and Epilepsy: Rasmussen's Syndrome.* Boston, MA: Butterworth-Heinemann, pp. 7–35.

Rasmussen T, Andermann F (1991) Rasmussen' syndrome: symptomatology of the syndrome of chronic encephalitis and seizures: 35-year experience with 51 cases. In: Lüders H (ed.) *Epilepsy Surgery.* New York: Raven Press, pp. 173–8.

Rasmussen T, Olszewski J, Lloyd-Smith D (1958) Focal seizures due to chronic localized encephalitis. *Neurology* 8:435–45.

Robitaille Y (1991) Neuropathologic aspects of chronic encephalitis. In: Andermann F (ed.) *Chronic Encephalitis and Epilepsy: Rasmussen's Syndrome.* Boston, MA: Butterworth-Heinemann, pp. 79–110.

Rogers SW, Andrews PI, Gahring LC, *et al.* (1994) Autoantibodies to glutamate receptor GluR3 in Rasmussen's encephalitis. *Science* 265:648–51.

So N, Gloor P (1991) Electroencephalographic and electrocorticographic findings in chronic encephalitis of the Rasmussen type. In: Andermann F (ed.) *Chronic Encephalitis and Epilepsy: Rasmussen's Syndrome.* Boston, MA: Butterworth-Heinemann, pp. 37–45.

Villani F, Spreafico R, Farina L, *et al.* (2001) Positive response to immunomodulatory therapy in an adult patient with Rasmussen's encephalitis. *Neurology* 56:248–50.

Villemure J-G (1997) Hemispherectomy techniques: a critical review. In: Tuxhorn I, Holthausen H, Boenigk H (eds.) *Pediatric Epilepsy Syndromes and their Surgical Treatment.* London: John Libbey, pp. 729–38.

Vincent A, Buckley C, Schott JM, *et al.* (2004) Potassium channel antibody-associated encephalopathy: a potentially immunotherapy-responsive form of limbic encephalitis. *Brain* 127:701–12.

Wiendl H, Bien CG, Bernasconi P, *et al.* (2001) GluR3 antibodies: prevalence in focal epilepsy but no specificity for Rasmussen's encephalitis. *Neurology* 57:1511–14.

Chapter 82

Systemic lupus erythematosus and other collagen vascular diseases

Rolando Cimaz and Andrea Taddio

Introduction: the causal diseases

Definitions and epidemiology

Systemic lupus erythematosus (SLE) is a prototypic auto-immune disease with variable clinical manifestations, characterized by widespread inflammation of blood vessels and connective tissue. The presence of antinuclear antibodies (ANA), especially antibodies to native (double-stranded) DNA (dsDNA) is characteristic. It is a rare disease with an incidence among adults of 2.0 per 100 000 per year; few studies on children estimate an annual incidence between 0.36 and 0.6 per 100 000 with a higher rate in girls.

The term vasculitis indicates the presence of inflammation in a blood vessel wall. It includes a number of diseases which can be classified by the size of the vessels affected as: large-vessel vasculitis (giant cell arteritis, Takayasu's arteritis), medium-vessel vasculitis (polyarteritis nodosa; Kawasaki disease), and small-vessel vasculitis (Wegener granulomatosis, Churg–Strauss syndrome, microscopic polyangiitis, Henoch-Schönlein purpura, cryoglobulinemic vasculitis, cutaneous leukocytoclastic angiitis).

Scleroderma is a disorder characterized by an excessive accumulation of collagen in the skin and can be subdivided into localized and systemic forms. It is quite a rare disease with an incidence of 2.7 cases per 100 000 per year. Its pathogenesis is still unknown but dysfunction of the immune system plays a prominent role. Some authors consider the endothelial cell injury the central pathogenic event; endothelial cells and fibroblasts may present integrines on their surface facilitating mononuclear cell damage. Moreover an increased number of collagen-producing fibroblasts and a defect in the regulation of genes controlling apoptosis of fibroblasts have been reported.

Pathology, physiology, and clinical features

Systemic lupus erythematosus is the most common collagen vascular disease associated with epilepsy.

Except for drug-induced lupus, the etiology of SLE remains unknown. It is evident that SLE results from the interaction of both genetic and environmental factors. The end result is an immune dysregulation with the presence of autoreactive B and T lymphocytes causing several different clinical manifestations, many of which are antibody or immune complex mediated. Different pathogenic mechanisms may predominate in different aspects of the disease. Systemic lupus erythematosus ranges from an insidious chronic illness with a long history of intermittent signs and symptoms to an acute rapidly fatal disease. A common clinical feature is the cutaneous involvement, with a broad range of manifestations varying from the classic "butterfly" rash to livedo reticularis and purpura, to discoid lesions, nodules, and alopecia as expression of chronic skin disease. Lupus nephritis is present in a large proportion of patients with SLE, and is a major determinant of long-term outcome together with central nervous system (CNS) disease involvement, which remains a major cause of morbidity and mortality. Neuropsychiatric manifestations during the disease comprise mostly mood and cognitive disorders, seizures, anxiety, peripheral neuropathy, cerebrovascular disease, and psychosis.

Other clinical manifestations include musculoskeletal disease (arthritis), mucosal involvement (oral and nasal septum ulcers), cardiac involvement (pericarditis, myocarditis, valvulitis), pleuropulmonary disease (pleural effusions, pulmonary hemorrhage), hematologic abnormalities (hemolytic anemia and thrombocytopenia), and gastrointestinal manifestations (e.g., pancreatitis, lupoid hepatitis).

Characteristically associated with SLE is antiphospholipid syndrome (APS). Diagnosis requires the presence of venous or arterial vascular thrombosis and the presence of antibodies directed against β_2-glycoprotein I-dependent phospholipids (such as anticardiolipin antibodies or lupus anticoagulant).

Since neurologic symptoms of SLE may have multiple causes, it is difficult to obtain precise prevalence figures for seizures. However, seizures are listed first on SLE activity indexes, which indicates their relevance.

The Causes of Epilepsy, eds. S. D. Shorvon, F. Andermann, and R. Guerrini. Published by Cambridge University Press. © Cambridge University Press 2011.

Various autoantibodies have also been implicated in the pathogenesis of neuropsychiatric SLE. Anti-ribosomal P antibodies have been first described as a good marker of CNS involvement, in particular of psychosis and depression, in SLE patients; however elevated levels are frequently seen in patients without CNS involvement, therefore their real utility remains controversial (Brey 2007). Their determination could be helpful only in differentiating an SLE-associated psychosis from other forms of psychosis when few other clinical manifestations of SLE are present.

Other brain-specific and antineuronal antibodies, such as anti-NR2 glutamate receptor antibodies and anti-N-methyl-D-aspartate (NMDA) receptor antibodies, have been demonstrated in patients with SLE, mostly associated with psychosis, depression, and cognitive impairment. Their real clinical importance has not been clearly elucidated and at the present time they should be considered as research tools only (Benseler and Silverman 2007).

One of the most intriguing issues in this field is the association of neuropsychiatric manifestations with antiphospholipid antibodies (aPL), which includes anticardiolipin antibodies (aCL), anti-β_2-glycoprotein I antibodies (anti-β_2GPI), and lupus anticoagulant (LA). These autoantibodies can lead to thrombosis of cerebral vessels, both arterial and venous, but a non-thrombotic, immune-mediated neurologic impairment has also been associated with aPL. The contribution of animal models to the understanding of the pathogenesis of neurolupus has been of invaluable help; an example of such a model utilizes immunization of BALB/c mice with monoclonal human anticardiolipin antibodies. These mice not only displayed elevated levels of circulating aPL, anti-β_2 GPI, and anti-endothelial cell antibodies, but were also impaired neurologically when compared to controls.

A direct neuromodulatory effect of aPL could be mediated by antibody–neuroantigen interactions, as growing evidence suggests direct binding of aPL to brain tissue and endothelium, and some aPL have also been demonstrated to bind directly to cat brain. Although some studies supported a direct aPL reactivity to nervous structures, it is still not clear whether such a binding can be mediated by β_2GPI-dependent pathogenic autoantibodies alone. The neuropathogenic potential of aPL, of direct interest to epilepsy pathogenesis, was confirmed by demonstration that immunoglobulin (IgG) from APS patients have been shown to be able to render directly permeable and depolarize brain synaptoneurosomes. Finally, aPL may bind neurotransmitters such as adenosine triphosphate (ATP), thereby interfering with neuronal functions, and it has been postulated that they may have a direct effect on seizure genesis through inhibition of the γ-aminobutyric acid (GABA) receptor–ion channel complex (Cimaz et al. 2006).

Epilepsy in systemic lupus erythematosus and in other connective tissue disorders
Frequency of epilepsy

Neuropsychiatric involvement is one of the most common clinical features of SLE, with a variable incidence reported between 15% and 75% in adults and between 20% and 85% in children. Some papers report that approximately 40% of children have CNS involvement as a presenting sign of the disease, while in approximately 70% of children the CNS manifestations will occur within the first year of disease (Yu et al. 2006).

The spectrum of neuropsychiatric manifestations in patients with CNS involvement is wide and includes: aseptic meningitis, cerebrovascular disease, demyelinating syndrome, headache, myelopathy, acute confusional state, anxiety, cognitive dysfunction, mood disorder, and psychosis.

Seizures seem to be the most frequent neuropsychiatric manifestation, both at disease onset and during SLE evolution, with a variable frequency ranging from 40% to 85% (Jacques-Spinosa et al. 2007).

The prevalence of epilepsy in the main published reports is summarized in Table 82.1.

Whilst the occurrence of epileptic seizures in SLE is well established, there is less clear evidence concerning the frequency of epilepsy in primary APS. In one large study, the frequency of epilepsy in primary and secondary antiphospholipid syndrome, and associated features that would suggest risk factors for epilepsy in APS, was assessed. The clinical features of patients with APS who had epilepsy were analysed and compared to the clinical features of non-epileptic APS patients. Of 538 APS patients, 46 (8.6%) had epilepsy. Epilepsy was more prevalent among APS secondary to SLE compared to primary APS (13.7% vs. 6%; $p = 0.05$). The multivariate logistic regression analysis found CNS thromboembolic events as the most significant factor associated with epilepsy, with an odds ratio (OR) of 4.05 (95% confidence interval [CI] 2.05–8), followed by SLE (OR 1.4, 95% CI 1.2–4.7), and cardiac valvular vegetations (OR 2.87, 95% CI 1–8.27). This study concluded that epilepsy is common in APS and most of the risk seems to be linked to vascular disease as manifested by extensive CNS involvement, heart valvulopathy, livedo reticularis, and to the presence of SLE (Shoenfeld et al. 2004).

Seizures have also been described during different vasculitides such as Kawasaki disease (Tabarki et al. 2001), Henoch-Schönlein purpura (Chien-Lang et al. 2000), Wegener granulomatosis (von Scheven et al. 1998); however involvement of the CNS in these diseases is less common than in SLE. Among other connective tissue diseases, localized scleroderma is, for the most part, a benign condition with clinical manifestations limited to the skin and subdermal tissues; however, a recent report (Zulian et al. 2005) evaluated the prevalence of extracutaneous manifestations in a large cohort of 750 children, finding that almost 25% of patients with juvenile localized scleroderma had at least one extracutaneous manifestation during the course of the disease. Neurologic involvement was present in 4.4% of patients; the most common neurologic abnormalities included mainly seizures followed by recent-onset headache, peripheral neuropathy, and CNS vasculitis. Interestingly, neurologic involvement was particularly found in patients with linear scleroderma with hemifacial atrophy of the face, known as Parry–Romberg syndrome. In adults

Table 82.1 Epilepsy prevalence in the main published reports on patients affected by systemic lupus erythematosus

No. of patients	F : M	Epilepsy, no. of patients (%)	Mean age, years (range)	aPL association	Reference
221	–	21 (9.5)	–	YES	Herranz et al. (1994)
340	–	24 (7)	–	YES	Toubi et al. (1995)
195	9:1	28 (14)	32.6 ± 7.5	YES	Mikdashi et al. (2005)
519	–	60 (11.6)	–	YES	Appenzeller et al. (2004)
1200	–	142 (6.9)	–	NO	Gonzalez-Duarte et al. (2008)
137	5.5:1	4 (3)	13.0 (3.1–17.7)	–	Avcin et al. (2008)
188	5:1	23 (12.2)	–	YES	Shoenfeld et al. (2004)
323	20.5:1	27 (8.3)	43.1 ± 12.6	YES	Sanna 2002
25	7:1	16 (64)	12.2 ± 3.8	–	Quintero del Rio 2000
185	5.8:1	54 (29.1)	13.2 ± 3	NO	Yu et al. (2006)
47	3:1	17 (36.2)	11.4 ± 2.6	NO	Spinosa et al. (2007)

patients, intractable epilepsy can be part of the spectrum of disease in linear scleroderma (Kister et al. 2008).

Risk factors for epilepsy

Although the risk factors for epilepsy are not well known, seizures seem to be correlated with the presence of aPL antibodies. A British group from St. Thomas's hospital in London initially published two articles dealing with aPL and CNS lupus, including epilepsy (Herranz et al. 1994; Toubi et al. 1995). In the first paper the authors tried to determine whether, in a cohort of 221 SLE patients, the occurrence of seizures was correlated with circulating aPL, and concluded that epilepsy as a primary neuropsychiatric event was significantly associated with moderate-to-high titers of IgG aCL. In the second study, 96 out of 340 unselected SLE patients had CNS manifestations not attributed to any cause other than SLE, and 24 of them had epilepsy. Of the 53 patients who underwent a brain magnetic resonance imaging (MRI) study, 33 exhibited small high-density lesions suggestive of vasculopathy and 26 of them were positive for aPL. These two papers underlined one of the possible mechanisms for seizure occurrence in SLE, i.e., aPL-mediated, ischemic changes and this has been confirmed by several additional studies. Although this association is now well established, the presence of multiple comorbidities and the high baseline presence of aPL in SLE make comparisons between different studies difficult, and incidence data even more difficult to obtain. Subsequently, Mikdashi et al. found that 28 of 195 patients with SLE had epileptic seizures during the course of their disease, while recurrence of seizures, i.e., epilepsy, was observed in 12 of them (Mikdashi et al. 2005). Certain clinical features at baseline were independent predictors of seizures, while higher disease activity at baseline, concurrent multiple neuropsychiatric SLE manifestations, and male gender were predictive of epilepsy. Again, the problems with this kind of study is that even if the seizures were defined as due to no

other cause than SLE, this disease in itself can be the origin of seizures by a multitude of mechanisms, making interpretations very difficult. A similar study in a large cohort evaluated the frequency and risk factors of epileptic seizures in 519 patients with SLE. Again, isolated seizures were frequent but their recurrence was rare, since 60 patients with epileptic seizures were identified but only seven had recurrent attacks (all with antiphospholipid antibody syndrome) (Appenzeller et al. 2004). Therefore, it appears that one of the major mechanisms for seizures and epilepsy in lupus is mediated by aPL.

In a recent single-center retrospective cohort study (Avcin et al. 2008), the titers of autoantibodies were determined in 137 children, but the presence of autoantibodies did not differ between the subgroup of SLE patients with seizures and those without epilepsy. Moreover in a Finnish study (Ranua et al. 2004) in which the presence of autoantibodies was determined in a large cohort of almost 1000 patients with epilepsy, aCL antibodies were found in 4.5%, but also in a similar percentage of a control group of 580 healthy subjects. It is therefore possible that the mere presence of those antibodies may not be sufficient to induce clinical manifestations, but that additional factors, possibly SLE-linked, may be necessary. In this study, as well as in others, duration of epilepsy, frequency of seizures, and poor disease control were associated with increased aPL positivity. This observation raises the question whether autoantibodies may be the effect, rather than the cause, of seizures, since it is known that seizures can activate cytokine and autoantibody production. Another point worth mentioning is the possible interference with antiepileptic medications, some of which may induce the production of autoantibodies, sometimes complicating the understanding of the association between the two disorders. It is in fact known that in many cases of drug-induced lupus the offending drug is an anticonvulsant.

In SLE, the risk of disease is influenced by complex genetic and environmental contributions: for example, alleles including HLA-DRB1, IRF5, and STAT4 are established susceptibility genes. More recently, new genetic loci for SLE have been described: a promoter-region allele associated with reduced expression of B lymphoid tyrosine kinase and increased expression of C8orf13 (chromosome 8p23.1), and variants on chromosome 16p11.22, near the genes encoding integrin alpha M (ITGAM, or CD11b) and integrin alpha X (ITGAX). A genetic predisposition for specific system involvements is also possible, which may also be relevant to epilepsy. Indeed, in a recent study Bautista et al. (2008) used a covariate-based linkage analysis to detect a potential genetic locus on chromosome 15 influencing the development of seizures in individuals with SLE. The authors hypothesized that the phenotypic heterogeneity seen in SLE may reflect an underlying genetic heterogeneity, and studied a large number of multiplex SLE families for seizure susceptibility with the genotyping of microsatellite markers. A potential susceptibility locus on chromosome 15 was detected. Seizures that were associated with known risk factors such as drugs or metabolic derangements (e.g., uremia, ketoacidosis, or electrolyte imbalance) were excluded. Moreover in this series there was no difference in aPL positivity in patients with and without seizures. Finally, the authors state that some individuals may have had seizures unrelated to the diagnosis of SLE.

Types of epilepsy, characteristics, treatment, and prognosis

Seizures are rarely the presenting symptom of SLE; they often appear in the course of the disease, typically during flare-up of systemic or CNS lupus (Koppel 2008). Seizures contribute to poor outcome when they occur in children (Rood et al. 1999) and in a study they doubled the rate of mortality when found with nephritis in adults. Both focal and generalized seizures occur in SLE. In one series of 91 patients with SLE, 22% had experienced generalized seizures and only 5% had focal attacks (Futrell et al. 1992). Generalized seizures can either represent the only manifestation of brain involvement in CNS lupus or may represent an expression of hypertensive or metabolic encephalopathy. Focal seizures have been variously attributed to cerebrovascular complications, abscess, or meningitis while status epilepticus has been reported especially as a preterminal event (West et al. 1995). Treatment with antiepileptic drugs (AEDs) is not necessarily needed if a precipitant factor for seizures can be identified and treated. However, if frequent seizures occur, short-term AED treatment can be necessary until the lupus flare-up is controlled. Although drug-induced lupus has been reported with the use of various AEDs, it is unlikely that treating a patient with SLE with an AED will exacerbate the underlying disorder (Cimaz and Guerrini 2008).

Diagnostic tests

The diagnosis of SLE (and of the other connective tissue disorders) is generally a clinical one, supported by laboratory tests. With regard to neurologic involvement, radiologic

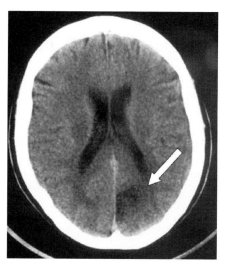

Fig. 82.1. Brain CT scan of a 13-year-old girl who presented with sudden right temporal hemianopsia. The figure shows an ischemic lesion of the left occipital cortex. The patient, who was diagnosed with SLE, subsequently developed intractable epilepsy.

techniques may be extremely helpful. Neurocognitive impairment, even if not directly associated with epilepsy, but more generally with neurologic involvement, is present in a high percentage of adult patients; however a few reports have been published on pediatric SLE showing a relatively high rate of abnormalities on testing, and longer disease duration was associated with lower cognitive function.

Although computed tomography (CT) can be helpful in assessing patients suspected of having cerebral hemorrhage, stroke, pseudotumor cerebri, and sinus thrombosis, MRI scans are superior in detecting early lesions and lesions secondary to small vessel involvement. Lesions seen on MRI are frequently small, multifocal, and bilateral with high signal intensity. Brain biopsy studies have shown that the MRI abnormalities represented a small vessel vasculitis. Although large-vessel CNS vasculitis is rarely seen, the yield on MR angiogram is generally considered to be equivalent to conventional cerebral angiogram. Overall, MRI is the preferred study in patients with suspected CNS involvement and CT scans have a more limited role. Benseler and Silverman suggest that in patients with seizures, brain MRI should be rapidly performed to search for intracranial hemorrhage, ischemia, or other brain lesions. However, although about 75% of patients with active disease will exhibit some sort of MRI abnormality, there does not seem to be a distinctive pattern associated with seizure occurrence (Benseler and Silverman 2007) (Figs. 82.1, 82.2). The same applies to electroencephalographic (EEG) investigations, as epileptiform abnormalities are often observed in SLE patients without seizures and may be absent in those with seizures. The role of HMPAO-labeled technetium-99 cerebral single photon emission computed tomography (SPECT) scans is still debated, since abnormal SPECT scans have been reported in up to 40% of patients without overt CNS involvement. A diffusely abnormal SPECT scan can be highly sensitive for diffuse CNS involvement, although specificity is low. These scans have little value in monitoring CNS disease activity, as studies in both pediatric and adult SLE populations have

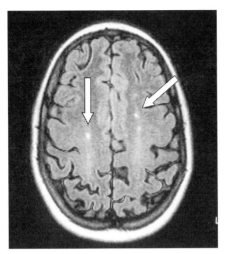

Fig. 82.2. Magnetic resonance imaging scan. Centrum semiovale diffuse gliosis and demyelination in a 9-year-old patient affected by SLE and who presented with seizures.

shown that SPECT abnormalities persist following resolution of clinical disease.

Principles of management

Most experts advocate treatment of CNS involvement with monthly intravenous pulse cyclophosphamide and cortico-steroids (usually pulse methylprednisolone). However, there has not been many large controlled studies of therapy in pediatric or adult CNS SLE. In the first pediatric SLE (pSLE) study all five children who received either azathioprine or cyclophosphamide in addition to prednisone had a good recovery, while two out of 11 patients treated with prednisone alone died and three other patients had residual neurological defects (Yancey *et al.* 1991). A treatment regimen based on high-dose daily prednisone and monthly pulses of both cyclo-phosphamide and methylprednisolone was associated with improvement in all 10 patients, with complete recovery in six (Baca *et al.* 1999). More recently no significant difference was found in outcome between 10 patients treated with cyclophosphamide when compared with seven patients treated with azathioprine (Olfat *et al.* 2004). However, the cyclophosphamide-treated patients tended to have more extensive disease. Some authors suggest that cyclophospha-mide should be reserved for patients who relapsed on steroids alone, but even in this case only half of the patients seemed to have full recovery. Taken together, these studies in pSLE suggest that patients with significant CNS involvement should be treated with a combination of high-dose steroids and an immunosuppressant agent. A safer profile with the same response rate with mycophenolate mofetil in comparison with cyclophosphamide was recently presented; however, these data still need to be confirmed.

In adults, the general experience is almost the same: high-dose corticosteroids plus intravenous pulse cyclopho-sphamide are recommended for cerebral vasculopathy with epilepsy; IVIG and plasma exchange can be considered for any CNS manifestations unresponsive to previous treatment. The role of newer immunosuppressive agents including ritux-imab remains to be determined.

References

Appenzeller S, Cendes F, Costallat LT (2004) Epileptic seizures in systemic lupus erythematosus. *Neurology* 63:1808–12.

Avcin T, Benseler S, Tyrrell P, Cucnik S, Silverman E (2008) A follow-up study of antiphospholipid antibodies and associated neuropsychiatric manifestations in 137 children with systemic lupus erythematosus. *Arthritis Rheum* 59:206–13.

Baca V, Lavalle C, García R, *et al.* (1999) Favorable response to intravenous methylprednisolone and cyclophosphamide in children with severe neuropsychiatric lupus. *J Rheumatol* 26:432–9.

Bautista JF, Kelly JA, Harley JB, Gray-McGuire C (2008) Addressing genetic heterogeneity in complex disease: finding seizure genes in systemic lupus erythematosus. *Epilepsia* 49:527–30.

Benseler SM, Silverman ED (2007) Neuropsychiatric involvement in pediatric systemic lupus erythematosus. *Lupus* 16:564–71.

Brey RL (2007) Neuropsychiatric lupus. *Bull NYU Hosp Jt Dis* 65:194–9.

Chien-Liang C, Yee-Hsuan C, Chan-Yao W, Ping-Hong L, Hsiao-Min C (2000) Cerebral vasculitis in Henoch–Schoenlein purpura: a case report with sequential magnetic resonance imaging changes and treated with plasmapheresis alone. *Pediatr Nephrol* 15:276–8.

Cimaz R, Meroni PL, Shoenfeld Y (2006) Epilepsy as part of systemic lupus erythematosus and systemic antiphosphoplipid syndrome (Hughe syndrome). *Lupus* 15:191–7.

Cimaz R, Guerrini R (2008) Epilepsy in lupus. *Lupus* 17:777–9.

Futrell N, Schultz LR, Millikan C (1992) Central nervous system disease in patients with systemic lupus erythematosus. *Neurology* 42:1649–57.

González-Duarte A, Cantú-Brito CG, Ruano-Calderón L, Garcia-Ramos G (2008) Clinical description of seizures in patients with systemic lupus erythematosus. *Eur Neurol* 59:320–3.

Herranz MT, Rivier G, Khamashta MA, Blaser KU, Hughes GR (1994) Association between antiphospholipid antibodies and epilepsy in patients with systemic lupus erythematosus. *Arthritis Rheum* 37:568–71.

Jaques-Spinosa M, Bandeira M, Noronha Liberalesso PB, *et al.* (2007) Clinical, laboratory and neuroimage findings in juvenile systemic lupus erythematosus presenting involvement of the nervous system. *Arq Neuropsiquiatr* 65:433–9.

Kister I, Inglese M, Laxer RM, Herbert J (2008) Neurologic manifestations of localized scleroderma: a case report and literature review. *Neurology* 71:1538–45.

Koppel BS (2008) Connective tissue diseases. In: Engel J Jr. and Pedley TA (eds.) *Epilepsy: A Comprehensive Textbook.* Philadelphia, PA: Lippincott Williams and Wilkins, pp. 2653–60.

Mikdashi J, Krumholz A, Handwerger B (2005) Factors at diagnosis predict subsequent occurrence of seizures in systemic lupus erythematosus. *Neurology* 64:2102–7.

Olfat MO, Al-Mayouf SM, Muzaffer MA (2004) Pattern of neuropsychiatric manifestations and outcome in juvenile systemic lupus erythematosus. *Clin Rheumatol* **23**:395–9.

Quintero del Rio AI (2000) Neurologic symptoms in children with systemic lupus erythematosus. *J Child Neurol* **15**:803–7.

Ranua J, Luoma K, Peltola J, *et al.* (2004) Anticardiolipin and antinuclear antibodies in epilepsy: a population-based cross-sectional study. *Epilepsy Res* **58**:13–18.

Rood MJ, ten Cate R, van Suijlekom-Smit LWA, *et al.* (1999) Childhood-onset systemic lupus erythematosus. *Scand J Rheumatol* **28**:222–6.

Sanna G, Bertolaccini ML, Cuadrado MJ, *et al.* (2003) Neuropsychiatric manifestations in systermic lupus erythematosus: prevalence and association with antiphospholipid antibodies. *J Rheumatol* **30**:985–92.

Shoenfeld Y, Lev S, Blatt I, *et al.* (2004) Features associated with epilepsy in the antiphospholipid syndrome. *J Rheumatol* **31**:1344–8.

Spinosa MJ, Bandeira M, Liberalesso PB, *et al.* (2007) Clinical laboratory and neuroimage findings in juvenile systemic lupus erythematosus presenting involvement of the central nervous system. *Arg Neuropsiquiatr* **65**:433–9.

Tabarki B, Mahdhaoui A, Selmi H, Yacoub M, Essoussi AS (2001) Kawasaki disease with predominant central nervous system involvement. *Pediatr Neurol* **25**:239–41.

Toubi E, Khamashta MA, Panarra A, Hughes GR (1995) Association of antiphospholipid antibodies with central nervous system disease in systemic lupus erythematosus. *Am J Med* **99**:397–401.

Von Scheven E, Lee C, Berg BO (1998) Pediatric Wegener's granulomatosis complicated by central nervous system vasculitis. *Pediatr Neurol* **19**:317–19.

West SG, Emlen W, Wener MH, Kotzin BL (1995) Neuropsychiatric lupus erythematosus: a 10-year prospective study on the value of diagnostic tests. *Am J Med* **99**:153–63.

Yancey CL, Doughty RA, Athreya BH (1981) Central nervous system involvement in childhood systemic lupus erythematosus. *Arthritis Rheum* **24**:1389–95.

Yu H-H, Lee J-H, Wang L-C, Yang Y-H, Chiang B-L (2006) Neuropsychiatric manifestations in pediatric systemic lupus erthematosus: a 20-year study. *Lupus* **16**:651–7.

Zulian F, Vallongo C, Woo P, *et al.* (2005) Localized scleroderma in childhood is not just a skin disease. *Arthritis Rheum* **52**:2873–81.

Chapter

83 Inflammatory and immunological diseases of the nervous system

Michael P. T. Lunn

Epilepsy is relatively common as a manifestation of systemic autoimmune diseases such as systemic lupus erythematosus and vasculitis and these are dealt with in previous chapters. There are a number of emerging, central nervous system (CNS) predominant autoimmune diseases, which present as a "limbic" or more diffuse encephalitis or encephalopathy, and the epilepsies can be a major feature of the presentation of these.

These rare disorders are probably underdiagnosed and are the subject of this chapter. Initially they were thought to be predominantly paraneoplastic, but increasingly non-malignant and treatable entities are being established. This chapter will cover the condition commonly known as Hashimoto encephalopathy and the treatment-responsive encephalopathies associated with antibodies to neuronal antigens. This is an expanding group of disorders in which novel antigenic targets with serum and CNS antibodies are being identified. Epilepsy has also been associated with the inflammatory bowel diseases (ulcerative colitis, Crohn disease, and celiac disease), although this association is more contentious. They will be discussed here for completeness.

Limbic encephalitis

Background and history

Limbic encephalitis (LE) is an inflammatory disorder of the CNS which is now best identified and described by the clinical presentation. Early descriptions were of a rare condition, which associated cancer with CNS inflammation limited to the limbic system. Limbic encephalitis has broadened to include benign and malignant neoplasm associated disorders as well as conditions where no neoplasm is identifiable. The anatomical extent of inflammation often reaches beyond the limbic system and a number of antibodies are associated with some of the many emerging phenotypes. Furthermore, LE is probably not as rare as previously thought. There are no reliable epidemiological data but 3–5% of patients with small-cell lung cancer, 15–20% with thymomas, and 3–10%

with B cell or plasma cell neoplasms may develop a paraneoplastic syndrome (Dalmau and Rosenfeld 2008) of which a significant but unknown number will be LE.

The first description of LE is attributed to Brierley (1960) who described three patients with a "subacute limbic encephalitis of later life, mainly affecting the limbic areas." Although one of these patients had confirmed bronchial carcinoma, and in another it was suspected, the authors felt it was unlikely the encephalitis and malignancy were related. Lord Brain's description of Hashimoto encephalitis (Brain *et al.* 1966) associated an encephalitis with a serum antibody for the first time. From the 1980s until the present, increasing numbers of paraneoplastic antibodies have been described, associated with a series of recognizable homogeneous clinical presentations and occurring in the context of first malignant tumors (e.g., anti-Hu antibodies in association with small-cell carcinoma of the lung) and non-malignant tumors (e.g., anti-NMDA [*N*-methyl-D-aspartate] antibodies associated with ovarian teratomas).

Clinical features

Limbic encephalitis refers to a series of phenotypically overlapping conditions (see Table 83.1 and below). The common clinical feature of LE is impairment of short-term memory, but often memory for autobiographical events is preserved. Usually the presentation is acute or subacute over days to weeks. Limbic involvement also manifests with hallucinations and complex partial and secondary generalized seizures and sleep disturbance. The severe anterograde amnesia contributes to the psychiatric symptomatology with anxiety, depression, irritability, and personality changes, or more rarely agitation and delusional or paranoid behavior. However, since widespread cortical areas are involved in different sorts of LE, additional clinical features may be present that confuse the clinical presentation, but in some cases may positively identify the likely pathogenic antibody (see below).

The differential diagnosis includes viral (particularly herpes simplex) encephalitis, Sjögren syndrome, syphilis,

The Causes of Epilepsy, eds. S. D. Shorvon, F. Andermann, and R. Guerrini. Published by Cambridge University Press. © Cambridge University Press 2011.

Table 83.1 Limbic encephalitis (LE) syndromes: distinguishing features, investigations, and treatment

	"Classical" intracellular antibodies, e.g., Hu, Ma-2	Extracellular antibodies, e.g., VGKC	Antibodies to NMDAR	Antibodies to other cell membrane antigens
Selective antibody reactivity to hippocampal neurons	No – antibodies react to all neurons of neuraxis	Moderate – some react with cerebellar and cerebral cortex	Intense – cerebrospinal fluid contains high antibody titer	Intense – also molecular layer of cerebellum
Cerebrospinal fluid inflammatory changes	Frequent	Infrequent or mild	Frequent	Frequent
Oligoclonal bands	Frequent	Infrequent or absent	Frequent – antibodies may only be detected in cerebrospinal fluid	No data
Hyponatremia	No, except in association with SCLC	Frequent	No	No
Distinguishing symptoms additional to LE	See individual antibodies in text	Neuromyotonia, Morvan syndrome	Psychiatric symptoms, decreased consciousness, autonomic dysfunction, stereotypies and dyskinesia	Infrequent – usually "pure" LE
Magnetic resonance imaging findings	Mesial temporal high signal FLAIR (typical)	Typical	25% of cases typical findings. Normal. Increased FLAIR signal in cerebral or cerebellar cortex; transient meningeal enhancement	Typical. Sometimes focal cortical high signal
Response to tumor removal or immunotherapy	Infrequent – sometimes good response to testicular removal in Ma2	Frequent; steroids and IVIG/PEx	Frequent; teratoma removal, IVIG, steroids, PEx, cyclophosphamide, rituximab	Tumor resection plus typical immunosuppression
Antibody titer response to treatment	Poor clinical correlation – may persist	Decreases with clinical improvement	Decreases or disappears with clinical improvement	Decreases with clinical improvement

Abbreviations: FLAIR, fluid attenuated inversion recovery; IVIG, intravenous immunoglobulin; NMDAR, N-methyl-D-aspartate receptor; PEx, plasma exchange; SCLC, small cell lung cancer; VGKC, voltage-gated potassium channel.

systemic lupus erythematosus, Hashimoto encephalitis (see below), Korsakoff syndrome, toxic/metabolic encephalitides, glioma, and metastasis.

Epilepsy

Epilepsy is common to all of the limbic encephalitides and occurs in almost all cases. Seizures may be very subtle varying from short atypical absences to short simple partial seizures, to more typical psychomotor or temporal lobe complex partial seizures that may secondarily generalize. The electroencephalogram (EEG) is almost always abnormal (Lawn *et al.* 2003) with unilateral or bilateral epileptic activity in the temporal lobes or generalized slowing. Clinical events may or may not be associated with EEG abnormality.

Investigations

Electroencephalography, magnetic resonance imaging (MRI) scanning, and examination of the cerebrospinal fluid (CSF) are all useful investigations in a patient presenting with LE. The EEG in LE is nearly always abnormal. The MRI scan shows high signal fluid attenuated inversion recovery (FLAIR) abnormalities in the temporal lobes in 70–80% of patients (Lawn *et al.* 2003) and these may be unilateral or bilateral. Seldom do these lesions enhance. Abnormal MRI imaging has an important differential which includes herpes simplex and other infective encephalitides. Normal MRI imaging does not exclude the diagnosis. The CSF is often tested at this stage and in 70–80% this is abnormal. It should be noted that the CSF in some of the emerging non-neoplasm-associated LE cases may be normal. A mildly raised cell count (<100 cells/mm^3, usually lymphocytes), a moderately raised protein, and a normal glucose would be most common. Positive oligoclonal bands may be found. In voltage-gated potassium channel (VGKC) antibody mediated LE concentrations of protein and cell counts may be lower. The CSF should be tested for the presence of viruses by polymerase chain reaction (PCR) if infective encephalitis remains of concern.

In most cases a neoplasm must be considered. Neurological symptoms precede the discovery of a neoplasm in two-thirds of cases (Lawn *et al.* 2003). At present high-resolution computed tomography (CT) scanning of the chest, abdomen, and pelvis, probably with fluorodeoxyglucose positron emission tomography (FDG-PET) is recommended, even though this may also be negative. However PET may show temporal-lobe hypermetabolism, even if the MRI is normal.

Testing serum for the presence of antibodies may help to confirm the presence of a paraneoplastic LE, direct investigation towards a particular malignant or tumor-containing tissue, promote continued vigilance for the appearance of an occult malignancy, or suggest a non-neoplasm-associated LE. These antibodies will be discussed individually below. Testing for antibodies to neuronal antigens is available in larger immunology centers.

The presence of an anti-neuronal antibody in the serum in the absence of a clinical LE or other neurological condition does not mean that a neoplasm is present or that the patient has a paraneoplastic condition (Table 83.2). Whereas the presence of an LE-associated serum antibody was once strongly associated with the presence of a tumor (e.g., in anti-Hu-associated LE with small-cell carcinoma of the lung), emerging syndromes have a lesser degree of association with malignancy. For example, VGKC antibodies are associated with malignancy in fewer than 30% of cases (Dalmau and Rosenfeld 2008). Therefore, a better way to consider antibodies is in relation to their target antigen, particularly whether they are present on the cell surface or intracellular (Table 83.2). Diseases with antibodies to cell-surface antigens are easier to model in animal and in vitro systems, are thought to be predominantly B-cell driven, and, in general, respond reasonably to treatment. Those associated with antibodies to intracellular antigens probably have T cells directed to the same antigens. These are less easy to model and provide supportive evidence for pathogenesis. Cytotoxicity is more prominent and hence these syndromes respond less well to treatment, especially if delayed.

Limbic encephalitis associated with intracellular antigens

Hu/ANNA-1

One of the Hu antigens, HuD, is expressed in small-cell lung cancer (SCLC). Seventy-five percent of patients with SCLC have Hu antibodies. Anti-Hu antibodies associate with a wide range of paraneoplastic neurological phenotypes including cerebellar degeneration, sensory and motor neuronopathies, and autonomic failure. Only 10% of patients with anti-Hu have LE. However, the anti-Hu LE is often complicated by other aspects of the Hu syndrome such as cerebellar degeneration or a sensory neuronopathy and thus these features help to support a diagnosis. Limbic encephalitis responds relatively well to treatment, although the overall prognosis for an anti-Hu-associated syndrome is poor.

Ma-2

The LE associated with Ma-2 often presents with coexistent brainstem and hypothalamic dysfunction. Eye movement abnormalities (vertical gaze paresis and nystagmus), hyperthermia, weight gain, diabetes insipidus, hypnagogic hallucinations, hypersomnolence, cataplexy, and gelastic seizures may all present in conjunction with LE. In men under the age of 50, Ma-2 LE is highly associated with intratubal germ cell tumors which may be microscopic. Orchidectomy is recommended even if the tumor is not visible. This may result in resolution or significant improvement of the symptoms. Otherwise about 30% of patients improve with immunosuppression.

CRMP-5

Limbic encephalitis associated with collapsin-response-mediator protein 5 (CRMP-5) is rare. The manifestations of CRMP-5-associated disease are very diverse and include cerebellar syndromes, retinopathy, uveitis, and cranial nerve, root, or peripheral nerve involvement.

Amphiphysin

Amphiphysin is a synaptic-vesicle-associated protein which resides close to the synaptic membrane. Antibodies to amphiphysin are highly associated with breast cancer. The typical amphiphysin-associated syndrome is "stiff-person syndrome" or a paraneoplastic LE in which seizures can occur. Myelopathy and cerebellar ataxia have also been described.

Glutamic acid decarboxylase

Antibodies to glutamic acid decarboxylase (GAD) are common in type I diabetes but in high titer are also associated with stiff person syndrome. Anti-GAD antibodies react strongly with GABAergic neurons on rat cerebellum but their exact mechanism of pathogenesis in vivo is not known. Four of 19 patients described by Solimena *et al.* (1990) with stiff person syndrome had epilepsy. Eight of 51 patients with partial epilepsy were found to have anti-GAD antibodies, of whom two had very high titers and one had had resistant seizures for more than 30 years (Peltola *et al.* 2000). Aggressive immunosuppression with cyclophosphamide may be required and may be successful (Kanter *et al.* 2008).

Table 83.2 Serum antibodies in limbic encephalitis syndromes

Antibody	Target antigen	Antigen location[a]	Malignancies associated	Frequency of malignancy	Response to treatment
Hu/ANNA-1	RNA binding protein	i/c	SCLC, other	High (>75% SCLC)	Poor
CRMP-5/antiCV2 (may coexist with Hu or Zic)	Collapsin-response-mediator protein 5	i/c	SCLC, thymoma	90%	Thymoma associated cases may respond well
Ma-2	mRNA associated	i/c	Testis, non-SCLC, other solid tumor	Men <50, almost 100% testis. Older men and women less frequent	30%–35% improve
Amphyphysin (may coexist with Hu and VGKC)	Synaptic vesicle associated protein	Cytoplasmic membrane	Breast, SCLC		Poor
GAD	Glutamic acid decarboxylase	i/c	None	N/A	Good in some
VGKC	Voltage-gated potassium channel	e/c	SCLC	20–30%	Good
NMDAR	NR1/NR2 heteromers of N-methyl-D-aspartate receptor	e/c	Ovarian teratoma	65%	Good
Other neuropil	Various including glycine receptor	Various	SCLC, thymoma	Unknown	Good/variable

Notes:
[a]i/c, intracellular; e/c, extracellular. Other abbreviations as in Table 83.1.

Limbic encephalitis associated with extracellular antigens

Voltage-gated potassium channels

Buckley *et al.* (2001) reported two cases of reversible LE associated with voltage gated potassium channel (VGKC) antibodies. Many more have now been described. There is a male predominance. Seizures occur in up to 90%, particularly in the acute phase, but some may be subtle simple motor or complex partial seizures that are easily missed, but typical when seen. Myotonia is often found and, with sleep disturbances, hallucination, and autonomic dysfunction may be referred to as Morvan syndrome. Headache, drowsiness, and loss of consciousness are not generally features. Variations in clinical presentation are attributed to varying specificities of the VGKC antibodies to different Shaker-type potassium channel subgroups (Kleopa *et al.* 2006).

Hyponatremia is very common, occurring in 12 of 17 cases in the early series (Thieben *et al.* 2004; Vincent *et al.* 2004). The CSF may be completely normal; a mild pleocytosis only is more usually found. The MRI scan often shows bilateral mesial temporal lobe high signal.

Neoplasms are rarely found in cases of VGKC-associated LE but SCLC, thymoma, and prostate cancer have all been associated. Treatment with high-dose methylprednisolone, plasma exchange, and/or intravenous immunoglobulin (IVIG) may be very effective and associated with decreases in titer of the serum antibody.

N-methyl-D-aspartate receptor

The LE associated with N-methyl-D-aspartate receptor (NMDAR) is a severe but treatment-responsive condition that once seen is not forgotten (Dalmau *et al.* 2007). Most patients are young women who present with a prodrome of flu-like illness followed by personality change, delusions, and thought disorder associated with anterograde amnesia. Many become stuporose or comatose with periods of staring, stereotypical movements, and catatonic posturing, interspersed with generalized or complex partial seizures.

Most patients have an ovarian teratoma, and 70% of these are benign. However, males also present and may have no identifiable malignancy. Teratomata may only be found by more traditional imaging methods (CT/transvaginal ultrasound) as benign teratomata may be silent to PET examination.

Hyponatremia does not occur in these patients. Most have a CSF pleocytosis and oligoclonal bands and the anti-NMDAR antibodies may only be found in the CSF, so both serum and CSF must be tested. The assay is of limited availability at present (Oxford in the UK, Pennsylvania in USA).

Identification and removal of the tumor combined with immunosuppression, plasma exchange, and/or IVIG often result in dramatic but not necessarily full recovery.

Other antibodies in limbic encephalitis

Antibodies associated with previously unexplained idiopathic limbic encephalitis continue to be described. Antibodies to glycine receptors (Hutchinson *et al.* 2008), adenylate kinase 5 (Tuzun and Dalmau 2007), BR serine/threonine kinase 2 (Sabater *et al.* 2005), and other unknown antigens have all been described.

Treatment

Paraneoplastic and non-paraneoplastic LE is relatively rare and phenotypically diverse, driven by the individual antibody reactivities above. As a result no randomized controlled trials of treatment have been performed. Patients with a longer duration of symptoms or more severe disease respond less well to intervention. In general patients with pathogenic antibodies to cell-surface antigens respond more favorably to treatment. For example, over 80% of patients with VGKC antibodies will respond to therapy. Patients with antibodies to intracellular antigens (possibly T-cell-dependent mechanisms) respond less well; only 35% of patients with antibodies to Ma-2 respond. Where a malignancy is identified, outcomes for treatments are generally less good. Early identification and removal of the tumor however can result in substantial and sometimes prolonged improvement in cell-surface and intracellular-antigen-related conditions (Fadul *et al.* 2005; Shimazaki *et al.* 2007). Medical therapy may have to be instituted to stabilize a patient enough for surgery.

Accepted medical treatments for surface-antigen-related LE are high-dose steroids, plasma exchange, and/or IVIG, which are sometimes given in combination (Dalmau and Rosenfeld 2008). These practices are supported by evidence from case reports and small series only. Cyclophosphamide may be added to resistant cases, usually those that are mediated by antibodies to intracellular antigens. Rituximab has been used successfully in some cases (anti-NMDA, anti-Hu, and anti-Yo related) but as yet its role is uncertain. The use of tacrolimus and other oral immunosuppressives has been described with variable results. All immunosuppressive regimens may result in substantial toxicity in their own right.

Symptomatic treatments including anticonvulsants, antidepressants, neuroleptics, physiotherapy, and occupational therapy should be used as necessary.

Epilepsy associated with antibodies to neuronal antigens without encephalopathy

A number of reports exist in the literature associating serum antibodies to neuronal cell surface antigens with drug-resistant epilepsy syndromes. Some appear to be responsive to immune modulation and hence tentative causative associations are drawn. However these patients are rare and the significance of the antibodies remains uncertain.

(1) *Voltage-gated potassium channel antibodies.* Antibodies to voltage-gated potassium channels (VGKC) were described in 6% of female patients with long-standing drug-resistant epilepsy (Majoie *et al.* 2006). These patients were indistinguishable from the other patients in the group, but

had no other features of an LE syndrome. The significance of these antibodies remains to be determined.

(2) *Voltage-gated calcium channel antibodies.* Antibodies to voltage-gated calcium channels (VGCC) typically occur in patients with Lambert–Eaton myasthenic syndrome (LEMS). One patient with low titers of VGCC antibodies and drug-resistant epilepsy was reported by Majoie *et al.* (2006). The significance of this association is uncertain.

(3) *Anti-GM1 antibodies.* Bartolomei and colleagues (1996) described four patients from a group of 64 tested who had immunoglobulin G or M (IgG or IgM) (or both) serum antibodies to GM1 ganglioside. All patients had cryptogenic partial epilepsy syndromes that were drug-resistant and associated with psychiatric abnormalities. Two responded to IVIG. Theoretically anti-GM1 antibodies could interfere with membrane channel function by binding to glycolipid–protein complexes in membrane rafts. However this clinical finding has not been duplicated or repeated and so its significance remains uncertain.

(4) *Others.* Antibodies to Glu-R3 and Munc 18–1 associated with Rasmussen encephalitis are discussed elsewhere.

In cases of drug-resistant epilepsy it may be appropriate to carry out limited and targeted testing for serum antibodies of this sort. If found, and especially if at high titer, then immunomodulatory therapy may be tried. However no firm recommendations can be given as the area is evidence free.

Hashimoto encephalopathy or steroid-responsive encephalopathy associated with autoimmune thyroiditis

The index disease for this group of immune-mediated epilepsy syndromes is the entity known as Hashimoto encephalopathy or steroid-responsive encephalopathy associated with autoimmune thyroiditis (SREAT). This was first described by Lord Brain (Brain *et al.* 1966) in a patient with an encephalopathy and a hypothyroid chronic lymphocytic thyroiditis. Cases have also been described with euthyroid and hyperthyroid states and it appears that the unifying feature is high serum levels of anti-thyroid peroxidase (anti-TPO) antibodies (formerly known as microsomal antibodies). The pathogenic relevance of the antibodies is unknown (see below). The other feature is that a significant proportion, but by no means all, appear to be responsive to steroids hence the recently suggested acronym SREAT (Castillo *et al.* 2006). It was suggested by these authors that the steroid non-responsive patients had other pathogeneses, confirmed in four of 12 patients with non-SREAT who underwent postmortems prior to study publication. Interestingly the index case of Brain *et al.* did not respond to steroids but remitted spontaneously.

SREAT is rare. In a recent review of the literature only 105 cases fitting their definition were found. Because of its rarity and diversity accurate information on clinical features, pathogenesis, and treatment is from case reports and small series only.

Epilepsy in SREAT

Seizures are common in SREAT (60–70%), but occur as part of a diverse symptom complex (Chong *et al.* 2003; Castillo *et al.* 2006). Castillo *et al.* defined their patients as follows: encephalopathy, presence of anti-thyroid antibodies, euthyroid status, no evidence of toxic, metabolic, or infectious process, no evidence of other antibody-mediated encephalopathy, no neuroimaging findings to explain encephalopathy, with (SREAT) or without (non-SREAT) complete or near complete return to normality following corticosteroid treatment. In the context of this tight definition, 60% (12/20) of patients had seizures, classified as generalized (10), partial (7) or both (5). Patients may present with seizures or in status epilepticus.

Presentation of SREAT

The encephalopathy of SREAT is highly variable in its presentation leading to initial diagnoses of stroke, Creutzfeldt–Jakob disease, viral encephalitis, Lewy body disease, psychosis, Alzheimer disease, or migraine in almost all cases before the correct diagnosis is reached. There is an excess of females (4 : 1) and a wide range of presenting ages (9–78 years).

The usual tempo of presentation is subacute. All patients have cognitive impairment, usually of a fluctuating or relapsing–remitting nature. In addition aphasia, tremor, myoclonus, gait ataxia, sleep disorders, headache, lateralized motor and sensory deficits, and psychosis have all been described. The neurological signs can be very variable, including cognitive, corticospinal, extrapyramidal, and sensory with stupor or coma in some.

Pathogenesis of SREAT

Anti-thyroid antibodies occur in a wide variety of autoimmune conditions, and in 5–20% of older females without a clinical correlate. There is no known binding of anti-thyroid antibodies to brain and indeed anti-TPO and anti-thyroglobulin antibodies have no known biological activity. T-cell mechanisms mediate most of the pathology of the thyroiditis. As a result their pathogenic relevance has been called into question. However it is probable that other antibodies to brain antigens have yet to be found in this group and anti-thyroid antibodies reflect the presence of antibodies to a broader set of epitopes.

In six published patients histopathological material was obtained; the results are described for five (one postmortem and four brain biopsy specimens). One specimen was normal but the other four had a vasculopathy, with lymphocytic infiltration of veins or small arterioles leading to gliosis and microglial activation in one. This implication of this is that a steroid-responsive vasculopathy with a possible humoral basis is responsible for the features of the disease.

Diagnosis of SREAT

The diagnosis of SREAT is clinical, based upon the recognition of the features above and supported by the presence of high titers of anti-thyroid antibodies. Infective and metabolic causes should be ruled out. The EEG examination is abnormal in almost 100% of cases, usually with diffuse slowing, but in some cases mesial temporal seizure discharges have been described. The CSF protein is high in 75–85% of patients, usually with few cells although 5% may have >100 cells/mm^3. Imaging studies are inconsistent. Normal, minimally abnormal, or atrophic brains are most often reported but widespread white matter disease and dural enhancement are also described.

Anti-thyroid antibodies are by definition abnormal. These can be anti-thyroid peroxidase or anti-thyroglobulin antibodies and although the titer is very often high, the titer does not correlate with clinical presentation or response to treatment. Patients may present with clinical or subclinical hypo- or hyperthyroidism.

Treatment of SREAT

No trials or uniform guidelines are available to inform therapeutic decisions. Lord Brain's index case did not respond to treatment with prednisone and remitted spontaneously. However, in the literature review of Hashimoto encephalopathy from Chong *et al.* (2003), 69 patients were treated with steroid (24 also with thyroxine), of whom 66 improved. In Castillo's series (Castillo *et al.* 2006), all patients responded to steroid by definition. Fifteen returned to normal, five having mild residual neurologic deficits. Intravenous methylprednisolone induction followed by oral prednisolone at a dose of 1 mg/kg would seem to be an appropriate starting dose for therapy, tapering after 4–6 weeks. Relapses occur and have been treated with re-exposure to methylprednisolone and steroid sparing agents such as azathioprine, methotrexate, cyclophosphamide, and IVIG.

Seizures may remit as the encephalopathy is treated. Acute treatment of status epilepticus may be required initially but continued control may be difficult without additional immunosuppressive treatment.

Inflammatory bowel disease

Inflammatory bowel disease is a term that traditionally refers to ulcerative colitis (UC) and Crohn disease. Both are chronic relapsing inflammatory diseases of the gut which have well-defined anatomical distribution and histopathological and epidemiological features. In neither is a pathogenesis really understood, although UC is more often associated with other autoimmune diseases. In this respect it is likened to celiac disease. Crohn disease is typified by granulomatous inflammation, likened to Johne disease in farm animals, which is caused by *Mycobacterium paratuberculosis*, and hence an infective pathogenesis is thought more likely. Celiac disease might also be considered under the generic heading of inflammatory bowel disease, and is better understood. Inflammation of the small intestine is induced by prolamins in wheat barley and rye (gliadins, hordeins, and secalins).

Neither UC nor Crohn disease is especially common. Ulcerative colitis has a prevalence of between 8 and 12 per 100 000 and Crohn disease between 5 and 7 per 100 000 population. Celiac disease has a strong genetic susceptibility and in affected populations the prevalence may be extremely high, notably the west of Ireland where the prevalence is 1 in 300; in Europe the prevalence ranges from between 1 in 6000 to 1 in 1500.

All three conditions have been associated with neurological complications, of which epilepsy is one. The evidence for this association however is not strong and the association is a rare one. In both UC and Crohn disease it is supported largely by case reports and small series. Other extraintestinal manifestations are more common. For example, erythema nodosum, uveitis, arthropathy, liver disease, and pericarditis are associated with UC, and amyloid, renal stones, and complications of malabsorption are seen in Crohn disease. Other organ specific autoimmune diseases and systemic lupus erythematosus are commonly associated with celiac disease.

Epilepsy in inflammatory bowel disease

The point prevalence of epilepsy is approximately 0.5% to 1% of the population. Ulcerative colitis and Crohn's disease are less common, but it is not surprising that a number of patients have both conditions coexisting. Two studies suggested that seizures occurred in between 5% and 50% of patients with inflammatory bowel disease (IBD). However neither of these figures has emerged in a full publication and there has been no subsequent confirmation. In another study, the point prevalence of epilepsy in a cohort of 638 patients with IBD was 1.9%, but of these 12 patients, ten had structural or metabolic causes for their epilepsy and two had epilepsy pre-dating their IBD by more than 15 years (Lossos et al. 1995). There are therefore no good epidemiological data to support a link between UC or Crohn disease and epilepsy.

The epidemiological association of celiac disease with epilepsy is a little stronger. Between 3.5% and 5.5% of patients with celiac disease have epilepsy, and conversely between 0.8% and 2.5% of patients with epilepsy in four other studies had celiac disease (Bushara 2005). The described association of epileptogenic occipital calcifications with epilepsy and celiac disease in a number of Italian studies has been replicated elsewhere in a small series (Sammaritano et al. 1988).

Pathogenesis of epilepsy

The pathogenesis of epilepsy in IBD is as unclear as the epidemiological association. It is likely that a number of diverse factors contribute, there being no one clear outstanding mechanism.

Immunological mechanisms have been postulated, but with little support. Elsehety and Bertorini (1997) reported that six of 15 patients with epilepsy related to Crohn disease improved with immunotherapy and postulated a small vessel central and peripheral nervous system vasculopathy to link the diseases and improvement. Vasculitis has been postulated in two other studies, diagnosed by imaging only (Masaki et al. 1997) or simply suggested in the other. The rarity of these cases with unusual mechanisms makes them unlikely. More probable pathogenic mechanisms are the systemic complications of IBD itself. These include cerebral thromboembolism, hypomagnesemia and hypocalcemia, fluid shifts, and hypoxia, all more common in severely unwell patients or those undergoing bowel surgery. It is not surprising that immunotherapy directed at the improvement of an inflammatory disease with resultant reinstatement of homeostasis might improve the results of its disturbance.

A single animal study has provided support to links between IBD and epilepsy. In a mouse model of intestinal inflammation, mice were found to have lower seizure thresholds during the period of bowel inflammation, and this was attributable to endogenous opioid and not nitric oxide release (Riazi et al. 2004). Once again, however, this supports a susceptibility mechanism rather than a pathogenesis.

In celiac disease, gluten exclusion diets have been reported to improve seizure control and reduce (but not stop) need for medication in many case reports (Bushara 2005). The occurrence of occipital calcifications in patients with celiac disease remains clear and it is likely that these might be epileptogenic.

Diagnosis of inflammatory bowel diseases

Celiac disease presents with diarrhea, abdominal pain, weight loss, and the biochemical and hematological consequences of malabsorption. These may all be reflected in simple biological tests. There is often steatorrhea, and hydrogen breath tests may identify bacterial overgrowth. Immunoglobulin A (IgA) antibodies to endomysium, gliadin, and reticulin are all highly sensitive and specific. With dietary exclusion, antibodies may become undetectable. Duodenal biopsies showing villous atrophy and inflammatory infiltration of the lamina propria are the gold standard for diagnosis.

Ulcerative colitis and Crohn disease also present with abdominal pain and malabsorption syndromes. The diarrhea in UC is frequently bloody, and the pain of Crohn disease may more frequently be in the right iliac fossa. There are no clear serological tests for either UC or Crohn disease although protoplasmic-staining antineutrophil cytoplasmic antibodies (p-ANCA) are associated with UC and anti-*Saccharomyces cerevisiae* antibodies (ASCA) with Crohn disease. Barium follow-through studies and CT/MRI imaging of the abdomen are able to demonstrate narrowed segments of gut with thickened inflamed walls and fistulae in Crohn disease which may be directly visualized with the colonoscope along with patchy skip lesions of macroscopic inflammation. Granulomatous infiltration of the bowel wall at these sites is diagnostic. The inflammation seen in UC is not specific to the diagnosis.

Treatment of inflammatory bowel diseases

The treatment of the underlying Crohn disease, UC, or celiac disease is likely to lead to a restitution of physiological and nutritional homeostasis, a decrease in systemic inflammation and an improvement in coexistent epilepsy. In all cases adequate balanced nutritional and fluid support is essential which may be in the form of elemental diets in severe cases. In celiac disease exclusion of glutens is the primary treatment; a small number of patients may require steroid or steroid-sparing agents but they are unusual. In UC and Crohn disease remission is achieved with systemic and/or local steroid in conjunction with oral immunosuppressant/steroid sparing agents, most commonly azathioprine, ciclosporin, mesalazine, sulphasalazine, and Pentasa. Infliximab may be used in UC. Surgery is occasionally necessary and in these circumstances patients may be particularly vulnerable to seizures.

Treatment of epilepsy

No specific recommendations for epilepsy treatment in IBD apply. Patients with IBD should be treated to achieve remission from their gastrointestinal disease and normalize nutrition. Where absorbative capacity is limited by short gut or inflammation parenteral therapies may have to be considered. There is no evidence to support the use of any specific therapies for epilepsy in IBD.

References

Bartolomei F, Boucraut J, Barrie M, *et al.* (1996) Cryptogenic partial epilepsies with anti-GM1 antibodies: a new form of immune-mediated epilepsy? *Epilepsia* 37:922–6.

Brain L, Jellinek EH, Ball K (1966) Hashimoto's disease and encephalopathy. *Lancet* 2:512–14.

Brierley JB (1960) Subacute encephalitis of later adult life mainly affecting the limbic areas. *Brain* 83:357–68.

Buckley C, Oger J, Clover L, *et al.* (2001) Potassium channel antibodies in two patients with reversible limbic encephalitis. *Ann Neurol* 50:73–8.

Bushara KO (2005) Neurologic presentation of celiac disease. *Gastroenterology* 128(4 Suppl 1):S92–7.

Castillo P, Woodruff B, Caselli R, *et al.* (2006) Steroid-responsive encephalopathy associated with autoimmune thyroiditis. *Arch Neurol* 63:197–202.

Chong JY, Rowland LP, Utiger RD (2003) Hashimoto encephalopathy: syndrome or myth? *Arch Neurol* 60:164–71.

Dalmau J, Rosenfeld MR (2008) Paraneoplastic syndromes of the CNS. *Lancet Neurol* 7:327–40.

Dalmau J, Tuzun E, Wu HY, *et al.* (2007) Paraneoplastic anti-*N*-methyl-D-aspartate receptor encephalitis associated with ovarian teratoma. *Ann Neurol* 61:25–36.

Elsehety A, Bertorini TE (1997) Neurologic and neuropsychiatric complications of Crohn's disease. *South Med J* 90:606–10.

Fadul CE, Stommel EW, Dragnev KH, Eskey CJ, Dalmau JO (2005) Focal paraneoplastic limbic encephalitis presenting as orgasmic epilepsy. *J Neurooncol* 72:195–8.

Hutchinson M, Waters P, McHugh J, *et al.* (2008) Progressive encephalomyelitis, rigidity, and myoclonus: a novel glycine receptor antibody. *Neurology* 71:1291–2.

Kanter IC, Huttner HB, Staykov D, *et al.* (2008) Cyclophosphamide for anti-GAD antibody-positive refractory status epilepticus. *Epilepsia* 49:914–20.

Kleopa KA, Elman LB, Lang B, Vincent A, Scherer SS (2006) Neuromyotonia and limbic encephalitis sera target mature Shaker-type K$^+$ channels: subunit specificity correlates with clinical manifestations. *Brain* 129:1570–84.

Lawn ND, Westmoreland BF, Kiely MJ, Lennon VA, Vernino S (2003) Clinical, magnetic resonance imaging, and electroencephalographic findings in paraneoplastic limbic encephalitis. *Mayo Clin Proc* 78:1363–8.

Lossos A, River Y, Eliakim A, Steiner I (1995) Neurologic aspects of inflammatory bowel disease. *Neurology* 45:416–21.

Majoie HJ, de Baets M, Renier W, Lang B, Vincent A (2006) Antibodies to voltage-gated potassium and calcium channels in epilepsy. *Epilepsy Res* 71:135–41.

Masaki T, Muto T, Shinozaki M, Kuroda T (1997) Unusual cerebral complication associated with ulcerative colitis. *J Gastroenterol* 32:251–4.

Peltola J, Kulmala P, Isojarvi J, *et al.* (2000) Autoantibodies to glutamic acid decarboxylase in patients with therapy-resistant epilepsy. *Neurology* 55:46–50.

Riazi K, Honar H, Homayoun H, *et al.* (2004) Intestinal inflammation alters the susceptibility to pentylenetetrazole-induced seizure in mice. *J Gastroenterol Hepatol* 19:270–7.

Sabater L, Gomez-Choco M, Saiz A, Graus F (2005) BR serine/threonine kinase 2: a new autoantigen in paraneoplastic limbic encephalitis. *J Neuroimmunol* 170:186–90.

Sammaritano N, Andermann F, Melanson D, *et al.* (1988) The syndrome of intractable epilepsy, bilateral occipital calcifications, and folic acid deficiency. *Neurology* 38(Suppl 1):239.

Shimazaki H, Ando Y, Nakano I, Dalmau J (2007) Reversible limbic encephalitis with antibodies against the membranes of neurons of the hippocampus. *J Neurol Neurosurg Psychiatry* 78:324–5.

Solimena M, Folli F, Aparisi R, Pozza G, De CP (1990) Autoantibodies to GABA-ergic neurons and pancreatic beta cells in stiff-man syndrome. *N Engl J Med* 322:1555–60.

Thieben MJ, Lennon VA, Boeve BF, *et al.* (2004) Potentially reversible autoimmune limbic encephalitis with neuronal potassium channel antibody. *Neurology* 62:1177–82.

Tuzun E, Dalmau J (2007) Limbic encephalitis and variants: classification, diagnosis and treatment. *Neurologist* 13:261–71.

Vincent A, Buckley C, Schott JM, *et al.* (2004) Potassium channel antibody-associated encephalopathy: a potentially immunotherapy-responsive form of limbic encephalitis. *Brain* 127:701–12.

Chapter 84

Psychiatric disorders

Brent Elliott and John O'Donavan

Introduction

A chapter on the psychiatric causes of epilepsy might at first glance be expected to restrict itself to a discussion on the proconvulsant actions of antidepressant and antipsychotic drugs or to the acute and chronic effects of illicit drug misuse. There are however several other areas of interest, most notably the possibility of a "bidirectional relationship" between certain psychiatric disorders and seizures. It is well known that patients with epilepsy are at increased risk of developing psychiatric disorders, but what is now emerging is a picture in which psychiatric disorders themselves may increase the risk of subsequently developing epilepsy, worsen seizure control, or directly precipitate seizures. In this chapter we provide a review of the available literature, in regard to the following "causal conditions": (1) stress; (2) depression; (3) illicit psychoactive drug misuse; (4) psychotropic medication (antidepressants and antipsychotics); (5) autistic spectrum disorders; (7) Tourette syndrome; and (8) attention deficit hyperactivity disorder (ADHD).

The causal conditions

Stress

Definition

Stress is clearly a difficult concept to define; most commonly it is used in the metaphorical sense to describe an emotional state that occurs secondary to challenges occurring in everyday life. Stress in the biological sense refers to the consequences of the failure of a human or animal body to respond appropriately to emotional or physical threats, whether actual or imagined (Selye 1959).

The concept of stress is acknowledged (although not defined) in the *International Statistical Classification of Diseases and Related Health Problems*, 10th Revision (ICD-10) (World Health Organization 1992) under the category "Reaction to severe stress and adjustment disorders" (F43). An acute stress reaction is a transient disorder that develops in an individual without any other apparent mental disorder in response to

exceptional physical and/or mental stress and that usually subsides within hours or days. The effects of particular stressors on an individual vary, and individual vulnerability and coping capacity are known to play a significant role.

Stress as a seizure precipitant

Stress is frequently identified as a precipitant of seizures by patients with epilepsy. Nakken *et al.* (2005) for example found the most frequently reported precipitants to be emotional stress, sleep deprivation, and tiredness. In a separate study of patients with juvenile myoclonic epilepsy the most common precipitants included stress (83%), sleep deprivation (77%), specific thoughts/mental concentration (23%), and speaking out in public (11%) (Da Silva Sousa *et al.* 2005).

Despite these subjective reports the exact nature of the relationship is not clear. Haut *et al.* (2007) did not find an association between stress and the likelihood of a seizure the next day, whilst Thapar *et al.* (2009) found that it was depression that mediated the relationship between stress, seizure recency (time since last seizure), and seizure frequency. It has been suggested that certain perceived triggers may be misattributed to the precipitation of seizures due to an underlying psychological predisposition (M.R. Sperling *et al.* 2008). These workers found that self-perception of seizure precipitants was significantly related to seizure control, anxiety level, and external health locus of control.

Despite these findings there is good evidence from animal studies that supports a possible causal link between stress and seizures.

Prenatal and early postnatal stress in rats

Prenatal stress in rats increases both seizure vulnerability and anxiety. Edwards *et al.* (2002), for example, found that both early and mid/late gestation prenatal stress significantly lowered the after-discharge threshold and increased the rate of kindled seizure development in infant, 14-day-old rat offspring, as compared to non-stressed controls. These effects are more pronounced in infancy but may also extend into adulthood, with Frye and Bayon (1999) demonstrating that adult

The Causes of Epilepsy, eds. S. D. Shorvon, F. Andermann, and R. Guerrini. Published by Cambridge University Press. © Cambridge University Press 2011.

rats exposed to prenatal stress tend to have more partial seizures and significantly more tonic–clonic seizures (following administration of 3α, 5α-tetrahydroprogesterone prior to testing for kainic-acid-induced ictal activity) that were of longer duration than no prenatal stress rats.

Postnatal stress and gender also appear to play a role. Salzberg et al. (2007) found that rats exposed to early postnatal maternal separation (180 min/day) displayed significantly increased anxiety at 7 weeks when compared with rats who received early handling and brief separation (15 min/day). When implanted with bipolar electrodes in the left amygdala, female rats required fewer stimulations following maternal separation than early handling to reach the fully kindled state. They concluded that early maternal separation leads to a persisting vulnerability to limbic epileptogenesis in females, increases anxiety in both sexes, and involves gender-specific factors such as hormones.

There is also evidence that links repeated psychosocial or restraint stress with structural changes in the hippocampus. Magarinos et al. (1997) measured ultrastructural parameters associated with mossy fiber–CA3 synapses in control and 21-day restraint stressed rats. Terminals from stressed animals showed a marked rearrangement of vesicles, with more densely packed clusters localized in the vicinity of active zones. Restraint stress also increased the area of the mossy fiber terminal occupied by mitochondrial profiles and consequently a larger localized energy-generating capacity. A single stress session did not produce these changes.

The cellular effects of stress, in particular the role of corticotrophin releasing hormone, corticosteroids, and neurosteroids on the hippocampus and epilepsy are detailed in a review by Joels. He found that stress hormones rapidly enhance CA1/CA3 hippocampal activity. At the same time corticosterone starts gene-mediated events which enhance calcium influx several hours later. This serves to normalize activity but also imposes a risk for neuronal injury if and when neurons are concurrently strongly depolarized, e.g., during a seizure. Under repetitive stress and/or early life stress hormonal influences on inhibitory tone (via γ-aminobutyric acid [GABA] receptors) are diminished; instead enhanced calcium influx and increased excitation become more important (Joels 2008).

Stress occurring in adult life in humans

In human observational studies, the most common experimental stressors have been combat-related. Moshe et al. (2008), for example, examined the effects of occupational stress (physical and mental) in new military recruits with no previous history of epilepsy or with epilepsy in remission for over 2 years. They found the incidence of seizures, (in patients with no seizure history) to be higher in those soldiers assigned to combat units as compared with maintenance units or administrative units (relative risk = 1.29, 95% confidence interval [CI] 1.03–1.62) but there was no difference in seizure recurrence between groups. Neufeld et al. (1994) examined the effect of stress (in the form of SCUD missile attacks) on seizure frequency, in 100 adult patients with epilepsy during the 1991 Persian Gulf War. An increase in generalized seizure frequency was seen in eight patients; in only four of these were the seizures directly related to the sounding of an alarm. Of the remaining four, disturbed sleep and being off medication at the time of the seizure were the main contributory factors. They concluded that epilepsy control was only weakly affected by this quite significant external stress.

Klein and van Passel (2005), however, examined the effect of 9/11 attack-related emotional stress on seizures among 66 adult patients with epilepsy from the Georgetown University Hospital epilepsy clinic (3 miles [about 5 km] from the Pentagon). Twenty-eight of 66 patients (42%) were stressed by the attack: 13 (19.6%) mildly, 11 (16.6%) moderately, and 4 (6%) severely. Six patients were directly affected by the attack (e.g., a family member died or the patient was in a building that was threatened). The authors found that this stressful event was associated with seizure exacerbation (defined as a 50% increase in seizure frequency) in only a small proportion (in this case 12%) of exposed patients with epilepsy, but in a higher proportion (29%) in patients stressed by the event and in 50% of patients directly affected by the event. They conclude that magnitude of stress (plus individual vulnerability) may therefore be important in determining whether or not stress is associated with seizure exacerbation.

Cognitive/emotional triggers for seizures

Woods and Gruenthal (2006) present a case report of a 32-year-old woman with primary generalized epilepsy who described absence events precipitated by talking about childhood sexual abuse, her epilepsy, or her father's difficulty with schizophrenia. During video/electroencephalograph (EEG) monitoring 30 absence seizures were recorded, 28 of which occurred while discussing one of these three precipitants.

Diagnosis

We were unable to identify any studies that attempted to correlate scores on a "stress" rating scale with the risk of seizure. From the above discussion there are several factors that are likely to confound this relationship such as anxiety levels, seizure control, and an external health locus of control. The relationship may also be accounted for by comorbid depression and this should be screened for as described below.

One scale that is available to quickly quantify stress is the Epilepsy Stressor Inventory – Revised (Snyder 1993). This is short (22 items) and easy to administer with a high internal consistency (alpha of 0.93) and a test–retest reliability of 0.76.

Treatment

If comorbid anxiety and depression exist then antidepressants may be required. As will be seen later in the section on psychotropic drugs and seizures, the selective serotonin reuptake inhibitors (SSRIs) and mirtazepine may in fact have antiepileptic effects. We were unable to identify any human trials of antidepressants in the treatment of stress (although antiglucocorticoid antidepressants are in development); however, an interesting animal study is provided by Pericic *et al.* (2005) who were able to demonstrate that fluoxetine given acutely or repeatedly shows anticonvulsant properties against convulsions induced in unstressed and swim-stressed mice by the GABAA receptor antagonist picrotoxin.

It might seem intuitive that psychological interventions aimed at treating "stress" such as relaxation therapy, biofeedback, and cognitive behavioral therapy may improve seizure control and/or quality of life in patients with epilepsy. Despite this expectation a *Cochrane Review* assessing whether the treatment of epilepsy with psychological methods is effective in reducing seizure frequency and/or leads to a better quality of life has recently been published. The authors concluded that "in view of methodological deficiencies and limited number of individuals studied, we have found no reliable evidence to support the use of these treatments and further trials are needed" (Ramaratnam *et al.* 2008).

Links between stress and depression

Much of the current psychiatric research into depression (in patients without epilepsy) focuses on the concept of gene × environment interactions. In this model stressful life events are thought to interact with a particular genotype to precipitate depression in vulnerable individuals. One example of this work includes a classic paper by Caspi *et al.* (2003), who investigated the effect of a functional polymorphism in the promoter region of the serotonin transporter (5-HT T) gene on the influence of stressful life events in mediating depression. They found that individuals with one or two copies of the short allele of the 5-HT T promoter polymorphism exhibited more depressive symptoms, diagnosable depression, and suicidality in relation to stressful life events than individuals homozygous for the long allele.

The same group also examined the effect of work stress (psychological job demands, work decision latitude, low work social support, physical work demands) on the risk of developing major depressive disorder or generalized anxiety disorder. They found that participants exposed to high psychological job demands (excessive workload, extreme time pressures) had a twofold risk of major depressive disorder or generalized anxiety disorder compared to those with low job demands in individuals without any pre-job history of diagnosis or treatment for either disorder (Melchior *et al.* 2007). Whilst this area remains a topic of much debate the concept of individual vulnerability to developing depression in response to stress is likely to be important for patients with epilepsy, as will be explained below.

Depression

Introduction

The justification for including depression in a chapter on the causes of epilepsy lies in the fact that there may be a bidirectional relationship between the psychiatric disorder and the epilepsy itself. This is not a new idea; Hippocrates wrote that "melancholics ordinarily become epileptics, and epileptics melancholics" (Lewis 1934) whilst more recently, Sir William Gowers (1901) observed that "suicide although not a certainty is often a probable indication of a morbid family tendency and some weight must be given to it as an indication of a disposition to a disease of which epilepsy may be the result even when it has an immediate exciting cause".

Recent work supports these early observations. The main findings are:

(1) Adults with late-onset epilepsy (>54 years) are 3.7 times more likely to have a history of depression than controls (Hesdorffer *et al.* 2000).

(2) Those with new-onset epilepsy are seven times more likely to have a history of depression than controls and the risk may be even higher (as much as 17-fold) in focal epilepsy (Forsgren and Nystrom 1990).

(3) Children with new-onset epilepsy are four times more likely to have had a depressive episode prior to the first seizure (Hesdorffer *et al.* 1999).

(4) Adults and children over 10 years of age with a first unprovoked seizure or newly diagnosed epilepsy are five times more likely to have a history of attempted suicide (Hesdorffer *et al.* 2006). In this study, attempted suicide increased subsequent seizure risk even after adjusting for age, sex, alcohol intake, major depression, and number of symptoms of depression suggesting the increased risk may be due to "recurrence of pre-morbid suicidal behavior" (Elliott *et al.* 2009).

Clinical presentation/definitions

For everyday clinical convenience it is useful to divide affective disorders in patients with epilepsy into periictal (preictal, ictal, and postictal) and interictal categories. It is the interictal disorders with which we are concerned here.

In ICD-10, a depressive episode (F32) is characterized by a lowering of mood which varies little from day to day, is unresponsive to circumstances, and may be accompanied by so-called "somatic" symptoms, such as loss of interest and pleasurable feelings, waking in the morning several hours before the usual time, depression that is worst in the morning, psychomotor agitation or retardation, loss of appetite and/or weight, and loss of libido. There is usually a reduction in energy and decrease in activity. The capacity for enjoyment, interest, and concentration is reduced, and marked tiredness after even minimum effort is common. Self-esteem and self-confidence are almost always reduced and some ideas of guilt or worthlessness are often present. Depending upon the number and severity of the symptoms, a depressive episode may be specified as mild, moderate, or severe. The *Diagnostic and Statistical Manual of Mental Disorders*, 4th edn (DSM-IV) (American Psychiatric Association 1995) also specifies that the symptoms should be present on most days for a minimum period of 2 weeks.

595

The ICD-10 category of recurrent depressive disorder (F33) is characterized by repeated episodes of depression, without any history of independent episodes of mood elevation and increased energy (mania).

Prevalence

Lifetime prevalence for a major depressive episode in the general population ranges between 3.7% and 6.7%. In patients with epilepsy rates range from 11% (current depression) to 62% (lifetime-to-date depressive disorder) with an estimated mean of 30% across studies (Gaitatzis *et al.* 2004; Barry *et al.* 2008). Prevalence may be lower (3–9%) in patients with good seizure control (Kanner 2003).

Diagnosis

Ordinarily the diagnosis of depression is made on the basis of a patient meeting criteria for a depressive syndrome as per ICD-10 or DSM-IV; however, there are depressive syndromes in epilepsy that do not meet standardized operational criteria (Mendez *et al.* 1986). Furthermore, the diagnosis of depression in this particular patient group is complicated by the fact that atypical presentations are common and certain symptoms (e.g., problems with sleep, appetite, libido, cognition, or memory) may be interpreted as side effects of antiepileptic drugs.

Gilliam and colleagues have attempted to address this issue by developing and validating. The Neurological Disorders Depression Inventory for Epilepsy (NDDI-E) (Gilliam *et al.* 2006). It takes only 3 min to complete, has been validated in patients with epilepsy, and a score of ≥15 has a specificity of 90% and sensitivity of 81% for a diagnosis of major depression. Other potentially useful rating scales include the Beck Depression Inventory (BDI-II) (Beck *et al.* 1996) which takes about 5 min to complete and has also been validated in epilepsy; scores over 20 indicate moderate to severe depression (Elliott *et al.* 2009).

Treatment

Antidepressants

There is a clear need for randomized placebo controlled studies of antidepressants in patients with epilepsy. In the only published controlled study Robertson and Trimble (1985) found higher-dose amitriptyline (150 mg/day) to be effective. Specchio *et al.* (2004) in an open label uncontrolled study were able to show a marked improvement in depression in 39 patients treated with citalopram 20 mg/day. Finally, Kuhn *et al.* (2003) analyzed post hoc data from 2 years of treatment of 75 inpatients with major depression and temporal lobe epilepsy. They compared citalopram, mirtazepine, and reboxetine, finding these drugs to be equally efficacious. There were no serious adverse events or drug interactions.

The largest clinical antidepressant trial to date, the NIMH STAR-D (sequenced treatment alternatives to relieve depression) trial, was recently completed (Trivedi *et al.* 2006). Whilst STAR-D was not carried out specifically in patients with epilepsy, the results, when combined with data from patients with epilepsy, suggest that a simple and evidence-based pathway for the treatment of depression in this patient group would be to start treatment with citalopram, and then if remission of symptoms is not achieved to progress through sertraline, mirtazepine, and venlafaxine.

Cognitive behavioral therapy

It is likely that affective disorders respond better to a combination of pharmacotherapy and psychological therapy than to either modality alone. Cognitive behavioral therapy (CBT) usually involves 12–16 sessions with a specially trained psychologist or psychiatrist during which a patient's unhelpful beliefs about themselves and the world they interact with are explored. The behaviors that result from these beliefs may act to reinforce the depressed state. In the therapy these views are challenged, alternative possibilities explored, and a more helpful set of attitudes and beliefs encouraged.

Electroconvulsive therapy

Epilepsy is not a contraindication to electroconvulsive therapy (ECT); in fact there is good evidence that ECT actually increases seizure threshold. The use of ECT has declined significantly in routine clinical psychiatric practice but it is still used (albeit rarely) in patients with severe depression, treatment-resistant mania, and very rarely in psychosis.

Mental and behavioral disorders secondary to psychoactive substance misuse

A variety of commonly used recreational drugs can act either directly or indirectly to cause seizures. In the UK these include opioids, stimulants (cocaine, amphetamine, methylenedioxymethamphetamine), marijuana, benzodiazepines, barbiturates, club drugs (phencyclidine and ketamine), hallucinogens, and inhalants. The role of alcohol is considered in detail in Chapter 95 and will not be discussed here.

Opioids

The endogenous opiates, enkephalin and endorphin, are derived from their peptide precursors pro-opiomelanocortin (POMC), proenkephalin, and prodynorphin and then stored in opiate neurons in the arcuate nucleus. These neurons project to the nucleus accumbens and ventral tegmental area where the endogenous opiates are released and exert their role in mediating reinforcement and pleasure in reward circuitry. The most important receptor subtypes are the mu, delta, and kappa opiate receptors. Exogenous opiates (e.g., heroin) act on these same receptors, particularly at mu sites, to produce a brief euphoria followed by a profound sense of tranquillity (Stahl 2008).

The pharmacological basis of opioid-induced seizures in not clear and opioids are variably proconvulsant or anticonvulsant depending on species, seizure model, rate of administration and particular agent (e.g., mu-, delta-, or kappa-agonist).

Seizures are not a feature of withdrawal (except in neonates), but may occur in overdose (along with pinpoint pupils and respiratory depression). Since the latter presentation is so unusual concomitant cocaine, alcohol withdrawal, or central nervous system (CNS) infection should be looked for (Brust 2007). Past or current heroin use has been identified as a risk factor for new-onset seizures independent of head trauma, infection, stroke, ethanol, or other drugs in a case–control study. The risk was greatest if heroin had been used on the day of the seizure and persisted even after a year of abstinence (Ng *et al.* 1990).

Stimulants

Cocaine blocks monoamine reuptake by the dopamine transporter thereby augmenting the effects of catecholamine neurotransmitters, and increasing dopaminergic stimulation, at critical brain sites. Cocaine also blocks serotonin and norepinephrine reuptake, a feature associated with the "kindling" phenomenon (Zagnoni and Albano 2002).

Seizures are common among first-time cocaine users; as many as 40% may be affected (Lowenstein *et al.* 1987). In retrospective studies the frequency of cocaine-associated seizures varies from 1% to 8% (Zagnoni and Albano 2002); however, one autopsy study showed that 36% of 36 fatalities related to cocaine had seizures before death (Pascual-Leone *et al.* 1990). Single generalized motor seizures are the most common, but multiple seizures and status epilepticus occur immediately or in less than 2 hr after ingestion and coincide with peak blood levels (Zagnoni and Albano 2002). Focal seizures suggest a structural lesion such as cocaine-related intracerebral hemorrhage and status epilepticus following cocaine use is often refractory to conventional anticonvulsant therapy (Brust 2007). Seizures appear to be more likely to occur after smoking crack than after snorting cocaine hydrochloride, and this is probably a dosing effect. There is also some animal evidence that prenatal exposure to cocaine may increase later susceptibility to seizures (Keller and Snyder-Keller 2000).

Amphetamine-like drugs include amphetamine, methamphetamine, dextroamphetamine, and methylphenidate, and their role in causing seizures appears less strong than that of cocaine (Hanson *et al.* 1999; Zagnoni and Albano 2002). Their mechanism of action is via an increase in presynaptic release of dopamine. They tend to cause seizures in the setting of overdose (fever, hypertension, cardiac arrhythmias, delirium, or coma) and this effect is mediated by the stimulation of N-methyl-D-aspartate (NMDA) receptors and the inhibition of GABAA receptors. They rarely induce epileptic seizures at therapeutic doses, but seizures may occur after the first dosing (Zagnoni and Albano 2002; Brust 2007).

Methylenedioxymethamphetamine (MDMA, "ecstasy") has both stimulant and hallucinogenic effects. Seizures appear to be the most common clinical CNS complication after ingestion of ecstasy; the pathophysiology of these appears to be related to severe hyponatremia (Hedetoft and Christensen 1999). Caffeine at high doses can also induce epileptic seizures because of its adenosine-

receptor-antagonizing properties but it can also act on the cerebral vasculature to reduce blood flow (Zagnoni and Albano 2002).

Marijuana

Marijuana was actually used to treat epilepsy in the nineteenth century, with Gowers reporting that "I have administered [it] in many cases, and with the effect of delaying the paroxysms and mitigating their severity in some individuals" (Gowers 1881). Despite conflicting results on the effect of marijuana on seizure threshold its use would seem to be quite common among patients with epilepsy. Gross *et al.* (2004), for example, found that 21% of their patients with epilepsy (in a tertiary care center) had used marijuana in the past year, with the majority of active users reporting beneficial effects on seizures.

Gordon and Devinsky (2001) provide a detailed review on the safety of marijuana use in patients with epilepsy. The mechanisms by which marijuana or the cannabinoids alter seizure threshold is not clear and may involve a functional connectivity between cannabinoid and NMDA receptors, a change in the level of catecholamine neurotransmitters, or an effect on thalamocortical projections, altering seizure threshold by increasing seizure synchronicity. They highlight that marijuana and its active cannabinoids (in particular cannabidiol) may have antiepileptic effects, but these may be specific to partial or tonic–clonic seizures. Marijuana use may also transiently impair short-term memory, and thereby increase non-compliance with antiepileptic drugs, and marijuana use or withdrawal could also potentially trigger seizures in susceptible patients. They conclude that there are currently insufficient data to determine whether occasional or chronic marijuana use influences seizure frequency.

Sedative hypnotics

These include barbiturates, benzodiazepines, and the Z-drug hypnotics, all of which are positive allosteric modulators for GABA-A receptors. Barbiturates are the least safe in overdose, are more frequently subject to abuse and dependence, and produce more dangerous withdrawal reactions. Downregulation of GABA receptors is probably a major mechanism of seizures during barbiturate and benzodiazepine withdrawal, following which seizures and delirium tremens can occur. This usually happens within 24 hr of stopping a short-acting agent and within several days of stopping a long-acting agent. Seizures tend to be dose-related and are unlikely in patients taking recommended therapeutic doses (Brust 2007).

Withdrawal seizures have also been described with a number of non-barbiturate/non-benzodiazepine sedatives including meprobamate, chloral hydrate, and zolpidem. Seizures can also be a feature of recreational antihistamine use and γ-hydroxbutyrate intoxication can lead to myoclonus and seizures (Brust 2007).

Club drugs (phencyclidine and ketamine)

Phencyclidine and ketamine are antagonists at NMDA receptors, causing NMDA hypoactivity which in turn leads to disinhibiton of dopamine release. Intoxicated patients may display features of catatonia (excitement alternating with stupor/catalepsy), psychosis, and disorientation. They may also be aggressive with raised blood pressure and enlarged non-reactive pupils (Zagnoni and Albano 2002). In a review of 1000 cases of phencyclidine toxicity there were 26 grand mal seizures and five cases of status epilepticus (McCarron et al. 1981).

Hallucinogens

The most popular agents are peyote cactus containing mesca-line, mushrooms containing psilocybin, and the synthetic ergot compound D-lysergic acid diethylamide (LSD). In the review by Zagnoni and Albano psychedelic compounds were found only rarely to induce epileptic seizures (Zagnoni and Albano 2002; Brust 2007).

Indirect mechanisms

Recreational drug use can also act indirectly to produce seizures; assault or accidents can result in cerebral trauma, intravenous drug use may result in systemic and CNS infection (e.g., HIV), there is an increased risk of ischemic or hemorrhagic stroke, e.g., with cocaine, and metabolic complications such as hypoglycemia and hyponatremia may also occur (Brust 2007).

Treatment

In the UK treatment for drug addiction is overseen by the National Treatment Agency for Substance Misuse (NTA). There are a variety of both statutory and voluntary sector agencies providing rehabilitation for drug users. The National Health Service (NHS) provides clients (with pre-dominantly opiate, alcohol, stimulant, and benzodiazepine dependence) with "walk in" access to Specialist Addiction Services. Management is based on principles of engaging and retaining the client in treatment over the long term and focuses on the provision of both substitute prescribing and psychological treatment.

At the time of writing substitute prescribing is largely limited to opiate users. Opiate receptors can readapt to normal if given the chance to do so. In practice this usually requires the client to be switched from heroin (usually intravenous or smoked) to prescribed methadone or buprenorphine which can then be slowly tapered. Some users find that they need regular substitute maintenance therapy rather than gradual downward dose titration until they are psychologically prepared for change.

There are at present no substitutes available for stimulant users. There may be a cocaine vaccine (TA-CD) in the future and modafenil is also being tested in this regard. Various antipsychotics including olanzapine, and in particularly D2 partial antagonists such as aripiprazole are also being tested. Experimental treatments include D3 receptor partial antagonists or antagonists and long-lasting dopamine releasers. Naltrexone is also being investigated. *N*-acetyl-cysteine acts on the cysteine–glutamatergic exchange mechanism to reduce craving and interest in cocaine. Rimonabant, a "marijuana antagonist," may be a potential therapeutic agent in various types of drug abuse, from cigarette smoking to alcoholism to marijuana. It has not yet been approved in the USA by the Food and Drug Administration (FDA) due to concerns about the possibility that long-term use might increase suicidal ideation (Stahl 2008).

Psychological treatments

The strongest evidence is for CBT approaches including motivational interviewing, relapse prevention, and community reinforcement/contingency management:

Motivational interviewing –– This is a brief (two to six sessions) CBT approach, where the therapist takes the position of a collaborative partner, rather than an expert. Both the benefits and costs of the drug use to the individual are explored in detail with the intention that patients persuade themselves that change is desirable (Wanigaratne et al. 2005).

Relapse prevention –– This is one of the main CBT approaches used in the UK. Relapse prevention strategies include: (1) identifying high-risk situations and triggers for craving; (2) developing strategies to limit exposure to high-risk situations; (3) developing skills to manage cravings and other painful emotions without using substances; (4) learning to cope with lapses; (5) learning how to recognize, challenge, and manage unhelpful or dysfunctional thoughts about substance use; (6) developing an emergency plan for coping with high-risk situations when other skills are not working; (7) learning to recognize how one is "setting oneself up" to use substances; (8) generating pleasurable sober activities and relationships, building a life worth living, and attaining a lifestyle balance (Wanigaratne et al. 2005).

Contingency management –– Contingency management, also known as "voucher-based therapy," remains controversial in the UK. Its aim is to encourage positive behavior by providing reinforcing consequences when a client meets treatment goals (i.e., not using illicit drugs) and by withholding these positive consequences when the client uses drugs. Often, the positive reinforcement for behavior change is a voucher that can be exchanged for consumer goods of the client's choice (Wanigaratne et al. 2005).

Iatrogenic effects: proconvulsant effects of psychotropic drugs

The fear of increasing seizure frequency can lead to clinicians avoiding the use of psychotropic medication in patients with epilepsy. In general these fears are somewhat misplaced and the "take-home" message should be that psychiatric disorders in this particular patient group need to be identified and appropriately treated. Most of the more modern antidepressants are by and large safe to use in epilepsy although the risk associated with antipsychotics, in particular clozapine, may be slightly higher. This area is briefly reviewed below but for a detailed review see Pisani *et al.* (2002).

When imipramine was first introduced to the market in 1958 a number of case reports soon followed linking the drug to epileptic seizures. The activating effect of this and other tricyclic antidepressants on the EEG in patients both with and without epilepsy as well as data from studies performed on animals reinforced this belief. In some studies the incidence of seizures during antidepressant therapy ranged from 0.1% to 0.6%, seven times greater than the incidence of first unprovoked seizure in the general population. There is however enormous variability in seizure incidence between studies; for example, in one study including a total of about 8000 patients the estimated seizure risk for imipramine was approximately tenfold greater than that for amitriptyline. Conversely a seizure incidence of 2% was observed in a sample of 200 patients receiving amitriptyline and no seizures occurred in another group of 200 patients receiving imipramine (Pisani *et al.* 2002). Notwithstanding this variability a further problem relates to the fact that much of this work relates to tricyclic antidepressants which are now much less frequently used.

The incidence of seizures in people without epilepsy treated with SSRIs, noradrenergic and specific serotonergic antidepressants (NaSSA), and serotonin and noradrenaline reuptake inhibitors (SNRI) is actually significantly lower than would be expected in the general population (citalopram <0.3%, sertraline 0.0%, fluoxetine 0.2%, duloxetine 0.0%, mirtazepine 0.04%, venlafaxine 0.1%) with the exception of bupropion immediate release (IR) (Alper *et al.* 2007). Serotonin has been shown to inhibit epileptiform activity in rat hippocampal CA1 neurons via 5-hydroxytryptamine 1A receptor activation, and depresses excitatory postsynaptic potentials in a concentration-dependent manner (Lu and Gean 1998). Fluoxetine (Favale *et al.* 1995) and citalopram (Favale *et al.* 1995; Specchio *et al.* 2004) have been reported to produce antiepileptic effects in open-label studies of non-depressed epileptic patients reducing seizure frequency by as much as 35–64% and it may be that seizures that occur after starting SSRIs are merely reflecting the increased risk of seizures associated with the depressive disorder (Kanner and Blumer 2007). Assuming the incidence of unprovoked seizures in the general population is 60 per 100 000 patient exposed years (PEY; the cumulative time in years that a patient is exposed to a drug or placebo), the reported incidence of seizures of 1116.7 per 100 000 PEY in patients treated with placebo in antidepressant clinical trials reviewed by Alper *et al.* (2007) represents approximately 19 times the rate seen in the general population.

Since tricyclic (particularly high-dose) and tetracyclic antidepressants are felt to pose a greater level of risk, some references recommend avoiding these agents altogether if at all possible, although they have been used to good effect with no exacerbation of seizures in some studies (Blumer and Altshuler 1998). Bupropion (contraindicated in epilepsy according to manufacturer's prescribing information), clomipramine,

amoxapine, and maprotiline pose the highest risk and should be avoided in epilepsy given the wide variety of alternatives available.

Almost all available antipsychotics are mildly epileptogenic, with seizure incidence rates (in patients who previously had not had seizures) ranging from approximately 0.1% to approximately 1.5% (the incidence of a first unprovoked seizure in the general population is 0.07% to 0.09%) (Pisani *et al.* 2002). Changes in the EEG seem to occur in about 7% of patients treated with antipsychotic drugs, but in most cases are of little clinical consequence (Benkert and Hippius 1998). In one recent review seizure incidence for the different atypical antipsychotics was given as 0.3% for risperidone and 0.9% for olanzapine and quetiapine. Another study found that a set of all antipsychotics (olanzapine, quetiapine, clozapine, risperidone, ziprasidone, and aripiprazole) was not significantly associated with an increased risk of seizures after the removal of both olanzapine and clozapine from the group (Alper *et al.* 2007).

Seizures related to olanzapine (which has a chemical structure related to clozapine) have been reported, with Camacho *et al.* (2005), for example, describing a case of myoclonic status in a 54-year-old woman with probable Alzheimer disease. The risk with clozapine appears to increase in a dose-dependent manner from 1.0% with low doses (<300 mg/day) to 2.7% with moderate doses and 4.4% with high dose (600–900 mg/day) treatment (Alldredge 1999). Pacia and Devinski (1994) in a post-marketing study of more than 5000 patients on clozapine showed a lower rate (1.3%) with no dose dependency, and when Langosch and Trimble (2002) treated six patients with epilepsy and severe psychosis with clozapine, none showed an increase and in three there was a substantial reduction in seizure frequency. Wong and Delva (2007) found that tonic–clonic seizures were the most frequently reported seizure type with myoclonic and atonic seizures accounting for around one-quarter.

The fear of eliciting additional seizures has led to what we consider exaggerated caution in antidepressant and antipsychotic drug use, and in patients co-medicated with antiepileptic drugs (as is almost always the case in patients with epilepsy) the risk of an increase in seizures is low. In clinical practice, this becomes an important issue mainly in those who are seizure-free, in whom the recurrence of seizures has a generally greater impact. Seizures would appear to be a dose-dependent adverse effect and with regard to dose titration the maxim "start low, go slow" probably applies. Other important factors that play a role include the individual's inherited seizure threshold as well as acquired seizureogenic conditions (e.g., febrile convulsions, brain damage, epilepsy, etc.) (Pisani *et al.* 2002).

Tourette syndrome

Gilles de la Tourette syndrome (GTS) is a childhood-onset neuropsychiatric condition characterized by motor and vocal tics for a period of at least 1 year with a maximum remission during that year of 2 months. The motor and vocal tics do not need to occur simultaneously. Patients present with motor tics at 5–7 years of age and develop vocal tics later at around 11–13 years. There is a high prevalence of comorbid ADHD (30–80%) and obsessive–compulsive disorder (20–60%) in GTS. Impulse control disorders, self-harm behaviors, and mood disorders are also more common in the GTS population (Singer 2005).

The natural history of the disease is to peak in early adolescence and improve during adult life but not remit entirely, and the comorbidities of GTS tend to cause more distress over time than the tics (Singer, 2005). Tics wax and wane over time, increase with stress, are suppressible, exhibit rebound after suppression, and are suggestible. Less frequently echo phenomena are seen and coprophenomena occurs rarely with rates of approximately 30% in a specialist clinic (Robertson 2000). Prevalence of GTS is about 1%; there is a 3.5 : 1 male-to-female ratio and a strong association with pervasive developmental disorders with 4.6% of 7288 GTS patients in the GTS international database consortium having a pervasive developmental disorder (Burd *et al.* 2009). The cause of GTS is unknown but polygenic inheritance is likely and there is monozygotic concordance of 53% in comparison to 17% in dizygotic twins; there is also strong evidence that the GTS spectrum including ADHD and obsessive–compulsive disorder occur with greater frequency in families of GTS patients (Singer 2005). A large-scale international study for the relevant genes in GTS failed to find specific genes but did find evidence of linkage on chromosome 2p (Tourette Syndrome Association International Consortium for Genetics 2007). The pathophysiology of GTS is complex but abnormalities in corticostriatal-thalamocortical circuitry as a consequence of disordered dopaminergic systems, potentially under frontal cortical control, have been suggested (Baym *et al.* 2008).

Relationship with epilepsy

There are several mechanisms by which GTS is likely to be comorbid with epilepsy:

(1) Among GTS patients, 4.6% have autism spectrum disorder, and prevalence of epilepsy in the latter disorder is 30%. (Burd *et al.* 2009; Tuchman *et al.* 2009).

(2) D1CT-7 mice which exhibit D1+ upregulation resulting in increased forebrain glutamate and seizures provide a good animal model for GTS (Campbell *et al.* 2000).

(3) GTS involves aberrant cortical neurodevelopment. (Church *et al.* 2009).

Epilepsy associated with GTS tends to present in the context of ASD and a multitude of other psychiatric problems including ADHD, mental retardation, impulsivity, and rarely psychosis. There are no studies of the prevalence of GTS in populations with epilepsy but a recent study examining psychiatric comorbidity of 53 children with idiopathic epilepsy found that 5% of the epilepsy group had a tic disorder in comparison to one of the control group (Jones *et al.* 2007).

Diagnostic tests

Diagnosis of GTS is clinical; there are no biological tests and the EEG is normal (Neufeld *et al.* 1990). The distinction between myoclonus and a tic is crucial; this should be possible clinically but appropriate neurophysiology can help the diagnosis. The role of anti-basal-ganglia antibodies and the PANDAS (pediatric autoimmune neuropsychiatric disorders associated with streptococcal infection) hypothesis remains debated (Singer 2005).

Treatment

Treating GTS patients with epilepsy is a complex matter, and specialist multidisciplinary care is advisable. Treatment goals are seizure freedom and symptomatic control of the GTS. The tics tend to improve with time but the associated symptoms of obsessionality and ADHD cause long-term disability (Bloch *et al.* 2006). Treatment involves combined pharmacotherapy and behavioral modification. Tics respond to antipsychotics or dopamine modulators including high-potency D2 blockers, atypical antipsychotics, and aripiprazole. Comorbidities such as obsessive–compulsive disorder and depression benefit from SSRIs and ADHD symptoms from psychostimulants (Srour *et al.* 2008) There are case reports of antiepileptic drugs including carbamazepine, phenobarbitone, and lamotrigine precipitating GTS, but the mechanism is unknown (Sotero de Menezes *et al.* 2000). In severe GTS which fails to respond to conventional therapies functional neurosurgery may be considered; multiple approaches have been tried but currently deep brain stimulation is preferred (Servello *et al.* 2008). There is a single case report of GTS improving via coincidental vagus nerve stimulation implant for epilepsy (W. Sperling *et al.* 2008). Behavioral therapy using habit reversal training and response inhibition are integral to treatment.

Austistic spectrum disorders

The core features of autism and related disorders (ASD) are qualitative abnormalities in reciprocal social interactions, patterns of communication, and a restricted stereotyped repetitive repertoire of interests and activities. The disorders are subdivided into the following categories: typical autism, atypical autism, Rett syndrome, Asperger syndrome, disintegrative disorder, and pervasive developmental disorder, unspecified (see Table 84.1). Rett syndrome is dealt with elsewhere (see Chapter 34) and will not be considered further here. Due to phenotypic and etiological variability they might be better considered as the autisms in a manner analogous to the epilepsies (Tuchman *et al.* 2009). Although mental retardation is not listed as a diagnostic criterion, the prevalence of mental retardation in ASD is up to 70% (Tuchman and Rapin 2002).

The prevalence of ASD has been estimated at 5–6 per 1000 in younger children in the UK and prevalence rates have been increasing, arguably due to changes in diagnostic practice (Timimi 2004).

Table 84.1 Abridged ICD-10 diagnostic criteria for autistic spectrum disorders

ICD-10 number and category	Diagnostic criteria
F84 Childhood autism	Abnormal or impaired development manifest before the age of 3 years.
	Abnormal functioning in all three areas of (1) reciprocal social interaction, (2) communication both verbal and non-verbal, and (3) restricted stereotyped, repetitive behavior.
F84.1 Atypical autism	Abnormal or impaired development may be manifest before or after 3 years of age.
	Abnormal functioning as for autism but does not fulfil the diagnostic criteria for abnormality in all three areas.
	Atypical autism may be diagnosed as atypical in age of onset in which case the age of onset is after 3 years of age but the other criteria of abnormal reciprocal social interaction, communication, and restricted behavior is fulfilled or it may be atypical in both age of onset and symptoms.
F84.2 Rett syndrome	Normal development until about 5–6 months followed by deceleration of head growth between 5 months and 4 years and loss of acquired purposeful hand skills between 5 and 30 months of age that is associated with concurrent communication dysfunction, severe aphasia, development of motor disorder, and stereotyped midline hand movements.
F84.3 Disintegrative disorder	Normal development to 2 years followed by a loss of previously acquired skills at the onset of the disorder including language, play, social skills, continence, and motor skills. There is qualitatively abnormal social functioning.
F84.5 Asperger syndrome	No clinically significant delay in language or cognition to 2 years of age. There may be motor clumsiness. Single words must be used by 2 years of age and phrases by 3 years or earlier. There are qualitative abnormalities in reciprocal social interaction, unusually intense circumscribed interests or restricted repetitive and stereotyped pattern of behavior. The disorder is not attributable to other pervasive developmental disorder or psychiatric disorder.
F84.9 Pervasive developmental disorder, unspecified	This is a residual diagnostic catergory for disorders that fit the general description of a pervasive developmental disorder but the criteria for a specific subtype cannot be met.

Relationship with epilepsy

A meta-analysis of the prevalence of epilepsy in ASD suggested a figure of 21.8% in ASD with intellectual disability and 8% in ASD with normal intellect (Amiet *et al.* 2008), but rates of up to 38% have been reported (Danielsson *et al.* 2005). The male-to-female ratio in autism is 3.5 : 1 or higher but in ASD associated with epilepsy the ratio changes to 2 : 1 possibly due to the fact that although ASD is less common in girls when it occurs it tends to be more severe and more often associated with intellectual disability (Amiet *et al.* 2008).

Autism by definition begins before 3 years of age and onset of epilepsy in ASD occurs most frequently before 5 years of age with another peak around adolescence (Tuchman and Rapin 2002). One long-term prospective study of 120 patients with ASD found median age of epilepsy onset at 3.5 years of age in the severely mentally retarded group and 7.2 years in the mild or moderately retarded group. The lifetime prevalence was 38% and remission of epilepsy only occurred in 16%. Partial seizures occurred in 73% but the authors acknowledged diagnostic difficulties due to semiology and absence of investigations (Danielsson *et al.* 2005). It is accepted that prevalence of epilepsy increases with age, length of follow-up, decreasing IQ, cerebral palsy, and secondary autism cases (Tuchman and Rapin 2002).

Unprovoked seizures in the first year of life are associated with a 1 in 20 chance of developing an ASD and infantile spasms are associated with average odds ratios of 5.53 for development of a later ASD (Saemundsen *et al.* 2007, 2008). Of 107 children attending a tertiary epilepsy center 32% scored in the diagnostic range on an ASD screening questionnaire (Clarke *et al.* 2005), and the 1999 British Child and Adolescent Mental Health Survey found a prevalence rate of 16% of ASD/pervasive developmental disorder in their group with complicated epilepsy (Davies *et al.* 2003).

Establishing seizure type in ASD is difficult. A video EEG study of 32 patients with ASD referred for diagnosis found that not one of 15 recorded events was ictal but the semiology was typical for complex partial or absence seizures (Kim *et al.*

601

2006). All seizure types have been reported in ASD with epilepsy with greatest frequency of partial seizures but this must be interpreted cautiously.

The pathophysiology of epilepsy in ASD is complex, reflecting different etiologies and mechanisms. The disorder shares pathological features with epilepsy including abnormalities in the limbic system, decreases in GABA activity, and cortical dysgenesis (Palmen *et al.* 2004). Current research suggests that pathological neurodevelopment occurs under influence of several genes which results in synaptic disruption, alterations in GABA interneuron function, and more grossly in altered cortical–subcortical pathways resulting in features of autism and susceptibility to seizures (Tuchman *et al.* 2009).

Regression and the relationship between autism and Landau–Kleffner syndrome

About 30% of ASD children experience "autistic regression" which is the loss of previously acquired language and social skills. The exact cause for autistic regression is not known but epilepsy has been suggested as a cause. There are plausible reasons to invoke epilepsy, including the known deleterious effects of seizures on the brain, the fact that epilepsy can independently alter cognitive and behavioral outcomes in children, the high prevalence of epilepsy in ASD, and similarities between autistic regression and Landau–Kleffner syndrome (Ballaban-Gil and Tuchman 2000). However, there are difficulties with Landau–Kleffner syndrome as a model for autistic regression: age of onset is later (5–7 years) than in autistic regression normally (between 2 and 3 years), the language disturbance of Landau–Kleffner syndrome is not the same as the combined language and social decline in ASD, the EEG findings are dissimilar, and Landau–Kleffner syndrome as strictly defined is a very rare condition whereas autistic regression is not (Tuchman 2006). A recent study examining rates of regression in a representative sample of 255 children with ASD found 28 with definite regression and 10 with lower-level regression. Of the 28 with definite regression, 26/28 had an ASD. The rate of regression was 30% in narrowly defined autism as opposed to 8% in the broad ASD group. Baird *et al.* (2008) did not find epilepsy to be a relevant factor, thus suggesting that regression is a function of the core autism phenotype.

Diagnostic tests

Excepting Rett syndrome (genetic diagnosis), ASDs are diagnosed on history and examination. Parents can correctly detect abnormalities of development from the age of about 18 months and an accurate clinical diagnosis can be made from 2 years onwards (Baird *et al.* 2003). The American Academy of Neurology guideline suggests that children who are not babbling or pointing by 12 months, have no single words by 16 months, and no two-word spontaneous phrases by 24 months should be assessed by means of audiological examination and screening for lead poisoning if pica is present.

Screening via questionnaire such as the CHAT (Childhood Assessment of Autism Tool) should be administered although there are concerns about the sensitivity of the test which has been reported as 35% (Baird *et al.* 2003).

Testing for underlying etiology via neuroimaging, chromosomal analysis, and metabolic screens should be guided by the individual presentation. The yield is low in the absence of mental retardation and clinical signs of the condition being sought (Baghdadli *et al.* 2006). Routine EEG in all patients is not indicated and its use in regression is still debated (Fong *et al.* 2008).

Treatment

Poor communication skills, intellectual disability, and co-occurrence of "seizure mimics" in ASD can make the clinical evaluation of seizures difficult. This is further complicated by the difficulty obtaining investigations and even when investigations are obtained, interpreting the results correctly (Kim *et al.* 2006). Accurate collateral history from family, carers, and nursing staff is crucial.

Treatment of the epilepsy is otherwise standard with the proviso that children in the ASD population are vulnerable to medication side effects. There are no pharmacological treatments for the core deficits in ASD.

Attention deficit hyperactivity disorder

Attention deficit hyperactivity disorder is a childhood-onset illness characterized by severe inattention, hyperactivity, and impulsivity. Depending on what constellation of symptoms are present the disorder can be further classified into three types: (1) combined inattentive, hyperactive, and impulsive (80%), (2) predominantly inattentive (10–15%), and (3) impulsive (5%). By definition the symptoms must not occur exclusively as a consequence of a pervasive developmental disorder, schizophrenia, or other psychotic disorder, must occur in all situations, and must be present before 7 years of age (Rappley 2005).

The prevalence of the disorder varies from 3% to 7% and shows a marked sex bias of 2.5–9 : 1 boy : girl. It is strongly genetically transmitted with heritability estimated at up to 80% but other factors such as low birth weight, brain injury, maternal smoking, and exposure to lead have also been implicated (Rappley 2005). The suggested pathophysiogy involves altered neurotransmission of dopamine and norepinephrine in frontostriatal circuitry (Stanley *et al.* 2008). The natural history of ADHD is to improve as the child matures but it is also recognized in adults with a prevalence of 4.4% reported. However, the concept of adult ADHD is still controversial due to the disputed validity of applying diagnostic criteria from a childhood illness to an adult population (Kessler *et al.* 2006).

Relationship with epilepsy

The prevalence of ADHD in children with epilepsy is increased fivefold from 3–7% to 14–38% (Plioplys *et al.* 2007). The type of ADHD associated with epilepsy differs epidemiologically to standard ADHD. The predominant subtype in primary ADHD is mixed (80%) but in ADHD associated with epilepsy it is inattentive and the sex ratio equalizes (Aldenkamp et al. 2006). Onset of ADHD pre-dates onset of epilepsy; a population-based case–control study from Iceland found that children with new-onset seizures were 2.5 times more likely to have prior symptoms of ADHD than the control group but the association was only statistically significant for the inattentive subtype (Hesdorffer et al. 2004). This finding has been reproduced subsequently in a study of 75 children with new-onset idiopathic epilepsy where ADHD pre-dated epilepsy in 31.5% compared to the control group rate of 6% and once again the inattentive subtype was most common (Hermann et al. 2007). This suggests that ADHD and epilepsy arise from common biological mechanisms with ADHD symptoms predating the epilepsy. As severity of epilepsy increases so does prevalence of ADHD symptoms, with over 60% of a treatment refractory group showing symptoms of ADHD, but how much was due to ictal and treatment effects versus true ADHD comorbidity is not clear (Sherman et al. 2007).

The pathophysiology of ADHD in epilepsy has only just begun to be investigated but increased frontal lobe gray matter and decreased brainstem volume have been reported, suggesting problems with cortical pruning as a possible mechanism common to both (Hermann et al. 2007). ADHD with epilepsy responds to methylphenidate suggesting that there is a dopamine abnormality as in primary ADHD (Torres et al. 2008).

Diagnostic tests

Diagnosis of ADHD is clinical and based upon fulfilling the DSM-IV criteria (Rappley 2005). Symptoms must be pervasive which makes collateral history from parents, teachers, and others essential. Several rating scales exist such as the ADHD Rating Scale-IV, Conner's and CBCL (child behavior checklist), all of which are useful as screening instruments but not *diagnostic* and were not designed for use in a population with epilepsy. Diagnosing ADHD in association with epilepsy requires an appreciation of both conditions and how they might interact. ADHD is frequently comorbid with other psychiatric illnesses but particularly anxiety, affective disorders, tic disorders, and childhood oppositional disorders (Rappley 2005). Adult ADHD is frequently comorbid with affective disorders, substance misuse, and personality disorder (Kessler et al. 2006). It goes without saying that diagnosis should be made by a specialist in the area.

Treatment

The first priority is effective treatment of the epilepsy and, once this is achieved, making sure that the observed ADHD symptoms are not cognitive side effects from anticonvulsants. Certain anticonvulsants are more often cited as offenders but it is best to assess each case individually. Rating scales can be useful to baseline symptoms and monitor treatment response (Dunn and Kronenberger 2005). Pharmacological therapies for ADHD in epilepsy are derived from treatment of primary ADHD where they have proven effectiveness and safety. However, ADHD with epilepsy is a different population. The trials that have been done are generally open-label with small numbers and underpowered to determine changes in seizure frequency unless seizures are occurring frequently. However, from the evidence available to date it appears that methylphenidate is safe to use cautiously in ADHD with epilepsy in the pediatric population (Torres et al. 2008) and there is preliminary evidence that it is safe in adults also (Kessler et al. 2006).

References

Aldenkamp AP, Arzimanoglou A, Reijs R, Van Mil S. (2006) Optimizing therapy of seizures in children and adolescents with ADHD. *Neurology* **67**:S49–51.

Alldredge BK (1999) Seizure risk associated with psychotropic drugs: clinical and pharmacokinetic considerations. *Neurology* **53**(5 Suppl 2): S68–75.

Alper K, Schwartz KA, Kolts RL, Khan A (2007) Seizure incidence in psychopharmacological clinical trials: an analysis of Food and Drug Administration (FDA) summary basis of approval reports. *Biol Psychiatry* **62**:345–54.

American Psychiatric Association (1995) *Diagnostic and Statistical Manual of Mental Disorders*, 4th edn. Washington, DC: American Psychiatric Association.

Amiet C, Gourfinkel-An I, Bouzamondo A, et al. (2008) Epilepsy in autism is associated with intellectual disability and gender: evidence from a meta-analysis. *Biol Psychiatry* **64**:577–82.

Baghdadli A, Beuzon S, Bursztejn C, et al. (2006) [Clinical guidelines for the screening and the diagnosis of autism and pervasive developmental disorders.] *Arch Pediatr* **13**:373–8.

Baird G, Cass H, Slonims V (2003) Diagnosis of autism. *Br Med J* **327**:488–93.

Baird G, Charman T, Pickles A, et al. (2008) Regression, developmental trajectory and associated problems in disorders in the autism spectrum: the SNAP study. *J Autism Dev Disord* **38**:1827–36.

Ballaban-Gil K, Tuchman R (2000) Epilepsy and epileptiform EEG: association with autism and language disorders. *Ment Retard Dev Disabil Res Rev* **6**:300–8.

Barry JJ, Lembke A, Gisbert PA, Gilliam F (2008) Affective disorders in epilepsy. In: Ettinger AB, Kanner AM (eds.) *Psychiatric Issues in Epilepsy: A Practical Guide to Diagnosis and Treatment*, 2nd edn. Philadelphia, PA: Lippincott Williams & Wilkins, pp. 203–47.

Baym CL, Corbett BA, Wright SB, Bunge SA (2008) Neural correlates of tic severity and cognitive control in children with Tourette syndrome. *Brain* **131**:165–79.

Beck AT, Steer RA, Ball R, Ranieri W (1996) Comparison of Beck Depression Inventories -IA and -II in psychiatric outpatients. *J Pers Assess* **67**:588–97.

Benkert O, Hippius H (1998) *Kompendium der psychiatrischen Pharmackotherapie*. Berlin: Springer-Verlag.

Bloch MH, Peterson BS, Scahill L, et al. (2006) Adulthood outcome of tic and obsessive–compulsive symptom severity in children with Tourette syndrome. *Arch Pediatr Adolesc Med* **160**:65–9.

Blumer D, Altshuler LL (1998) Affective disorders. In: Engel J, Pedley TA (eds.) *Epilepsy: A Comprehensive Textbook.* Philadelphia, PA: Lippincott-Raven, pp. 2083–99.

Brust JCM (2007) Alcohol and drug abuse. In: Engel J, Pedley TA, Aicardi J, Dichter MA, Moshé SL (eds.) *Epilepsy: A Comprehensive Textbook*, 2nd edn Philadelphia, PA: Lippincott Williams and Wilkins, pp. 2683–7.

Burd L, Li Q, Kerbeshian J, Klug MG, Freeman RD (2009) Tourette syndrome and comorbid pervasive developmental disorders. *J Child Neurol* **24**:170–5.

Camacho A, García-Navarro M, Martínez B, Villarejo A, Pomares E (2005) Olanzapine induced myoclonic status. *Clin Neuropharmacol* **28**:145–7.

Campbell KM, Veldman MB, McGrath MJ, Burton FH (2000) TS+OCD-like neuropotentiated mice are supersensitive to seizure induction. *NeuroReport* **11**:2335–8.

Caspi A, Sugden K, Moffitt TE, *et al.* (2003) Influence of life stress on depression: moderation by a polymorphism in the 5-HTT gene. *Science* **301**:291–3.

Church JA, Fair DA, Dosenbach NU, *et al.* (2009) Control networks in pediatric Tourette syndrome show immature and anomalous patterns of functional connectivity. *Brain* **132**:225–38.

Clarke DF, Roberts W, Daraksan M, *et al.* (2005) The prevalence of autistic spectrum disorder in children surveyed in a tertiary care epilepsy clinic. *Epilepsia* **46**:1970–7.

Da Silva Sousa P, Lin K, Garzon E, Sakamoto AC, Yacubian EM (2005) Self perception of factors that precipitate or inhibit seizures in juvenile myoclonic epilepsy. *Seizure* **14**:340–6.

Danielsson S, Gillberg IC, Billstedt E, Gillberg C, Olsson I (2005) Epilepsy in young adults with autism: a prospective population-based follow-up study of 120 individuals diagnosed in childhood. *Epilepsia* **46**:918–23.

Davies S, Heyman I, Goodman R (2003) A population survey of mental health problems in children with epilepsy. *Dev Med Child Neurol* **45**:292–5.

Dunn DW, Kronenberger WG (2005) Childhood epilepsy, attention problems, and ADHD: review and practical considerations. *Semin Pediatr Neurol* **12**:222–8.

Edwards HE, Dortok D, Tam J, Won D, Burnham WM (2002) Prenatal seizure thresholds and the development of kindled seizures in infant and adult rats. *Horm Behav* **42**:437–47.

Elliott B, Amarouche M, Shorvon SD (2009) The psychiatric features of epilepsy and their management. In: Shorvon SD, Perucca E, Engel J (eds.) *The Treatment of Epilepsy*, 3rd edn. Oxford, UK: Blackwell Publishing, pp. 273–87.

Favale E, Rubino V, Mainardi P, Lunardi G, Albano C (1995) Anticonvulsant effect of fluoxetine in humans. *Neurology* **45**:1926–7.

Favale E, Audenino D, Cocito L, Albano C (2003) The anticonvulsant effect of citalopram as an indirect evidence of serotonergic impairment in human epileptogenesis. *Seizure* **12**:316–18.

Fong CY, Baird G, Wraige E (2008) Do children with autism and developmental regression need EEG investigation in the absence of clinical seizures? *Arch Dis Childh* **93**:998–9.

Forsgren L, Nystrom L (1990) An incident case-referent study of epileptic seizures in adults. *Epilepsy Res* **6**:66–81.

Frye CA, Bayon LE (1999) Prenatal stress reduces the effectiveness of the neurosteroid 3 alpha, 5 alpha-THP to block kainic-acid-induced seizures. *Dev Psychobiol* **34**(3):227–34.

Gaitatzis A, Trimble MR, Sander JW (2004) The psychiatric comorbidity of epilepsy. *Acta Neurol Scand* **110**:207–20.

Gilliam FG, Barry JJ, Hermann BP, *et al.* (2006) Rapid detection of major depression in epilepsy: a multicentre study. *Lancet Neurol* **5**:399–405.

Gordon E, Devinsky O (2001) Alcohol and marijuana: effects on epilepsy and use by patients with epilepsy. *Epilepsia* **42**:1266–72.

Gowers WR (1881) *Epilepsy and Other Chronic Convulsive Disorders.* London: Churchill.

Gowers WR (1901) *Epilepsy and Other Chronic Convulsive Diseases: Their Causes, Symptoms and Treatment.* London: Churchill.

Gross DW, Hamm J, Ashworth NL, Quigley D (2004) Marijuana use and epilepsy: prevalence in patients of a tertiary care epilepsy center. *Neurology* **62**:1924–5.

Hanson GR, Jensen M, Johnson M, White HS (1999) Distinct features of seizures induced by cocaine and amphetamine analogs. *Eur J Pharmacol* **377**:167–73.

Haut SR, Hall CB, Masur J, Lipton RB (2007) Seizure occurrence: precipitants and prediction. *Neurology* **69**:1905–10.

Hedetoft C, Christensen HR (1999) Amphetamine, ecstasy and cocaine: clinical aspects of acute poisoning. *Ugeskr Laeger* **161**:6907–11.

Hermann B, Jones J, Dabbs K, *et al.* (2007) The frequency, complications and etiology of ADHD in new onset pediatric epilepsy. *Brain* **130**:3135–48.

Hesdorffer DC, Ludvigsson P, Hauser A, *et al.* (1999) Depression is a risk factor for epilepsy in children. *Epilepsia* **39**(Suppl 6):222.

Hesdorffer DC, Hauser WA, Anneqers JF, Cascino G (2000) Major depression is a risk factor for seizures in older adults. *Ann Neurol* **47**:246–9.

Hesdorffer DC, Ludvigsson P, Olafsson E, *et al.* (2004) ADHD as a risk factor for incident unprovoked seizures and epilepsy in children. *Arch Gen Psychiatry* **61**:731–6.

Hesdorffer DC, Hauser WA, Olafsson E, Ludvigsson P, Kjartansson O (2006) Depression and suicide attempt as risk factors for incident unprovoked seizures. *Ann Neurol* **59**:35–41.

Joels M (2008) Stress, the hippocampus, and epilepsy. *Epilepsia* **50**:586–97.

Jones JE, Watson R, Sheth R, *et al.* (2007) Psychiatric comorbidity in children with new onset epilepsy. *Dev Med Child Neurol* **49**:493–7.

Kanner AM (2003) When did neurologists and psychiatrists stop talking to each other? *Epilepsy Behav* **4**:597–601.

Kanner A, Blumer D (2007) Affective disorders. In: Engel J, Pedley T (eds.) *Epilepsy: A Comprehensive Textbook*, 2nd edn. Philadelphia, PA: Lippincott Williams and Wilkins, pp. 2123–38.

Keller RW Jr. Snyder-keller A (2000) Prenatal cocaine exposure. *Ann NY Acad Sci* **909**:217–32.

Kessler RC, Adler L, Barkley R, *et al.* (2006) The prevalence and correlates of adult ADHD in the United States: results from the National Comorbidity Survey Replication. *Am J Psychiatry* **163**:716–23.

Kim HL, Donnelly JH, Tournay AE, Book TM, Filipek P (2006) Absence of seizures despite high prevalence of epileptiform EEG abnormalities in children with autism monitored in a tertiary care center. *Epilepsia* **47**:394–8.

Klein P, van Passel L (2005) Effect of stress related to the 9/11/2001 terror attack on seizures in patients with epilepsy. *Neurology* **64**:1815–16.

Kuhn KU, Quednow BB, Thiel M, *et al.* (2003) Antidepressive treatment in patients with temporal lobe epilepsy and major depression: a prospective study with three different antidepressants. *Epilepsy Behav* **4**:674–9.

Langosch JM, Trimble MR (2002) Epilepsy, psychosis and clozapine. *Hum Psychopharmacol* **17**:115–19.

Lewis AJ (1934) Melancholia: a historical review. *J Ment Sci* **80**:1–42.

Lowenstein DH, Massa SM, Rowbotham MC, *et al.* (1987) Acute neurologic and psychiatric complications associated with cocaine abuse. *Am J Med* **83**:841.

Lu KT, Gean PW (1998) Endogenous serotonin inhibits epileptiform activity in rat hippocampal CA1 neurons via 5-hydroxytryptamine1A receptor activation. *Neuroscience* **86**:729–37.

Magarinos AM, Verdugo JM, McEwen BS (1997) Chronic stress alters synaptic terminal structure in hippocampus. *Proc Natl Acad Sci USA* **94**:14 002–8.

McCarron MM, Schulze BW, Thompson GA, Conder MC, Goetz WA (1981) Acute phencyclidine intoxication: incidence of clinical findings in 1000 cases. *Ann Emerg Med* **10**:237–42.

Melchior M, Caspi A, Milne BJ, *et al.* (2007) Work stress precipitates depression and anxiety in young, working women and men. *Psychol Med* **37**:1073–4.

Mendez MF, Cummings JL, Benson DF (1986) Depression in epilepsy: significance and phenomenology. *Arch Neurol* **43**:766–70.

Moshe S, Shilo M, Chodick G, *et al.* (2008) Occurrence of seizures in association with work related stress in young male army recruits. *Epilepsia* **49**:1451–6.

Nakken KO, Solaas MH, Kjeldsen MJ, *et al.* (2005) Which seizure-precipitating factors do patients with epilepsy most frequently report? *Epilepsy Behav* **6**:85–9.

Neufeld MY, Berger Y, Chapman J, Korczyn AD (1990) Routine and quantitative EEG analysis in Gilles de la Tourette's syndrome. *Neurology* **40**:1837–9.

Neufeld MY, Sadeh M, Cohn DF, Korczyn AD (1994) Stress and epilepsy: the Gulf War experience. *Seizure* **3**:135–9.

Ng SKC, Brust JCM, Hauser WA, Sugger M (1990) Illicit drug use and the risk of new onset seizures. *Am J Epidemiol* **132**:47–57.

Pacia SV, Devinsky O (1994) Clozapine-related seizures: experience with 5629 patients. *Neurology* **44**:2247–9.

Palmen SJ, van Engeland H, Hof PR, Schmitz C (2004) Neuropathological findings in autism. *Brain* **127**:2572–83.

Pascual-Leone A, Dhuna A, Altafullah I, Anderson DC (1990) Cocaine induced seizures. *Neurology* **40**:404.

Pericic D, Lazic J, Svob Strac D (2005) Anticonvulsant effects of acute and repeated fluoxetine treatment in unstressed and stressed mice. *Brain Res* **1033**:90–5.

Pisani F, Oteri G, Costa C, Di RG, Di PR (2002) Effects of psychotropic drugs on seizure threshold. *Drug Saf* **25**:91–110.

Plioplys S, Dunn DW, Caplan R. (2007) 10-year research update review: psychiatric problems in children with epilepsy. *J Am Acad Child Adolesc Psychiatry* **46**:1389–402.

Ramaratnam S, Baker GA, Goldstein LH (2008) Psychological treatments for epilepsy. *Cochrane Database Syst Rev*: CD002029.

Rappley MD (2005) Clinical practice: attention deficit-hyperactivity disorder. *N Engl J Med* **352**:165–73.

Robertson MM (2000) Tourette syndrome, associated conditions and the complexities of treatment. *Brain* **123**:425–62.

Robertson MM (2008a) The prevalence and epidemiology of Gilles de la Tourette syndrome. I. The epidemiological and prevalence studies. *J Psychosom Res* **65**:461–72.

Robertson MM (2008b) The prevalence and epidemiology of Gilles de la Tourette syndrome. II. Tentative explanations for differing prevalence figures in GTS, including the possible effects of psychopathology, etiology, cultural differences, and differing phenotypes. *J Psychosom Res* **65**:473–86.

Robertson MM, Trimble MR (1985) The treatment of depression in patients with epilepsy: a double-blind trial. *J Affect Disord* **9**:127–36.

Saemundsen E, Ludvigsson P, Hilmarsdottir I, Rafnsson V (2007) Autism spectrum disorders in children with seizures in the first year of life: a population-based study. *Epilepsia* **48**:1724–30.

Saemundsen E, Ludvigsson P, Rafnsson V (2008) Risk of autism spectrum disorders after infantile spasms: a population-based study nested in a cohort with seizures in the first year of life. *Epilepsia* **49**:1865–70.

Salzberg M, Kumar G, Supit L, *et al.* (2007) Early postnatal stress confers enduring vulnerability to limbic epileptogenesis. *Epilepsia* **49**:2079–85.

Selye H (1959) *The Stress of Life.* New York: McGraw-Hill.

Servello D, Porta M, Sassi M, Brambilla A, Robertson MM (2008) Deep brain stimulation in 18 patients with severe Gilles de la Tourette syndrome refractory to treatment: the surgery and stimulation. *J Neurol Neurosurg Psychiatry* **79**:136–42.

Sherman EM, Slick DJ, Connolly MB, Eyrl KL (2007) ADHD, neurological correlates and health-related quality of life in severe pediatric epilepsy. *Epilepsia* **48**:1083–91.

Singer HS (2005) Tourette's syndrome: from behavior to biology. *Lancet Neurol* **4**:149–59.

Snyder M (1993) Revised Epilepsy Stressor Inventory. *J Neurosci Nurs* **25**:9–13.

Sotero de Menezes MA, Rho JM, Murphy P, Cheyette S (2000) Lamotrigine-induced tic disorder: report of five pediatric cases. *Epilepsia* **41**:862–7.

Specchio LM, Iudice A, Specchio N, *et al.* (2004) Citalopram as treatment of depression in patients with epilepsy. *Clin Neuropharmacol* **27**:133–6.

Sperling MR, Schilling CA, Glosser D, Tracy JI, Asadi-Pooya AA (2008) Self-perception of seizure precipitants and their relation to anxiety level, depression and health locus of control in epilepsy. *Seizure* **17**:302–7.

Sperling W, Reulbach U, Maihofner C, Kornhuber J, Bleich S (2008) Vagus nerve stimulation in a patient with Gilles de la Tourette syndrome and major depression. *Pharmacopsychiatry* **41**:117–18.

Srour M, Lesperance P, Richer F, Chouinard S (2008) Psychopharmacology of tic disorders. *J Can Acad Child Adolesc Psychiatry* **17**:150–9.

Stahl SM (2008) *Essential Psychopharmacology: Neuroscientific Basis and Practical Applications*, 3rd edn.

Cambridge, UK: Cambridge University Press.

Stanley JA, Kipp H, Greisenegger E, *et al.* (2008) Evidence of developmental alterations in cortical and subcortical regions of children with attention-deficit/hyperactivity disorder: a multivoxel in vivo phosphorus 31 spectroscopy study. *Arch Gen Psychiatry* **65**:1419–28.

Thapar A, Kerr M, Harold G (2009) Stress, anxiety, depression, and epilepsy: investigating the relationship between psychological factors and seizures. *Epilepsy Behav* **14**:134–40.

Timimi S (2004) Diagnosis of autism: current epidemic has social context. *Br Med J* **328**:226.

Torres AR, Whitney J, Gonzalez-Heydrich J (2008) Attention-deficit/hyperactivity disorder in pediatric patients with epilepsy: review of pharmacological treatment. *Epilepsy Behav* **12**:217–33.

Tourette Syndrome Association International Consortium for Genetics (2007) Genome scan for Tourette disorder in affected-sibling-pair and multigenerational families. *Am J Hum Genet* **80**:265–72.

Trivedi MH, Rush AJ, Wisniewski SR, *et al.* (2006) Evaluation of outcomes with citalopram for depression using measurement-based care in STAR*D: implications for clinical practice. *Am J Psychiatry* **163**(1):28–40.

Tuchman R (2006) Autism and epilepsy: what has regression got to do with it? *Epilepsy Curr* **6**:107–11.

Tuchman R, Rapin I (2002) Epilepsy in autism. *Lancet Neurol* **1**:352–8.

Tuchman R, Moshe SL, Rapin I (2009) Convulsing toward the pathophysiology of autism. *Brain Dev* **31**:95–103.

Wanigaratne S, Davis P, Pryce K, Brotchie J (2005) *The Effectiveness of Psychological Therapies on Drug Misusing Clients.* London: National Treatment Agency for Substance Misuse.

Wong J, Delva N (2007) Clozapine-induced seizures: recognition and treatment. *Can J Psychiatry* **52**:457–63.

Woods RJ, Gruenthal M (2006) Cognition-induced epilepsy associated with specific emotional precipitants. *Epilepsy Behav* **9**:360–2.

World Health Organization (1992) ICD-10: *International Statistical Classification of Diseases and Related Health Problems* vol. 1. Geneva: World Health Organization.

Zagnoni PG, Albano C (2002) Psychostimulants and epilepsy. *Epilepsia* **43**(Suppl 2):28–31.

Chapter 85

Multiple sclerosis and other acquired demyelinating diseases

Mark R. Manford

Epidemiology of multiple sclerosis

Multiple sclerosis (MS) is the commonest acquired demyelinating disease of the central nervous system and is characterized by a relapsing–remitting or progressive course. Its distribution is worldwide, but there is significant geographic variation (Compston and Confavreux 2006). For example, the prevalence of MS ranges from 10 in 100 000 in Hawaii to 177 in 100 000 in the Northwestern states of the USA. In general, the further from the equator, the higher the risk of MS but this is complicated by racial variation and by the effects of migration. Individuals who migrate as an adult tend to take the risk of their country of origin with them but those who migrate when young acquire the risk of their new home. The female to male ratio for MS is about 2 : 1 and the peak age of onset is between the ages of 20 and 40 years; it is rare below the age of 16 or above the age of 65. The genetic component to MS has long been recognized (Sawcer 2008), with around 15% of patients having a first-degree relative with the condition. The strongest recognized association is with the HLA-DR2 allele but more recently an association has also been recognized with the interleukin 7 receptor. Numerous environmental factors have also been linked to MS with varying degrees of evidence, including infectious agents such as Epstein–Barr virus, human herpesvirus 6, and other factors such as sunlight.

Pathology of multiple sclerosis

The characteristic lesion of MS is the plaque (Laussmann and Wekerle 2006), in which axons are preserved but their myelin is lost and there is an astrocytic scar. In the acute phase, there are inflammatory changes with infiltration, predominantly of T lymphocytes of both CD4 and CD8 types. Macrophages are also present and when they contain fragments of myelin are the hallmark of an actively demyelinating plaque. In very aggressive lesions, and as inflammation recurs, axonal loss ensues, which is manifest both pathologically and on magnetic resonance imaging (MRI) as shrinkage of pathways, for example in spinal cord atrophy. Loss of function may be due to the acute inflammatory process itself, axonal loss, conduction block following demyelination, or failure of remyelination.

Clinical patterns of multiple sclerosis

Multiple sclerosis is characterized clinically by two major patterns; relapsing–remitting neurological deficits and a progressive neurological deficit. The phenotype comprises these components in different degrees (Fig. 85.1) with the commonest pattern being a young adult patient presenting with the relapsing–remitting form and going on to a secondary progressive form, sometimes with continuing relapses. Relapses are usually characterized by new deficits evolving over days and improving over weeks (Table 85.1). It is believed that the relapsing–remitting course is due to acute inflammatory lesions and this is strongly supported by MRI evidence, showing contrast enhancement in active plaques. The progressive phase may comprise a progressive tetraparesis, ataxic syndrome, with bulbar involvement and cognitive decline, which is sometimes severe. About 15% of patients present with a progressive deficit without clear relapses, most commonly as a progressive spinal cord syndrome. Mean age of onset of the relapsing–remitting form is 29 years and of the progressive form 38 years and the median survival of patients with MS is approximately 30 years after onset.

The diagnosis of multiple sclerosis

The key diagnostic investigation in MS is MRI scanning, which is abnormal in 95% of patients. However, the sensitivity and specificity of the technique depends on the clinical situation and the modality used. Typical cerebral lesions are high signal on T2-weighted sequences (Fig. 85.2) and are in the periventricular regions. In acute lesions there may be enhancement with gadolinium. In clinical practice, the commonest radiological differential diagnosis is with cerebrovascular disease, but unlike in MS, ischemic lesions are rare in the corpus callosum and spinal cord. In the cerebrospinal fluid (CSF) of about 95% of patients with MS, there are oligoclonal bands of

The Causes of Epilepsy, eds. S. D. Shorvon, F. Andermann, and R. Guerrini. Published by Cambridge University Press. © Cambridge University Press 2011.

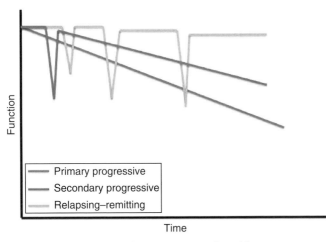

Fig. 85.1. Clinical patterns of deteriorating neurological function in patients with multiple sclerosis.

Legend:
- Primary progressive
- Secondary progressive
- Relapsing–remitting

Time

Function

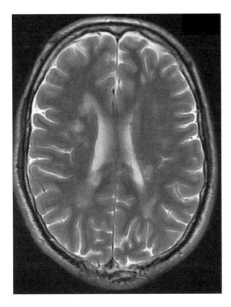

Fig. 85.2. T2-weighted MRI scan of a patient with MS, showing typical periventricular location of white matter lesions

Table 85.1. Common patterns of clinical involvement in multiple sclerosis

Optic neuritis	Variable visual loss especially affecting central and color vision
Spinal cord	Paraparesis or tetraparesis with prominent sensory and bladder symptoms
Brainstem	Ataxia, vertigo, and diplopia with limb weakness, tremor
Cerebellum	Ataxia and tremor
Cerebral hemisphere	Hemiparesis and cognitive changes (uncommon in early disease)

immunoglobulin G (IgG), unmatched in blood. They are only occasionally found in other inflammatory conditions, infections, tumors, or paraneoplastic syndromes. The third arm of testing is visual evoked potentials, which may show typical changes of delayed conduction with preserved amplitude in up to 70% of patients with MS, even if they have no history of clinical optic nerve disease.

Poser criteria for a clinically definite diagnosis of MS (Poser *et al.* 1983) required two or more clinical attacks supported by clinical evidence or one attack could be supported by paraclinical evidence, for example a delayed visual evoked potential. With the advent of MRI, it was felt that imaging could provide evidence of dissemination, and was incorporated into new criteria for diagnosis (McDonald *et al.* 2001); either if a new gadolinium-enhancing lesion appeared at least 3 months after clinical presentation or if an appropriate, new T2 lesion appeared at least 3 months after an initial scan, which was within 3 months of presentation. A different definition is

needed for those patients with primary progressive MS, but these patients may also have radiological evidence of dissemination. Oligoclonal bands in the CSF provide additional laboratory support for patients with a single clinical lesion, progressive illness, or non-diagnostic MRI. The differential diagnosis includes a wide range of conditions which may have a relapsing–remitting course, for example neurosarcoidosis, other progressive lesions such as spinal cord tumors, or conditions that may mimic the radiological appearance of MS, such as cerebrovascular disease. Additional investigations are aimed at excluding these alternatives.

Epilepsy in multiple sclerosis

A number of studies have analysed the frequency of seizures in MS (Ghezzi *et al.* 1990; Engelsen and Grøning 1997; Moreau *et al.* 1998; Olaffson *et al.* 1999; Sokić *et al.* 2001; Nyquist *et al.* 2002; Nicoletti *et al.* 2003) and have found varying results, ranging from no increase in prevalence compared to the background prevalence (Nyquist *et al.* 2002) to a frequency of 7.8% (Sokić *et al.* 2001). Methodological differences may account for some of the variability; some studies include patients with a pre-existing diagnosis of epilepsy and others specifically exclude patients if seizure onset was prior to MS diagnosis. Whilst this may be a pragmatic way of excluding patients whose seizures are unlikely to be causally linked to MS, other authors have described patients in whom seizures were the first presentation of MS, and one study (Gambardella *et al.* 2003) described four patients with apparently typical MRI appearance of MS and positive CSF oligoclonal bands, in whom focal temporal lobe type seizures were the only manifestation of their illness during follow-up of 4 to 10 years. This is somewhat problematic since although they may have had epilepsy they do not fulfill conventional criteria for MS as they had no clinical deficit other than their seizures. Some studies also include a single seizure in the context of MS, which would not satisfy the usual definition of epilepsy. The broad conclusion from all the studies is that there is probably an increase of two- to threefold in the frequency of seizures amongst patients with definite MS. All studies report both focal seizures and tonic–clonic seizures, presumed secondarily generalized, with the ratio varying from one- to two-thirds focal seizures. The

A

B

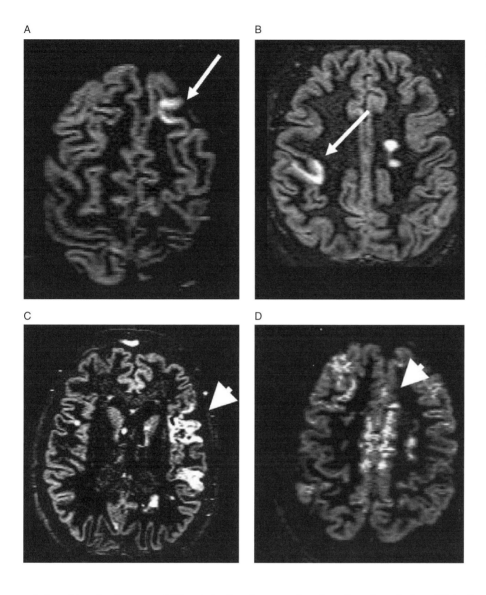

C

D

Fig. 85.3. Double inversion recovery MRI showing prominent, serpiginous changes in the cerebral cortex, consistent with demyelinating cortical lesions, in four patients with epilepsy and MS. (Reproduced with permission from Calabrese *et al.* 2008.)

relationship of seizures to MS activity has been explored and most studies report that about one-third of seizures occur in the context of an acute relapse of MS, sometimes taking the form of focal status epilepticus, usually focal motor status. These acute symptomatic seizures often cease with remission of the relapse and do not require long-term treatment. Neuroimaging may show an obvious acute, enhancing MS lesion (Thompson *et al.* 1993) which is concordant with the clinical seizure localization or electroencephalogram (EEG). Some authors have tried to correlate lesion distribution with epilepsy. Since MS is a disease of myelin and epilepsy is a cortical disturbance, they have looked for and generally found involvement of the cerebral cortex in patients with MS and epilepsy (Thompson *et al.* 1993; Moreau *et al.* 1998). Only one of these studies had controls with MS and no epilepsy (Calabrese *et al.* 2008). They examined 20 patients with seizures and matched controls, in their cohort of 800 patients with MS using a double inversion recovery sequence on MRI, which is said to increase the detection of intracortical lesions (Fig. 85.3). They

found that 85% of patients with seizures had demonstrable intracortical lesions compared to 49% of controls and on average had four times as many intracortical lesions, as well as a greater total intracortical lesion volume load.

Interictal EEG abnormalities are probably more common than in most adult-onset epilepsy, with focal sharp waves, spikes, and generalized spike–wave complexes reported in the majority of patients. There may be some selection bias as some studies excluded patients who did not have diagnostic EEG abnormalities, in order to differentiate from non-epileptic paroxysmal events in MS. The commonest of these are brief tonic spasms, which affect about 4% of patients with MS and occur many times per day in a cluster, and which often subside spontaneously after weeks or months. Other manifestations are transient somatosensory phenomena, transient ataxia, or aphasia. They are thought to be due to ephaptic transmission between demyelinated nerves and are usually abolished by low doses of membrane-stabilizing agents such as carbamazepine, which is generally much more effective than it is for focal seizures.

Treatment of multiple sclerosis

The treatment of multiple sclerosis falls into three broad categories. First, symptomatic treatment of the neurological complications of MS, which includes a wide range of medication and the full gamut of non-medical treatment of disability. Baclofen is an anti-spasticity agent, which has been recognized occasionally to be proconvulsive; the risk is highest for severely disabled patients, in whom it is being used as a continuous intrathecal infusion. Depression is common in MS and most patients will receive antidepressants at some point, which also carry a small risk of triggering seizures. Second, treatment of acute relapses is with high-dose corticosteroids such as methyl-prednisolone 1000 mg daily for 3 days; the short duration means that adverse effects of glucocorticoids on the central nervous system are very rare in clinical practice. Third, disease-modifying therapies, including beta-interferon, glatari-mer acetate, natalizumab, and mitoxantrone. Seizures are reported as an occasional adverse reaction to beta-interferon and natalizumab. Numbers are too small for satisfactory evidence regarding particular treatment or prognosis of seizures associated with MS but in the limited case series, the prognosis for remission appears to be good. About 1 in 5000 to 1 in 1000 patients treated with natalizumab for MS may develop with progressive multifocal leukoencephalopathy, a viral infection which itself primarily affects white matter and may manifest with seizures, sometimes at presentation (see Chapter 67).

Other acquired demyelinating diseases

A much less common demyelinating condition is acute disseminated encephalomyelitis (ADEM) (Hynson *et al.* 2001; Tenembaum *et al.* 2002), which is a monophasic illness, generally recognized to be a post-infectious syndrome, with a recent preceding infection or immunization recognized in about three-quarters of affected individuals. It usually affects children and may be fulminant and even rapidly fatal, especially in its fortunately very rare, hemorrhagic form. ADEM is an acute monophasic illness, usually reaching its peak within 1 week of onset. It is characterized by severe neurological deficits, including hemiparesis, spinal cord and optic nerve involvement. Altered consciousness is much more common than in MS and focal or generalized seizures have been reported in up to 35% of cases, sometimes as a presenting feature. The MRI characteristically

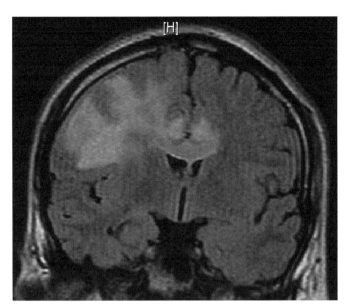

Fig. 85.4. Fluid attenuated inversion recovery MRI of a 25-year-old man with a fulminant presentation with ADEM, showing a large white matter lesion crossing the corpus callosum with significant mass effect. The patient was critically ill in a coma.

shows much larger lesions with mass effect (Fig. 85.4) but the appearance may be indistinguishable from MS. Oligoclonal bands are absent from the CSF.

Marchiafava–Bignami disease is a very rare, non-inflammatory disorder of myelin affecting alcoholics, characterized by abnormalities of the corpus callosum and cerebral white matter (Heinrich *et al.* 2004). Its cause is not clear but it may be related to thiamine deficiency or sodium abnormalities analagous to central pontine myelinolysis. It presents with a prodrome of days to weeks of ataxia and cognitive symptoms, evolving into coma and seizures. General support leads to partial recovery, often leaving a cerebral disconnection syndrome.

Neuromyelitis optica or Devic disease is an uncommon, severe relapsing demyelinating condition with a predilection for the spinal cord and optic nerves. It has recently, in the majority of patients, been associated with antibodies to aquaporin-4, the commonest water channel in the central nervous system, and this marker has led to the diagnosis being made more frequently. The phenotype is consequently expanding, but seizures are not generally a feature of this condition.

References

Calabrese M, de Stefano N, Atzori, M, *et al.* (2008) Extensive cortical inflammation is associated with epilepsy in multiples sclerosis. *J Neurol* **255**:581–6.

Compston A, Confavreux C (2006) The distribution of multiple sclerosis. In: Compston A, Confavreux C, Lassman H, *et al.* (eds.) *McAlpine's Multiple Sclerosis*,

4th edn. London: Churchill Livingstone, pp. 69–112.

Engelsen BA, Grøning M (1997) Epileptic seizures in patients with multiple sclerosis: is the prognosis of epilepsy underestimated? *Seizure* **6**:377–82.

Gambardella A, Valentino P, Labate A, *et al.* (2003) Temporal lobe epilepsy as a unique manifestation of multiple sclerosis. *Can J Neurosci* **30**:228–32.

Ghezzi A, Montanini R, Basso PF, *et al.* (1990) Epilepsy in multiple sclerosis. *Eur Neurol* **30**:218–30.

Heinrich A, Tunge U, Khaw AV (2004) Clinicoradiologic subtypes of Marchiafavi–Bignami disease. *J Neurol* **251**:1050–9.

Hynson JL, Kornber AJ, Coleman LT, *et al.* (2001) Clinical and neuroradiologic features of acute disseminated encephalomyelitis in children. *Neurology* **56**:1308–12.

Kinnunen E, Wikström J (1986) Prevalence and prognosis of epilepsy in patients with multiple sclerosis. *Epilepsia* **27**:729–33.

Lasussman H, Wekerle H (2006) The pathology of multiple sclerosis. In: Compston A, Confavreux C, Lassman H, (eds.) *McAlpine's Multiple Sclerosis*, 4th edn. London: Churchill Livingstone, pp. 557–600.

McDonald WI, Compston A, Gilles Edan G, *et al.* (2001) Recommended diagnostic criteria for multiple sclerosis: guidelines from the International Panel on the Diagnosis of Multiple Sclerosis. *Ann Neurol* **50**:121–7.

Miller D, McDonald WI, Smith K (2006) The diagnosis of multiple sclerosis. In: Compston A, Confavreux C, Lassman H,

et al. (eds.) *McAlpine's Multiple Sclerosis*, 4th edn. London: Churchill Livingstone, pp. 347–88.

Moreau T, Sochurkova D, Lemesle M, *et al.* (1998) Epilepsy in patients with multiple sclerosis: radiological and clinical correlations. *Epilepsia* **39**:893–6.

Nicoletti A, Sofia V, Biondi R, *et al.* (2003) Epilepsy and multiple sclerosis in Sicily: a population-based study. *Epilepsia* **44**:1445–8.

Nyquist PA, Cascino G, McLelland, Annegers JF, Rodriguez M (2002) Incidence of seizures in patients with multiple sclerosis: a population-based study. *Mayo Clin Proc* **77**:910–12.

Olafsson E, Benedikz J, Hauser WA (1999) Risk of epilepsy in patients with multiple sclerosis: a population-based study in Iceland. *Epilepsia* **40**:745–7.

Poser CM, Paty DW, Scheinberg L, *et al.* (1983) New diagnostic criteria for multiple sclerosis: guidelines for research protocols. *Ann Neurol* **13**:227–31.

Sawcer SJ (2008) The complex genetics of multiple sclerosis. *Brain* **131**:3118–31.

Sokić DV, Stojsavljević N, Drulović J, *et al.* (2001) Seizures in multiple sclerosis. *Epilepsia* **42**:72–9.

Tenembaum S, Chamoles N, Fejerman N (2002) Acute disseminated encephalomyelitis: a long-term follow-up study of 84 pediatric patients. *Neurology* **59**:1224–31.

Thompson AJ, Kermode AG, Moseley IF, MacManus DG, McDonald WI (1993) Seizures due to multiple sclerosis: seven patients with MRI correlations. *J Neurol Neurosurg Psychiatry* **56**:1317–20.

Chapter

Hydrocephalus and porencephaly

Pierangelo Veggiotti and Federica Teutonico

Hydrocephalus
Clinical forms and epidemiology

Hydrocephalus is defined as the condition in which the volume of cerebrospinal fluid (CSF) is increased in all part of the intracranial fluid spaces, and in which the increased volume is not due to primary atrophy or dysgenesis of the brain. The incidence of hydrocephalus is not perfectly known – the usually reported incidence of 3 per 1000 live births applies only to congenital cases. In recent years, systematic fetal ultrasonography during pregnancy has modified our knowledge of the incidence of congenital hydrocephalus: in Sweden Fernell *et al.* (1994) found a mean prevalence with onset in the first year of life of 0.53 per 1000 during 1967–82, with an increasing trend from 0.48 in 1967–70 to 0.63 in 1979–82. The origin of hydrocephalus differed between preterm and term infants: in term infants the origin was considered to be prenatal in 70%, perinatal in 25%, and postnatal in 5%.

Hydrocephalus represents a heterogeneous group of clinical conditions that can be classified according to different elements: type of onset (acute vs. chronic), etiology, or age of onset. The most common causes of antenatal hydrocephalus include malformations of the CSF pathways or, more extensively, the brain, and abnormal events during pregnancy (infections, intra- or periventricular hemorrhage, trauma).

Infantile hydrocephalus is chiefly caused by bacterial meningitis, parasitic infections, and malformation syndrome such as the Dandy–Walker syndrome. Many causes of fetal hydrocephalus are also major causes of infantile hydrocephalus since they can become manifest after the first year of life. Childhood hydrocephalus commonly results from tumors in the posterior fossa, sellar and suprasellar areas, infections, and hemorrhage.

Clinical features

The clinical manifestations of hydrocephalus also differ with age. The chief clinical signs suggestive of congenital hydrocephalus include abnormally increased head circumference, tense and large anterior fontanelle, splayed sutures, and scalp vein distension. Sometimes congenital hydrocephalus can manifest with irritability, drowsiness, or unexplained vomiting. Kirkpatrick *et al.* (1989) reported that among 51 patients, hydrocephalus was asymptomatic in 49% of cases.

Acute infantile hydrocephalus can manifest with lethargy, stupor, vomiting, and oculomotor nerve palsy (Racette *et al.* 2004). In older children the clinical symptoms of hydrocephalus can be acute or subacute and include headache, nausea, vomiting, and progressive disturbances in vigilance. Chronic cases may manifest with slowly progressive neurological signs such as disturbances of behavior, neuropsychological regression, ataxia, and pyramidal signs.

Epilepsy in hydrocephalus

Epilepsy is not commonly reported as the presenting symptom of hydrocephalus and has been described more frequently in patients with shunts than in those who have not undergone surgery. Ines and Markand (1977) and Di Rocco *et al.* (1985) found the frequency of seizures to be respectively 18.2% and 14% pre-surgery. Bourgeois *et al.* (1999) studied a series of 802 children with hydrocephalus and emphasized the difference in the severity of epilepsy between patients in whom seizures developed before shunting and those in whom seizures developed afterwards. In the post-shunt group most children (80%) had recurrent unprovoked seizures and their condition was poorly controlled with medication.

Interestingly, there was a peak incidence of seizure occurrence around the time of shunt insertion, with the majority being observed in the days immediately preceding shunt insertion. In the pre-shunt period, an increase in seizure activity is probably triggered by increased intracranial pressure and/or parenchymal damage consequent to decompensated hydrocephalus.

The relationship between epilepsy and hydrocephalus is complex. In most children hydrocephalus is part of a clinical picture usually characterized by several neurological disabilities, e.g., cerebral palsy, motor problems, and mental retardation; epilepsy can be one of the symptoms of this encephalopathy of varying etiology.

The Causes of Epilepsy, eds. S. D. Shorvon, F. Andermann, and R. Guerrini. Published by Cambridge University Press. © Cambridge University Press 2011.

The presence of neuroradiological abnormalities, in particular cerebral malformations and parenchymal lesions caused by infections represent the main predisposing factors for seizures in hydrocephalic children. The existence of birth injuries is another significant risk factor for the development of seizures. The incidence of epilepsy tends to be lower in children affected by mielomeningocele and/or spina bifida, in whom seizures occur only if cerebral abnormalities demonstrated by structural neuroimaging are present.

Epilepsy is reported to be commonly associated with shunt-treated hydrocephalus. Several authors have described an increased incidence of seizures after shunt implantation, ranging from 24% to 71% (Graebner and Celesia 1973; Hosking 1974; Ines and Markand 1977; Dan and Wade 1986; Venes and Dauser 1987; Johnson et al. 1996; Bourgeois et al. 1999). The trauma of catheter placement and the subsequent presence of a foreign body within the substance of the brain are potential causes of seizures and electroencephalogram (EEG) abnormalities.

The relation between the onset of epilepsy and the insertion of a ventricular catheter through the cerebral mantle is controversial. The development of epilepsy after shunt placement for hydrocephalus could be directly related to shunt implantation (Copeland et al. 1982; Venes and Dauser 1987). The influence of the ventricular catheter has been explored by studying EEG abnormalities which have been frequently found in patients in whom shunts have been placed. In the series of Bourgeois et al. (1999) – a group of patients with epilepsy in whom no radiological abnormalities were found on computed tomography (CT) or magnetic resonance imaging (MR) – a detailed analysis of EEG findings was performed before and after shunt insertion. Focal EEG abnormalities, which appeared after shunt placement and were localized to the same region of it, were found in 40% of cases. Also, Veggiotti et al. (1998) observed focal EEG abnormalities presenting on the same side as the shunt in 95% of their cases. The same finding was reported by Caraballo et al. (2008) in all patients of their series but not confirmed by other authors (Klepper et al. 1998; Ben Zeev et al. 2004).

Veggiotti et al. (1998) described the specific morphological characteristics of the epileptiform abnormalities detected in their patients, showing a wide amplitude (about 300 μV), and correlated this particular electrical signal with a defect in cortical gyration and organization caused by hydrocephalus. The hypothesis advanced was that hydrocephalus itself might affect the structural organization of the cortex, causing atrophy and thinning, and likely provoking cytological alterations and disruption of the normal cortical architecture sufficient to interfere with the genesis of the electrical signal. All these alterations might be attributed to increased CSF pressure which, owing to the effect of compression, could upset both the normal horizontal pattern of cortical cells and the normal orientation of the dipoles.

Shunt complications – both infective and mechanical – predispose to epilepsy and represent important risk factors for the occurrence of seizures in hydrocephalic children. However, Bourgeois et al. (1999) found that seizures alone were the presenting symptom of shunt dysfunction in only 8% of their series. This percentage was higher (28%) in children with a previous history of epilepsy.

Johnson et al. (1996) confirmed that shunt dysfunction may predispose to epileptic seizures in addition to the presence of the shunt catheter. Other authors (Agrawal and Durity 2006) reported that the occurrence of seizures in post-shunted hydrocephalus might be the only clinical manifestation of intracranial hypotension due to a shunt dysfunction. They postulated that this condition could be more common in shunted children than generally thought and the development of postural seizures in patients with a patent shunt should arouse the suspicion of intracranial hypotension. Nevertheless, Klepper et al. (1998) reported that epilepsy is not influenced by the number of shunt revisions in their series and concluded that epilepsy in hydrocephalus is related to the underlying encephalopathy rather than to surgical intervention.

Apart from the controversial hypothesis about the possible cause of epilepsy, it is universally accepted that the prognosis for seizure control in hydrocephalic children is poor. Epilepsy is frequently correlated with poor cognitive outcome and negative effects on psychological, social, and educational aspects in hydrocephalic children. It is mandatory to take all reasonable precautions to reduce the risk of infections and to avoid shunt dysfunction, since these are predisposing factors reported to be associated with seizure development.

All types of seizure have been described to be associated with hydrocephalus, with a prevalence of focal simple motor seizures. The prognosis of epilepsy is strongly influenced by the development of a pharmacoresistant condition which is reported to range from 35% to 75% of cases. In the series of Bourgeois et al. (1999), only 70 of 255 patients had antiepileptic medication discontinued and 21 of them suffered a relapse within 6 months of ceasing therapy. Noetzel and Blake (1992) reported that mental retardation and central nervous system malformations are important predictors of poor seizure control.

The presence of a medically refractory epilepsy in these children negatively impacts on their cognitive and neuropsychological development. One intriguing point concerns the correlation between hydrocephalus and the occurrence of continuous spike and waves during sleep (CSWS). Veggiotti et al. (1998) first described the presence of CSWS in six patients with shunted hydrocephalus, suggesting that the appearance of learning and cognitive disturbances in hydrocephalic children might be derived not only from neurosurgical problems linked to a possible chronic malfunctioning of the ventriculoperitoneal shunt system but also from the occurrence of a CSWS. The authors stressed that use of some antiepileptic drugs, such as carbamazepine and phenobarbital, might induce the onset of a similar electrical pattern and consequently the withdrawal of them followed by the introduction of specific medication, such as clobazam, ethosuximide, and sulthiame, could positively influence the evolution of these patients. The demonstration of the CSWS in hydrocephalic children has been reported by other authors (Battaglia et al. 2004; Ben Zeev et al. 2004; Caraballo et al. 2008).

Even if there is no clear evidence about which factors may influence the onset of CSWS in patients with hydrocephalus, all authors stress that accurate video-EEG monitoring during sleep is advised in patients with hydrocephalus to facilitate detection of CSWS and thus prevent the negative neuro-psychological effects caused by this condition.

Porencephaly

Clinical forms

The term porencephaly is used for any cavitating hemispheric lesion but it is best to restrict its use to circumscribed necrosis that occurs before the adult features of the hemisphere are manifest. Most porencephalic lesions involve both the gray and white matter. Multicystic encephalomalacia or multicystic encephalopathy is another term used to define multiple cavities that involve large parts of the cerebral hemispheres. These cavities affect either the white and the gray matter but also the cortex and basal ganglia, and are usually located predominantly in the territories of the anterior and middle cerebral arteries. The diagnosis is mostly postnatal and the status of infants at birth is often normal.

Clinical features

In patients with multicystic encephalopathy and porencephaly, MRI represents the modality of choice to define the extent of the lesion. Hemiparesis occurs in 25–35% of surviving infants with unilateral cerebral lesion. The likelihood of hemiparesis is nearly 100% if the distribution of the stem of the middle cerebral artery is affected.

Cognitive function is impaired after unilateral infarctions in approximately 25–50% of patients.

Epilepsy in porencephaly

Epilepsy also occurs in approximately 10–30% of infants with porencephalic lesions (Volpe 2008). The prognosis of epilepsy is variable and strongly influenced by the extent of the lesion. Epilepsy is usually characterized by the occurrence of partial seizures; partial motor seizures are the most frequent type in these patients. Focal seizures are the main seizure type in this group of patients with a prevalence of focal motor seizures. Patients are usually responsive to medical therapy, even if seizures related to prenatal lesions tend to be more resistant to medical treatment than those related to lesions of perinatal origin.

The typical EEG pattern in this group of patients is characterized by asymmetric background activity and focal slow and epileptiform activity over the areas identified as abnormal on neuroimaging. Epileptiform discharges can also be observed in patients who have no seizures and can persist even after seizure control is achieved. Even if epilepsy can be managed medically in most cases, approximately 6–7% of cases become refractory to treatment. In this group, all children presented with a severe epileptic syndrome starting almost invariably during the first year of life. The onset is often characterized by the occurrence of West syndrome followed by the development of pharmacoresistant focal epilepsy.

Veggiotti *et al.* (1999) and Guzzetta *et al.* (2006) reported a group of pharmacoresistant patients with a porencephalic lesion presenting with unilateral CSWS. These cases presented with partial seizures refractory to medical treatment, cognitive decline, and worsening of spontaneous movements in the hemibody contralateral to CSWS activity lasting for a few hours after night-time sleep. These symptoms improved later in the day.

Since both seizures and CSWS appear resistant to medical treatment, a surgical approach is a valid therapeutic option in these patients (Figs. 86.1, 86.2). The type of surgical approach

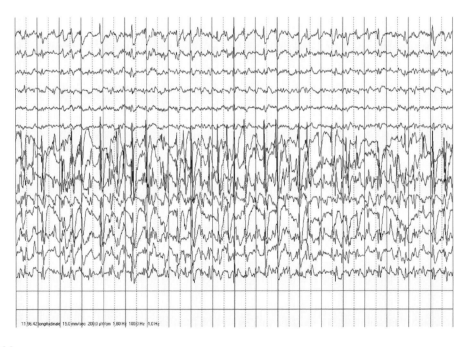

Fig. 86.1. Unilateral CSWS in a patient with a left congenital porencephalic lesion (before surgery).

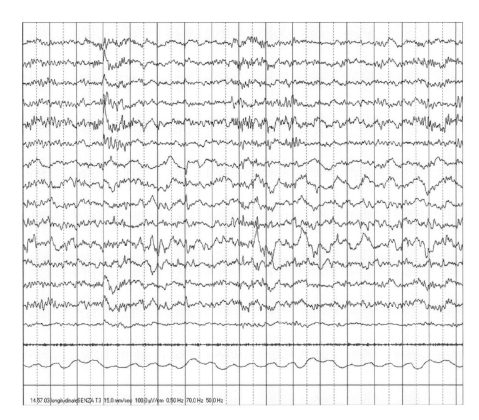

Fig. 86.2. The EEG pattern in a patient with a left congenital porencephalic lesion (after hemispherectomy).

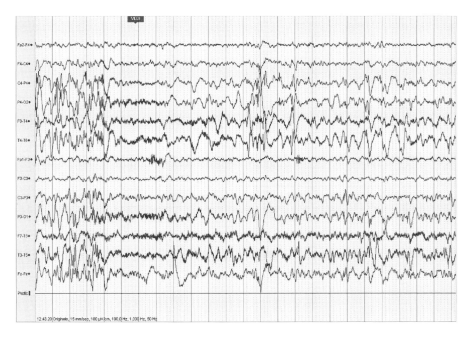

Fig. 86.3. Ictal pattern of "subtle" focal seizures in multicystic encephalomalacia.

can be different: partial hemispherectomy is usually performed but a cortical resection with excision of multiple lobes or of the porencephalic lesion itself may be indicated in patients presenting with a mild hemiparesis or preserved visual field (Guzzetta *et al.* 2006). Other authors propose a cortical resection guided by intraoperative electrocorticography to localize the epileptogenic focus when multiple seizure type and diffuse scalp EEG abnormalities are present (Iida *et al.* 2005).

In the literature (Battaglia *et al.* 2009), patients with porencephaly-related epilepsy who underwent surgery had an excellent seizure outcome and a cognitive improvement.

One intriguing problem is the association of congenital extratemporal porencephaly and hippocampal sclerosis. Ho *et al.* (1997) reported that mesial temporal sclerosis often coexists with porencephaly and is responsible for the epileptogenic activity when electroclinical data are demonstrated to be

A

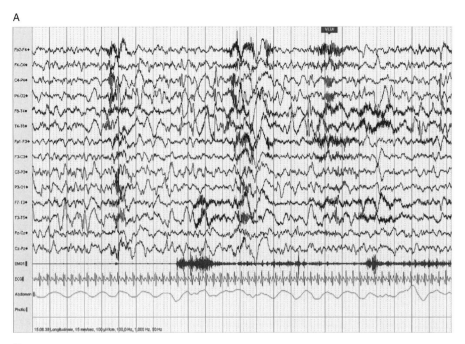

Fig. 86.4. (A) "Subtle" spasms and (B) typical spasms in multicystic encephalomalacia.

B

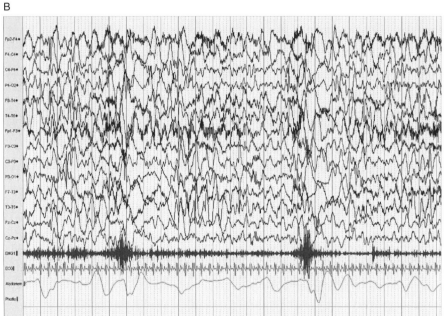

concordant. This finding could explain the development of medically refractory epilepsy in some patients and should indicate a more careful electroclinical study.

The excellent results of surgery have great implications for the clinical treatment of this group of patients and a more selective surgical approach such as temporal lobectomy might represent a valid option instead of hemispherectomy. The more likely mechanism to explain the dual pathology is a common ischemic pathogenesis for the two lesions. While the cause of mesial temporal sclerosis is still unclear, an ischemic mechanism for the pathogenesis of porencephaly is well established.

Multicystic encephalomalacia

Multicystic encephalomalacia represents a severe clinical condition characterized by impaired neurological status, seizures, and apathy with onset soon after birth. The neurological disorder consists of hemiparesis or more often tetra- or quadriparesis. Psychomotor development is severely impaired. Seizures are often focal motor at onset, characterized by "subtle" clinical manifestations (eye and/or head deviation, mild hypertonus) which are not recognized by parents. The use of video-EEG monitoring is mandatory to detect the aforementioned seizures. The ictal EEG is characterized by attenuation with superimposed brief bursts of fast activity (5–10 s), sometimes prevalent on one cerebral hemisphere (Fig. 86.3). Seizures occur frequently during the day and negatively influence the psychomotor development of these children. Seizures are not well controlled by the most commonly used antiepileptic drugs and tend to persist unchanged over the first months of life. The EEG shows multifocal abnormalities that evolve into a hypsarrhythmia pattern after approximately 5–7 months. At this time, typical spasms become evident but "subtle" seizures can still be present (Fig. 86.4).

The EEG can reveal a focal or lateralized epileptiform activity associated with a hypsarrhythmia pattern.

This group of patients is often refractory to medical treatment with adrenocorticotrophic hormone and vigabatrin, and complete seizure control is never achieved even after the use of different therapeutic agents (benzodiazepines, lamotrigine, ketogenic diet). The prognosis of epilepsy is poor: spasms tend to persist over time or evolve into "polymorphic" seizures typical of other epileptic encephalopathies (such as Lennox–Gastaut syndrome).

References

Agrawal D, Durity FA (2006) Seizure as a manifestation of intracranial hypotension in a shunted patient *Pediatr Neurosurg* **42**:165–7.

Aicardi J (2009) Hydrocephalus and nontraumatic pericerebral collections. In: Aicardi J (ed.) *Diseases of the Nervous System in Childhood*. London: MacKeith Press, pp. 185–209.

Battaglia D, Acquafondata C, Lettori D, *et al.* (2004) Observation of continuous spike-waves during slow sleep in children with myelomeningocele. *Childs Nerv Syst* **20**:462–7.

Battaglia D, Veggiotti P, Lettori D, *et al.* (2009) Functional hemispherectomy in children with epilepsy and CSWS due to unilateral early brain injury including thalamus: sudden recovery of CSWS *Epilepsy Res* **87**:290–8.

Ben Zeev B, Kivity S, Pshitizki Y, *et al.* (2004). Congenital hydrocephalus and continuous spike wave in slow-wave sleep: a common association? *J Child Neurol* **19**:129–34.

Bourgeois M, Sainte-Rose C, Cinalli G, *et al.* (1999) Epilepsy in children with shunted hydrocephalus. *J Neurosurg* **90**:274–81.

Caraballo RH, Bongiorni L, Cersòsimo R, *et al.* (2008) Epileptic encephalopathy with continuous spikes and waves during sleep in children with shunted hydrocephalus: a study of nine cases. *Epilepsia* **49**:1520–7.

Copeland GP, Foy PM, Shaw MDM (1982) The incidence of epilepsy after ventricular shunting operations. *Surg Neurol* **17**:279–81.

Dan NG, Wade MJ (1986) The incidence of epilepsy after ventricular shunting procedures. *J Neurosurg* **65**:19–21.

Di Rocco C, Iannelli A, Pallini R, Rinaldi A (1985) Epilepsy and its correlation with cerebral ventricular shunting procedures in infantile hydrocephalus. *J Pediatr Neurosci* **1**:255–63.

Fernell E, Hagberg H, Hagberg B (1994) Infantile hydrocephalus epidemiology: an indicator of enhanced survival. *Arch Dis Childh Fetal Neonatol Ed* **70**:F123–8.

Graebner RW, Celesia GG (1973) EEG findings in hydrocephalus and their relation to shunting procedures. *Electroencephalogr Clin Neurophys* **35**:517–21.

Guzzetta F, Battaglia D, Di Rocco C, Caldarelli M (2006) Symptomatic epilepsy in children with poroencephalic cysts secondary to perinatal middle cerebral artery occlusion. *Childs Nerv Syst* **22**:922–30.

Ho SS, Kuzniesky RI, Gilliam F, *et al.* (1997) Congenital poroencephaly and hippocampal sclerosis: clinical features and epileptic spectrum *Neurology* **49**:1382–8.

Hosking GP (1974) Fits in hydrocephalic children. *Arch Dis Childh* **49**:633–5.

Ines DF, Markand ON (1977) Epileptic seizures and abnormal electroencephalographic findings in hydrocephalus and their relation to the shunting procedures. *Electroencephalogr Clin Neurophysiol* **42**:761–8.

Iida K, Otsubo H, Arita K, Andermann F, Olivier A (2005) Cortical resection with electrocorticography for intractable porencephaly-related partial epilepsy. *Epilepsia* **46**:76–83.

Johnson DL, Conry J, O'Donnell R (1996) Epileptic seizures as a sign of cerebrospinal fluid shunt malfunction. *Pediatr Neurosurg* **24**:223–8.

Kirkpatrick M, Engelman H, Minns RA (1989) Symptoms and signs of progressive hydrocephalus. *Arch Dis Childh* **64**:124–8.

Klepper J, Büsse M, Strassburg HM, Sörensen N (1998) Epilepsy in shunt-treated hydrocephalus. *Dev Med Child Neurol* **40**:731–6.

Low C, Garzon E, Carrete H Jr., *et al.* (2007) Early destructive lesions in the developing brain: clinical and electrographic correlates. *Arq Neuropsiquiatr* **65**:416–22.

Noetzel MJ, Blake JN (1992) Seizures in children with congenital hydrocephalus: long-term outcome. *Neurology* **42**:1277–81.

Prayson RA, Hannahoe BM (2004). Clinicopathologic findings in patients with infantile hemiparesis and epilepsy. *Hum Pathol.* **35**:734–8.

Racette BA, Esper GT, Antenor J, *et al.* (2004) Pathophysiology of parkinsonism due to hydrocephalus. *J Neurol Neurosurg Psychiatry* **75**:1617–19.

Veggiotti P, Beccaria F, Papalia G, *et al.* (1998) Continuous spikes and waves during sleep in children with shunted hydrocephalus. *Childs Nerv Syst* **14**:188–94.

Veggiotti P, Beccaria F, Guerrini R, Capovilla G, Lanzi G (1999). Continuous spike-and-wave activity during slow-wave sleep: syndrome or EEG pattern? *Epilepsia* **40**:1593–601.

Venes JL, Dauser RC (1987). Epilepsy following ventricular shunt placement. *J Neurosurg* **66**:154–5.

Volpe JJ (2008) Hypoxic–ischemic encephalopathy: clinical aspects. In: *Neurology of the Newborn*, 5th edn. Philadelphia, PA: Saunders Elsevier, pp. 400–480.

Chapter

87

Alzheimer disease and other neurodegenerative diseases

Sigmund Jenssen and Kandan Kulandaivel

Alzheimer disease and other neurodegenerative dementias

Definition and epidemiology

Dementia is a clinical process characterized by loss of function in multiple cognitive domains. DSM-IV diagnostic criteria require memory impairment and at least one of the following: aphasia, apraxia, agnosia, or a disturbance of executive function. The cognitive impairments must be severe enough to cause a decline in social and occupational functioning. The decline must also be from a previously higher level of functioning. Finally, the diagnosis of dementia cannot be made if the cognitive deficits occur exclusively during the course of delirium. Dementia can present primarily with disordered personality and executive function rather than memory deficit as in frontal temporal dementia and a cognitive decline from a previous higher level can be noticed in high functioning individuals before there are problems in social functioning.

Alzheimer disease (AD) is the most common cause of dementia, accounting for more than half of all dementia patients. It affects approximately 4.5 million people in the United States. Age is the most important risk factor. The prevalence increases exponentially, affecting 5% of those older than 60 years of age and almost 30% of those over 85 (Kokmen 1989; McDowell *et al.* 1994). Alzheimer disease has a major economic impact since it hampers the productivity of both patients and care-givers. It is one of the most common illnesses requiring nursing home placement. The lifetime risk of developing AD is estimated to be between 12% and 17% (Cooper 1991). Risk factors for developing late-onset AD are apolipoprotein E-4 allele (APOE-4), female gender, low education, family history of AD, cerebrovascular disease, history of significant head trauma, hypertension, elevated homocysteine levels, high fat intake, and diabetes mellitus. Early-onset AD is caused by genetic mutations. Three of these are known and all are of autosomic dominant inheritance. Mutated genes are located on chromosomes 21, 14, and 1 and their respective protein products are amyloid precursor protein, presenilin 1, and presenilin 2. On the other hand, lifestyle features like physical exercise, social activities, and cognitively simulating activities may protect against developing AD.

Pathology, physiology, and clinical features of dementia

Neurodegenerative dementia affects predominantly either the cortical structures or the subcortical structures at onset, or both of these systems to a similar degree. In the "cortical" type, higher cognitive processes are primarily affected while the speed of processing and other neurological functions like dexterity, balance, and bulbar functions remain normal. The most typical condition here is AD. "Subcortical" types have typically relatively well-preserved higher functions while the speed of processing is severely impaired, often with abnormalities in the motor system, balance, and cranial nerves. Typical for this group is the dementia of Parkinson disease (PD), progressive supranuclear palsy, and Huntington disease. The degenerative process will eventually affect both cortical and subcortical systems producing a combination of cognitive and motor impairment. Some dementias affect both systems at onset, such as Lewy body dementia (LBD). Degeneration of the frontal lobes also typically present with deficits of processing and judgment. Epilepsy is not a typical feature of the subcortical dementia types.

In AD we find neuronal loss and two types of pathological protein aggregates: cortical neuritic plaques and neurofibrillary tangles. The plaques have a central core of beta amyloid, an insoluble polypeptide derived from the abnormal cleavage of a neuronal membrane protein called amyloid precursor protein (APP). The amyloid cascade hypothesis states that the deposition of amyloid is the initial pathogenic process that subsequently leads to AD. Plaques presumably lead to microglial activation, associated inflammatory response, and free radical formation. Tau-positive neurites then develop around the amyloid core resulting in neuritic plaques. These protein aggregates are formed by abnormal hyperphosphorylated Tau, a microtubule-associated protein which stabilizes microtubules. When Tau becomes hyperphosphorylated,

The Causes of Epilepsy, eds. S. D. Shorvon, F. Andermann, and R. Guerrini. Published by Cambridge University Press. © Cambridge University Press 2011.

microtubules are destabilized and this leads to disruption of the axonal transport and eventually neuronal death (Maccioni et al. 2001).

Symptoms of AD are both cognitive and behavioral. There is insidious, progressive loss of recent episodic memory, with relative preservation of short-term and semantic memory. Language function declines later on. The patient has initially no significant motor dysfunction and the personality is preserved. Behavioral symptoms include personal neglect, apathy, paranoid ideations, and hallucinations. Frontal release signs like snout reflex, palmomental reflex, grasp, and rooting reflex are present in late stages with falls and anorexia. Death results from intercurrent infection.

Epilepsy in Alzheimer disease and other types of dementia

Frequency of epilepsy

Epilepsy is diagnosed as a rule after two or more spontaneous seizures. Advanced age increases the risk of both epilepsy and dementia. Stroke is another factor that sets the elderly up for seizures. The incidence of any type of first seizure in those aged more than 60 years is 127 per 100 000, more than twice the incidence in persons aged 40–59 years.

Dementing illnesses account for 7–17% of elderly patients with epilepsy (Hauser 1992; Mendez and Lim 2003). One study showed 5–10 times greater risk in patients with dementia than in a reference population (Hauser 1986; Hesdorffer et al. 1996).

Risk factors for developing epilepsy

Seizures can occur at any stage of AD but tend to occur in the late stages, around six or more years after the onset of dementia. The patients with the highest risk of seizures are those with AD starting at a younger age (50–59 years), who exhibit poor cognition and have focal epileptiform activity in the EEG (Amatniek et al. 2006). The three autosomal dominant genes that cause early-onset AD are associated with increased risk of seizures. The APOE-4 allele, a well-known risk factor for late-onset AD which 15% of the general population carries, does not in itself increase the risk of seizures in dementia.

The mechanisms of epilepsy in dementia are the subject of increasing research. The dementing process may cause a selective loss of inhibitory neurons that encourages the formation of epileptogenic foci producing seizures. Alzheimer disease and temporal lobe epilepsy (TLE) share several clinical and imaging features. Both conditions have memory deficits that are accompanied by cell loss in the hippocampus. Epileptogenesis in AD correlates with lower counts of pyramidal cells in the cortical layers 3–4 of parietal (area 7) and parahippocampal gyri (area 28), especially in those patients with generalized

motor seizures (Jack et al. 2000). Hippocampal atrophy can also be a predictor of seizures in AD. Although similar structures and systems are affected, the patterns of degeneration are rather different in the two diseases. There is for example CA1 degeneration in the hippocampus of both AD and TLE patients, but the granule cell layer is typically well preserved in AD and greatly diminished in TLE. The extracellular deposition of beta amyloid could be epileptogenic independent of cell loss. Patients with Down syndrome, most of whom carry an extra copy of the APP gene, develop early-onset AD and 84% of these have clinical seizures (see Chapter 39) (Lai and Williams 1989). The deposition of beta amyloid in the hippocampus in APP transgenic mice, which have histological and clinical changes typical for AD, can cause spontaneous non-convulsive seizures and even hippocampal hyperexcitability as measured by depth electrodes without any obvious clinical changes on inspection (Palop et al. 2007).

Two other dementias in which seizures form a common part of the clinical picture are LBD and vascular dementia. The pathological hallmark of LBD apart from diffuse cerebral atrophy are disseminated "Lewy bodies," composed mainly of an alpha synuclein protein distributed in the cortex and midbrain (McKeith et al. 2004). Clinical clues to the presence of LBD as opposed to AD are delirium, movement disorders, psychosis, and seizures. There is little information on seizure types and treatment response particular for LBD. Patients with LBD have pronounced variability in the localization of slowing in the electroencephalogram (EEG) which is possibly related to the severe cholinergic deficit observed in these patients causing synaptic instability (Roks et al. 2008).

Vascular dementia is caused by repeated strokes, both cortical and subcortical. The clinical course is characterized by the appearance of multiple neurological deficits affecting both motor movements and higher cognitive functions. Seizures occur focally in this condition and the risk of developing epilepsy is highest in patients with large cortical or hemorrhagic strokes. Repeated seizures following an ischemic stroke promote increased cognitive impairment in patients with vascular dementia. Pre-existing dementia increases the risk of late seizures after stroke (occurring more than a week after stroke), but not of early seizures (occurring within a week of stroke). Interestingly recent studies have found that only 4% of autopsies of patients with vascular dementia show pure vascular dementia, while the great majority also have pathological changes consistent with especially AD.

Creutzfeldt–Jakob disease (CJD) is the most common of the human transmissible spongiform encephalopathies (prion diseases). The prion diseases appear to result from the intracellular accumulation of a prion protein which is an abnormal conformation of a cellular protein. The sporadic form of CJD is typically diagnosed in people between 50 and 70 years of age. In the course of the disease, patients develop a rapidly progressive dementia and combinations of other neurological signs, including seizures, myoclonus, and motor, sensory, visual, and autonomic deficits. Epilepsia partialis continua, convulsive status epilepticus, and complex partial status epilepticus have been reported as presenting symptoms of CJD. Myoclonus, often provoked by startle, is present in more than 80% of patients. The neurological status deteriorates rapidly leading to death within 1 year of clinical onset. Elevation of 14–3–3 protein in the cerebrospinal fluid can support the diagnosis of CJD. The EEG can reveal periodic sharp wave complexes. Magnetic resonance imaging (MRI) is the most sensitive test, and can show signal abnormality prominent in the cortical ribbon, caudate, and putamen (Johnson and Gibbs 1998; Mastrianni 2004).

Special characteristics of epilepsy in dementia and old age

In elderly patients, new-onset epilepsy is most often focal in type and most seizures take the form of complex partial seizures, with possible secondary generalization, but motor movement and convulsions get less frequent with age (Hiyoshi and Yagi 2000). Seizures become both briefer and more non-specific, while the duration of the postictal state increases. Not uncommonly, intermittent or constant seizure activity is detected on the EEG of elderly patients with dementia and acute mental status changes (Sheth *et al.* 2006), indicating that epileptic activity might more often cause prolonged confusion than time-limited seizures. Auras and automatisms are less common and ictal confusion can be protracted, with waxing and waning blurring the difference between so-called ictal and interictal periods (Ramsay *et al.* 2004). Some of the differences in clinical presentation have been thought to be due to the higher frequency of seizures with an extratemporal focus when compared to the younger adults. All these factors contribute to making the diagnosis more difficult.

No single test can make up for the lack of good history-taking. This is particularly difficult in demented patients because they often have difficulty remembering and communicating prior events. Many patients live alone or in institutions and have limited social interaction so the episodes are often unwitnessed. To complicate matters further, elderly patients are more prone to other conditions that can be confused with seizures. These include syncope and presyncope, cardiac arrhythmias, transient ischemic attacks, and metabolic and psychiatric disorders.

In adults, the EEG can sometimes provide definitive information, since in younger age groups the specificity of interictal or ictal epileptiform activity in the EEG is high. This is not so clear-cut in elderly demented patients. Subclinical rhythmic discharges in the adult (SREDA) can be misinterpreted as focal seizures and periodic epileptiform discharges (PEDS) do not necessarily mean seizures. The sensitivity of the EEG, on the other hand, is even lower in the elderly than in younger age groups. Only 26–35% of patients above the age of 65 developing epilepsy had a positive first EEG in one study (Drury and Beydoun 1998). The decrease in sensitivity of standard EEG makes video-EEG monitoring a useful, and

often underutilized, tool. Several studies have highlighted the importance of video-EEG in this age group and its beneficial effect on management (Keranen *et al.* 2002). Neuroimaging, blood work, and spinal fluid examination mainly serve to detect symptomatic causes that then are helpful in the treatment and management.

Diagnostic tests for dementia

Dementia in the overwhelming majority is caused by an irreversible degenerative process. Reversible types of dementia are considered to be relatively uncommon, accounting now for less than 1% of cases (Clarfield 2003). Recent practice parameters of the American Academy of Neurology (Knopman *et al.* 2001) recommend neuroimaging (non-contrast computed tomography [CT] or MRI) as well as screening for vitamin B_{12} deficiency and hypothyroidism in all patients with new onset dementia. The purpose is to detect reversible and potentially treatable conditions; however, neuroimaging can also help in verifying the type of dementia (Table 87.1). Genetic screening is only recommended in the case of early-onset dementia. Neuropsychological evaluation is helpful in evaluating for type of dementia. The NINCDS–ADRDA Alzheimer Criteria are among the most used in the diagnosis and estimate the likelihood that a patient suffers from AD (McKhann *et al.* 1984):

(1) Definite AD – Clinical features of probable AD confirmed with autopsy.
(2) Probable AD – Patients between 40–90 years, deficits in two or more areas of cognition (including memory), confirmed by clinical and neuropsychological evaluation and not associated with delirium or other illnesses.
(3) Possible AD – Dementia syndrome with atypical onset or progression of unknown etiology.
(4) Unlikely AD – Dementia syndrome with sudden onset, focal neurologic signs, seizures, or gait disturbance.

Principles of management

It is important to remove any precipitating cause of seizures, such as metabolic disorders, adverse drug reaction, or drug withdrawal.

Treatment is usually initiated after a second seizure. The mainstay of epilepsy treatment in the patient with dementia is anticonvulsant medication. The goal is seizure freedom with the fewest side effects possible, especially cognitive side effects. Research into the treatment of epilepsy in demented patients is limited. Information on the tolerability and efficacy of antiepileptic drugs (AED) in elderly patients in general, and related to pharmacokinetics and mechanisms of action could be helpful when choosing AED and dose (Tables 87.2, 87.3).

The ideal AED for use in this setting most likely needs to have several characteristics. A lack of pharmacologic interactions is important because elderly patients are exposed to many other medications directed at other comorbidities (Table 87.2). In one study, elderly patients were taking on average between 7 and 13 other medications. Several of the first-generation AEDs interact with many of commonly used medications including: coumadin, statins, antidepressants, antiretrovirals, calcium-channel blockers, digoxin, and theophylline.

Enzyme cytochrome P-450-inducing AEDs such as phenytoin, carbamazepine, and phenobarbital, as well as the hepatic inhibitor valproic acid, have all been associated with osteoporosis. These same agents have been found to increase homocysteine levels, which is a known risk factor for stroke and myocardial infarction.

The pharmacokinetic characteristic that best predicts tolerability of AED in the elderly patient is protein binding. Low protein levels can result in an elevation of the pharmacologically active free fraction of drugs that are heavily protein-bound, leading to side effects or intoxication. Most measurements of serum levels assess the total amount of the drug in serum rather than the free fraction. The distribution of highly protein-bound drugs is also affected by other factors that alter protein binding of the drug. Decreases in the lean : fat ratio with advancing age reduces the volume of distribution, and can affect lipid-soluble drug concentrations. Decreases in gastric motility and absorption and progressive loss of gastric parietal cells can affect gastric absorption. Decreased hepatic metabolism or renal clearance with advancing age also can affect the metabolism of AEDs.

Antiepileptic drugs with a short half-life will require medication to be taken several times a day which can be challenging in an elderly person with defective memory function, although this is less of a problem in institutionalized patients.

Drugs have stronger pharmacodynamic effects in the elderly in general, in some cases possibly due to a reduction in the number of drug receptors.

Dementia leads in most cases to loss of brain volume and to reduced cognitive reserve. Sedation is usually not a desirable side effect, but in some agitated patients can be beneficial. A mood-stabilizing effect can be beneficial for some patients.

Table 87.1 Overview of the causes of dementia

Reversible dementia without persisting deficits	Reversible dementia with persisting deficits	Degenerative dementia
Depression	Vascular dementia	Alzheimer disease
Hypoxia (e.g., from anemia, decreased cardiac output, lung disease)	Alcoholic dementia	Frontotemporal dementias
Electrolyte imbalance (e.g., hyponatremia)	Trauma (e.g., dementia pugilistica)	Huntington disease
Hepatic insufficiency	Syphilis (i.e., general paresis)	Parkinson disease
Endocrine disease (e.g., hyperthyroidism, Addison disease, Cushing disease)	Some intoxications (e.g., lead)	Lewy body dementia
Some intoxications (e.g., therapeutic drugs)	Vitamin B_{12} deficiency (e.g., long-standing)	Multiple sclerosis
Vitamin B_{12} deficiency (e.g., of short duration)	Normal pressure hydrocephalus	Creutzfeldt–Jakob disease
Normal pressure hydrocephalus (e.g., of short duration)	Postencephalitic dementia	Human immunodeficiency virus dementia
	Anoxic dementia	Progressive supranuclear palsy
		Amyotrophic lateral sclerosis

Table 87.2 Interactions between medications for Alzheimer disease and antiepileptic drugs

Alzheimer medications	Phenytoin	Carbamazepine	Phenobarbital	Benzodiazepine	Valproic acid	Oxcarbazepine	Levetiracetam	Topiramate	Gabapentin	Lamotrigine	Zonisamide	Pregabalin
Donepezil (D)	↓	↓	↓	–[a]	–	↓	–	–	–	–	–	–
Galantamine (G)	↓	↓	↓	–	–	↓	–	–	–	–	–	–
Rivastigmine (R)	none[b]	none	none	none	none	none	none	none	none	none	–	none
Tacrine (T)	none	none	none	none	none	none	none	none	none	none	–	none
Memantine (M)	none	none	none	none	none	none	none	none	none	none	–	none

Notes:
[a] No interaction detected.
[b] No information available.

Table 87.3 Systematic comparison of antiepileptic drugs

Drug	Metabolism	Excretion	Protein binding	Dosing[a]	Main adverse effects	Important drug interactions
Phenytoin	Hepatic CYP (enzyme inducer)	Biliary	80–95%	qid/bid	Osteopenia, conduction block	Warfarin, cyclosporin, digoxin, tricyclic antidepressants, sertraline, fluoxetine, ticlopidine, propranolol, metoprolol, diltiazem, verapamil, nimodipine, felodipine, AED
Carbamazepine	Hepatic CYP (enzyme inducer)	Biliary	75%	bid/tid	Hyponatremia, conduction block	Warfarin, fluoxetine, tricyclic antidepressants, sertraline, ticlopidine, propranolol, metoprolol, simvastatin, diltiazem, verapamil, nimodipine, felodipine, AED
Valproic acid	Hepatic glucuronidation (enzyme inhibitor)	Biliary	75–90%	bid/tid	Tremor, parkinsonism, pancreatitis	AED
Phenobarbital	Hepatic CYP (enzyme inducer)	Biliary	45–50%	qid/bid	Sedation, osteopenia	Warfarin, tricyclic antidepressants, propranolol, metoprolol, nimodipine, felodipine, AED
Lamotrigine	Hepatic glucuronidation	Renal	50%	bid	Sedation	Sertraline
Gabapentin	Not metabolized	Renal	Not bound	tid/qid	Somnolence, weight gain	None
Oxcarbazepine	Hepatic glucuronidation (weak CYP enzyme inducer)	Renal	35–50%[b]	bid	Hyponatremia	Verapamil, felodipine
Topiramate	Hepatic (weak enzyme inducer)	Renal	20%	bid	Cognitive decline, nephrolithiasis	Digoxin
Levetiracetam	Minimal non-hepatic	Renal	Not bound	bid	Behavioral effects	None
Zonisamide	Hepatic	Renal	50%	qid/bid	Nephrolithiasis, fatigue, somnolence, ataxia	AED
Pregabalin	Not metabolized	Renal	Not bound	bid/tid	Dizziness, somnolence	None

CYP, cytochrome p450.
Notes:
[a]bid, twice a day; qid, four times a day; tid, three times a day.
[b]Protein binding of racemic MHD, oxcarbazepine's active metabolite.

Antiepileptic drugs can even be used as a hypnotic, especially if most seizures are nocturnal, but again the decrease in alertness can easily outweigh the benefits (Mendez and Lim 2003; Jenssen and Schere 2010).

Large studies that shed light on the prognosis of epilepsy in elderly demented patients are lacking. One report on new-onset epilepsy in 117 elderly patients, with and without dementia, indicated that 62% of patients became seizure-free on their first AED. The number increased to 79% after changes in AEDs. Of these, 93% were taking only one AED. Patients attaining remission were more likely to have had fewer pre-treatment seizures than those who did not obtain full seizure control. No AED was more likely to confer seizure freedom than any other (Tsolaki *et al.* 2000).

Another open-label study showed 61% of elderly patients (with or without dementia) were rendered seizure-free on one AED, but 27% had significant side effects. To date, there are no comparisons of AED treatment versus placebo in elderly patients. It is not known whether treatment should be started after one or more seizures and for how long. Since seizures are frequently of focal onset, patients are considered to have high risk of recurrence, and many will receive lifelong treatment without much empirical evidence of the value of this.

Status epilepticus, most often of the non-convulsive type, needs to be treated gently in most cases avoiding respiratory suppression and endotracheal intubation if possible.

Epilepsy can have negative consequences on the dementia, including a decline in cognitive abilities, reduced autonomy, greater risk of injury, and a higher mortality rate (Volicer *et al.* 1995). The clinician therefore needs to have a high suspicion of seizures, look for precipitating causes, choose the AED and dose judiciously, and monitor for side effects.

References

Amatniek JC, Hauser WA, DelCastillo-Castaneda C, *et al.* (2006) Incidence and predictors of seizures in patients with Alzheimer's disease. *Epilepsia* **47**:867–72.

Clarfield AM (2003) The decreasing prevalence of reversible dementias: an updated meta-analysis. *Arch Intern Med* **163**:2219–29.

Cooper B (1991) The epidemiology of primary degenerative dementia and related neurological disorders. *Eur Arch Psychiatry Clin Neurosci* **240**:223–33.

Drury I, Beydoun A (1998) Interictal epileptiform activity in elderly patients with epilepsy. *Electroencephalogr Clin Neurophysiol* **106**:369–73.

Hauser WA (1986) Seizures and myoclonus in patients with Alzheimer's disease. *Neurology* **36**:1226–30.

Hauser WA (1992) Seizure disorders: the changes with age. *Epilepsia* **33**:S6–14.

Hesdorffer DC, Hauser WA, Annegers JF, Kokmen E, Rocca WA (1996) Dementia and adult-onset unprovoked seizures. *Neurology* **46**:727–30.

Hiyoshi T, Yagi K (2000) Epilepsy in the elderly. *Epilepsia* **41**:31–5.

Jack CR, Petersen RC, Xu Y, *et al.* (2000) Rates of hippocampal atrophy correlate with change in clinical status in aging and AD. *Neurology* **55**:484–90.

Jenssen S, Schere D (2010) Treatment and management of epilepsy in the elderly

demented patient. *Am J Alz Dis other Demen* **25**:18–26.

Johnson R, Gibbs C (1998) Creutzfeldt–Jakob disease and related transmissible spongiform encephalopathies. *N Engl J Med* **339**:1994–2004.

Keranen T, Rainesalo S, Peltola J (2002) The usefulness of video-EEG monitoring in elderly patients with seizure disorders. *Seizure* **11**:269–72.

Knopman DS, DeKosky ST, Cummings JL, *et al.* (2001) Practice parameter: diagnosis of dementia (an evidence-based review). Report of the Quality Standards Subcommittee of the American Academy of Neurology. *Neurology* **56**:1143–53.

Kokmen E (1989) Prevalence of medically diagnosed dementia in a defined United States population: Rochester, Minnesota, January 1, 1975. *Neurology* **39**:773–6.

Lai F, Williams RS (1989) A prospective study of Alzheimer disease in Down syndrome. *Arch Neurol* **46**:849–53.

Maccioni RB, Muñoz JP, Barbeito L (2001) The molecular bases of Alzheimer's disease and other neurodegenerative disorders. *Arch Med Res* **32**:367–81.

Mastrianni J (2004) Prion diseases. *Clin Neurosci Res* **3**:469–80.

McDowell I, Hill G, Lindsay J, *et al.* (1994) Canadian Study of Health and Aging: study methods and prevalence of dementia. *Can Med Ass J* **150**:899–912.

McKeith I, Mintzer J, Aarsland D, *et al.* (2004) Dementia with Lewy bodies. *Lancet Neurol* **3**:19–28.

McKhann G, Drachman D, Folstein M, *et al.* (1984) Clinical diagnosis of Alzheimer's disease: report of the NINCDS–ADRDA Work Group under the auspices of Department of Health and Human Services Task Force on Alzheimer's Disease. *Neurology* **34**:939–44.

Mendez MF, Lim GTH (2003) Seizures in elderly patients with dementia: epidemiology and management. *Drugs Aging* **20**:791–803.

Palop JJ, Chin J, Roberson ED, *et al.* (2007) Aberrant excitatory neuronal activity and compensatory remodeling of inhibitory hippocampal circuits in mouse models of Alzheimer's disease. *Neuron* **55**:697–711.

Ramsay R, Rowan A, Pryor F (2004) Special considerations in treating the elderly patient with epilepsy. *Neurology* **62**:24–9.

Roks G, Korf E, van der Flier W, Scheltens P, Stam C (2008) The use of EEG in the diagnosis of dementia with Lewy bodies. *Br Med J* **79**:377.

Sheth RD, Drazkowski JF, Sirven JI, Gidal BE, Hermann BP (2006) Protracted ictal confusion in elderly patients. *Arch Neurol* **63**:529–32.

Tsolaki M, Kourtis A, Divanoglou D, Bostanzopoulou M, Kazis A (2000) Monotherapy with Lamotrigine in patients with Alzheimer's disease and seizures. *Am J Alz Dis other Demen* **15**:74–9.

Volicer L, Smith S, Volicer BJ (1995) Effect of seizures on progression of dementia of the Alzheimer type. *Dementia* **6**:258–63.

Chapter

88

Introduction to the concept of provoked epilepsy

Simon D. Shorvon, Renzo Guerrini, and Frederick Andermann

The fact that seizures can be "provoked" has of course been long recognized. The precipitation by light was recorded by Pliny and by Apuleius, and by the nineteenth century, cases of epilepsy induced by stress, startle, sensory stimulation, shock, noise, sexual activity and masturbation, eating, reading, and music, for instance, were well recorded. Following Tissot (1770), most authorities for the next hundred years at least tended to divide the causes of epilepsy into two categories: (a) underlying causes (syn. predisposing causes), and (b) "exciting" or provoking causes (see Chapter 2). Exciting causes were often described in relation to reflex action, and these were systematically explored by Marshall Hall (who coined the term) (Hall 1850), Brown-Séquard, and Hughlings Jackson amongst others. Jackson described a number of provoked seizures, including one case in which seizures were induced by a tap on the head. Gowers (1885) described cases of epileptic seizures induced by "light, voluntary movement and sudden muscular tension." In experimental animals, seizure provocation by touch was first demonstrated by Amantea (1921), by light by Clementi (1929), and by noise by Morgan and Morgan (1939). Pavlov's demonstration on conditional reflexes stimulated further research and Gastaut described conditioned-reflex epilepsy in 1956. Gastaut and his colleagues also made early studies of photic-induced seizures, and the first experiments in the photosensitive baboon, *Papio papio*, were made by Naquet in Gastaut's unit in 1956 (Beaumanoir 1995). In any book dealing with etiology, the provoking causes of seizures are important. In our etiological classification, provoked seizures are divided, if somewhat arbitrarily, into two categories: seizure precipitants and reflex seizures.

Seizure precipitants

In many types of epilepsy, both idiopathic and symptomatic, seizures are more likely to occur at times of stress, menstruation, sleep deprivation, fever, alcohol intake/withdrawal, metabolic disturbance, hypoglycemia, and so on. These are commonly known as "seizure precipitants" (although, as stressed below, they can be considered in reality as "causes"), and are widely accepted.

Epilepsy has a multifactorial causation and of course the differentiation of "underlying cause" from a "seizure precipitant" is simply one of degree. Spratling succinctly put this in 1904: if it takes 100 points to induce a seizure in an individual, a predisposition could contribute 60 points and an exciting cause 40 points, whereas if the predisposition contributed only 40 points, it would require an exciting cause to have 60 points in order to reach the "seizure point" (Spratling 1904). In a study of 500 drug-resistant patients, Aird (1983) concluded that in 17% seizure-inducing factors made a significant contribution to the occurrence of seizures and that manipulating these factors in these cases could greatly improve seizure control in such patients. It makes sense therefore to consider seizure precipitants as much a cause as any other, and the view that these are not "proper" causes makes little sense, and whether a precipitant accounts for 10%, 50%, or 70% of Spratling's "100 points" makes little difference. An example, in a case of post-traumatic epilepsy in which seizures are "precipitated" by stress, the distinction between cause and precipitant is a matter of degree only. In the authors' opinion, both stress and previous trauma have to be considered causes – even if of unequal potency or importance. Even if it were possible (which it is not) to measure the "number of points," any dividing line between "cause" and "precipitation" is always arbitrary.

Reflex epilepsy

To understand this term, it is important to account for its historical context. In Chapter 1, some aspects of the history of reflex theories of epilepsy are outlined. The original meaning and usage of the term, as espoused by Marshall Hall, Brown-Séquard, and Jackson, for instance, was physiological and they considered that many epilepsies had a "reflex" origin in the sense that there were "nervous reflexes" which affected brain excitation. The term reflex was used in relation to many "seizure precipitants." This concept was widely held, and notable contributions were the work of Muskens (1928), heavily influenced by Sherrington (who wrote the foreword to the English edition of his book), and then by Pavlov and others.

The Causes of Epilepsy, eds. S. D. Shorvon, F. Andermann, and R. Guerrini. Published by Cambridge University Press. © Cambridge University Press 2011.

However, in recent years, the original, rather mechanistic, meaning has been modified, and reflex epilepsy is now differentiated from less specific "seizure precipitants." The physiology remains largely obscure and what is clear is that mechanisms more complex than simple "reflexes" underpin the seizures, and in both cortical and many other types subcortical or brainstem structures are involved.

In current usage, the term refers to epilepsies in which there is an external trigger. Definition is difficult and it is interesting to note that in the monograph by Forster (1977) devoted to the topic, no definition is even attempted. Gastaut in 1989 defined reflex epilepsies as those in which all seizures, or a large part of them, are reliably provoked by naturally occurring or artificial stimulation of a certain receptor or group of receptors. For the purposes of this book, a working definition of reflex epilepsy might be: *an epilepsy in which seizures are reliably provoked by a specific identifiable environmental trigger.* This does not imply that such individuals can not also have seizures which occur spontaneously.

Currently, the reflex epilepsies are commonly subdivided into two categories:

(a) Simple reflex epilepsies – where the seizures are precipitated by simple sensory stimuli, e.g., flashing lights, startle, etc. Photosensitive epilepsy is by far the most common type and has been extensively studied (not least in recent times by Kasteleijn-Nolst Trenité and co-workers) (Zifkin and Kasteleijn-Nolst Trenité 2000; de Kovel *et al.* 2010), and stimulation parameters that are highly specific are sometimes found in these epilepsies (Wilkins *et al.* 2004).

(b) Complex reflex epilepsy – where the stimuli are more complex. Examples include musicogenic epilepsy, in which sometimes a highly specific piece of music triggers the seizure (as reported for instance in the classic paper of Critchley in 1937), seizures induced by thinking, reading, eating, spatial or other highly specific cognitive tasks, or hot-water epilepsy.

The epilepsies can be either focal or generalized, as for instance in some photosensitive and some reading epilepsies. This is a nosological gray area. Internal triggers, such as the effects of menstruation or fatigue, are not usually included in the category of provoked seizures (although they were in the nineteenth century). Some stimuli straddle both simple and complex categories, for instance reading or hot-water epilepsy. The line between etiology, common precipitants, and "reflex epilepsy" is not easy to draw, and to do so is to apply largely arbitrary criteria. A not uncommon situation in idiopathic generalized epilepsy is for seizures sometimes to be precipitated by visual stimuli, sometimes by lack of sleep, and sometimes to occur spontaneously. The mode of visual precipitation in such an individual is exactly the same as in a person who has reflex epilepsy, exclusively due to visual stimuli.

Acute symptomatic seizures

This is a rather unfortunate concept. It was first widely applied in 1970, in the landmark epidemiological work from Rochester, Minnesota. The term was devised to differentiate such seizures from "remote symptomatic" and "idiopathic" epilepsy (the latter term previously meaning "no cause found," and not in its current usage as suggesting a genetic cause). It then fell largely from fashion for obvious reasons, but recently the Epidemiology Commission of the International League Against Epilepsy (ILAE) convened a subgroup to reconsider the definition of acute symptomatic seizures for epidemiological studies. This group has defined an acute symptomatic seizure as "a clinical seizure occurring at the time of a systemic insult or in close temporal association with a documented brain insult" (Hauser *et al.* 2009). There are two main problems with the term used in this way.

The first problem is that of heterogeneity. The term includes two quite different phenomena – the "early seizures" related to an acute brain damage and also the seizures that result from a reversible provocation such as electrolyte disturbance or alcohol intoxication. In the opinion of the authors, it makes no sense to include both categories, which differ so much clinically, physiologically, and pathologically. The underlying premise is that there is something fundamentally different about these seizures and those of "genuine epilepsy." In some situations this is clearly the case. For instance, in seizures occurring immediately after a head injury ("early seizures"), the physiology is quite different from that in chronic post-traumatic epilepsy which may not occur until a period of months or years has passed during which time the progressive changes underpinning the post-traumatic seizures have developed ("late seizures"). In early seizures, the epilepsy may be caused by contusions, hemorrhage, metabolic change, endocrine change, hypotension, etc. – all mechanisms that have nothing in common with the late seizures in post-traumatic epilepsy. Similar considerations apply to the "early seizures" in stroke, infection, or neonatal hypoxic–ischemic brain injury for instance.

However, lumping together cases of "early seizures," with other cases where provoked seizures occur in acute brain injury without any obvious acute brain pathology is problematic. Seizures that are due to reversible environmental triggers such as metabolic change or fever (seizure precipitants as defined above) have no known physiological difference from those of patients with epilepsy who experience seizures provoked by the same cause (or indeed from individuals who do not have seizures when exposed to the same precipitant). In some cases, it has been shown for instance that a genetic predisposition is also demonstrable (e.g., in febrile seizures). In effect, these seizures are surely simply "provoked seizures" in patients with a predisposition to epilepsy, and reflect the interplay of the provoking factor and the individual "seizure threshold".

The second problem with the current usage is the extremely arbitrary nature of the criteria for inclusion, and indeed of the list of included conditions. Why, for instance, in the ILAE scheme is the period for categorizing a seizure as "acute symptomatic" within 1 week of trauma and stroke, but longer (not specified) for a subdural hematoma or infection? Why are parasitic infections included but congenital toxoplasmosis excluded? Alcohol withdrawal seizures are included but not alcohol-induced seizures. Why are not "reflex seizures" due to environmental triggers such as visual stimulation not included although seizures induced by hypoglycemia are included?

Furthermore, in some publications too the term has even been extended to include seizures which lead to the diagnosis of progressive conditions such as tumors (primary and secondary) which obviously makes no sense (Annegers et al. 1995).

In the metabolic conditions, arbitrary cut-off levels are cited for inclusion as "acute symptomatic epilepsy" despite the fact that there is individual variation in susceptibility ("seizure threshold"), that much depends on the homeostatic mechanisms and the context of the metabolic perturbation, and also that the rate of change of metabolic factors is probably as important as the extent of change itself.

It is for these reasons that the classification of epilepsy into remote symptomatic, acute symptomatic, and idiopathic seizures has now been largely abandoned. In the authors' opinion, if the term is to be retained, it should be restricted to the physiologically distinct "early seizures" after acute brain injury, which, mechanistically, are clearly completely different from any subsequent consequential chronic epilepsy.

Mechanisms of provoked epilepsies

The mechanism of seizure provocation has been the subject of study at least since the time of Marshall Hall and Jackson. Various theories have enjoyed periods of fashion, but to date none provides a comprehensive understanding of the processes involved. It is indeed clear that mechanisms differ, and the mechanisms of epileptogenesis are not likely to be the same in the epilepsies exacerbated by menstrual factors, the early seizures after severe acute brain insults, or the seizures provoked by photic stimulation. Most of the scientific work has focused for obvious reasons, on the seizures in reflex epilepsies, as these seizures can be reliably provoked and therefore studied in laboratory conditions and also because there are a number of suitable animal models. These are discussed in more detail in Chapter 96. Here a few points are made that place this section in context.

First, it is clear that genetic factors can play an important role, but these are usually complex. The phenomenon of photic-induced seizures, for instance, is heavily genetically determined, but even in very large kindreds, the identification of single causative genetic abnormalities has evaded detection (Fig. 88.1). Recent studies of hot-water epilepsy, another striking genetically determined human reflex epilepsy, have demonstrated linkage to different genes in families but no identifiable variant in any specific gene (Ratnapriya 2009a,b).

Experimental models, for instance, the photosensitive baboon Papio papio or the audiogenic DBA/2 mouse, have an equally unknown genetic basis. At an anecdotal level, families are encountered in whom other or additional provoking factors (such as stress or menstruation) are encountered in close relatives, suggesting that provocation generally may have a partial genetic basis, but no clear data exist on this point.

Second, it is also clear that non-genetic factors are also important. Examples are the startle-induced seizures which are not uncommon in prefrontal lesional epilepsies due to acquired or congenital causes, or the temporal lesions underpinning cases of eating epilepsy (Bakker et al. 2006). Partial seizures can be induced by sensory stimuli in patients with localized lesions in the precentral gyrus, as was clearly demonstrated by Jackson and Gowers, and more recently reviewed by Vignal and colleagues (1998).

Third is the question of the anatomical substrate of reflex seizures. There has been considerable interest in the past in the involvement of subcortical structures in the generation of reflex seizures (notably the involvement of brainstem and basal ganglia) and there is no doubt from the elegant work of Naquet and colleagues that such structures are involved in the sometimes extended circuitry which underpins some reflex seizures (see Naquet & Valin [1995] for a discussion of this work). However, most recent studies have focused on hyperexcitability of the cortex, as the fundamental mechanism of provoked seizures (Harding 2004). This can itself be localized, for instance in the occipital lobe in photic-induced seizures, or the temporal lobes in musicogenic seizures or in eating epilepsy, or in the central region in somatosensory-evoked seizures or in the prefrontal regions in startle-induced attacks (Ferlazzo et al. 2005). Eating epilepsy is a type of "reflex" epilepsy which can be seen in both idiopathic generalized epilepsy syndromes and also in focal epilepsies. Similarly photic-induced epilepsy is common in idiopathic generalized epilepsy syndromes, in progressive myoclonic epilepsy syndromes, and in congenital or acquired focal occipital lobe epilepsies (Guerrini & Genton 2004).

Fourth is the observation that provocation of seizures seems particularly common in the various sub-syndromes of idiopathic generalized epilepsy. This applies to reflex epilepsy syndromes as well as to the provocation by lack of sleep, menstrual effects, alcohol, and stress. These seizures are usually generalized even if the provocation only stimulates a localized region of the brain, for example photic-induced seizures. There is no need to evoke focal structural abnormalities and the evidence of any focal abnormality in the idiopathic syndromes is anyway extremely weak.

Finally, there is the issue of the neurochemical basis and specificity of therapy. It is clear that certain drugs have profound effects on some types of reflex epilepsy. The remarkable suppression of photosensitivity by valproate or levetiracetam and the absence of any effect by carbamazepine is an example. Similarly, GABAergic drugs seem particularly effective in the

A

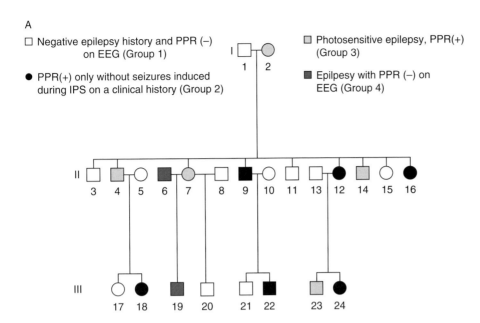

☐ Negative epilepsy history and PPR (–) on EEG (Group 1)

● PPR(+) only without seizures induced during IPS on a clinical history (Group 2)

☐ Photosensitive epilepsy, PPR(+) (Group 3)

■ Epilpesy with PPR (–) on EEG (Group 4)

Fig. 88.1. (A) Family tree of large family with photosensitive epilepsy. (B) Haplotype analysis of chromosome 1 showing lack of linkage (From Lo 2010.)

B

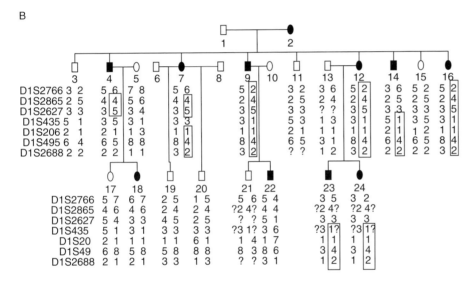

photosensitive baboon *Papio papio* and the audiogenic mouse models. In other types, particularly in focal lesional epilepsy, provoked seizures respond well to a wider range of drugs, and in particular to carbamazepine.

It is clear from the above that seizure provocation may occur in genetic and acquired epilepsy, in focal or generalized epilepsy, have multiple anatomical and neurochemical bases and does not map easily across conventional seizure type or syndromic classifications. This is partly the reason for considering these syndromes separately in the etiologically based classification outlined in Chapter 2 and for devoting a separate section to these epilepsies in this book.

References

Annegers JF, Hauser WA, Lee JR, Rocca WA (1995) Incidence of acute symptomatic seizures in Rochester, Minnesota, 1935–1984. *Epilepsia* **36**:327–33.

Amantea F (1921) Über experimentelle beim Versuchstier infolge afferenter Reize erzeugte Epilepsie. *Arch Ges Physiol Berl* **188**:287–97.

Aird RB (1983) The importance of seizure-inducing factors in the control of refractory forms of epilepsy. *Epilepsia* **24**:567–83.

Bakker MJ, van Dijk JG, van den Maagdenberg AM, Tijssen MA Startle syndromes. *Lancet Neurol* 5:513–24.

Beaumanoir A (1995) History of reflex epilepsy. In: Zifkin B, Andermann F, Beaumanoir A, Rowan J (eds.) *Reflex Epilepsies and Reflex Seizures*. Philadelphia, PA: Lippincott-Raven, pp. 1–4.

Clementi A (1929) Stricninizzasione della sfera corticale visiva ed epilessia sperimentale da stimuli luminosi. *Arch Fisiol* **27**:356–87.

Critchley M (1937) Musicogenic epilepsy. *Brain* **60**:13–27.

de Kovel CG, Pinto D, Tauer U, *et al.* (2010) Whole-genome linkage scan for epilepsy-related photosensitivity: a mega-analysis. *Epilepsy Res* **89**:286–94.

Ferlazzo E, Zifkin BG, Andermann E, Andermann F (2005) Cortical triggers in generalized reflex seizures and epilepsies. *Brain* **128**:700–10.

Forster FM (1977) *Reflex Epilepsy, Behavioral Therapy, and Conditional Reflexes.* Springfield, IL: Charles C. Thomas.

Gastaut H (1989) Synopsis and conclusions of the International Colloquium on Reflex Seizures and Epilepsies, Geneva, 1988. In: Beaumanoir A, Gastaut H, Naquet R (eds.) *Reflex Seizures and Reflex Epilepsies.* Geneva: Editions Médecine et Hygiène, pp. 497–507.

Gowers WR (1885) *Epilepsy and Other Chronic Convulsive Disorders: Their Causes, Symptoms and Treatment.* London: Churchill.

Guerrini R, Genton P (2004) Epileptic syndromes and visually induced seizures. *Epilepsia* **45**(Suppl 1):14–18.

Hall M (1850) *Synopsis of the Distaltic Nervous System.* London: Joseph Mallet.

Harding G (2004) The reflex epilepsies with emphasis on photosensitive epilepsy. *Clin Neurophysiol* **57**(Suppl):433–8.

Hauser W, Beghi E, Carpio A, *et al.* (2009) Recommendation for a definition of Acute Symptomatic Seizure. *Epilepsia* **51**:671–5.

Lo C (2010) Genetics in epilepsy. Ph.D. thesis, University College London.

Morgan CT, Morgan JD (1939) Auditory induction of an abnormal pattern of behavior in rats. *J Comp Physiol* **27**:505–8.

Muskens LJJ (1928) *Epilepsy: Comparative Pathogenesis, Symptoms and Treatment.* London: Bailliere, Tindall and Cox.

Naquet RG, Valin A (1995) Experimental models of reflex epilepsy. In: Zifkin B, Andermann F, Beaumanoir A, Rowan J (eds.) *Reflex Epilepsies and Reflex Seizures.* Philadelphia, PA: Lippincott-Raven, pp. 15–28.

Ratnapriya R, Satishchandra P, Kumar SD, *et al.* (2009a) A locus for autosomal dominant reflex epilepsy precipitated by hot water maps at chromosome 10q21.3–q22.3. *Hum Genet* **125**:541–9.

Ratnapriya R, Satishchandra P, Dilip S, Gadre G, Anand A (2009b) Familial autosomal dominant reflex epilepsy triggered by hot water maps to 4q24–q28. *Hum Genet* **126**:677–83.

Spratling W (1904) *Epilepsy and Its Treatment.* Philadelphia, PA: WB Saunders.

Tissot SA (1770) *Traité de l'épilepsie. Faisant le tome troisième du traité des nerfs et de leurs maladies.* Lausanne: Antoine Chapuis.

Vignal JP, Biraben A, Chauvel PY, Reutens DC (1998) Reflex partial seizures of sensorimotor cortex (including cortical reflex myoclonus and startle epilepsy). *Adv Neurol* **75**:207–26.

Wilkins AJ, Bonanni P, Porciatti V, Guerrini R (2004) Physiology of human photosensitivity. *Epilepsia* **45**(Suppl 1):7–13.

Zifkin BG, Kasteleijn-Nolst Trenité D (2000) Reflex epilepsy and reflex seizures of the visual system: a clinical review. *Epilept Disord* **2**:129–36.

Chapter

Fever

89

Thomas P. Bleck

Fever and seizures

Fever was described as a manifestation of disease in extant medical texts dating back to the sixth century BC. The authors of these works often incorporated fever into their theoretic frameworks of medicine; some, such as Hippocrates, came to understand fever as a defense mechanism against some forms of disease. Measuring body temperature came much later, and was firmly established in 1868 by Wunderlich. He demonstrated that body temperature varied throughout the day, and that there is a normal range in the general population of healthy people (Mackowiak 2010). Recent studies suggest that the majority of oral temperatures in normal subjects spans a range from 36 to 38 °C (97 to 100.4 °F). However, the study of clinical temperature abnormalities should be based on rectal temperature or other estimates of core temperature, such as blood, bladder, or esophageal temperature. These estimates are approximately 0.5 °C (1°F) higher than oral temperatures.

The balance between heat generation and heat clearance is controlled by the hypothalamus; despite substantial study, the precise nuclei involved in temperature sensing and regulation remain debated. Blood temperature in the hypothalamus is the major afferent signal, but other inputs modulate this, including skin temperature on the cheeks and hands; warming these areas helps to prevent shivering during therapeutic attempts to lower temperature. The integration of these thermal inputs produces an estimate of core temperature. Hypothalamic nuclei provide a setpoint against which the sensed core temperature is compared, and they mediate thermoregulatory behaviors. The setpoint can be altered by a variety of stimuli; most research has focused on circulating pyrogens, such as tumor necrosis factor α and various interleukins. Antipyretic drugs, such as non-steroidal anti-inflammatory agents, work in part by lowering the setpoint.

A core temperature below the setpoint prompts behaviors that generate heat (e.g., shivering), seek warmth (e.g., moving to a warmer location), and conserve heat (e.g., putting on warmer clothes). The autonomic nervous system causes cutaneous vasoconstriction (to limit heat loss to the environment). When the core temperature exceeds the setpoint, the opposite behaviors and autonomic effects occur; in addition, sweating leads to heat loss by evaporation.

Exposure to excessively hot environments may exceed the ability of the organism to keep the core temperature within the normal range. Moderate increases in core temperature may result in volume depletion because of excessive sweating. When the core temperature reaches about 40 °C (104 °F) because of high environmental temperature, otherwise healthy humans may develop heatstroke. In this condition, the mechanisms promoting heat loss and behaviors intended to decrease heat exposure fail. Convulsions are among the neurologic manifestations of heatstroke; however, epilepsy does not appear to be a sequel of this disorder. Central stimulant intoxication, caused by abuse of substances such as cocaine and the numerous congeners of amphetamine, can produce a phenomenologically similar condition (Devlin and Henry 2008). Other drug-related conditions, such as neuroleptic malignant syndrome, serotonin syndrome, and malignant hyperthermia, can produce life-threatening elevations of core temperature, but do not appear to be antecedents of epilepsy.

The mechanisms by which hyperthermia itself produces seizures remain uncertain. Increasing temperature in general increases ion traffic through channels, and may therefore move neuronal membrane potentials closer to their firing threshold. A specific effect on Na(V)1.2 sodium channels in the initial segment appears very likely, however, and may eventually yield a target for a trial of preventive therapy (Thomas *et al.* 2009). Changes in firing rates with increasing temperature are easily observable in individual neurons in slices or cultures, but its effects on networks of excitatory and inhibitory systems are less predictable. Excitatory amino acid systems are probably the most affected (Morimoto *et al.* 1995). In some experimental systems, hyperthermia appears to have profound effects on inhibitory transmitters, shifting the balance of these systems in favor of seizures

The Causes of Epilepsy, eds. S. D. Shorvon, F. Andermann, and R. Guerrini. Published by Cambridge University Press. © Cambridge University Press 2011.

(González-Ramírez *et al.* 2005). Some of the positive and negative cytokine mediators of fever also have direct effects on neuronal excitability (Bartfai *et al.* 2007). Hyperthermia may interfere with the production of proteins that protect neurons from injury, such as members of the heat shock protein series (Krueger *et al.* 1999).

Fever commonly produces tachypnea out of proportion to the increase in metabolic acid production associated with illness, resulting in a respiratory alkalosis that may be profound. This respiratory alkalosis is itself epileptogenic in experimental models, especially in immature animals (Morimoto *et al.* 1996). The relative contribution of other metabolic disorders that may accompany febrile illness, such as hypoosmolality, is uncertain.

The relationship of these physiologic aspects of fever to the genesis of febrile seizures in humans is uncertain. In animal models that produce prolonged seizures in the setting of fever, about a third of the surviving animals develop epilepsy characterized by complex partial seizures that occur without fever (Dubé *et al.* 2009). Although clinicians have long harbored the suspicion that prolonged febrile seizures are somehow related to the development of mesial temporal sclerosis with subsequent intractable epilepsy, this relationship remains unclear pending the analysis of the long-term follow-up of patients in a prospective study of prolonged febrile seizures (Shinnar *et al.* 2008).

The excessive motor activity of generalized convulsions, especially generalized convulsive status epilepticus (GCSE), can raise core temperature. The near ubiquity of fever in patients during GCSE often leads to the conclusion that an infection, such as meningitis or encephalitis, is present. Epidemiologic considerations are important; for example, cerebral malaria is an important differential diagnostic consideration when patients are, or have been, in areas endemic for this condition. While these conditions are important in the differential diagnosis, the presence of fever must not dissuade the clinician from searching for other non-infectious etiologies. In GCSE, the core temperature may rise above 40 °C (104 °F), causing additive neuronal damage to that already caused by the epileptic status. Non-convulsive status epilepticus (NCSE) can also cause an increase in core temperature, presumably by alteration of the hypothalamic setpoint. Rare cases of NCSE in which fever occurs without any notable motor activity have been reported (Semel 1987).

Further complicating the differential diagnosis of fever and seizures is the increasing recognition of non-infectious encephalitides as causes of seizures or status. Autoimmune and paraneoplastic conditions need to be considered, especially in patients with focal areas of fluid-attenuated inversion recovery (FLAIR)/T2 increase on magnetic resonance imaging (Bleck 2010). When these abnormalities occur in the mesial temporal regions in a febrile patient, herpes simplex encephalitis is an important consideration, and treatment with acyclovir is reasonable until the result of a polymerase chain reaction test for herpes simplex DNA is available.

The dehydration associated with febrile illnesses may also lead to cerebral venous thromboses, either septic or due to increased viscosity or a hypercoagulable state. These patients often present with seizures in addition to other manifestations of venous obstruction, frequently in the setting of hemorrhagic venous infarctions. A high index of suspicion is necessary for this diagnostic possibility, which is typically investigated with magnetic resonance venography.

Hemorrhagic cerebrovascular disorders, especially aneurysmal subarachnoid hemorrhage, are sometimes associated with convulsions, especially at the time of presentation. These patients frequently develop fever during their course, although infectious causes must always be sought. Many of these patients have fever without evidence of infection and are thus considered to have "central fever." A growing number of reports document the development of subclinical seizures in patients with either subarachnoid or intracerebral hemorrhage; these seizures are associated with worse neuropsychological outcomes among survivors, and with more cerebral edema in those with parenchymal hematomata (Vespa *et al.* 2003). While fever and the non-convulsive seizures are often coincident, the relationship, if any, between them remains to be elucidated. Modern neurocritical care practice usually involves strict temperature control for these patients, attempting to enforce normothermia. However, the influence of this practice on the incidence of seizures remains to be determined.

Fever may also be a consequence of seizures, rather than an antecedent (Rossetti *et al.* 2007). This complicates the analysis of the relationship between them, especially when febrile seizures are suspected, since the seizure frequently serves as the first stimulus to check the patient's temperature.

Central stimulant intoxication produces both seizures and hyperthermia. The total pathologic brain effects of the seizures and the temperature elevation are probably more than additive (Tor-Agbidye *et al.* 2001), and argue for therapies that rapidly control both seizures and fever.

Epilepsies related to fever

Ancient physicians described a connection between fever and disease, but prior to the nineteenth century seizures brought on by fever were thought to be manifestations of the various etiologies of fever (e.g., infections) in children rather than a potential consequence of the rise in core temperature. The concept of febrile seizures as a benign entity emerged in the early years of the twentieth century. Although the usage is incorrect, any seizure occurring in proximity to a fever (measured or inferred) is often mislabeled a febrile seizure. For both clinical and epidemiologic reasons, the clinician should distinguish true febrile seizures from other seizure types that may be triggered by fever, followed by fever, or share a common etiology with the fever.

A febrile seizure is currently defined by a consensus panel of the National Institutes of Health as "an event in infancy or early childhood, usually occurring between three months and five years of age, associated with fever but without evidence of intracranial infection or defined cause. Seizures with fever in children who have suffered a previous nonfebrile seizure are excluded." (Nelson and Ellenberg 1981) Febrile seizures are divided into simple and complex types. Simple febrile seizures are apparently generalized seizures lasting less than 15 min; complex febrile seizures, in contrast, involve one or more of the following characteristics: longer duration, partial (focal) features, or recurrance within 24 hr (Camfield *et al.* 2008). Febrile status epilepticus (FSE) is defined by duration exceeding 30 min. In a recent epidemiologic study, the median age of patients with FSE was 1.3 years, the mean peak temperature 39.5 °C (103.2 °F), and the median duration of seizure activity 68 min (Shinnar *et al.* 2008).

Between 2% and 5% of children experience at least one febrile seizure. That seizure is complex in up to a third of cases, which raises concern for the subsequent development of mesial temporal sclerosis and later epilepsy. Almost half the children experiencing a febrile seizure will have at least one more. The likelihood of recurrence is greater in children with a family history of febrile seizures. The genetics of febrile seizures are poorly understood, but there is a two- to fourfold increase in their likelihood when a relative is affected.

When a child's first seizure is accompanied by a fever, the question of a central nervous system (CNS) infection is paramount. The factors involved in deciding whether a lumbar puncture is necessary are beyond the scope of this chapter. Similarly, decisions regarding the need for neurodiagnostic studies require a careful history and physical examination. The American Academy of Pediatrics (1996) has provided some guidance.

The rate of core temperature rise is often said to correspond to the likelihood that a febrile seizure will occur; the same is also conjectured for other types of seizures that may occur in the setting of fever. However, there is little evidence to illuminate these contentions in either direction. Since the seizure is frequently the event that leads parents to measure the child's temperature, actual knowledge of the fever pattern is rare.

Information linking particular organisms to febrile seizures is sparse with the exception of human herpesvirus 6 (HHV-6) infection (Barone *et al.* 1995). When the onset of fever is followed by a typical rash (with or without seizures), this infection is termed roseola, but the rash may not appear or may be evanescent. Since the fever of roseola tends to rise abruptly to a relatively high value in children who were not previously ill, this may help to explain the above noted association with the rate of rise. However, the discovery of HHV-6 DNA in the cerebrospinal fluid of several children with otherwise typical febrile seizures argues for an actual CNS infection in these cases.

The clinician must distinguish febrile seizures from other types of seizures that may be triggered by fever. There are some epilepsies for which febrile exacerbation is characteristic, such as generalized epilepsy with febrile seizures plus, and severe myoclonic epilepsy of infancy (Dravet syndrome).

However, as may be surmised from the pathophysiologic discussion in the preceding section, either fever itself or the accompanying respiratory alkalosis may trigger seizures in patients with many types of epilepsy.

Principles of management

Febrile seizures

Aside from physical measures to prevent harm and decrease the risk of aspiration, simple febrile seizures themselves are self-limited events that do not require therapy. A search for a precipitating infection may reveal a condition that requires treatment. Most parents will already have begun antipyretic therapy and simple external cooling measures, although their efficacy is unknown.

The duration of complex febrile seizures that might mandate abortive therapy to prevent the development of status epilepticus is unknown. In a broad population of children, including some with febrile seizures, seizures that had already lasted for 12 min were unlikely to terminate spontaneously (Shinnar *et al.* 2001), suggesting that this is a reasonable time at which to intervene; typically this involves administration of a benzodiazepine, although this has not been specifically studied in the population of patients with febrile seizures.

There does not appear to be an advantage to chronic administration of anticonvulsant drugs in these children.

Conventional methods of fever management

Time-honored means of fever control, including antipyretic drugs and the application of cool damp clothes to exposed areas of skin, are frequently used in an attempt to lower core temperature in a patient with seizures. Whether they have any effect on the likelihood of immediate seizure recurrence in children with febrile seizures is unknown.

Lowering the temperature of patients who are markedly febrile in the setting of status epilepticus involves termination of seizure activity as well as external cooling and treatment of any underlying condition producing fever, such as infection. High doses of anticonvulsant drugs typically result in poikilothermia. Neuromuscular junction (NMJ) blockade is rarely needed beyond a brief period to facilitate endotracheal intubation, but could be considered when seizures are difficult to control and the core temperature remains high. However, NMJ blockade is not a substitute for aggressive anticonvulsant administration, including general anesthetic agents if needed, in convulsive status patients regardless of core temperature.

Newer methods of therapeutic temperature regulation

Recognition of the deleterious effects of elevated temperature in acute neurologic diseases such as acute stroke and coma after cardiac arrest led to the development of a variety of therapeutic devices for the control of core temperature.

A variety of external devices that rely upon facilitated transfer of heat from the skin to cooling pads are now available. These devices include a connection for an indwelling thermometer, either bladder or rectal, in order to create a feedback loop to keep the core temperature within a narrow desired range (typically 33 °C for neurologic applications).

Intravascular closed-loop cooling systems are also available. They provide more rapid cooling and better control of core temperature, but require placement of cooling catheters in central veins (Diringer 2004). The fastest way to achieve target temperature is by the rapid infusion of chilled saline or saline slurry (Vanden Hoek *et al.* 2004).

Hypothermia for refractory status epilepticus

Induced hypothermia is gaining attention as a potential therapy for refractory status epilepticus. Diringer and colleagues reported on four patients in whom reducing core temperature to 31–35 °C resulted in marked diminution or elimination of seizures when more conventional anticonvulsant therapy had failed (Corry *et al.* 2008). Lowering temperature appeared to suppress seizures only symptomatically, however, as they recurred when the patients were allowed to rewarm. Nonetheless, this treatment might allow the clinician time for another therapeutic approach to work.

References

American Academy of Pediatrics (1996) Provisional Committee on Quality Improvement, Subcommittee on Febrile Seizure. Practice parameter: the neurodiagnostic evaluation of the child with a first simple febrile seizure. *Pediatrics* **97**:769–72.

Barone SR, Kaplan MH, Krilov LR (1995) Human herpesvirus-6 infection in children with first febrile seizures. *J Pediatr* **127**:95–7.

Bartfai T, Sanchez-Alavez M, Andell-Jonsson S, *et al.* (2007) Interleukin-1 system in CNS stress: seizures, fever, and neurotrauma. *Ann N Y Acad Sci* **1113**:173–7.

Bleck TP (2010) Less common etiologies of status epilepticus. *Epilepsy Curr* **10**:31–3.

Camfield CS, Camfield PR, Neville BG (2008) Febrile seizures. In: Engel JE, Pedley T (eds.) *Epilepsy: A Comprehensive Textbook*, 2nd edn. Philadelphia, PA: pp. 659–64.

Corry JJ, Dhar R, Murphy T, Diringer MN (2008) Hypothermia for refractory status epilepticus. *Neurocrit Care* **9**:189–97.

Devlin RJ, Henry JA (2008) Clinical review: Major consequences of illicit drug consumption. *Crit Care* **12**:202 (http://ccforum.com/content/12/1/202).

Diringer MN (2004) Neurocritical Care Fever Reduction Trial Group. Treatment of fever in the neurologic intensive care unit with a catheter-based heat exchange system. *Crit Care Med* **32**:559–64.

Dubé CM, Brewster AL, Baram TZ (2009) Febrile seizures: mechanisms and relationship to epilepsy. *Brain Dev* **31**:366–71.

González-Ramírez M, Orozco S, Salgado H, Feria A, Rocha L (2005) Hyperthermia-induced seizures modify the $GABA_A$ and benzodiazepine receptor binding in immature rat brain. *Cell Mol Neurobiol* **25**:955–71.

Kondo K, Nagafuji H, Hata A, Tomomori C, Yamanishi K (1993) Association of human herpesvirus 6 infection of the central nervous system with recurrence of febrile convulsions. *J Infect Dis* **167**:1197–200.

Krueger AM, Armstrong JN, Plumier J, Robertson HA, Currie RW (1999) Cell specific expression of Hsp70 in neurons and glia of the rat hippocampus after hyperthermia and kainic acid-induced seizure activity. *Brain Res Mol Brain Res* **71**:265–78.

Mackowiak PA (2010) Temperature regulation and the pathogenesis of fever. In: Mandell GM, Bennett JE, Dolin R (eds.) *Principles and Practice of Infectious Diseases*, 7th edn. New York: Churchill, Livingstone, pp. 765–78.

Morimoto T, Kida K, Nagao H, *et al.* (1995) The pathogenic role of the NMDA receptor in hyperthermia-induced seizures in developing rats. *Brain Res Dev Brain Res* **84**:204–7.

Morimoto T, Fukuda M, Aibara Y, Nagao H, Kida K (1996) The influence of blood gas changes on hyperthermia-induced seizures in developing rats. *Brain Res Dev Brain Res* **92**:77–80.

Nelson KB, Ellenberg JH (eds.) *Febrile Seizures*. New York: Raven Press.

Rossetti AO, Tosi C, Despland PA, Staedler C (2007) Post-ictal fever: a rare symptom of partial seizures. *Eur J Neurol* **14**:586–90.

Semel JD (1987) Complex partial status epilepticus presenting as fever of unknown origin. *Arch Intern Med* **147**:1571–2.

Shinnar S, Berg AT, Moshe SL, Shinnar R (2001) How long do new-onset seizures in children last? *Ann Neurol* **49**:659–64.

Shinnar S, Hesdorffer DC, Nordli DR Jr., *et al.* (2008) Phenomenology of prolonged febrile seizures: results of the FEBSTAT study. *Neurology* **71**:170–6.

Thomas EA, Hawkins RJ, Richards KL, *et al.* (2009) Heat opens axon initial segment sodium channels: a febrile seizure mechanism? *Ann Neurol* **66**:219–26.

Tor-Agbidye J, Yamamoto B, Bowyer JF (2001) Seizure activity and hyperthermia potentiate the increases in dopamine and serotonin extracellular levels in the amygdala during exposure to d-amphetamine. *Toxicol Sci* **60**:103–11.

Vanden Hoek TL, Kasza KE, Beiser DG, *et al.* (2004) Induced hypothermia by central venous infusion: saline ice slurry versus chilled saline. *Crit Care Med* **32**(9 Suppl):S425–31.

Vespa PM, O'Phelan K, Shah M, *et al.* (2003) Acute seizures after intracerebral hemorrhage: a factor in progressive midline shift and outcome. *Neurology* **60**:1441–6.

Chapter

90

The menstrual cycle and catamenial epilepsy

Andrew G. Herzog

Definition, patterns, and prevalence of catamenial epilepsy

Seizures do not occur randomly in the majority of men and women with epilepsy (Tauboll *et al.* 1991). They tend to cluster in over 50% of cases (Tauboll *et al.* 1991; Fowler *et al.* 2006). The clusters, in turn, may occur with temporal rhythmicity in a significant proportion of men (29%) and women (35%) with epilepsy (Almqvist 1955). When the periodicity of seizure exacerbation aligns with the menstrual cycle, it is commonly known as catamenial epilepsy (Herzog *et al.* 1997). The concept of catamenial epilepsy is strengthened by the finding that the periodicities of seizure occurrence vary with the ovulatory status of the menstrual cycle (Tauboll *et al.* 1991; Quigg *et al.* 2008) and that catamenial epilepsy may be significantly more common with a left-sided unilateral temporal epileptic electroencephalogram (EEG) focus as compared to a right-sided temporal focus (Kalinin and Zheleznova 2007; Quigg *et al.* 2009). Catamenial seizure exacerbation may be attributable to (1) the neuroactive properties of steroid hormones and (2) the cyclic variation in their serum levels (Herzog *et al.* 1997).

Physiological endocrine secretion during the menstrual cycle influences the occurrence of seizures (Fig. 90.1). In ovulatory cycles, seizure frequency shows a statistically significant positive correlation with the serum estradiol/progesterone ratio (Backstrom 1976). This ratio is highest during the days prior to ovulation and menstruation and is lowest during the early and mid-luteal phase (Backstrom 1976). The premenstrual exacerbation of seizures has been attributed to the rapid withdrawal of the antiseizure effects of progesterone (Backstrom 1976; Herzog *et al.* 1997). Mid-cycle exacerbations may be due to the preovulatory surge of estrogen, unaccompanied by any rise in progesterone until ovulation occurs (Laidlaw 1956; Backstrom 1976; Herzog *et al.* 1997). Seizures are least common during the mid-luteal phase when progesterone levels are highest (Laidlaw 1956; Backstrom 1976; Herzog *et al.* 1997) except in

anovulatory cycles in which the mid-cycle surge in estrogen still occurs, albeit not as high as in ovulatory cycles, but unaccompanied by any substantial increase in progesterone levels (Herzog *et al.* 1997).

Herzog *et al.* (1997, 2004) have presented statistical evidence in prospective investigations to support the concept of catamenial epilepsy and the existence of at least three distinct patterns of seizure exacerbation in relation to the menstrual cycle (Fig. 90.1): (1) perimenstrual (C1: Day −3 to 3) and (2) periovulatory (C2: Day 10 to −13) in normal cycles, and (3) luteal (C3: Day 10 to 3) in inadequate luteal phase cycles. In these cycles, Day 1 is the first day of menstrual flow and ovulation is presumed to occur 14 days before the subsequent onset of menses (Day −14). These three patterns can be demonstrated simply by (1) charting menses and seizures and (2) obtaining a mid-luteal phase serum progesterone level to distinguish between normal and inadequate luteal phase cycles (<5 ng/mL).

While the precise definition of catamenial epilepsy remains arbitrary, one may maximize the efficiency of distinguishing between women whose seizure occurrence shows a high versus low degree of hormonal sensitivity by using the points of inflection of the S-shaped distribution curves that define the relationship between the severity of seizure exacerbation and the number of women who have exacerbation (Herzog *et al.* 1997, 2004) (Fig. 90.2). These points are calculated to be between 1.5 to twofold increase in average daily seizure frequency during the phases of exacerbation relative to the baseline phases for all three types of catamenial exacerbation. We propose the use of these points of inflection values in seizure frequency for the designation of catamenial epilepsy. By this criterion, approximately one-third of women with intractable partial epilepsy would qualify for the designation of having catamenial epilepsy (Herzog *et al.* 1997, 2004). Adoption of a standard albeit arbitrary nomenclature may provide greater uniformity to study designs for the investigation of the pathogenesis and treatment of catamenial seizure exacerbation.

The Causes of Epilepsy, eds. S. D. Shorvon, F. Andermann, and R. Guerrini. Published by Cambridge University Press. © Cambridge University Press 2011.

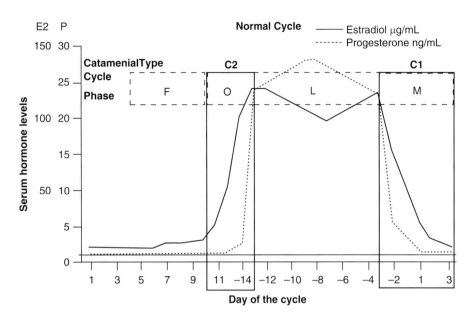

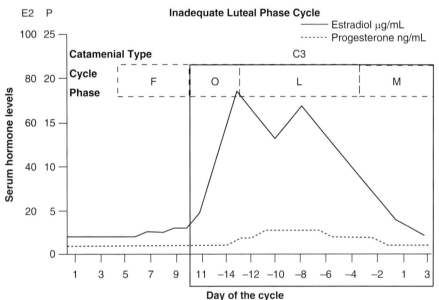

Fig. 90.1. Three patterns of catamenial epilepsy: perimenstrual (C1) and periovulatory (C2) exacerbations during normal ovulatory cycles and entire second half of the cycle (C3) exacerbation during inadequate luteal phase cycles where Day 1 is the first day of menstrual flow and Day-14 is the day of ovulation.

Pathophysiology

Neuroactive properties of reproductive steroids

The steroid hormones estradiol and progesterone do not only regulate the reproductive system but also modulate the excitability of the central and peripheral nervous systems. Catamenial epilepsy, the cyclic exacerbation of seizures in relation to the menstrual cycle, may represent the net effect of cyclically varying concentrations of neuroexcitatory and neuroinhibitory reproductive steroids on a hormonally sensitive epileptic substrate. There is considerable scientific evidence at molecular biological, neuronal, experimental animal, and clinical levels to indicate that reproductive steroids have neuroactive properties that play an important role in the pathophysiology of epilepsy

and the pattern of seizure occurrence. Steroids act in the brain by direct membrane-mediated (short latency) effects as well as receptor-mediated genomically mediated (long latency) effects (Paul and Purdy 1992; McEwen 1994). Additionally, there is considerable evidence to suggest that certain epileptic brain substrates such as the amygdala and the cerebral cortex (Marcus 1966) show exquisitely sensitive short latency electrophysiological responses to the systemic or topical application of neuroactive steroids. While acknowledging that hormones have very complex effects that vary with their isomers (e.g., α and β estradiol), concentrations and receptor subunits, as well as with their durations and sites of action, this chapter will present a model in which estradiol generally has neuroexcitatory and proconvulsant effects whereas progesterone has

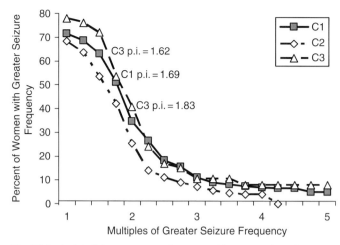

Fig. 90.2. A plot of the percentage of women with greater seizure frequency during phases of seizure exacerbation in each of the three patterns of catamenial epilepsy (C1, C2, and C3) versus multiples of greater seizure frequency yielded three descending S-shaped curves. Points of inflection (p.i.) were calculated for optimal distinction between women with high and low susceptibility to menstrual cycle and, presumably, hormonal influences on seizure occurrence and for the designation of catamenial epilepsy.

reduced metabolites with potent neuroinhibitory and anticonvulsant effects, a model that appears to be most consistent with clinical observations.

Estradiol

Estradiol exerts direct excitatory effects at the neuronal membrane, where it augments N-methyl-D-aspartate (NMDA)-mediated glutamate receptor activity (Smith 1989; Wong and Moss 1992). This enhances the resting discharge rates of neurons in a number of brain areas, including the hippocampus (Smith 1989; Wong and Moss 1992) where estradiol increases excitability of the hippocampal CA1 pyramidal neurons and induces repetitive firing in response to Schaffer collateral stimulation (Wong and Moss, 1992).

Estradiol also affects inhibitory neurotransmission. Estradiol receptors are found in inhibitory γ-aminobutyric acid (GABA) ergic interneurons. In a rodent model, estradiol transiently decreases inhibitory GABA boutons and synapses, at 24–48 hr, and then, by 72 hr, restores the number of GABA synapses and inhibitory tone in rats (Rudick and Woolley 2001). The resulting combined increase in excitatory synapses and restoration of inhibitory synapses leads to a wider dynamic range of neuronal responses and may contribute to the synchrony of firing that is important to the occurrence of seizures.

Estradiol also modulates neuronal excitability by regulating neuronal development and plasticity. Estradiol receptors colocalize with brain-derived neurotrophic factor (BDNF) and can increase BDNF gene expression in the hippocampus and cerebral cortex (Allen and McCarson 2005). BDNF has proconvulsant properties that may promote seizure occurrence (Scharfman *et al.* 2003). Estradiol increases the density of spines and excitatory, NMDA-receptor-containing synapses

on the spines of apical dendrites of hippocampal CA1 pyramidal neurons via a post-transcriptional mechanism (Woolley and McEwen 1994). The dendritic spine density on these neurons correlates positively with the levels of circulating estradiol during the estrous cycle of the rat and is decreased by oophorectomy (Woolley and McEwen 1994). Estradiol may thus further increase excitatory input to the CA1 neurons.

Estradiol may affect neuronal excitability by cytosolic neuronal estrogen receptor-mediated, genomically dependent mechanisms. Receptors are particularly abundant in the temporolimbic system, especially in the medial and cortical amygdaloid nuclei, and occur in much fewer numbers in the hippocampal pyramidal cell layer and the subiculum (Pfaff and Keiner 1973). Estrogen receptor-containing neurons colocalize with other neurotransmitters, including GABA (Finn and Gee 1993). By regulating the expression of genes affecting the activity, release and postsynaptic action of different neurotransmitters and neuromodulators, estrogens may act to increase the excitability of neurons, which concentrate estradiol. For instance, estradiol lessens inhibitory neurotransmission by decreasing GABA synthesis in the corticomedial amygdala by reducing the activity of glutamic acid decarboxylase (Wallis and Luttge 1980), and enhances brain epileptogenic muscarinic neurotransmission by increasing choline acetyl transferase and acetylcholine (Luine *et al.* 1986).

In adult experimental animals, the thresholds of limbic seizures in female rats fluctuate during the estrus cycle inversely to estradiol levels (Rudick and Woolley 2001). Physiological doses of estradiol activate spike discharges (Logothetis and Harner 1960; Marcus *et al.* 1966; Wong and Moss 1992) and lower the thresholds of seizures induced by electroshock, kindling, pentylenetetrazol, kainic acid, ethyl chloride, and other agents and procedures (Logothetis and Harner 1960; Marcus *et al.* 1966; Nicoletti *et al.* 1985). The topical brain application, as well as intravenous systemic administration, of estradiol in rabbits produces a significant increase in spontaneous electrically recorded paroxysmal spike discharges (Marcus *et al.* 1966). The increase is seen within a few seconds of application to suggest a direct membrane rather than a genomic effect and is more dramatic in animals with pre-existent cortical lesions (Logothetis and Harner 1960; Marcus *et al.* 1966). The role of estrogen, however, may be more complex since there is also evidence in some models that estradiol can raise seizure thresholds in the hippocampal region and provide neuroprotection against seizure-induced injury (Veliskova *et al.* 2000).

Clinically, Logothetis *et al.* (1959) showed that intravenously administered conjugated estrogen clearly activated epileptiform discharges in 11 of 16 women and was associated with clinical seizures in four.

Progesterone

Progesterone has reduced neuroactive metabolites, most notably tetrahydroprogesterone (allopregnanolone, AP) that exert direct membrane-mediated inhibitory effects by potentiating $GABA_A$-mediated chloride conductance (Majewska et al. 1986; Paul and Purdy 1992; Gee et al. 1995). At physiological (nanogram) concentrations, AP acts allosterically at an extrasynaptic site to facilitate $GABA_A$-mediated chloride channel opening and prolong the inhibitory action of GABA on neurons (Majewska et al. 1986; Paul and Purdy 1992; Gee et al. 1995; Maguire et al. 2005). At higher pharmacological (micromolar) concentrations, AP also has a direct action at the synaptic $GABA_A$ receptor to induce chloride currents (Paul and Purdy 1992; Gee et al. 1995). AP is one of the most potent ligands of $GABA_A$ receptors in the central nervous system, with affinities similar to those of the potent benzodiazepine, flunitrazepam, and approximately a thousand times higher than pentobarbital (Paul and Purdy 1992; Gee et al. 1995). The parent steroid, progesterone, enhances GABA-induced chloride currents only weakly and only in high concentrations (Paul and Purdy 1992). Plasma and brain levels of AP parallel those of progesterone in rats. In women, plasma levels of AP correlate with progesterone levels during the menstrual cycle and pregnancy (Paul and Purdy 1992). However, brain activity of progesterone and AP is not dependent solely on ovarian and adrenal production, as they are both synthesized de novo in the brain (Cheney et al. 1995). Their synthesis is region-specific and includes the cortex and the hippocampus (Cheney et al. 1995).

Allopregnanolone and a number of other endogenous and synthetic pregnane steroids have a potent anticonvulsant effect in bicuculine-, metrazol-, picrotoxin-, pentylenetetrazol-, pilocarpine-, and kainic-acid-induced seizures and against status epilepticus, but are ineffective against electroshock and strychnine-induced seizures (Majewska et al. 1986; Kokate et al. 1994, 1996). The anticonvulsant properties of AP resemble those of the benzodiazepine clonazepam (Majewska et al. 1986; Finn and Gee 1993; Kokate et al. 1996). It is less potent than clonazepam but may have lower relative toxicity (Kokate et al. 1994, 1996). The anticonvulsant effect of AP is greater in female rats in the diestrus 1 part of the ovulatory cycle (equivalent to human mid-luteal phase when progesterone levels are high) than in estrus (equivalent to ovulation when estrogen levels are high) or in the male (Maguire et al. 2005). Enhanced mid-luteal efficacy at the $GABA_A$ receptor may be related to progesterone-induced enhanced formation of the δ $GABA_A$ receptor subtype (Maguire et al. 2005). Rapid withdrawal of progesterone in late diestrus makes the $GABA_A$ receptor insensitive to benzodiazepine, but not AP, perhaps as the result of a decrease in the benzodiazepine-sensitive synaptic $GABA_A$ receptors (Smith et al. 1998). This effect can be blocked by inhibiting the formation of the α4-subunit of the $GABA_A$ receptor (Smith et al. 1998; Maguire et al. 2005).

Progesterone may act via genomic mechanisms to influence the enzymatic activity controlling the synthesis and release of various neurotransmitters and neuromodulators produced by progesterone receptor-containing neurons (McEwen 1994). Progesterone binds specific cytosolic receptors not only to produce its own characteristic effects but also to lower estrogen receptor numbers and thereby antagonize estrogen actions (Hsueh et al. 1976).

Chronic progesterone exposure decreases the number of hippocampal CA1 dendritic spines and excitatory synapses faster than the simple withdrawal of estrogen, counteracting the stimulatory effects of estradiol (Woolley and McEwen 1994). Progesterone and AP have also been shown to have neuroprotective effects on hippocampal neurons in kainic-acid-induced seizure models (Frye 1995).

In most adult female animal models, progesterone depresses neuronal firing (Landgren et al. 1978), and lessens spontaneous and induced epileptiform discharges (Woolley and Timiras 1962; Landgren et al. 1978; Nicoletti et al. 1985; Smith et al. 1987; Frye 1995). It retards kindling and decreases seizure occurrence (Woolley and Timiras 1962; Landgren et al. 1978; Nicoletti et al. 1985; Smith et al. 1987; Frye 1995).

Backstrom et al. (1984) found that intravenous infusion of progesterone, sufficient to produce luteal phase serum levels, was associated with a significant decrease in interictal spike frequency in four of seven women with partial epilepsy.

Hormonal treatment
Progestogen therapy

The term "progestogen" refers to the broad class of progestational agents. These include progesterone (i.e., naturally occurring progesterone) and progestins (i.e., synthetic progestational agents). Progestogen treatment (Tables 90.1, 90.2) has taken two forms: (1) cyclic progesterone therapy which supplements progesterone during the luteal phase and withdraws it gradually premenstrually and (2) suppressive therapy in which the goal is to suppress the menstrual cycle which is generally accomplished using injectable progestins or gonadotropin releasing-hormone analogues.

Cyclic progesterone therapy

In contrast to published cyclic oral progestin investigations that did not result in significant reduction of seizure frequency (Dana Haeri and Richens 1983; Mattson et al. 1984), two open-label trials of adjunctive progesterone therapy for women with catamenial epilepsy did result in clinically important and statistically significant reductions in seizure occurrence (Table 90.2) (Herzog, 1986, 1995). In one investigation of women who had inadequate luteal phase cycles with catamenial exacerbation of intractable complex partial seizures, six of eight women experienced improved seizure control with a 68% decline in average monthly seizure frequency over 3 months for the whole group (Herzog 1986). In a subsequent open trial of adjunctive cyclic progesterone versus the optimal antiseizure medication alone in 25 women (14 with inadequate luteal phase or anovulatory cycles and 11 with normal cycles and perimenstrual seizure exacerbation), 18 (72%) experienced fewer seizures with an overall average monthly decline of 54% for complex partial and 58% for secondary generalized

Table 90.1 Investigational sex hormone treatments of women with epilepsy

Investigational treatments	Dosage	Potential adverse effects
Progesterone lozenges	Days 14–25: ½–1 lozenge tid; Days 26–27: ¼–½ lozenge tid; Day 28: ¼ lozenge tid	Sedation, depression, breast tenderness, vaginal bleeding, constipation, exacerbation of asthma, weight gain
Depomedroxyprogesterone	150–250 mg IM q 1–3 months	As above plus delay of months to 2 years in recovery of ovulatory cycles during which time seizure numbers may increase sometimes beyond baseline
Gonadotrophin-releasing hormone analog	Leuprolide: 3.75 mg IM q 4 weeks; 11.25 mg IM q 12 weeks	Menopausal symptoms unless concomitant estradiol and progesterone supplement is administered
Clomiphene	Days 5–9: 25–50 mg daily	Ovarian overstimulation syndrome and pelvic pain

Table 90.2 Adjunctive cyclic progestogen therapy

	Medroxyprogesterone (Herzog 1984)	Progesterone suppositories (Herzog 1986)	Progesterone lozenges (Herzog 1995)	Progesterone lozenges: 3-year follow-up (Herzog 1999)
Regimen	5–10 mg q.d. days 15–28 of cycle	100–200 mg. t.i.d. days 15–28 of cycle	100–200 mg. t.i.d. days 15–28 of cycle	100–200 mg. t.i.d. days 15–28 of cycle
Assessment	@ 3 months	@ 3 months	@ 3 months	@ 3 years
Subjects	24	8	25	15 of original 25
Number improved	10 (42%)	6 (75%)	18 (72%)	15 (100%; 60% overall)
Seizure frequency	−10%	−68%*	−54%** CPS −58%* SGMS	−62%** CPS −74%** SGMS

Notes:
*, $p < 0.05$.
**, $p\ 0 < .01$.
CPS, complex partial seizures; SGMS, secondary generalized motor seizures.

motor seizures over 3 months (Herzog 1995). Progesterone was more efficacious when administered during the entire second half of the cycle, rather than just premenstrually, and then tapered and discontinued gradually over three or four days at the end of the cycle (Herzog 1995). Failure to taper gradually premenstrually can result in rebound seizure exacerbation. At 3 years, the average daily seizure frequency per patient showed that the 15 women who remained on cyclic progesterone therapy and their original antiepileptic drugs continued to show improved seizure control in comparison to their own baseline (Table 90.2 – 3-year follow-up) (Herzog 1999). Three women were entirely seizure free. Four had total seizure reductions of 75–99%. Eight had reductions of 50–74%. Complex partial seizures in these 15 were lower by a statistically significant 62% (baseline: 0.328, 3-year follow-up: 0.125; $p < 0.01$); secondary generalized motor seizures, by 74% (baseline: 0.148, 3-year follow-up: 0.038; $p < 0.01$). Antiepileptic drug serum levels continued to show no significant change. The three remaining women who continued on progesterone therapy had 10–50% improvement at the end of the original investigation at 3 months and were not considered further because they changed antiepileptic drugs.

By way of critique, the weakness of these preliminary progesterone investigations is that they were not placebo-controlled or blinded. The favorable 3-year follow-up results are biased by analysis of only 15 of the original 25 subjects. These 15 who remained on the original treatment regimen are more likely to represent those who had the most favorable response. There are reasons, however, to consider that the results of the present investigation may represent more than placebo effects.

(1) Few placebo studies, including our own progestin trial that used a similar methodology, and could be used, therefore, as a retrospective control, show favorable response in more than 50% of subjects.

(2) Few placebo treatments have resulted in greater than 50% seizure reduction.

(3) While placebo effects generally wear off over a few months, substantial and statistically significant improvements in the present investigation persisted after 3 years in the majority of subjects (Herzog 1999).

Another argument against the placebo explanation is that the beneficial effect of progesterone can be eliminated by the concomitant use of a reductase inhibitor which presumably blocks the reduction of progesterone to its potent GABAergic metabolite AP (Herzog and Frye 2003). Finally, there is transcranial magnetic stimulation evidence that progesterone may increase inhibition in the brain premenstrually (Herzog *et al.* 2001). A prospective multicenter, randomized, double-blind, placebo-controlled investigation of cyclic, adjunctive progesterone therapy in the management of women with catamenially exacerbated, intractable localization related epilepsy is now under way (Herzog *et al.* 2004; Fowler *et al.* 2006).

Natural progesterone is available as an extract of soy in lozenge form in variable dosages ranging from 25 to 200 mg and should be administered three times daily because of its brief half-life of about 4–6 hr (Herzog, 1986, 1995, 1999). The daily regimen to achieve physiological luteal range serum levels measured 4 hr after administration ranges from 50–200 mg, taken three times daily, with the usual optimal daily dose ranging from 300 to 600 mg (Herzog 1986, 1995, 1999). The maintenance dosage and regimen should be individualized and based on a combination of clinical response and serum progesterone levels between 20 and 40 ng/mL. Progesterone is also available in micronized form in an oral capsule preparation that may also exert similar antiseizure effects although formal investigations to this effect are lacking. Theoretically, it is possible that first pass through the liver using the oral micronized form may result in the delivery of different concentrations of progesterone and its neuroactive metabolite to the brain.

Adverse effects occur with overdosage and include sedation, emotional depression, and asthenia (Herzog 1986, 1995, 1999). Progesterone use may also occasionally be associated with breast tenderness, weight gain, and irregular vaginal bleeding, and sometimes constipation. The vehicle used to dissolve progesterone for suppository use may rarely be responsible for the development of an allergic rash. Discontinuation of the hormone or lowering of the dosage resolves these side effects (Herzog 1986, 1995, 1999).

Drug interactions are an important consideration. Higher progesterone dosages may be required to achieve luteal range levels in women who take antiseizure medications because carbamazepine, phenytoin, and barbiturates are known to enhance the hepatic metabolism of gonadal and adrenal steroid hormones as well as to increase hormonal binding to serum proteins (Herzog and Frye 2003). Progesterone use has been associated with changes in antiseizure medication levels in some cases but this effect has been sporadic and not in a predictable direction. Therefore, total and possibly free serum antiseizure medication levels should be checked regularly during concomitant hormonal therapy.

Progestin therapy

Parenteral depomedroxyprogesterone may lower seizure frequency when it is given in sufficient dosage to induce amenorrhea (Zimmerman *et al.* 1973; Mattson *et al.* 1984). In one open-label study of 14 women with refractory partial seizures and normal ovulatory cycles, parenteral depomedroxyprogesterone administration in doses large enough to induce amenorrhea (i.e., 120–150 mg every 6–12 weeks) resulted in a 39% seizure reduction (Mattson *et al.* 1984). It was unclear whether the effect was due to direct anticonvulsant activity of medroxyprogesterone or to the hormonal consequences of the induced amenorrhea. One patient who had absence rather than partial seizures did not improve. Side effects included those encountered with natural progesterone. Depot administration, however, is also commonly associated with hot flushes, irregular breakthrough vaginal bleeding, and a lengthy delay of 6 to 24 months in the return of regular ovulatory cycles (Mattson *et al.* 1984). Long-term hypoestrogenic effects on cardiovascular and emotional status need to be considered with chronic use. Bone density is only partially maintained.

Oral synthetic progestins administered cyclically or continuously have not proven to be an effective therapy for seizures in clinical investigations (Dana Haeri and Richens 1983; Mattson *et al.* 1984) although individual successes with continuous daily oral use of norethistrone and combination pills have been reported (Hall 1977).

Gonadotrophin-releasing hormone analog therapy

Bauer *et al.* (1990) used triptorelin, a synthetic gonadotrophin-releasing hormone (GnRH) analog (3.75 mg), in a controlled release depot form intramuscularly every 4 weeks for an average of 11.8 months in 10 women (aged 20–50) with catamenial seizures intractable to high therapeutic doses of carbamazepine, diphenylhydantoin, phenobarbital, and valproic acid in monotherapy or combined. They remained on a stable dose of the anticonvulsant throughout the period of treatment with triptorelin. They reported that three patients became seizure-free; four showed a decrease in seizure frequency of up to 50%. In one the duration of seizures was shortened; two had no therapeutic effect. These results were attained within the first 2 months of starting triptorelin. The study was not controlled and longer-term follow-up was not available for some of the patients. Serum luteinizing hormone and estrogen were measured in one patient before and during the second month of triptorelin treatment; and as expected showed marked inhibition of luteinizing hormone and estrogen production. All the women became amenorrheic. Eight of the ten patients experienced hot flushes, headache, or weight gain.

Haider and Barnett (1991) reported on their use of goserelin 3.6 mg subcutaneously every 4 weeks in a 41-year-old woman who had had frequent catamenial status epilepticus despite therapeutic anticonvulsant drug levels which also did not respond to levonorgestrel/ethinyl estradiol. They reported a decrease in frequency from ten admissions for status epilepticus to three over a similar period.

Gonadotrophin-releasing hormone analogs basically create a medical oophorectomy. Common side effects are flushing, vaginal dryness, and dyspareunia. Serious long-term risks include osteoporosis and cardiovascular disease. Reid and Gangar (1992) suggested the addition of medroxyprogesterone acetate and conjugated estrogens to goserelin to prevent this while still abolishing most of the cyclical fluctuations of ovarian hormones. Although neither Bauer et al. (1992) nor Haider and Barnett (1991) reported exacerbation of seizures with GnRH analogs, Herzog (1991) found that during the first 3 weeks, when there is an initial stimulation of estrogen before its production is inhibited, some women experienced such a marked exacerbation of their seizures and auras that they could not tolerate further use of GnRH analog.

References

Allen AL, McCarson KE (2005) Estrogen increases nociception-evoked brain-derived neurotrophic factor gene expression in the female rat. *Neuroendocrinology* **81**:193–9.

Almqvist R (1955) The rhythm of epileptic attacks and its relationship to the menstrual cycle. *Acta Psychiatr Neurol Scand* **30**(Suppl 105):1–116.

Backstrom T (1976) Epileptic seizures in women related to plasma estrogen and progesterone during the menstrual cycle. *Acta Neurol Scand* **54**:321–47.

Backstrom T, Zetterlund B, Blom S, Romano M (1984) Effects of intravenous progesterone infusions on the epileptic discharge frequency in women with partial epilepsy. *Acta Neurol Scand* **69**:240–8.

Bauer J, Wildt L, Flugel D, Stefan H (1992) The effect of a synthetic GnRH analogue on catamenial epilepsy: a study in ten patients. *J Neurol* **239**:284–6.

Cheney DL, Uzunov D, Costa E, Guidotti A (1995) Gas chromatographic-mass fragmentographic quantitation of 3a-hydroxy-5a-pragnan-20-one (allopregnanolone) and its precursors in blood and brain of adrenalectomized and castrated rats. *J Neurosci* **15**:4641–50.

Dana Haeri J, Richens A (1983) Effect of norethistrone on seizures associated with menstruation. *Epilepsia* **24**:377–81.

Finn DA, Gee KW (1993) The influence of estrus cycle phase on neurosteroid potency at the GABA$_A$ receptor complex. *J Pharmacol Exp Ther* **265**:1374–9.

Fowler K, Massaro J, Harden C, et al. (2006) Distribution of seizure occurrence in women with epilepsy: preliminary data analysis in a prospective multicenter investigation. *Epilepsia* **47**:1–7.

Frye CA (1995) The neurosteroid 3a-5a-THP has antiseizure and possible neuroprotective effects in an animal model of epilepsy. *Brain Res* **696**:113–20.

Gee KW, McCauley LD, Lan NC (1995) A putative receptor for neurosteroids on the GABA receptor complex: the pharmacological properties and therapeutic potential of epalons. *Crit Rev Neurobiol* **9**:207–27.

Haider Y, Barnett DB (1991) Catamenial epilepsy and goserelin. *Lancet* **338**:1530.

Hall SM (1977) Treatment of menstrual epilepsy with a progesterone-only oral contraceptive. *Epilepsia* **18**:235–6.

Herzog AG (1984) Treatment of seizures with medroxyprogesterone acetate: a preliminary report. *Neurology* **34**:1255–8.

Herzog AG (1986) Intermittent progesterone therapy and frequency of complex partial seizures in women with menstrual disorders. *Neurology* **36**:1607–10.

Herzog AG (1991) Reproductive endocrine considerations and hormonal therapy for women with epilepsy. *Epilepsia* **32**:S27–33.

Herzog AG (1995) Progesterone therapy in complex partial and secondary generalized seizures. *Neurology* **45**:1660–2.

Herzog AG (1999) Progesterone therapy in women with epilepsy: a 3-year follow-up. *Neurology* **52**:1917–18.

Herzog AG, Frye CA (2003) Seizure exacerbation associated with inhibition of progesterone metabolism. *Ann Neurol* **53**:390–1.

Herzog AG, Klein P, Ransil BJ (1997) Three patterns of catamenial epilepsy. *Epilepsia* **38**:1082–8.

Herzog AG, Friedman MN, Freund S, Pascual-Leone A (2001) Transcranial magnetic stimulation evidence of a potential role for progesterone in the modulation of premenstrual cortico-cortical inhibition in a woman with catamenial seizure exacerbation. *Epilepsy Behav* **2**:367–9.

Herzog AG, Harden CL, Liporace J, et al. (2004) Frequency of catamenial seizure exacerbation in women with localization-related epilepsy. *Ann Neurol* **56**:431–4.

Hsueh AJW, Peck EJ, Clark JH (1976) Control of uterine estrogen receptor levels by progesterone. *Endocrinology* **98**:438–44.

Kalinin VV, Zheleznova EV (2007) Chronology and evolution of temporal lobe epilepsy and endocrine reproductive function in women: relationships to side of focus and cateminality. *Epilepsy Behav* **11**:185–91.

Kokate TG, Svensson BE, Rogawski MA (1994) Anticonvulsant activity of neurosteroids: correlation with γ-aminobutyric acid-evoked chloride current potentiation. *J Pharmacol Exp Ther* **270**:1223–9.

Kokate TG, Cohen AL, Karp E, Rogawski MA (1996) Neuroactive steroids protect against pilocarpine- and kainic acid-induced limbic seizures and status epilepticus in mice. *Neuropharmacology* **35**:1049–56.

Laidlaw J (1956) Catamenial epilepsy. *Lancet* **271**:1235–7.

Landgren S, Backstrom T, Kalistratov G (1978) The effect of progesterone on the spontaneous interictal spike evoked by the application of penicillin to the cat's cerebral cortex. *J Neurol Sci* **36**:119–33.

Logothetis J, Harner R (1960) Electrocortical activation by estrogens. *Arch Neurol* **3**:290–7.

Logothetis J, Harner R, Morrell F, Torres F (1959) The role of estrogens in catamenial exacerbation of epilepsy. *Neurology (Minneap)* **9**:352–60.

Luine VN, Renner KJ, McEwen BS (1986) Sex-dependent differences in estrogen regulation of choline acetyltransferase are altered by neonatal treatments. *Endocrinology* **119**:874–8.

Maguire JL, Stell BM, Rafizadeh M, Mody I (2005) Ovarian cycle-linked changes in GABA$_A$ receptors mediating tonic inhibition alter seizure susceptibility and anxiety. *Nat Neurosci* **8**:797–804.

Majewska MD, Harrison NL, Schwartz RD, Barker JL, Paul SM (1986) Steroid hormone metabolites are barbiturate-like modulators of the GABA receptor. *Science* **232**:1004–7.

Marcus EM, Watson CW, Goodman PL (1966) Effects of steroids on cerebral electrical activity. *Arch Neurol* **15**:521–32.

Mattson RH, Cramer JA, Caldwell BV, Siconolfi BC (1984) Treatment of seizures with medroxyprogesterone acetate: preliminary report. *Neurology (Cleveland)* **34**:1255–8.

McEwen BS (1994) How do sex and stress hormones affect nerve cells? *Ann N Y Acad Sci* **743**:1–16.

Nicoletti F, Speciale C, Sortino MA, *et al.* (1985) Comparative effects of estradiol benzoate, the antiestrogen clomiphene citrate, and the progestin medroxyprogesterone acetate on kainic acid-induced seizures in male and female rats. *Epilepsia* **26**:252–7.

Paul SM, Purdy RH (1992) Neuroactive steroids. *FASEB Lett* **6**:2311–22.

Pfaff DW, Keiner M (1973) Estradiol-concentrating cells in the rat amygdala as part of a limbic-hypothalamic hormone-sensitive system. In: BE Eleftheriou (ed.) *The Neurobiology of the Amygdala*. New York: Plenum Press, 1973, pp. 775–92.

Quigg M, Fowler KM, Herzog AG (2008) Progesterone Trial Study Group. Circalunar and ultralunar periodicities in women with partial seizures. *Epilepsia* **49**:1081–5.

Quigg M, Smithson SD, Fowler KM, Sursal T, Herzog AG (2009) Progesterone Trial Study Group. Laterality and location of seizure foci influence catamenial seizure expression in women with partial epilepsy. *Neurology* **73**:223–7.

Reid B, Gangar KF (1992) Catamenial epilepsy and goserelin. *Lancet* **339**:253.

Rudick CN, Woolley CS (2001) Estrogen regulates functional inhibition of hippocampal CA1 pyramidal cells in the adult female rat. *J Neurosci* **21**:6532–43.

Scharfman HE, Mercurio TC, Goodman JH, Wilson MA, MacLusky NJ (2003) Hippocampal excitability increases during the estrous cycle in the rat: a potential role for brain-derived neurotrophic factor. *J Neurosci* **23**:11641–52.

Smith SS (1989) Estrogen administration increases neuronal responses to excitatory amino acids as a long term effect. *Brain Res* **503**:354–7.

Smith SS, Waterhouse BD, Woodward DJ (1987) Sex steroid effects on extrahypothalamic CNS. II. Progesterone, alone and in combination with estrogen, modulates cerebellar responses to amino acid neurotransmitters. *Brain Res* **422**:52–62.

Smith SS, Gong QH, Hau F-C, *et al.* (1998) GABA$_A$ receptor α4 subunit suppression prevents withdrawal properties of an endogenous steroid. *Nature* **392**:926–30.

Tauboll E, Lundervold A, Gjerstad L (1991) Temporal distribution of seizures in epilepsy. *Epilepsy Res* **8**:153–65.

Teresawa E, Timiras P (1968) Electrical activity during the estrous cycle of the rat; cyclic changes in limbic structures. *Endocrinology* **83**:207–76.

Veliskova J, Velisek L, Galanopoulou AS, Sperber EF (2000) Neuroprotective effects of estrogens on hippocampal cells in adult female rats after status epilepticus. *Epilepsia* **41**(Suppl 6):S30–5.

Wallis CJ, Luttge WG (1980) Influence of estrogen and progesterone on glutamic acid decarboxylase activity in discrete regions of rat brain. *J Neurochem* **34**:609–13.

Wong M, Moss R (1992) Long-term and short-term electrophysiological effects of estrogen on the synaptic properties of hippocampal CA1 neurons. *J Neurosci* **12**:3217–25.

Woolley CS, McEwen BS (1994) Estradiol regulates hippocampal dendritic spine density via an *N*-methyl-d-aspartate receptor-dependent mechanism. *J Neurosci* **14**:7680–7.

Woolley CS, Timiras PS, (1962) Estrous and circadian periodicity and electroshock convulsions in rats. *Am J Physiol* **202**:379–82.

Zimmerman AW, Holden KR, Reiter EO, Dekaban AS (1973) Medroxyprogesterone acetate in the treatment of seizures associated with menstruation. *J Pediatr* **83**:959–63.

Chapter

Sleep

91

Liborio Parrino, Giulia Milioli, Fernando De Paolis, Andrea Grassi, Gioia Gioi,
and Mario Giovanni Terzano

Introduction

The variations of arousal level across the 24-hr rhythm play an important role in the modulation of epileptic events. The sleep–wake cycle, and particularly the conditions of instability that occur during sleep, significantly affect the appearance of interictal electroencephalogram (EEG) discharges and epileptic seizures. This interaction, either in the sense of inhibition or, more frequently, in the direction of activation, relies on the characteristics of the epileptic syndrome (type of attacks, clinical course, etiology), on the time of day, and on the structural components of sleep (falling asleep, EEG arousal, rapid eye movement (REM) sleep, non rapid eye movement (NREM) stages). In particular, the two neurophysiological states that characterize sleep (NREM and REM) have opposite consequences on interictal abnormalities and on ictal manifestations.

Several 24-hr studies have investigated the influence of vigilance states on the occurrence of epileptic manifestations, showing that epileptic manifestations more likely appear when the level of vigilance is low (relaxation, drowsiness, sleep) and unstable (arousal fluctuations) and that frequency and morphology of epileptiform EEG patterns may depend on sleep stages.

Accordingly, the relationship between sleep and epilepsy is closely related to the basic mechanisms underlying the sleep–wake continuum.

Circadian rhythms and epilepsy

The endogenous circadian system is an important modulator of the sleep–wake rhythm. The circadian oscillator is located in the suprachiasmatic nuclei of the anterior hypothalamus and, independently of other factors, potentiates wakefulness at one phase of the diurnal cycle and facilitates sleep at the opposite phase (Fig. 91.1). This autonomous pacemaker determines the sleep propensity in relation to other biological functions and, in particular, to the rhythmicity of deep body temperature. Laboratory studies have demonstrated that the timing of peaks and troughs of sleep propensity during the day is highly correlated with the thermal curve: besides the high sleep propensity during nocturnal hours (primary sleep gate concomitant to the descending branch of deep body temperature), a less prominent peak of sleep propensity is observed in mid-afternoon (secondary sleep gate), about 10 hr after the temperature minimum clock time. In contrast, besides the trough of sleep propensity in the late morning (ascending branch of deep body temperature), there is a period of low sleep propensity in the early evening (forbidden zones for sleep), about 8 hr before the temperature minimum time.

Although sleep may modulate epileptogenicity through cortical excitation or other mechanisms, its contribution to circadian seizure patterns varies with the pathophysiology of the underlying epileptic syndrome (and above all with the localization of the epileptic focus) because of the differing sensitivity of brain regions to circadian modulation. Both experimental epilepsy models (Shouse *et al.* 1996) and studies in symptomatic partial epilepsies (Quigg 2000) provide the clearest evidence that the main vigilance states differentially facilitate seizures depending on the location of the epileptic foci. In particular, kindling models of partial epilepsy have proportionately more seizures during wakefulness compared to generalized seizure models (Shouse *et al.* 1996); seizures of patients with extratemporal lobe epilepsies are distributed in a pattern not statistically distinguishable from a uniform 24-hr rate, while seizures of patients with mesial temporal lobe epilepsy show a peak of occurrence in the mid-to-late portion of the light phase of the day (Quigg 2000).

In experimental models of limbic epilepsy spontaneous seizures occur predominantly during the light half of the cycle. This daily pattern persists when epileptic rats are allowed to free-run in constant darkness. In this condition without time cues, seizures continue to recur in an identical pattern, endogenously mediated by the circadian rhythm of body temperature (Quigg *et al.* 2000). Other physiological cyclic functions (i.e., body temperature, hypothalamic–pituitary–adrenal axis, hypothalamic–pituitary–gonadal axis) might be equally important in the modulation of seizure occurrence (Quigg

The Causes of Epilepsy, eds. S. D. Shorvon, F. Andermann, and R. Guerrini. Published by Cambridge University Press. © Cambridge University Press 2011.

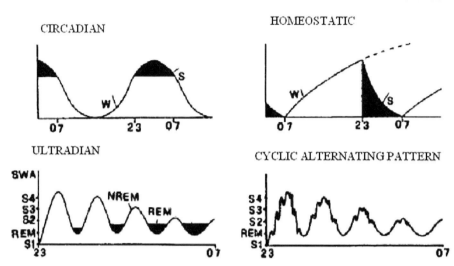

NEUROPHYSIOLOGICAL PROCESSES OF SLEEP REGULATION

Fig. 91.1. The four basic mechanisms of sleep regulation. The clock time is reported on the *x*-axis. W, wakefulness; S, sleep; SWA, slow-wave activity; REM, rapid eye movement sleep; S1 stage 1, S2 stage 2, S3 stage 3, S4 stage 4 of NREM (non rapid eye movement) sleep.

2000). Moreover, the pattern of EEG activity may be deeply influenced by the increased engagement in physical and mental performances during the diurnal hours. In other words, the genuine distribution of EEG bursts over the 24-hr period can be obscured by several masking factors. This masking hypothesis can be tested by having patients suffering from epilepsy lie in bed under constant conditions and instructing them to refrain from any type of activity. Then the distribution of EEG paroxysms might reveal a different picture.

Homeostatic process

The variations of sleep propensity over time are not only an effect of the biological clock but are also influenced by the subject's prior sleep–wake history. Extensive studies on sleep deprivation (SD) have shown a positive relationship between the duration of pre-sleep wakefulness and the spectral energy enhancement of slow-wave activities (0.5–4 Hz). In effect, sleep stages 3 and 4 are mostly concentrated in the early portions of sleep, while they are practically absent in the final hours. The priority of recuperation of stages 3 and 4 (slow-wave sleep or SWS) after sleep onset and the progressive decline of deep sleep along the night suggests the involvement of a compensatory mechanism based on the accumulation while awake of some unknown factor, which undergoes a sort of dissipative process during sleep. In short, prolonged wakefulness hastens sleep onset and proportionally potentiates slow-waves activities, regardless of the circadian phase (Dijk *et al.* 1990). The increased intensity of sleep after prolonged wakefulness indicates that the characteristics of sleep recovery respond to mechanisms of homeostatic regulation.

It is known that increased depth of sleep is associated with increased interictal epileptiform discharges (IEDs): NREM sleep has been shown by most authors to activate IEDs in patients with partial epilepsy, with the maximal spiking rates occurring during the deeper stages (SWS) of sleep, and less

frequently, to occur during the lighter sleep stages 1 and 2 (Malow *et al.* 1997).

The effect of sleep on IEDs in partial epilepsies of extratemporal lobe origin is not as well characterized as in temporal lobe epilepsy. In children with benign epilepsy of childhood with rolandic spikes, maximal spike rates are related to deeper stages of sleep and in general to the first cycle (Clemens and Majoros 1987). Sammaritano and Saint-Hilaire (1998) observed maximal spiking rates during SWS of NREM sleep in three patients with extratemporal lobe epilepsy referred for presurgical evaluation.

As clarified above, SD increases slow-wave activity. As a result, it may have an overall activating effect on epileptic phenomena. Rodin *et al.* (1962) noted high-voltage paroxysmal activity in the EEG of normal subjects after 120 hr of SD and concluded that "prolonged loss of sleep is associated with increased cerebral irritability which may result in epileptic-like manifestations in certain predisposed individuals." Further studies showed that sleep-deprived EEG activates epileptiform abnormalities in 30–50% of people with epilepsy. This activation method has a high specificity. On the basis of these observations, SD became established as an activating method to elicit epileptiform activity in EEGs.

There is no general agreement on the question as to whether SD in epileptic patiens has a genuine activating effect on EEG, or whether it acts through sleep induction. However same studies support the premise that SD may activate IEDs independently of the activating effects of sleep (Fountain *et al.* 1998).

NREM–REM sleep cycle

A third mechanism of sleep regulation is the NREM–REM cycling characterized by periods of sustained high-voltage, slow-wave synchronized EEG patterns (NREM sleep) that are periodically replaced by sustained periods of low-voltage, fast-wave desynchronized EEG rhythms (REM sleep). The NREM–REM cycle is conventionally composed of a descending branch (from light to deep NREM sleep), a trough (the deepest stage of the sleep cycle), and an ascending branch (from the deepest NREM stage to REM sleep). Experimental investigation has shown that the intrinsic alternation between NREM and REM sleep is under the control of an oscillatory process generated by a particular rhythmicity of neurotransmission and by the reciprocal interaction between two neuronal groups with REM-on and REM-off activities (Hobson et al. 1975).

The two main sleep states have different physiological components and contrasting effects on generalized ictal and interictal discharges. The hypothalamic and brainstem generators of sleep and arousal have diffuse ascending and descending projections (Jones 1994) that give rise to a number of distinguishing physiological characteristics, called components, and that influence the likelihood that an electrographic or clinical seizure will occur. The most salient state-specific components affecting epilepsy seem to be the degree to which cellular discharge patterns are synchronized and the alterations in anti-gravity muscle tone (Cohen and Dement 1970; Shouse et al. 1996).

During NREM, virtually every cell in the brain discharges synchronously (Steriade et al. 1993). Synchronous synaptic effects, whether excitatory or inhibitory, could augment the magnitude and propagation of postsynaptic responses, including epileptic discharges. Background EEG effects seem to be exacerbated by sudden surges of afferent stimulation associated with transient, synchronous phasic arousal events. Generalized seizures, particularly generalized tonic–clonic or myoclonic convulsions, tend to occur during NREM sleep or transitional arousal periods characterized by background EEG synchronization, often with phasic events which include sleep EEG transients such as sleep spindles, k-complexes, and ponto-geniculo-occipital (PGO) waves. In the majority of patients with primary generalized epilepsy (PGE) frequent brief bursts of spikes, polyspikes, and spike–wave-like discharges are associated with k-complexes or spindles which are specific phasic EEG patterns of NREM sleep.

In contrast, REM sleep, with its asynchronous cellular discharge patterns (Jones 1994) and skeletal motor paralysis, is resistant to propagation of epileptic EEG potentials and to clinical motor accompaniment (Shouse et al. 1989) even though spontaneous phasic activity and focal EEG seizure discharges persist at this time and may be evoked by photic stimulation. While anti-gravity muscle tone is preserved in NREM sleep and waking, thus permitting seizure-associated movement, profound lower motor neuron inhibition occurs in REM, creating virtual paralysis and preventing seizure-related movement.

These conclusions are supported by other experimental and clinical findings indicating that substrates of state-specific components rather than integrity of the state per se can be salient determinants of seizure propagation regardless of the epileptic syndrome. Agents that synchronize the EEG, such as cholinergic or noradrenergic antagonists, have pro-convulsant effects. Conversely, agents that desynchronize the EEG discourage epileptic EEG discharge propagation. Finally, pharmacologic manipulations that induce atonia, such as carbachol infusion into the brainstem, also block clinical motor accompaniment (Velasco and Velasco 1982).

Collectively, these findings confirm that neural cell discharge patterns and alterations in muscle tone can affect electrographic and clinically evident seizure manifestations in different epileptic syndromes (Shouse et al. 1990). Phasic activity can provoke epileptiform discharges, but the extent of epileptic EEG discharge propagation and clinical motor accompaniment depend upon tonic EEG and motor sleep components.

Cyclic alternating pattern and epilepsy
Physiological bases

The cyclic alternating pattern (CAP) is a periodic EEG activity of NREM sleep, characterized by sequences of transient electrocortical events that are distinct from background EEG activity and recur at up to 1 min intervals. This is the EEG translation of a sustained arousal oscillation between activation (phase A) and inhibition (phase B) that translates the condition of neurophysiological instability (Terzano et al. 2001). The complementary pattern, defined as non-CAP (NCAP) and consisting of a rhythmic EEG background, with few, randomly distributed arousal-related phasic events, represents, on the contrary, a stable sleep condition. Intensive though subwakening perturbation delivered during NCAP determines the prompt appearance of a CAP sequence. Variations during CAP involve to different degrees muscle tone, heart rate, and respiratory activity, which increase during phase A and decrease during phase B (Terzano and Parrino 1993). On the contrary, NCAP sleep periods are associated with stable neurovegetative activities.

Three subtypes of A phases corresponding to different levels of neurophysiological activation can be distinguished (Fig. 91.2).

Subtypes A1 A phases with synchronized EEG patterns (sequences of k-complexes or delta bursts), associated with mild or trivial polygraphic variations.

Subtypes A2 A phases with desynchronized EEG patterns preceded by or mixed with slow high-voltage waves (k-complexes with alpha and beta activities, k-alpha, arousals with slow wave synchronization), linked with a moderate increase of muscle tone and/or cardiorespiratory rate.

Subtypes A3 A phases with desynchronized EEG patterns alone (transient activation phases or arousals) or exceeding two-thirds of the phase A length, and coupled with a remarkable enhancement of muscle tone and/or cardiorespiratory rate.

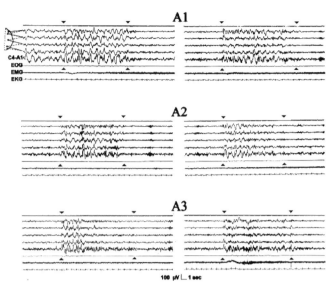

Fig. 91.2. Phase A subtypes of cyclic alternating pattern (CAP). The black triangles mark the start and the end of phase A, with a progressive increase of the fast low-amplitude portion of the phase from the A1 subtype to the A3 subtype (see text for more details).

In the physiological architecture of sleep, the A1 subtypes prevail in the build-up and maintenance of deep NREM sleep, while the A2 and A3 subtypes dominate in light sleep that precedes the onset of desynchronized REM sleep.

CAP time is the temporal sum of all CAP sequences and can be calculated throughout total NREM sleep. The percentage ratio of CAP time to sleep time is referred to as CAP rate. In human sleep CAP rate is an index of arousal instability which shows a particular evolution along the lifespan (mean values in preschool-aged children 26%; school-aged children 33%; teenagers 43%; young adults 32%; middle-aged 38%; elderly 55%), and correlates with the subjective appreciation of sleep quality (the higher the CAP rate the poorer the sleep quality).

CAP and interictal discharges

Pioneering contributions in the early 1990s (Terzano *et al.* 1991, 1992) focused attention on the dynamic relationship between epileptic paroxysms and EEG phasic events during sleep. These studies confirmed sleep as a major physiological activator of epileptic manifestations, highlighting the relevance of arousal instability as an important triggering factor. In PGE, IEDs are commonly activated during unstable sleep, with the number of EEG paroxysms per minute of sleep significantly higher during CAP compared to the NCAP. Phase A has a significant activation influence, while phase B exerts a powerful and prolonged inhibitory effect especially if we consider that its mean duration (16 s) is twice the phase A length (8 s).

Identical CAP-related influences are found in juvenile myoclonic epilepsy, yet in the presence of a lower all-night amount of EEG discharges (Gigli *et al.* 1992). Compared to normal controls, the occurrence of IEDs in patients with PGE has no remarkable consequences on sleep macrostructure, but produces significant effects on arousal stability, as epileptic patients show higher CAP rate values (Terzano *et al.* 1992). Within the epileptic group, the CAP cycles that include at least one IED are significantly longer than those without IEDs. The selective lengthening of CAP cycles (only those with IEDs) and the increase of CAP rate support the hypothesis that CAP and IED share common anatomical pathways and behave as a concerted pattern that links a regular physiological phenomenon (CAP) to a random pathological event (IED). In the dynamic interplay between EEG spiking and arousal modulation, the CAP sequence (especially its activating swings) triggers the paroxysmal burst, while the latter may in turn promote the generation of a phase A or increase the instability of sleep up to full wakefulness. Though extremely short-lived, the IEDs are an activating event traveling along the same pathways of normal cerebral communication. The reciprocal support of the two activating processes determines the high probability of a simultaneous occurrence of both phenomena. Accordingly, the low amount of arousal-related phasic events that characterizes the NCAP condition makes this an unfavorable background for epileptic discharges.

Moreover, in PGE, 70% of all the phase A subtypes are A1, 24% are A2, and 6% are A3. The equivalent distribution of interictal discharges throughout the three phase A subtypes clearly indicates that none of the A phase subtypes plays an attractive or repulsive action on PGE paroxysms. However, when the position of PGE interictal abnormalities within each phase A subtype is determined, it can be seen that there is a striking preference for the portions characterized by EEG synchrony. In effect, the EEG paroxysms tend to occur throughout the entire length of subtypes A1 (totally expressed by EEG synchronized patterns), while the interictal discharges are mostly concentrated in the initial portions of the A2 and in the A3 subtypes that almost invariably start with a k-complex or a delta burst (Fig 91.3).

A powerful activating effect of CAP-related events has been described also for temporal lobe epilepsy with a spike frequency significantly higher in phase A than in phase B (Loh *et al.* 1997). This study also revealed an intermediate activating effect of NCAP between phase A and phase B.

Patients with focal lesional frontotemporal epilepsy show significant IED differences between CAP and NCAP, between phase A and phase B, and between phase A and NCAP, but not between phase B and NCAP. As occurs for PGE, the presence of focal lesional IEDs impairs the stability of sleep.

Ninety-one per cent of secondarily generalized focal lesional bursts are collected in CAP, while 96% of all the EIDs found in CAP occur during phase A (Terzano *et al.* 1991).

On the contrary, despite the high burst frequency during NREM, in benign epilepsy with rolandic spikes (BERS), the discharges are not modulated by the arousal-related mechanisms of CAP.

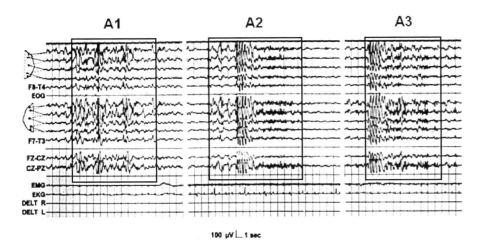

Fig. 91.3. Interictal spike-and-wave discharges during NREM sleep in primary generalized epilepsy (PGE). The EEG paroxysms can occur in any of the three phase A subtypes of CAP. While the paroxysms tend to occur throughout the entire length of subtypes A1 (totally expressed by slow oscillation), they are mostly concentrated in the initial portions of subtypes A2 and A3 that almost invariably begin with a k-complex or a delta burst. EOG, eye movements; EMG, chin muscle; EKG, heart rate. The phase A subtypes of CAP are in the boxes.

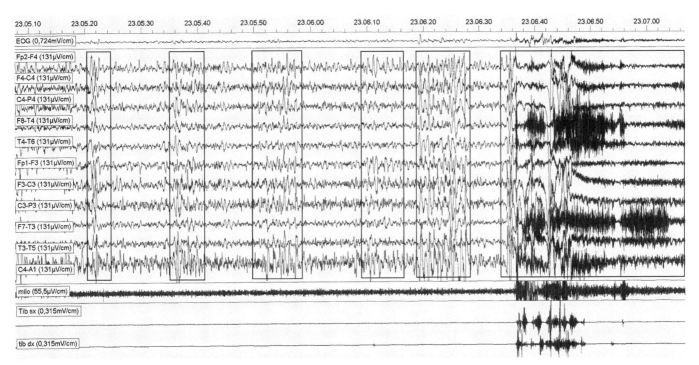

Fig. 91.4. A CAP sequence in slow wave sleep that heralds the onset of a major episode in a patient with nocturnal frontal lobe epilepsy. The motor event is preceded by a brief discharge of the same high-voltage EEG waves that compose the previous A phases of the CAP sequence (in black boxes). Milo, chin muscle; Tib sx, left tibialis anterior muscle; tib dx, right tibialis anterior muscle.

The CAP-independence of BERS cannot exclude a possible relation between interictal discharges and other microstructural events, in particular EEG features such as sleep spindles which are generally separate from the CAP (especially phase A) patterns. A spectral EEG-polysomnography study in nine patients with BERS showed a significant positive correlation between IEDs during sleep and sigma (12–16 Hz) activity (Nobili et al. 1999).

According to this result, the occurrence of IEDs during non-REM sleep may depend on a number of complex factors including the degree of integration between the epileptogenic focus and the neurophysiological circuits involved in the production of phasic events. Consolidated data indicate that some basic elements of CAP, in particular k-complexes and delta bursts, are generated in the thalamocortical circuits in which a pivotal role is played by the thalamic reticular nucleus. The activation of EEG discharges could interfere with the function of these pathways. Hypothetically, in PGE and in frontal lobe epilepsy (FLE) the firing area and these thalamocortical circuits coincide (in PGE) or extensively overlap (in FLE), and this could explain why in these types of epilepsy the EEG abnormalities are significantly triggered during phase A. In functional epilepsy such as BERS, the focus is probably detached from the CAP-related mechanisms. Accordingly,

CAP rate is increased in the sleep recordings of PGE and FLE, even without nocturnal ictal manifestations. In contrast, CAP rate values show slight variations in BERS in which IEDs are associated with spindling activity which abounds during NCAP.

CAP and ictal manifestations

Although the continuum from subclinical EEG paroxysms to clinical seizures is still incompletely understood, there is general agreement on the assumption that sleep instability facilitates both interictal and ictal phenomena. The close relationship between CAP and spike occurrence actually finds extensive confirmation in sleep-related seizures. In a study conducted on patients with focal epilepsy, 43 out of 45 nocturnal partial motor seizures occurred during NREM sleep. Among the NREM seizures, 42 appeared in CAP ($p <$ 0.0001) and always during a phase A (Terzano et al. 1991). The following investigation confirmed that 83% of temporal lobe seizures recorded in stage 2 NREM sleep occurred during CAP with a predominant activating action manifested by phase A (Dinner 1995).

In patients with nocturnal frontal lobe epilepsy (NFLE), major episodes lasting between 10 and 60 s are often preceded by a prolonged CAP sequence which reflects a condition of sustained arousal instability (Fig. 91.4). CAP also modulates the recurrence of repetitive minor motor events which show a 20–40-s periodicity and occur in close temporal relation with the A phases of CAP. Accordingly, sleep in NFLE is extremely unstable with high amounts of CAP rate (Parrino et al. 2006).

In conclusion, epilepsy research continues to look at sleep mainly as a practical method of activation of both interictal and ictal events. Besides the consolidated knowledge on sleep vs. wakefulness and NREM sleep vs. REM sleep, major attention should be paid to the circadian, and homeostatic processes as well as to the conditions of stable and unstable sleep. In particular, CAP analysis should be commonly applied in all sleep studies as a sensitive procedure for exploring the dynamic EEG interplay between physiological phasic events and paroxysmal abnormalities.

References

Clemens B, Majoros E (1987) Sleep studies in benign epilepsy of childhood with rolandic spikes. II. Analysis of discharge frequency and its relation to sleep dynamics. *Epilepsia* **28**:24–7.

Cohen HB, Dement WC (1970) Prolonged tonic convulsions in REM deprived mice. *Brain Res* **22**:421–2.

Dijk DJ, Beersma DG, Brunner DP, Daan S, Borbély AA (1990) Spectral analysis of day sleep in humans. In: Horne JA (ed.) *Sleep'90*. Bochum: Pontenagel Press, pp. 324–8.

Dinner DS (1995) Mesial temporal lobe epilepsy. *J Clin Neurophysiol* **12**:1–14.

Fountain NB, Kim JS, Lee SI (1998) Sleep deprivation activates epileptiform discharges independent of the activating effects of sleep. *J Clin Neurophysiol* **15**:69–75.

Gigli GL, Calia E, Marciani MG, et al. (1992) Sleep microstructure and EEG epileptiform activity in patients with juvenile myoclonic epilepsy. *Epilepsia* **33**:799–804.

Hobson JA, McCarley RW, Wyzinski PW (1975) Sleep cycle oscillation: reciprocal discharge by two brainstem neuronal groups. *Science* **189**:55–8.

Jones BE (1994) Basic mechanism of sleep wake states. In: MH Kryger, T Roth, WC Dement (eds.) *Principles and Practice of Sleep Disorders Medicine*, vol. 2.

Philadelphia, PA: WB Saunders, pp. 145–62.

Loh NK, Dinner DS, Arunkumar G, Foldvary N, Ahuja M (1997) Relation of interictal epileptiform activity to sleep microarchitecture in temporal-lobe epilepsy. *Epilepsia* **38**(Suppl 8):119.

Malow BA, Kushwaha R, Lin X, Morton KJ, Aldrich MS (1997) Relationship of interictal epileptiform discharges to sleep depth in partial epilepsy. *Electroencephalogr Clin Neurophysiol* **102**:20–6.

McCarley RW, Hobson JA. (1975) Neuronal excitability modulation over the sleep cycle: a structural and mathematical model. *Science* **189**:58–60.

Nobili L, Ferrillo F, Baglietto MG, et al. (1999) Relationship of sleep interictal epileptiform discharges to sigma activity (12–16 Hz) in benign epilepsy of childhood with rolandic spikes. *Clin Neurophysiol* **110**:39–46.

Parrino L, Halasz P, Tassinari CA, Terzano MG (2006) CAP, epilepsy and motor events during sleep: the unifying role of arousal. *Sleep Med Rev* **10**:267–85.

Quigg M (2000) Circadian rhythms: interactions with seizures and epilepsy. *Epilepsy Res* **42**:43–55.

Quigg M, Clayburn H, Straume M, Menaker M, Bertram EH III (2000) Effects of circadian regulation and rest-activity state on spontaneous seizures

in a rat model of limbic epilepsy. *Epilepsia* **41**:502–9.

Rodin EA, Luby ED, Gottlieb JS (1962) The electroencephalogram during prolonged experimental sleep deprivation. *Electroencephalogr Clin Neurophysiol* **14**:544–51.

Sammaritano MR, Saint-Hilaire JM (1998) Contribution of interictal spiking during sleep to localization of extratemporal epileptic foci. *Epilepsia* **39**:75.

Shouse MN, Siegel JM, Wu MF, Szymusiak R, Morrison AR. (1989) Mechanisms of seizure suppression during rapid-eye-movement (REM) sleep in cats. *Brain Res* **505**:271–82.

Shouse MN, King A, Langer J, et al. (1990) Basic mechanisms underlying seizure-prone and seizure-resistant sleep and awakening states in feline kindled and penicillin epilepsy. In: Wada JA (ed.) *Kindling*, vol. 4, New York: Plenum Press, pp. 313–27.

Shouse MN, da Silva AM, Sammaritano M (1996) Circadian rhythm, sleep, and epilepsy. *J Clin Neurophysiol* **13**:32–50.

Steriade M, McCormick DA, Sejnowski TJ (1993) Thalamocortical oscillations in the sleeping and aroused brain. *Science* **262**:679–85.

Terzano MG, Parrino L (1993) Clinical applications of cyclic alternating pattern. *Physiol Behav* **54**:807–13.

Terzano MG, Parrino L, Spaggiari MC, Barusi R, Simeoni S (1991)

Discriminatory effect of cyclic alternating pattern in focal lesional and benign rolandic interictal spikes during sleep. *Epilepsia* **32**:616–28.

Terzano MG, Parrino L, Anelli S, Boselli M, Clemens B (1992) Effects of generalized interictal EEG discharges on sleep stability: assessment by means of cyclic alternating pattern. *Epilepsia* **33**:317–26.

Terzano MG, Parrino L, Sherieri A, *et al.* (2001) Atlas, rules, and recording techniques for the scoring of cyclic alternating pattern (CAP) in human sleep. *Sleep Med* **2**:537–53.

Velasco M, Velasco F (1982) Brain stem regulation of cortical and motor excitability: effects on experimental focal motor seizures. In: Sterman MB, Shouse MN, Passouant P (eds.) *Sleep and Epilepsy*. New York: Academic Press, pp. 53–61.

Chapter

92

Metabolic and endocrine-induced seizures

Bernhard J. Steinhoff

Definitions and epidemiology

According to the international classification of epileptic syndromes (ILAE 1989) situation-related epileptic seizures (Gelegenheitsanfälle) belong to the group of special syndromes. They are defined as seizures that are almost exclusively explained by the seizure-provoking circumstances. In other words: if these seizure-provoking circumstances are avoided the epileptic seizure would not occur in the individual case. Among potential seizure-provoking conditions, metabolic causes such as non-ketotic hyperglycemia and eclampsia are explicitly cited, along with other causes of situation-related seizures such as alcohol and drugs.

In addition to situation-related seizures due to metabolic or endocrine factors, there is a wide variety of metabolic and endocrine disorders that may be associated with seizures and become manifest mainly in children. Endogenous or exogenous potential precipitants of isolated seizures are also reported in two-thirds of patients with chronic epilepsies. However, in these patients seizures also occur independently of such specific triggering circumstances (Frucht *et al.* 2000).

The purpose of this chapter is to summarize the most relevant metabolic and endocrine circumstances that can trigger isolated situation-related or acute symptomatic seizures. These disorders are also important factors in facilitating seizures in individuals with epileptic syndromes in general. A brief summary of metabolic syndromes of childhood that are typically associated with seizures follows. The reader should refer to the chapters addressing these diseases specifically to get more detailed information.

There are few investigations that address the epidemiology of metabolic and endocrine triggering seizures. However, metabolic factors for acute symptomatic seizures, which occur in 29 to 39 persons per 100 000 per year, are amongst the most common causes of seizures, along with traumatic brain injury, cerebrovascular disease, drug withdrawal, and infarctions (Hauser and Beghi 2008).

Pathology, physiology, and clinical features

Epilepsies with underlying inherited metabolic causes show a clear preponderance during childhood. Most of these disorders have a poor prognosis. Usually patients show severe additional neurological symptoms and mental retardation. These conditions include peroxisomal, mitochondrial disorders, lysosomal disorders, neurotransmitter defects, aminoacidopathies, organic acidopathies, carbohydrate metabolic disorders, inborn disturbances of glycolization, and impairment of the metabolism of purine or pyridoxine (Kruse *et al.* 2004). Metabolic errors that cause epileptic seizures include hypoglycemia, pyridoxine-dependency, non-ketotic hyperglycinemia, organic acidurias, folinic acid responsive seizures, urea cycle defects, neonatal adrenoleukodystrophy, Zellweger syndrome, holocarboxylase synthase deficiency, molybdenum cofactor deficiency and sulfite oxidase deficiency, glucose transporter 1 deficiency, creatine deficiency, biotinidase deficiency, aminoacidopathies, organic acidurias, the infantile form of neuronal ceroid lipofuscinosis (NCL 1), the late infantile and the juvenile form of neuronal ceroid lipofuscinosis (NCL 2, NCL 3), mitochondrial disorders, lysosomal storage disorders, and progressive myoclonus epilepsies (Wolf *et al.* 2005). Metabolic causes for seizures encompass lack of energy, intoxication, impaired neuronal function in storage disorders, and disturbances of neurotransmitter systems with excess of excitation or lack of inhibition (Wolf *et al.* 2005). The understanding of the underlying molecular genetics is growing rapidly (Pearl *et al.* 2005) and these conditions are considered elsewhere in this volume.

The epidemiologically most important causes of acute symptomatic seizures in adulthood are alcohol and drugs (Vassella and Fröscher 2004) (see Chapters 94 and 95). Metabolic and – to a lesser extent – endocrine causes of seizures in adulthood still play an important role (Frucht *et al.* 2000; Vassella and Fröscher 2004). Among type 1 diabetes patients, 40% are reported to have had at least one hypoglycemic coma or seizure (Jacobson *et al.* 2007). Conversely, seizures as a complication of diabetes in adulthood are reported only occasionally

The Causes of Epilepsy, eds. S. D. Shorvon, F. Andermann, and R. Guerrini. Published by Cambridge University Press. © Cambridge University Press 2011.

in the literature and are certainly much less common than in children or in the rare inherited causes of hypoglycemia such as the hyperinsulinism–hyperammonemia syndrome (Monali *et al.* 2005; Vriesendorp *et al.* 2006; Bahi-Buisson *et al.* 2008). Other endocrinological causes of seizures are mainly related to thyroid and sex hormones. Hypothyroidism may occasionally cause situation-related seizures (Tachman and Guthrie 1984; Bryce and Poyner 1992). There are reports of thyrotoxicosis, or thyroxine intake, inducing seizures (Li Voon Chung *et al.* 2000; Aydin *et al.* 2004). It is generally accepted that estrogen is a pro-convulsant (Scharfman and MacLusky 2006) due to modifying effects both at excitatory and inhibitory central nervous receptor systems (Frye 2008). This may result in catamenial epilepsy. There are no reliable predictors for the course of epilepsies during pregnancy (Zahn *et al.* 1998). With wide variability, increases of the seizure frequency were reported in up to 35%, decreases in up to 22%, but in most instances the seizure frequency remains stable (Steinhoff 2008a). In some women, the menopause appears to be a risk factor for new-onset epilepsies (Abbasi *et al.* 1999). Although there have been case reports of a beneficial effect of hormonal replacement therapy on seizure frequency (Peebles *et al.* 2000), it is usually considered to be a risk factor for increased seizure occurrence which has been emphasized by a recent randomized placebo-controlled trial (Harden 2003; Harden *et al.* 2006; Steinhoff 2008b). The most important metabolic and endocrine precipitants are summarized in Table 92.1.

Metabolic causes of epileptic seizures should always be considered if seizures occur during catabolic states like vomiting and limited food intake during febrile infections. Pathophysiologically, in these situations there may be an endogenous overload with amino acids that cannot be metabolized sufficiently. In other instances alternative pathways via long- and medium-chain fatty acids may be impaired in case of a glucose deficiency, especially if specific impairments of metabolism existed that were previously unknown.

Inborn errors of metabolism usually lead to clinical symptoms some time after birth, but are responsible for prenatally acquired disturbances of organogenesis. Thus, the presence of dysmorphic features should suggest an underlying inborn error of metabolism (Leonard and Morris 2006).

Diagnostic tests

Appropriate diagnostic tests and specific therapeutic consequences are well described elsewhere (Buist *et al.* 2002; Pearl *et al.* 2005; Wolf *et al.* 2005).

Seizure types are rarely specific for certain metabolic disorders, nor for electroencephalogram (EEG) findings (Wolf *et al.* 2005). The most characteristic seizure types are myoclonic seizures and generalized tonic–clonic seizures. Other seizure types are rare. Epilepsia partialis continua is seen with Alpers disease and other mitochondrial disorders (Wolf *et al.* 2005). Generalized tonic–clonic seizures are the most frequent seizure type in situation-related seizures of adulthood that

Table 92.1 Metabolic and endocrine precipitants of epileptic seizures

Energy deficiency

- Hypoglycemia
- GLUT-1 deficiency
- Respiratory chain deficiency
- Creatine deficiency

Disequilibrium of electrolytes

- Hypercalcemia
- Hypocalcemia
- Hypomagnesiemia
- Hyponatremia
- Hypernatremia

  Hypernatremic dehydration

  Iatrogenic hypernatremia

Disturbance of neurotransmitter system

- Non-ketotic hyperglycinemia, γ-aminobutyric acid (GABA) transaminase deficiency, succinic semialdehyde dehydrogenase deficiency

Impaired neuronal function

- Storage disorders

Associated brain malformation

- Peroxisomal disorders, *O*-glycosylation defects

Intoxications

- Endogenous

  Urea cycle defects

  Hepatic encephalopathy

  Hyperammonemia

- Exogenous

  Drugs, chemical, and biological ingredients

Porphyria

Vitamin/co-factor dependency

- Pyridoxine and pyridoxal phosphate dependent epilepsy, folinic-acid-responsive epilepsy, biotinidase deficiency

Eclampsia

Hormonal causes

- Hypothyroidism
- Thyrotoxicosis
- Progesterone

Miscellaneous

- Congenital disorders of glycosylation, serine biosynthesis deficiency, inborn errors of brain excitability (ion channel disorders)

Source: Modified from Vassella and Fröscher (2004), Kurlemann (2004), and Wolf *et al.* (2005).

result from metabolic or endocrine causes. However, in patients with focal epilepsy aggravation of complex partial seizures and non-convulsive status epilepticus due to metabolic reasons are also occasionally described (Steinhoff and Stodieck 1993; Okazaki *et al.* 2007). In addition, de novo non-convulsive status epilepticus in the elderly can be due to metabolic factors (Thomas and Gelisse 2009).

The determination of glucose and electrolytes should be carried out in all patients, as well as prophylactic therapy with vitamin B$_6$ and folate. Pyridoxine-dependent seizures are usually drug-resistant and are instantly and completely suppressed by intravenous infusion of vitamin B$_6$. Early diagnosis and therapy are crucial, since a severe residual encephalopathy can be avoided. Usually the syndrome requires lifelong substitution, and the condition will relapse if vitamin B$_6$ is discontinued. The mean period before the reoccurrence of seizures is 5 days. The reintroduction of vitamin B$_6$ suppresses seizures reliably (Haenggeli *et al.* 1991). Whereas the genetic mechanisms of pyridoxine-sensitive seizures are still not identified, folinic-acid-responsive seizures that usually require substitution with folate (Djukic 2007) have been shown to occur due to α-aminoadipic semialdehyde dehydrogenase deficiency, associated with pathogenic mutations in the *ALDH7A1* gene. Interestingly, recently it was reported that such patients may also benefit from pyridoxine application so that the pragmatic approach to give both pyridoxine and folinic acid was proposed (Gallagher *et al.* 2009). Furthermore, patients are identified whose epileptic seizures were unresponsive to pyridoxine or anticonvulsant drugs but responded to pyridoxal phosphate (Bagci *et al.* 2008).

Some metabolic disorders such as phenylketonuria are routinely identified by screening (Wilcken and Wiley 2008). Specific neurological signs or symptoms, dysmorphic stigmata, or other non-neurological clinical findings can help diagnostically. To assist early diagnosis without unnecessary costs, it is essential to seek advice from an appropriate laboratory on the performance of diagnostic tests (Leonard and Morris 2006). In some instances cerebrospinal fluid, muscle, or skin biopsy is necessary.

Hypoglycemia as a cause of epileptic seizures may be masked by the postictal glucose increase in serum. In suspicious cases, a lumbar puncture may be justified in order to measure the cerebrospinal fluid–serum glucose ratio. Glucose transporter deficiency is suggested if this ratio is below 0.35. Hypoglycemia and hypocalcemia are the most frequent metabolic cause of epileptic seizures in the newborn, and account for 5% of all seizures (Kurlemann 2004). Hypocalcemic seizures should be considered if agitation, carpopedal spasms, or laryngeal spasms are noticed. Not infrequently hyperreflexia is seen.

Along with the intrinsic epileptogenic role of porphyrins, hyponatremia is considered to contribute to the elevated risk of epileptic seizures in porphyria (Solinas and Vajda 2004).

Patients with non-ketotic hyperglycinemia suffer from a severe encephalopathy of the newborn, epileptic seizures that mostly consist of bilateral myoclonic jerks, hiccups, apnea, and marked hypotonia. The underlying cause is a deficiency of the glycine detoxification system, a multienzyme complex at the inner mitochondrial membranes in liver, kidneys, brain, and placenta. Glycine acts as an excitatory neurotransmitter at the *N*-methyl-D-aspartate (NMDA) receptor (Kurlemann 2004).

Sulfite oxidase deficiency syndromes are associated with a severe infantile encephalopathy and may be diagnosed by the detection of sulfite in fresh urine. Whereas patients with isolated sulfite oxidase deficiency show normal uric acid serum levels, uric acid is markedly reduced if the sulfite oxidase deficiency results from a lack of molybdenum pterine complex that affects the xanthine metabolism as well (Kurlemann 2004).

Hypertonic or hypotonic but not isotonic dehydration may cause epileptic seizures. Hypertonic dehydration (sodium serum levels above 145 mmol/L) usually occurs in neonates. Agitation, strident yelling, lethargy, stupor, cramps, tachypnea, and pasty skin are the main clinical symptoms. Hyperglycemia often occurs. Epileptic seizures are often seen during iatrogenic rehydration if this is performed too rapidly and causes brain edema. Hypotonic dehydration (sodium serum levels below 132 mmol/ L) usually leads to more prominent symptoms (lethargy, stupor, coma, or shock symptoms). The most important causes are gastrointestinal loss of water and electrolytes associated with intake of hypotonic solutions, nephropathies, diuretics, and reduced levels of mineralocorticoids.

Dialysis disequilibrium syndrome is caused by brain edema after rapid hemodialysis and may present with headache, nausea, vomiting, cramps, tremor, impaired consciousness, and seizures (Patel *et al.* 2008).

Table 92.2 summarizes briefly the common neurometabolic investigations in patients with epileptic seizures.

Principles of management

Epilepsies that result from metabolic disorders are usually drug-resistant. The underlying disease often does not allow survival into adult life (Steinhoff 2006). A classical example of such a severe underlying disease is neuronal ceroid lipofuscinosis (Kruse *et al.* 2004).

In other instances prompt supplementation, for example with vitamin B$_6$ or folinic acid, may instantly lead to permanent relief and is therefore used routinely in children with ongoing seizures. Patients with a biotinidase deficiency syndrome frequently present seizures alone or with other neurological symptoms or cutaneous findings. They benefit from the replacement of biotine (Wolf *et al.* 1985). Defects of serine biosynthesis require serine supplementation (Wolf *et al.* 2005). In glucose transporter deficiency, the ketogenic diet is the first-line treatment (Boles *et al.* 1999, De Vivo *et al.* 2002). In case of glutaric aciduria type 1 metabolic compensation has to accompany conventional antiepileptic drug treatment (Wolf *et al.* 2005).

Table 92.2 Diagnostic investigation of patients with epileptic seizures and suspected metabolic origin

Indications	In case of progressive encephalopathies, drug-resistant epilepsy of unknown etiology, extrapyramidal movement disorders, muscle hypotonia, external ophthalmoplegia, oculogyral crisis, disturbance of body temperature regulation, hypersalivation
Blood	Blood cell count, blood gas analysis, electrolytes, glucose, ammonium, biotinidase, uric acid, lactate, pyruvate, amino acids including homocysteine, tandem mass spectrometry screening (synchronous detection of aminoacidopathies, disorders of fatty acid oxidation, carnitine metabolism, and organic acidurias); additional determinations in case of hypoglycemia in childhood: β-hydroxybutyrate, free fatty acids, insulin, growth hormone
Urine	Lactate, ketones, amino acids, organic acids, purine, pyrimidine, sulfite test
Cerebrospinal fluid (CSF)	Cell count, protein, lactate, pyruvate, CSF–serum ratio <0.35 in case of GLUT-1 deficiency, CSF–serum ratio >0.6 in case of non-ketotic hyperglycinemia, CSF–serum ration <0.2 in case of serine synthese deficiency, biogene amines and metabolites

Sources: After Kurlemann (2004) and Wolf *et al.* (2005).

Patients with hypertonic dehydration should be cautiously rehydrated to avoid seizures. A rehydration period of 36 to 48 hr with a target sodium level of 135 mmol/L is recommended (Vassella and Fröscher 2004). In hypotonic dehydration, prompt treatment of shock is essential. In seizures caused by hypocalcemia, calcium gluconate is used at a dosage of approximately 1 mg/kg in children (Vassella and Fröscher 2004).

In adults with metabolic or endocrine-induced seizures it is obvious that the underlying cause should be identified and treated if apparent. If not, the exceptional circumstances that were responsible for the situation-related seizure should be avoided thereafter. On the other hand, it is crucial not to rely only on laboratory abnormalities that might explain the seizure. Other potential causes for epilepsy should be ruled out so that early treatment is not delayed.

References

Abbasi F, Krumholz A, Kittner SJ, Langenberg P (1999) Effects of menopause on seizures in women with epilepsy. *Epilepsia* **40**:205–10.

Aydin A, Cemeroglu AP, Baklan B (2004) Thyroxine-induced hypermotor seizure. *Seizure* **13**:61–5.

Bagci S, Zschocke J, Hoffmann GF, *et al.* (2008) Pyridoxal phosphate-dependent neonatal epileptic encephalopathy. *Arch Dis Child Fetal Neonatal ed* **93**:F151–2.

Bahi-Buisson N, Roze E, Dionisi C, *et al.* (2008) Neurological aspects of hyperinsulinism-hyperammonaemia syndrome. *Dev Med Child Neurol* **50**:945–9.

Boles RG, Seashore MR, Mitchell WG, *et al.* (1999) Glucose transporter type 1 deficiency: a study of two cases with video-EEG. *Eur J Pediatr* **158**:978–83.

Bryce GM, Poyner F (1992) Myxoedema presenting with seizures. *Postgrad Med J* **68**:35–6.

Buist NR, Dulac O, Bottiglieri T, *et al.* (2002) Metabolic evaluation of infantile epilepsy: summary recommendations of the Amalfi Group. *J Child Neurol* **17**(Suppl 3):S98–102.

De Vivo DC, Leary L, Wang D (2002) Glucose transporter 1 deficiency syndrome and other glycolytic

defects. *J Child Neurol* **17**(Suppl 3): S15–23.

Djukic A (2007) Folate-responsive neurologic disease. *Pediatr Neurol* **37**:387–97.

Frucht MM, Quigg M, Schwaner C, Fountain NB (2000) Distribution of seizure precipitants among epilepsy syndromes. *Epilepsia* **41**:1534–9.

Frye CA (2008) Hormonal influences on seizures: basic neurobiology. *Int Rev Neurobiol* **83**:27–77.

Gallagher RC, Van Hove JL, Scharer G, *et al.* (2009) Folinic acid-responsive seizures are identical to pyridoxine-dependent epilepsy. *Ann Neurol* **65**:550–6.

Haenggeli CA, Girardin E, Paunier L (1991) Pyridoxine-dependent seizures, clinical and therapeutic aspects. *Eur J Pediatr* **150**:452–5.

Harden CL (2003) Menopause and bone density issues for women with epilepsy. *Neurology* **61**(Suppl 2):S16–22.

Harden CL, Herzog AG, Nikolov BG, *et al.* (2006) Hormone replacement therapy in women with epilepsy: a randomized, double-blind, placebo-controlled study. *Epilepsia* **47**:1447–51.

Hauser WA, Beghi E (2008) First seizure definitions and worldwide incidence and mortality. *Epilepsia* **49**(Suppl 1):8–12.

International League Against Epilepsy (1989) Commission on Classification and Terminology. Proposal for revised classification of epilepsies and epileptic syndromes. *Epilepsia* **30**:389–99.

Jacobson AM, Musen G, Ryan CM, *et al.* (2007) Diabetes Control and Complications Trial/Epidemiology of Diabetes Interventions and Complications Study Research Group. Long-term effect of diabetes and its treatment on cognitive function. *N Engl J Med* **356**:1842–52.

Kruse B, Tuxhorn I, Wörmann F (2004) Symptomatische Epilepsien im Kindesalter. In: Fröscher W, Vassella F, Hufnagel A (eds.) *Die Epilepsien: Grundlagen, Klinik, Behandlung*, 2nd edn. Stuttgart: Schattauer, pp. 60–72.

Kurlemann G (2004) Gezielte Abklärung von Stoffwechseldefekten. In: Fröscher W, Vassella F, Hufnagel A (eds.) *Die Epilepsien: Grundlagen, Klinik, Behandlung*, 2nd edn. Stuttgart: Schattauer, pp. 395–410.

Leonard JV, Morris AA (2006) Diagnosis and early management of inborn errors of metabolism presenting around the time of birth. *Acta Paediatr* **95**:6–14.

Li Voon Chong JS, Lecky BR, Macfarlane IA (2000) Recurrent encephalopathy and generalized seizures associated with relapses of thyrotoxicosis. *Int J Clin Pract* **54**:621–2.

Monami M, Mannucci E, Breschi A, Marchionni N (2005) Seizures as the only clinical manifestation of reactive hypoglycaemia: a case report. *Endocrinol Invest* **28**:940–1.

Okazaki M, Ito M, Kato M (2007) Effects of polydipsia-hyponatremia on seizures in patients with epilepsy. *Psychiatry Clin Neurosci* **61**:330–2.

Patel N, Dalal P, Panesar M (2008) Dialysis disequilibrium syndrome: a narrative revire. *Semin Dial* **21**:493–8.

Pearl PL, Bennett HD, Lhademian Z (2005) Seizures and metabolic disease. *Curr Neurol Neurosci Rep* **5**:127–33.

Scharfman HE, MacLusky NJ (2006) The influence of gondadal hormones on neuronal excitability, seizures, and epilepsy in the female. *Epilepsia* **47**:1423–40.

Solinas C, Vajda FJ (2004) Epilepsy and porphyria: new perspectives. *J Clin Neurosci* **11**:356–61.

Steinhoff BJ (2006) Optimizing therapy of seizures in patients with endocrine disorders. *Neurology* **67**(Suppl):S23–7.

Steinhoff BJ (2008a) Pregnancy, epilepsy and anticonvulsants. *Dialogues Clin Neurosci* **10**:63–75.

Steinhoff BJ (2008b) AED treatment in postmenopausal women. In: Panayiotopoulos CP, Crawford P, Tomson T (eds.) *The Educational Kit on Epilepsies*, vol. **4**. Oxford, UK: Medicinae, pp. 184–8.

Steinhoff BJ, Stodieck SRG (1993) Temporary abolition of seizure activity by flumazenil in a case of valproate-induced non-convulsive status epilepticus. *Seizure* **2**:261–5.

Tachman ML, Guthrie GP Jr. (1984) Hypothyroidism: diversity of presentation. *Endocr Rev* **5**:456–65.

Thomas P, Gelisse P (2009) Non-convulsive status epilepticus. *Rev Neurol (Paris)* **165**:380–9. (In French.)

Vassella F, Fröscher W (2004) Spezielle Syndrome Kurlemann. In: Fröscher W, Vassella F, Hufnagel A (eds.) *Die Epilepsien: Grundlagen, Klinik, Behandlung*, 2nd edn. Stuttgart: Schattauer, pp. 213–23.

Vriesendorp TM, DeVries JH, van Santen S, *et al.* (2006) Evaluation of short-term consequences of hypoglycaemia in an intensive care unit. *Crit Care Med* **34**:2714–18.

Wilcken B, Wiley V (2008) Newborn screening. *Pathology* **40**:104–15.

Wolf B, Heard GS, Weissbecker KA, *et al.* (1985) Biotinidase deficiency: initial clinical features and rapid diagnosis. *Ann Neurol* **18**:614–17.

Wolf NI, Bast T, Surtees R (2005) Epilepsy in inborn errors of metabolism. *Epilepti Disord* **7**:67–81.

Zahn CA, Morrell MJ, Collins SD, Labiner DM, Yerby MS (1998) Management issues for women with epilepsy: a review of the literature. *Neurology* **51**:949–56.

Chapter

93

Electrolyte and sugar disturbances

Bindu Menon and Simon D. Shorvon

Disturbances of electrolytes or sugar are a relatively common precipitant of seizures in clinical practice, and occur in a variety of settings (Castilla-Guerra *et al.* 2006). The risk of a seizure depends on the type of electrolyte disturbance, the cause, the rate at which the normal equilibrium is perturbed, and the degree of the perturbation. Here we will provide a brief overview of the commonest electrolyte disturbances resulting in seizures – those of sodium, glucose, calcium, and magnesium. Disorders of potassium homeostasis also very occasionally result in seizures and will be also briefly mentioned.

A few general points are worth making. Where seizures are precipitated, this is often within the context of an encephalopathy, and associated with other neurological signs such as drowsiness, confusion, headache, and stupor. Encephalopathy is typical of disorders of sodium and osmolality, hypercalcemia, and hypermagnesemia. Conversely hypocalcemia and hypomagnesemia produce neuronal irritability. The electroencephalogram (EEG) has, since its inception in 1937, been well recognized to be affected by hypoglycemia and electrolyte disturbance, but there is little specificity especially in an encephalopathic setting where non-specific slowing progresses to high-voltage delta activity. Although periodic epileptiform discharges, triphasic waves, and other epileptic abnormalities are described in some encephalopathic situations, they are uncommon. The EEG in hypercalcemia is more specific. The seizures themselves can be generalized or less often focal (the latter particularly in non-ketotic hyperglycemia).

The seizures in electrolyte disturbance are generally successfully resolved by reversing the disturbance and do not recur in the longer term unless permanent cerebral damage is caused. They are thus categorized, within an etiological classification, as "seizure precipitants." Treatment should generally focus on reversing the perturbation rather than using antiepileptic drugs, which anyway are often ineffective in the setting of electrolyte disturbance (Table 93.1).

Hyponatremia

Hyponatremia is usually defined as a reduction in plasma sodium concentration below 136 mmol/L (Adrogue and Madias 2000a)

although different institutional laboratories have slightly differing values based on the population means of that institution.

It is a common electrolyte disturbance, affecting 2.5% of hospitalized patients (Anderson *et al.* 1985), but the differential diagnosis and management are often challenging. Sodium is the predominant extracelluar cation and the main determinant of serum osmolality and extracellular fluid volume. The effects of the disturbance on brain function are responsible for the morbidity and mortality in hyponatremia.

Etiology

Hyponatremia is the reflection of excessive total body water relative to total body sodium content. Depending on the plasma osmolality, hyponatremia can be hypovolemic, euvolemic, or hypervolemic. Hypovolemic hyponatremia occurs most commonly in: gastrointestinal losses (diarrhea or vomiting), other losses (for instance with burns), renal losses (for instance with diuretic therapy, mineralocorticoid deficiency, osmotic diuresis, salt-losing nephropathies). Euvolemic hyponatremia occurs most commonly in: Addison disease, hypothyroidism, the syndrome of inappropriate antidiuretic hormone secretion, drug therapy (notably diuretic, oxcarbazepine and carbamazepine, tolbutamide, oxytocin, antidepressants), and primary polydipsia (especially psychogenic polydipsia). Hypervolemic hyponatremia occurs most commonly in: cirrhosis, heart failure, acute and chronic kidney disease, and nephrotic syndrome. In epilepsy practice, chronic hyponatremia due to carbamazepine or oxcarbazepine therapy is by far the most common cause of hyponatremia but is seldom if ever severe enough to cause seizures.

Psychogenic polydipsia is also a notable cause of hyponatremia encountered in neurological clinics. Hyponatremia caused by polydipsia appears to be a risk factor for aggravation of habitual seizures in patients with epilepsy (Okazaki *et al.* 2007).

Pathophysiology

The blood–brain barrier separates the brain from the systemic circulation, and lipid-insoluble substances do not gain entry. The glial cells and the vascular endothelial cells form a tight

---

The Causes of Epilepsy, eds. S. D. Shorvon, F. Andermann, and R. Guerrini. Published by Cambridge University Press. © Cambridge University Press 2011.

Table 93.1 Disturbances of electrolytes and sugar

Electrolyte	Normal values[a]	Condition in which seizures occur	Frequency of seizures[b]	Level at which seizures typically develop[b]
Sodium	136–145 mEq/L	Hyponatremia	29% (acute) 4% (chronic)	<115 mEqL
		Hypernatremia	n/k	>160 mEq/L
Calcium	8.5–10.5 mEq/L	Hypocalcemia	20–25%	5–6 mg/dL
		Hypercalcemia	Uncommon	>13.5 mEq/L
Glucose	126–200 mg/dL	Hypoglycemia	Common	<40 mg/dL
		Hyperglycemia	25%	>600 mg/dL[c]
Magnesium	1.7–2.2 mg/dL	Hypomagnesemia	n/k	<0.8 mEq/L
		Hypermagnesemia	Seizures are very rare	n/a
Potassium	3.5–5.0 mEq/L	Hypokalemia	Seizures are very rare	n/a
		Hyperkalemia	Seizures are very rare	n/a

Notes:
[a] Typical values, but these vary slightly in different institutional laboratories.
[b] These are indicative values only (taken from individual papers cited in the text). Other factors also influence the occurrence of seizures and the levels at which seizures occur such as the rate of change of electrolyte values, the cause of the disturbance, and the clinical setting.
[c] In non-ketotic hyperglycemia.
n/a, data not available; n/k, not known.

junction making the blood–brain barrier a complex entity. The intracellular and extracellular fluids maintain equal osmolality. When plasma osmolality is reduced, the equilibrium is maintained by either intracellular solutes passing out or water from extracellular space passing in and diluting the intracellular solutes (Fraser and Arieff 1997). If the solute extrusion is not adequate, water will continue to enter the brain to maintain equilibrium resulting in increased intracranial pressure and cerebral edema leading to seizures, coma, or death. This edema starts the process of extrusion of intracellular solutes via the Na–K ATPase pump in sodium channels which are the main mechanisms for protecting against cerebral edema and decreasing brain osmolality. After this the brain water content progressively decreases without any change in the brain electrolyte content (Sterns et al. 1989). This is explained by loss of organic osmolytes, which are intracellular, osmotically active solutes that normally contribute substantially to the osmolality of cell water and that do not adversely affect cell functions when their concentrations change. If brain electrolytes were lost without loss of brain organic osmolytes, the increase in brain water content would be much greater (Sterns et al. 1993).

The changes described above can result in acute brain swelling and thus tentorial herniation, and these are risks of acute hyponatremia. The adaptive processes result in the movement of water from the interstitial space to the cerebrospinal fluid and then the systemic circulation, and the egress of osmolytes from cerebral cells. If the decline in sodium is slow, these adaptive processes prevent edema, but in acute hyponatremia and where levels are very low, these processes are overwhelmed (Adrogue and Madias 2000a). The same processes apply (in reverse) on rehydration and again if this is too fast, the osmotic demyelination syndrome occurs resulting in permanent cerebral damage. The seizures in hyponatremia have several mechanisms. In vitro experiments have shown that low osmolarity and decreased Na$^+$ concentration increases neuronal excitability. Furthermore in acute hyponatremia, cerebral edema can cause a decrease in cerebral perfusion pressure. The hypo-osmolar ionic disturbances can increase cellular excitability and facilitate epileptic activity (Schwartzkroin et al. 1998). The rapid correction of serum sodium in chronic hyponatremia can precipitate the osmotic dysmyelination syndrome which can be associated with seizures in 1% of patients (Ellis 1995). This is precipitated because the process of recovery of osmolytes during correction is slower than during loss (Sterns and Silver 2006).

Clinical features

The major symptoms of hyponatremia relate to central nervous system dysfunction, and are much more common in rapid falls in serum sodium or when the levels fall very low. The symptoms are more severe the greater the degree of brain edema. Symptoms include headache, confusion, seizures, weakness, restlessness, nausea, and vomiting. Seizures are a serious development and require urgent attention. The factors responsible for seizures are: the rate of change, the absolute level in serum sodium, and the duration of the abnormal serum sodium levels. Seizures in hyponatremia are most commonly encountered in acute hyponatremia, where the sodium decreases over less than 48 hr, and this reflects the rapidity with which the brain adapts to the reduced osmolality. Convulsions typically occur with serum sodium concentrations of less than 115 mEq/L but if the decrease in sodium is rapid then it may occur at higher serum values (Boggs 1997). In one early study, patients with acute hyponatremia (defined as less than 12 hr duration) had a 29% incidence of seizures and a 50% mortality rate, largely attributable to hyponatremia, whereas patients with chronic hyponatremia (3 or more days in duration) had a 4% incidence of seizures and a 6% mortality rate with no deaths attributable to hyponatremia (Arieff et al. 1976). Children are at particular risk from cerebral edema in hyponatremia as their brain-to-skull ratio is larger (Castilla-Guerra et al. 2006). Gender is also a factor with women said to have a 25-fold higher risk of permanent neurological damage or death from hyponatremia than men (Castilla-Guerra et al. 2006).

Seizures are occasionally the presenting feature in hyponatremia and can be partial or generalized. Grand mal seizures are a typical manifestation of advanced hyponatremia (Fraser and Arieff 1997).

Seizures may sometimes occur iatrogenically due to the too-rapid correction of hyponatremia. Seizures can also be part of a more widespread osmotic demyelination syndrome (previously sometimes known as central pontine or extrapontine myelinolysis) also due to too rapid a correction (Lin and Po 2008), but can occur with as slow an increase in plasma sodium as 8–12 mEq/24 hr (Adrogue and Madias 2000a). The risk of the osmotic demyelination syndrome is also greater in patients with coexisting comorbidities such as liver disease or alcoholism.

Diagnosis

Laboratory tests in all acute seizures should include serum electrolytes and where indicated serum and urine osmolality. Other investigations depend on the underlying cause.

Hyponatremia can also affect the EEG. Low sodium levels (116 mg/dL or lower) initially produce posterior slowing followed by more diffuse delta activity. Other EEG abnormalities that have been recorded include triphasic waves and periodic lateralized epileptiform discharges during the course of recovery from hyponatremia (Ellis and Lee 1977; Itoh et al. 1994).

Treatment

The usual approach to hyponatremia is the replacement of water and sodium in hypovolemic hyponatremia with normal saline, fluid restriction and sometimes a diuretic in hypervolemic hyponatremia, and by the treatment of the cause in euvolemic hyponatremia. Seizures usually are resistant to anticonvulsants.

Urgent intervention is unnecessary if the hyponatremia is slight (>125 mEq/L) and symptoms are mild, or if moderate (110–125 mmol/L) but without clinical symptoms.

If the hyponatremia is severe (<110 mmol/L; effective osmolality <238 mOsm/kg) active therapy is usually needed.

Too rapid a correction of even mild hyponatremia carries the risk of precipitating the osmotic demyelination syndrome. Sodium should be corrected no faster than 0.5 mEq/L/hr in the first few hours of treatment, except in life-threatening severe hyponatremia or where seizures or neurological symptoms are present.

If neurological symptoms are present (e.g., confusion, lethargy, seizures, coma), most recommend that the serum sodium is raised faster, but still at a rate of less than 1 mEq/L/hr (2 mEq/L/hr for the first 2 to 3 hr if seizures are occurring). Hypertonic (3%) saline (containing 513 mEq Na/L) may be occasionally used, under the close supervision of a metabolic team, if seizures are recurrent or intractable. Up to 100 mL/hr of hypertonic saline can be administered over 4 to 6 hr in amounts sufficient to raise the serum sodium 4 to 6 mEq/L (which depends on calculating the total sodium deficit).

In all cases, the rise of sodium should not exceed 10 mEq/L over the first 24 hr to avoid the osmotic demyelination syndrome.

Hypernatremia

Hypernatremia is defined as a serum sodium level exceeding 145 mmol/L, and is much less common than hyponatremia.

Etiology

As with hyponatremia, hypernatremia can be hypovolemic, euvolemic, or hypervolemic. The common causes of hypovolemic hypernatremia include: net water loss due to inadequate water intake, excessive losses of water from the urinary tract (or gastrointestinal loss) or extreme sweating. The commonest cause of euvolemic hypernatremia is diabetes insipidus. The common causes of of hypervolemic hypernatremia are the intake of hypertonic fluid or mineralocorticoid excess (Conn syndrome or Cushing syndrome).

Pathophysiology

The presence of hypernatremia indicates a relative deficit of body water in relation to body sodium content. Thirst is stimulated with plasma sodium concentration above 145 mEq/L, resulting in ingestion of water. Antidiuretic hormone release from hypothalamic osmoreceptors and renal reabsorption prevent further loss of water. These normal physiological responses help bring plasma sodium back to normal. The water moves from the brain intracellular to the extracellular compartment. Excess loss can cause brain shrinkage which can predispose to vascular damage and intracerebral and/or subarachnoid hemorrhage. Cerebral processes then act to restore lost water by gaining solutes. This however does not correct hyperosmolality. Histologically, elevation of the plasma sodium by more than 30 mmol/L in less than 24 hr can lead to cellular necrosis, cerebral demyelinating lesions, and hypoxic ischemic changes in multiple areas of the brain (Arieff and

657

Ayus 1996). The brain shrinkage in severe hyponatremia can be severe and result in rupture of cerebral veins and subarachnoid hemorrhage, which itself can cause seizures.

Clinical features

The major symptoms of hypernatremia are those of encephalopathy. Neurologic signs generally develop with serum sodium concentrations >160 mEq/L (Riggs 1989), but symptoms are more common and more severe when the changes in serum sodium concentration are rapid. Chronic hypernatremia and slow rises in sodium are much more likely to be asymptomatic even to levels in excess of 170 mEq/L. Values above 180 mEq/L are often fatal. Initial symptoms may be anorexia, restlessness, irritability, lethargy, muscle weakness, and nausea. Neurological symptoms include confusion, stupor, coma, and seizures. These require urgent attention. Seizures can also be precipitated iatrogenically if the hypernatremia is corrected too rapidly. Indeed, the most common setting in which convulsions occur in relation to hypernatremia is when a patient is treated with aggressive hypotonic fluids in the setting of prolonged hyperosmolality, which may cause cerebral edema, leading to coma, convulsions, and death. These seizures can be generalized or partial.

Treatment

The aim of therapy is to replace body water and restore osmotic homeostasis and brain volume, but at a rate that does not cause complications. The speed of correction depends on the clinical urgency, and also whether the hypernatremia was acute or chronic. Replacement with hypotonic saline or dextrose is usual, with fluids given orally in non-acute situations. Intravenous fluids can be given in more urgent situations. Plasma sodium concentration should be reduced by 1 mmol/L/hr with acute hypernatremia, but in less urgent situations, the rate of correction should not exceed 0.5 mmol/L/hr (Kahn et al. 1979). Seizures do not require anticonvulsant therapy. Cautious correction of hypernatremia with half-isotonic saline may reduce the likelihood of convulsions occurring during treatment. Because of the risk of brain edema, the volume of infusate should be restricted by the amount required to correct hypertonicity and this can be calculated according to body weight (Adrogue and Madias 2000b).

Hypoglycemia

Abnormalities of glucose levels can cause seizures. As glucose is the only fuel for the brain with minimal storage capacity, the brain is vulnerable to glucose changes. Hypoglycemia is defined arbitrarily as blood glucose of less than 50 mg/dL (2.8 mmol/L) with neuroglycopenic symptoms, or less than 40 mg/dL (2.2 mmol/L) in the absence of symptoms (Carroll et al. 2003). It is a very potent precipitant of seizures (and well recognized for many years, from the earliest days of EEG; Lennox for instance studied EEG changes in epilepsy by inducing hypoglycemia with insulin in his own cousin).

Etiology

The seizures in hypoglycemia usually occur in the setting of diabetes, as a complication of insulin or oral hypoglycemia therapy. However, hypoglycemia also occurs in insulinoma, primary hypothalamic dysfunction, sepsis, severe alcoholism, hypothyroidism, Addison disease, fasting, after gastric surgery, or in terminal cancer. Deliberate or accidental injection of insulin or oral hypoglycemics can also be a cause of hypoglycemic seizures, and cases are sometimes encountered in a forensic setting.

Pathophysiology

Glucose is the primary energy substrate of the brain. In hypoglycemic states, there is initially reversible dysfunction caused by elevated NH3 and depressed γ-aminobutyric acid (GABA) and lactate levels. Irrreversible hypoglycemic brain damage can occur in a pattern similar to that in cerebral hypoxemia, affecting particularly the cerebral cortex, hippocampus, striatum, and cerebellum; and hypoxia and hypoglycemia may cause cerebral damage via common pathways.

Clinical features

The initial symptoms of hypoglycemia include sweating, a feeling of hunger, fatigue, weakness, and tremor, and these can progress to confusion, erratic or bizarre behavior, stupor, coma, and seizures. Hypoglycemic seizures usually occur at serum glucose <40mg/dL. The essential biochemical abnormality is critical lowering of blood glucose. Diabetic children below 6 years of age can have frequent hypoglycemic episodes, with 90% of these episodes manifesting as seizures (Davis et al. 1997). Insulinoma may present with all forms of seizures and with refractory epilepsy (O'Sullivan and Redmond 2005). As with other endocrine disturbances, the rate of fall is important, and chronic hypoglycemia is associated with a much lower rate of seizures. Hypoglycemic seizures can be generalized or focal or take the form of myoclonic attacks.

Hypoglycemia itself can cause erratic behavior, which can be misdiagnosed as seizure activity (Dion et al. 2004; Graves et al. 2004). Typically, though, hypoglycemic attacks are longer-lasting, have a slow prodrome, and take a more bizarre form than epileptic seizures.

Diagnosis

Hypoglycemia needs to be considered in any patient presenting with seizures. The EEG may show increasing slowing of the background while increasing hypoglycemia shows diffuse slowing. Theta frequencies replace alpha frequencies at levels of 50 to 80 mg/dL, but the EEG may show theta and delta activity with intermittent rhythmic delta activity below 40 mg/dL (Davis 1943). Occasionally there may be sharp waves coinciding with seizures. There is not clear-cut correlation between clinical observations, EEG appearance, and biochemical values, and there are marked individual variations.

Treatment

Antiepileptic drugs have no role and treatment should be directed at reversing the hypoglycemia. Treatment is urgent and takes the form of rapid intravenous administration of 50% dextrose. There is no place for slow correction. Antiepileptic drugs are sometimes needed for long-term therapy if hypoglycemic brain damage has occurred and epilepsy is a not infrequent sequel of this.

Hyperglycemia

Elevated levels of blood sugar can cause seizures, although less frequently than low levels. A syndrome in which seizures seem particularly common is non-ketotic hyperosmolar hyperglycemia (NKHH) characterized by severe hyperglycemia, hyperosmolality, and dehydration with minimal or no ketoacidosis. This is a complication of diabetes. The most common presenting symptom is repetitive seizures which can be generalized or focal. One of the authors (BM) sees hyperglycemic seizures in NKHH more commonly than hypoglycemic seizures, and these usually take the form of partial seizures or EPC. Focal seizures in hyperglycemia were first reported in 1965 (Maccario et al. 1965). Seizures are much less common in diabetic keotacidosis with hyperglycemia.

Pathophysiology

Experimental (Chwechter et al. 2003) and human studies (Huang et al. 2008) have suggested that glucose may have a proconvulsant effect. Hippocampal and neocortical neurons also have ATP-sensitive potassium channels which are responsible for increasing neuronal excitability in hyperglycemic environments (Miki and Seino 2005) Further GABA levels decrease thereby lowering the seizure threshold in non-ketotic hyperosmolar states (Guisado and Arieff 1975). Seizures are rare in diabetic ketoacidosis as ketones are available for brain energy utilization and hence GABA levels remain elevated, increasing the threshold for seizure activity. Focal seizures might also be due to underlying focal cerebral ischemia (Singh and Strobos 1980).

Clinical features

Seizures may be the presenting neurological symptom in patients with NKHH. Epilepsia partialis continua and partial motor seizures are the most common form. Epilepsia partialis continua occurs when the serum glucose level is between 600 and 800 mg/dl and in the early stages when the patient is alert (Singh and Strobos 1980). A study has proposed the cut-off point for plasma glucose (>16.11 mmol/L) and plasma osmolarity (>288 mOsm/kg) (Tiamkao et al. 2003). Twenty-five percent of patients with NKHH develop seizures, of which 19% are focal motor seizures, and 6% present with repetitive focal motor seizures as their initial symptom prior to the onset of coma (Singh and Strobos 1980). Seizure clustering and recurrence is more common in diabetic patients than in non-diabetic patients

(Huang et al. 2008). Occasionally patients in NKHH may have focal motor seizures which are reflex or posture-induced as a presenting feature. Status epilepticus (Singh and Strobos 1980; Huang et al. 2005) and occipital seizures with visual phenomenology (Harden et al. 1991) are also not uncommon.

Diagnosis

The diagnosis is made by biochemical measurement. However, magnetic resonance imaging (MRI) is also worthwhile in patients who present with seizures and are diagnosed as having NKHH, as imaging abnormalities may occur (Singh and Strobos 1980) and these can be transient (Raghavendra et al. 2007). The EEG may be normal with mild hyperglycemia. Later fast activity and focal epileptiform discharges may be present (Gibbs et al. 1940). Delta activity may be seen with very low glucose levels.

Treatment

Focal seizures associated with NKHH are refractory to anticonvulsant treatment and respond best to insulin and rehydration. It is advisable to avoid phenytoin because it has been implicated in the precipitation of diabetic ketoacidosis, can exacerbate hyperglycemia in NKHH (Guisado and Arieff 1975), and may even aggravate seizures (Carter et al. 1981). If the diagnosis is made early a complete recovery without sequelae can be expected.

Hypocalcemia

Hypocalcemia is defined as a plasma calcium level of <8.5 mg/dL. Seizures are a prominent feature and hypocalcemia is often a medical emergency.

Etiology

Hypocalcemia can occur in a number of different settings. The most common are: vitamin D deficiency, hypoparathyroidism and pseudohypoparathyroidism, and renal disease. Other causes include: acute pancreatitis, septic shock, iatrogenic causes (notably the enzyme-inducing antiepileptic drugs such as phenytoin and rifampicin), hyperphosphatemia, and magnesium depletion. High calcitonin concentrations do not usually result in hypocalcemia.

Pathophysiology

A homeostatic mechanism to keep the calcium in the normal range requires an integrated action of parathyroid hormone, vitamin D, and, to some extent, calcitonin. There is increased neuromuscular excitability. In case of failure of any of these there will be a sustained fall in calcium. Several theories have been suggested to explain epileptogenesis in hypocalcemia, including neuronal membrane excitability changes, hypertensive encephalopathy, and hypercalcemia-induced vasoconstriction (Kaplan 1998). Mechanisms of epileptogenesis studied in rat models with low calcium show that CA1 of the hippocampus is involved with ephaptic transmission. Hypocalcemia may also lower the excitation threshold for seizures if the patient has pre-existing subclinical epilepsy.

Clinical features

Hypocalcemia is usually symptomatic. The associated signs of congenital hypoparathyroidism or type 1A pseudohypoparathyroidsim may be present. The commonest symptoms are muscle cramps, tetany, skin changes (in chronic hypocalcemia), and seizures. Hyperreflexia and Chvostek and Trousseau signs may be present. Seizures occur at calcium levels between 5–6 mg/dL. Hypocalcemia much more commonly results in seizures than hypercalcemia. Hypocalcemic seizures are typically generalized, but partial motor or sensory seizures occur in 20% of patients and atypical absence seizures are also reported. Focal seizures are said not necessarily to correlate with localized cerebral abnormalities. Hypomagnesemia and hypokalemia are common in hypocalcemia (Boggs 1997). Absence status has been described but is rare (Vignaendra and Frank 1977). Seizures may be the presentation in the emergency department in 20–25% of patients presenting with hypocalcemia (Gupta 1989) and in 30–70% of patients with symptomatic hypoparathyroidism, usually with tetany, altered mental status, and hypocalcemia.

Diagnosis

The diagnosis is by biochemical estimations. The differentiation of conditions causing abnormal vitamin D, parathyroid hormone, and calcitonin levels is outside the scope of this book, and can be complex requiring careful assessment.

Electroencephalographic abnormalities can occur and revert back to normal after calcium is restored. Severe hypercalcemia shows EEG slowing and generalized spike burst. Paroxysmal epileptiform discharges are noted in hypocalcemia-induced seizures (Glaser and Levy 1959).

Treatment

In the acute situation, with seizures, treatment of hypocalcemia should be immediate to reduce the associated morbidity and mortality (Desai et al. 1988). Parenteral therapy with intravenous calcium gluconate can rapidly relieve symptoms and provide time for the underlying cause to be evaluated and treated definitively. In chronic hypocalcemia, especially in the absence of seizures, correction of the underlying cause and supplementation with calcium, vitamin D, or vitamin D analogs may be sufficient depending on the clinical setting.

Hypercalcemia

Hypercalcemia is defined as total serum calcium concentration >10.5 mEq/L (2.6 mmol/L). It is much more common than hypocalcemia in clinical practice, but seizures are a less prominent symptom.

Etiology

Hypercalcemia is usually caused by abnormally high bone reabsorption, and there are many causes of this including: primary hyperparathyroidism, malignancy, granulomatous disease, acute and chronic renal failure, immobilization, vitamin D or A toxicity, and hyperthyroidism. It can also result from excessive calcium absorption such as in sarcoidosis and other granulomatous diseases, or milk-alkali syndrome. It can also result from drug therapy with such drugs as lithium, theophylline, and thiazides, and from other endocrine disturbances such as Addison disease, hypothyroidism, and Cushing disease or from the rare genetic syndrome of familial hypocalcuric hypercalcemia.

Clinical features and pathophysiology

Patients are often asymptomatic in mild hypercalcemia. Symptoms, when they do occur, are initially predominantly gastrointestinal: constipation, vomiting, anorexia, abdominal pain, ileus. Severe hypercalcemia may then cause neurological symptoms including confusion, delirium, psychosis, stupor, and coma. Other symptoms include muscle weakness and renal stones. Severe hypercalcemia (>13.5 mEq/L) can cause seizures though these are uncommon. Seizures can very rarely also occur in chronic hypercalcemia (Bauermeister et al. 1967; Hauser et al. 1989). A "parathyroid storm" can present with acute seizures and coma (Sallman et al. 1981). Focal seizures have been ascribed to clotting of small blood vessels within the brain (Bauermeister et al. 1967). Hypercalcemic hypertensive encephalopathy and vasoconstriction may be a cause of seizures (Chen et al. 2004). Seizures can also occur as part of the posterior reversible encephalopathy syndrome, which can be associated with hypercalcemia.

Diagnosis

The diagnosis is by biochemical measurement and these may include (depending on cause): serum calcium, parathyroid hormone, phosphate, alkaline phosphatase, other electrolytes, urea, and protein immunoelectrophoresis. Imaging may be needed diagnostically. The EEG shows theta activity, fast activity, and bursts of delta and theta slowing which are seen at calcium levels about 13 mg/100 mL, with spikes and sharp waves. With further rises in calcium levels, there may be increased background frontal slowing, paroxysmal theta/delta bursts, and triphasic waves (Moore 1967; Allen et al. 1970; Swash and Rowan 1972; Nagashima and Kupota 1981).

Treatment

Acute treatment includes rapid hydration (at a rate between 200 and 5000 mL/hr) and the use of intravenous hypocalcemic agents such as bisphosphonates. Once rehydration has been achieved, furosemide 40 mg is usually given. In chronic hypercalcemia, treatment is usually directed at the underlying cause though oral bisphosphonates can be given.

Hypomagnesemia

Hypomagnesemia occurs when the serum magnesium level falls below 1.2 mEq/L. The incidence of magnesium deficiency in intensive care unit patients is 20–65% and this is a common electrolyte disturbance in hospitalized patients (Reinhart and Desbine 1985; Ryzen et al. 1985). The serum magnesium level does not necessarily reflect the whole body level as only 2% of body magnesium is extracellular, and concentrations also vary from organ to organ. Magnesium deficiency is often associated with calcium deficiency and the symptomatology can reflect a combination of both deficiencies.

Etiology

The usual causes are: dietary deficiency, perturbations of calcium metabolism, drug-induced deficiencies, primary hypomagnesemia, stress hypomagnesemia, alcoholism, renal disease, parathyroid disease, pregnancy (pre-eclampsia/eclampsia), gastrointestinal disease (diarrhea or small-bowel bypass), diabetic ketoacidosis, and various congenital and genetic inborn errors of metabolism.

Clinical features

The common symptoms are very similar to those of hypocalcemia. These include: anorexia, vomiting, lethargy, weakness, and personality change. As with hypocalcemia, Chvostek and Trousseau signs can occur. Neurological signs develop particularly when there is associated hypocalcemia. Severe hypomagnesemia can result in generalized tonic–clonic or multifocal seizures, especially in children and in critically ill patients. Seizures and other neurologic symptoms are typically encountered when the serum magnesium concentration falls to <0.8 mEq/L (Riggs 2002). Chronic magnesium deficiency is also recorded as a rare cause of intractable seizures (Nuytten et al. 1991). Seizures also release catecholamines, which in turn lower the magnesium level, so a low magnesium level in the setting of acute seizures can be the result as well as the cause of the seizures.

Treatment

Rapid correction of magnesium levels with intravenous magnesium salt solutions are needed if seizures are present (Fishman 1965). The usual therapy is with 50% magnesium sulfate which contains 1 g/2 mL. It is usual to give 2–4 g over 5–10 min and then repeat this if seizures persist up to a total of 10 g over the next 6 hr. Slow intravenous bolus can be given if renal function is normal

Hypermagnesemia

Hypermagnesemia does not cause seizures. The usual cause is renal failure, and the symptoms are those of hypotension and respiratory and cardiac depression. Treatment is calcium gluconate and hemodialysis may be required.

Hypokalemia

The normal serum potassium level is between 3.5 and 5.0 mEq/L, varying slightly between laboratories. Hypokalemia is a very rare cause of seizures.

Etiology

There are many causes of a low potassium level, but the most common are vomiting, diarrhea, Cushing syndrome, or laxative or diuretic therapy. Other causes include Fanconi syndrome, hypomagnesemia, hyperthyroidism, insulin, and some drug therapies (including terbulatine and theophylline).

Clinical features

The commonest features are muscle weakness, cramps and twitches, and abnormalities of cardiac rhythm. Very rarely seizures and other neurological signs develop, but these are not a major feature and when seizures do occur these are either with very low potassium levels or related to comorbidities or other electrolyte disturbances. The lack of seizures is surprising, considering the importance of potassium channels in cerebral function and the fact that rare genetically determined epilepsies are due to potassium channel defects.

Treatment

Usually therapy with oral potassium supplements is sufficient. In very severe hypokalemia, including hypokalemia complicated by seizures, intravenous potassium should be given.

Hyperkalemia

Hyperkalemia does not cause seizures. The usual causes are increased ingestion of potassium, renal disease, severe burns, diabetes, or metabolic acidosis. The major risk is of cardiac arrhythmia. Very severe hyperkalemia is treated with calcium, insulin, and glucose, and by dialysis.

References

Adrogue HJ, Madias NE (2000a) Hyponatremia. *N Engl J Med* **342**:1493–9.

Adrogue HJ, Madias NE (2000b) Hypernatremia. *N Engl J Med* **342**:1581–9.

Allen EM, Singer FR, Melamed D (1970) Electroencephalographic abnormalities in hypercalcemia. *Neurology* **20**:15–22.

Anderson RJ, Chung HM, Kluge R, Schrier RW (1985) Hyponatremia: a prospective analysis of its epidemiology and the pathogenetic role of vasopressin. *Ann Intern Med* **102**:164–8.

Arieff AI, Ayus JC (1996) Pathogenesis and management of hypernatremia. *Curr Opin Crit Care* **2**:405–82.

Arieff AI, Llach F, Massry SG (1976) Neurological manifestations and morbidity of hyponatremia: correlation with brain water and electrolytes. *Medicine (Baltimore)* **55**:121–9.

Bauermeister DE, Jennings ER, Cruse DR, Sedgwick Vde M (1967) Hypercalcemia with seizures: a clinical paradox. *J Am Med Ass* **201**:132.

Boggs JG (1997) Seizures in medically complex patients. *Epilepsia* **38**(Suppl 4): S55–9.

Carroll MF, Burge MR, Schade DS (2003) Severe hypoglycemia in adults. *Revi Endocr Metab Disord* **4**:149–57.

Carter BL, Small RE, Mandell MD, Starkman MY (1981) Phenytoin induced hyperglycemia. *Am J Hosp Pharm* **38**:1508–12.

Castilla-Guerra L, del Carmen Fernandez-Moreno M, Lopes-Chozas JM, Fernandez-Bolanos R (2006) Electrolyes disturbances and seizures. *Epilepsia* **47**:1990–8.

Chen TH, Huang CC, Chang YY, *et al.* (2004) Vasoconstriction as etiology of hypercalcemia-induced seizures. *Epilepsia* **45**:551–4.

Chwechter EM, Veliskova J, Velisek L (2003) Correlation between extracellular glucose and seizure susceptibility in adult rats. *Ann Neurol* **53**:91–101.

Davis EA, Keating B, Byrne GC, Russell M, Jones TW (1997) Hypoglycemia: incidence and clinical predictors in a large population based sample of children and adolescents with IDDM. *Diabetes Care* **20**:22–5.

Davis PA (1943) Effect on the electroencephalogram of changing the blood sugar level. *Arch Neurol Psychiatr* **49**:186–94.

Desai TK, Carlson RW, Geheb MA (1988) Prevalence and clinical implications of hypocalcemia in acutely ill patients in a medical intensive care setting. *Am J Med* **84**:209–14.

Dion MH, Cossette P, St-Hilaire JM, Rasio E, Nguyen DK (2004) Insulinoma misdiagnosed as intractable epilepsy. *Neurology* **62**:1443–5.

Ellis JM, Lee SI (1977) Acute prolonged confusion in later life as an ictal state. *Epilepsia* **19**:119–28.

Ellis SJ (1995) Severe hyponatremia: complications and treatment. *Q J Med* **88**:905–9.

Fishman RA (1965) Neurological aspects of magnesium metabolism. *Arch Neurol* **12**:562–9.

Fraser CL, Arieff AI (1997) Epidemiology, pathophysiology, and management of hyponatremic encephalopathy. *Am J Med* **102**:67–77.

Gibbs FA, Williams D, Gibbs EL (1940) Modification of the cortical frequency spectrum by changes in CO_2, blood sugar and O_2. *J Clin Neurophysiol* **3**:49–58.

Glaser G, Levy LL (1959) Seizures and idiopathic hypoparathyroidism: a clinical–electroencephalographic study. *Epilepsia* **1**:454–65.

Graves TD, Gandhi S, Smith SJ, Sisodiya SM, Conway GS (2004) Misdiagnosis of seizures: insulinoma presenting as adult-onset seizure disorder. *J Neurol Neurosurg Psychiatry* **75**:1091–2.

Guisado R, Arieff A (1975) Neurologic manifestations of diabetic comas: correlation with biochemical alterations in the brain. *Metabolism* **24**:665–79.

Gupta MM (1989) Medical emergencies associated with disorders of calcium homeostasis. *J Ass Physicians India* **37**:629–31.

Harden CL, Rosenbaum DH, Daras M (1991) Hyperglycemia presenting with occipital seizures. *Epilepsia* **32**:215–20.

Huang CW, Hsieh YJ, Pai MC, Tsai JJ, Huang CC (2005) Non-ketotic hyperglycemia-related epilepsia partialis continua with ictal unilateral parietal hyperperfusion. *Epilepsia* **46**:1843–4.

Huang CW, Tsai JJ, Ou HY, *et al.* (2008) Diabetic hyperglycemia is associated with the severity of epileptic seizures in adults. *Epilepsy Res* **79**:71–7.

Hauser GJ, Gale AD, Fields AI (1989) Immobilization hypercalcemia: an unusual presentation with seizures. *Pediatr Emerg Care* **5**:105–7.

Kahn A, Bracket E, Blum D (1979) Controlled fall in natremia and risk of seizures in hypertonic dehydration. *Intens Care Med* **5**:27–31.

Kaplan PW (1998) Reversible hypercalcemia cerebral vasoconstriction with seizures and blindness: a paradigm for eclampsia? *Clin Electroencephalogr* **29**:120–3.

Lin CM, Po HL (2008) Extrapontine myelinolysis after correction of hyponatremia presenting as generalized tonic seizures. *Am J Emerg Med* **26**:632–6.

Maccario M, Messis CP, Vastola F (1965) Focal seizures as a manifestation of hyperglycemia without ketoacidosis. *Neurology* **15**:195–206.

Miki T, Seino S (2005) Roles of K ATP channels as metabolic sensors in acute metabolic changes. *J Mol Cell Cardiol* **38**:917–25.

Moore JMB (1967) The electroencephalogram in hypercalcemia. *Arch Neurol* **17**:34–51.

Nagashima C, Kupota S (1981) Parathyroid epilepsy with continuous EEG abnormalities. *Clin Electroencephalogr* **12**:133–8.

Nuytten D, Van Hees J, Meulemans A, Carton H (1991) Magnesium deficiency as a cause of acute intractable seizures. *J Neurol* **238**:262–4.

Okazaki M, Ito M, Kato M (2007) Effects of polydipsia–hyponatremia on seizures in patients with epilepsy. *Psychiatry Clin Neurosci* **61**:330–2.

O'Sullivan SS, Redmond J (2005) Insulinoma presenting as refractory late-onset epilepsy. *Epilepsia.* **46**:1690–1.

Raghavendra S, Ashalatha R, Thomas SV, Kesavadas C (2007) Focal neuronal loss, reversible subcortical focal T2 hypointensity in seizures with a nonketotic hyperglycemic hyperosmolar state. *Neuroradiology* **49**:299–305.

Reinhart RA, Desbine NA (1985) Hypomagnesemia in patients entering the ICU population. *Crit Care Med* **13**:506–7.

Riggs J (1989) Neurologic manifestations of fluid and electrolyte disturbances. *Neurol Clin* **7**:509–23.

Riggs J (2002) Neurologic manifestations of fluid and electrolyte disturbances. *Neurol Clin* **20**:227–39.

Ryzen E, Wagers PW, Singer FR, Rude RK (1985) Magnesium deficiency in a medical ICU population. *Crit Care Med* **13**:19–21.

Sallman A, Goldberg M, Wombolt D (1981) Secondary hyperparathyroidism manifesting as acute pancreatitis and status epilepticus. *Arch Intern Med* **141**:1549–50.

Schwartzkroin PA, Baraban SC, Hochman DW (1998) Osmolarity, ionic flux, and changes in brain excitability. *Epilepsy Res* **32**:275–85.

Singh BM, Strobos RJ (1980) Epilepsia partialis continua associated with nonketotic hyperglycaemia: clinical and biochemical profile of 21 patients. *Ann Neurol* **8**:155–60.

Sterns RH, Silver SM (2006) Brain volume regulation in response to hypo-osmolality and its correction. *Am J Med* **119**(Suppl 1):S12–16.

Sterns RH, Thomas DJ, Herndon RM (1989) Brain dehydration and neurologic deterioration after rapid correction of hyponatremia. *Kidney Int* **35**:69–75.

Sterns RH, Baer J, Ebersole S, *et al.* (1993) Organic osmolytes in acute hyponatremia. *Am J Physiol* **264**:F833–6.

Swash M, Rowan J (1972) Electroencephalographic criteria of

hypocalcemia and hypercalcemia. *Arch Neurol* **26**:218–28.

Tiamkao S, Pratipanawatr T, Tiamkao S, *et al.* (2003) Seizure in nonketotic hyperglycemic. *Seizure* **12**:409–10.

Vignaendra V, Frank AO (1977) Absence status in a patient with hypocalcemia. *Electroencephalogr Clin Neurophysiol* **43**:429–33.

Chapter

Drug-induced seizures

94

Aidan Neligan

Drug-induced seizures can arise in the setting of acute drug withdrawal or drug toxicity, or as a consequence of medication use for acute illness in patients with no prior history of seizures. Seizure exacerbation can also occur in people with a prior history of epilepsy as a result of the addition of an antiepileptic medication that exacerbates seizure control or by medication that alters the metabolism of antiepileptic medications.

To establish a causative association between a drug exposure and a subsequent seizure several conditions have been proposed (Ruffmann *et al.* 2006):

(1) Temporal relationship: the timing of the drug exposure must precede the seizure with the probability of causation stronger the shorter the time interval between the two events.

(2) Strength: the risk of subsequent seizures is higher in those with the drug exposure compared to non-exposed individuals, and the higher the difference in the exposure the stronger the association.

(3) Consistency: the effect (seizures) should be reproducible in different populations and under different conditions.

(4) Biological gradient: the risk of seizures should be demonstrably increased at increasing doses.

(5) Biological plausibility: a plausible biological mechanism should exist for the drug exposure and seizure induction.

While many drugs in overdose can cause seizures, as evidenced by the large number of single case reports of drug-induced seizures or status epilepticus, we will focus only on drugs shown consistently to increase the risk of seizures.

Epidemiology

It is difficult to assess accurately the incidence of drug-induced seizures as most reports are retrospective studies from single institutions and large epidemiological studies focusing on the problem are lacking. In a series of 32 812 consecutively monitored medical inpatients, none of whom had identified risk factors for seizures, 26 (0.8 per 1000) had drug-induced seizures with the most common causes being intravenous penicillin (5), insulin (4), and lignocaine (4) (Porter and Jick 1977).

A previous report from the same group found that drug-induced seizures occurred in 17 of 12 617 medical patients (1.3 per 1000) with the principal identified causes being the same as in the later study (Boston Collaborative Surveillance Program 1972). In a 10-year period, 53 cases of drug-induced seizures were identified, accounting for 1.7% of all seizures (out of 3155 cases) in San Francisco. Of the identified cases, half (27) were as a result of suicide attempts (27), 18 were as a result of intoxication from prescribed medication, and six cases were as a result of recreational drug abuse. All but two of the seizures were generalized and eight were episodes of status epilepticus. Isoniazid (10) and psychotropic drugs (15) were the most commonly identified precipitants, which were also the commonly used drugs in suicide attempts (Messing *et al.* 1984). In a retrospective review of all cases of new-onset generalized seizures presenting to the emergency department of a New York hospital over a 4-year period, 17 of 279 cases (6.1%) were felt to be drug-related with cocaine intoxication (35%), benzodiazepine withdrawal (29%), and bupropion (24%) the major causes (Pesola and Avasarala 2002).

The incidence of acute symptomatic seizures as a result of drug toxicity in Rochester (Minnesota) between 1935 and 1984 was 2.2 per 100 000 with the highest rates in those aged ≥75 years. Commonly cited causes were carbon monoxide poisoning and acetylsalicyclic acid overdose (Annegers *et al.* 1995).

In a retrospective hospital review of patients admitted with a diagnosis of status epilepticus over a 10-year period, 12 of the 67 cases with no prior history of epilepsy were due to drug toxicity, of which the causative drugs were cocaine (6), theophylline (3), amphetamine (2), isoniazid (2), and isoetharine (1) (Lowenstein and Alldredge 1993). In contrast in a prospective population-based study of status epilepticus, the number of cases of status epilepticus due to drug toxicity was less then 5% (DeLorenzo *et al.* 1996).

The Causes of Epilepsy, eds. S. D. Shorvon, F. Andermann, and R. Guerrini. Published by Cambridge University Press. © Cambridge University Press 2011.

Table 94.1 Commonly cited epileptogenic drugs

Analgesics

Meperidine

Tramadol

Anesthetics

Lignocaine

Propofol

Sevoflurane

Antidepressants

Clomipramine

Amitriptyline (TCAs)

Imipramine

Maprotiline

Amoxapine

Bupropion

Antipsychotics

Clozapine

Olanzapine

Quetiapine

Phenothiazines (chlorpromazine)

Lithium

Drugs of abuse

Cocaine

Amphetamines

Phencyclidine (PCP)

MDMA ("ecstasy")

Chemotherapeutics/immunosuppressants

Cyclosporin

Chlorambucil

Iphosphamide

Busulphan

Antiepileptic drugs

Phenytoin

Carbamazepine

Gabapentin

Lamotrigine

Tiagabine

Vigabatrin

Respiratory drugs

Isoniazid

Theophylline

Anitbacterials

Penicillins (IV)

Mefloquine

Imipenem–cilastatin

Ciprofloxacin

Antivirals

Zidovudine

Withdrawal

Benzodiazepines

Barbiturates

Baclofen

Alcohol

Miscellaneous

Iodinated contrast media

A retrospective review of all cases referred to the California poison center over a 2-year period (1988–1989) identified 191 cases of drug-induced seizures with cyclic antidepressants (tricyclic antidepressants [TCAs], amoxapine, fluoxetine) (29%), cocaine and other stimulants (29%), diphenhydramine and other antihistamines (7%), and theophylline and isoniazid (5%) each being the main causes (Olson *et al.* 1994). Comparison with figures from 1981 showed a significant increase in the proportion of seizures caused by cocaine (29% vs. 4%). A further review was carried out at the same center in 2003 of all cases of drug- or poison-induced seizures, affording an opportunity to examine the changing epidemiology of drug-induced seizures over time from the same geographical region (Thundiyil *et al.* 2007). Of 529 identified cases associated with seizures, 386 were felt to be drug-related of which the leading causes were bupropion (23%), diphenhydramine (8.3%), TCAs (7.7%), tramadol (7.5%), amphetamines (6.9%), isoniazid and venlaflaxine (5.9% each), cocaine (4.9%), various antipsychotics (4.7%), MDMA ("ecstasy") (3.4%), and other antidepressants (excluding bupropion and the TCAs) (9.3%). Attempted suicide was the cause of 65.5% of cases and 14.8% were due to drug abuse while only 9.6% of cases were the result of accidental or unintentional overdose. The majority of cases resulted in a single seizure (68.6%) while 3.6% presented with status epilepticus.

When compared with the previous study (Olson *et al.* 1994), there was a statistically significant decrease in seizures caused by TCAs even though there was an increase in antidepressant-induced seizures overall. There was a decreasing trend in stimulant-induced seizures, and this was particularly marked for cocaine-induced seizures. There were no cases of theophylline-induced seizures (Thundiyil *et al.* 2007).

Table 94.2 A mnemonic for causes of drug- and toxin-induced seizures

OTIS CAMPBELL
Organophosphates
Tricyclic antidepressants
Isoniazid, **I**nsulin
Sympathomimetics
Cocaine, **C**lozapine
Amphetamines, **A**ntiepileptics
Methylxanthines (theophylline, caffeine)
Phencyclidine (PCP)
Benzodiazepine/**B**arbiturate withdrawal
Ethanol withdrawal
Lidocaine
Lithium

Psychotropic medications

Psychotropic medications, namely the antidepressants, the antipsychotics, and mood stabilizers, have long been recognized as being potentially epileptogenic and as such have been subject to several reviews (Rosenstein *et al.* 1993; Pisani *et al.* 2002; Lee *et al.* 2003). It has been long recognized that the antidepressants cause drug-induced seizures by lowering seizure threshold particularly at supratherapeutic levels (Swinkels *et al.* 2005). Because of this, many physicians are reluctant to use antidepressant medication in people with epilepsy. This is unfortunate as the risk is low and psychiatric comorbidities are common in people with epilepsy (Gaitatzis *et al.* 2004), leading some to hypothesize a common biochemical pathophysiology for epilepsy and depression (Kanner 2006). It should also be borne in mind that the protection inferred by antiepileptic medication is much greater then the potential epileptogenic effect of psychotropic medication.

Antidepressants

Seizures have been reported to occur in 0.1% to approximately 1.5% of patients treated at therapeutic doses of the most common antidepressants and antipsychotics, with the incidence of seizures increasing to 4% up to 30% in overdose (Pisani *et al.* 2002). While knowledge of the relative risk of seizures with individual drugs in overdose is important, it is of far greater importance to know the relative risks of seizure at commonly used therapeutic doses. The most commonly implicated drugs are the TCAs clomipramine, maprotiline, amoxapine and bupropion. In contrast the selective serotonin reuptake inhibitors (SSRIs) appear to have low epileptogenic potential. However caution must be applied when interpreting reports of high seizure incidence with antidepressants as many

are based on small sample sizes with much smaller incidence rates seen with larger sample sizes (Pisani *et al.* 1999).

In a retrospective review there was a 0.1% incidence of seizures with imipramine and a 0% incidence with amitriptyline at a daily dose of ≤200 mg, increasing to 0.6% and 0.06% respectively at higher doses (Peck *et al.* 1983). Similarly in a prospective study of 1704 patients on either imipramine, amitriptyline, or doxepin the incidence of seizures was 0.0–0.7% (Jick *et al.* 1983).

While a risk of 0.4% of seizures (25 of 6100 patients) was reported in clinical trials with maprotiline, a second-generation tetracyclic antidepressant, only 229 seizures were noted with 920 000 prescriptions in the UK (0.025% per month exposure) with seizures more common with doses >150 mg/day (Dessain *et al.* 1986). In a 3-year retrospective review of 1313 cases of overdose with cyclic antidepressants at the Maryland Poison Center, seizures were more common with amoxapine (24.5%) and maprotiline (12.2%) compared with other TCAs (3.0%) or trazaodone (0%) (Wedin *et al.* 1986).

The proconvulsant potential of maprotiline is thought to be due to its strong lipophilic activity leading to high levels in the central nervous system with selective blockage of noradrenaline reuptake (Baumann and Maitre 1979). A dose-related risk of seizures is also associated with clomipramine, a tertiary TCA. In 4160 patients with clomipramine there was a 0.5% incidence of seizures, increasing to 1.66% with daily doses >250 mg (Rosenstein *et al.* 1993). It also seems that seizures are more common in patients with obsessive compulsive disorder treated with clomipramine then with patients with depression (DeVeaugh-Geiss *et al.* 1992). Compared to other drugs, overdose with TCAs is associated with high mortality (Olson *et al.* 1994).

Bupropion, a monocyclic inhibitor of dopamine, which is an antidepressant and smoking cessation drug, has been shown to have a clear dose-related risk of seizures with a seizure incidence of 0.4% at doses ≤450 mg/day, increasing to 2.2% at doses >450 mg/day in 4262 patients treated with bupropion (Davidson 1989). Seizures occurred in 15% of 2424 intentional overdoses with bupropion compared with less then 1% in unintentional exposures (Belson and Kelley 2002).

The SSRIs appear to have low epileptogenic potential even in overdose. Of the four cases of fluoxetine-associated seizures in the series by Olson *et al.* (1994), all occurred with co-ingestion of other potentially proconvulsant medication. Indeed no seizures occurred in a series of 234 cases of fluoxetine overdose (Borys *et al.* 1992).

Alper *et al.* reviewed the data from all Food and Drug Administration (FDA) phase II and III trials in the USA between 1985 and 2004 involving a total of 75 873 patients treated with psychotropic medication to determine the seizure incidence in psychopharmacological clinical trials (Alper *et al.* 2007). The authors calculated the standardized incidence ratio (SIR) for each drug and class of drugs. The SIR = 1 if the number of observed seizures with the active drug was equal to that seen with placebo. Within each class of drugs (antidepressants, anti-anxiety, antipsychotics) the drugs were subdivided into two categories (groups I and II) to denote high and low seizure incidence. The antidepressant group included bupropion IR (intermediate release) (group I), and citalopram, fluoxetine, venlaflaxine, bupropion SR (slow release), paroxetine, nefazadone, mirtazapine, escitalopram, duloxetine, and sertraline. The SIR for all the antidepressants was 0.48 (95% confidence interval [CI] 0–36–0.61) implying that the seizure incidence was lower relative to placebo. The SIR decreased further to 0.31 (95% CI 0.21–0.43) with the exclusion of bupropion IR. Bupropion IR was the only antidepressant associated with a significantly increased risk of seizures with an SIR of 1.58 (95% CI 1.03–2.32) (26 seizures with 4419 exposures).

Such findings imply that contrary to commonly held perceptions the antidepressants are broadly anticonvulsant rather then proconvulsant. It is possible that some patients may have been on antiepileptic medication (either for a pre-existing diagnosis or as mood stabilizers) thus contributing to the lower then expected frequency of seizures. However this is unlikely to account for the total anticonvulsant effect. Such findings are supported by the fact that fluoxetine has been shown to enhance the anticonvulsant potency of several antiepileptic drugs through selective metabolic inhibition of the cytochrome P450 (CYP450) system (Leander 1992; Favale *et al.* 1995; Lee *et al.* 2003).

It should be noted that there was a relatively high rate of seizures in the placebo groups for all psychotropic medication trials, which suggests that psychiatric illness is itself associated with increased seizure risk.

Antipsychotics

The risk of seizures with the typical antipsychotics was recognized early following the advent of the phenothiazine chlorpromazine in the 1950s. In a follow-up study over 4.5 years of 859 patients without epilepsy treated with phenothiazines, spontaneous seizures occurred in 10 patients (1.2%) (seven with chlorpromazine, one each with trifluoperazine, thioridazine, and prochlorperazine). All but one of the seizures on chlorpromazine occurred at daily doses $\geq$1000 mg giving a seizure incidence of 0.5% and 9% for <1000 mg/day and $\geq$1000 mg/day (Logothetis 1967).

Clozapine, an atypical antipsychotic, demonstrates a clear dose-related risk of seizures, and has the highest risk of drug-induced of all the antipsychotic medications. In 1418 patients treated with clozapine over a 16-year period, seizures occurred in 41 (2.9%), with a cumulative risk of seizures of 10% at 3 years. The seizure frequency was 4.4% in patients on $\geq$600 mg/day, 2.7% with a dose of 1.6% 300–599 mg/day, and 1% on <300 mg/day (Devinsky *et al.* 1991). In the first 6-month post-marketing phase seizures occurred in 71 (1.3%) of 5629 patients treated with clozapine. Seizure incidence was 1.9% with doses $\geq$600 mg/day, 0.8% with 300–599 mg/day, and 1.6% with <300 mg/day. When patients with a previous

history of seizures were excluded (16), the seizure frequencies were 0.9% (<300 mg/day), 0.8% (300–599 mg/day), and 1.5% ($\geq$600 mg/day) (Pacia and Devinsky 1994). It is postulated that the epileptogenic potential of clozapine may be due to its relatively weak antidopaminergic action combined with its selectivity for mesolimbic and reduced affinity for striatal dopamine receptors (Baldessarini and Frankenburg 1991).

An increased risk of seizures has also been reported with olanzapine and quetiapine.

In premarketing studies of olanzapine, the seizure frequency was 0.9% (22/2500) and several cases reports of seizures with olanzapine have been reported including one case of fatal status epilepticus (Wyderski *et al.* 1999). Similarly in the premarketing data on quetiapine, seizures occurred in 0.8% (18/2387). In a 5-year retrospective of all cases of acute quetiapine overdose reported to the California Poison Center, 945 cases of quetiapine overdoes were identified, of whom seizures occurred in 22 patients (2%), which was similar to the number of seizures caused by overdose of all other antipsychotics seen during the same time period (22 /744, 2%) (Ngo *et al.* 2008).

Alper *et al.* (2007) found that the antipsychotics were associated with a significantly increased incidence of seizures (SIR = 2.05, 95% CI 1.74–2.40), which remained significant following the exclusion of clozapine (SIR = 1.35, 95% CI 1.09–1.66) but was not significant following the exclusion of both clozapine and olanzapine, (SIR = 1.18, 95% CI 0.92–1.49). Of all psychotropic drugs, clozapine was associated with the highest seizure incidence (61/1742) (SIR = 9.50, 95% CI 7.27–12.20). Both olanzapine (23/2500) and quetiapine (18/2387) were also associated with an increased risk of seizures (SIR = 2.50, 95% CI 1.58–3.74 and SIR = 2.05, 95% CI 1.21–3.23 respectively). In contrast the other antipsychotics (ziprasidone, aripiprazole, and risperidone), as a group, were not associated with a significantly increased incidence of seizures.

Other psychotropic drugs

Seizures with lithium intoxication are common particularly when levels exceed 3.0 mEq/L although seizures have been reported in patients on lithium at therapeutic levels. The Obsessive Compulsive Disorder treatment group was associated with increased seizures (SIR = 2.55, 95% CI 0.74–2.51) but not after clomipramine was excluded from the analysis (SIR = 1.44, 95% CI 0.74–2.51). Clomipramine was associated with a significantly increased incidence of seizures (25/3519) (SIR = 4.08, 95% CI 2.64–6.02) (Alper *et al.* 2007).

Antibiotics

Seizures have been reported with several classes of antibiotics particularly the penicillins, the cephalosporins, the carbapanems (β-lactam antibiotics), and the fluoroquinolones. It appears that seizures induced by all antibiotics are the result of binding (direct or indirect antagonism) to γ-aminobutyric acid (GABA) GABA$_A$ receptors (Wallace 1997).

In the Boston Collaboration study, seizures occurred in 4 out of 1245 (0.32%) patients given intravenous penicillins, with no seizures occurring in 2398 patients who received oral or intramuscular penicillin or its derivatives (Porter and Jick 1977). In a multicenter randomized controlled trial of intravenous ciprofloxacin versus imipenem–cilastatin (an carbapenem antibiotic given with cilastin to prevent nephrotoxicity) for the treatment of severe pneumonia, seizures occurred in 1% (3/202) of those on ciprofloxacin, with the seizure occurring >1 week after the drug was discontinued in 2/3 patients. In contrast seizures occurred in 6% (11/200) of patients on imipenem, all of which occurred during active treatment (Fink et al. 1994).

In several large surveillance studies examining the incidence of seizures on imipenem/cilastatin seizure frequency appears to be much lower, varying between 0.2% and 0.9% (Ruffmann et al. 2006).

In experimental models the most potent proconvulsant antibiotics were cefazolin, benzylpenicillin, ceftezole, and aztreonam (DeSarro et al. 1989).

Identified risk factors for antibiotic-induced seizures are: age extremes, renal insufficiency, previous seizures or central nervous system deficit, cardiopulmonary bypass surgery, and sepsis or bacterial endocarditis. The risk is also determined by mode of administration with high-dose antibiotics given intravenously or intrathecally carrying a high risk and oral or intramuscularly administered antibiotics a very low risk. Co-administration with other drugs, namely other antibiotics, theophylline, cilastatin, and non-steroidal anti-inflammatories (with the fluoroquinolones), increases the risk (Franson et al. 1995; Wallace 1997).

Tramadol

Tramadol is a centrally acting analgesic which is a weak μ-opioid receptor agonist and also inhibits serotonin and noradrenaline reuptake (Potschka et al. 2000). While seizures have been reported with tramadol at therapeutic doses, seizures are much commoner at supratherapeutic levels (Kahn et al. 1997). In a retrospective multicenter site review of tramadol overdoses over a 2.5-year period, 190 cases were identified. Seizures occurred in 13.7%. The dose associated with seizures was 200 mg with 84.6% of seizures occurring within 6 hr of taking tramadol. On analysis the risk of seizures was higher in males, chronic use, suicide attempts or intentional abuse, and tachycardia (Marquardt et al. 2005). In a prospective study of all cases of tramadol overdose reported to seven poison centers over a 10-month period, 87 cases of tramadol overdose (alone) were identified. Seizures occurred in seven (8%) with the lowest dosage associated with seizures being 500 mg (Spiller et al. 1997).

Isoniazid

Isoniazid, an antituberculosis treatment, is a common cause of drug-induced seizures, particularly in intentional overdose (Messing et al. 1984). The metabolite of isoniazid inhibits pyridoxine phosphokinase causing pyridoxine (vitamin B_6) deficiency, the activated form of which is required for the formation of GABA (by the conversion of glutamic acid by glutamic acid decarboxylase). Seizures caused by isoniazid are believed to be due to reduced levels of GABA (Wills and Erickson 2006). In a retrospective study of all cases of isoniazid poisoning in a single center over a 5-year period, 52 of the 270 cases identified were reviewed, all of whom were associated with seizures. Given that <20% of cases of isoniazid poisoning were reviewed, it is clear that isoniazid poisoning does not inevitably lead to seizures. It does however underline the high potential of seizures in cases of isoniazid overdose (Panganiban et al. 2001). Isoniazid has a narrow therapeutic range with a recommended dose of 5 mg/kg in adults and 10 to 15 mg/kg in children, and problems can arise particularly in children due to inadvertent overdosing (Rubin et al. 1983; Wallace 1997). Isoniazid-induced seizures should be treated with a gram-to-gram equivalent of intravenous pyridoxine to the isoniazid digested, particularly as isoniazid-induced status epilepticus is particularly difficult to treat with conventional antiepileptic regimens (Wallace 1997).

Theophylline

Theophylline is well recognized as a cause of seizures and status epilepticus in both intentional and accidental overdoses. In a literature review of cases of theophylline overdose over a 12-year period, 399 cases were identified in whom seizures occurred in 99 (25%), of which 33 occurred as a result of intentional overdose and 66 in iatrogenic toxicity. For those with theophylline overdose, only one patient had seizures with a serum concentration less than 60 mg/L, with the mean peak and baseline serum level being 138 mg/L and 119 mg/L respectively. In contrast the mean theophylline serum level in 21 patients with iatrogenic toxicity was 45 mg/L (Paloucek and Rodvold 1988). The tendency of seizures to occur at much lower serum levels in chronic overmedication compared to acute overdose was also noted by Olson et al. (1985). While most theophylline-related seizures occur as a result of high toxic levels, seizures can occur at therapeutic levels (10–20 mg/L) or low toxic, particularly in children and the elderly on theophylline therapy (Franson et al. 1995). In a series of 12 patients (mean age 67.2 years) who experienced seizures while taking theophylline, serum levels ranged between 14 and 35 mg/L; seven of these developed focal or generalized status epilepticus, leading the authors to recommend that theophylline should be maintained at serum levels of 10–15 mg/L particularly in the elderly and those with previous central nervous system disease (Bahls et al. 1991). Theophylline-induced seizures may be related to its antagonism at the adenosine receptor but also possibly to inhibition of GABA and depletion of pyridoxine (Wills and Erickson 2006).

Intravenous contrast media

Seizures have been reported in patients after intravenous iodinated contrast media while undergoing radiological examination. In a series of 15 226 patients undergoing cranial computed tomography (CT), 29 had medium-induced seizures, giving an incidence of 0.19%, all of which were brief in duration with no episodes of status epilepticus. There was a previous history of seizures in 22/29 and 15/29 (52%) had evidence of an enhancing intracranial mass while a further 8/29 (28%) had focal intracranial pathologies, suggesting that medium-induced seizures occur primarily in patients with an identifiable epileptic focus. All seizures were brief and easily controlled with no episodes of status epilepticus (Nelson et al. 1989). Similarly in the series of 1418 patients studied by Scott (1980), seven (0.49%) had seizures following administration of intravenous contrast medium. Five of these had no prior history of seizures and CT revealed evidence of intracranial foci in five patients. While no cases of status epilepticus were reported in either of these series, it is possible that subtle cases of convulsive status epilepticus or non-convulsive status epilepticus, which has been reported following intravenous contrast administration (Lukovits et al. 1996), may have been missed.

Other drugs

Seizures have been reported with the anesthetic agents propofol, sevolfurane and lidocaine (Ruffmann et al. 2006). Propofol, which acts on the $GABA_A$ receptors and is used in the treatment of refractory status epilepticus, has also been associated with seizures with the majority occurring during the induction of or withdrawal from anesthesia (Walder et al. 2002). The chemotherapy agent chlorambucil has been reported to cause seizures in children while the immunosuppressant cyclosporine and interferon-α have also been associated with seizures (Ruffmann et al. 2006).

Seizures can occur in the setting of drug withdrawal, in particular with benzodiazepines and barbiturates, and also baclofen. Baclofen, which acts on the $GABA_A$ receptor, has also been reported to cause non-convulsive status epilepticus (Zak et al. 1994).

A list of drugs commonly associated with status epilepticus are listed in Table 94.3.

Cocaine and other stimulants

Reational drugs can cause seizures, in particular cocaine and the stimulants like amphetamines and phencyclidine. In a review of 49 cases of recreational drug-induced seizures seen over a 12-year period, cocaine (predominantly intranasal and intravenous) was implicated in 32 (65%), amphetamine (predominantly intravenous) in 11 (22%), heroin in 7 (14%), and phencyclidine in 4 (8%). All seizures were generalized. These were single episodes in 36 (74%), multiple seizures in 7 (14%), and status epilepticus in 2 (4%). Almost all patients (48/49,

Table 94.3 Drugs most commonly associated with status epilepticus

Antiepileptic drugs	Respiratory drugs
Carbamazepine	Isoniazid
Lamotrigine	Theophylline
Tiagabine[a]	
Sodium valproate (toxicity)	
Vigabatrin	**Miscellaneous**
	Baclofen
Antibiotics (cephalosporins)	Flumazenil
Cefepime[a]	Lithium[a]
Ceftazidime[a]	
Chemotherapeutic agents	
Ifosfamide[a]	
Cisplatin	
Tacrolimus	

Note:
[a]Most commonly associated with non-convulsive status epilepticus.

98%) left hospital without any neurological sequelae, while one patient who had intranasal-cocaine-induced status epilepticus had mild neurological deficits on discharge (Alldredge et al. 1989).

In a retrospective review of 474 patients seen with complications due to acute cocaine intoxication, 403 had no prior history of seizures, of whom 32 (7.9%) had experienced an acute seizure within 90 min of cocaine use. Seizures were almost three times as common in women, with black women (23.7%) having the highest frequency of cocaine-induced seizures. Seizures most commonly occurred following intravenous or crack cocaine administration, compared to nasally inhaled cocaine, possibly due to higher serum and brain levels.

In the 73 patients with a history of non-cocaine-related seizures, seizures occurred in 12 (16.9%) within 90 min of cocaine administration, which were similar in semiology to the previous episode in all but one case (Pascual-Leone et al. 1990).

In a retrospective review of all emergency department and hospital admissions over a 2-year period, 1900 admissions were related to complications of cocaine use, and 58 patients (3%) had seizures, with crack cocaine (36) being the most commonly implicated mode of administration. Of these 14 (24%) had a prior history of non-cocaine-related seizures while another 17 (33%) had other identifiable seizure risk factors. Similarly 6% of 844 admissions for epilepsy or seizures were cocaine-related (Koppel et al. 1996). The risk of cocaine-induced is highest with rapid methods of administration (i.e., intravenous and crack cocaine) which appears to be mediated by cocaine's effect on serotonin (5-HT) transmission (O'Dell et al. 2000).

Phencyclidine

Acute intoxication with phencyclidine (PCP, "angel dust"), whose effects are mediated by antagonism at the N-methyl-d-aspartate (NMDA) receptor, is characterized by significant behavioral problems, aggression, hallucinations, and psychosis in addition to physical signs like hyperthermia, hypertension, nystagmus, rhabdomyolsis, and seizures (Wills and Erickson 2006). In a prospective study of 1000 cases of phencyclidine intoxication, generalized seizures occurred in 26 (2.6%) and status epilepticus in another five (0.5%) (McCarron et al. 1981).

Antiepileptic medication and worsening seizures

It has long been recognized that the addition of a new anti-epileptic drug (AED) may lead to a paradoxical increase in seizures, the appearance of new seizure types, or even status epilepticus, and this topic has been the subject of several reviews (Bauer 1996; Perucca et al. 1998; Somerville 2002; Chaves and Sander 2005). In some cases, it is difficult to establish whether the addition of a new AED is really the cause of worsening seizures, as the seizures may represent the natural course of the epilepsy in the face of an ineffective medication. Moreover many episodes of seizure exacerbation occur in the context of the addition of a new AED with the simultaneous withdrawal of another AED, which may be the real cause of the exacerbation.

Seizure aggravation following an AED may be a non-specific manifestation of drug intoxication/overdose or AED-induced encephalopathy, or it may be specific to the particular AED, for example as an inappropriate choice in the context of a particular epileptic syndrome or seizure type. Deterioration in seizure control or the appearance of a new seizure type may also be a paradoxical effect of an AED which is usually effective and an appropriate choice for that seizure type or epileptic syndrome.

The older AEDs particularly, have been most commonly associated with paradoxical increase in seizures as a result of toxicity. This is particularly true of phenytoin which because of non-linear pharmacokinetics is at higher risk of inadvertent toxicity. Levy and Fenichel (1965) classically described three cases of phenytoin encephalopathy associated with increased seizures, changing seizure semiology, and associated hemiparesis which all resolved upon discontinuation of phenytoin. Indeed increase in seizure frequency may be the only clinical manifestation of toxicity (Troupin and Ojemann 1975). Intoxication with AEDs may also manifest as both convulsive and non-convulsive status epilepticus. Reports of seizure aggravation or AED-induced status epilepticus have been reported with most AEDs, for example carbamazepine (Stommel et al. 1992; Neufeld 1993), valproate with which increasing seizures may be a sign of underlying hepatic toxicity (Eeg-Olofsson and Lindskog 1982; Konig et al. 1994), lamotrigine (Trinka et al. 2002; Dinnerstein et al. 2007,

pregabalin (Knake et al. 2007), and levetiracetam (Nakken et al. 2003; Pustorino et al. 2007);

Tiagabine, which blocks the reuptake of GABA into neurons and glial cells, has been implicated in the causation of status epilepticus (Kellinghaus et al. 2002), particularly non-convulsive status epilepticus, even in patients without a prior diagnosis of epilepsy (Jette et al. 2006; Vollmar and Noachtar 2007). It has been postulated that non-convulsive status epilepticus caused by tiagabine may be due to complete inhibition of GABA reuptake at high doses leading to GABA depletion in the presynaptic neurons (Trinka et al. 1999).

A review of clinical trial data provided by the manufacturers of three new AEDs (tiagabine, topiramate, and levetiracetam) has been carried out to determine whether a paradoxical increase in seizure frequency was more likely on an AED compared to placebo. Analysis demonstrated that the addition of tiagabine, levetiracetam, or topiramate did not lead to an increase in seizures compared to placebo. Indeed an increase in seizure frequency was significantly less likely to occur in patients taking topiramate or levetiracetam compared to placebo. A doubling of seizure frequency was more likely with patients taking placebo but this did not reach statistical significance (Somerville 2002). Indeed in a review of the safety data of tiagabine from clinical trials, the authors concluded that treatment with tiagabine at recommended doses did not increase the risk of status epilepticus in patients with partial seizures (Shinnar et al. 2001).

Seizure aggravation as a specific drug effect

The risk of exacerbation of seizures due to the addition of a new AED underlines the importance of syndromic classification, for many cases occur specifically in the idiopathic generalized epilepsies. Both carbamazepine and less frequently phenytoin have been shown to potentially increase seizures in the idiopathic generalized epilepsies, particularly in childhood absence epilepsy and juvenile myoclonic epilepsy (Perucca et al. 1998; Chaves and Sander 2005). In a retrospective analysis of patients with juvenile myoclonic epilepsy, carbamazepine exacerbated seizures in 68% (65% without phenytoin) and phenytoin exacerbated seizures in 38% (29% without carbamazepine) (Genton et al. 2000). Osorio et al. (2000) reported a series of patients with idiopathic generalized epilepsy of which absence seizures were a component who presented in absence status epilepticus. In patients being treated with either phenytoin or carbamazepine at the time of status, absence status epilepticus proved more refractory to standard treatment (intravenous high-dose benzodiazepines) compared to cases of patients not on either carbamazepine or phenytoin. The authors concluded that the presence of carbamazepine or phenytoin was the primary cause of the refractory absence status epilepticus which was only controlled following the withdrawal of carbamazepine or phenytoin.

Treatment with an inappropriate agent in idiopathic generalized epilepsy may result in absence status epilepticus or myoclonic status epilepticus, often with atypical features. In a retrospective review of all patients (14) with idiopathic generalized epilepsy, misclassified as either having cryptogenic partial epilepsy or unclassified generalized epilepsy who developed video-documented status epilepticus over an 8-year period, all were taking at least potentially aggravating AEDs (all were on carbamazepine with 50% on polytherapy with either phenytoin, vigabatrin, or gabapentin). The final correct diagnosis were juvenile absence epilepsy in six, juvenile myoclonic epilepsy in four, epilepsy with grand mal on awakening in two, and childhood absence epilepsy in two. Five patients developed typical absence status epilepticus, five developed atypical absence status epilepticus, and four developed myoclonic status epilepticus (one with typical and three with atypical features). Identified potential aggravating causes were the initiation of carbamazepine, vigabatrin, or gabapentin, increase in carbamazepine or phenytoin, and the reduction of the dose of phenobarbital. The status epilepticus was brought under control following removal of the precipitating agent (Thomas *et al.* 2006).

Carbamazepine-induced seizure aggravation has also been reported with patients with atonic seizures, benign idiopathic partial epilepsy, and unspecified seizure types (Perucca *et al.* 1998). Seizure aggravation and status epilepticus has been reported in children with Lennox–Gastaut syndrome treated with benzodiazepines (clonazepam, clobazam, or intravenous diazepam) (Tassinari *et al.* 1972; Chaves and Sander 2005).

Vigabatrin like other GABAergic agents (tiagabine and gabapentin) can exacerbate seizures in idiopathic generalized epilepsy, particularly absence and myoclonic seizures (Perucca *et al.* 1998).

Oxcarbazepine, like carbamazepine, has been shown to cause an increase in seizure frequency or appearance of new seizure types and should be avoided in idiopathic generalized eplilepsy (Gelisse *et al.* 2004).

Valproate is rarely associated with seizure aggravation except in the context of valproate-induced encephalopathy. Despite being the treatment of choice, valproate has been reported with the worsening of absence seizures in a small group of children (Lerman-Sagie *et al.* 2001). Levetiracetam has occasionally been associated with seizure exacerbation (Nakken *et al.* 2003; Chaves and Sander 2005), and also has been associated with the appearance of de novo drop attacks in one patient after starting the drug (Chaves and Sander 2005).

In a review of 21 patients with severe myoclonic epilepsy of infancy (Dravet syndrome) treatment with lamotrigine resulted in seizure deterioration in 80% (17) with 33% having an increase in myoclonic seizures (Guerrini *et al.* 1998). Lamotrigine has also been associated with the development of myoclonic status epilepticus in a girl with Lennox–Gastaut syndrome at high doses after initial seizure improvement on lower doses (Guerrini *et al.* 1999). Lamotrigine has also been reported to worsen seizures and induce negative myoclonus in a patient with idiopathic rolandic epilepsy (Cerminara *et al.* 2004). Lamotrigine may also cause worsening of myoclonic seizures in patients with juvenile myoclonic epilepsy (Chaves and Sander 2005).

References

Alldredge BK, Lowenstein DH, Simon RP (1989) Seizures associated with recreational drug abuse. *Neurology* **39**:1037–9.

Alper K, Schwartz KA, Kolts RL, *et al.* (2007) Seizure incidence in psychopharmacological clinical trials: an analysis of Food and Drug Administration (FDA) summary basis of approval reports. *Biol Psychiatry* **62**:345–54.

Annegers JF, Hauser WA, Lee JR, *et al.* (1995) Incidence of acute symptomatic seizures in Rochester, Minnesota, 1935–1984. *Epilepsia* **36**:327–33.

Bahls FH, Ma KK, Bird TD (1991) Theophylline-associated seizures with "therapeutic" or low toxic serum concentrations: risk factors for serious outcome in adults. *Neurology* **41**:1309–12.

Baldessarini RJ, Frankenburg FR (1991) Clozapine: a novel antipsychotic agent. *N Engl J Med* **324**:746–54.

Bauer J (1996) Seizure-inducing effects of antiepileptic drugs: a review. *Acta Neurol Scand* **94**:367–77.

Baumann PA, Maitre L (1979) Neurobiochemical aspects of maprotiline (Ludiomil) action. *J Int Med Res* **7**:391–400.

Belson MG, Kelley TR (2002) Bupropion exposures: clinical manifestations and medical outcome. *J Emerg Med* **23**: 223–30.

Borys DJ, Setzer SC, Ling LJ, *et al.* (1992) Acute fluoxetine overdose: a report of 234 cases. *Am J Emerg Med* **10**:115–20.

Boston Collaborative Surveillance Program (1972) Drug-induced convulsions. *Lancet* **2**:677–9.

Cerminara C, Montanaro ML, Curatolo P, *et al.* (2004). Lamotrigine-induced seizure aggravation and negative myoclonus in idiopathic rolandic epilepsy. *Neurology* **63**:373–5.

Chaves J, Sander JW (2005) Seizure aggravation in idiopathic generalized epilepsies. *Epilepsia* **46** Suppl **9**: 133–9.

Davidson J (1989) Seizures and bupropion: a review. *J Clin Psychiatry* **50**:256–61.

DeLorenzo RJ, Hauser WA, Towne AR, *et al.* (1996) A prospective, population-based epidemiologic study of status epilepticus in Richmond, Virginia. *Neurology* **46**:1029–35.

DeSarro A, De Sarro GB, Ascioti C, *et al.* (1989) Epileptogenic activity of some beta-lactam derivatives: structure–activity relationship. *Neuropharmacology* **28**: 359–65.

Dessain EC, Schatzberg AF, Woods BT, *et al.* (1986) Maprotiline treatment in depression: a perspective on seizures. *Arch Gen Psychiatry* **43**:86–90.

DeVeaugh-Geiss J, Moroz G, Biederman J, *et al.* (1992) Clomipramine hydrochloride in childhood and adolescent obsessive–compulsive disorder: a multicenter trial. *J Am Acad Child Adolesc Psychiatry* **31**:45–9.

Devinsky O, Honigfeld G, Patin J (1991) Clozapine-related seizures. *Neurology* **41**:369–71.

Dinnerstein E, Jobst BC, Williamson PD (2007) Lamotrigine intoxication provoking status epilepticus in an adult with localization-related epilepsy. *Arch Neurol* **64**:1344–6.

Eeg-Olofsson O, Lindskog U (1982) Acute intoxication with valproate. *Lancet* 1:1306.

Favale E, Rubino V, Mainardi P, *et al.* (1995) Anticonvulsant effect of fluoxetine in humans. *Neurology* 45:1926–7.

Fink MP, Snydman DR, Niederman MS, *et al.* (1994) Treatment of severe pneumonia in hospitalized patients: results of a multicenter, randomized, double-blind trial comparing intravenous ciprofloxacin with imipenem-cilastatin. *Antimicrob Agents Chemother* 38:547–57.

Franson KL, Hay DP, Neppe V, *et al.* (1995) Drug-induced seizures in the elderly: causative agents and optimal management. *Drugs Aging* 7:38–48.

Gaitatzis A, Trimble MR, Sander JW (2004) The psychiatric comorbidity of epilepsy. *Acta Neurol Scand* 110:207–20.

Gelisse P, Genton P, Kuate C, *et al.* (2004) Worsening of seizures by oxcarbazepine in juvenile idiopathic generalized epilepsies. *Epilepsia* 45:1282–6.

Genton P, Gelisse P, Thomas P, *et al.* (2000) Do carbamazepine and phenytoin aggravate juvenile myoclonic epilepsy? *Neurology* 55:1106–9.

Guerrini R, Belmonte A, Parmeggiani L, *et al.* (1999) Myoclonic status epilepticus following high-dosage lamotrigine therapy. *Brain Dev* 21:420–4.

Guerrini R, Dravet C, Genton P, *et al.* (1998) Lamotrigine and seizure aggravation in severe myoclonic epilepsy. *Epilepsia* 39:508–12.

Jette N, Cappell J, VanPassel L, *et al.* (2006) Tiagabine-induced nonconvulsive status epilepticus in an adolescent without epilepsy. *Neurology* 67:1514–15.

Jick H, Dinan BJ, Hunter JR, *et al.* (1983) Tricyclic antidepressants and convulsions. *J Clin Psychopharmacol* 3:182–5.

Kahn LH, Alderfer RJ, Graham DJ (1997) Seizures reported with tramadol. *J Am Med Ass* 278:1661.

Kanner AM (2006) Epilepsy, suicidal behavior, and depression: do they share common pathogenic mechanisms? *Lancet Neurol* 5:107–8.

Kellinghaus C, Dziewas R, Ludemann P (2002) Tiagabine-related non-convulsive status epilepticus in partial epilepsy: three case reports and a review of the literature. *Seizure* 11:243–9.

Knake S, Klein KM, Hattemer K, *et al.* (2007) Pregabalin-induced generalized myoclonic status epilepticus in patients with chronic pain. *Epilepsy Behav* 11:471–3.

Konig SA, Siemes H, Blaker F, *et al.* (1994) Severe hepatotoxicity during valproate therapy: an update and report of eight new fatalities. *Epilepsia* 35:1005–15.

Koppel BS, Samkoff L, Daras M (1996) Relation of cocaine use to seizures and epilepsy. *Epilepsia* 37:875–8.

Leander JD (1992) Fluoxetine, a selective serotonin-uptake inhibitor, enhances the anticonvulsant effects of phenytoin, carbamazepine, and ameltolide (LY201116). *Epilepsia* 33:573–6.

Lee KC, Finley PR, Alldredge BK (2003) Risk of seizures associated with psychotropic medications: emphasis on new drugs and new findings. *Expert Opin Drug Saf* 2:233–47.

Lerman-Sagie T, Watemberg N, Kramer U, *et al.* (2001) Absence seizures aggravated by valproic acid. *Epilepsia* 42:941–3.

Levy LL, Fenichel GM (1965) Diphenylhydantoin activated seizures. *Neurology* 15:716–22.

Logothetis J (1967) Spontaneous epileptic seizures and electroencephalographic changes in the course of phenothiazine therapy. *Neurology* 17:869–77.

Lowenstein DH, Alldredge BK (1993) Status epilepticus at an urban public hospital in the 1980s. *Neurology* 43:483–8.

Lukovits TG, Fadul CE, Pipas JM, *et al.* (1996) Nonconvulsive status epilepticus after intravenous contrast medium administration. *Epilepsia* 37:1117–20.

Marquardt KA, Alsop JA, Albertson TE (2005) Tramadol exposures reported to statewide poison control system. *Ann Pharmacother* 39:1039–44.

McCarron MM, Schulze BW, Thompson GA, *et al.* (1981) Acute phencyclidine intoxication: incidence of clinical findings in 1000 cases. *Ann Emerg Med* 10:237–42.

Messing RO, Closson RG, Simon RP (1984) Drug-induced seizures: a 10-year experience. *Neurology* 34:1582–6.

Nakken KO, Eriksson AS, Lossius R, *et al.* (2003) A paradoxical effect of levetiracetam may be seen in both children and adults with refractory epilepsy. *Seizure* 12:42–6.

Nelson M, Bartlett RJ, Lamb JT (1989) Seizures after intravenous contrast media for cranial computed tomography. *J Neurol Neurosurg Psychiatry* 52:1170–5.

Neufeld MY (1993) Exacerbation of focal seizures due to carbamazepine treatment in an adult patient. *Clin Neuropharmacol* 16:359–61.

Ngo A, Ciranni M, Olson KR (2008) Acute quetiapine overdose in adults: a 5-year retrospective case series. *Ann Emerg Med* 52:541–7.

O'Dell LE, Kreifeldt MJ, George FR, *et al.* (2000) The role of serotonin(2) receptors in mediating cocaine-induced convulsions. *Pharmacol Biochem Behav* 65:677–81.

Olson KR, Benowitz NL, Woo OF, *et al.* (1985) Theophylline overdose: acute single ingestion versus chronic repeated overmedication. *Am J Emerg Med* 3:386–94.

Olson KR, Kearney TE, Dyer JE, *et al.* (1994) Seizures associated with poisoning and drug overdose. *Am J Emerg Med* 12:392–5.

Osorio I, Reed RC, Peltzer JN (2000) Refractory idiopathic absence status epilepticus: a probable paradoxical effect of phenytoin and carbamazepine. *Epilepsia* 41:887–94.

Pacia SV, Devinsky O (1994) Clozapine-related seizures: experience with 5629 patients. *Neurology* 44:2247–9.

Paloucek FP, Rodvold KA (1988) Evaluation of theophylline overdoses and toxicities. *Ann Emerg Med* 17:135–44.

Panganiban LR, Makalinao IR, Corte-Maramba NP (2001) Rhabdomyolysis in isoniazid poisoning. *J Toxicol Clin Toxicol* 39:143–51.

Pascual-Leone A, Dhuna A, Altafullah I, *et al.* (1990) Cocaine-induced seizures. *Neurology* 40:404–7.

Peck AW, Stern WC, Watkinson C (1983) Incidence of seizures during treatment with tricyclic antidepressant drugs and bupropion. *J Clin Psychiatry* 44:197–201.

Perucca E, Gram L, Avanzini G, *et al.* (1998) Antiepileptic drugs as a cause of worsening seizures. *Epilepsia* 39:5–17.

Pesola GR, Avasarala J (2002) Bupropion seizure proportion among new-onset generalized seizures and drug related seizures presenting to an emergency department. *J Emerg Med* 22:235–9.

Pisani F, Oteri G, Costa C, *et al.* (2002) Effects of psychotropic drugs on seizure threshold. *Drug Saf* 25:91–110.

Pisani F, Spina E, Oteri G (1999) Antidepressant drugs and seizure susceptibility: from in vitro data to clinical practice. *Epilepsia* **40** (Suppl 10): S48–56.

Porter J, Jick H (1977) Drug-induced anaphylaxis, convulsions, deafness, and extrapyramidal symptoms. *Lancet* **1**:587–8.

Potschka H, Friderichs E, Loscher W (2000) Anticonvulsant and proconvulsant effects of tramadol, its enantiomers and its M1 metabolite in the rat kindling model of epilepsy. *Br J Pharmacol* **131**:203–12.

Pustorino G, Spano M, Sgro DL, et al. (2007) Status gelasticus associated with levetiracetam as add-on treatment. *Epilept Disord* **9**:186–9.

Rosenstein DL, Nelson JC, Jacobs SC (1993) Seizures associated with antidepressants: a review. *J Clin Psychiatry* **54**:289–99.

Rubin DH, Carbone J, Fong B, et al. (1983) Chronic isoniazid poisoning: case report and recommendations for usage of the drug. *Clin Pediatr (Philadelphia)* **22**:518–19.

Ruffmann C, Bogliun G, Beghi E (2006) Epileptogenic drugs: a systematic review. *Expert Rev Neurother* **6**:575–89.

Scott WR (1980) Seizures: a reaction to contrast media for computed tomography of the brain. *Radiology* **137**:359–61.

Shinnar S, Berg AT, Treiman DM, et al. (2001) Status epilepticus and tiagabine therapy: review of safety data and epidemiologic comparisons. *Epilepsia* **42**:372–9.

Somerville ER (2002) Aggravation of partial seizures by antiepileptic drugs: is there evidence from clinical trials? *Neurology* **59**:79–83.

Spiller HA, Gorman SE, Villalobos D, et al. (1997) Prospective multicenter evaluation of tramadol exposure. *J Toxicol Clin Toxicol* **35**:361–4.

Stommel EW, Bihler J, Swenson R, et al. (1992) Carbamazepine encephalopathy. *Neurology* **42**:705.

Swinkels WA, Kuyk J, van Dyck R et al. (2005) Psychiatric comorbidity in epilepsy. *Epilepsy Behav* **7**:37–50.

Tassinari CA, Dravet C, Roger J, et al. (1972) Tonic status epilepticus precipitated by intravenous benzodiazepine in five patients with Lennox–Gastaut syndrome. *Epilepsia* **13**:421–35.

Thomas P, Valton L, Genton P (2006) Absence and myoclonic status epilepticus precipitated by antiepileptic drugs in idiopathic generalized epilepsy. *Brain* **129**:1281–92.

Thundiyil JG, Kearney TE, Olson KR (2007) Evolving epidemiology of drug-induced seizures reported to a Poison Control Center System. *J Med Toxicol* **3**:15–19.

Trinka E, Moroder T, Nagler M, et al. (1999) Clinical and EEG findings in complex partial status epilepticus with tiagabine. *Seizure* **8**:41–4.

Trinka E, Dilitz E, Unterberger I, et al. (2002) Non-convulsive status epilepticus after replacement of valproate with lamotrigine. *J Neurol* **249**:1417–22.

Troupin AS, Ojemann LM (1975) Paradoxical intoxication: a complication of anticonvulsant administration. *Epilepsia* **16**:753–8.

Vollmar C, Noachtar S (2007) Tiagabine-induced myoclonic status epilepticus in a nonepileptic patient. *Neurology* **68**:310.

Walder B, Tramer MR, Seeck M (2002) Seizure-like phenomena and propofol: a systematic review. *Neurology* **58**:1327–32.

Wallace KL (1997) Antibiotic-induced convulsions. *Crit Care Clin* **13**:741–62.

Wedin GP, Oderda GM, Klein-Schwartz W, et al. (1986) Relative toxicity of cyclic antidepressants. *Ann Emerg Med* **15**:797–804.

Wills B, Erickson T (2006) Chemically induced seizures. *Clin Lab Med* **26**:185–209.

Wyderski RJ, Starrett WG, Abou-Saif A (1999) Fatal status epilepticus associated with olanzapine therapy. *Ann Pharmacother* **33**:787–9.

Zak R, Solomon G, Petito F, et al. (1994) Baclofen-induced generalized nonconvulsive status epilepticus. *Ann Neurol* **36**:113–14.

Chapter

95

Alcohol- and toxin-induced seizures

Michelle J. Shapiro and Andrew J. Cole

Definitions and epidemiology of toxin-induced seizures

Seizures are a common consequence of toxin exposure. To attribute a seizure to toxin exposure, there must be a clear exposure to the implicated toxin at a dose, in a manner, and with a temporal relationship that is known to cause seizures. Alternative or confounding causes, such as head trauma or metabolic derangements, must be excluded. Finally, the patient's overall clinical presentation must be in keeping with the expected consequences of the toxin. Further support for a toxin-induced symptomology comes when symptoms stabilize or improve once the exposure has ceased or been removed. Little is known about the overall rates of toxin-induced seizures, but drugs appear to be the most common cause of seizures in this category (Olson *et al.* 1994).

Epilepsy associated with toxin-induced seizures

Whereas seizures are a common consequence of toxin exposure, epilepsy as a result of toxin exposure is rare. Toxin-induced seizures, typically generalized in their phenomenology, are by definition provoked and therefore do not contribute to the diagnosis of epilepsy per se. None the less, some toxins, for example domoic acid or carbon monoxide (see below), may cause acute seizures, chronic epilepsy, or both as a consequence of toxin exposure.

Diagnosis of toxin-induced seizures

A wide variety of toxins have the ability to cause seizures (see Table 95.1). With the exception of more common causes, such as alcohol withdrawal, the diagnosis of toxin-induced seizures generally requires a high degree of suspicion on the part of the clinician. A detailed history often provides the important clue. Particular attention should focus on the type, route, dose, and duration of potential or known toxin exposures. The patient's occupation and hobbies, symptoms in family members or co-workers, and a history of substance abuse should all be surveyed. On examination, in addition to vital signs, general and neurological examination, it is important to look for more specific signs that might be related to specific toxins. The physician should examine for odors on the patient's breath and clothes, since many toxins have pathognomonic odors. Cyanide, for example, produces an odor of bitter almonds and camphor the odor of mothballs. One should also assess skin and urine color, look for skin lesions and track marks, and nailbed signs such as Mee's lines (seen in arsenic, thallium, and other poisonings). Finally, the physician should evaluate for possible toxin-associated syndromes, such as the cholinergic syndrome comprising hypersalivation, excessive sweating and lacrimation, diarrhea, bronchorrhea, wheezing, urinary incontinence, and tenesmus that occurs with organophosphate exposure

Basic investigations of toxin-induced seizures include standard blood tests (complete blood count, electrolytes, glucose, calcium, magnesium, creatinine, blood urea nitrogen, liver function tests), urine toxicology, electrocardiogram, electroencephalogram (EEG), and brain imaging. Assessment of anion and osmolar-gap is crucial, as this can reveal a toxic exposure to ethanol, ethylene glycol, or methanol amongst others. Brain imaging is important in part to look for confounding causes of seizures such as head trauma, intracranial hemorrhage, or abscess. Depending on the type of exposure, other investigations may be necessary, including chest X-ray, blood gas, nerve conduction studies, or urine heavy-metal screen.

Treatment of toxin-induced seizures

The immediate treatment of toxin-induced seizures resembles that of any acute seizure and begins with ABC (airway, breathing, circulation), followed by glucose assessment and replacement, and the use of anticonvulsant medications starting with benzodiazepines, and followed by administration of longer-lasting anticonvulsants in situations where the toxin is not rapidly cleared. Phenytoin is often the drug of choice,

The Causes of Epilepsy, eds. S. D. Shorvon, F. Andermann, and R. Guerrini. Published by Cambridge University Press. © Cambridge University Press 2011.

Table 95.1. Examples of toxins that can cause seizures

Metals	Alcohols and glycol
Thallium	Ethanol withdrawal
Lead	Methanol
Arsenic	Ethylene glycol
Silver	Propylene glycol
Nickel	**Industrial and environmental toxins**
Tin	Carbon monoxide
Copper	Carbon disulfide
Mercury	Methyl bromide
Biotoxins	**Hydrocarbons**
Scorpion sting	Toluene
Gyromitrin mushrooms	Camphor
Domoic acid (shellfish)	Acetone
Coelenterates (jellyfish and anemones)	Benzene
Venomous fish (including stingrays, weever fish, and stonefish)	Ethyl ether
Herbals/plants	**Insecticides/repellents**
Chinese cucumber (compound Q or *Trichosanthes kirilowii*)	DDT
Ma Huang (*Ephedra*)	Lindane (benzene hexachloride)
Water hemlock	Rotenone
Belladonna	DEET
Angel's trumpet	**Drugs of abuse**
Jimsonweed	Crack/cocaine
Christmas rose	Phencyclidine (PCP)
Jerusalem cherry	Lysergic acid diethylamide (LSD)
Chinaberry	3,4-methylenedioxymethamphetamine (MDMA or "ecstasy")
Bleeding hearts	**Nerve agents**
Carolina jasmine	Tabun (GA)
Nicotine	Sarin (GB)
Wormwood (absinthe)	Soman (GD)
	Cyclosarin (GF)
	VX

though it has shown decreased efficacy in some settings such as alcohol withdrawal and cocaine-induced seizures (Alldredge *et al.* 1989; Derlet and Albertson 1990). Some toxin exposures may also require additional intervention such as whole-bowel irrigation, the use of activated charcoal, chelation therapy, or specific antidotes such as antivenins.

Poison control centers are a great source of information and aid in the treatment of toxin exposures. In many countries, access to these centers is available on the web. The American Association of Poison Control Centers can be found at www.aapcc.org or by calling their hotline at 1–800–222–1222. The Canadian site is www.capcc.ca. From these main locations, local poison control centers can easily be found.

In the following sections we highlight several toxins of interest either because of their mechanism of action or their importance from a public health point of view.

Alcohol

It is unclear whether or not alcohol intoxication or exposure on its own can lead to seizures (Gordon and Devinsky 2001). On the other hand, alcohol withdrawal may be the most frequent cause of toxin-induced seizure encountered in clinical practice. This is particularly true in urban centers where up to 10% of status epilepticus cases may be directly related to alcohol use (Alldredge and Lowenstein 1993). Most alcohol withdrawal seizures are generalized tonic–clonic attacks that occur within 6–48 hr after cessation of alcohol use. Seizures may be followed by delirium tremens. Longer periods of alcohol abuse increase the risk of withdrawal seizures (Kosten and O'Connor 2003). Alcoholic patients often have confounding causes for seizures including head trauma, subdural hematoma, stroke, abscess, meningitis, and metabolic derangements. In patients treated with antiepileptic medication, induction of metabolic pathways or non-compliance may be issues as well. Rates of seizures due to alcohol withdrawal have been estimated as high as 24% among alcoholics (Chan 1985) making this a major public health issue.

The EEGs in alcoholic patients with and without seizures are largely normal, though ictal and interictal epileptiform discharges have been described (Krauss and Niedermeyer 1991). The most common EEG finding is a low-voltage (<25 μV) tracing that persists in hyperventilation and sleep. This finding correlates with cortical atrophy seen on brain imaging in chronic alcoholic patients. Reports of increased photosensitivity during acute alcohol withdrawal, while often discussed, had not been convincingly validated (Hauser *et al.* 1988). Alcohol withdrawal may exacerbate periodic lateralized epileptiform discharges (PLEDs) seen with chronic focal cerebral lesions (Van Sweden and Niedermeyer 1991). Finally, Niedermeyer has described a syndrome of subacute alcoholic encephalopathy involving focal seizures, transient cortical deficits, and PLEDs (Niedermeyer *et al.* 1991).

Alcohol (ethanol) is a central nervous system (CNS) depressant that produces tolerance and dependence in humans. Alcohol dependence causes a downregulation of γ-aminobutynic acid (GABA) GABA$_A$ receptors and therefore a decrease in their postsynaptic density, resulting in decreased inhibitory synaptic strength. In addition, ethanol has

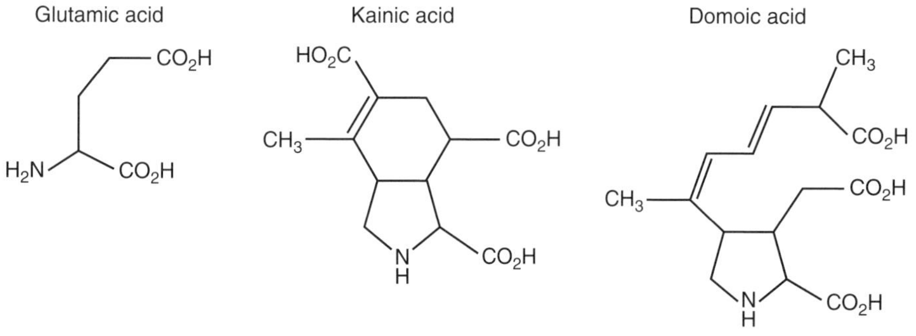

Glutamic acid   Kainic acid   Domoic acid

Fig. 95.1. Chemical structures of glutamic acid, kainic acid, and domoic acid.

inhibitory effects on N-methyl-D-aspartate (NMDA) receptors, leading to upregulation. The subsequent increased excitation may be an additional mechanism of alcohol withdrawal seizures. On an anatomic level, there is some evidence that alcohol withdrawal seizures may be mediated in part by the brainstem, especially the inferior colliculus (Rogawski 2005).

Immediate treatment for alcohol withdrawal seizures generally starts with benzodiazepines. Although these have been shown to be effective in humans (Ntais *et al.* 2005) phenytoin has in fact been shown to have decreased efficacy in this setting, except in the treatment of status epilepticus (Alldredge and Lowenstein 1993). Valproic acid or topiramate may be better choices. Longer-term prophylaxis is problematic in this patient population because of frequent non-compliance. Animal models indicate that NMDA receptor antagonists could have a role in this setting (Stepayan *et al.* (2008), but human studies are not available.

Domoic acid

Domoic acid is a toxin that accumulates in marine organisms, particularly those that feed on phytoplankton. It has been found in many sea creatures including scallops, squid, cuttlefish, sea lions, and octopus amongst others. In late 1987, an outbreak of domoic acid poisoning occurred in Canada. Contaminated mussels from Prince Edward Island produced gastrointestinal and neurologic consequences in many who consumed them. Afflicted individuals suffered from vomiting, diarrhea, or abdominal cramps within 24 hr of mussel consumption and/or neurological signs and symptoms including confusion, disorientation, memory loss, coma, or seizures within 48 hr of consumption. In 107 patients reviewed by Trish *et al.* (1990), the time to first symptom after mussel consumption ranged from 15 min to 38 hr (mean 5.5 hr). Eighteen percent of patients were hospitalized, 16 of whom had medical records available for review. Eight of the 16 patients had seizures. The EEGs showed localized epileptogenic abnormalities in two patients, and generalized slowing in nine. Temporal lobe epilepsy with complex partial seizures developed 1 year after domoic acid intoxication in one patient who had suffered complex partial status epilepticus progressing to generalized convulsions at the time of poisoning (Cendes *et al.* 1995).

Domoic acid is an excitotoxin structurally related to kainic acid and glutamate (Fig. 95.1). It has action at both AMPA and kainic acid receptors in the CNS, but is three to four times more potent than kainic acid. Although both domoate and kainate produce a large physiological response in CA3 hippocampal neurons, they appear to have independent actions in CA1 (Sari and Kerr 2001). Grossly, domoic acid produces damage and necrosis primarily in hippocampus and amygdala. The hippocampal damage is similar to that of kainic acid toxicity, with neuronal loss in the H_3, H_4, and H_5 regions more so than in H_1, and relative sparing of H_2. Necrosis or damage in the dentate gyrus is often present as well (Teitelbaum *et al.* 1990). In other words, domoate intoxication produces a pathological picture highly reminiscent of severe hippocampal sclerosis.

Treatment for domoic acid exposure is supportive and no antidote is available. Seizures should be treated symptomatically. Of note, the patient that developed complex partial status epilepticus following domoic acid exposure did not respond to phenytoin but did well with phenobarbital in the acute setting (Cendes *et al.* 1995).

Carbon monoxide

Carbon monoxide (CO) is the leading cause of death by poisoning in the United States. Accidental CO deaths may be caused by house fires, car and boat exhaust, indoor heating systems, stoves, and water heaters. Of note, rates of accidental deaths caused by CO have declined in the last two decades, in part due to the use of catalytic converters (Kao and Nanagas 2004). Poisoning by CO is also a common cause of death by suicide.

Acutely, CO poisoning may produce headache, nausea, vomiting, blurred vision, confusion, chest pain, syncope, dysrhythmias, hypotension, rhabdomyolysis, pulmonary edema, myocardial infarction, cardiac arrest, seizures, and coma. Some patients manifest a cherry-red skin color (Ernst and Zibrak 1998). Seizures typically occur with severe poisoning, but focal seizures have been reported as a presenting symptom (Durnin 1987). It is estimated that up to one-third of CO exposures go undiagnosed due to the fact that the symptoms mimic various other disorders. Delayed neurological symptoms occur in up to 47% of patients from 2 to 40 days after exposure, including memory loss, confusion, ataxia, seizures, hallucinations,

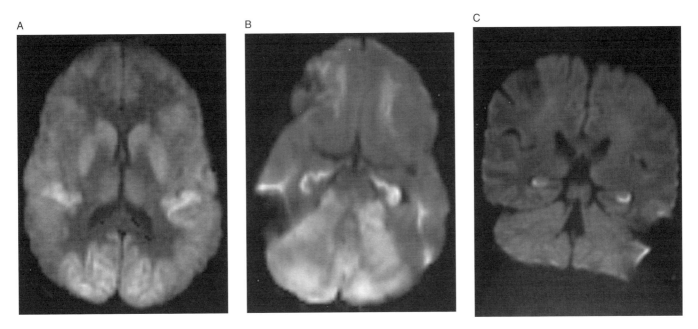

Fig. 95.2. Magnetic resonance imaging demonstrating the diversity of lesions seen after CO poisoning. All images obtained using fluid attenuated inversion recovery (FLAIR) sequences. Note diffuse cerebral edema and characteristic hyperintensity of the globus pallidus bilaterally (A), extensive cerebellar involvement in a child with CO poisoning (B), and bilateral hippocampal involvement (C). Each image is from a different patient.

parkinsonism, and psychosis (Kao and Nanagas 2004). Finally, while anecdotal evidence has led to the hypothesis that chronic exposure to low concentrations of CO over days or months may result in mild neurological symptoms including headache, lethargy, and reduced intellectual function, there are no definitive studies or conclusive evidence to support this hypothesis (Townsend and Maynard 2002).

Carbon monoxide has a 200-fold greater affinity for hemoglobin than oxygen, and binds to hemoglobin to form carboxyhemoglobin (CO–Hgb) causing a left shift in the oxyhemoglobin dissociation curve. A small increase in CO partial pressure causes a large increase in the amount of CO–Hgb formed. Additionally, CO disrupts oxidative metabolism by binding to heme-proteins such as cytochrome aa_3. It binds to myoglobin, likely reducing oxygen availability, and impairs cellular respiration through the inactivation of mitochondrial enzymes and oxygen radicals that disrupt electron transport. It produces an inflammatory response that may result in reperfusion injury. Other actions include vasodilatation resulting from the stimulation of guanylyl cyclase and the subsequent increase of c-GMP, as well as vasodilation and oxidative damage caused by nitric oxide and other oxygen free radicals (Thom 2005).

When acute CO poisoning is suspected, serum carboxyhemoglobin levels should be measured. Baseline CO–Hgb levels are higher in smokers than in non-smokers. Mild symptoms occur with levels <15%, while levels of >60–70% are generally fatal. Metabolic acidosis correlates with the severity of exposure. Importantly, pulse oximetry may be inaccurate, since pulse oximeters do not distinguish between carboxyhemoglobin and oxyhemoglobin. Carbon monoxide exposure

characteristically causes high intensity T2 signal abnormalities in the globus pallidus bilaterally, but also causes injury to white matter, cortex, and hippocampi (Kao and Nanagas 2004) (Fig. 95.2).

Acute CO poisoning is generally treated with hyperbaric oxygen if available; however, its efficacy is uncertain. Treatment with high-flow oxygen under normal pressure should be initiated immediately upon recognition of acute CO exposure. Seizures in this setting should be treated symptomatically.

Lead

Lead poisoning may occur with exposures including welding, grinding and sandblasting of lead-coated surfaces, battery manufacturing and recycling, smelting of lead ores, wounds from lead-containing bullets or shotgun pellets (especially when these reside in joint spaces within the body), ingestion of lead paint chips or lead objects such as fishing weights (especially in children), smoking adulterated marijuana, drinking home-distilled alcohol, boiling water or keeping food in lead-containing vessels, and eating from lead-glazed ceramics. Lead poisoning may cause headache, nausea, vomiting, constipation, renal failure, motor neuropathy, cognitive impairment, ataxia, seizures, and coma. Seizures associated with lead poisoning are generally seen in the setting of lead encephalopathy, a potentially life-threatening event that occurs more frequently in children than in adults. Lead encephalopathy is typically seen after high-dose lead exposure (>80–100 μg/L). Seizures are usually generalized but can be focal, and occur in up to 75% of patients with lead encephalopathy (Kosnett 2005). In one study, just over half of the children who survived

A

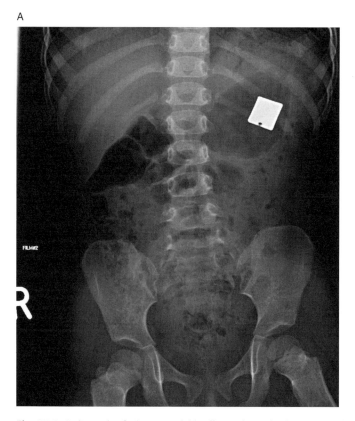

B

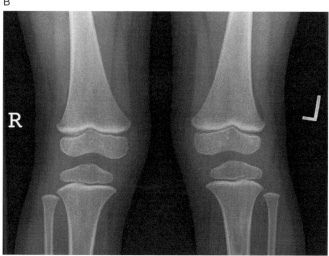

Fig. 95.3. Radiographic findings in a child suffering chronic lead poisoning. Abdominal X-ray demonstrates metal object swallowed by a 3-year-old child (A). Long bone X-ray demonstrates classical "lead lines" in the same child, resulting from lead poisoning (B).

lead encephalopathy went on to develop epilepsy (Perlstein and Attala 1966).

Lead toxicity is primarily the result of lead interfering with the cellular and membrane actions of calcium, leading to increased levels of calcium in the cytoplasm of many cells, and resulting in abnormal neurotransmission. Lead is known to inhibit heme synthesis, resulting in anemia. Lead also interferes with a number of proteins and enzymes, including those related to DNA binding. Finally, lead may be involved in neuronal apoptosis. Pathologically, lead encephalopathy results in various changes including diffuse astrocytosis, petechial hemorrhages, foci of necrosis, swelling of endothelial cells, and a perivascular proteinacous exudate (Schochet and Gray 2004).

If lead poisoning is suspected, blood lead levels should be measured. The complete blood count will likely reveal a microcytic hypochromic anemia, and a peripheral blood smear may demonstrate basophilic stippling of erythrocytes. Blood urea nitrogen and creatinine as well as liver function tests may be elevated. With encephalopathy, there is generally an increased opening pressure on lumbar puncture with an elevated protein, and a normal or mildly elevated white cell count in cerebrospinal fluid. Brain magnetic resonance imaging (MRI) may demonstrate diffuse cerebral edema, but focal cerebellar edema can also be seen. In children, bone radiographs may show thick transverse opacities at the ends of long bones, also known as "lead lines" (Fig. 95.3). Bone lead levels can give a measurement of long-term exposure. Occasional patients may also have a blue line along the gums, a so-called "gingival lead line."

Acute lead poisoning is treated with whole-bowel irrigation, gastric lavage, or cathartics, but lead colic and constipation may inhibit their effectiveness. Chelation therapy with agents such as calcium edetate, dimercaprol, or both may be necessary. Since lead is excreted primarily by the kidney, it is important to monitor urine output, especially in patients with lead encephalopathy and a decreased level of consciousness. Increased intracranial pressure in lead encephalopathy may respond to mannitol and hyperventilation. First-line treatment for seizures in the acute setting is with benzodiazepines, whereas standard anticonvulsants are used for chronic treatment.

Sarin

Liquid nerve agents, such as sarin (isopropyl methylphosphonofluoridate), are potent and deadly substances used in chemical warfare. In 1995, thousands of people were injured and at least eight killed when liquid sarin was released on several lines of the Tokyo subway system. Numerous troops were also exposed to sarin at the end of the Gulf War in 1991.

A   B   C

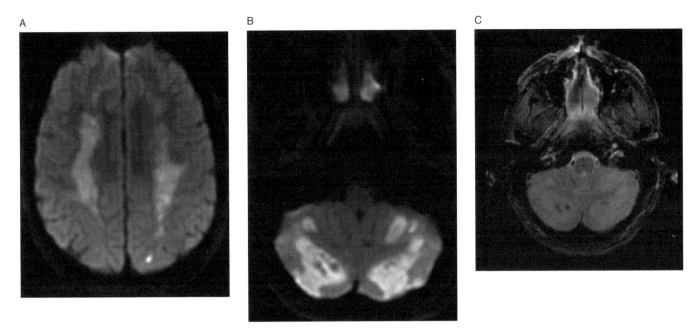

Fig. 95.4. Magnetic resonance imaging demonstrating the diversity of lesions seen with cocaine abuse. All images are from the same patient. Diffusion weighted image demonstrates restricted diffusion in the cerebral white matter bilaterally (A) and in the cerebellar hemispheres (B). Gradient echo image demonstrates punctuate magnetic susceptibility indicating hemorrhage in the cerebellum (C).

Nerve agents such as sarin are cholinesterase inhibitors, and result in cholinergic crisis. Their effect is very similar to that of the organophosphate insecticides. Sarin is extremely volatile as a liquid and quickly evaporates at room temperature, thus exposure is usually in the form of a vapor. Sarin exposure causes miosis, blurred vision, rhinorrhea, salivation, bronchorrhea and bronchospasm, nausea, vomiting, abdominal pain, diarrhea, tachycardia, bradycardia, hypotension, hypertension, fasciculations, flaccid paralysis, coma, seizures, and central apnea. Seizures can develop within seconds of exposure, and status epilepticus sometimes ensues. Rats that endured 30 min of sarin-induced seizures manifest severe damage to the hippocampus, piriform cortex, and thalamic nuclei (Gilat *et al.* 2005).

Diagnosis of nerve agent exposure is achieved primarily by history and physical examination. Miosis is a helpful sign in distinguishing this type of exposure from other toxins such as cyanide (Newmark 2008). Long-term, low-level exposure can cause decreased white matter volume and atrophy on MRI (Heaton *et al.* 2007).

Treatment of sarin exposure begins with decontamination. Supportive care with particular attention to respiratory status is important. Atropine should be used as an anticholinergic, and can be administered either intramuscularly or intravenously. Total doses as high as 15–20 mg may be needed in severe exposures. Oximes can also be used, but may only be available through poison control centers. Unfortunately, status epilepticus induced by sarin may not respond to standard antiepileptic drugs such as phenytoin, phenobarbital, valproic acid, or carbamazepine. Benzodiazepines should be used in this setting, preferably midazolam (Newmark 2008).

Cocaine

Cocaine is an amphetamine narcotic and a common drug of abuse. It can be ingested by snorting, intravenous injection, or smoking the freebase form as crack. It has a legitimate medical application as a local anesthetic and is still used in neurology in the diagnosis of Horner syndrome. Cocaine abuse reached its peak in the 1980s, but the widespread use of crack since that time has contributed to an increased overall morbidity and mortality amongst users.

Seizures related to isolated cocaine use are typically generalized and dose-related. They are seen more frequently with intravenous and crack use. Cocaine can also cause a number of focal central nervous system abnormalities such as trauma, stroke, hemorrhage, and vasculitis. In these cases when seizures arise, they tend to be focal and related to the site of the lesion, and may be remote from acute drug use. Cocaine use is known to exacerbate pre-existing epilepsy (Pascual-Leone *et al.* 1990). Seizures have also been well documented as a preterminal manifestation of cocaine overdose, especially in cases of "body packing" in which people hide large quantities of drugs in body cavities. Finally, cocaine readily crosses the placenta and can be a cause of seizures in neonates. Seizures associated with cocaine abuse are common. One study found that 7.9% of people with cocaine-related admissions to a county medical center had seizures, but this increased to 16.9% in those with pre-existing epilepsy. A more recent large retrospective review found that seizures occurred in 3% of cocaine-related admissions, while 6% of people with seizure-related admissions admitted to cocaine use (Koppel *et al.* 1996).

Cocaine inhibits the reuptake of monoamines including dopamine, norepinephrine, and serotonin. In addition, cocaine has been reported to block voltage-gated sodium channels. The mechanism whereby cocaine intoxication causes seizures is not clearly understood, however, it is known that stimulation of D_1 dopamine receptors facilitate cocaine-induced seizures, while D_1 receptor antagonists inhibit them. Serotonin 5-HT$_2$ receptor antagonists also inhibit cocaine-induced seizures and selective serotonin reuptake inhibitors facilitate them. Beta-blockers such as propranolol have been known to enhance cocaine-induced seizures. Finally, GABA$_A$ stimulation and NMDA antagonism have been shown to have a protective affect against cocaine-induced seizures (Lason 2001).

Diagnosis of acute cocaine toxicity is made by history and physical examination. A sympathomimetic toxic syndrome may be present, including dilated pupils, hypertension, tachycardia, tachypnea, hyperthermia, and agitated delirium. The patient's clinical symptoms should guide the investigations (Fig. 95.4). Note that cocaine can cause a variety of cardiac, pulmonary, gastrointestinal, and renal manifestations.

Medication treatment of acute cocaine-induced seizures should start with benzodiazepines. Much like with alcohol-withdrawal seizures, phenytoin has been found to have reduced efficacy in this setting (Derlet and Albertson 1990), thus an alternative longer-acting antiepileptic medication may be preferred. Presumably as the result of ischemic injury related to cocaine-associated vasculitis, a substantial number of patients with a history of cocaine abuse may be at risk for developing chronic epilepsy. Nonetheless, there is no data to support chronic treatment with anticonvulsants after presentation with seizures in the setting of acute intoxication with cocaine.

References

Alldredge BK, Lowenstein DH (1993) Status epilepticus related to alcohol abuse. *Epilepsia* 34:1033–7.

Alldredge BK, Lowenstein DH, Simon RP (1989) Placebo-controlled trial of intravenous diphenylhydantoin for short-term treatment of alcohol withdrawal seizures. *Am J Med* 87:645–8.

Cendes F, Andermann F, Carpenter S, *et al.* (1995) Temporal lobe epilepsy caused by domoic acid intoxication: evidence for glutamate receptor-mediated excitotoxicity in humans. *Ann Neurol* 37:123–6.

Chan AW (1985) Alcoholism and epilepsy. *Epilepsia* 26:323–33.

Derlet RW, Albertson TE (1990) Anticonvulsant modification of cocaine-induced toxicity in the rat. *Neuropharmacology* 29:255–9.

Durnin C (1987) Carbon monoxide poisoning presenting with focal epileptiform seizures. *Lancet* 1(8545):1319.

Ernst A, Zibrak JD (1998) Carbon monoxide poisoning. *N Engl J Med* 339:1603–8.

Gilat E, Kadar T, Levy A, *et al.* (2005) Anticonvulsant treatment of sarin-induced seizures with nasal midazolam: an electrographic, behavioral, and histological study in freely moving rats. *Toxicol Appl Pharmacol* 209:74–85.

Gordon E, Devinsky O (2001) Alcohol and marijuana: effects on epilepsy and use by patients with epilepsy. *Epilepsia* 42:1266–72.

Hauser WA, Ng SK, Brust JC (1988) Alcohol, seizures, and epilepsy. *Epilepsia* 29(Suppl 2):S66–78.

Heaton KJ, Palumbo CL, Proctor SP, *et al.* (2007) Quantitative magnetic resonance brain imaging in US army veterans of the 1991 Gulf War potentially exposed to sarin and cyclosarin. *Neurotoxicology* 28:761–9.

Kao LW, Nanagas K (2004) Carbon monoxide poisoning. *Emerg Med Clin N Am* 22:985–1018.

Koppel BS, Samkoff L, Daras M (1996) Relation of cocaine use to seizures and epilepsy. *Epilepsia* 37:875–8.

Kosnett MJ (2005) Lead. In: Brent J, Wallace KL, Burkhart KK, *et al.* (eds.) *Critical Care Toxicology: Diagnosis and Management of the Critically Poisoned Patient*. Philadelphia, PA: Elsevier Mosby, pp. 821–36.

Kosten TR, O'Connor PG (2003) Management of drug and alcohol withdrawal. *N Engl J Med* 348:1786–95.

Krauss GL, Niedermeyer E (1991) Electroencephalogram and seizures in chronic alcoholism. *Electroencephalogr Clin Neurophys* 78:97–104.

Lason W (2001) Neurochemical and pharmacological aspects of cocaine-induced seizures. *Pol J Pharmacol* 53:57–60.

Newmark J (2008) Neurologic aspects of chemical and biological terrorist threats. *Continuum Lifelong Learning Neurol* 14:150–78.

Niedermeyer E, Freund G, Krumholz A (1981) Subacute encephalopathy with seizures in alcoholics: a clinical electroencephalographic study. *Clin Electroencephalogr* 12:113–29.

Ntais C, Pakos E, Kyras P, Ioannidis JP (2005) Benzodiazepines for alcohol withdrawal. *Cochrane Database Syst Rev* 20:CD005063.

Olson KR, Kearney TE, Dyer JE, *et al.* (1994) Seizures associated with poisoning and drug overdose. *Am J Emerg Med* 12:565–8.

Pascual-Leone A, Dhuna A, Altafullah I, Anderson DC (1990) Cocaine-induced seizures. *Neurology* 40:404–7.

Perlstein MA, Attala R (1966) Neurological sequelae of plumbism in children. *Clin Pediatr* 5:292–298.

Rogawski MA (2005) Update on the neurobiology of alcohol withdrawal seizures. *Epilepsy Curr* 5:225–30.

Sari P, Kerr DS (2001) Domoic acid-induced hippocampal CA1 hyperexcitability independent of region CA3 activity. *Epilepsy Res* 47:65–76.

Schochet SS, Gray F (2004) Acquired metabolic disorders. In: Gray F, De Girolami U, Poirier J (eds.) *Escourolle and Pourier Manual of Basic Neuropathology*. Philadelphia, PA: Butterworth-Heinemann, pp. 197–217.

Stepayan TD, Farook JM, Kowalski A, *et al.* (2008) Alcohol withdrawal-induced hippocampal neurotoxicity in vitro and seizures in vivo are both reduced by memantine. *Alcohol Clin Exp Res* 32:2128–35.

Teitelbaum JS, Zatorre RJ, Carpenter S, *et al.* (1990) Neurologic sequelae of domoic acid intoxication due to the ingestion of contaminated mussels. *N Engl J Med* **322**:1781–7.

Thom SR (2005) Carbon monoxide. In: Brent J, Wallace KL, Burkhart KK, *et al.* (eds.) *Critical Care Toxicology: Diagnosis and Management of the Critically Poisoned Patient*. Philadelphia, PA: Elsevier Mosby, pp. 975–85.

Townsend CL, Maynard RL (2002) Effect on health of prolonged exposure to low concentrations of carbon monoxide. *Occup Environ Med* **59**:708–11.

Trish MP, Bedard L, Kosatsky T, *et al.* (1990) An outbreak of toxic encephalopathy caused by eating mussels contaminated with domoic acid. *N Engl J Med* **322**:1775–80.

Van Sweden B, Niedermeyer E (1999) Toxic encephalopathies. In: Niedermeyer E, Lopes De Silva F (eds.) *Electroencephalography: Basic Principles, Clinical Applications, and Related Fields*. Baltimore, MD: Lippincott Williams and Wilkins, pp. 692–701.

Chapter

96

How reflex mechanisms cause epilepsy

Benjamin Zifkin and Frederick Andermann

"The unexpected happens by necessity. The surprise is built in."
Krenek (1962)

In a work devoted to the causes of epilepsy, a discussion of reflex seizures must tread carefully. It should be emphasized from the outset that the stimuli of reflex seizures are not causes of epilepsy, any more than concrete causes buildings. A seizure triggered by a flashing television screen would not have occurred then without the screen, but the predisposition to have seizures, the epilepsy, is not caused by the screen.

Reflex seizures were known long before the advent of the electroencephalogram (EEG), particularly with visual stimuli. In the mid twentieth century, early EEG studies of reflex seizures triggered by flashing light investigated the clinical and EEG responses to stroboscopic white flash stimulation, especially as an age- and sex-related phenomenon. The advent of television, especially in Europe with its slower 50 Hz screens, led to reports of seizures induced by the television set; these subjects were usually photosensitive. The discovery that some photosensitive patients were also sensitive to striped patterns led to major advances. Arnold Wilkins and colleagues at the Montreal Neurological Hospital and at the epilepsy centre at Heemstede, the Netherlands, were able to identify those properties of patterns such as the orientations, spatial frequencies and their relative size within the visual field that were most likely to trigger seizures and thus to deduce that this sensitivity arose in the primary visual cortex (Wilkins *et al.* 1975, 1980, 1981; Binnie *et al.* 1985).

Most clinical attention was devoted to epileptic sensitivity to unpatterned intermittent white light flash stimulation delivered by a stroboscope in the EEG laboratory (Kasteleijn-Nolst Trenité 1989) and to the closely related problem of seizures triggered by environmental visual stimulation, especially television screens. Most articles on other forms of reflex seizures reported only elementary attempts to document the relation of the stimulus to the seizures and to determine what characteristics of the trigger events could be responsible

for them. The methods that the Anglo-Dutch school developed for visual stimuli could be adapted to other reflex seizures, with detailed statistical methods and explorations of the triggers. More widespread use of intensive EEG monitoring, computed tomography (CT) scanning and then magnetic resonance imaging (MRI) enabled better characterization of the nature of the effective stimulus and of the cerebral localization and pathways of seizure genesis. These studies usually focused on single patients or small groups, especially with seizures triggered by visual stimuli, spatial thought, reading, programming and performing motor tasks, or hearing music. Occasionally other opportunities arose: seizures caused by television screens and later by video games became notorious and guidelines were developed to prevent the broadcasting of screen content likely to provoke seizures. A mass outbreak of triggered seizures was possible if these were not implemented or followed, including those not previously known to be photosensitive, and indeed occurred in Japan in response to a cartoon (Wilkins *et al.* 2005). Hundreds of Japanese children had seizures when a popular program broadcast a sequence of bright flashing colors. This outbreak also led to renewed interest in the effects of colored light stimulation: photosensitivity is usually assessed with white light. Parra *et al.* (2007) examined whether color modulation could be an independent factor in human epileptic photosensitivity. They concluded that "colour sensitivity follows two different mechanisms: one, dependent on colour modulation, plays a role at lower frequencies (5–30 Hz). Another, dependent on single-colour light intensity modulation, correlates to white light sensitivity and is activated at higher frequencies."

The genetics of reflex seizures has been studied for some time. Familial cases of photosensitivity and of reading epilepsy have been known for years but no single gene has been reliably associated with any type of reflex seizure other than in single families or in small groups though susceptibility genes have been suggested (Mulley *et al.* 2005; Pinto *et al.* 2005; Dibbens *et al.* 2007; Nobile *et al.* 2009).

The general principles of the genesis of reflex seizures have been reviewed by Zifkin and Andermann (2010). Several reflex

The Causes of Epilepsy, eds. S. D. Shorvon, F. Andermann, and R. Guerrini. Published by Cambridge University Press. © Cambridge University Press 2011.

stimuli which are subserved by localized cortical areas or by functional networks can cause clinically bilateral or generalized EEG paroxysmal activity or seizures, often in patients with underlying idiopathic generalized epileptic syndromes (Ferlazzo *et al.* 2005). Sensitivity to these triggers does not require any evident brain lesion or handicap. Using photosensitivity as an example, for this is the commonest type and the most extensively studied, generalized epileptiform activity and clinical seizures can be activated by the localized occipital trigger. Studies in photosensitive patients who are also pattern sensitive suggest that generalized seizures and EEG paroxysmal activity can occur in these subjects if normal excitation of abnormally sensitive visual cortex involves a certain "critical mass" of cortical area with synchronization and subsequent spreading of excitation (Wilkins *et al.* 1975, 1980, 1981; Binnie *et al.* 1985). Wilkins *et al.* (1982) suggested that a similar mechanism involving recruitment of a critical mass of parietal rather than visual cortex is responsible for generalized seizures induced by thinking or by spatial tasks. Subsequently, studies of seizures precipitated by combined thought and action appeared in Japanese journals. These were described in English-language book chapters under the unfamiliar term "praxis-induced seizures" (Inoue *et al.* 1994); and a large and important study by Matsuoka *et al.* (2000) clarified many questions, and seemed to confirm and expand the ideas in a Montreal series collected by Frederick Andermann and reported by Goossens *et al.* (1990). More recently, Matsuoka *et al.* (2005) reported that writing, spatial construction, and written calculation were the most effective triggers, all involving a combination of spatial thought and use of the hands. Praxis induction and seizures induced by thinking appear almost exclusively in idiopathic generalized epilepsies as they are now understood, and particularly in juvenile myoclonic epilepsy (JME), although seizures induced by thinking can occur with no motor component in the stimulus or the response. Tasks that can trigger seizures in patients with seizures induced by thinking involve the processing of spatial information and possibly sequential decisions. The generalized seizures and EEG discharges may depend on initial involvement of parietal or, possibly, frontal cortex and subsequent generalization. The cerebral representation of calculation and spatial thought involves a bilateral functional network activated by such tasks (Stanescu-Cosson *et al.* 2000). The EEG responses in praxis-induced seizures consist of bisynchronous spike or polyspike-and-wave bursts at times predominant over centroparietal regions. In its milder forms, such as the morning myoclonic jerk of the arm manipulating a utensil, this phenomenon resembles cortical reflex myoclonus as part of a "continuum of epileptic activity centered on the sensorimotor cortex" (Vignal *et al.* 1998). It also appears to be another manifestation of triggering of a generalized or bilateral epileptiform response by a local or functional trigger, in this case requiring participation of the rolandic region of one or both hemispheres which may be regionally hyperexcitable in juvenile

myoclonic epilepsy (Wolf 1994). The seizures of idiopathic generalized epilepsy may involve only selected thalamocortical networks (Blumenfeld 2003), a concept initially proposed by Gastaut (1950) for some partial epilepsies. Patients with seizures induced by thinking or by praxis are only rarely sensitive to reading. Even so, studies of reading epilepsy also suggest that increased task difficulty, complexity, or duration increases the chance of EEG or clinical activation (Christie *et al.* 1988; Wolf *et al.* 1998). The importance of coexisting juvenile myoclonic epilepsy has been mentioned in conferring sensitivity to a variety of cortical triggers: whether or not juvenile myoclonic epilepsy is a truly generalized epilepsy or something like a regional or network hyperexcitability involving sensorimotor cortex is not clear. Evidence is accumulating that it is a model of a "system" epilepsy (see for example Inoue and Zifkin 2004, Lin *et al.* 2009a,b). This possibility also arises from computational studies, for example those of Lopes da Silva and colleagues (2003) which hearken back to the alumina cream epileptic focus model of Wyler and Ward (1980). The nature of epilepsies customarily regarded as generalized is more and more called into question, and studies of reflex seizures have led to these questions being posed and have provided essential evidence toward better understanding of these disorders (Binnie 2004).

Other reflex seizure triggers are however usually associated with lesional epilepsies and clinically focal seizures, often in patients with known focal epilepsy. These typically involve perisylvian somatosensory or motor cortex as in seizures precipitated by sensory stimuli such as brushing the teeth or eating, proprioceptive stimuli, and some cases of reading epilepsy. Temporolimbic lesions may be found or suspected in cases of seizures triggered by music or in some cases by eating.

Sensitivity to visual stimuli was relatively easy to study. The EEG manifestations are usually clear-cut, the patients are generally young and cooperative without motor or intellectual handicap, and this form of sensitivity is relatively common, especially in girls. However, the localization of visual function to the relatively small occipital lobes and adjacent cortex was potentially misleading and may have obscured the essential idea that the cortical representations of the complex activities triggering these reflex seizures were not localized to one area, nor were they necessarily contiguous, but were networks of functionally linked areas. In reading epilepsy, Wolf (1994) observed that seizure evocation would depend on involvement of the multiple processes used for reading, an activity involving both hemispheres, with a functional rather than a topographic anatomy. "Maximal interactive neuronal performance is at least a facilitating factor."

In the last 10 years, improved morphologic and functional imaging of dysplastic brain lesions and functional brain networks have opened new areas of extraordinarily fruitful study in epilepsy, and these methods have also been applied to reflex seizures.

Functional MRI has shown the distribution of cortical networks activated by many mental activities in normal controls and also in patients with reflex seizures. Activities such as calculation, reading, and music have been studied in controls, in subjects with brain lesions, and in some with reflex seizures (e.g., Naldi *et al.* 2008; Nieder and Dehaene 2009; Salek-Haddadi *et al.* 2009). Magnetic source localization has shown localization of epileptiform activity in some cases, for example in startle epilepsy (García-Morales *et al.* 2009), in which the causative lesion is not always obvious.

References

Binnie CD (2004) Evidence of reflex epilepsy on functional systems in the brain and "generalized epilepsy". In: Wolf P, Inoue Y, Zifkin B (eds.) *Reflex Epilepsies: Progress in Understanding.* Montrouge, France: John Libbey Eurotext, pp. 7–14.

Binnie CD, Findlay J, Wilkins AJ (1985) Mechanisms of epileptogenesis in photosensitive epilepsy implied by the effects of moving patterns. *Electroencephalogr Clin Neurophysiol* **61**:1–6.

Blumenfeld H (2003) From molecules to networks: cortical/subcortical interactions in the pathophysiology of idiopathic generalized epilepsy. *Epilepsia* **44**(Suppl 2):7–15.

Christie S, Guberman A, Tansley BW, *et al.* (1988) Primary reading epilepsy: investigation of critical seizure-provoking stimuli. *Epilepsia* **29**:288–93.

Dibbens LM, Ekberg J, Taylor I, *et al.* (2007) NEDD4-2 as a potential candidate susceptibility gene for epileptic photosensitivity. *Genes Brain Behav* **6**:750–5.

Ferlazzo E, Zifkin BG, Andermann E, Andermann F (2005) Cortical triggers in generalized reflex seizures and epilepsies. *Brain* **128**:700–10.

García-Morales I, Maestú F, Pérez-Jiménez MA, *et al.* (2009) A clinical and magnetoencephalography study of MRI-negative startle epilepsy. *Epilepsy Behav* **16**:166–71.

Gastaut H (1950) Évidences électrographiques d'un mécanisme sous-cortical dans certaines épilepsies partielles: la signification clinique des secteurs aréo-thalamiques. *Rev Neurol* **83**:396–401.

Goossens LAZ, Andermann F, Andermann E, Rémillard GM (1990) Reflex seizures induced by calculation, card or board games, and spatial tasks: a review of 25 patients and delineation of the epileptic syndrome. *Neurology* **40**:1171–6.

Inoue Y, Zifkin B (2004) Praxis induction and thinking induction: one or two mechanisms? In: Wolf P, Inoue Y, Zifkin B (eds.) *Reflex Epilepsies: Progress in Understanding.* Montrouge, France: John Libbey Eurotext, pp. 41–55.

Inoue Y, Seino M, Kubota H, *et al.* Epilepsy with praxis-induced seizures. In: Wolf P (ed.) *Epileptic Seizures and Syndromes.* London: John Libbey, pp. 81–92.

Kasteleijn-Nolst Trenité DG (1989) Photosensitivity in epilepsy: electrophysiological and clinical correlates. *Acta Neurol Scand* **125**(Suppl):31–49.

Krenek E (1962) Extents and limits of serial techniques. In: Lang PH (ed.) *Problems of Modern Music: The Princeton Seminar in Advanced Musical Studies.* New York: Norton, WW, pp. 83–91.

Lin K, Carrete H Jr., Lin J, *et al.* (2009a) Magnetic resonance spectroscopy reveals an epileptic network in juvenile myoclonic epilepsy. *Epilepsia* **50**:1191–200.

Lin K, Jackowski AP, Carrete H Jr., *et al.* (2009b) Voxel-based morphometry evaluation of patients with photosensitive juvenile myoclonic epilepsy. *Epilepsy Res* **86**:138–45.

Lopes da Silva FH, Blanes W, Kalitzin SN, *et al.* (2003) Dynamical diseases of brain systems: different routes to epileptic seizures. *IEEE Trans Biomed Eng* **50**:540–8.

Matsuoka H, Takahashi T, Sasaki M, *et al.* (2000) Neuropsychological EEG activation in patients with epilepsy. *Brain* **123**:318–30.

Matsuoka H, Nakamura M, Ohno T, *et al.* (2005) The role of cognitive-motor function in precipitation and inhibition of epileptic seizures. *Epilepsia* **46**(Supp 1):17–20.

Mulley JC, Scheffer IE, Harkin LA, Berkovic SF, Dibbens LM (2005) Susceptibility genes for complex epilepsy. *Hum Mol Genet* **14**:R243–9.

Naldi I, Cortelli P, Bisulli A, *et al.* (2008). Videopolygraphic and functional MRI study of musicogenic epilepsy: a case report and literature review. *Epilepsy Behav* **13**:685–92.

Nieder A, Dehaene S (2009) Representation of number in the brain. *Ann Rev Neurosci* **32**:185–208.

Nobile C, Michelucci R, Andreazza S, *et al.* (2009) LGI1 mutation in autosomal dominant and sporadic lateral temporal epilepsy. *Hum Mutat* **30**:530–6.

Parra J, Lopes da Silva FH, Stroink H, Kalitzin S (2007). Is colour modulation an independent factor in human visual photosensitivity? *Brain* **130**:1679–89.

Pinto D, Westland B, de Haan GJ, *et al.* (2005) Genome-wide linkage scan of epilepsy-related photoparoxysmal electroencephalographic response: evidence for linkage on chromosomes 7q32 and 16p13. *Hum Mol Genet* **14**:171–8.

Salek-Haddadi A, Mayer T, Hamandi K, *et al.* (2009) Imaging seizure activity: a combined EEG/EMG-fMRI study in reading epilepsy. *Epilepsia* **50**:256–64.

Stanescu-Cosson R, Pinel P, van De Moortele PF, *et al.* (2000) Understanding dissociations in dyscalculia: a brain imaging study of the impact of number size on the cerebral networks for exact and approximate calculation. *Brain* **123**:2240–55.

Vignal J-P, Biraben A, Chauvel PY, *et al.* (1998) Reflex partial seizures of sensorimotor cortex (including cortical reflex myoclonus and startle epilepsy). In: Zifkin BG, Andermann F, Beaumanoir A, Rowan AJ (eds.) *Reflex Epilepsies and Reflex Seizures.* Philadelphia, PA: Lippincott-Raven, pp. 207–26.

Wilkins AJ, Andermann F, Ives J (1975) Stripes, complex cells and seizures: an attempt to determine the locus and nature of the trigger mechanism in pattern-sensitive epilepsy. *Brain* **98**:365–80.

Wilkins AJ, Binnie CD, Darby CE (1980) Visually induced seizures. *Prog Neurobiol* **15**:85–117.

Wilkins AJ, Binnie CD, Darby CE (1981) Interhemispheric differences in photosensitive epilepsy. I. Pattern sensitivity threshold. *Electroencephalogr Clin Neurophysiol* **52**:461–8.

Wilkins AJ, Zifkin B, Andermann F, *et al.* (1982) Seizures induced by thinking. *Ann Neurol* **11**:608–12.

Wilkins AJ, Emmett J, Harding GFA (2005) Characterizing the patterned images that precipitate seizures and optimizing guidelines to prevent them. *Epilepsia* **46**:1212–18.

Wolf P, Mayer T, Reker M (1998) Reading epilepsy: report of five new cases and further considerations on the pathophysiology. *Seizure* 7:271–9.

Wolf P (1989) Reflex epilepsies and syndrome classification: an argument for considering primary reading epilepsy as an idiopathic localization-related epilepsy. In: Beaumanoir A, Gastaut H, Naquet R (eds.) *Reflex Seizures and Reflex Epilepsies*. Geneva: Éditions Médecine et Hygiène, pp. 283–8.

Wolf P (1994) Regional manifestation of idiopathic epilepsy: introduction. In: Wolf P (ed.) *Epileptic Seizures and Syndromes*. London: John Libbey, pp. 265–7.

Wyler AR, Ward AA Jr. (1980) Epileptic neurons. In: Lockard JS, Ward AA Jr. (eds.) *Epilepsy: A Window to Brain Mechanisms*. New York: Raven, pp. 51–68.

Zifkin B, Andermann F (2010) Epilepsy with reflex seizures. In: Wyllie E, Cascino GD, Gidal B, Goodkin H (eds.) *Wyllie's Treatment of Epilepsy: Principles and Practice*, 5th edn. North Wales, PA: Springhouse Publishing, pp. 305–16.

Chapter

97

Visual stimuli, photosensitivity, and photosensitive epilepsy

Dorothée Kasteleijn-Nolst Trenité, Laura Cantonetti, and Pasquale Parisi

Photosensitivity

Definitions

Photosensitivity or visual sensitivity is abnormal sensitivity to light stimuli, detected usually with electroencephalography (EEG) as a paroxysmal reaction to intermittent photic stimulation (IPS).

Photosensitivity is a broad term and is used both for (a) epileptiform EEG discharges and (b) epileptic seizures, evoked by visual stimuli. Several types of visual stimuli are known of which flickering sunlight or IPS, TV, videogames, and striped patterns are the most common.

A photoparoxysmal EEG response is a localized or generalized epileptiform EEG reaction to IPS or stimulation with other stimuli; see Figs. 97.1 and 97.2 for examples of both types of photoparoxysmal responses (PPR).

Photosensitivity is customarily divided into three groups: patients with visually induced seizures only, patients with photosensitivity and some other epileptic disorder, and asymptomatic individuals with PPR as an isolated finding (Kasteleijn-Nolst Trenité et al. 2001). During follow-up patients may shift from asymptomatic and from visually induced seizures only to the other categories.

Some photosensitive patients can evoke generalized epileptiform discharges by fast eyelid fluttering and upward gaze or simply by eye closure: they are called auto- or self-inducers. There is some overlap with eyelid myoclonia with absences (EMA or EMEA) and self-induction (Striano et al. 2009).

In this chapter we make a distinction between the epileptiform EEG responses to IPS, the PPRs (patients are photosensitive), and the seizures provoked by visual stimuli in daily life (visually induced seizures).

Epidemiology

Photoparoxysmal responses in healthy children and aircrew candidates

In healthy children without any abnormality in the clinical history, a prevalence of 1.4% PPRs has been found in Scandinavian countries and in Brazil (Herrlin 1954; Kasteleijn-Nolst Trenité et al. 2003). Roy et al. (2003) found a rate of 0.7% of PPRs in male candidates for aircrew.

Photoparoxysmal responses in epilepsy patients

Several studies have been performed in epilepsy patients to determine the prevalence of PPR. In Caucasians, the prevalence of generalized PPR ranges between 5% and 10% with a clear maximum at adolescence (Wolf and Goosses 1986, Kasteleijn-Nolst Trenité 1989). In Japan and India the prevalence of PPRs is much lower at 1–2% (Saleem et al. 1994; Shiraishi et al. 2001). The incidence of PPRs also varies in the different ethnic groups: De Graaf found in South Africa that 0.4% of blacks, 4% of coloreds, and 5.2% of whites showed a PPR (De Graaf 1992). Neither sunshine duration, sunlight intensity, nor the amount of pigmentation of the eyelids and retina (albino black people) can account for this difference (Danesi 1985; Familusi et al. 1998); thus PPRs seem to depend primarily on genetic factors. Because the prevalence of epilepsy in the various countries is roughly similar, PPRs are thought to be a separate trait, adding to or modifying the other epilepsy genes. This is confirmed by twin studies (Daly and Bickford 1951) and family EEG studies by the German group of Doose (Doose et al. 1969; Doose and Waltz 1993). Family EEG studies give a sibling risk ratio as high as 50% when siblings with at least one parent with a PPR are systematically studied between 5 and 15 years of age (Waltz 1994).

In nearly all studies on photosensitivity and independent of the IPS methodology used, a clear predominance of females has been found, amounting to 60% of patients (Herrlin 1954; Jeavons and Harding 1975; Wolf and Goosses 1986; Kasteleijn-Nolst Trenité 1989; Obeid et al. 1991; Familusi et al. 1998).

Visually induced seizures in a general population

After the reporting of generalized tonic–clonic epileptic seizures (GTCS) during *Nintendo*-videogaming in the UK in 1992, a nationwide prospective study was undertaken to determine the incidence of TV- and videogame-induced seizures (Quirk et al. 1995). The annual incidence of cases of visually

The Causes of Epilepsy, eds. S. D. Shorvon, F. Andermann, and R. Guerrini. Published by Cambridge University Press. © Cambridge University Press 2011.

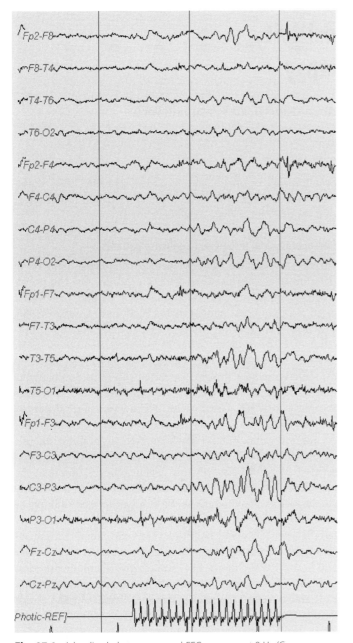

Fig. 97.1. A localized photoparoxysmal EEG response at 8 Hz (Grass PS-33 photic stimulator) with eyes open in a female adolescent. EEG settings: amplification 7–10 µV/mm, high-frequency filter 70 Hz, time constant 0.3 s, and paper speed 30 mm/s.

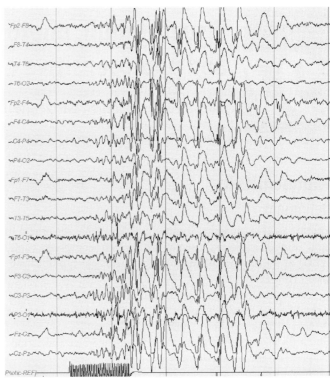

Fig. 97.2. A generalized photoparoxysmal EEG response at 40 Hz (Grass PS-33 photic stimulator) with eyes open in a female adolescent. EEG settings: amplification 7–10 µV/mm, high-frequency filter 70 Hz, time constant 0.3 s, and paper speed 30 mm/s.

sensitive epilepsy and PPRs, as determined in this study in newly diagnosed epilepsy patients over a 3-month period, was conservatively estimated to be 1.1 per 100 000, representing approximately 2% of all new cases of epilepsy. If the age range was restricted to 7–19 years, the annual incidence rose to 5.7 per 100 000 (10% of all new cases). Since not all the patients had an EEG recorded and different IPS methods were used, an estimate had to be made.

An epidemiological survey held after the TV transmission in Japan of a Pokémon cartoon with flashing colored images gave the following results: 80% of the Japanese children had watched the program and 67 (6.1%) of them had shown neurological problems: 10 (0.9%) had seizure symptoms during the program; 28 (2.6%) had complaints like headache, nausea, blurred vision, or vertigo around the cartoon broadcasting time, and in 29 children (2.7%) the symptoms and signs started within 30 min of the cartoon (Furusho *et al.* 2002). The children with seizures were older (over 8 years old) and more often had an individual or family history of seizures. A clear PPR was found in only three of the 10 children who had reported seizures. In research carried out by the Japanese Ministry of Health, in a survey including older children and adolescents, up to 10.4% of viewers had symptoms and 1.4% seizures. In children it is sometimes difficult to make a distinction between migraine and epilepsy; headache can be the only sign of an epileptic event (Parisi *et al.* 2007).

Clinical features and pathophysiology of disease
Clinical features

Photosensitivity can be found in all epilepsy types (albeit more in the generalized epilepsies than the partial ones). Dependent on the epilepsy type with which it is connected, the visually evoked reflex seizure type is an absence, myoclonic, partial simple, or partial complex seizure (Kasteleijn-Nolst Trenité *et al.* 2001). Photosensitive patients can clinically roughly be divided in two types: (1) those with predominantly myoclonic jerks and 2) those with "absence" type of seizures (including occipital seizures and other partial seizure types). The first category of patients is generally fully aware of the jerks and the causal relationship with visual stimuli like flashing lights and TV screens. Typically, myoclonic jerks occur in the eyelids, neck, shoulders, and arms and are basically symmetrical. Secondary GTCSs occur frequently and especially after sleep deprivation and stress.

The second category of patients does not notice any seizures unless a GTCs has occurred. It is usually only through circumstantial evidence (seizures occur for example always while watching TV at a close distance) that the seizures are considered as reflex ones.

Although noticeable by the patient, occipital seizures with loss of vision and nausea develop gradually and are usually not easily recognized as being induced by visual stimuli. After a relatively long period, this symptomatology can also be followed by loss of consciousness and finally a GTCS. These so-called photosensitive occipital seizures are found predominantly in children.

Pathophysiology

The different types of visually evoked seizures reflect the underlying pathophysiology; different seizure types are found between patients.

Visually sensitive patients have normal vision (Kasteleijn-Nolst Trenité 1989). They have an abnormal cortical reaction to certain visual stimuli. Activation of the visual cortex depends on triggering a critical mass of cortical neurons, synchronization of the physiologic activation, and spreading to other cortical areas, often following preferential pathways (Wilkins et al. 1979). Both magno- and parvocellular mechanisms are involved (Harding & Fylan 1999).

Abnormal visual contrast gain control may be underlying the abnormal cortical response to visual stimuli (Porciatti et al. 2000).

Of particular interest in understanding the pathophysiology of photosensitivity is the crossroad between migraine, epilepsy, and photosensitivity (Parisi et al. 2007, 2008; Parisi 2009).

Links and overlap between epilepsy, migraine, and photosensitivity

The close association between migraine and idiopathic benign childhood epilepsy and especially with the occipital lobe epilepsies has been well recognized, and a differential diagnosis in some particular case still represents a challenge (Guerrini et al. 1998; Parisi et al. 2007; Piccioli et al. 2009). Occipital epilepsies and migraine have visual aura preceding headache and other autonomic symptoms in common. In both, the visual aura's symptoms and signs can be elicited by bright and flashing lights, and can be either positive (flicker scotoma, hallucinations) or negative (temporary loss of vision) in nature (Piccioli et al. 2009).

Wendorff and Juchniewicz (2005) found that the prevalence of PPR in 263 migraine patients aged 7–18 years was high and was most frequently found in the group below 12 years of age with migraine with aura (17.6%); in 7/12 headache was exclusively provoked by visual stimuli.

In families with both migraine and epilepsy, it is more likely that epileptic photosensitivity plays an important role (Piccioli et al. 2009); in a recently described case of a 14-year-old photosensitive girl with status migrainosus for 3 days, only after intravenous administration of diazepam did the complaints disappear (Parisi et al. 2007). It appeared that the "migraine" status was provoked by prolonged television viewing (a new, large-screen television) and visiting an exhibition with much color and contrast. This relatively long delay of epileptic phenomena after visual stimulation is rather typical for occipital photosensitive epilepsies and in this case the headache is thus a photosensitive occipital seizure.

In summary, it is important to make EEG recordings with standardized IPS in cases in which the headache might be clearly triggered by visual stimuli and especially if both epilepsy and migraine occur within the family.

Genetics

Evidence for a genetic component for PPR comes from twin and family studies: (1) monozygotic twin pairs showed an almost 100% concordance and (2) a sibling risk ratio of 20% or even 50% has been found when siblings with at least one affected parent were studied between the age of 5 and 15 years (Waltz et al. 2000).

There is consensus that PPR is a heritable epilepsy-related EEG trait with an autosomal dominant mode of inheritance with reduced penetrance. Two independent genome-wide linkage screens have been conducted in multiplex PPR families with identification of the four PPR loci 7q31 and 16p13 (Pinto et al. 2005) and 6p21 and 13q31 (Tauer et al. 2005). It is possible that the ascertainment of Dutch and French PPR families with prominent myoclonic idiopathic generalized epilepsy background have resulted in the selection of a specific set of PPR genes (on 7q32 and 16p13), involved in the predisposition of that particular seizure type. The German sample was predominantly of absence type. Although the PPR endophenotype concept assumes that the underlying genetic liability of endophenotypes is less complex and easier to elucidate than the liability of complex phenotypes, such as idiopathic generalized epilepsy, many genes may interact at many levels, leading to activation of multiple neuronal circuits, which results in phenotypic variations (Pinto et al. 2007).

Epilepsy in photosensitivity
Frequency of epilepsy in the disease
Photoparoxysmal responses and clinical epilepsy

Up until now, the lifetime relationship between the EEG finding of a PPR and the clinical diagnosis of epilepsy or visual sensitivity, manifesting itself as myoclonic jerks, absence seizures, or simple and complex partial seizures in daily life, is not known; no long-term follow-up studies have been done in persons with and without epilepsy, but with a PPR. Therefore, it is not possible to predict the occurrence of epileptic seizures over a lifetime in someone with a PPR.

However, several retrospective studies in rather unselected EEG populations have been performed: some 75–77% of subjects with a generalized PPR have a history of epilepsy (Jayakar and Chiappa 1990; So et al. 1993).

In a prospective study in an epilepsy center, 94 of 100 patients with a generalized PPR outlasting the flash-stimulus had a seizure history, compared to 84 of those without a PPR. In these 94 IPS-positive patients, 55 (59%) had a clear history of visually induced seizures in daily life (Kasteleijn-Nolst Trenité 1989).

Although Reilly and Peters (1973) emphasized the predictive value of an epileptiform response that continues after the train of flashes, others did not find a difference in outcome between those with and without self-sustaining PPRs (Jayakar and Chiappa 1990; Nagarajan et al. 2003).

Photoparoxysmal responses and epilepsy types

Photoparoxysmal responses have been found albeit predominantly in idiopathic generalized epilepsy, in all epilepsy types, including progressive epilepsy types like Lafora and Unverricht–Lundborg (Kasteleijn-Nolst Trenité et al. 2001) and mesial temporal lobe epilepsy (Fiore et al. 2003). They are more often found among those with an idiopathic generalized epilepsy (60%) than among those with a focal epilepsy (30%), compared to 15% idiopathic generalized epilepsy and 60% focal epilepsies in control patients without any PPR and matched for age and sex (Kasteleijn-Nolst Trenité 1989)

Among the different idiopathic generalized epilepsy syndromes, the highest prevalence of a PPR is found in juvenile myoclonic epilepsy (30%) followed by childhood absence epilepsy (18%), and juvenile absence epilepsy (8%) (Wolf and Goosses 1986; Shiraishi et al. 2001). Relatively often a PPR is found in the catastrophic epilepsy syndromes, although studies on the prevalence are lacking. See Table 97.1 for an overview of the prevalence of PPRs in the various epilepsy syndromes and its peculiarities.

Photoparoxysmal responses and clinical signs in the EEG laboratory

Observational studies as early as 1953 described in detail the overall spectrum of clinical signs and symptoms that could be evoked by IPS in 27 photosensitive children between 2 and 13 years of age, six of whom were mentally retarded: absence seizures; myoclonic jerks in the arms, head, eyelids, or upper limbs; speech arrest; turning of the eyes to the left or right side or a GTCS after head-turning to the left with build-up of occipital epileptiform activity on the right side with generalization afterwards. Two children only had complaints of dizziness (Daly and Bickford 1951).

A more recent video-EEG study in children and adolescents again revealed clinical signs in all photosensitive patients with a generalized PPR (Piccioli et al. 2003). Interestingly the clinical signs during videogame playing were similar to the PPRs evoked by IPS.

About only half of photosensitive children, adolescents, and adults are aware of IPS-evoked clinical signs (Kasteleijn-Nolst Trenité et al. 1987).

Self-induction

A very specific phenomenon in photosensitivity is self-induction or auto-induction; some patients can deliberately evoke epileptiform discharges and seizures. Patients may be compulsively drawn to sources of flicker or pattern stimulation such as TV screens, or they may induce attacks with maneuvers producing visual stimulation such as repeated eye-rolling and eyelid flicker. Although mentally retarded patients show this behavior more bluntly and are more easily recognized as such, this self-stimulation occurs equally in normal intelligent children and adults (for examples see Kasteleijn-Nolst Trenité 1989). Pleasurable sensations and stress relief are the most common reasons for self-stimulation. Recognition of such a sensation may help in differentiating EMA from self-induced seizures.

Risk factors
Daily life

Besides more general precipitating factors like stress and sleep deprivation, visually sensitive reflex seizures are provoked by a variety of natural and artificial visual stimuli. Among the most provocative and best recognized are: flickering sunlight shining through trees, discothèque lights, old TV sets, special TV and computer programs with colored and white flashing lights, and certain video games. Less well known are dysfunctioning fluorescent lighting and striped or dotted black-and-white patterns like in Venetian blinds, rolling walkways, clothes, and buildings.

Modern displays like liquid crystal, organic, and polymer light-emitting diodes, and plasma-driven panels all generate their light output in a different way, and it depends on the size of the screen, the contrast, and luminance as to whether these will provoke seizures in photosensitive patients (Kasteleijn-Nolst Trenité et al. 2004). The amount and variety of provocative visual stimuli in daily life is still increasing; the likelihood of a photosensitive patient getting a reflex seizure is for that reason very high.

Laboratory

The most common and routinely used provocative factor in the EEG laboratory is stroboscopic light flashing at between 2 and 60 Hz. The most important physical characteristics are modulation depth of the light (the proportional change in luminance with each flash), the frequency of the modulation in Hz, average luminance (intensity), and wave length (color);

Table 97.1. Overview of the prevalence and peculiarities concerning occurrence of photoparoxysmal EEG responses in the various syndromes; the data are derived from studies as well as clinical descriptions within the various articles, since there are very limited evidence-based data on the prevalence of photosensitivity in most syndromes

Syndromes	Prevalence of PPR including pattern %	Peak age of photosensitivity in years	Peculiarities
Generalized epilepsies			
(1) Idiopathic generalized epilepsies (IGE)			
(a) Benign myoclonic epilepsy of infancy	10		
(b) Childhood absence epilepsy	13–18	8–12	
(c) Juvenile absence epilepsy	8	12–20	
(d) Juvenile myoclonic epilepsy	30	12–25	Photosensitivity strongest in the early morning
(e) GTCS on awakening	4–10	?	
(f) IGE with practice-induced seizures, including primary reading epilepsy	60	?	Pattern sensitivity
(g) Visually sensitive IGE, including eyelid myoclonias with absences	100	8–30	
(2) Cryptogenic generalized epilepsies			
(a) Epilepsy with myoclonic–astatic seizures (Doose syndrome)	?	?	
(3) Symptomatic generalized epilepsies			
(a) Progressive myoclonus epilepsies			
Neuronal ceroidlipofuscinosis	20	3–25	Giant evoked potentials to single flashes
Lafora disease	100	10–16	PPR especially at low flash frequencies early morning
Unverricht–Lundborg disease	50	10–16	PPR especially at low flash frequencies early morning
Myoclonus epilepsy with ragged red fibers (MERRF)	?	?	Giant evoked potentials to single flashes
(b) Gaucher (type III, neuronopathic form)	?	?	One case described
(c) Other forms	?	?	
Localization-related epilepsies			
(1) Idiopathic partial epilepsies			
(a) Idiopathic photosensitive occipital lobe epilepsy	100		Visual hallucinations, delay between visual stimulation and seizures
(2) Symptomatic and cryptogenic partial epilepsies	?	?	
Undetermined epilepsies			
(a) Severe myoclonic epilepsy of infancy (Dravet syndrome)	40	2–4	Often self-induction of seizures and pattern sensitivity
Situation-related and occasional seizures			
(a) Strong provocative visual stimuli in patients with latent visual sensitivity	100	10–30	Family history of photosensitivity
(b) Alcohol withdrawal, drugs, vitamins, toxic drugs	Individual cases	?	Temporarily PPRs
(c) Trauma, concussion	?	childhood	Temporarily PPRs

Source: Based on Kasteleijn-Nolst Trenité *et al.* (2001).

Table 97.2 Scoring table of photosensitivity ranges per patient and per time point

Flash frequency (/s)	1	2	6	9	10	12	15	18	20	23	25	30	40	50	60
Hz →															
Eye condition ↓															
Eye closure	–	–	+	0	0	0	0	0	0	0	0	0	+	–	–
Eyes closed	–	–	±	+	0	0	0	0	0	0	0	+	–	–	–
Eyes open	–	–	–	±	±	±	+	0	0	+	±	–	–	–	–

Notes:
Name: PH Photo. Concomitant medication: valproate 1000 mg, lamotrigine 50 mg. Date of EEG: 12–3–2009, time: 13.05. Photosensitivity ranges:
Eye closure 6–40 Hz; Eyes closed 9–30 Hz; Eyes open 15–23 Hz.+, generalized epileptiform activity; ±, localized epileptiform activity; –, no pathological reaction; 0, frequency not tested.

these determine the likelihood of evoking PPRs (Takahashi 1999). Striped patterns with high contrast and a spatial frequency of 4 cycles per degree are provocative in about 30% of the patients (Wilkins *et al.* 1979). Only in specialized laboratories are these patterns tested in photosensitive patients (Brinciotti *et al.* 1994).

Treatment and prognosis
Non-pharmacological treatment

Avoidance of potentially provocative visual stimuli seems advisable for all patients and can be the only treatment in those who are sensitive to a relatively narrow frequency range. Others, who notice their provoked jerks, can be instructed to look away from the stimulus or to close or cover one eye when the stimulus occurs unexpectedly. Monocular occlusion by covering the orbit of one eye with the palm of a hand is a very effective measure to reduce the epileptogenic effects of flicker and striped patterns. In general, it is important to keep a distance from TV sets and to lower the contrast and luminance of TV and computer programs. In some very sensitive patients it may be necessary to remove environmental sources like old TV sets, old fluorescents bulbs, or striped patterns in clothing or buildings, either at home or at school. Discothèques, arcades, and pop concerts should especially be avoided, since alcohol intake, stress, and sleep deprivation are additional factors in lowering the seizure threshold.

Wearing very dark polarized glasses is as effective as closing one eye. For use inside home and buildings, blue light-colored glasses are a good alternative for many patients (Capovilla *et al.* 1999).

Drug treatment

The choice of drug treatment will depend on the likelihood of getting seizures evoked by visual stimuli; it depends on age, photosensitivity range, frequency and severity of seizures, and the type of epileptic syndrome as well as on the environment in which the patient lives.

Valproate is most effective; 85% of the visually sensitive patients will become seizure-free with valproate (Covanis *et al.*

1982; Harding and Jeavons 1994). Alternatives are levetiracetam and lamotrigine (Specchio *et al.* 2006). Second-best alternatives to valproate are clobazam and ethosuximide.

Treatment effects can be monitored by determining the photosensitivity range before and after drug treatment. During adolescence, the prescribed dosage should be increased not only because of the increase in body weight, but especially due to an increase in the photosensitivity itself. Therapy should in general be maintained until the age of about 25 years. Intermittent photic stimulation in the laboratory will then help in predicting the relapse rate after partial or total withdrawal of the drug. If the photosensitivity range is increased, the medication should not be diminished further to prevent the occurrence of GTCSs.

Special attention is needed in treating self-inducing patients: a prescription of high-dosage valproate as soon as self-induction behavior is diagnosed in childhood might suppress the sensitivity so effectively that the compulsive behavior stops and stays away. Older self-inducing photosensitive patients may refuse treatment or not comply with it.

Diagnostic tests

Intermittent photic stimulation

Photosensitivity is discovered or confirmed with an EEG investigation with IPS, provided a high-quality photo stimulator is used (flash frequency range of 2–60 Hz and luminance of 100 cd/m^2 per flash (Kasteleijn-Nolst Trenité *et al.* 1999). Many commercial and cheap stimulators are not capable of delivering this range of flash rates and cannot do so with sufficient and consistent flash intensity.

Because of the important role of the TV screen itself in triggering seizures independent of program content, routine IPS should include stimulation at frequencies of 50–60 flashes/s depending on the local AC frequency, and the corresponding 25 or 30 flashes/s rate. Some degenerative disorders with photosensitivity at the earlier stages of the disease like Lafora and Unverricht–Lundborg are associated with abnormal responses to slow rates and stimulation protocols should include rates of 1 and 2 flashes/s.

Patients are most sensitive to IPS at active eye closing and this eye condition should be tested besides the routinely performed eyes closed and eyes open condition.

A photosensitivity range for each patient can be determined by eliciting the upper and lower limits of sensitivity to IPS for that patient. The photosensitivity range is relatively stable for each patient and can be regarded as a measure of epileptogenicity.

Due to a standardized IPS procedure (short delivery of flashes, determination of threshold frequencies, for which the patient shows an epileptiform EEG response and simultaneous recording of the EEG and observation of the patient) the likelihood of provoking prominent clinical seizures is in this way extremely low. In Table 97.2 such an example is given of the determination of photosensitivity ranges in the three eye conditions in a patient.

Especially when the patient is seated, concomitant clinical signs like (eyelid) myoclonias and self-induction behavior can be observed.

Imaging techniques such as MEG, functional magnetic resonance imaging (fMRI), positron emission tomography (PET), and MRS have so far been used for scientific purposes only. An extensive clinical history with emphasis on the detection of possible provocative visual factors is the most valuable approach.

References

Brinciotti M, Matricardi M, Pelliccia A, Trasatti G (1994) Pattern sensitivity and photosensitivity in epileptic children with visually induced seizures. *Epilepsia* **35**:842–9.

Capovilla G, Beccaria F, Romeo A, *et al.* (1999) Effectiveness of a particular blue lens on photoparoxysmal response in photosensitive epileptic patients. *Ital J Neurol Sci* **20**:161–6.

Covanis A, Gupta AK, Jeavons PM (1982) Sodium valproate: monotherapy and polytherapy. *Epilepsia* **23**:693–710.

Daly D, Bickford RG (1951) Electroencephalographic studies of identical twins with photo-epilepsy. *Electroencephalogr Clin Neurophysiol* **3**:245–9.

Danesi MA (1985) Geographical and seasonal variations in the incidence of epileptic photosensitivity. *Electroencephalogr Clin Neurophysiol* **61**:S216.

De Graaf AS, Lombard, CJ, Claassen DA (1995) Influence of ethnic and geographic factors on the classic photoparoxysmal response in the electroencephalogram of epilepsy patients. *Epilepsia* **36**:219–23.

Doose H, Waltz S (1993) Photosensitivity: genetics and clinical significance. *Neuropediatrics* **24**:249–55.

Doose H, Gerken H, Volzke E, Volz C (1969) Investigations on the genetics of photosensitivity. *Electroencephalogr Clin Neurophysiol* **27**:625.

Familusi JB, Adamolekun B, Olayinka BA, Muzengi D, Levy LF (1998) Electroencephalographic photosensitivity among Zimbabwean youths. *Ann Trop Paediatr* **18**:267–74.

Ferlazzo E, Magaudda A, Striano P, *et al.* (2007) Long-term evolution of EEG in Unverricht–Lundborg disease. *Epilepsy Res* **73**:219–27.

Filocamo M, Mazzotti R, Stroppiano M, *et al.* (2004) Early visual seizures and progressive myoclonus epilepsy in neuronopathic Gaucher disease due to a rare compound heterozygosity. *Epilepsia* **45**:1154–7.

Fiore LA, Valente K, Gronich G, Ono CR, Buchpiguel CA (2003) Mesial temporal lobe epilepsy with focal photoparoxysmal response. *Epilept Disord* **5**:39–43.

Furusho J, Suzuki M, Tazaki I, *et al.* (2002) A comparison survey of seizures and other symptoms of Pokemon phenomenon. *Pediatr Neurol* **27**:350–5.

Guerrini R, Bonanni P, Parmeggiani L, *et al.* (1998) Induction of partial seizures by visual stimulation: clinical and electroencephalographic features and evoked potentials studies. *Adv Neurol* **75**:159–78.

Harden A, Pampiglione G (1982) Neurophysiological studies (EEG, ERG, VEP, SEP) in 88 children with so-called neuronal ceroid-lipofuscinosis. In: Armstrong D, Koppang N, Rider JA (eds.) *Ceroid-Lipofuscinoses (Batten's Disease)*. Amsterdam: Elsevier, pp. 61–70.

Harding GFA, Fylan F (1999) Two visual mechanisms of photosensitivity. *Epilepsia* **40**:1446–51.

Harding GFA, Jeavons M (1994) *Photosensitive Epilepsy*, 2nd edn. London: MacKeith Press.

Herrlin KM (1954) EEG with photic stimulation: a study of children with manifest or suspected epilepsy. *Electroencephalogr Clin Neurophysiol* **6**:573–89.

Jayakar P, Chiappa KH (1990) Clinical correlations of photoparoxysmal responses. *Electroencephalogr Clin Neurophysiol* **75**:251–4.

Jeavons PM, Harding GFA (1975) *Photosensitive Epilepsy*. London: Heinemann.

Kasteleijn-Nolst Trenité DGA (1989) Photosensitivity in epilepsy: electrophysiological and clinical correlates. *Acta Neurol Scand* **80**:S25(1–150).

Kasteleijn-Nolst Trenité DGA, Binnie CD, Meinardi H (1987) Photosensitive patients: symptoms and signs during intermittent photic stimulation and their relation to seizures in daily life. *J Neurol Neurosurg Psychiatry* **50**:1546–9.

Kasteleijn-Nolst Trenité DGA, Binnie CD, Harding GFA, *et al.* (1999) Medical technology assessment, photic stimulation: standardization of screening methods. *Neurophysiol Clin* **29**:318–24.

Kasteleijn-Nolst Trenité DG, Guerrini R, Binnie CD, Genton P (2001) Visual sensitivity and epilepsy: a proposed terminology and classification for clinical and EEG phenomenology. *Epilepsia* **42**:692–701.

Kasteleijn-Nolst Trenité DG, Silva LCB, Manreza MLG (2003) Prevalence of photoparoxysmal EEG responses in normal children and adolescents in Teofile Otoni, Brazil: 2001–2002. *Epilepsia* **44**(Suppl. 8):48.

Kasteleijn-Nolst Trenité DG, Van Der Beld G, Heynderickx I, Groen P (2004) Visual stimuli in daily life. *Epilepsia* **45**(Suppl 1):2–6.

Nagarajan L, Kulkarni A, Palumbo-Clark L, *et al.* (2003) Photoparoxysmal responses in children: their characteristics and clinical correlates. *Pediatr Neurol* **29**:222–6.

Obeid T, Daif AK, Waheed G, *et al.* (1991) Photosensitive epilepsies and photoconvulsive responses in Arabs. *Epilepsia* **32**:77–81.

Parisi P (2009) Why is migraine rarely, and not usually, the sole ictal epileptic manifestation? *Seizure* **18**:309–12.

Parisi P, Kasteleijn-Nolst Trenité DGA, Piccioli M, *et al.* (2007) A case with atypical childhood occipital epilepsy "Gastaut type": an ictal migraine manifestation with a good response to intravenous diazepam. *Epilepsia* **48**:2181–6.

Parisi P, Piccioli M, de Sneeuw S, *et al.* (2008) Redefining headache diagnostic criteria as epileptic manifestation. *Cephalalgia* **28**:408–9. Author reply 409.

Piccioli M, Parisi P, Tisei P, *et al.* (2009) Ictal headache and visual sensitivity. *Cephalalgia* **29**:194–203.

Piccioli M, Ricci S, Vigevano F, *et al.* (2003) Visual sensitive children: symptoms and signs during intermittent photic stimulation and video game playing. *Epilepsia* **44**:(Suppl 9):307.

Pinto D, Westland B, de Haan GJ, *et al.* (2005) Genome-wide linkage scan of epilepsy-related photoparoxysmal electroencephalographic response: evidence for linkage on chromosomes 7q32 and 16p13. *Hum Mol Genet* **14**:171–8.

Pinto D, Kasteleijn-Nolst Trenité DG, Cordell HJ, *et al.* (2007) Explorative two-locus linkage analysis suggests a multiplicative interaction between the 7q32 and 16p13 myoclonic seizures-related photosensitivity loci. *Genet Epidemiol* **31**:42–50.

Porciatti V, Bonanni P, Fiorentini A, Guerrini R (2000) Lack of cortical contrast gain control in human photosensitive epilepsy. *Nat Neurosci* **3**:259–63.

Quirk JA, Fish DR, Smith SJ, *et al.* (1995) Incidence of photosensitive epilepsy: a prospective national study. *Electroencephalogr Clin Neurophysiol* **95**:260–7.

Reilly EL, Peters JF (1973) Relationship of some varieties of electroencephalographic photosensitivity to clinical convulsive disorders. *Neurology* **23**:1050–7.

Roy AK, Pinheiro L, Rajesh SV (2003) Prevalence of photosensitivity: an Indian experience. *Neurol India* **51**:241–3.

Saleem SM, Thomas M, Jain S, Maheshwari MC (1994) Incidence of photosensitive epilepsy in unselected Indian epileptic population. *Acta Neurol Scand* **89**:5–8.

Santavuori P, Rapola J, Nuutila A, *et al.* (1991) The spectrum of Jansky–Bielschowsky disease. *Neuropediatrics* **22**:92–6.

Shiraishi H, Fujiwara T, Inoue Y, Yagi K (2001) Photosensitivity in relation to epileptic syndromes: a survey from an epilepsy center in Japan. *Epilepsia* **42**:393–7.

So EL, Ruggles KH, Ahmann PA, Olson KA (1993) Prognosis of paroxysmal response in nonepileptic patients. *Neurology* **43**:1719–22.

Specchio LM, Gambardella A, Giallonardo AT, *et al.* (2006) Open label, long-term, pragmatic study on levetiracetam in the treatment of juvenile myoclonic epilepsy. *Epilepsy Res* **71**:32–9.

Striano S, Capovilla G, Sofia V, *et al.* (2009) Eyelid myoclonia with absences (Jeavons syndrome): a well-defined idiopathic generalized epilepsy syndrome or a spectrum of photosensitive conditions? *Epilepsia* **50**(Suppl 5):15–19.

Takahashi T (1999) Activation methods. In: Niedermeyer E, Lopes da Silva F (eds.) *Electroencephalography: Basic Principles, Clinical Applications and Related Fields,* (4th edn.) Baltimore, MD: Williams & Wilkins, pp. 261–84.

Tassinari CA, Bureau-Paillas M, Dalla Bernardina B, *et al.* (1978) Lafora disease. *Rev Electroencephalogr Neurophysiol Clin* **8**:107–22.

Tauer U, Lorenz S, Lenzen KP, *et al.* (2005) Genetic dissection of photosensitivity and its relation to idiopathic generalized epilepsy. *Ann Neurol* **57**:866–73.

Waltz S (1994) Photosensitivity and epilepsy: a genetic approach, In: Malafosse A, Genton P, Hirsch E, *et al.* (eds.) *Idiopathic Generalized Epilepsies: Clinical, Experimental and Genetic Aspects* London: John Libbey, pp. 317–28.

Waltz S, Stephani U (2000) Inheritance of photosensitivity. *Neuropediatrics* **31**:82–5.

Wendorff J, Juchniewicz B (2005) Photosensitivity in children with idiopathic headaches. *Neurol Neurochir Pol* **39**(4 Suppl 1):S9–16.

Wilkins AJ, Darby CE, Binnie CD (1979) Neurophysiological aspects of pattern-sensitive epilepsy. *Brain* **102**:1–25.

Wolf P, Goosses R (1986) Relation of photosensitivity to epileptic syndromes. *J Neurol Neurosurg Psychiatry* **49**:1386–91.

Chapter

98

Startle-induced (and other sensory-induced) epilepsy

Jean-Pierre Vignal, Sandrine Aubert, and Patrick Chauvel

The startle reaction is defined as "an immediate reflex response to sudden, intense stimulation" (Landis and Hunt 1939). Startle seizures are motor seizures (tonic, clonic, myoclonic, or atonic) triggered by a sudden, more or less intense, stimulation. In the classification of the International League Against Epilepsy (1989), they have been described as bilateral tonic seizures, usually symptomatic, and categorized as partial symptomatic epilepsies. Startle seizures have been reported in a wide spectrum of lesional etiologies, from atrophic cortical lesions to cortical dysplasias. In the particular case of infantile hemiplegia they characterize a well-circumscribed syndrome (Alajouanine and Gastaut 1955; Chauvel *et al.* 1987, 1992).

Startle epilepsy with infantile hemiplegia

Startle seizures are characterized by a bilateral tonic contraction, predominating on the paretic side when asymmetric, and comprising head and trunk flexion, rising of flexed or extended upper limbs, extension of lower limbs, eye closure, and facial contraction. They are so brisk that they usually provoke a fall. Deviation of the head, ipsilateral to the paretic side, facial flushing, urination, and late mood alteration (euphoria or crying) can also be associated with the seizure. Duration is short (10–20 s). Rarely, seizures start with focal clonic jerks of the paretic upper limb. In half the cases, consciousness is not impaired during the seizure. Besides startle seizures spontaneous attacks with roughly similar semiology but starting sometimes with somatosensory signs may occur. Seizures are frequent and usually occur every day. The scalp-recorded, triggered and spontaneous, attacks consist of flattening and fast low-voltage discharge, either diffuse or involving frontoparietal regions (Fig. 98.1). This discharge is preceded by a high-amplitude evoked spike of larger amplitude at the vertex. In a few cases, the ictal electroencephalogram (EEG) is obscured by muscle artifacts. Triggering modalities are usually auditory but can also be somatosensory (unexpected shock to the hemiparetic side, stumbling of the paretic foot or an obstacle) or visual

(sudden irruption of an object into the patient's visual field). The effective stimuli should be unexpected but not necessarily intense. A low-intensity and unexpected noise can be sufficient in some patients. Habituation is possible when repeated stimuli occur.

Startle seizures usually occur in children having ante-, peri-, or early postnatal lesions (before 2 years of age), of infectious, ischemic, or undetermined origin. Neurological examination always shows a unilateral motor deficit, spasticity, or hemianesthesia, and in half the children an intellectual deficit. Age at seizure onset is variable, between 5 months and 16 years (Chauvel *et al.* 1992). Atrophic lesions, frequently porencephaly, in the frontoparietal regions associated with a hemicerebral atrophy reflect widespread lesions involving the suprasylvian lateral cortex but sparing the most medial and dorsal cortex (Fig. 98.2).

Stereo-electroencephalographic (SEEG) recordings have demonstrated an essential role of the pre-motor cortex, especially the supplementary motor area (SMA), and of the motor cortex in generating startle seizures (Bancaud *et al.* 1967, 1975; Chauvel *et al.* 1992). In most cases, the fast low-voltage discharge (FLVD) simultaneously involves motor and premotor cortices with preferential secondary spread bilaterally to the medial frontal cortex. Rarely, the FLVD has a more restricted spatial distribution, limited to the medial frontocentral cortex or to the SMA (Fig. 98.3).

The triggering stimulus of startle seizures is an unexpected stimulus but one that would not as readily elicit a startle reaction in normal subjects. In other words, the threshold of reaction is abnormally low in startle seizure patients, reflecting a default of inhibition. The startle reaction in normal humans comprises eye closure, elevation of the upper limbs and flexion of the neck, trunk, and upper and lower limbs (Brown *et al.* 1991). The pattern of muscular involvement at onset of startle seizures is different from the pattern observed in physiological startle (Chauvel *et al.* 1992). In animals, the generators of the startle reaction are localized in the bulbo-pontine reticular formation (Leitner *et al.* 1980) which is under the control of upper cortical centers. In the physiological startle reflex, an afferent facilitatory control from the cortical

The Causes of Epilepsy, eds. S. D. Shorvon, F. Andermann, and R. Guerrini. Published by Cambridge University Press. © Cambridge University Press 2011.

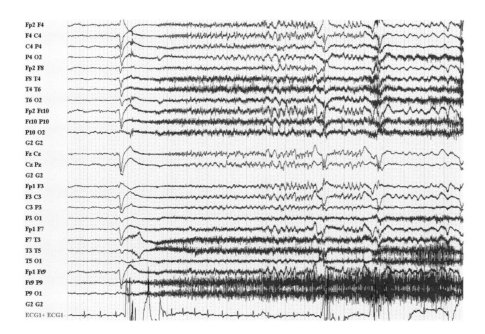

Fig. 98.1. Startle seizure: bilateral tonic seizure triggered by an unexpected sound. The electro-encephalogram (EEG) consisted of bilateral fast discharges, preceded by a high-amplitude evoked spike maximal at the vertex.

A

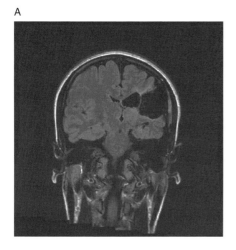

B

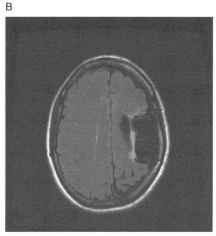

Fig. 98.2. Cerebral magnetic resonance image (MRI) of an 18-year-old woman showing a large porencephalic cyst involving the left frontoparietal region.

sensory areas is exerted onto the reticular pontine nuclei (Ascher 1965). It has also been demonstrated in patients that cortical lesions, for instance in the superior temporal gyrus, lead to a decreased amplitude of the audiospinal facilitation mediating the startle reaction (Ho *et al.* 1987; Liegeois-Chauvel *et al.* 1989). Briefly, the sensory area facilitates startle in the modality in which it is elicited. In contrast, the corticospinal motor system could exert inhibitory control on the startle reflex (Voordecker *et al.* 1997; Oguro *et al.* 2001). It is not unlikely that startle seizures in patients with widespread cortical lesions frequently involving underlying white matter, especially the pyramidal tract, could be triggered after an initial exaggerated startle reflex. The precipitating stimulus would induce such a reflex and thus a bilateral motor contraction predominating in the hemiplegic side, reflecting activation of an abnormally facilitated subcortical loop. In addition, proprioceptive reafferentation from the muscles first involved at seizure onset, directly projecting to hyperexcitable motor and premotor cortices through a transcortical reflex loop, would then trigger the motor seizure itself (Chauvel *et al.* 1992).

These epilepsies are usually medically intractable. In cases with massive hemiplegia a focal resection of the cortex involved in the epileptogenic zone may be indicated. Intracerebral recordings (SEEG) are required to delineate the epileptogenic zone (Chauvel *et al.* 1992). The presurgical investigations must first ensure that the lesion and the epileptogenic zone area are strictly unilateral, then delineate the extent of the epileptogenic zone in the affected hemisphere, so as to determine the surgical strategy (tailored cortectomy, lobectomy, hemispherotomy, etc.). Surprisingly, in a number of cases, the epileptogenic zone size can be far less extensive than the lesion. In the patient illustrated in Fig. 98.3, whatever the

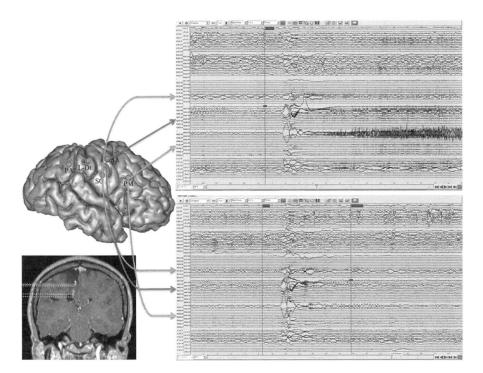

Fig. 98.3. Two startle seizures recorded with depth electrodes in the same patient (GC). Top: the seizure, triggered by a sudden sound, is characterized by arrest of speech, slight flexion of the neck, bilateral elevation of both arms, predominant on the left, with abduction of the left arm, and slight deviation of the head to the left, then extension and abduction of the left leg. Bottom: with same triggering, the clinical semiology is limited to flexion of the neck and elevation–abduction of the left arm. The two seizures are initiated by a huge slow spike, then a fast discharge in the right SMA and anterior medial premotor cortex, with a slower rhythmic discharge in the ipsilateral precentral cortex, and bilateral spread to the postcentral cortex. The different duration of the two seizures, but the same propagation, illustrates the mode of organization of startle seizures in the pericentral areas.

duration of the seizure, its spread remained limited to the motor and medial premotor cortex on the damaged side.

Startle seizures and other epileptic syndromes

Startle seizures triggered by an unexpected sensory stimulation have also been reported in Lennox–Gastaut syndrome, Down syndrome, Reye syndrome, Sturge–Weber syndrome, mitochondrial disease, Angelman syndrome, Tay–Sachs disease, and dysplastic lesions (Nakamura *et al.* 1975; Aguglia *et al.* 1984; Guerrini *et al.* 1990; Manford *et al.* 1996; Tibussek *et al.* 2006, Ferlazzo *et al.* 2009). These startle seizures were usually characterized by: (1) focal or generalized tonic motor signs, with a possible focal somatosensory onset (Manford *et al.* 1996); (2) generalized or axial tonic signs; (3) generalized atonic manifestations; (4) myoclonic manifestations; (5) generalized tonic–clonic signs; and (6) atypical absences in some cases. Seizures could be triggered by sudden sounds, somatosensory stimuli (unexpected touch), and visual stimuli (sudden irruption into the visual field). Spontaneous seizures were always observed. Frequency of seizures was especially high (often more than one a day).

Startle seizures are actually not specific for any epileptic syndrome but may be observed in various diseases and in a wide spectrum of cerebral lesions from an area of dysplasia to widespread bilateral cortico-subcortical lesions. The triggering mechanism is not clearly elucidated. Given the multiplicity of causes, multiple mechanisms are possible. In cases of widespread cerebral lesions, motor reactions triggered by an unexpected but not intense stimulus frequently occur without following seizures (Tibussek *et al.* 2006). One might hypothesize a default of inhibition secondary to a lesion within the subcortical loop of the startle reaction (nucleus reticularis pontis caudalis) and also a mechanism close to the abovementioned proprioceptive reafferentation to hyperexcitable motor and premotor cortices, as recently suggested in Down syndrome (Ferlazzo *et al.* 2009).

Cutaneous stimulation in the trigger zone and movement-induced seizures

These seizures are rare, constituting 1.1% of patients recorded between 1992 and 1996 in a video-EEG monitoring unit (Vignal *et al.* 1998). The description of these epilepsies is therefore based on only a few published case reports.

Seizures elicited by cutaneous stimulation of a trigger zone start with localized paresthesiae such as tingling sensations. These sensations spread according to a Bravais–Jacksonian march preceding the tonic (more rarely clonic) motor signs which are initially focal and sometimes rapidly become bilateral. Seizures end with focal tonic–clonic signs. Duration is short, usually less than 40 s. Secondary tonic–clonic generalizations are rare. Usually, there is no loss of contact, and occurrence of speech arrest depends on the involvement of the motor frontal opercular cortex. Associated spontaneous seizures are common. The localization of ictal somatosensory or somatomotor signs is closely related to the localization of the trigger zone, which is a spatially restricted cutaneous region whose stimulation by shock, rubbing, or tapping elicits dysesthesiae. These dysesthesiae may remain focal or spread and be followed by somatomotor signs; they can also occur

A 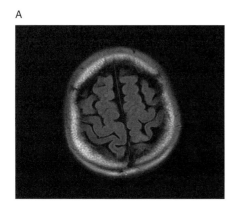 B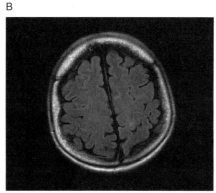

Fig. 98.4. Cerebral MRI of a 58-year-old woman, showing a fluid attenuated inverse recovery (FLAIR) hypersignal localized in the left paracentral lobe suggestive of focal cortical dysplasia. Seizures were diagnosed at 10 years of age and are characterized by initial tingling in the right foot spreading to the whole right lower limb followed by tonic manifestations. Seizures could be triggered by rubbing the right foot.

spontaneously in this zone. These ictal dysesthesiae are related to brief and repeated fast discharges localized in the primary sensory cortex (Vignal *et al.* 1998). The trigger zone can be localized in a limb, the trunk, or the face. To be efficient, the stimulus must usually be repeated but does not necessarily have to be unexpected. It can also be evoked by the sole mental representation of the triggering stimulus as reported by Goldie and Green (1959) in a patient having a parietal angioma who could trigger a seizure by rubbing the right side of the face, and also by the simple thought of this rubbing. Seizures starting with facial paresthesiae followed by hemifacial motor signs, head deviation, and salivation can be triggered by teeth brushing (Holmes *et al.* 1982; O'Brien *et al.* 1996). In these cases, gums were the trigger zone.

The somatosensory onset is determined by a hyperexcitability of the primary sensory cortex. This localization within the postcentral gyrus was confirmed by intracranial recordings (Penfield and Erickson 1941; Forster *et al.* 1949, Vignal *et al.* 1998). Vignal *et al.* (1998) showed close temporal correlations between transient FLVD recorded from intracerebral electrodes within this cortex and tingling sensations evoked by repeated cutaneous stimulations. This type of seizure is related to focal lesions of variable etiology (dysplasia, vascular, etc.) (Fig. 98.4). To facilitate seizures triggered by cutaneous stimulation, patients associate a movement of the nearby joint with the stimulation of the cutaneous trigger zone.

These seizures triggered by movements must be distinguished from familial kinesigenic paroxysmal choreoathetosis initially described by Mount and Reback (1940) (Vignal *et al.* 1998). These are provoked by sudden movement and are never associated with spontaneous attacks. Patients have normal interictal and ictal EEGs, and a natural history typically characterized by a childhood onset, juvenile worsening, and a favorable outcome during adulthood. Gastaut and Tassinari (1966) reported seizures provoked by unexpected movement in patients with startle epilepsy. There are however also seizures triggered by voluntary and expected movement. These seizures are characterized by focal somatosensory and somatomotor signs involving initially the joint whose movement triggered the seizure. Somatosensory signs usually precede

motor signs which are usually tonic and then tonic–clonic. Rarely motor signs can inaugurate the seizure, are first focal, and secondarily spread (Falconer *et al.* 1963; Santiago *et al.* 1989; Pierelli *et al.* 1997). Initial myoclonic jerks (Kochen 1989) and even atonic seizures in patients with widespread bilateral cerebral lesions (Oller-Daurella and Oller 1989) have been reported. The triggering movement can be voluntary or passive, single or repeated. Physiologically, any movement requires the activation of premotor and motor cortices and produces a proprioceptive reafferentation volley towards the primary sensory cortex and motor and premotor cortices. Two mechanisms have been invoked to explain the ictal triggering effect of movement: the first considers that the physiological features of preparation for movement involves progressive firing of premotor and motor cortex neurons which, in these cases, are hyperexcitable (Gabor 1974; Pierelli *et al.* 1997); the second considers that proprioceptive afferent volleys are the main stimuli inducing long-loop reflex activation of the motor cortex (Santiago *et al.* 1989; Vignal *et al.* 1998). Both mechanisms are possible according to the cases and to the type of triggering movement. They might also be operating concurrently.

Startle epilepsies and other reflex epilepsies with seizures evoked by sensorimotor stimuli are not defined by their etiologies but rather by the mode of triggering of their seizures. However, at least for startle seizures, the perinatal ischemic stroke has been a prominent etiological factor. The decrease in startle occurrence is explained by the same epidemiological features as for other syndromes starting in infancy, electively depending on early treatment of recurrent seizures, and prevention of hypoxic/hypometabolic shock and of status epilepticus complicating febrile convulsions (Chauvel *et al.* 1992). However, the reason why all motor or sensorimotor seizures originating from the primary sensorimotor areas are not reflex-induced (although the hypothesized pathophysiological mechanisms are present) is still unknown. Nevertheless, this could suggest that early damage to the cerebral cortex (and thalamocortical loops) with functional reorganization of the multimodal afferents to the motor cortices is a necessary condition.

References

Aguglia U, Tinuper P, Gastaut H (1984) Startle-induced epileptic seizures. *Epilepsia* 25:712–20.

Alajouanine T, Gastaut H (1955) La syncinésie-sursaut et l'épilepsie-sursaut à déclenchement sensoriel ou sensitif inopiné. *Rev Neurol* 93:29–41.

Ascher P (1965) La réaction de sursaut du chat anesthésié au chloralose. Ph.D.thesis, Université, Louis-Jean, Gap, France.

Bancaud J, Talairach J, Bonis A (1967) Physiopathologie des épilepsies-sursaut (à propos d'une épilepsie de l'AMS). *Rev Neurol* 117:441–53.

Bancaud J, Talairach J, Lamarche M, Bonis A, Trottier S (1975) Hypothèses neurophysiopathologiques sur l'épilepsie-sursaut chez l'homme. *Rev Neurol* 131:559–71.

Brown P, Rothwell JC, Thomson PD, *et al.* (1991) New observations on the normal auditory startle reflex in man. *Brain* 114:1891–902.

Chauvel P, Vignal JP, Liegeois-Chauvel C, *et al.* (1987) Startle epilepsy with infantile brain damage: the clinical and neurophysiological rationale for surgery. In: Wieser HG, Elger CE (eds.) *Presurgical Evaluation of Epileptics.* Berlin: Springer-Verlag, pp. 306–7.

Chauvel P, Trottier S, Vignal JP, Bancaud J (1992) Somatomotor seizures of frontal lobe origin. *Adv Neurol* 57:707–32.

Falconer MA, Driver MV, Serafetinides EA (1963) Seizures induced by movement. Report of case relieved by operation. *J Neurol Neurosurg Psychiatry* 26:300–7.

Ferlazzo E, Adjien CK, Guerrini R, *et al.* (2009) Lennox-Gastaut syndrome with late-onset and prominent reflex seizures in trisomy 21 patients. *Epilepsia* 50:1–9.

Forster MF, Penfield W, Jasper H, Madow L (1949) Focal epilepsy, sensory precipitation and evoked cortical potentials. *Electroenceph Clin Neurophysiol* 1:349–56.

Gabor AJ (1974) Focal seizures induced by movement without sensory feedback mechanisms. *Electroenceph Clin Neurophysiol* 36:403–8.

Gastaut H, Tassinari CA (1966) Triggering mechanisms in epilepsy: the electroclinical point of view. *Epilepsia* 7:86–138.

Goldie L, Green JA (1959) A study of the psychological factors in a case of sensory reflex epilepsy. *Brain* 82:505–24.

Guerrini R, Genton P, Bureau M, Dravet C, Roger J (1990) Reflex seizures are frequent in patients with Down syndrome and epilepsy. *Epilepsia* 31:406–17.

Ho KJ, Kileny P, Paccioretti D, McLean DR (1987) Neurologic, audiologic, and electrophysiologic sequelae of bilateral temporal lobe lesions. *Arch Neurol* 44:982–7.

Holmes GL, Blair S, Eisenberg E, *et al.* (1982) Tooth-brushing induced epilepsy. *Epilepsia* 23:657–61.

International League Against Epilepsy (1989) Proposal for revised classification of epilepsies and epileptic syndromes. *Epilepsia* 30:389–99.

Kochen S (1989) Reflex epilepsy induced by movement: a case report. In: Beaumanoir A, Gastaut H, Naquet R (eds.) *Reflex Seizures and Reflex Epilepsies.* Geneva: Editions medicine et hygiene, pp. 115–17.

Landis C, Hunt WA (1939) *The Startle Pattern.* New York: Farrar and Rinehart.

Leitner DS, Powers AS, Hoffman HS (1980) The neural substrate of the startle response. *Physiol Behav* 25:291–7.

Liegeois-Chauvel C, Morin C, Mussolino A, Bancaud J, Chauvel P (1989) Evidence for a contribution of the auditory cortex to audiospinal facilitation in man. *Brain* 112:375–91.

Manford MR, Fish DR, Shorvon SD (1996) Startle provoked epileptic seizures: features in 19 patients. *J Neurol Neurosurg Psychiatry* 61:151–6.

Mount LA, Reback S (1940) Familial paroxysmal choreoathetosis: preliminary report on a hitherto undescribed syndrome. *Arch Neurol Psychiat* 44: 841–7.

Nakamura M, Kanai H, Miyamoto Y (1975) A case of Sturge–Weber syndrome with startle epilepsy. *Brain Nerve* 27:325–9.

O'Brien TJ, Hogan RE, Sedal L, Murrie V, Cook MJ (1996) Tooth-brushing epilepsy: a report of a case with structural and functional imaging and electrophysiology demonstrating a right frontal focus. *Epilepsia* 37:694–7.

Oguro K, Aiba H, Hojo H (2001) Different responses to auditory and somaesthetic stimulation in patients with an excessive startle: a report of pediatric experience. *Clin Neurophysiol* 112:1266–72.

Oller-Daurella L, Oller FVL (1989) Seizures induced by volontary mouvements. In: Beaumanoir A, Gastaut H, Naquet R (eds.) *Reflex Seizures and Reflex Epilepsies.* Geneva: Editions medicine et hygiene, pp. 139–46.

Penfield W, Erickson TC (1941) *Epilepsy and Cerebral Localization.* Springfield, IL: Charles C. Thomas.

Pierelli F, Di Gennero G, Gherardi M, Spanelda F, Marciani MG (1997) Movement-induced seizures: a case report. *Epilepsia* 38:941–4.

Santiago M, Sampaio MJF, Keating J (1989) Movement-induced epilepsy: a study of two cases. In: Beaumanoir A, Gastaut H, Naquet R (eds.) *Reflex Seizures and Reflex Epilepsies.* Geneva: Editions medicine et hygiene, pp. 139–46.

Tibussek D, Wohlrab G, Boltshauser E, Schmitt B (2006) Proven startle-provoked epileptic seizures in childhood: semiologic and electrophysiologic variability. *Epilepsia* 46:1050–8.

Vignal JP, Biraben A, Chauvel P, Reutens DC (1998) Reflex partial seizures of sensorimotor cortex (including cortical reflex myoclonus and startle epilepsy). *Adv Neurol* 75:207–26.

Voordecker P, Mavroudakis N, Blecic S, Hildebrand J, Zegers de Beyl D (1997) Audiogenic startle reflex in acute hemiplegia. *Neurology* 49:470–3.

Primary reading epilepsy

Matthias Koepp

The causal disease

Definition

Reading epilepsy (RE) was first described by Bickford *et al.* (1956), who distinguished "primary" or "specific" RE, with seizures only in relation to reading, from a "secondary," non-specific variety with seizures when reading but under other conditions as well. The primary–specific variety is the only reflex syndrome accepted by the Commission on Classification and Terminology of the International League Against Epilepsy as an age-related idiopathic localization-related epilepsy syndrome (ILAE 1989).

Epidemiology

Reading epilepsy is a relatively rare but possibly often under-diagnosed condition. Since a first meta-analysis of 111 published cases in 1992, a further 63 cases have been reported with three larger case series from the Bethel Centre (Wolf *et al.* 1992, 1998), Mayo Clinic (Radhakrishnan *et al.* 1995), and London (Koutroumanidis *et al.* 1998) in addition to several single case reports. It is a syndrome with male preponderance (1.8 : 1) and a strong genetic component with a positive family history in about 40% of cases (Wolf 1992).

Clinical features

The age of onset is adolescence and young adulthood, long after reading skills have been acquired. Patients with RE report jaw jerking or clicking usually after reading for some time but no spontaneous seizures. Jaw jerks are the hallmark of RE but many other, distinct types of reading-induced ictal symptoms have been described: abrupt loss of consciousness, absences, paroxysmal alexia or dyslexia, and prolonged stuttering. In other cases, seizures are characterized by initial visual symptoms consisting of elementary visual hallucinations (e.g., sensation of spots before the eyes) or complex visual hallucinations with an impression of movement and palinopsia (e.g., words becoming distorted and incomprehensible). Seizures characteristically may progress to generalized seizure activity, if the patient continues to read.

Precipitating factors

Reading is a complex cognitive process including visual analysis, memory functions, and grapheme-to-phoneme conversion, more or less followed by articulation and acoustic monitoring. Debate continues as to precisely which cognitive step or component of the reading process is epileptogenic but it is obvious that there is significant variability amongst patients, with eye movements, comprehension, emotional content, speech production, and proprioceptive feedback all being reported as effective triggers (see Wolf 1992 for review). Other linguistic tasks, i.e., reading, speaking, and writing, have been reported to result in similar seizures characterized by involuntary jaw jerks, sometimes followed by staring. It is unclear whether this represents a separate syndrome, also called language-induced epilepsy (Geschwind and Sherwin 1967), or whether it represents part of a spectrum of language-related epilepsies, as these other linguistic modalities are also effective in some patients with a diagnosis of RE (Katsounis 1988; Salek-Haddadi *et al.* 2009).

Pathomechanism

Recruitment of a "critical mass" of language-related areas with synchronization and subsequent spreading of excitation in response to the epileptogenic stimulus could precipitate a clinical seizure. Increasing the complexity of epileptogenic stimuli may facilitate such recruitment. Task difficulty, complexity, emotional content, or duration enhance the chances of electrographic or clinical activation in RE, suggesting maximal neuronal interaction to be at least a facilitating factor (Koepp *et al.* 1998b). This recruitment may involve the participation and interaction of several cortical and subcortical structures activated by reading or the emotional content of the reading material (mesiotemporal/amygdala/limbic structures). It may rely on both existing and reorganized functional links between brain regions and need not be confined

---

The Causes of Epilepsy, eds. S. D. Shorvon, F. Andermann, and R. Guerrini. Published by Cambridge University Press. © Cambridge University Press 2011.

to physically contiguous brain sites or established neuronal links. This would be consistent with the concept of variable hyperexcitability at multiple cortical and subcortical levels potentially allowing for any combination of asymmetric or symmetric, generalized, regional, and focal discharges. This concept is also consistent with the heterogeneity of clinical phenomena encountered in RE (Radhakrishnan *et al.* 1995) and the variable efficacy of various, in particular emotionally charged, linguistic stimuli as seizure triggers (Koutroumanidis *et al.* 1998).

Specific characteristics

The positioning of RE as a localization-related epilepsy seems not unambiguous. Electro-clinical data strongly suggest several similarities between RE and juvenile myoclonic epilepsy (JME):

- several cases were published recently who had RE and JME independently (Radhakrishnan *et al* 1995; Mayer *et al.* 2006; Salek-Haddadi *et al.* 2009);
- linguistic activities (e.g., reading) are effective in inducing epileptic discharges in JME (Matsuoka *et al.* 2000);
- periorofacial reflex myoclonia induced by reading was observed in a subset of patients with JME (Mayer *et al.* 2006);
- Age-related onset, seizure phenomenology with myoclonic jerks, non-lesional (idiopathic) origin, positive family history with other idiopathic generalized epilepsies, and positive pharmacologic response to valproate and levetiracetam.

Consequently, primary RE is now considered a reflex epilepsy syndrome without specifying whether it is focal or generalized (Engel 2001).

Periorofacial reflex myoclonia are found in different epileptic syndromes and their semiology is not fundamentally different, where they indicate restricted local epileptic activity. They remain often undiagnosed because the patients are not aware that they are a symptom and fail to report them. In many patients with RE and JME, reflex epileptic traits are present temporarily during a certain age period.

The relationship of supposedly "generalized" discharges to the regional expression of bilateral or unilateral clinical symptoms remains controversial (Wolf *et al.* 1998). The thalamus and a complex reciprocal thalamocortical network are thought to be critically important in generalized seizures. In view of the extensive thalamocortical and corticothalamic connections, and the wide range of motor, sensory, and higher-order functions subserved by the thalamus, it is reasonable to assume that the widespread thalamic connection may be crucial for seizure propagation in RE: abnormally increased activity in some areas of the brain (language areas) can lead to functional inhibition (speech arrest) or disinhibition (orofacial reflex myoclonus) in remotely located brain structures, presumably through transsynaptic mechanisms.

Treatment and prognosis

Seizures can be controlled satisfactorily by avoiding the trigger(s), and quite a few patients with RE decide not to take any antiepileptic drug but to prevent generalized tonic–clonic seizures by reacting to the myoclonic seizures and stopping reading. Never to be able to read more than short passages is a significant drawback in literate societies. Thus most patients decide to take antiepileptic drugs. Of these, valproate or clonazepam are the most commonly used. In an interesting family with all affected members displaying electroencephalographic (EEG) features of idiopathic generalized epilepsy, all responded to levetiracetam (Valenti *et al.* 2006). Not surprisingly, in those few reported patients with prolonged alexia suggestive of a "partial variant" (Koutroumanidis *et al.* 1998), valproate and clonazepam were not effective but carbamazepine led to a significant improvement.

The prognosis of RE is good. Even if untreated, seizures usually remain strictly bound to precipitation by reading or whatever related additional stimulus may individually be active. Spontaneous seizures were not observed in any of the 111 cases reported by Wolf (1992).

Diagnostic tests

Neurophysiology: electroencephalography

The absence of interictal epileptiform EEG abnormalities in RE is a common finding, not an unusual one in idiopathic epilepsies. The ongoing activity is normal. Ictally, RE is characterized by evoked paroxysmal rhythmic theta activity or spikes over either one or both frontocentral, centroparietal, or temporoparietal regions in spite of the rather uniform clinical correlates (jaw jerk). They are most commonly bilateral with unilateral accentuation, whereas unilateral or focal discharges are seen less frequently. Lateralization to the language-dominant hemisphere is more common than to the non-dominant side.

Prolonged partial seizures are associated with a wide variety of activity, either with bursts of slow activity over the left temporal area (Koutroumanidis *et al.* 1998), with left occipital transients (Chavany *et al.* 1956) or fast rhythmic discharge localized at the left parieto-occipital region (Gastaut and Tassinari 1966).

Neuroimaging

Structural neuroimaging is usually normal. However, one group reported a local structural abnormality in two out of three patients with an unusual gyrus branching anteriorly off the left central sulcus suggesting that the spikes in RE spread from working memory areas into adjacent motor cortex, activating a cortical subcortical circuit (Archer *et al.* 2003). In a more recent study, we did not find any structural abnormalities, neither individually nor in the group analysis of nine patients with RE (Salek-Haddadi *et al.* 2009).

Functional neuroimaging, using functional magnetic resonance imaging (fMRI), single photon emission computed tomography (SPECT), and positron emission tomography (PET), allows the localization of changes in cerebral blood flow, metabolism, and neurotransmitter levels that accompany changes in neural activity. Ictal investigations are difficult to perform due to the paroxysmal nature of the epilepsies but RE has attracted a recent surge in such investigations: RE is an ideal model to examine peri-ictal changes, the neuronal systems that underlie the specific seizure-provoking trigger, and their relationship to epileptiform activity, because of the possibility of reliably inducing seizures within the scanner environment without significant movement artifacts (jaw jerks only).

In a 16-year-old female patient with RE, a spike-triggered fMRI study showed increased activity, related to individual spikes in the left posterior middle frontal gyrus, that colocalizes with the brain regions activated by the working memory component of the reading task, and also bilateral motor cortical and subcortical activity in the bilateral inferior central sulcus and bilateral globus pallidus (Archer et al. 2003). In the so-far largest series of RE with nine patients (Salek-Haddadi et al. 2009), ictal fMRI revealed activations within cortical (right medial frontal gyrus) and subcortical (left putamen) areas during reading-induced seizures. Whilst there were no gross abnormalities in cognitive or motor organization, most of the cortical areas were either in close proximity or directly overlapping with the areas activated by cognitive and motor functions.

Ictal radioisotope studies are limited by the low temporal resolution in SPECT and PET. Ictal SPECT with [^{99m}Tc]hexamethylpropylene amine oxime (HMPAO) in a 14-year-old Japanese boy revealed hyperperfusion in both frontal lobes, more notable in the left, and also within the left temporal lobe. Meaningful interpretation of the findings was difficult as the healthy control also showed left frontotemporal hyperperfusion albeit to a lesser degree and extent. The ictal EEG in this patient was characterized by bilateral spike–wave complexes with a left frontotemporal predominance and in a similar distribution to the ictal SPECT findings.

Koepp et al. (1998a) found direct in vivo PET evidence for the dynamic multifocal release of endogenous opioids during and following reading-induced partial seizures in areas known to be involved in reading, visual processing, and word recognition. The most significant affected areas during reading-induced seizures were in close proximity to areas found to be hypoactive in the same patients in areas of the brain involved in normal reading (Salek-Haddadi et al. 2009). These cortical and subcortical areas may both represent hyperexcitable cortex and constitute part of the normal reading network. This leads to the hypothesis that there are networks of cortical areas concurrently subserving both cognitive functions and epileptic activity (Miyamato et al. 1995; Koepp et al. 1998a,b; Archer et al. 2003). Understanding hyperexcitable networks and their role in epilepsy is of increasing clinical relevance.

Principles of management

Despite recent advances in diagnostic technology, RE is a prime example of the need to emphasize careful history-taking for environmental precipitating factors in seizure disorders. The introduction of more effective treatment with valproate in the 1970s, and more recently levetiracetam, for many similar seizure disorders and the subsequent widespread use of these medications may have deterred physicians from asking about triggering factors and patients from volunteering such information. In this context, I would like to conclude with a quotation from Bickford (1954):

> Clinicians (should) be constantly on the alert for precipitating factors in their patients' seizures. In many instances, these will not be discovered unless specific questions are asked covering the various categories of precipitation … The electroencephalographer will also miss the diagnosis in these cases, unless he is prepared to record the electroencephalogram under varied conditions of stress in contrast to the classical recording condition of relaxation and the more recent recommendation of sedation and sleep … I firmly believe that simple but detailed studies of individual patients of this kind are more likely to lead us to an understanding of epilepsy than the ill-digested statistical conglomerations of clinical and electroencephalographic data that presently clutter and choke our scientific journals.

References

Archer JS, Briellmann RS, Syngeniotis A, Abbott DF, Jackson GD (2003) Spike-triggered fMRI in reading epilepsy: involvement of left frontal cortex working memory area. *Neurology* **60**:415–21.

Bickford RG (1954) Sensory precipitation of seizures. *J Michigan State Med Soc* **53**:1018–20.

Bickford RG, Whelan JL, Klass DW, et al. (1956) Reading epilepsy: clinical and electroencephalographic studies of a

new syndrome. *Trans Am Neurol Ass* **81**:100–2.

Chavany JA, Fischgold H, Messimy R, et al. (1956) Clinical and EEG aspects of a case of epilepsy electively induced by reading. *Rev Neurol* **95**:381–7.

Engel J Jr. (2001) A proposed diagnostic scheme for people with epileptic seizures and with epilepsy: report of the ILAE Task Force on Classification and Terminology. *Epilepsia* **42**:796–803.

Gastaut H, Tassinari CA (1966) Triggering mechanisms in epilepsy: the

electroclinical point of view. *Epilepsia* **2**:85–138.

Geschwind N, Sherwin I (1967). Language-induced epilepsy. *Arch Neurol* **16**:25–31.

International League Against Epilepsy (1989) Proposal for revised classification of epilepsies and epileptic syndromes. *Epilepsia* **30**:389–99.

Kartsounis LD (1988) Comprehension as the effective trigger in a case of primary reading epilepsy. *J Neurol Neurosurg Psychiatry* **51**:128–30.

Koepp MJ, Richardson MP, Brooks DJ, *et al.* (1998a) Focal cortical release of endogenous opioids during reading-induced seizures. *Lancet* **352**:952–5.

Koepp MJ, Hansen ML, Pressler RM, *et al.* (1998b) Comparison of EEG, MRI and PET in reading epilepsy: a case report. *Epilepsy Res* **29**:251–7.

Koutroumanidis M, Koepp MJ, Richardson MP, *et al.* (1998) The variants of reading epilepsy: a clinical and video-EEG study of 17 patients with reading-induced seizures. *Brain* **121**:1409–27.

Matsuoka H, Takahashi T, Sasaki M, *et al.* (2000) Neuropsychological EEG activation in patients with epilepsy. *Brain* **123**:318–30.

Mayer TA, Schroeder F, May TW, Wolf PT (2006) Perioral reflex myoclonias: a controlled study in patients with JME and focal epilepsies. *Epilepsia* **47**:1059–67.

Miyamoto A, Takahashi S, Tokumitsu A, Oki J (1995) Ictal HMPAO-single photon emission computed tomography findings in reading epilepsy in a Japanese boy. *Epilepsia* **36**:1161–3.

Radhakrishnan K, Silbert PL, Klass DW (1995) Reading epilepsy: an appraisal of 20 patients diagnosed at the Mayo Clinic, Rochester, Minnesota, between 1949 and 1989, and delineation of the epileptic syndrome. *Brain* **118**:75–89.

Salek-Haddadi A, Mayer T, Hamandi K, *et al.* (2009) Imaging seizure activity: a combined EEG/EMG-fMRI study in reading epilepsy. *Epilepsia* **50**:256–64.

Valenti MP, Rudolf G, Carre S, *et al.* (2006) Language-induced epilepsy, acquired stuttering, and idiopathic generalized epilepsy: phenotypic study of one family. *Epilepsia* **47**:766–72.

Wolf P (1992) Reading epilepsy. In: Roger J, Bureau M, Dravet C, *et al.* (eds.) *Epileptic Syndromes in Infancy, Childhood and Adolescence* 2nd edn. Montrouge, France: John Libbey Eurotext, pp. 281–98.

Wolf P, Mayer T, Reker M (1998) Reading epilepsy: report of five new cases and further considerations on the pathophysiology. *Seizure* **7**:271–9.

Chapter

100

Auditory-induced epilepsy

Carlo Di Bonaventura and Frederick Andermann

Definitions

Auditory-induced epilepsy is a particular clinical condition in which epileptic seizures are induced by an acoustic stimulus, which is often unexpected and varies from a simple noise to more structured sounds. From a nosological point of view, these conditions usually encompass several different entities; consequently the term "auditory-induced epilepsy" is used to refer not to a specific epileptic syndrome, but to those clinical contexts in which seizures evoked by any acoustic trigger recur as the predominant epileptic manifestation. Some of these conditions, such as those rare syndromes in which seizures are precipitated by specific sensory stimulations, may be included in the general chapter on reflex epilepsy (Zifkin and Zatorre 1998; Engel 2001). As in other forms of reflex epilepsy, any attempt to classify auditory-induced seizures on the basis of the stimulus type is likely to be unsatisfactory and questionable. Indeed, a "pure" acoustic trigger does not exist in the majority of cases, seizures usually being elicited by a complex and highly elaborate stimulus that involves not only the acoustic system, but also other components (e.g., somatosensory, vegetative, psychic–cognitive) as well as their related underlying structures. In a highly simplified, functional classification, auditory-induced (or audiogenic) reflex epilepsy may be subdivided in two different subtypes (Avanzini 2003) The first, more "simple" subtype, is "startle epilepsy," a condition in which seizures are related to a normal startle reflex that evokes a secondary pathological abnormality; the second, more "complex" subtype, is a condition in which seizures are usually related to more integrated stimuli (such as music) that induce an ictal cortical response.

Seizure types and precipitating stimuli

Following the simplified scheme proposed in this chapter, the ictal clinical features and related precipitating stimuli can be divided in two main subgroups. The first, more general group, comprising startle epilepsy (or startle-induced seizure), is characterized by symmetric or asymmetric tonic seizures evoked by sudden noise. In the second group, comprising other forms of auditory-induced epilepsy, seizures are triggered by a wider sample of stimuli, ranging from simple noise to more complex stimuli, such as music, sounds, voices, and the telephone. The latter group is almost exclusively made up of partial epilepsies; seizures are usually focal and are predominantly characterized by symptoms pointing to the involvement of lateral or mesial temporal structures, isolated or followed by loss of contact and/or secondary generalization.

Startle epilepsy

Although startle epilepsy is included in the proposed syndrome classification (Engel 2001), it may more realistically be considered as a heterogeneous condition in which the main feature is the occurrence of startle-induced seizures (Alajouanine and Gastaut 1955; Wilkins et al. 1986; Meinck 2006). Indeed, the etiology, electroencephalographic (EEG) correlates, and brain structural abnormalities of startle epilepsy vary. Its prevalence is very low, and onset occurs in childhood or early adolescence. Most patients suffer from congenital or infantile, focal or diffuse brain damage (usually occurring within the first 2 years) with consequent spastic hemi-, di-, or tetraplegia associated with mental retardation (Fig. 100.1). Spontaneous seizures are very common. Startle-induced seizures are often described in patients with Down syndrome (Guerrini et al. 1990), though they may be observed in other encephalopathies. As in the common startle reflex, unexpected sudden noise is the most effective means of evoking the seizures: indeed, a prerequisite for inducing the event is the surprise effect of the stimulus, the method used being less important. However, in some patients seizures can be evoked by other stimuli, such as somatosensory and, occasionally, visual triggers. As mentioned before, epileptic seizures are a secondary pathological brief response (up to 30 s) to a normal startle reflex; typical features consist of axial tonic seizures with uni- or bilateral limb posturing (frequently causing falls), turning of the head, and speech arrest. Concomitant signs, including autonomic manifestations, automatisms, laughter, and jerks, may occur. In many cases, consciousness is at least partly preserved. Other ictal patterns, such as absences, atonic seizures, and generalized

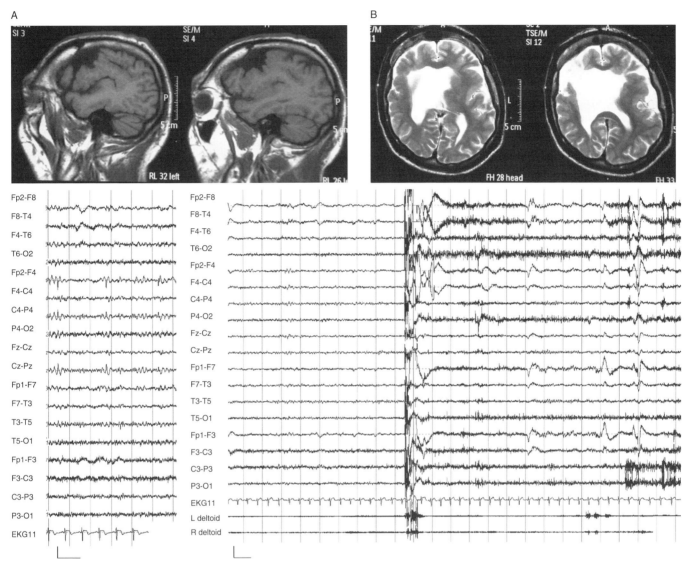

Fig. 100.1. A 30-year-old patient affected by mental retardation and startle epilepsy. (A) MR image documents a complex cortical development malformation (bilateral frontal polymicrogyria predominantly in the right hemisphere, where an open-lip schizencephaly is also evident). (B) In the same patient, the interictal EEG (left panel) shows sharp wave abnormalities well localized in the right frontocentral regions; the ictal EEG (right panel) documents an asymmetric brief tonic seizure evoked by the acoustic stimulus. The EMG clearly shows the first muscular component, corresponding to the startle reflex, followed by brief tonic activity in the deltoids with left predominance, related to the secondary epileptic seizure (as often occurs, the EEG tracing is completely obscured by the muscular artifacts).

seizures, are less common. Interictal EEG usually shows abnormalities related to underlying brain pathology. The ictal EEG pattern consists of an initial vertex discharge often characterized by a flattening or low-voltage fast activity arising from the motor or premotor cortex and spreading extensively to mesial frontal, parietal, and contralateral frontal regions (Bancaud *et al.* 1975; Manford *et al.* 1996; Vignal *et al.* 1998). Ictal EEG may, however, often be difficult to interpret because it is obscured by marked electromyogram (EMG) activity. The pathophysiology of this condition is not completely understood. Pre-existing spontaneous seizures, which are often drug-resistant and occur at a high frequency, may facilitate the mechanisms leading to startle epilepsy, probably by means of a kindling process. As suggested by electroclinical and neuroimaging findings in most cases, both spontaneous and startle-induced seizures reflect a primary

involvement of the motor cortex, particularly in the supplementary motor area (Bancaud *et al.* 1975; Vignal *et al.* 1998). Which components of the normal startle reflex, which is primarily organized in the brainstem, actually trigger the cortical pathological "response" in the motor and premotor areas is not yet clear (Meinck 2006). However, it may be argued that muscular tonic activation may, via a corollary or reafferent discharge or via the vegetative and emotional components of the startle reflex, induce the seizures. Neuroimaging studies typically reveal frontal or frontoparietal lesions or malformations on one or both sides (Sáenz-Lopez *et al.* 1984; Manford *et al.* 1996).

Seizures are drug-resistant and the prognosis poor, though this depends on the severity of the underlying pathologies. Unilateral startle seizures reportedly respond better to carbamazepine, and bilateral ones to clonazepam, clobazepam and lamotrigine than to other anticonvulsants (Aguglia *et al.* 1984; Faught 1999). Surgery has been proposed in selected cases to control startle epilepsy associated with infantile hemiplegia (Oguni *et al.* 1998).

More "complex" auditory-induced epilepsies

Some rare conditions are characterized by seizures induced by more integrated auditory stimulations. A wide spectrum of noises and sounds have been reported to induce more complex seizures (Dreifuss 1998), while some clinical conditions, such as musicogenic epilepsy and telephone-induced epilepsy, have been proposed as specific reflex syndromes.

Musicogenic epilepsy

Musicogenic epilepsy is characterized by seizures induced by listening to certain sounds, typically music (Critchley 1977) (Fig. 100.2A). Seizures can occur while the subjects are exposed to music, with triggers including listening, playing a piece, or merely thinking about it. The stimulus is usually highly stereotyped and often exclusive for each patient: it can range from an elaborate musical piece to a more simple sound. Since affective and emotional factors appear to be significantly involved, many authors have suggested that the pathogenesis of musicogenic epilepsy is causally related more closely to the emotions produced by music than to pure auditory content (Wieser *et al.* 1997). The seizures are usually of the simple or complex partial type. When recognizable, ictal subjective manifestations include vegetative, affective, or psychic symptoms, and may be followed by staring, loss of contact, automatisms, and secondary generalization. Most patients also have spontaneous seizures and reflex seizures, which often start more than a year after the onset of the spontaneous attacks (Wieser *et al.* 1997). Interictal EEG usually shows epileptiform abnormalities in the temporal lobes, while ictal EEG often documents discharges arising from the same structures, sometimes with a right hemisphere predominance (Wieser *et al.* 1997; Tayah *et al.* 2006).

The neurological examination and structural magnetic resonance imaging (MRI) are normal in the vast majority of patients reported to suffer from idiopathic or cryptogenic (probably symptomatic) partial epilepsy.

Although the temporal lobe is considered to be frequently implicated, the anatomical structures responsible for producing musicogenic seizures have not been clearly demonstrated. This condition is currently known to be a heterogeneous syndrome with multiple seizure onset areas and a complex epileptogenic network. Indeed, the difficulties encountered in defining the anatomical and pathophysiologycal substrates of musicogenic epilepsy are likely to depend on the complexity of the anatomo-functional basis of music processing. This concept appears to be supported by data from depth electrode studies and functional neuroimaging studies based on different techniques, including positron emission tomography (PET), single photon emission computed tomography (SPECT), and functional MRI (fMRI)

(Creutzfeldt and Ojemann 1989; Johnsrude *et al.* 2002). Musical stimuli may have widespread effects on neuronal activity in human temporal lobes (Creutzfeldt and Ojemann 1989; Liegeois-Chauvel *et al.* 1991), with the different components of music having varying effects, even with specialized lateralization and localization. Data from neuroimaging studies also confirm that different structures are involved in the music processing functional network, which extends well beyond the classical auditory cortex of Heschl's gyrus. Indeed, the multiple tonotopically organized sections render this area particularly sensitive to pure tones, and consequently insufficient for higher-order pattern perception. By contrast, more complex musical stimuli activate several bilateral cortical and subcortical structures with right hemisphere predominance (Zifkin and Zatorre 1998), which are functionally connected with the primary area. Some functional neuroimaging studies, performed during the seizures, have documented a dysfunction and abnormal activation in the temporolimbic structures (Wieser *et al.* 1997; Morocz *et al.* 2003; Cho *et al.* 2007); more recent EEG/fMRI studies have documented a wider, more diffuse epileptogenic network.

In predisposed patients, the musical trigger may evoke an abnormal response of the hyperexcitable cortical areas, which are stimulated to varying extents. The epileptic discharge may recruit other functionally connected areas, some of which (e.g., limbic and insular structures) are physiologically responsible for the emotional and psychic contents of music processing (Stewart *et al.* 2006). The involvement of these specific areas amply justifies the ictal clinical pattern, which is often characterized by temporomesial typical findings.

Telephone-induced and other hearing-induced epilepsies

Telephone-induced epilepsy is a form of reflex epilepsy in which the seizures are exclusively induced by answering the telephone (both fixed and mobile) (Michelucci *et al.* 2004) (Fig. 100.2B). Answering the telephone is a complex and elaborate auditory stimulus in which hearing the "calling voice" constitutes the effective precipitating factor. Similarly to musicogenic epilepsy, the auditory trigger in this condition is a highly integrated stimulus that comprises various components, including not only the specific features of the voice but also the strain involved in recognizing the caller as well as emotional and surprise factors. Reports of telephone-induced seizures are somewhat exceptional, as are those of other similar forms described as voice-induced seizures or "heard-word" epilepsy (reported specific triggers include the voices of certain radio announcers and direct speaking with the patient) (Forster *et al.* 1969; Tsuzuki and Kasuga 1978).

In all these cases, the epileptogenic network is presumed to include the structures activated by the stimulus, i.e., the auditory temporal areas and other associative regions functionally connected with these areas. Auditory information processing and the related psychic and emotional contents may be considered as the "password" to this network, which is consequently activated.

The clinical semiology in the small number of patients reported to have telephone-induced epilepsy is characterized

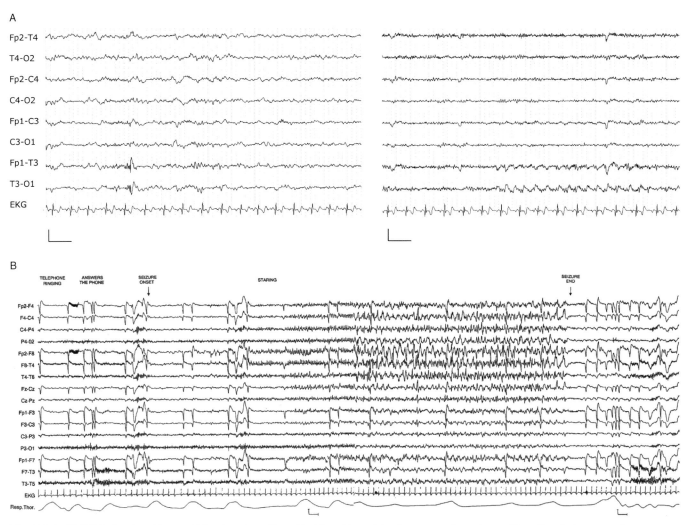

Fig. 100.2. (A) EEG findings in a 29-year-old female patient affected by idiopathic partial epilepsy presenting seizures with auditory features sometimes precipitated by listening to sounds and music. The ambulatory 24-hr EEG documents epileptiform abnormalities localized in the left temporal lobe (left panel) and a brief seizure involving the same lobe (right panel): in her diary, the patient described "an air pocket in her ears … mostly on the right side…". (B) EEG tracing documenting a telephone-induced seizure in a patient affected by lateral temporal partial epilepsy. Answering the telephone induced a seizure arising from the right temporal lobe: low-amplitude, fast activity in this region is followed by rhythmic spiking activity involving the right temporoparietal areas with further spreading; polygraphic traces show early ictal tachycardia and irregular thoracic breathing. Clinically, the patient presented a staring expression and postictal prolonged aphasia. (Reproduced from Michelucci *et al.* [2004], with permission of the author and the journal *Epilepsia* (Blackwell Publishing Inc.)

by auditory, dysphasic, and vertiginous symptoms, though complex partial and secondary generalized seizures have also been described. When available, the EEG documents focal seizures arising from the temporal lobe. As regards the etiology of these seizures, patients usually have a normal neurological examination and a normal MRI. A benign evolution that is controlled well by means of appropriate medication is often described. Some of the reported characteristics support the "idiopathic" nature of these epilepsies, pointing to a diagnosis of autosomal dominant lateral temporal lobe epilepsy (ADLTE), a familial condition often associated with mutations of the Epitempin (*LGI1*) gene (Morante-Redolat *et al.* 2002). This hypothesis has recently been confirmed in a sporadic case with telephone-induced seizures in which a de novo mutation of the *LGI1* gene (Michelucci *et al.* 2007) was identified. A further interesting finding that lends support to the idiopathic nature of this condition is the frequent occurrence of auditory-induced seizures in members of some families with ADTLE (with or without *LGI1* mutations).

References

Aguglia U, Tinuper P, Gastaut H (1984) Startle-induced epileptic seizures. *Epilepsia* 25:712–20.

Alajouanine T, Gastaut H (1955) Synkinesis-startle and epilepsy startle triggered by unexpected sensory and sensitive factors. I. Anatomical and clinical data on 15 cases. *Rev Neurol* 93:29–41.

Avanzini G (2003) Musicogenic seizures. *Ann N Y Acad Sci* **999**: 95–102.

Bancaud J, Talairach J, Lamarche M, Bonis A, Trottier S (1975)

Neurophysiopathological hypothesis on startle epilepsy in man. *Rev Neurol* **131**:559–71.

Cho JW, Seo DW, Joo EY, *et al.* (2007) Neural correlates of musicogenic epilepsy: SISCOM and FDG–PET. *Epilepsy Res* **77**:169–73.

Creutzfeldt O, Ojemann G (1989) Neuronal activity in the human lateral temporal lobe. III. Activity changes during music. *Exp Brain Res* **77**:490–8.

Critchley M (1977) Musicogenic epilepsy. In: Critchley M, Hensen RA (eds.) *Music and the Brain.* London: Heinemann, pp. 344–53.

Dreifuss FE (1998) Classification of reflex epilepsies and reflex seizures. In: Zifkin BG, Andermann F, Beaumanoir A, *et al.* (eds.) *Reflex Epilepsies and Reflex Seizures.* Philadelphia, PA: Lippincott-Raven, pp. 5–13.

Engel J Jr. (2001) A proposed diagnostic scheme for people with epileptic seizures and with epilepsy: report of the ILAE Task Force on Classification and Terminology. *Epilepsia* **42**:796–803.

Faught E (1999) Lamotrigine for startle-induced seizures *Seizure* **8**:361–3.

Forster FM, Hansotia P, Cleeland CS, Ludwig A (1969) A case of voice-induced epilepsy treated by conditioning. *Neurology* **19**:325–31.

Genc BO, Genc E, Tastekin G, Iihan N (2001) Musicogenic epilepsy with ictal single photon emission computed tomography (SPECT): could these cases contribute to our knowledge of music processing? *Eur J Neurol* **8**:191–4.

Guerrini R, Genton P, Bureau M, Dravet C, Roger J (1990) Reflex seizures are frequent in patients with Down syndrome and epilepsy. *Epilepsia* **31**:406–17.

Johnsrude IS, Giraud AL, Frackowiak RSJ (2002) Functional imaging of the auditory system: the use of positron emission tomography. *Audiol Neurootol* **7**:251–7.

Liegeois-Chauvel C, Musolino A, Chauvel P (1991) Localization of the primary auditory area in man. *Brain* **114**:139–51.

Manford MR, Fish DR, Shorvon SD (1996) Startle-provoked epileptic seizures: features in 19 patients. *J Neurol Neurosurg Psychiatry* **61**:151–6.

Meinck HM (2006) Startle and its disorders. *Neurophysiol Clin* **36**:357–64.

Michelucci R, Gardella E, de Haan GJ, *et al.* (2004) Telephone-induced seizures: a new type of reflex epilepsy. *Epilepsia* **45**:280–3.

Michelucci R, Mecarelli O, Bovo G, *et al.* (2007) A de novo *LGI1* mutation causing idiopathic partial epilepsy with telephone-induced seizures. *Neurology* **68**:2150–1.

Morante-Redolat JM, Gorostidi-Pagola A, Piquer-Sirerol S, *et al.* (2002). Mutations in the *LGI1*/Epitempin gene on 10q24 cause autosomal dominant lateral temporal epilepsy. *Hum Mol Genet* **11**:1119–28.

Morocz IA, Karni A, Haut S, Lantos G, Liu G (2003) fMRI of triggerable aurae in musicogenic epilepsy. *Neurology* **60**:705–9.

Oguni H, Hayashi K, Usui N, Osawa M, Shimizu H (1998) Startle epilepsy with infantile hemiplegia: report of two cases improved by surgery. *Epilepsia* **39**:93–8.

Rosenow F, Luders HO (2000) Hearing-induced seizures. In: Luders HO, Noachtar S (eds.) *Epileptic Seizures: Pathophysiology and Clinical Semiology.* New York: Churchill Livingstone, pp. 580–4.

Sáenz-Lopez E, Herranz FJ, Masdeu JC (1984) Startle epilepsy: a clinical study. *Ann Neurol* **16**:16–78.

Stewart L, von Kriegstein K, Warren JD, Griffiths TD (2006) Music and the brain: disorders of musical listening. *Brain* **129**:2533–53.

Tayah TF, Abou-Khalil B, Gilliam FG, *et al.* (2006) Musicogenic seizures can arise from multiple temporal lobe foci: intracranial EEG analyses of three patients. *Epilepsia* **47**:1402–6.

Tsuzuki H, Kasuga I (1978) Paroxysmal discharges triggered by hearing spoken language. *Epilepsia* **19**:147–54.

Vignal JP, Biraben A, Chauvel PY, Reutens DC (1998) Reflex partial epilepsy of sensorimotor cortex (including cortical reflex myoclonus and startle epilepsy). *Adv Neurol* **75**:207–26.

Wieser HG, Hungerbühler H, Siegel AM, Buck A (1997) Musicogenic epilepsy: review of the literature and case report with ictal single photon emission computed tomography. *Epilepsia* **38**:200–7.

Wilkins DE, Hallett M, Weiss MM (1986) Audiogenic startle reflex of man and its relationship to startle syndromes. *Brain* **109**:561–73.

Zifkin BG, Zatorre R (1998) Musicogenic epilepsy. In: Zifkin BG, Andermann F, Beaumanoir A, Rowan AJ (eds.) *Reflex Epilepsies and Reflex Seizures.* Philadelphia, PA: Lippincott-Raven, pp. 273–81.

Chapter

101

Focal reflex seizures – with emphasis on seizures triggered by eating

Benjamin Zifkin, Guy M. Rémillard, and Frederick Andermann

Reflex seizures that begin as clinical and electroencephalographic focal seizures can be triggered by many different events. Usually a patient is sensitive to one type of stimulus or to a group of related stimuli, and the triggered seizures occur in patients with known epilepsy and apparently spontaneous seizures. Thus these reflex seizures are only rarely classified as epileptic syndromes, and are usually considered as seizure types, classified according to the triggering stimulus in the current classification proposal (Engel 2001).

Table 101.1 shows many triggers with examples of typical effective stimuli and localizations.

Reflex seizure etiology in these cases depends on the localization of the lesion and on its relations with surrounding or functionally linked tissue. This is no surprise: in the 1920s and 1930s, Clementi showed how the creation of focal epileptogenic lesions in canine sensory cortices would lead to reflex seizures triggered by the appropriate afferent stimulation initially in visual cortex (Clementi 1929) and then in other regions. In human reflex seizures, acquired disorders such as traumatic or ischemic lesions and congenital or early lesions such as gross or subtle disorders of cortical development can be found. These seizures may occur with other spontaneous seizures which can be intractable and the tissue pathology of resected tissue has been reported in some cases. Malone *et al.* (2008) provide a recent example of intractable epilepsy with reflex triggering and dysplastic cortex which was not seen preoperatively despite modern imaging. Techniques beyond current magnetic resonance imaging (MRI) may also be useful. Magnetic source localization has shown localization of epileptiform activity in some cases, for example in startle epilepsy (García-Morales *et al.* 2009), in which the causative lesion is not always obvious.

The roles of dysplastic lesions and of subtle cortical malformations in causing focal seizures have become more obvious since they have been detectable preoperatively in many cases with modern neuroimaging; previously such patients appeared to have normal brains when only computed tomography (CT) scanning was available (for example see Manford *et al.* 1996), and progress in the field will probably mean that more such cases can be identified.

Quite complex seizure triggers may also exist in these disorders, such as for some musicogenic seizures and in isolated case reports, such as a patient whose seizures were triggered by thinking of his childhood home (Martinez *et al.* 2000).

The occurrence of a reflex seizure at some moment is not a function of its etiology alone. Wilkins *et al.* (1982) suggested that reflex seizure genesis was related to the recruitment of sufficient epileptogenic tissue by the stimulus to form a critical mass of hyperexcitable cortex. While the clinical trigger was one that promoted the formation of this, other factors could inhibit it, such as level of awareness, or competing tasks that were subsumed by other cortical areas. The occurrence of a seizure thus depends on constantly changing dynamic cortical activities. Lopes da Silva *et al.* (2003) noted that:

> critical parameters may gradually change with time,
> in such a way that the attractor can deform either gradually
> or suddenly, with the consequence that the distance between
> the basin of attraction of the normal state and the separatrix
> tends to zero. This can lead, eventually, to a transition
> to a seizure … In the special cases of reflex epilepsy,
> the leap between the normal ongoing attractor and
> the ictal attractor is caused by a well-defined external
> perturbation.

Seizures induced by somatosensory stimulation

Seizures may be induced by tapping or rubbing individual regions of the body (Vignal *et al.* 1998). These are partial seizures, often with initial localized sensory symptoms and tonic features, and typically occur in patients with lesions involving postrolandic cortex. A well-defined trigger zone may be found over some area of the skin. Some patients may report triggers such as brushing the teeth. Evaluation for epileptogenic lesions is required as for other cases of focal epilepsy.

Table 101.1 Triggers with examples of typical effective stimuli and localizations

Clinical trigger and seizure type: all may generalize secondarily	Typical effective stimuli	Region or system subserving the trigger
Predominantly non-limbic		
Induction by somatosensory stimuli, rubbing skin: tonic motor, usually with initial localized aura	Touching, rubbing, or pricking skin, often with a well-defined trigger zone, typically unilateral	Primary or secondary somatosensory cortex
Startle epilepsy: sudden startle, altered tone, supplementary motor seizure, may fall	Startle	Gross or subtle frontal or perirolandic lesions
Seizures with eating, tooth-brushing: aura, focal motor, or absence-like seizure	Eating, tooth-brushing, other oral sensory stimuli	Perisylvian lesions
Seizures with proprioceptive stimuli: typically focal motor	Walking, movement of limbs	Postcentral or paracentral lesions
Often limbic		
Seizures with eating: focal absence-like	Eating, taste of food	Temporal ± frontal limbic
Seizures induced by experiential thought: focal absence-like, focal motor	Recall of trigger thought	Temporal limbic
Musicogenic seizures: focal absence-like, focal motor	Music	Temporal limbic and non-limbic

Seizures induced by eating

Boudouresques and Gastaut (1954) first described eating epilepsy in four patients who experienced seizures after a heavy meal. Gastric distension may have been at least partly responsible for the attacks (Poirier and Gastaut 1964). This presentation has turned out to be unusual: most such seizures occur early in a meal and are unrelated to gastric distension (Loiseau *et al.* 1986). An extraordinarily high frequency of these attacks in Sri Lanka (Senanayake 1990) appears due to the inclusion of all attacks occurring from 30 min before to 30 min after eating;

many of these would not be considered to be reflex seizures. The clinical characteristics are usually stereotyped in individual patients but there are few common features among patients. Some patients have seizures at the very sight or smell of food, whereas others have them only in the middle of a meal or shortly afterwards. In some patients, the seizures may be associated with the emotional or autonomic components of eating; in others, they are associated with sensory afferents from tongue or pharynx. These seizures have also been documented in young children, in whom they can be mistaken for gastroesophageal reflux (Plouin *et al.* 1989).

Periodic spasms have been triggered by eating in a patient with bilateral opercular dysplasia and motor deficits (Labate *et al.* 2006) and in another report in two children with unspecified pathology (Nakazawa *et al.* 2002).

Seizures associated with eating are almost always related to symptomatic or cryptogenic focal epilepsy. They can be related to temporolimbic and to extratemporal perisylvian lesions. Rémillard and colleagues (1998) surmised in adults that patients with these seizures and temporolimbic epilepsy are activated by eating from the beginning of their seizure disorder and continue to have most seizures with meals. In contrast, patients with localized extralimbic, usually postcentral, seizure onset develop reflex activation of focal seizures later in their course, with less constant triggering by eating and more prominent spontaneous seizures. These patients typically have more obvious lesions and findings on neurologic examination. Late-onset opercular reflex seizures induced by movements of the jaw and mouth have been reported (Biraben *et al.* 1999) and we have observed such seizures in a patient with bilateral perisylvian syndrome as also reported by Kishi *et al.* (1999).

The mechanism of eating-related epilepsy is unclear. Interaction among several areas, including the insula and hypothalamus, has been suggested but it is not clear what are the necessary and sufficient regions for seizure occurrence. Oral automatisms have been evoked in patients by extraoperative stimulation of the mesial temporal lobe, the cingulate gyrus, the right mesial superior frontal gyrus, and the frontal opercular cortex (Maestro *et al.* 2008; Unnwongse *et al.* 2009). Afferents involved in eating enter the brain through the trigeminal and vagal systems. Patients with extralimbic cortical lesions seem much like others with perisylvian lesions and focal reflex seizures with triggers such as brushing the teeth or other forms of tactile or proprioceptive stimulation. When the abnormal cortex is located in regions responding to proprioceptive and other sensory afferents (especially lingual, buccal, or pharyngeal) activated by the extensive sensory input generated by a complex behavior such as eating, patients may be more sensitive to the physical manipulation of food, texture, temperature, and chewing. It is also of interest that Rosenzweig and Manford (2008) reported a patient with apparent seizures induced by eating in a patient with a lesion of the medulla involving the dorsal vagal nucleus and the nucleus tractus solitarius, and that vagal nerve stimulation has been reported to be particularly effective in intractable seizures triggered by eating (Cukiert *et al.* 2009).

Focal onset seizures with visual stimulation

Sensitivity to flashing light is often associated with epilepsy syndromes such as juvenile myoclonic epilepsy, now regarded as a generalized epilepsy. Intermittent photic stimulation can also induce clear-cut partial seizures originating in one occipital lobe (reviewed by Hennessy and Binnie 2000). Environmental triggers include television and videogames. Many of these patients have idiopathic photosensitive occipital lobe epilepsy, a relatively benign, age-related syndrome without spontaneous seizures, although cases with occipital lesions have been reported, including in patients with celiac disease. The visual stimulus triggers initial visual symptoms that may be followed by versive movements and motor seizures; however, migraine-like symptoms of throbbing headache, nausea, and sometimes vomiting are common and can lead to delayed or incorrect diagnosis.

Startle epilepsy and proprioceptive-induced seizures

Startle epilepsy involves seizures induced by sudden and unexpected stimuli. Typically lateralized and tonic, the seizures are often associated with developmental delay, gross neurologic signs such as hemiplegia, and cerebral lesions. Computed tomography scans often show unilateral or bilateral mesial frontal lesions (Aguglia et al. 1984) and seizures typically arise from lesioned frontal areas. These are often intractable and patients may have other intractable seizures as well. For these reasons, aggressive and early surgical treatment has been suggested in patients with infantile hemiplegia (Anan et al. 2009).

Seizures induced by proprioceptive stimulation are seen with movement of an arm or leg, fingers, or toes. They are focal and although they may be related to a lesion, they may arise as a transient finding with acute metabolic encephalopathy or typically non-ketotic hyperglycemia, and resist treatment until the underlying disorder is effectively treated. Although they may appear to be induced by movement, studies in animals and humans suggest that proprioceptive afferents to somatosensory cortex are the likely triggers of these events (Arseni et al. 1967; Chauvel and Lamarche 1975).

Musicogenic seizures

Musicogenic epilepsy consists of seizures provoked by hearing music (see also Chapter 100). The music that triggers seizures often is remarkably patient-specific and no consistently epileptogenic features of musical sound can be identified. A startle effect is not required. Many patients have spontaneous attacks as well. Some attacks can be provoked by music and by non-musical sounds, such as ringing or whirring noises. In some patients, an effective musical stimulus often induces emotional and autonomic manifestations before the clinical seizure begins. Patients may report triggers with personal emotional significance and often report that they have an interest in music or some musical training. The seizures thus seem to be very different from the audiogenic seizures of mice, which will not be further considered here. Musicogenic seizures are usually associated with non-dominant temporal epileptiform activity. Right anterior and mesial hyperperfusion during ictal single photon emission computed tomography (SPECT) has been documented and ictal onsets and spread studied with positron emission tomography (PET), functional MRI, and invasive electrodes have implicated the right mesial temporal region initially, with involvement of lateral temporal regions, Heschl's gyrus, the insula, and the frontal cortex (Pittau et al. 2008; Marrosu et al. 2009; Mehta et al. 2009). Temporal and premotor cortices may be functionally linked and interact closely in both the perception and production of music in normal subjects (reviewed by Zatorre et al. 2007) and these patterns may be important in the origin and spread of these seizures.

References

Aguglia U, Tinuper P, Gastaut H (1984) Startle-induced epileptic seizures. *Epilepsia* **25**:712–20.

Anan M, Kamida T, Abe E, *et al.* (2009) A hemispherotomy for intractable startle epilepsy characterized by infantile hemiplegia and drop attacks. *J Clin Neurosci* **16**:1652–5.

Arseni C, Stoica I, Serbanescu T (1967) Electroclinical investigations on the role of proprioceptive stimuli in the onset and arrest of convulsive epileptic paroxysms. *Epilepsia* **8**:162–70.

Biraben A, Scarabin JM, de Toffol B, Vignal JP, Chauvel P (1999) Opercular reflex seizures: a case report with stereo-

electroencephalographic demonstration. *Epilepsia* **40**:655–63.

Boudouresques J, Gastaut H (1954) Le mécanisme réflexe de certaines épilepsies temporales. *Rev Neurol* **90**:157–8.

Chauvel P, Lamarche M (1975) Analyse d'une 'épilepsie du mouvement' chez un singe porteur d'un foyer rolandique. *Neurochirurgie* **21**:121–37.

Clementi A (1929) Stricninizzazione della sfera corticale visiva ed epilessia sperimentale da stimoli luminosi. *Arch Fisiol* **27**:356–87.

Cukiert A, Mariani PP, Burattini JA, *et al.* (2009) Vagus nerve stimulation might have a unique effect in reflex eating seizures. *Epilepsia*. **51**:301–3.

Engel J Jr. (2001) A proposed diagnostic scheme for people with epileptic seizures and with epilepsy: report of the ILAE Task Force on Classification and Terminology. *Epilepsia* **42**:796–803.

García-Morales I, Maestú F, Pérez-Jiménez MA, *et al.* (2009). A clinical and magnetoencephalography study of MRI-negative startle epilepsy. *Epilepsy Behav* **16**:166–71.

Gastaut H, Poirier F (1964) Experimental, or "reflex," induction of seizures: report of a case of abdominal (enteric) epilepsy. *Epilepsia* **5**:256–70.

Genc BO, Genc E, Tastekin G, Iihan N (2001) Musicogenic epilepsy with ictal single photon emission computed tomography (SPECT): could these cases contribute to our knowledge of music processing? *Eur J Neurol* **8**:191–4.

Hennessy M, Binnie CD (2000) Photogenic partial seizures. *Epilepsia* **41**:59–64.

Kishi T, Moriya M, Kimoto Y, Nishio Y, Tanaka T (1999) Congenital bilateral perisylvian syndrome and eating epilepsy. *Eur Neurol* **42**:241–3.

Labate A, Colosimo E, Gambardella A, *et al.* (2006) Reflex periodic spasms induced by eating. *Brain Dev* **28**:170–4.

Loiseau P, Guyot M, Loiseau H, Rougier A, Desbordes P (1986) Eating seizures. *Epilepsia* **27**:161–3.

Lopes da Silva F, Blanes W, Kalitzin SN, *et al.* (2003) Epilepsies as dynamical diseases of brain systems: basic models of the transition between normal and epileptic activity. *Epilepsia* **44**(Suppl 12):72–83.

Maestro I, Carreño M, Donaire A, *et al.* (2008) Oroalimentary automatisms induced by electrical stimulation of the fronto-opercular cortex in a patient without automotor seizures. *Epilepsy Behav* **13**:410–12.

Malone S, Miller I, Jakayar P, *et al.* (2008) MRI-negative frontal lobe epilepsy with ipsilateral akinesia and reflex activation. *Epilept Disord* **10**:349–55.

Manford MR, Fish DR, Shorvon SD (1996) Startle provoked epileptic seizures: features in 19 patients. *J Neurol Neurosurg Psychiatry* **61**:151–6.

Marrosu F, Barberini L, Puligheddu M, *et al.* (2009) Combined EEG/fMRI recording in musicogenic epilepsy. *Epilepsy Res* **84**:77–81.

Martinez O, Reisin R, Zifkin BG, Andermann F, Sevlever G (2000) Evidence for reflex activation of experiential complex partial seizures. *Neurology* **56**:121–3.

Mehta AD, Ettinger AB, Perrine K, *et al.* (2009) Seizure propagation in a patient with musicogenic epilepsy. *Epilepsy Behav* **14**:421–4.

Nakazawa C, Fujimoto S, Watanabe M, *et al.* (2002). Eating epilepsy characterized by periodic spasms. *Neuropediatrics* **33**:294–7.

Pittau F, Tinuper P, Bisulli F, *et al.* (2008) Videopolygraphic and functional MRI study of musicogenic epilepsy: a case report and literature review. *Epilepsy Behav* **13**:685–92.

Plouin P, Ponsot C, Jalin C (1989) Eating seizures in a three-year-old child. In: Beaumanoir A, Gastaut H, Naquet R (eds.) *Reflex Seizures and Reflex Epilepsies.* Geneva: Editions médecine et hygiène, pp. 309–13.

Rémillard GM, Zifkin BG, Andermann F (1998) Seizures induced by eating. In: Zifkin BG, Andermann F, Beaumanoir A, Rowan AJ (eds.) *Reflex Epilepsies and Reflex Seizures.* Philadelphia, PA: Lippincott-Raven, pp. 227–40.

Rosenzweig I, Manford M (2008) Trouble at dinner: an unusual case of eating-induced seizures. *J Neurol Neurosurg Psychiatry* **79**:335–7.

Senanayake N (1990) Eating epilepsy: a reappraisal. *Epilepsy Res* **5**:74–9.

Unnwongse K, Lachhwani D, Tang-Wai R, *et al.* (2009) Oral automatisms induced by stimulation of the mesial frontal cortex. *Epilepsia* **50**:1620–3.

Vignal J-P, Biraben A, Chauvel PY, *et al.* (1998) Reflex partial seizures of sensorimotor cortex (including cortical reflex myoclonus and startle epilepsy). In: Zifkin BG, Andermann F, Beaumanoir A, Rowan AJ (eds.) *Reflex Epilepsies and Reflex Seizures.* Philadelphia, PA: Lippincott-Raven, pp. 207–26.

Wilkins AJ, Zifkin B, Andermann F, McGovern E (1982) Seizures induced by thinking. *Ann Neurol* **11**:608–12.

Zatorre RJ, Chen JL, Penhune VB (2007) When the brain plays music: auditory–motor interactions in music perception and production. *Nat Rev Neurosci* **8**:547–58.

Hot-water epilepsy

Chapter

102

P. Satishchandra, S. Sinha, and A. Anand

Introduction

Seizures precipitated by a specific sensory stimulus are described as reflex or sensory epilepsy. Reflex epilepsy is interesting not only because it is an intriguing neurobehavioral phenomenon, but also for the insights it provides into the pathophysiology of epilepsy. Penfield was the first to use the term "sensory precipitation of seizures" in 1941 as a seizure-inducing mechanism, rather than the cause (Gastaut 1973). One such reflex epilepsy, hot-water epilepsy (HWE), is precipitated by the stimulus of bathing in hot water poured over the head (Mani *et al.* 1968, 1974; Subrahmanyam 1972; Szymonowicz and Meloff 1978; Satishchandra *et al.* 1985, 1988; Satishchandra 2003). It is also variously known as water-immersion epilepsy or bathing epilepsy (Mofenson *et al.* 1965; Velmurugendran 1985; Shaw *et al.* 1988; Lenoir *et al.* 1989).

History

Though HWE was first described in 1945 from New Zealand (Allen 1945), there have since been case reports from all round the world: Australia (Keipert 1969), the USA (Stensman and Ursing 1971), Canada (Szymonowicz and Meloff 1978), the UK (Parsonage *et al.* 1976), Japan (Kurata 1979; Morimoto *et al.* 1985), and Turkey (Bebek *et al.* 2001). However, it is particularly in the southern parts of India that a large number of cases of HWE have been reported (Mani *et al.* 1968, 1974; Satishchandra *et al.* 1985, 1988; Satishchandra 2003). A cohort of 279 HWE cases from the National Institute of Mental Health and Neuro Sciences (NIMHANS), a university hospital and tertiary care center, has been evaluated over a 4-year period (1980–1983) (Satishchandra *et al.* 1988). The detailed initial clinical description and subsequent studies on this geographically specific epilepsy syndrome have been carried out by two researchers: K. S. Mani and P. Satishchandra, both from the same geographical region and institute.

Prevalence

A house-to-house Bangalore urban–rural neuroepidemiologic survey (BURN) of 102557 persons reported that HWE accounts for 6.9% of all epilepsies in this community. Another prevalence study conducted in a rural community reported a prevalence rate of 60 per 100 000 (Gururaj and Satishchandra 1992). Mani and colleagues published an epidemiologic study from Yelandur, a rural area near Mysore in Karnataka, and reported a prevalence rate of 255 per 100 000 (Mani *et al.* 1998). The classification proposed by the International League Against Epilepsy (ILAE) in 2001 included HWE as a form of reflex epilepsy (Engel 2001).

Phenotypic description

Most often HWE is precipitated during a customary bath in south India where a hot-water head bath is taken once every 3–7 days or so. The temperature of the hot water is 40–45 °C (ambient temperature: 25–30 °C). Usually hot water from a bucket is poured over the head. Episodes of HWE are usually precipitated by this bathing ritual. Less frequently, HWE has also been reported in individuals using a shower or bathtub in various other parts of the world.

Although HWE has been reported in a number of adults from our center, children are relatively more frequently affected (Mani *et al.* 1968, 1974; Satishchandra *et al.* 1985, 1988; Satishchandra 2003). Males seem to be affected more frequently than females (2–2.5 : 1). Generally, the frequency of these seizures depends on the frequency of the head baths. At a later stage in the natural history, 5–10% of HWE patients develop seizures even during a body bath when water is not poured over the head. The most common semiology of hot-water-induced seizures is complex partial with or without secondary generalization. It is characterized by a dazed look, sense of fear, irrelevant speech, and visual and auditory hallucinations with complex automatisms. About one-third of all reported cases have primary generalized tonic–clonic seizures.

These have been witnessed in the laboratory and have been documented on video in a few instances (Stensman and Ursing 1971; Kurata 1979; Satishchandra 2003). About 10% of HWE patients, who experience intense desire or pleasure, continue to pour hot water over the head until they lose consciousness,. These cases could be considered to have "self-induced HWE" (Satishchandra et al. 1988). The seizures last for 30 s to 3 min and occur either at the beginning or at the end of the bath. Interestingly, a small proportion of patients also report seizures during cold-water baths, and these episodes can coexist with HWE, or occur as an independent phenomenon, in a later part in the natural history. Spontaneous non-reflex epilepsy occurs a few years later in 16–38% of HWE patients (Subrahmanyam 1972; Mani et al. 1974; Satishchandra et al. 1988; Satishchandra 2003). A history of epilepsy among family members has been reported in 7–22.6% of cases. There are no neurologic deficits observed in these patients.

Electroencephalographic features

The interictal scalp electroencephalogram (EEG) is usually normal, but 15–20% show diffuse abnormalities (Subrahmanayam 1972; Mani et al. 1974; Satishchandra et al. 1985, 1988; Satishchandra 2003). Lateralized or localized spike discharges in the anterior temporal regions have been reported in a few isolated cases (Szymonowicz and Meloff 1978; Miyao et al. 1982). Ictal EEG recording has technical limitations and is difficult to obtain. However, seven reports in the literature provide information on the ictal EEG during provocation in water-immersion epilepsy. These studies report: left temporal rhythmic delta activity (Stensman and Ursing 1971), sharp and slow waves in the left hemisphere bilateral spikes (Parsonage et al. 1976), and temporal abnormalities (Shaw et al. 1988; Lenoir et al. 1989). Simultaneous split-screen video-EEG recording in one patient with "bathing" epilepsy showed delta waves starting from the right hemisphere with rapid secondary generalization (Roos and Van Diyk 1988).

Pathogenesis

The exact pathogenesis of this unusual form of reflex epilepsy remains unknown. Stensman and Ursing (1971) have suggested that HWE is precipitated by complex tactile and temperature-dependent stimuli. It has been possible to provoke seizures in the laboratory by pouring hot water over the heads of these patients: however, hot towels, sauna, or blowing hot air on the head do not induce seizures, suggesting that the triggering stimuli are complex and would involve a combination of factors such as (a) contact of the scalp with hot water, (b) temperature of the water, and (c) a specific cortical area of stimulation. As complex partial seizures are the commonest seizure type, and as the ictal EEG has demonstrated focal activity in the temporal or frontal lobe, Szymonowicz and Meloff (1978) suggested that there could be a structural lesion in the temporal lobe. However, neuroimaging in patients with HWE has not shown any focal structural lesions. Even if such a

lesion were present, it is still not clear whether the mechanism of seizures depends on increased neuronal excitability in the lesion or involvement of lower centers such as the hypothalamus or both (Parsonage et al. 1976). Shankar and Satishchandra (1994) reported pathological findings in three patients with HWE. In 11–27% of HWE patients from India, a clinical history of febrile convulsions, before the development of this reflex epilepsy, has been reported (Subrahmanyam 1972; Mani et al. 1974; Satishchandra et al. 1988; Satishchandra 2003). This association has not so far been noted from other parts of world.

Repeated exposure of the head of adult rats to hot water (45 °C) induced experimental seizures, which are comparable to kindling by repeated stimulation with sub-threshold electrical current. Klauenberg and Sparber (1984) called this *hyperthermic kindling*. Ullal et al. (1996) postulated that the similar phenomenon of hyperthermic kindling might be responsible for the development of HWE in humans. To understand the pathophysiological and pharmacological mechanisms underlying HWE, an experimental animal model that mimics the precipitating stimulus, the ictal events, and the EEG features has been developed (Satishchandra et al. 1993; Ullal et al. 1995, 1996, 2006). Hyperthermic kindling was demonstrated in this model by repeated hot-water stimulation. Translating this information to the human, Satishchandra et al. (1995) recorded the body temperature through a thermistor placed in the auditory canal in susceptible persons with HWE during a hot-water head bath and noted a rapid rise in temperature of 2–3 °F (1.1–1.7 °C) within a short span of 2 min. It takes 10–12 min for this temperature to return to the normal baseline, once the bath is completed. This compares to an increase of 0.5–0.6 °F (0.27–0.33 °C) noted in normal healthy volunteers, which returns to the baseline temperature immediately, at the end of the bath. This suggests that a special form of induced hyperthermia-like phenomenon could be responsible for causing HWE in susceptible individuals (Satishchandra et al. 1995). Patients with HWE seem extremely sensitive to the *rapid* increase in temperature occurring during hot-water head baths, which precipitates seizures. This aberrant thermoregulatory response may be genetically determined, and further work in this direction is currently underway.

Functional imaging

In the absence of apparent structural changes in magnetic resonance imaging (MRI) of HWE patients it is likely that functional neuronal changes underlie seizures. We conducted a study of interictal and ictal single photon emission computed tomography (SPECT) scans in ten HWE patients who had recurrent pure HWE, by using an ethylene cysteine dimer (ECD). All HWE individuals had MRI and interictal scalp EEG. Interictal ^{99m}Tc SPECT scans were performed initially in all these patients by using a single-head scanner. Patients were then stimulated with hot-water head baths. Five (50%) patients who had HWE in the laboratory were given intravenous ^{99m}Tc ECD at the onset of the ictal event, and peri-ictal SPECT scans were repeated. These were subtracted from the corresponding interictal SPECT scans. These studies demonstrated ictal hypermetabolic uptake in the medial temporal structures and hypothalamus on the left in three, and on the right in two patients, with spread to the opposite hemisphere. This suggests functional involvement of these structures in triggering HWE (Satishchandra *et al.* 2001).

Genetics

Although familial clustering and positive family histories seen in about 10–23% of HWE patients from southern India have long suggested a genetic etiology of the disorder (Mani *et al.* 1974; Satishchandra *et al.* 1999; Sinha *et al.* 1999; Satishchandra 2003), studies towards identification of HWE genes have only recently been initiated. In an ongoing effort

to understand the molecular basis of HWE, we have examined seven HWE families (12, 14, 52, 150, 257, 227, and 261) with several members affected by the disorder, ascertained at NIMHANS. These studies have helped in the identification of two loci for HWE on chromosomes 10q21.3–q22.3 (Ratnapriya *et al.* 2009a) and 4q24–q28 (Ratnapriya *et al.* 2009b). Among the families analyzed, Family 150 was the largest and comprised four generations with 10 affected and 20 apparently unaffected members (Fig. 102.1). This family was recruited through proband III:10 who was diagnosed with HWE at the age of 15 years. His interictal EEG showed epileptiform discharges arising from the left temporal region of the brain. The HWE phenotype in Family 150 and six additional families (12, 14, 52, 227, 257, and 261) transmitted in an apparently autosomal dominant mode with incomplete penetrance. A whole-genome linkage analysis involving about 400 microsatellite DNA markers was carried out in Family

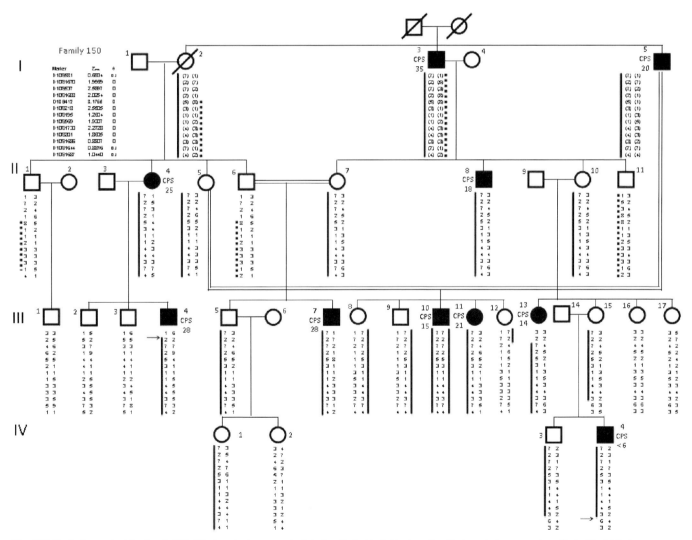

Fig. 102.1. Pedigree chart for Family 150. Filled symbols represent clinically affected individuals and unfilled symbols represent unaffected individuals. The roman numerals to the left of the pedigree denote generations and arabic numerals beside the symbols denote individuals. Fine mapping and haplotype analysis with 13 markers are shown. The HWE-associated haplotype is shaded. Age at onset is indicated beside symbols. Alleles in parentheses are inferred. Key recombinants (III:13 and IV:4) are indicated by arrows. CPS, complex partial seizures.

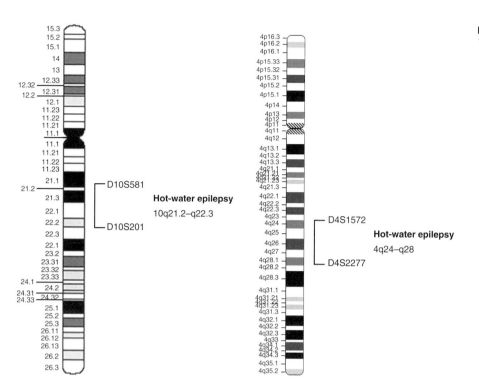

Fig. 102.2. Hot-water epilepsy loci at 10q21.2–q22.3 and 4q24–q28, respectively.

150 and parametric two-point logarithm of odds (LOD) scores were calculated considering autosomal dominant inheritance with 50–90% penetrance values, a disease allele frequency of 0.0001 and 1% phenocopy. Following the whole-genome analysis of Family 150, the highest two-point LOD score obtained was 3.17 at recombination faction (θ) = 0 and penetrance value of 60%, for the marker D10S412 at chromosomal region 10q21 (Fig. 102.2). Analysis of five additional HWE families mentioned above, for markers on chromosome 10, further strengthened the evidence of linkage to the same chromosomal region with three out of five families providing support for linkage to the same subchromosomal region. The markers D10S201 and D10S581 defined the boundaries of the critical genetic interval. In a similar study of Family 227 (Fig. 102.3), significant linkage was detected on chromosome 4q24–q28 (Fig. 102.2), with the highest two-point LOD score of 3.50 at recombination value (θ) of 0 for the marker D4S402. The markers D4S1572 and D4S2277 defined centromere-proximal and centromere-distal boundaries of this locus, respectively. The critical genetic interval spans about 24 megabases (Mb) of DNA.

Hot water triggering reflex epilepsy and high fever leading to febrile convulsions in children suggest apparently similar mechanisms. Genetic loci for familial febrile convulsions have been mapped to 2q23–q24, 3p24.2–p23, 5q14–q15, 5q31.1–q33.1, 6q22–q24, 8q13–q21, 18p11.2, 19p13, and 22q22 (Audenaert *et al.* 2006). However, the 10q21.3–q22.3 and 4q24–q28 loci identified for HWE (Fig. 102.2) are different from the loci implicated in febrile convulsions suggesting that HWE and febrile convulsions are independent clinical entities.

Reports of the high prevalence of HWE in south India suggest that there is a founder effect for the disorder. While the possibility of a recent common ancestor was excluded during interviews with members of the seven families, it remains to be determined whether families mapping at 10q21–22 have a distant ancestor in common. Analysis of high-resolution DNA markers in the region in these and additional families will help answer this question. Alternatively, HWE may be genetically heterogeneous and gene–environment interaction could explain the increased prevalence in southern India.

The identification of two genetic loci for HWE is an important step towards finding the responsible genes. The 15-Mb critical interval at 10q21.3–q22.3 and 24-Mb critical interval at 4q24–q28 harbor several genes known to be expressed in the human brain. Among the genes known from the 10q21.3–q22.3 region, the ones coding for ion channel proteins, *KCNMA1* and *VDAC2*, were the most obvious candidates for HWE, as epilepsies caused by mutations in ion channels are a large subset of monogenic epilepsies. Genes *SLC29A3* and *SLC25A16*, which are involved in regulation of neuronal ion flux, also map to this region. However, sequence analysis of these four genes did not identify a potentially causative coding mutation making involvement of these genes somewhat unlikely. Similarly, two genes, *SLC39A8* and *TRPC3*, at 4q24–q28 were examined for coding mutations but none were found. However, the possibility of variations in the gene copy number or in the transcript structures such as alternative spliced isoforms or promoter methylation at these genes need to be examined. Some insights about the genes, disturbances of which could cause temperature-dependent generation of

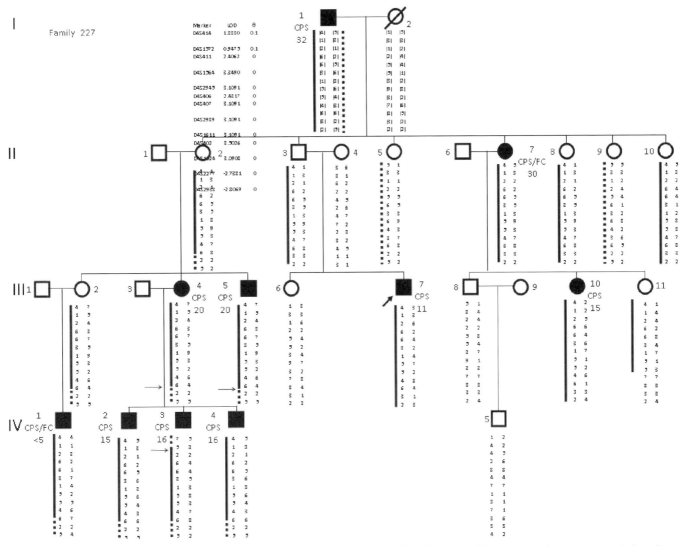

Fig. 102.3. Pedigree chart of Family 227. Key recombinant events in III:4, III:5, and IV:3 are indicated by arrows. Seizure types and age at onset are indicated beside symbols. CPS, complex partial seizures; FC, febrile convulsions.

seizures, have come from animal models. Temperature-sensitive, seizure-like phenotypes are also known to occur in *Drosophila* carrying mutations in *Shaker*, a gene known to code for sodium channel proteins (Jackson *et al.* 1984) Another *Drosophila* mutant, *Nubian*, displays temperature-dependent seizures due to a defect in phosphoglycerate kinase, an enzyme required for adenosine triphosphate (ATP) generation in the terminal stage of the glycolytic pathway (Wang *et al.* 2004). These findings suggest an involvement of diverse types of molecules in temperature-sensitive seizure phenotypes akin to hot-water epilepsy in humans. Interestingly, genes involved in nervous system development (*NEUROG3*), molecules involved in calcium signaling (*CAMK2G* and *MYOZ1*), cell cycle and apoptosis regulator (*CCAR1*), receptor of neuropeptide (*TACR2*), neuronal Ca^{2+}-binding proteoglycans (*SPOCK2*), and sphingolipid activator proteins (*PSAP*), map in the 10q21.3–q22.3 region and are potential candidates to be examined. Genes for neurodevelopment (*NEUROG2*, *ANK2*),

calcium signaling (*CAMK2D*), and the formation of myelin membranes (*UGT8*) are potentially strong candidates for being responsible for the disorder in the 4q24–q28 region. Further work in the analysis of these and other such genes to identify the gene responsible for HWE is in progress.

Management

Often HWE is managed in two ways: (a) using lukewarm water for a head bath or sponging with hot towels (Subrahmanayam 1972; Mani *et al.* 1974; Satishchandra *et al.* 1988; Satishchandra 2003) and (b) use of conventional antiepileptic drugs (AEDs) such as phenytoin or carbamazepine. Follow-up of 208 patients with HWE treated with conventional AEDs for a mean period of 14 ± 12.9 months (range 6–60 months) showed that in 60% seizures could be easily controlled, 18.3% had a 50% reduction in frequency, but others continued to have seizures at their last follow-up (Satishchandra *et al.* 1988).

It is interesting to note that 10% of these HWE patients exhibit compulsive behavior, that is, "self-induced HWE." From 16% to 38% of subjects with HWE continued to have seizures even during regular baths and developed non-reflex seizures during follow-up. This is indirect evidence for the phenomenon of hyperthermic kindling in humans, although the occurrence of kindling in humans is still controversial (Satishchandra *et al.* 1988; Satishchandra 2003). In view of the observation that HWE is a type of hyperthermic seizure akin to febrile convulsions, Satishchandra *et al.* (1998) evolved a newer method of intermittent oral prophylaxis with benzodiazepines. They advocated the use of 5–10 mg of oral clobazam 1.5–2 hr before a head bath and *not* every day. These patients do not require any other AEDs on a regular basis, thereby minimizing the cost and side effects of these AEDs. Conventional AEDs are to be used only if the patients develop non-reflex seizures apart from HWE (Satishchandra *et al.* 1998). Recently an analysis of 304 patients with HWE was carried out: (a) pure HWE ($n = 198$; 65.1%); (b) HWE plus ($n = 62$; 20.4%); and (c) defaulters ($n = 44$; 14.5%). Three-fourths of patients receiving intermittent clobazam (group a) showed an excellent response and additional AEDs might only be justified in the setting of poor therapeutic response and/or coexistent non-reflex epilepsy.

Acknowledgments

We thank Drs. G. R. Ullal, S. K. Shankar, K. G. Kallur, S. Dilip, and G. Gadre and Ms R. Rathnapriya for their association with research work on HWE at various stages.

References

Allen IM (1945) Observation on cases of reflex epilepsy. *N Z Med J* 44:135–42.

Audenaert D, Van Broeckhoven C, De Jonghe P (2006) Genes and loci involved in febrile seizures and related epilepsy syndromes. *Hum Mutat* 27:391–401.

Bebek N, Gurses C, Gokyigit A, *et al.* (2001) Hot-water epilepsy: clinical and electrophysiological findings based on 21 cases. *Epilepsia* 42:1130–4.

Engel J Jr. (2001) A proposed diagnostic scheme for people with epileptic seizures and with epilepsy: report of the ILAE Task Force on Classification and Terminology. *Epilepsia* 42:1–8.

Gastaut H (1973) *Dictionary of Epilepsy,* Part I. Geneva: World Health Organization.

Gururaj G, Satishchandra P (1992) Correlates of hot water epilepsy in rural south India: a descriptive study. *Neuroepidemiology* 11:173–9.

Jackson FR, Wilson SD, Strichartz GR, Hall LM (1984) Two types of mutants affecting voltage-sensitive sodium channels in *Drosophila melanogaster. Nature* 308:189–91.

Keipert JA (1969) Epilepsy precipitated by bathing: water-immersion epilepsy. *Aust Paediatr J* 5:244–7.

Klauenberg BJ, Sparber SBA (1984) Kindling-like effect inducted by repeated exposure to heated water in rats. *Epilepsia* 25:292–301.

Kurata S (1979) Epilepsy precipitated by bathing: a follow-up study. *Brain Dev (Domestic edn)* 11:400–5.

Lenoir P, Ranet J, Demeirleir L (1989) Bathing induced seizures. *Pediar Neurol* 5:124–5.

Mani KS, Gopalakrishnan PN, Vyas JN, *et al.* (1968) Hot-water epilepsy: a peculiar type of reflex epilepsy – a preliminary report. *Neurology* (*India*) 16:107–10.

Mani KS, Mani AJ, Ramesh CK (1974) Hot water epilepsy: a peculiar type of reflex epilepsy: clinical and electroencephalographic features in 108 cases. *Trans Am Neurol Ass* 99:224–6.

Mani KS, Rangan G, Srinivas HV, *et al.* (1998) The Yelandur study: a community-based approach to epilepsy in rural south India: epidemiological aspects. *Seizure* 7:281–8.

Miyao M, Tezuka M, Kuwajima K, *et al.* (1982) Epilepsy induced by hot water immersion. *Brain Dev* 4:158.

Mofenson HC, Weymuller CA, Greensher J (1965) Epilepsy due to water immersion: an unusual case of reflex sensory epilepsy. *J Am Med Ass* 191:600–1.

Morimoto T, Hayakawa T, Sugie H, *et al.* (1985) Epileptic seizures precipitated by constant light, movement in daily life and hot water immersion. *Epilepsia* 26:237–42.

Parsonage MJ, Moran JH, Exley KA (1976) So-called water immersion epilepsy. In: *Epileptology,* Proceedings of the 7th Internatational Symposium on Epilepsy. Stuttgart: Georg Thieme, pp. 50–60.

Ratnapriya R, Satishchandra P, Kumar D, *et al.* (2009a) A locus for autosomal dominant reflex epilepsy precipitated by hot water maps at chromosome 10q21.3–q22.3. *Hum Genet* 125:541–9.

Ratnapriya R, Satishchandra P, Dilip S, Gadre G, Anand A (2009b) Familial autosomal dominant reflex epilepsy triggered by hot water maps to 4q24–q28. *Hum Genet* 125:677–83.

Roos RAC, Van Diyk JE (1988) Reflex epilepsy induced by immersion in hot water. *Eur Neurol* 28:610.

Satishchandra P (2003) Hot-water epilepsy. *Epilepsia* 44(Suppl 1):29–32.

Satishchandra P, Shivaramakrishna A, Kaliaperumal VG (1985) Hot water epilepsy: a variant of reflex epilepsy in parts of South India. *J Neurol* 232(Suppl):212.

Satishchandra P, Shivaramakrishna A, Kaliaperumal VG, *et al.* (1988) Hot water epilepsy: a variant of reflex epilepsy in Southern India. *Epilepsia* 29:52–6.

Satishchandra P, Ullal GR, Shankar SK (1993) Experimental animal model for hot water epilepsy. *Epilepsia* 34(Suppl 2):101.

Satishchandra P, Ullal GR, Shankar SK (1995) Newer insight into the complexity of hot-water epilepsy. *Epilepsia* 36(Suppl 3):206–7.

Satishchandra P, Ullal GR, Shankar SK (1998) Hot water epilepsy. In: Zifkin BG, Andermann F, Beaumanoir A, *et al.* (eds). *Reflex Epilepsy and Reflex Seizures.* Philadelphia, PA: Lippincott-Raven, pp. 283–94.

Satishchandra P, Ullal GR, Sinha A, Shankar SK (1999) Pathophysiology and genetics of hot-water epilepsy. In: Berkovic S, Genton P, Marescaux C, Picard F (eds.) *Genetics of Focal Epilepsies: Clinical Aspects and Molecular Biology.* London: John Libbey, pp. 169–76.

Satishchandra P, Kallur KG, Jayakumar PN (2001) Inter-ictal and ictal ^{99m}Tc ECD SPECT scan in hot-water epilepsy. *Epilepsia* **42**(Suppl):158.

Shankar SK, Satishchandra P (1994) Autopsy study of brains in hot water epilepsy. *Neurology (India)* **42**:56–7.

Shaw NJ, Livingston JH, Minns RA, *et al.* (1988) Epilepsy precipitated by bathing. *Dev Med Child Neurol* **30**:108–11.

Sinha A, Ullal GR, Shankar SK, *et al.* (1999) Genetics of hot-water epilepsy: a preliminary analysis. *Curr Sci* **77**:1407–10.

Stensman R, Ursing B (1971) Epilepsy precipitated by hot water immersion. *Neurology* **21**:559–62.

Subrahmanayam HS (1972) Hot water epilepsy. *Neurology (India)* **20**(Suppl II):241–3.

Szymonowicz W, Meloff KL (1978) Hot water epilepsy. *Can J Neurol Sci* **5**:247–51.

Ullal GR, Satishchandra P, Shankar SK (1995) Seizure patterns, hippocampal and ictal temperature threshold with hyperthermic kindling in rats on hot-water stimulation. *Epilepsia* **36**(Suppl 3):552.

Ullal GR, Satishchandra P, Shankar SK (1996) Hyperthermic seizures: an animal model for hot-water epilepsy. *Seizure* **5**:221–8.

Ullal GR, Satishchandra P, Kalladka D, *et al.* (2006) Kindling and mossy fibre sprouting in the rat hippocampus. *Indian J Med Res* **124**:331–42.

Velmurugendran CU (1985) Reflex epilepsy. *J Neurol* **232**:212.

Wang P, Saraswati S, Guan Z, *et al.* (2004) A *Drosophila* temperature-sensitive seizure mutant in phosphoglycerate kinase disrupts ATP generation and alters synaptic function. *J Neurosci* **24**:4518–29.

Chapter 103

Reflex epilepsy with higher-level processing

Benjamin Zifkin and Frederick Andermann

The seizures of reflex epilepsy are reliably precipitated by some identifiable factor. The recent classification proposal (Engel 2001) defines *reflex epilepsy syndromes* as:

> syndromes in which all epileptic seizures are precipitated by sensory stimuli. Reflex seizures that occur in focal and generalized epilepsy syndromes that are also associated with spontaneous seizures, are listed as seizure types. Isolated reflex seizures can also occur in situations that do not necessarily require a diagnosis of epilepsy.

It admits few such syndromes: idiopathic photosensitive occipital lobe epilepsy, other visual sensitive epilepsies, primary reading epilepsy, and startle epilepsy. Others are defined as seizure types and a list provided of precipitating stimuli for reflex seizures. Reflex seizures are "objectively and consistently demonstrated to be evoked by a specific afferent stimulus or by activity of the patient. Afferent stimuli can be: elementary, i.e., unstructured (light flashes, startle, a monotone) or elaborate, i.e., structured. Activity may be *elementary*, e.g., motor (a movement); or *elaborate*, e.g., cognitive function (reading, chess playing), or both (reading aloud)" (Blume *et al.* 2001). Bearing this in mind, we would note that reflex seizures are more common than pure reflex epilepsies and the reflex seizures in disorders that cannot be called reflex epilepsy syndromes in the classification proposal do not differ from those triggered by the same stimuli in recognized epilepsy syndromes. Thus it is not clear that there is a difference in pathophysiology other than perhaps one of degree between reflex seizures and reflex epilepsy with the same trigger.

Reports of higher-level triggers such as calculation, reading, and thinking pre-date modern imaging and epilepsy monitoring. This chapter will consider seizures induced by thinking and action programming (planned action or praxis), reading and other language-related triggers, and some related stimuli. These share the characteristic that a specific stimulus can activate a bilateral or apparently generalized electroencephalographic (EEG) response and clinically generalized or bilateral seizures rather than only focal cortical events such as the focal reflex seizures (Clementi 1929) of animals with experimental cortical lesions.

Seizures induced by thinking or action programming

Seizures triggered by mental arithmetic were first documented as *epilepsia arithmetices* (Ingvar and Nyman 1962). A patient reporting that his seizures were triggered by mental arithmetic was studied extensively by Wilkins *et al.* (1982). This showed that spatial thought as well as more difficult calculation triggered seizures in this man. In this case, one might expect that the relatively specific nature of the tasks would have triggered focal epileptiform EEG abnormalities and possibly focal seizures. Instead they triggered bilateral spike-and-wave activity and brief absence attacks – generalized seizures. The patient did not have myoclonus and did not seem to have juvenile myoclonic epilepsy. Similarly, Binnie, Wilkins, and co-workers showed that pattern-sensitive epilepsy had a relatively localized occipital cortical trigger (Binnie *et al.* 1985), but that sensitivity to intermittent photic stimulation and to striped patterns also triggered bilateral or generalized EEG epileptiform activity and apparently generalized seizures. Studies of seizures precipitated by combined thought and action began to appear in Japanese journals at about this time. These were described in English language book chapters as "praxis-induced seizures" (Inoue *et al.* 1994). A large and important study by Matsuoka *et al.* (2000) clarified many of these questions, and seemed to confirm and expand the ideas that had been broached by Wilkins *et al.* (1982) in one patient and then in more detail in a series of patients reported by Goossens *et al.* (1990) some of whom could be triggered by purely mental tasks with no movement. Hand or finger movements without "action-programming activity" (defined by Matsuoka as "higher mental activity requiring hand movement" and apparently synonymous with praxis) are not effective triggers in praxis-induction: spatial thought and the intent to move are both necessary. Both praxis-induction and seizures induced by thinking appear almost exclusively in idiopathic generalized epilepsies as they are now understood, and particularly in juvenile myoclonic epilepsy, although seizures induced by thinking can occur with no motor component in the stimulus or the response. Other subjects report activation by drawing, but not typically by reading. The model of human pattern-sensitive epilepsy is of special interest in such seizures because it shows that generalized clinical events and generalized or bilateral EEG abnormalities can be activated by a specific functional stimulation with a known localization, in the case of pattern-sensitive epilepsy involving hyperexcitability of the primary visual cortex. This electroclinical pattern is found in many subjects with several types of reflex seizure triggers and idiopathic generalized epilepsy, without neurologic deficit or evident lesions on imaging, and who are, thus, presumed to have diffuse cortical hyperexcitability with a genetic component (Ferlazzo et al. 2005). The structures or networks that may be hyperexcitable or recruited to form a critical mass needed for a seizure to occur were earlier thought to be parietal in seizures induced by thinking. More recent studies on the cortical structures involved in manipulation of numbers and of calculation (Stanescu-Cosson et al. 2000; also reviewed in Ferlazzo et al. 2005) show that a more extensive bilateral functional network is involved. Spread to motor cortex or involvement of hyperexcitable motor cortex as may exist in juvenile myoclonic epilepsy can explain the observed myoclonic events, as discussed by Inoue and Zifkin (2004).

Reading epilepsy is characterized by orofacial reflex myoclonus triggered by reading, which the patients may report as jaw jerks, partial seizures which may become generalized convulsions, and in some patients, jerks of the arms and head with bilateral EEG discharges similar to those seen in juvenile myoclonic epilepsy (see also Chapter 99). Koutroumanidis et al. (1998) described the clinical and EEG variants of reading epilepsy. The seizures are usually easy to record if an EEG is performed during reading. If patients with jaw jerks continue to read, they may have a generalized seizure but patients with jaw jerks alone may not come to medical attention. Familial reading epilepsy is well documented but no responsible gene has been identified yet. Functional magnetic resonance imaging (fMRI) shows activations in most subjects in areas overlapping or adjacent to those physiologically activated during language and facial motor tasks, including subcortical structures, without significant lesions (Salek-Haddadi et al. 2009). Patients with primary reading epilepsy do not have other epileptic syndromes but some patients report activation by other language-related tasks such as recitation and writing, though not by calculation or spatial thought. Of interest in two subjects with seizures induced by writing, EEG responses were not always lateralized but the magnetoencephalograph localized the triggered dipoles to the dominant left centroparietal regions, even with only the thought of writing (Tanaka et al. 2006). Reading epilepsy, and language-induced seizures more generally, seem to be a further example of activation of a hyperexcitable functional network, which can produce seizures when sufficient critical mass is incorporated by adequate stimuli. Apart from the trigger, the seizures can be indistinguishable from those of an apparently generalized epilepsy. This form of reflex seizure genesis may rely on both existing and reorganized functional links between brain regions and need not be confined to physically contiguous brain sites or established neuronal links.

The pattern of praxis-induction fits well with juvenile myoclonic epilepsy, in which there is apparent regional hyperexcitability of sensorimotor cortex within an apparently generalized epileptic disorder (Wolf 1994). These and other observations in both reflex and spontaneous epileptogenesis (Binnie 2004) suggest that the postulated diffuse cortical hyperexcitability in idiopathic generalized epilepsy is not necessarily uniform; specific activities can activate specific cortical systems or functional networks spread over several cortical regions in one or both hemispheres and produce focal or regional discharges, or partial seizures, which may generalize. Kho et al. (2006) discussed the dissociation between drawing- and writing-induced seizures; this, in addition to the evidence from the seizures discussed above, suggests the existence of verbal and non-verbal hyperexcitable networks. The reflex seizures corresponding to these would be sensitive to triggers that activate networks preferentially lateralized to dominant and non-dominant hemispheres respectively.

An important question raised by the studies of these reflex seizures is "What is generalized about generalized epilepsy?" Does the prominence of juvenile myoclonic epilepsy in some of these patterns suggest that it is not a generalized disorder but a regional disorder of hyperexcitable frontocentral cortex susceptible to being triggered by different afferents from non-dominant and dominant hemispheres or by the hyperexcitability of a functional network? Whether or not juvenile myoclonic epilepsy is a truly generalized epilepsy or something like a regional or network hyperexcitability involving sensorimotor cortex is not clear. Evidence is accumulating that it is a model of "system" epilepsy (see for example Inoue and Zifkin 2004; Lin et al. 2009). At least some understanding of how the brain works in the useful yet somewhat artificial construct of generalized epilepsy has come from the study of reflex seizures but some difficult questions still await answers. These include how cognitive networks develop and can be modified in normal and epileptic brain, how these are under genetic control, and what antemortem structural abnormalities can be found with new imaging methods.

Treatments for these reflex seizures are medical and non-medical. General advice to avoid sleep deprivation and alcohol excess is given, especially since juvenile myoclonic epilepsy is typically worsened by sleep deprivation. Stimulus avoidance and stimulus modification are very useful and may allow treatment without medication if the reflex sensitivity is mild and the patient does not have juvenile myoclonic epilepsy. Guidelines exist in several countries to prevent the broadcasting of television images likely to trigger seizures in sensitive viewers (Wilkins et al. 2005). Increasing the distance from the television set, watching a small screen in a well-lighted room, using a remote control so that the set need not be approached, and monocular viewing or the use of polarized spectacles to block one eye are examples of stimulus modification that should provide protection from flashing or patterned screen content or environmental patterns. Colored spectacles may be useful in selected cases (Capovilla *et al.* 2006). Drug treatment is needed if these measures are impractical or unsuccessful, if sensitivity is severe, or if spontaneous attacks occur. The same is true in other reflex epilepsies. Patients with reading epilepsy may decline medication if they do not have generalized convulsive seizures. Avoiding reading carries obvious handicap. Several approaches to stimulus modification have been suggested, reviewed in Zifkin and Andermann (2010), in which drug treatment is also discussed. Antiepileptic drugs for generalized epilepsies are usually effective, especially when combined with non-medical approaches.

References

Binnie CD (2004) Evidence of reflex epilepsy on funtional systems in the brain and "generalized epilepsy". In: Wolf P, Inoue Y, Zifkin B (eds.) *Reflex Epilepsies: Progress in Understanding.* Montrouge, France: John Libbey Eurotext, pp. 7–14.

Binnie CD, Findlay J, Wilkins AJ (1985) Mechanisms of epileptogenesis in photosensitive epilepsy implied by the effects of moving patterns. *Electroencephalogr Clin Neurophysiol* **61**:1–6.

Blume WT, Luders HO, Mizrahi E, *et al.* (2001) Glossary of descriptive terminology for ictal semiology: report of the ILAE Task Force on Classification and Terminology. *Epilepsia* **42**:1212–18.

Capovilla G, Gambardella A, Rubboli G, *et al.* (2006) Suppressive efficacy by a commercially available blue lens on PPR in 610 photosensitive epilepsy patients. *Epilepsia* **47**:529–33.

Clementi A (1929) Stricninizzazione della sfera corticale visiva ed epilessia sperimentale da stimoli luminosi. *Arch Fisiol* **27**:356–87.

Engel J Jr. (2001) A proposed diagnostic scheme for people with epileptic seizures and with epilepsy: report of the ILEA Task Force on Classification and Terminology. *Epilepsia* **42**:796–803.

Ferlazzo E, Zifkin BG, Andermann E, Andermann F (2005) Cortical triggers in generalized reflex seizures and epilepsies. *Brain* **128**:700–10.

Goossens L A Z, Andermann F, Andermann E, Rémillard GM (1990) Reflex seizures induced by calculation, card or board games, and spatial tasks: a review of 25 patients and delineation of the epileptic syndrome. *Neurology* **40**:1171–6.

Ingvar DN, Nyman GE (1962) *Epilepsia arithmetices*: a new psychological trigger mechanism in a case of epilepsy. *Neurology* **12**:282–7.

Inoue Y, Zifkin B (2004) Praxis induction and thinking induction: one or two mechanisms? In: Wolf P, Inoue Y, Zifkin B (eds.) *Reflex Epilepsies: Progress in Understanding.* Montrouge, France: John Libbey Eurotext, pp. 41–55.

Kho KH, van den Bergh WM, Spetgens WPJ, Leijten FSS (2006) Figuring out drawing-induced epilepsy. *Neurology* **66**:723–6.

Koutroumanidis M, Koepp MJ, Richardson MP, *et al.* (1998) The variants of reading epilepsy: a clinical and video-EEG study of 17 patients with reading-induced seizures. *Brain* **121**:1409–27.

Lin K, Carrete H Jr., Lin J, *et al.* (2009) Magnetic resonance spectroscopy reveals an epileptic network in juvenile myoclonic epilepsy. *Epilepsia* **50**:1191–200.

Matsuoka H, Takahashi T, Sasaki M, *et al.* (2000) Neuropsychological EEG activation in patients with epilepsy. *Brain* **123**:318–30.

Salek-Haddadi A, Mayer T, Hamandi K, Symms M, *et al.* (2009) Imaging seizure activity: a combined EEG/EMG-fMRI study in reading epilepsy. *Epilepsia* **50**:256–64.

Stanescu-Cosson R, Pinel P, van De Moortele PF, *et al.* (2000) Understanding dissociations in dyscalculia: a brain imaging study of the impact of number size on the cerebral networks for exact and approximate calculation. *Brain* **123**:2240–55.

Tanaka N, Sakurai K, Kamada K, *et al.* (2006) Neuromagnetic source localization of epileptiform activity in patients with graphogenic epilepsy. *Epilepsia* **47**:1963–7.

Wilkins AJ, Andermann F, Ives J (1975) Stripes, complex cells and seizures: an attempt to determine the locus and nature of the trigger mechanism in pattern-sensitive epilepsy. *Brain* **98**:365–80.

Wilkins AJ, Zifkin B, Andermann F, *et al.* (1982) Seizures induced by thinking. *Ann Neurol* **11**:608–12.

Wilkins AJ, Emmett J, Harding GFA (2005) Characterizing the patterned images that precipitate seizures and optimizing guidelines to prevent them. *Epilepsia* **46**:1212–18.

Wolf P (1994) Regional manifestation of idiopathic epilepsy: introduction. In: Wolf P (ed.) *Epileptic Seizures and Syndromes.* London: John Libbey, pp. 265–7.

Zifkin B, Andermann F (2010) Epilepsy with reflex seizures. In: Wyllie E, Cascino GD, Gidal B, Goodkin H (eds.) *Wyllie's Treatment of Epilepsy: Principles and Practice*, 5th edn. North Wales, PA: Springhouse Publishing, pp. 305–16.

Chapter

104

Introduction – how status epilepticus is caused

Karthik Rajasekaran and Howard P. Goodkin

Status epilepticus (SE) is a term used to describe a prolonged, self-sustained seizure that may have overt, subtle, or no behavioral manifestations typically in association with a persistent ictal electroencephalographic (EEG) pattern. Given that patients who present in either convulsive or non-convulsive forms of SE are at risk for death or subsequent neurological morbidity, all forms of SE are considered a neurological emergency. Factors identified as potentially increasing the risk of mortality and morbidity include certain etiologies, age >60 years, and increasing seizure duration. Seizure duration is the most easily effected on presentation, and the prompt and early termination of SE is of utmost importance in improving outcome. Prompt, early termination is also important as the effectiveness of current first-line therapies is inversely related to seizure duration.

Clinical overview
Definition and classification

Status epilepticus can present in many forms but there is currently no single well-accepted, precise definition or classification system for SE. Widely used clinical definitions include non-specific terminology such as a "seizure of sufficient length of time or is repeated frequently enough to produce a fixed or enduring epileptic condition" (Gastaut 1983) or "a seizure that shows no clinical signs of arresting after a duration encompassing the great majority of seizures of that type in most patients or recurrent seizures without resumption of baseline central nervous system function" (ILAE 1989).

Other clinical definitions specify a time duration. Experimental animal studies demonstrate significant neurological damage occurring within 60 mins of continuous seizures, and for this reason the Working Group on Status Epilepticus of the Epilepsy Foundation of America (EFA) defined SE as more than 30 min of either continuous seizure activity or two or more sequential seizures without full recovery of consciousness between seizures (EFA 1993). In contrast, others, stressing the need for prompt treatment, have defined the seizure duration as short as 10 min (Treiman et al. 1998) or 5 min (Lowenstein et al. 1999).

Traditionally, the classification of SE has followed that of other seizure types and SE has been divided into partial (focal) and generalized forms. However, multiple alternative semiologically based classification systems have been proposed (Treiman and Delgado-Escueta 1980; Logroseino et al. 2001; Rona et al. 2005). These systems tend to divide SE into convulsive, non-convulsive, and simple focal forms. Non-convulsive SE comprises a broad group of continuous seizures in which convulsive movements are absent. This category may include episodes of SE that occur as the result of either a generalized (e.g., absence SE) or focal epileptic mechanism. For a more detailed discussion of SE classification, the reader is referred to excellent in-depth commentaries and reviews of this topic published elsewhere (Shorvon 1994, 2005; Luders et al. 1998).

Epidemiology

Derived epidemiological values for the incidence of SE will depend on several factors including the operational definition of SE employed, the type of study performed (e.g., prospective vs. retrospective), the population studied, and catchment area. Most of the current epidemiological studies have used a duration criteria of 30 min.

Based on a prospective, population-based study performed in Richmond, VA, USA, the incidence of SE was estimated at approximately 50 episodes of SE per year per 100 000 population (DeLorenzo et al. 1996). In comparison, a retrospective study defining the incidence in Rochester, MN, USA derived a lower value of 18.3 episodes per 100 000 population (Hesdorffer et al. 1998). Although direct comparison of these studies is limited due to differences in study design and SE classification, the excess of SE in the Richmond study appears to be partially accounted for by a difference in the racial composition of the catchment areas. In Europe, reported rates have ranged from 9.9 per 100 000 in Switzerland (Coeytaux et al. 2000) to 15.8 per 100 000 in Germany (Knake et al. 2001).

Status epilepticus is a disorder that occurs at the extremes of life. In the Richmond study, the highest incidence of SE

The Causes of Epilepsy, eds. S. D. Shorvon, F. Andermann, and R. Guerrini. Published by Cambridge University Press. © Cambridge University Press 2011.

occurred in children, primarily before 1 year of age, and adults older than 60 years of age. A similar bimodal distribution has also been observed in other studies (Wu *et al.* 2002; Chin *et al.* 2004).

Etiologies of status epilepticus

The range of etiologies of SE is wide. These include trauma, brain tumors, vascular diseases, infections, non-compliance with or change in antiepileptic drugs (AEDs), and alcohol withdrawal. In addition, as reviewed in Chapter 94, a variety of drugs can induce SE including several AEDs (e.g., tiagabine, phenytoin) and the benzodiazepine antagonist flumazenil.

To a large extent, etiology is age-dependent. In children, SE is often a consequence of fever and infection. In the prospective epidemiological study of convulsive SE among children in North London (NLSTEPSS) (Chin *et al.* 2006), prolonged febrile seizures and acute symptomatic etiologies (e.g., bacterial meningitis, viral central nervous system (CNS) infection, metabolic disturbances, head injury, and stroke) accounted for 50% of the SE episodes. In contrast, in adults, acute or remote cerebrovascular disease were the most common cause of SE in the Richmond study (DeLorenzo *et al.* 1996) and non-compliance with AEDs and alcohol withdrawal were the most common causes in another study reporting the incidence of SE in San Francisco (Lowenstein and Alldredge 1993).

Evaluation for the underlying etiology should be tailored to each individual patient's history and the results of the physical examination. Key points in the history include fever or other signs or symptoms of illness, recent or remote head trauma, intoxication or toxin exposure, and history of a chronic medical condition including risk factors for cerebrovascular disease. On presentation, each patient should have a serum glucose checked immediately to evaluate for the presence of hypoglycemia. Additional laboratory studies may include a complete blood count with differential, and measurements of electrolytes, calcium, phosphorous, magnesium, AED levels, a toxicology screen, an evaluation of the cerebrospinal fluid (CSF), neuroimaging computed tomography ([CT] or magnetic resonance imaging [MRI] scan), and EEG. It should be noted that SE can result in a leukocytosis or CSF pleocytosis even in the absence of infection. Following SE, Barry and Hauser (1994) found that four of 40 patients with epilepsy had an abnormal CSF white count that ranged from 5×10^6/L to 8×10^6/L. Although one of these patients had a history of head trauma and another was presumed to have a degenerative disease, the remaining two patients had idiopathic epilepsies. In the same study, the highest CSF white blood cell count after SE in the absence of an acute insult was 28×10^6/L. In patients in whom there is concern for an increase in intracranial pressure or mass lesion, emergent neuroimaging should precede the lumbar puncture. In those cases in which a lumbar puncture has to be deferred but in which there is a reasonable

possibility of infection, antibiotics or antiviral therapy should be given prior to the lumbar puncture. In addition to the above indications, neuroimaging should be obtained in all patients presenting with their first seizure and in cases where no definite etiology has been discovered. Many patients will not need an EEG as part of the evaluation. However, an EEG should be obtained when the diagnosis is in doubt, for instance when there is the possibility of pseudostatus epilepticus, or non-convulsive subtle SE in patients in whom there is no improvement in mental status following treatment of overt convulsive SE, or when non-convulsive SE is a possible cause of unexplained altered awareness (especially in the intensive care unit setting). The EEG is also of use in assisting in the treatment of refractory SE with high-dose suppressive therapy.

Additional details regarding the diagnostic assessment of the child with SE can be found in a recent American Academy of Neurology (AAN) practice parameter (Riviello *et al.* 2006).

Treatment

As the episode of SE progresses, brain compensatory mechanisms may fail, increasing the risk of neuronal injury (Lothman *et al.* 1990). As demonstrated in experiments performed on paralyzed and well-ventilated animals (Meldrum 1983; Nevander *et al.* 1985), even when systemic factors are well controlled, neuronal injury may still ensue. Therefore, a key goal in treating SE is to terminate the seizure as early as possible. The initiation of therapy for the underlying condition is also important to reduce the risk of neuronal injury.

Treatment of SE begins with the basic principles of neuroresuscitation (i.e., the ABCs – airway, breathing, circulation) followed by the initiation of drug therapies. The current drugs of first line in the treatment of SE are the benzodiazepines (e.g., lorazepam, diazepam, midazolam), phenytoin or its prodrug, fosphenytoin, and Phenobarbital (Lowenstein and Alldredge 1998; Riviello *et al.* 2006). Of these agents, a benzodiazepine is typically the drug of first choice. Current second-line treatments include intravenous sodium valproate and levetiracetam.

Treatment of SE should begin as soon as the diagnosis is made. Prehospital treatment with the benzodiazepines is associated with shorter seizure duration and a reduced likelihood of seizure recurrence in the emergency department (Alldredge *et al.* 2001).

The efficacy of the first-line agents in the treatment of SE was compared in the landmark Veterans Affair Cooperative Study for the treatment of SE (Treiman *et al.* 1998). In this study, the efficacy for the treatment of overt generalized convulsive SE was similar for lorazepam 0.1 mg/kg (65%), phenobarbital 15 mg/kg (58%), and diazepam 0.15 mg/kg plus phenytoin 18 mg/kg (56%). These three treatments were better than phenytoin 18 mg/kg alone (44%). The failure of phenytoin alone was partially the result of study design and the infusion time required to reduce the risk of cardiac depression and hypotension associated with the intravenous form of this medication. (The reader is referred to Chapter 106 for a further discussion of the treatment of convulsive status epilepticus.)

An important result of the Veterans Affairs Cooperative Study was the demonstration that treatment success was dependent on the duration of SE at the time treatment was initiated. Although the success rate in treating the overt generalized SE – episodes of SE with a median duration of 2.8 hr – was high and ranged from 44% to 65% dependent on treatment arm, efficacy in the treatment of more prolonged episodes of subtle SE – episodes of SE with a median duration of 5.8 hr – was much lower, ranging from only 7.7% in the phenytoin-alone group to 24.2% in the phenobarbital group. A time-dependent efficacy of treatment has been observed in several other studies (Eriksson *et al.* 2005; Chin *et al.* 2008) supporting the need for prompt treatment of all forms of SE.

Status epilepticus should be considered refractory when it persists for >1 hr despite adequate doses of conventional AEDs. Agents that have been used in the treatment of refractory SE include pentobarbital, midazolam, thiopental, lidocaine, inhalational anesthetics, chlormethiazole, etomidate, ketamine, magnesium, and propofol (Walker *et al.* 1995; Costello and Cole 2007). The prolonged use of propofol (>48 hr) has been associated with the induction of metabolic acidosis and death from propofol infusion syndrome (Vasile *et al.* 2003).

An outstanding question in the treatment of refractory SE is the degree of suppression required. In surveys performed in the US and Europe, the majority of respondents titrated treatment to a burst-suppression pattern on EEG with the goal of complete control of all seizures, electroclinical and electrographic (Claassen *et al.* 2003; Holtkamp 2003). However, there is some evidence that electrocerebral inactivity provides better seizure control than a burst-suppression pattern (Krishnamurthy and Drislane 1996, 1999). Treatment of refractory SE with high-dose suppressive therapy is typically maintained for up to 48 hr prior to tapering. If seizures recur, suppressive therapy is reinstituted. In some patients, suppressive therapy has been maintained for several months (Mirski *et al.* 1995; Sahin and Riviello 2001; Sahin *et al.* 2003).

Outcome

Fortunately, for many, SE occurs without consequence; however for others, SE results in death or potentially long-term neurological morbidity including cognitive impairment, behavioral problems, and epilepsy. In modern studies, mortality rates have ranged from 4% (Aicardi and Chevrie 1970) to 37% (Barry and Hauser 1993). In the Richmond study, a mortality of 25% was reported, a rate that approaches the mortality rates from gunshot wounds, major head trauma, and myocardial infarction (Towne *et al.* 1994).

Etiology is the most important predictor of outcome. Death is much more common when SE is due to acute brain injury (Claassen *et al.* 2002), and especially after stroke, cerebral hypoxia, or anoxia.

Overall, morbidity and mortality in children is much lower than that observed in adults. In the Richmond study, pediatric mortality was 3%. The overall adult (age >16 years) mortality was 26%; and, for those older than 60, mortality rose to 36%. In the Rochester study, approximately three-fourths of the deaths were observed in those older than 65 years. In the North London NLSTEPSS study, the overall mortality for convulsive SE in children was 3% (7/226): three children had bacterial meningitis, one glutaric aciduria type 1, and three had undiagnosed progressive neurodegenerative conditions.

Several studies also demonstrate that SE duration is also a factor. In the Richmond study, SE lasting longer than 60 min had a much higher mortality (32%) than SE lasting under 1 hr (2.7%). In the VA study, 65% of patients with prolonged subtle generalized convulsive SE died within 30 days of the episode compared to 27% of patients with shorter overt SE.

The mechanistic causes of status epilepticus

Fortunately, the majority of seizures stop spontaneously within several minutes of onset and the risk of morbidity and mortality associated with a single, brief seizure is low. However, for the prolonged seizures of SE, the mechanisms that normally result in seizure termination fail and the seizure becomes self-sustained. Failure in seizure termination could be due to changes in intrinsic properties of individual neurons that comprise a network or changes at the level of the network that leads to excessive excitation or reduced inhibition. While the former could be due to alterations in ion channels that control cellular excitability (e.g., K^+ channels) (Lugo *et al.* 2008), the latter could be an outcome of an imbalance between synaptically mediated excitatory and inhibitory neurotransmission and/or alterations in electrical coupling.

Most of our current knowledge on the basic mechanistic causes underlying SE are extrapolated from data obtained from experimental animal models of convulsive SE. Given that functional anatomy studies demonstrated that the hippocampus is a critical component of the neural network required for the induction and maintenance of SE (Kapur *et al.* 1989; Lothman 1991; VanLandingham *et al.* 1991), the majority of studies investigating the mechanistic causes of SE have focused on cellular and synaptic changes in this region.

GABAergic mechanisms in status epilepticus

The binding of γ-aminobutyric acid (GABA) to synaptic $GABA_A$ receptors results in fast synaptic inhibition via a conformational change in the receptor that facilitates hyperpolarizing Cl^- conductance. Low ambient concentrations of GABA in the extracellular space also maintain a persistent (tonic) form of inhibition by activation of extrasynaptic $GABA_A$ receptors.

The receptor is a heteromeric pentameric structure that belongs to the "Cys-loop" superfamily of ligand-gated ion channels. The $GABA_A$ receptors are formed from 16 subunit subtypes (Sieghart *et al.* 1999). The current consensus is that the majority of native $GABA_A$ receptors are assembled from two copies of an α-subunit; two copies of a β-subunit; and a single copy of either a γ-, δ-, or ε-subunit. Pharmacological and molecular biological studies have revealed that functional receptors present at the synapse have a γ2-subunit in their assembly, whereas receptors that contain a δ-subunit are exclusively extrasynaptic. The sensitivity of GABA$_A$ receptors to benzodiazepines – the first-line therapy in the treatment of SE due to enhancement of GABA$_A$ receptor-mediated inhibition – is dependent on the presence of the γ2-subunit in the receptor assembly (Sieghart 2006). In contrast, the presence of the δ-subunit renders the receptors insensitive to benzodiazepines (Saxena and Macdonald 1994).

Two distinct lines of evidence suggest that GABAergic-mediated inhibition is altered during SE. First, there is a correlation between a reduction in GABA-mediated inhibition and the genesis and maintenance of SE (Kapur and Lothman 1989; Kapur et al. 1989). Second, as reviewed above, the success of benzodiazepines, agents that enhance GABA-mediated inhibition, is inversely related to seizure duration, a relationship that has also been consistently observed in animal models of SE (Walton and Trieman 1988; Kapur and Macdonald 1997; Jones et al. 2002).

A reduction in GABA-mediated inhibition and the development of benzodiazepine pharmacoresistance during SE could potentially result from rapid modifications in the presynaptic release of GABA or from rapid modifications in the postsynaptic GABA$_A$ receptor population's response to GABA. A number of presynaptic factors could contribute to the mechanistic causes of SE including reduction in the rate of GABA release and a reduction in the probability of GABA release as the result of activation of presynaptic receptors including GABA$_B$ receptors, metabotropic glutamate receptors, or CB1 receptors. However, with the exception of a limited number of studies (Walton et al. 1990; Wasterlain et al. 1993; Sankar et al. 1997), the presynaptic plasticity of GABAergic transmission during SE remains largely unexplored.

Two studies were critical in demonstrating that there is a rapid modification in the postsynaptic GABA$_A$ receptor population. First, Kapur and Coulter (1995) acutely isolated CA1 pyramidal neurons from rats in chemoconvulsant-induced SE (SE-treated) and naive controls. The majority of SE-treated neurons were either unresponsive or less sensitive to GABA compared to the controls. Second, Kapur and Macdonald (1997) demonstrated that the allosteric modulation of GABA$_A$ receptors of SE-treated hippocampal dentate granule cells differed from controls.

Although these studies could not address whether there is a modification of the release of GABA from the presynaptic terminals of the interneuron or the site (synaptic or extrasynaptic) at which the modification in the receptor population occurs, they laid the groundwork for additional studies investigating the cause of the rapid modification in the postsynaptic GABA$_A$ receptor population.

Using an in vitro model of SE (Goodkin et al. 2005) and in vivo models of SE (Naylor et al. 2005; Goodkin et al. 2008;

Terunuma et al. 2008), subsequent studies have demonstrated that synaptic inhibition, but not extrasynaptic tonic inhibition, is reduced during SE. In addition, this reduction in synaptic inhibition is partially the result of a reduction in the surface expression of the benzodiazepine-sensitive GABA$_A$ receptors. In contrast, the surface expression of the benzodiazepine-insensitive GABA$_A$ receptors was not reduced.

These findings have implications for the treatment of SE. A subset of the benzodiazepine-insensitive GABA$_A$ receptors are sensitive to general anesthetics such as propofol and pentobarbital (Feng and Macdonald 2004; Feng et al. 2004); and the implications of these findings is that general anesthetics may need to be considered earlier in treatment protocols once benzodiazepine-pharmacoresistance has developed. Also, the use of neurosteroids, which mainly act on the δ-subunit-containing GABA$_A$ receptors, may be a potential future target in the treatment of SE.

Glutamatergic mechanisms in status epilepticus

Glutamate is the principal excitatory neurotransmitter that exerts its action via the ionotropic (α-amino-3-hydroxy-5-methyl-4-isoxazolepropionic acid [AMPA], N-methyl-D-aspartate [NMDA], and kainate) and metabotropic glutamate receptors. A role for glutamate in the initiation and maintenance of SE has been suggested based on experimental evidence that extracellular glutamate levels are elevated in hippocampus prior to (Millan et al. 1993), or following SE (Millan et al. 1991) and in association with a failure of glutamate uptake (Voutsinos-Porche et al. 2006).

Experimental evidence on the effects of NMDA receptor (NMDAR) blockade per se on terminating SE has varied depending on the regions studied, models (Borris et al. 2000; Martinand Kapur 2008), and the time of treatment (Mazarati and Wasterlain 1999). However, co-treatment with NMDAR antagonists and diazepam has revealed that NMDAR blockade can prevent the onset of refractoriness to diazepam (Rice and DeLorenzo 1999) and synergize the seizure terminating action of diazepam (Martin and Kapur 2008).

Despite observations in animal studies and clinical reports of successful use of NMDAR antagonists in refractory SE (Walker and Sander 1996; Bleck 2002; Pruss and Holtkamp 2008), the temporal alterations in synaptic glutamatergic neurotransmission during SE have not been investigated in detail. Data reported by Wasterlain and colleagues (Mazarati et al. 2006) suggest an association between enhanced immunoreactivity of the NMDA receptor NR1 subunit on the cell surface of dentate granule cells in hippocampal slices acutely obtained after 1 hr of chemoconvulsant-induced SE and enhanced frequency and amplitudes of NMDAR-mediated currents in recordings obtained from these cells.

AMPA receptors (AMPARs) are also involved in the initiation (Mazarati and Wasterlain 1999) and maintenance (Mikati et al. 1999) of SE. The effectiveness of topiramate in treating human refractory SE (Walker and Sander 1996; Towne et al.

2003; Perry *et al.* 2006) may in part be associated with its AMPAR antagonistic properties (Qian and Noebels 2003). Perhaps a more important role of AMPARs in SE may be related to the resultant neurotoxicity following changes in the AMPA receptor phenotype from calcium-impermeant (GluR2-containing AMPA receptors) to a calcium-permeant form (GluR2-lacking AMPA receptors) (Grooms *et al.* 2000). As is the case with NMDARs, the temporal changes in AMPAR mediated neurotransmission during SE remain unexplored.

Conclusion

Status epilepticus is an acute neurological emergency that most commonly occurs at the extremes of life and is associated with mortality and significant neurological sequelae. Diverse etiological factors underlie the occurrence of SE. Fever and infection are the principal etiologies in children and cerebrovascular disorders in adults. Emphasis is on prompt treatment to improve patient outcome, as drug refractoriness sets in as the duration of SE increases. Advances in experimental research suggest that, at the cellular level, alterations in the surface expression of receptors may contribute to the seizures' self-sustaining nature as the result of a net deficit in synaptic GABAergic inhibition and an excess of glutamatergic excitation. Further research on functional plasticity of neurotransmitter systems during SE is necessary before we uncover newer, effective mechanism-based drug targets to terminate SE.

Reference List

Aicardi J, Chevrie JJ (1970) Convulsive status epilepticus in infants and children: a study of 239 cases. *Epilepsia* **11**:187–97.

Alldredge BK, Gelb AM, Isaacs SM, *et al.* (2001) A comparison of lorazepam, diazepam, and placebo for the treatment of out-of-hospital status epilepticus. *N Engl J Med* **345**:631–7.

Barry E, Hauser WA (1993) Status epilepticus: the interaction of epilepsy and acute brain disease. *Neurology* **43**:1473–8.

Barry E, Hauser WA (1994) Pleocytosis after status epilepticus. *Arch Neurol* **51**:190–3.

Bleck TP (2002) Refractory status epilepticus in 2001. *Arch Neurol* **59**:188–9.

Borris DJ, Bertram EH, Kapur J (2000) Ketamine controls prolonged status epilepticus. *Epilepsy Res* **42**:117–22.

Chin RF, Neville BG, Scott RC (2004) A systematic review of the epidemiology of status epilepticus. *Eur J Neurol* **11**:800–10.

Chin RF, Neville BG, Peckham C, Bedford H, Wade A, Scott RC (2006) Incidence, cause, and short-term outcome of convulsive status epilepticus in childhood: prospective population-based study. *Lancet* **368**:222–9.

Chin RF, Neville BG, Peckham C, *et al.* (2008) Treatment of community-onset, childhood convulsive status epilepticus: a prospective, population-based study. *Lancet Neurol* **7**:696–703.

Coeytaux A, Jallon P, Galobardes B, Morabia A (2000) Incidence of status epilepticus in French-speaking Switzerland: EPISTAR. *Neurology* **55**:693–7.

Costello DJ, Cole AJ (2007) Treatment of acute seizures and status epilepticus. *J Intens Care Med* **22**:319–47.

Claassen J, Lokin JK, Fitzsimmons BF, Mendelsohn FA, Mayer SA (2002) Predictors of functional disability and mortality after status epilepticus. *Neurology* **58**:139–42.

Claassen J, Hirsch LJ, Mayer SA (2003) Treatment of status epilepticus: a survey of neurologists. *J Neurol Sci* **211**:37–41.

DeLorenzo RJ, Hauser WA, Towne AR, *et al.* (1996) A prospective, population-based epidemiologic study of status epilepticus in Richmond, Virginia. *Neurology* **46**:1029–35.

Epilepsy Foundation of America (1993) Treatment of convulsive status epilepticus: recommendations of the Epilepsy Foundation of America's Working Group on Status Epilepticus. *J Am Med Ass* **270**:854–9.

Eriksson K, Metsaranta P, Huhtala H, *et al.* (2005) Treatment delay and the risk of prolonged status epilepticus. *Neurology* **65**:1316–18.

Feng HJ, Macdonald RL (2004) Multiple actions of propofol on $\alpha\beta\gamma$ and $\alpha\beta\delta$ GABA$_A$ receptors. *Mol Pharmacol* **66**:1517–24.

Feng HJ, Bianchi MT, Macdonald RL (2004) Pentobarbital differentially modulates $\alpha1\beta3\delta$ and $\alpha1\beta3\gamma2L$ GABA$_A$ receptor currents. *Mol Pharmacol* **66**:988–1003.

Gastaut H (1983) Classification of status epilepticus. *Adv Neurol* **34**:15–35.

Goodkin HP, Yeh JL, Kapur J (2005) Status epilepticus increases the intracellular accumulation of GABA$_A$ receptors. *J Neurosci* **25**:5511–20.

Goodkin HP, Joshi S, Mtchedlishvili Z, Brar J, Kapur J (2008) Subunit-specific trafficking of GABA$_A$ receptors during status epilepticus. *J Neurosci* **28**:2527–38.

Grooms SY, Opitz T, Bennett MV, Zukin RS (2000) Status epilepticus decreases glutamate receptor 2 mRNA and protein expression in hippocampal pyramidal cells before neuronal death. *Proc Natl Acad Sci USA* **97**:3631–6.

Hesdorffer DC, Logroscino G, Cascino G, Annegers JF, Hauser WA (1998) Incidence of status epilepticus in Rochester, Minnesota, 1965–1984. *Neurology* **50**:735–41.

Holtkamp M, Masuhr F, Harms L, *et al.* (2003) The management of refractory generalised convulsive and complex partial status epilepticus in three European countries: a survey among epileptologists and critical care neurologists. *J Neurol Neurosurg Psychiatry* **74**:1095–9.

International League Against Epilepsy. (1989) Proposal for revised classification of epilepsies and epileptic syndromes. *Epilepsia* **30**:389–99.

Jones DM, Esmaeil N, Maren S, Macdonald RL (2002) Characterization of pharmacoresistance to benzodiazepines in the rat Li–pilocarpine model of status epilepticus. *Epilepsy Res* **50**:301–12.

Kapur J, Stringer JL, Lothman EW (1989) Evidence that repetitive seizures in the hippocampus cause a lasting reduction of GABAergic inhibition. *J Neurophysiol* **61**:417–26.

Kapur J, Lothman EW (1989) Loss of inhibition precedes delayed spontaneous seizures in the hippocampus after tetanic electrical stimulation. *J Neurophysiol* **61**:427–34.

Kapur J, Coulter DA (1995) Experimental status epilepticus alters GABA$_A$ receptor function in CA1 pyramidal neurons. *Ann Neurol* **38**:893–900.

Kapur J, Macdonald RL (1997) Rapid seizure-induced reduction of benzodiazepine and Zn^{2+} sensitivity of hippocampal dentate granule cell GABA$_A$ receptors. *J Neurosci* **17**:7532–40.

Knake S, Rosenow F, Vescovi M, *et al.* (2001) Incidence of status epilepticus in adults in Germany: a prospective, population-based study. *Epilepsia* **42**:714–18.

Krishnamurthy KB, Drislane FW (1999) Depth of EEG suppression and outcome in barbiturate anesthetic treatment for refractory status epilepticus. *Epilepsia* **40**:759–62.

Krishnamurthy KB, Drislane FW (1996) Relapse and survival after barbiturate anesthetic treatment of refractory status epilepticus. *Epilepsia* **37**:863–7.

Logroscino G, Hesdorffer DC, Cascino G, Annegers JF, Hauser WA (2001) Time trends in incidence, mortality, and case-fatality after first episode of status epilepticus. *Epilepsia* **42**:1031–5.

Lothman EW (1991) Functional anatomy: a challenge for the decade of the brain. *Epilepsia* **32**(Suppl 5):S3–13.

Lothman EW, Bertram EH, Kapur J, Stringer JL (1990) Recurrent spontaneous hippocampal seizures in the rat as a chronic sequela to limbic status epilepticus. *Epilepsy Res* **6**:110–18.

Lowenstein DH, Bleck T, Macdonald RL (1999) It's time to revise the definition of status epilepticus. *Epilepsia* **40**:120–2.

Lowenstein DH, Alldredge BK (1993) Status epilepticus at an urban public hospital in the 1980s. *Neurology* **43**:483–8.

Lowenstein DH, Alldredge BK (1998) Status epilepticus. *N Engl J Med* **338**:970–6.

Luders H, Acharya J, Baumgartner C, *et al.* (1998) Semiological seizure classification. *Epilepsia* **39**:1006–13.

Lugo JN, Barnwell LF, Ren Y, *et al.* (2008) Altered phosphorylation and localization of the A-type channel, Kv4.2 in status epilepticus. *J Neurochem* **106**:1929–40.

Martin BS, Kapur J (2008) A combination of ketamine and diazepam synergistically controls refractory status epilepticus induced by cholinergic stimulation. *Epilepsia* **49**:248–55.

Mazarati AM, Wasterlain CG (1999) *N*-methyl-D-asparate receptor antagonists abolish the maintenance

phase of self-sustaining status epilepticus in rat. *Neurosci Lett* **265**:187–90.

Mazarati AM, Liu H, Naylor D *et al.* (2006) Self-sustaining status epilepticus. In: Wasterlain CG, Treiman DM (eds.) *Status Epilepticus Mechanisms and Management*. Cambridge, MA: The MIT Press, pp. 209–28.

Meldrum BS (1983) Metabolic factors during prolonged seizures and their relation to nerve cell death. *Adv Neurol* **34**:261–75.

Mikati MA, Werner S, Gatt A, *et al.* (1999) Consequences of alpha-amino-3-hydroxy-5-methyl-4-isoxazolepropionic acid receptor blockade during status epilepticus in the developing brain. *Brain Res Dev Brain Res* **113**:139–42.

Millan MH, Chapman AG, Meldrum BS (1993) Extracellular amino acid levels in hippocampus during pilocarpine-induced seizures. *Epilepsy Res* **14**:139–48.

Millan MH, Obrenovitch TP, Sarna GS, *et al.* (1991) Changes in rat brain extracellular glutamate concentration during seizures induced by systemic picrotoxin or focal bicuculline injection: an in vivo dialysis study with on-line enzymatic detection. *Epilepsy Res* **9**:86–91.

Mirski MA, Williams MA, Hanley DF (1995) Prolonged pentobarbital and phenobarbital coma for refractory generalized status epilepticus. *Crit Care Med* **23**:400–4.

Naylor DE, Liu H, Wasterlain CG (2005) Trafficking of GABA$_A$ receptors, loss of inhibition, and a mechanism for pharmacoresistance in status epilepticus. *J Neurosci* **25**:7724–33.

Nevander G, Ingvar M, Auer R, Siesjo BK (1985) Status epilepticus in well-oxygenated rats causes neuronal necrosis. *Ann Neurol* **18**:281–90.

Perry MS, Holt PJ, Sladky JT (2006) Topiramate loading for refractory status epilepticus in children. *Epilepsia* **47**:1070–1.

Pruss H, Holtkamp M (2008) Ketamine successfully terminates malignant status epilepticus. *Epilepsy Res* **82**:219–22.

Qian J, Noebels JL (2003) Topiramate alters excitatory synaptic transmission in mouse hippocampus. *Epilepsy Res* **55**:225–33.

Rice AC, DeLorenzo RJ (1999) N-methyl-D-aspartate receptor activation regulates refractoriness of status epilepticus to diazepam. *Neuroscience* **93**:117–23.

Riviello JJ Jr., Ashwal S, Hirtz D, *et al.* (2006) Practice parameter: diagnostic assessment of the child with status epilepticus (an evidence-based review): report of the Quality Standards Subcommittee of the American Academy of Neurology and the Practice Committee of the Child Neurology Society. *Neurology* **67**:1542–50.

Rona S, Rosenow F, Arnold S, *et al.* (2005) A semiological classification of status epilepticus. *Epilept Disord* **7**:5–12.

Sahin M, Riviello JJ Jr. (2001) Prolonged treatment of refractory status epilepticus in a child. *J Child Neurol* **16**:147–50.

Sahin M, Menache CC, Holmes GL, Riviello JJ Jr. (2003) Prolonged treatment for acute symptomatic refractory status epilepticus: outcome in children. *Neurology* **61**:398–401.

Sankar R, Shin DH, Wasterlain CG (1997) GABA metabolism during status epilepticus in the developing rat brain. *Brain Res Dev Brain Res* **98**:60–4.

Saxena NC, Macdonald RL (1994) Assembly of GABA$_A$ receptor subunits: role of the delta subunit. *J Neurosci* **14**:7077–86.

Shorvon S (1994) *Status Epilepticus: Its Clinical Features and Treatment in Children and Adults*. Cambridge, UK: Cambridge University Press.

Shorvon S (2005) The classification of status epilepticus. *Epilept Disord* **7**:1–3.

Sieghart W, Fuchs K, Tretter V, *et al.* (1999) Structure and subunit composition of GABA$_A$ receptors. *Neurochem Int* **34**:379–85.

Sieghart W (2006) Structure, pharmacology, and function of GABA$_A$ receptor subtypes. *Adv Pharmacol* **54**:231–63.

Terunuma M, Xu J, Vithlani M, *et al.* (2008) Deficits in phosphorylation of GABA$_A$ receptors by intimately associated protein kinase C activity underlie compromised synaptic inhibition during status epilepticus. *J Neurosci* **28**:376–84.

Towne AR, Pellock JM, Ko D, DeLorenzo RJ (1994) Determinants of mortality in status epilepticus. *Epilepsia* **35**:27–34.

Towne AR, Garnett LK, Waterhouse EJ, Morton LD, DeLorenzo RJ (2003) The use of topiramate in refractory status epilepticus. *Neurology* **60**:332–4.

Treiman DM, Meyers PD, Walton NY, *et al.* (1998) A comparison of four treatments for generalized convulsive status epilepticus. Veterans Affairs

Status Epilepticus Cooperative Study Group. *N Engl J Med* **339**:792–8.

Treiman DM, Delgado-Escueta A (1980) Status epilepticus. In: Thompson RA, Green RA, Green JR (eds.) *Critical Care of Neurological and Neurosurgical Emergencies*. New York: Raven Press, pp. 53–99.

VanLandingham KE, Lothman EW (1991) Self-sustaining limbic status epilepticus. I. Acute and chronic cerebral metabolic studies: limbic hypermetabolism and neocortical hypometabolism. *Neurology* **41**:1942–9.

Vasile B, Rasulo F, Candiani A, Latronico N (2003) The pathophysiology of propofol infusion syndrome: a simple name for a complex syndrome. *Intensive Care Med* **29**:1417–25.

Voutsinos-Porche B, Koning E, Clement Y, *et al.* (2006) EAAC1 glutamate transporter expression in the rat lithium–pilocarpine model of temporal lobe epilepsy. *J Cereb Blood Flow Metab* **26**:1419–30.

Walker MC, Sander JW (1996) Topiramate: a new antiepileptic drug for refractory epilepsy. *Seizure* **5**:199–203.

Walker MC, Smith SJ, Shorvon SD (1995) The intensive care treatment of convulsive status epilepticus in the UK: results of a national survey and recommendations. *Anaesthesia* **50**:130–5.

Walton NY, Treiman DM (1988) Response of status epilepticus induced by lithium and pilocarpine to treatment with diazepam. *Exp Neurol* **101**:267–75.

Walton NY, Gunawan S, Treiman DM (1990) Brain amino acid concentration changes during status epilepticus induced by lithium and pilocarpine. *Exp Neurol* **108**:61–70.

Wasterlain CG, Baxter CF, Baldwin RA (1993) GABA metabolism in the substantia nigra, cortex, and hippocampus during status epilepticus. *Neurochem Res* **18**:527–32.

Wu YW, Shek DW, Garcia PA, Zhao S, Johnston SC (2002) Incidence and mortality of generalized convulsive status epilepticus in California. *Neurology* **58**:1070–6.

Causes of status epilepticus in children

Rod C. Scott

Convulsive status epilepticus (CSE) is the most common medical neurological emergency in childhood (Chin *et al.* 2006). It has been defined in many ways but the most common definition is of a seizure or series of seizures, during which full consciousness is not regained, that continues for at least 30 min. This is the definition that will be applied for the current chapter. The incidence of CSE in north London is approximately 18 per 100 000 children per year which equates to about 2000 lifetime first episodes per year in England and Wales (Chin *et al.* 2006). The incidence in Kenya is two to five times (Sadarangani *et al.* 2008) and in Japan approximately double (Nishiyama *et al.* 2007) the incidence in north London. The variability in estimates of incidence could be methodological but might also be a result of differences in etiologies, socioeconomic status (Chin *et al.* 2009), or ethnicity (DeLorenzo *et al.* 1996; Chin *et al.* 2009). The majority of CSE events during childhood occur in the first 5 years of life with the highest incidence in those children aged less than 1 year. There is a low mortality rate of 3–4% in developed countries (Chin *et al.* 2006), but is up to 15% in developing countries (Sadarangani *et al.* 2008).

Convulsive status epilepticus in children is important as it is associated with adverse outcomes including the development of subsequent epilepsy, learning impairments, and behavioral abnormalities (Raspall-Chaure *et al.* 2006). Although some of these adverse outcomes may be a direct consequence of brain injury associated with the electrical seizure discharges (Ben Ari 1985; Cavalheiro 1995; VanLandingham *et al.* 1998; Scott *et al.* 2002, 2003) it is likely that etiology is a more important determinant of outcome (Raspall-Chaure *et al.* 2006). Therefore it is essential that etiologies are identified and treated early as such a strategy may result in an important improvement in outcomes. See Fig. 105.1 for the spectrum of disorders associated with CSE in children.

There are not many epidemiological studies addressing CSE in children and those that there are largely relate to European and North American populations, although there are some data from Africa and from Japan. The majority of epidemiological studies were not established to investigate CSE specifically in children (Hauser *et al.* 1983; DeLorenzo *et al.* 1996; Chin *et al.* 2004). Although these studies are of importance, the proportion of ascertained patients who were children is small and therefore the primarily pediatric issues have not been a priority. There are however three population-based studies addressing CSE in children; one in north London (UK) known as the north London status epilepticus in childhood surveillance study (NLSTEPSS) (Chin *et al.* 2006), one based on the east coast of Kenya (Sadarangani *et al.* 2008) in the Kilifi district, and one in Okayama City, Japan (Nishiyama *et al.* 2007).

Although the number of epidemiological studies is small there is reasonable variety in geographical location and age groups, factors which may influence the range of causes of CSE. A finding that seems to be reasonably robust across geographical regions is that the children with CSE fall broadly into two groups: those who were previously neurologically normal and those with a previous neurological disorder. The proportion of children with CSE who were previously neurologically normal is about 50% in NLSTEPSS, 70% in Japan, and although a proportion is not explicitly stated it is the large majority of children in Kenya.

Etiology of convulsive status epilepticus in previously normal children

The most common etiology for CSE identified in children who were previously neurologically normal is a prolonged febrile seizure, i.e., CSE associated with fever that is not associated with a central nervous system (CNS) infection in children aged between 6 months and 5 years. Prolonged febrile seizures account for approximately one-third of episodes of CSE in the United Kingdom and Japan with upper respiratory tract infections and urinary tract infections frequently identified as the precipitating infection. The outcome following a prolonged febrile seizure is usually favorable (Nelson and Ellenberg 1978; Verity *et al.* 1993) although there is a relationship between prolonged febrile seizures, mesial temporal sclerosis, and subsequent temporal lobe epilepsy (Cendes *et al.* 1993; Murakami

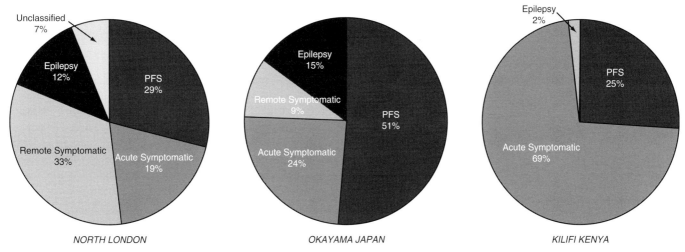

Fig. 105.1. Pie charts showing the distribution of causes of status epilepticus in children in three geographically disparate areas: north London, UK; Okayama, Japan; and Kilifi, Kenya. The data were extracted from the published papers on these studies. PFC, prolonged febrile convulsions; PFS, prolonged febrile seizures.

et al. 1996; Trinka *et al.* 2002). There continues to be controversy about whether prolonged febrile seizures can cause hippocampal injury which matures into mesial temporal sclerosis although there is increasing evidence in animal models (Ben Ari 1985; Lothman *et al.* 1989; Cavalheiro 1995) and in humans that such a pathophysiological sequence is possible (VanLandingham *et al.* 1998; Lewis *et al.* 2002; Scott *et al.* 2002, 2003). In humans the proportion of children who develop mesial temporal sclerosis is low and therefore identification of a biomarker that predicts later mesial temporal sclerosis would enable neuroprotective and antiepileptogenic strategies to be appropriately targeted. Early increases in T2-weighted signal in the hippocampus may provide such a biomarker (Provenzale *et al.* 2008).

Episodes of fever are almost universal in children, but the incidence of febrile seizures is only between 2% and 8% (Tsuboi *et al.* 1984; Verity *et al.* 1985), and of those only 5–10% are prolonged. This suggests that individual children who have febrile seizures have an underlying predisposition to febrile seizures, and that a proportion of children have a propensity for prolongation. As febrile seizures run in families it is likely that there is a genetic predisposition to febrile seizures, and at least nine genetic loci have been identified (Nakayama 2009). However, there is no evidence that any of these loci are associated with seizure prolongation and they have not associated with later development of mesial temporal sclerosis. There is however a modest association between a single-nucleotide polymorphism of the interleukin 1B gene (IL-1 beta-511T) (Kanemoto *et al.* 2000) and mesial temporal sclerosis but again it remains uncertain whether this single-nucleotide polymorphism is associated with prolongation of febrile seizures. Further study is therefore required for the understanding of the genetic basis of febrile seizures, their relationship with hippocampal injury, and the factors

(genetic, environmental, or both) that are associated with prolongation of the seizures.

The International League Against Epilepsy has proposed that prolonged febrile seizures should be considered to be acute symptomatic seizures as it is possible that children with prolonged febrile seizures could have an underlying CNS infection that has not been diagnosed. However, a classification system that includes CSE associated with what is probably a genetically determined predisposition to seizures given the correct environmental insult (fever) and which has a favorable outcome together with CSE that is due to a direct CNS insult (e.g., meningitis or encephalitis) and which may lead to adverse outcomes is likely to lead to confusion. Studies that do not separate febrile CSE and acute symptomatic CSE are likely to amplify erroneously the severity of outcome of febrile CSE and, conversely, to dilute the severity of acute neurological insults (Chin *et al.* 2006).

Acute symptomatic seizures make up the remainder of CSE in children who were previously neurologically normal. The majority of children with acute symptomatic CSE have CNS infections. Other causes include acute metabolic derangements (electrolyte imbalance, hypoglycemia, hypocalcemia, or hypomagnesemia), head injury, stroke, and drug use. Therefore, fever is common in previously normal children with CSE, but the outcomes are dependent upon the cause of the fever.

It may be difficult to decide which children have meningitis soon after termination of CSE because postictal children are likely to be poorly responsive and the children are likely to have received sedative medications as part of the treatment of CSE. Early treatment of meningitis however may improve outcomes. Approximately 10–15% of children in north London who have CSE associated with fever have a CNS infection and even though the distinction between prolonged febrile seizures and meningitis is often easy to make this may not be the case in all children, particularly those who are young (Chin *et al.* 2005). The high rate of CNS infection in children who have CSE associated with fever combined with the potential for missing the diagnosis leads to challenges in therapeutic decision making. It is common practice for antibiotics and/or antivirals to be administered early, during the time when prolonged febrile seizures may be difficult to distinguish from CNS infections, with re-evaluation of the child within the subsequent 48 hr when a clinical decision on the validity of the treatment initiated can be reconsidered. Currently there are no data evaluating the effectiveness of this type of strategy, but such an evaluation may be timely.

The relationships between CSE and fever are more complex in resource-poor countries than in developed countries. For example, malaria is common but so is a parasitemia in children who do not have clinical malaria. On this background it may be difficult to decide whether a child admitted with CSE associated with fever has a genetically determined prolonged febrile seizure which has been provoked by a malaria infection, cerebral malaria, or another infection such as bacterial meningitis or an upper respiratory tract infection. Bacterial meningitis is a strong predictor of mortality following CSE in Kilifi (Berkley *et al.* 2001; Sadarangani *et al.* 2008) which means that accurate diagnosis and strategies that minimize mortality are essential. Many hospitals in rural Africa do not have the resources that are available in Kilifi and children may need to travel long distances to medical services. Therefore primary prevention strategies that reduce the incidence of bacterial meningitis (e.g., vaccination) are more likely to reduce the mortality associated with CSE than aggressive therapy once the child reaches medical care.

The incidence of prolonged febrile seizures and of acute symptomatic CSE may also be influenced by the socioeconomic status of the children and families, and upon their ethnicity (Chin *et al.* 2009). In NLSTEPSS the children from more impoverished areas had a 5–7% increase in their risk for the above types of CSE for each 1 point change in their IMD2004 score, which is a measure of socioeconomic status used by the government of the UK for allocation of resources. This means that previously neurologically normal children from the most deprived areas are approximately six times more likely to have an episode of CSE when compared to those from the least deprived areas. An adult-based epidemiological study based in Richmond, Virginia suggested that there may also be ethnic differences in CSE with black populations having the highest incidence (DeLorenzo *et al.* 1995). This was not replicated in NLSTEPSS once socioeconomic status had been taken into account. However, Asian children did have a higher incidence of prolonged febrile seizures than white children even after adjustment. Further understanding of the factors responsible for the increased risk in at-risk populations may lead to novel primary prevention strategies that minimize the incidence of CSE in children.

Etiology of convulsive status epilepticus in children who were not previously neurologically normal

The second major group of children with CSE are those who have pre-existing neurological abnormalities. In this group of children CSE is classified as remote symptomatic (CSE in a child with a previously abnormal brain), acute on remote symptomatic (CSE in a child with a previously abnormal brain which occurs during an acute illness), and previous epilepsy (idiopathic and cryptogenic). The NLSTEPSS study was a surveillance study and therefore detailed information on the underlying brain disorder was not easily available (Chin *et al.* 2006). However, the majority of children had cerebral palsies most commonly related to hypoxic ischemic encephalopathy and prematurity. Acute on remote symptomatic CSE is often associated with upper respiratory tract infections but as with previously neurologically normal children it is important to consider bacterial meningitis as a potentially treatable underlying illness. In the study based in Japan there were children identified as having developmental brain abnormalities including lissencephaly and focal cortical dysplasia (Nishiyama *et al.* 2007). Other potential causes that have been identified include metabolic disorders such as Menke disease.

Convulsive status epilepticus in children can also occur in the context of previously diagnosed epilepsy. However, the episode of CSE could be the seizure on which the diagnosis is made, i.e., the CSE could be the second seizure that a child ever experiences and this leads to the diagnosis of epilepsy. There are children who are predisposed to having prolonged seizures and a small number who only have prolonged seizures. Previously diagnosed epilepsy is only identified in approximately 12% of children with a lifetime first episode of CSE. When a cohort of children with epilepsy is followed up then approximately 10% of those children will have an episode of CSE with a median time from diagnosis to CSE of 2.5 years (Berg *et al.* 2004). Younger age of onset, symptomatic etiology for the epilepsy, and previous episodes of CSE are the best predictors of which children are likely to have episodes of CSE. Children with severe epilepsy syndromes such as Lennox–Gastaut syndrome or Dravet syndrome commonly have episodes of CSE but these disorders are rare. These latter syndromes have also been associated with episodes of non-convulsive status epilepticus.

The concept of non-convulsive status epilepticus in children

The diagnosis, classification, and outcomes of non-convulsive status epilepticus (NCSE) in children continue to be a matter of debate, and therefore NCSE is defined broadly as a range of conditions in which electrographic seizure activity is prolonged and results in non-convulsive clinical symptoms (Walker *et al.* 2005). A time definition that is frequently used for NCSE is 30 min, which is the same as that commonly used to define CSE. This construct appears to work for CSE; after 30 min the seizure becomes self-sustaining, is more likely to cause brain injury, and is associated with systemic decompensation, i.e., hypotension, hypoglycemia, etc. (Chen and Wasterlain 2006). However, the construct is less applicable to NCSE as 30 min may not describe a point following which there are potential pathophysiological changes that separate NCSE from short seizures with similar clinical manifestations. Although this is a construct that is helpful in adult populations it is a difficult construct in children. The types of NCSE described in adults are not commonly seen in children, but frequent epileptic discharges that amount to NCSE in electrical terms are seen in other situations. Children with hypsarrhythmia, Panayiotopoulos syndrome, electrical status epilepticus in slow-wave sleep (ESES), benign rolandic epilepsy, Landau–Kleffner syndrome, and Lennox–Gastaut syndrome may all meet electrical criteria for NCSE but do not constitute a single pathophysiological entity and have enormously differing outcomes (Stores et al. 1995; Hoffmann-Riem et al. 2000). The etiologies of NCSE in children are fundamentally the causes of the epilepsy syndromes in which they are identified. Another complexity to understanding NCSE in children is the relationship between epileptic discharges and permanent adverse cognitive/behavioral outcomes which is referred to as epileptic encephalopathy (Stafstrom 2007). The relationships between frequency of epileptic discharges and outcome from the severe epilepsy syndromes in children are not very clear and it remains uncertain whether early and aggressive treatment of epileptic discharges in the electroencephalogram (EEG) significantly improves outcomes in the majority (Lux et al. 2005). Aggressive therapy with antiepileptic medications is not without risk and may also be associated with cognitive abnormalities, particularly when drugs are used in combinations. Therefore, when faced with a child who may have NCSE it is important to try and identify the underlying epilepsy syndrome, to be aware of the expected natural history, and to use antiepileptic medications judiciously with a clear view of how they may alter the expected natural history.

Conclusions

The primarily pediatric studies described above are important as they have highlighted differences in the causes of childhood CSE when compared to previously reported data on CSE that occurs in adult populations. The three main differences are that CSE in the context of epilepsy, cerebrovascular disease, and alcohol-related seizures are less common in children, whilst infections and prolonged febrile seizures are far more common. Etiology is the most important predictor of outcome and therefore early diagnosis and treatment of the underlying disorders may reduce the incidence of adverse outcomes. Improvements in socioeconomic status and appropriate targeting of at-risk populations may become important primary prevention strategies, but further research is required in this field before clinically relevant advice can be given.

References

Ben Ari Y (1985) Limbic seizure and brain damage produced by kainic acid: mechanisms and relevance to human temporal lobe epilepsy. *Neuroscience* **14**:375–403.

Berg AT, Shinnar S, Testa FM, et al. (2004) Status epilepticus after the initial diagnosis of epilepsy in children. *Neurology* **63**:1027–34.

Berkley JA, Mwangi I, Ngetsa CJ, et al. (2001) Diagnosis of acute bacterial meningitis in children at a district hospital in sub-Saharan Africa. *Lancet* **357**:1753–7.

Cavalheiro EA (1995) The pilocarpine model of epilepsy. *Ital J Neurol Sci* **16**:33–7.

Cendes F, Andermann F, Gloor P, et al. (1993) Atrophy of mesial structures in patients with temporal lobe epilepsy: cause or consequence of repeated seizures? *Ann Neurol* **34**:795–801.

Chen JW, Wasterlain CG (2006) Status epilepticus: pathophysiology and management in adults. *Lancet Neurol* **5**:246–56.

Chin RF, Neville BG, Scott RC (2004) A systematic review of the epidemiology of status epilepticus. *Eur J Neurol* **11**:800–10.

Chin RF, Neville BG, Scott RC (2005) Meningitis is a common cause of convulsive status epilepticus with fever. *Arch Dis Child* **90**:66–9.

Chin RF, Neville BG, Peckham C, et al. (2006) Incidence, cause, and short-term outcome of convulsive status epilepticus in childhood: prospective population-based study. *Lancet* **368**:222–9.

Chin RF, Neville BG, Peckham C, et al. (2009) Socioeconomic deprivation independent of ethnicity increases status epilepticus risk. *Epilepsia* **50**:1022–9.

DeLorenzo RJ, Pellock JM, Towne AR, Boggs JG (1995) Epidemiology of status epilepticus. *J Clin Neurophysiol* **12**:316–25.

DeLorenzo RJ, Hauser WA, Towne AR, et al. (1996) A prospective, population-based epidemiologic study of status epilepticus in Richmond, Virginia. *Neurology* **46**:1029–35.

Hauser WA (1983) Status epilepticus: frequency, etiology, and neurological sequelae. *Adv Neurol* **34**:3–14.

Hoffmann-Riem M, Diener W, Benninger C, et al. (2000) Nonconvulsive status epilepticus: a possible cause of mental retardation in patients with Lennox–Gastaut syndrome. *Neuropediatrics* **31**:169–74.

Kanemoto K, Kawasaki J, Miyamoto T, Obayashi H, Nishimura M (2000) Interleukin (IL)1beta, IL-1alpha, and IL-1 receptor antagonist gene polymorphisms in patients with temporal lobe epilepsy. *Ann Neurol* **47**:571–4.

Lewis DV, Barboriak DP, MacFall JR, et al. (2002) Do prolonged febrile seizures produce medial temporal sclerosis? Hypotheses, MRI evidence and unanswered questions. *Prog Brain Res* **135**:263–78.

Lothman EW, Bertram EH, Bekenstein JW, Perlin JB (1989) Self-sustaining limbic status epilepticus induced by "continuous" hippocampal stimulation: electrographic and behavioral characteristics. *Epilepsy Res* **3**:107–19.

Lux AL, Edwards SW, Hancock E, *et al.* (2005) The United Kingdom Infantile Spasms Study (UKISS) comparing hormone treatment with vigabatrin on developmental and epilepsy outcomes to age 14 months: a multicentre randomised trial. *Lancet Neurol* **4**:712–17.

Murakami N, Ohno S, Oka E, Tanaka A (1996) Mesial temporal lobe epilepsy in childhood. *Epilepsia* **37**(Suppl 3):52–6.

Nakayama J (2009) Progress in searching for the febrile seizure susceptibility genes. *Brain Dev* **31**:359–65.

Nelson KB, Ellenberg JH (1978) Prognosis in children with febrile seizures. *Pediatrics* **61**:720–7.

Nishiyama I, Ohtsuka Y, Tsuda T, *et al.* (2007) An epidemiological study of children with status epilepticus in Okayama, Japan. *Epilepsia* **48**:1133–7.

Provenzale JM, Barboriak DP, VanLandingham K, *et al.* (2008) Hippocampal MRI signal hyperintensity after febrile status epilepticus is predictive of subsequent mesial temporal sclerosis. *Am J Roentgenol* **190**:976–83.

Raspall-Chaure M, Chin RF, Neville BG, Scott RC (2006) Outcome of pediatric convulsive status epilepticus: a systematic review. *Lancet Neurol* **5**:769–79.

Sadarangani M, Seaton C, Scott JA, *et al.* (2008) Incidence and outcome of convulsive status epilepticus in Kenyan children: a cohort study. *Lancet Neurol* **7**:145–50.

Scott RC, Gadian DG, King MD, *et al.* (2002) Magnetic resonance imaging findings within 5 days of status epilepticus in childhood. *Brain* **125**:1951–9.

Scott RC, King MD, Gadian DG, Neville BG, Connelly A (2003) Hippocampal abnormalities after prolonged febrile convulsion: a longitudinal MRI study. *Brain* **126**:2551–7.

Stafstrom CE (2007) Neurobiological mechanisms of developmental epilepsy: translating experimental findings into clinical application. *Semin Pediatr Neurol* **14**:164–72.

Stores G, Zaiwalla Z, Styles E, Hoshika A (1995) Non-convulsive status epilepticus. *Arch Dis Childh* **73**:106–11.

Trinka E (2002) Childhood febrile convulsions: which factors determine the subsequent epilepsy syndrome? A retrospective study. *Epilepsy Res* **50**:283.

Tsuboi T (1984) Epidemiology of febrile and afebrile convulsions in children in Japan. *Neurology* **34**:175–81.

VanLandingham KE, Heinz ER, Cavazos JE, Lewis DV (1998) Magnetic resonance imaging evidence of hippocampal injury after prolonged focal febrile convulsions. *Ann Neurol* **43**:413–26.

Verity CM, Butler NR, Golding J (1985) Febrile convulsions in a national cohort followed up from birth. I. Prevalence and recurrence in the first 5 years of life. *Br Med J (Clin Res Ed)* **290**:1307–10.

Verity CM, Ross EM, Golding J (1993) Outcome of childhood status epilepticus and lengthy febrile convulsions: findings of national cohort study. *Br Med J* **307**:225–8.

Walker M, Cross H, Smith S, *et al.* (2005) Nonconvulsive status epilepticus: Epilepsy Research Foundation workshop reports. *Epilept Disord* **7**:253–96.

Chapter

106

The causes of convulsive status epilepticus in adults

Elizabeth J. Waterhouse and Peter W. Kaplan

Definition

Convulsive status epilepticus (CSE) has been recognized for centuries and its definition continues to evolve. In 1981, the International League Against Epilepsy and the World Health Organization defined status epilepticus (SE) as occurring "Whenever a seizure persists for a sufficient length of time, or is repeated frequently enough to produce an enduring epileptic condition." The imprecise duration described in this definition made its application in research difficult, and a definition published in 1993 proposed that SE consists of "more than 30 minutes of continuous seizure activity, or two or more sequential seizures without full recovery of consciousness between seizures" (Dodson et al. 1993).

The 30-min time designation was supported by animal studies and human data showing physiological deterioration occurring after about 30 min of seizure activity (Lothman 1990). While this definition has been widely used for research, an operational definition of CSE advocates administering intravenous treatment after only 5 min of seizure activity (Lowenstein et al. 1999). This definition is supported by a study that documented the duration of a generalized tonic–clonic (GTC) seizure to be about 1 min on average, and to rarely exceed 2 min (Theodore et al. 1994). Therefore, a seizure lasting more than several minutes is unlikely to be self-limited, and treatment is warranted for impending SE, in order to terminate ictal activity and reduce morbidity and mortality.

Status epilepticus, although representing an "enduring state" of seizures (of sorts), cannot easily be categorized as an epilepsy. It occupies a position, possibly, lying along the seizure–epilepsy continuum, and has not been treated in the literature as epilepsy per se. Our review will follow, rather, the non-syndromic approach to CSE, although clearly CSE can occur with many distinct epilepsy syndromes.

Epidemiology

Incidence

Most population-based studies of SE epidemiology have used the traditional 30-min definition of SE, and have reported an annual incidence ranging from 6.2–41 per 100 000 individuals for all ages and all types of SE, and a case fatality rate of 7.6–39% (DeLorenzo et al. 1996; Hesdorffer et al. 1998; Coeytaux et al. 2000; Knake et al. 2001; Wu et al. 2002; Vignatelli et al. 2003; Waterhouse 2005). Convulsive SE comprises 37–70% of all SE, and when it is considered separately from non-convulsive SE, its annual crude incidence rate is 3.6–30 per 100 000 (Waterhouse 2008).

Most of the studies referenced in this section included various types of SE, although the study by Wu et al. (2002) focused on convulsive SE alone. When considering all types of SE, the occurrence of SE across the lifespan is bimodal, peaking during the first year of life and in adults over the age of 60 years. The elderly have 3–10 times the incidence of SE than younger adults (Knake et al. 2001; Wu et al. 2002; Vignatelli et al. 2003).

Studies have shown varying results regarding SE incidence in males and females, with some reporting no difference in incidence between the sexes (Wu et al. 2002; Vignatelli et al. 2003) and others reporting a higher incidence in males (Hesdorffer et al. 1998; Coeytaux et al. 2000; Knake et al. 2001). Some of the reported differences may be due to the increased occurrence of cerebrovascular disease in men (Knake et al. 2001). Men may also have an increased risk of SE-associated death than women, although male gender is not an independent risk factor for mortality (Towne et al. 1994; Logroscino et al. 1997). Most of these studies have included all types of SE.

The incidence of SE in African-Americans is at least two times higher than in Caucasians, in all age groups (DeLorenzo et al. 1996; Wu et al. 2002). However, SE-associated mortality is lower in African-Americans (17%) than in Caucasians (31%) (DeLorenzo et al. 1996). This difference in mortality is likely due to confounding variables, however, as race is not an independent risk factor for mortality.

Causes of status epilepticus

The most common causes of SE are demonstrated in Fig. 106.1. In adults, the most common etiologies are low antiepileptic drug levels, remote symptomatic etiologies, and stroke

The Causes of Epilepsy, eds. S. D. Shorvon, F. Andermann, and R. Guerrini. Published by Cambridge University Press. © Cambridge University Press 2011.

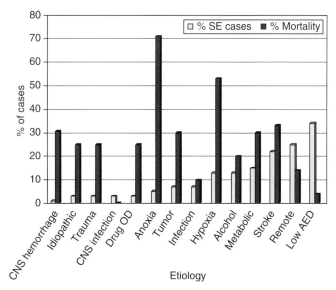

Fig. 106.1. The common causes of SE in adults are listed with associated mortality for each etiology. AED, antiepileptic drug(s); CNS, central nervous system; OD, overdose. (Based on data from DeLorenzo *et al.* [1995].)

(DeLorenzo *et al.* 1996). As will be discussed below, up to half of SE patients have a history of epilepsy. Subtherapeutic antiepileptic drug levels account for 34% of all SE, and has a relatively favorable prognosis. In the absence of another underlying brain lesion, SE due to low antiepileptic drug level is associated with a low mortality rate of 4–8.6% (Towne *et al.* 1994; DeLorenzo *et al.* 1995).

An acute symptomatic cause is the most common etiology of SE, accounting for 48–63% of all SE (Hesdorffer *et al.* 1998; Coeytaux *et al.* 2000). While SE occurs in 1.1–1.4% of patients with a first stroke (Labovitz *et al.* 2001; Velio *et al.* 2001), acute stroke is one of the most common acute symptomatic causes of SE, accounting for 14–22% of SE in adults (DeLorenzo *et al.* 1995; Knake *et al.* 2001). Remote stroke is also a major cause of SE in older adults. In a German study of SE in adults in whom the mean age was 65 years, remote stroke caused 36% of SE (Knake *et al.* 2001). In the Richmond, Virginia SE study, cerebrovascular disease (including acute and remote ischemic stroke and cerebral hemorrhages) was the etiology in 41% of SE in adults overall, and in 61% of SE in the elderly (DeLorenzo *et al.* 1995).

Mortality of status epilepticus

The overall mortality of SE is 22% (DeLorenzo *et al.* 1996). Mortality rates vary according to type of SE, but SE type is not an independent risk factor for mortality. There is a 30.5% mortality associated with all convulsive SE (including GTC and secondarily generalized GTC), and 22–47% for secondarily generalized SE (DeLorenzo *et al.* 1996; Logroscino *et al.* 1997; Hesdorffer *et al.* 1998). Myoclonic SE has the highest mortality of any type of SE, at 50–86%

(Hesdorffer *et al.* 1998; Vignatelli *et al.* 2003). Simple partial SE is associated with a mortality ranging from 17% to 24% (Waterhouse 2008).

A multivariate regression analysis of parameters contributing to SE mortality found three independent risk factors associated with SE mortality: advancing age, longer duration, and etiology (Towne *et al.* 1994). While mortality due to all types of SE combined is low in children (3%), it is 26% in adults, and increases steadily with each decade of age (DeLorenzo *et al.* 1996). Convulsive SE mortality in adults aged 60 and above is 38%, and it approaches 50% in those who are over 80 years of age (DeLorenzo *et al.* 1996).

Longer duration of SE is associated with a worse outcome (Aminoff and Simon 1980; Lowenstein and Alldredge 1993). In one study, prolonged or repetitive seizures lasting 10–29 min had a mortality of 3%, while SE lasting 30 min or longer had a mortality of 19%. Shorter seizure episodes were also significantly more likely to end spontaneously, without treatment (42% compared with 7%) (DeLorenzo *et al.* 1999). These statistics suggest that there may be underlying differences in the pathophysiology of shorter seizures compared with prolonged seizures. They also emphasize that the definition of SE used in a particular study may have a significant impact on the reported incidence and mortality.

Duration of SE is an independent predictor of SE mortality, and 1 hr is the threshold after which mortality rises steeply. Towne *et al.* (1994) reported that the mortality was 2.7% for SE lasting under 1 hr, and 32% for SE lasting at least 1 hr. With increasing duration, SE associated mortality continued to rise (Towne *et al.* 1994).

There are other parameters that contribute to ictal burden besides the total duration of an episode of SE. Status epilepticus may involve continuous convulsive activity, or intermittent convulsions with clinical unresponsiveness in between. Continuous convulsive SE has a significantly higher mortality than intermittent convulsive activity (31% vs. 19%) (Waterhouse *et al.* 1999).

The mortality of SE is dependent to a large degree on its underlying cause (see Fig. 106.1). Anoxia and hypoxia have the highest associated mortality, followed by acute brain insults (Hauser 1990; DeLorenzo *et al.* 1995; Knake *et al.*, 2001; Vignatelli *et al.* 2003). In a multivariate analysis, the only SE etiology that was *independently* associated with mortality was anoxia. Although SE has a relatively low mortality in the setting of low antiepileptic drug levels, this association was not statistically significant when confounding variables were considered (Towne *et al.* 1994).

The relative contributions of SE itself and its underlying etiology to mortality rates are difficult to separate. When stroke patients with SE were compared with a similar control group of stroke patients without SE, the mortality of SE in stroke patients was three times higher than the mortality of patients with stroke alone (Waterhouse *et al.* 1998). Stroke sizes did not significantly differ between the groups. A retrospective study of survivors of cardiac arrest, found that postanoxic SE was associated with death, independently of the type and length of cardiac arrest (Rossetti *et al.* 2007). These studies suggest that there is a synergistic effect of SE and certain etiologies on short-term mortality.

Long-term prognosis following SE may be also dependent on etiology. In a study by Logroscino *et al.* (2005), an increased risk of death for patients with SE was present even 10 years after an incident episode of SE, with a threefold increase in mortality compared to the general population. There were higher mortality rates for myoclonic SE, acute symptomatic SE, and prolonged SE lasting more than 24 hr, while the mortality rates for patients with cryptogenic or idiopathic SE did not significantly differ from the general population.

Pathophysiology

Many investigations of SE physiology have been performed with in vivo models, inducing seizures with chemical or electrical stimulation. These studies have demonstrated an early 30–60-min phase of SE, consisting of discrete convulsions, followed by a second phase during which seizures merge, and finally an electroclinical dissociation, with subtle or absent motor manifestations despite persistent electrographic (EEG) epileptiform activity. During the initial phase, ongoing seizures cause increased metabolic demands. Catecholamine release can lead to tachycardia, cardiac arrhythmias, hypertension, hyperpyrexia, and other autonomic changes. As seizures continue in the later phase, physiologic mechanisms are insufficient to compensate for metabolic demands, leading to decreased oxygenation, refractory seizures, and brain damage (Lothman 1990). Pharmacological paralysis of motor activity, supportive ventilation, and regulation of systemic and metabolic parameters did not protect against hippocampal neuronal damage (Meldrum *et al.* 1973; Blennow *et al.* 1978).

Initial seizure activity begins with an imbalance of excitatory and inhibitory influences. In animal models, longer-duration electrical stimulation, or higher doses of chemical proconvulsants, increase the likelihood of a single seizure progressing to SE. In humans, it is likely that there are numerous possible pathways to seizure onset, but one final common process – involving failure of γ-aminobutyric acid (GABA) inhibition and glutamate-mediated excitotoxicity – that leads to sustained seizures and neuronal damage (Hope and Blumenfeld 2005). The *N*-methyl-D-aspartate (NMDA) subtype of glutamate receptor, distributed primarily in the hippocampus, and to a lesser extent in the cortex, plays an important role in sustaining seizure activity in SE (Monaghan and Cotman 1985; Ozawa *et al.* 1998). The hippocampus may be particularly vulnerable to SE-induced neuronal injury because of its relatively high density of NMDA receptors, and because the use-dependent properties of these receptors within limbic circuits can lead to pathological repetitive depolarization. Mechanisms of neuronal damage include necrotic cell death, delayed cell death, and apoptosis (Fujikawa *et al.* 2000; Meldrum *et al.* 2003).

Clinical features

Convulsive SE of focal onset may start with alteration of consciousness, automatisms, asymmetric posturing, or focal clonic activity. The initial clinical manifestations are determined by the localization of the ictal activity in the brain. It may remain focal, or secondarily generalize. In adults, 27% of SE is generalized tonic–clonic at onset, and 69% is of focal onset. About 62% of those with focal onset have secondary generalization (DeLorenzo *et al.* 1996). Epilepsia partialis continua (EPC) is a form of focal motor SE in which there is focal, repeated clonic muscular twitching that occurs at regular intervals. Its duration varies, and it may last for many days or weeks.

Generalized convulsive SE is typically manifested as generalized tonic stiffening, followed by rhythmic jerking movements of the extremities that are usually symmetric. There is associated loss of consciousness. Clonic activity may persist continuously, or intermittently, but the patient's level of consciousness does not normalize between convulsions. Whether continuous or intermittent, clonic movements eventually attenuate, becoming less frequent and more subdued, while the patient's mental status remains impaired to a degree ranging from confusion to coma. It is important to recognize that SE has not necessarily ended when motor manifestations have ceased. Electroclinical dissociation is not uncommon, with EEG seizures continuing, while clinical manifestations of seizures are subtle or absent. Signs of subtle SE may include nystagmoid eye movements, or minimal twitching movements of the face or parts of the body (Treiman 1995). An EEG is required to differentiate postictal state from subtle or nonconvulsive SE.

Clonic SE and tonic SE are forms of generalized convulsive SE that occur primarily in children. Clonic SE consists of continuous generalized rhythmic jerking movements, and tonic SE, usually seen in the setting of Lennox–Gastaut syndrome, is associated with recurrent or continuous tonic contractions of the trunk, limbs, and/or face.

Myoclonic SE usually occurs in the setting of either myoclonic epilepsy or postanoxic brain injury. In patients with a primary generalized epilepsy, it is manifested as a prolonged series of myoclonic jerks that gradually increase in frequency and intensity, and may culminate in a GTC seizure. Patients with idiopathic generalized epilepsy and myoclonic SE may initially retain consciousness between recurrent myoclonic jerks, but awareness becomes altered as the SE progresses.

Ongoing or recurrent myoclonus following anoxic encephalopathy is usually classified as a type of convulsive SE, although some have debated that it should be placed in a category by itself – the clinical manifestation of a severe and often fatal brain injury. In the setting of anoxic encephalopathy, myoclonic SE appears as generalized, segmental, or multifocal myoclonic jerks occurring continuously or at intervals of one to several seconds. The EEG demonstrates a burst-suppression pattern, with a jerk corresponding to each burst, and the prognosis is poor (Jumao-as and Brenner 1990; Young *et al.* 1990; Krumholz *et al.* 1998).

Status epilepticus in the setting of epilepsy

It has been estimated that approximately 15% of epilepsy patients experience an episode of SE during their lifetimes (www.epilepsyfoundation.org). Convulsive SE may occur in the setting of epilepsy, or as a de novo manifestation of epilepsy.

Status epilepticus in previously diagnosed epilepsy

A history of epilepsy is present in 39–50% of people with SE (Waterhouse 2005). Sometimes SE is due to the epilepsy itself, but frequently, acute symptomatic causes are present concomitantly. The most common provoking factors in patients with epilepsy are medication non-compliance and subtherapeutic level of antiepileptic medication (Aminoff and Simon 1980).

Although non-convulsive SE occurs in the setting of idiopathic generalized epilepsies, convulsive SE is rare (Aminoff and Simon 1980; Shorvon and Walker 2005). Myoclonic SE or absence SE are reported to occur in one-third of cases of myoclonic absence epilepsy (Shorvon and Walker 2005). Myoclonic SE is less common in patients with juvenile myoclonic epilepsy, and usually occurs upon awakening (Panayiotopoulos *et al.* 1994). Myoclonic SE also may occur in association with progressive myoclonic epilepsies, although the frequency of its occurrence in these settings is not known. Convulsive SE may occur in adults with Lennox–Gastaut syndrome, and in those with epilepsy associated with ring chromosome 20, but non-convulsive SE is more common.

Status epilepticus as the initial manifestation of epilepsy

Status epilepticus presenting as the first manifestation of epilepsy is not uncommon. Approximately 12% of those who are ultimately diagnosed with epilepsy present with SE as their first manifestation (Hauser 1990; Hesdorffer *et al.* 1998). In some cases, SE is the cause of subsequent epilepsy, while in others it is the initial manifestation of an already established or innate decreased threshold for seizures.

In children, the risk of developing epilepsy following unprovoked SE does not significantly differ from the risk following a first unprovoked seizure (Meierkord 2007). However, in adults SE is associated with the subsequent development of chronic epilepsy, especially with acute symptomatic etiologies. Over a 10-year follow-up period, chronic epilepsy occurred in 42% of acute symptomatic SE cases and 13% of acute symptomatic seizure cases (Hesdorffer *et al.* 1998). Refractory SE is significantly more likely than non-refractory SE to be associated with subsequent epilepsy (Holtkamp *et al.* 2005). These findings suggest that the occurrence of SE contributes to epileptogenesis.

Causes of epilepsia partialis continua

Two types of EPC have been described: Type I, associated with non-progressive disorders, and Type II, associated with progressive central nervous system disorders and multiple seizure types (Bancaud *et al.* 1982). Type I EPC has been well documented in the setting of Russian spring–summer encephalitis, but also occurs in association with other infections such as tuberculosis, and AIDS. Other causes of Type I EPC include remote or acute stroke, vascular abnormalities, brain tumors, trauma, mitochondrial disorders, and metabolic disturbances, especially non-ketotic hyperglycemia and hyponatremia. Metrizamide, penicillin, and azlocillin-cefotaxime have been implicated as iatrogenic causes of Type I EPC. Type II EPC is typically associated with Rasmussen encephalitis. Sometimes EPC due to progressive lesions such as glioma may follow a Type II course (Schomer 2005).

Genetic factors

It is well known that genetic factors are associated with some forms of epilepsy, and that SE may occur as a result of these epilepsies. Genetic factors also play a role in determining the risk for SE. A study of 13 506 twin pairs in the Mid-Atlantic Twin Registry found that 22 monozygotic pairs and 44 dizygotic pairs included at least one twin with a history of SE. While none of the dizygotic twin pairs was concordant for SE, four of the monozygotic pairs were concordant, yielding a concordance rate of 0.31 for monozygotic and 0 for dizygotic twins. Among SE-concordant twins, there was variability of seizure type, epilepsy type, and age at SE onset, suggesting that genetic risk for SE is independent of the genes responsible for specific epilepsy types (Corey *et al.* 2004).

Social/geographic factors

Although a large proportion of people with epilepsy live in developing countries, there are limited data regarding SE in these regions. Case series and cohort studies suggest that SE is probably as common in developing countries as in Europe and North America. Potential barriers to optimal care for SE include geographic features such as terrain and weather conditions, which can cause delays in transportation, leading to treatment delay, and prolonged duration of SE. Social factors such as availability of emergency transportation, proximity of medical treatment, and availability of medication and diagnostic equipment in remote areas may have significant impact on timing of treatment and ultimate outcome.

In developing countries, infection is an important cause of SE in adults, while in the USA it is a common cause of SE in children, but not adults. In Africa, an infectious etiology is common, accounting for up to two-thirds of cases (Mbodj *et al.* 2000). A series of 99 SE patients in India found central nervous system infection in over half (Nair *et al.* 2009).

Social customs may also have an impact on SE etiology. In countries or ethnic groups in which alcohol use and dependence are limited, there is a lower incidence of alcohol-related SE. While alcohol has been reported to cause SE in 13% of cases of SE in urban American adults, it is an uncommon cause of SE in Chinese people living in Hong Kong (DeLorenzo et al. 1995; Hui et al. 2003).

Diagnostic tests

While convulsive SE is usually not difficult to recognize, there are other conditions, physiological and psychological, that can be mistaken for SE. Imitators of generalized convulsive SE include tremor, rigors, dystonia, rigidity, tetany, muscle spasms, clonus, shivering, periodic limb movements of sleep, restless legs syndrome, and myoclonus. Imitators of partial convulsive SE include hemifacial spasm, asymmetric tremor, myoclonic jerks, palatal myoclonus, tics, focal dystonia, paroxysmal nocturnal dyskinesia, and blepharospasm (Dworetsky and Bromfield 2005).

Electroencephalogram

The EEG is an essential tool in the diagnosis and management of SE. While convulsive SE is easily recognized, subtle forms of SE require EEG to establish the diagnosis. Focal onset of generalized seizures may sometimes be seen on EEG, or asymmetry of generalized ictal activity may suggest focal onset. During ongoing convulsive activity, the EEG typically shows a great deal of muscle artifact, although rhythmic EEG activity may sometimes be glimpsed in between muscular contractions or over midline electrodes. If a patient is intubated and mechanically ventilated, pharmacologic neuromuscular blockade can be used to abolish muscle artifact. Treiman described a sequence of five patterns of electrographic ictal discharges that are often observed during generalized convulsive SE: discrete electrographic seizures, waxing and waning, continuous, continuous with flat periods, and periodic epileptiform discharges on a relatively flat background (Treiman et al. 1990).

Epilepsia partialis continua may not be associated with an ictal discharge on scalp EEG, due to the small area of cortex involved. Cortical discharges may be seen with electrocorticography, or with back-averaged EEG recording that is triggered by a muscle jerk. Common EEG findings include lateralized slowing, lateralized asymmetric background slowing, or periodic lateralized epileptiform discharges (PLEDs).

Tonic SE usually consists of recurrent tonic seizures. The EEG initially demonstrates an abrupt change in the background, with generalized low-voltage fast activity. Sometimes this is preceded by a high-amplitude slow-wave discharge. As the seizure evolves, generalized rhythmic activity decreases in frequency and increases in amplitude, and there is muscle artifact.

In myoclonic SE due to idiopathic generalized epilepsy, the EEG shows bursts of generalized spike–wave or polyspike–wave discharges. When myoclonic SE occurs in the setting of anoxic brain injury, the EEG shows a burst-suppression pattern, with variable intervals of generalized suppression,

interrupted by bursts of higher-voltage mixed frequency activity. Bursts usually last a few seconds, and may include focal, multifocal, or generalized spikes or sharp waves. Typically, a myoclonic jerk accompanies each burst.

In addition to characterizing the SE, EEG is also used to monitor response to treatment. Following SE treatment, EEG should be used to confirm that SE has been terminated, and to monitor for subsequent subtle or non-convulsive seizures. In a study of SE patients whose clinical convulsions had stopped, 48% had electrographic seizures or non-convulsive SE recorded on EEG during the 24 hr following convulsive SE (DeLorenzo et al. 1998). Monitoring the EEG for recurrent seizures is advisable for all patients who do not recover rapidly and fully from SE. Monitoring is also advisable if periodic discharges are seen on the EEG, because these patterns can be seen as a late stage of SE, or in the setting of waxing and waning ictal activity.

Lumbar puncture

Lumbar puncture should be performed in SE patients with fever, suspected infection, or cases of unclear etiology. If either meningitis or encephalitis is suspected, empiric broad-spectrum treatment should be initiated immediately. Mild cerebrospinal fluid (CSF) pleocytosis, with white blood cell count of up to 28×10^6/L, has been described in cases of SE, even without acute neurological insult; however, pleocytosis should not be attributed to SE alone unless all other causes have been eliminated (Barry and Hauser 1994).

Neuron-specific enolase

Neuron-specific enolase is a marker of acute brain injury and blood–brain barrier dysfunction, and is elevated in CSF after SE. The highest concentrations were seen with non-convulsive forms of SE (DeGiorgio et al. 1999). Elevated serum neuron-specific enolase is a marker of poor prognosis following cardiopulmonary resuscitation (Zandbergen et al. 2006).

Immunological markers

Convulsive SE can rarely occur in patients with a variety of connective tissue disorders, central nervous system lupus, Sjogren disease, and Whipple disease, as well as paraneoplastic and non-paraneoplastic encephalitis. However, non-convulsive forms are the more frequent.

Neuroimaging

Interpretable neuroimaging studies cannot be obtained if a person has convulsions during the scan. Seizures should be treated with an intravenous benzodiazepine (see treatment section below), with attention to maintaining airway, and hemodynamic monitoring. As soon as seizures are controlled and the patient is stabilized, brain imaging should be obtained, to look for an acute or chronic lesion causing the SE. In the absence of EEG monitoring, paralysis with neuromuscular blockade should be avoided because it masks the clinical manifestations of seizures.

An initial head computed tomography (CT) scan will identify many, but not all, acute neurological causes of SE. Computed tomography accurately diagnoses most cases of acute intracranial hemorrhage, but it is not 100% sensitive for acute subarachnoid hemorrhage, acute stroke, or subtle lesions such as small metastases. Likewise, some remote symptomatic etiologies of seizures or SE – such as chronic strokes or major malformations – are easily seen on head CT, while subtle chronic lesions such as heterotopias, may require magnetic resonance imaging (MRI). The need for further imaging and diagnostic tests is determined by the differential diagnosis under consideration. Brain MRI, lumbar puncture, routine angiogram, MR angiography (MRA), MR venography (MRV), CT angiography (CTA), positron emission tomography (PET), or single photon emission computed tomography (SPECT) scan may offer additional information if the head CT is non-diagnostic.

Convulsive SE may also cause reversible and irreversible abnormalities on neuroimaging studies. Peri-ictal changes may include hippocampal swelling and sclerosis, migratory cortical lesions, abnormalities of the splenium, and posterior reversible leukoencephalopathy (Cole 2004).

Neuropsychological features

Status epilepticus occasionally occurs in the setting of psychiatric disorders, and may result from them indirectly. Hypoxic or anoxic encephalopathy following attempted suicide may be associated with SE. Status epilepticus following electroconvulsive therapy has also been described. Psychogenic water drinking with hyponatremia may cause SE. Pseudostatus epilepticus (pseudo-SE) has been documented, and when overlooked, may lead to iatrogenic complications (Pakalnis et al. 1991). Psychiatric diagnoses of conversion disorder, Munchausen syndrome, factitious disorder, or malingering are associated with pseudo-SE. The EEG during clinical pseudo-SE does not demonstrate electrographic seizure activity. Video correlation is helpful, as rhythmic artifacts may be challenging to interpret.

Although the high mortality associated with SE has been well documented, there is controversy over whether SE itself causes neuropsychological morbidity. Factors potentially confounding the study of this topic include pre-existing neurologic abnormalities relating to the underlying cause of SE, difficulties in diagnosing SE, systemic factors, and clinical variability of SE type and ictal burden. Helmstaedter reviewed studies of cognitive outcome of SE in adults, and acknowledged the difficulty in determining whether the SE itself, or its underlying etiology, causes subsequent cognitive changes that may be seen. He concluded that more severe mental impairments and clinical conditions appear to be a risk factor for sustaining SE, with less evidence that SE per se causes cognitive decline (Helmstaedter 2007). A study of 15 adult epilepsy patients who had IQ testing before and after SE found

that these patients did not show significant post-SE intellectual decline, when compared to a control population of epilepsy patients without SE (Adachi et al. 2005). However, non-convulsive SE has been demonstrated to be associated with cognitive decline by psychometric testing (Krumholz et al. 1995). Further study is needed to evaluate cognitive outcomes following SE.

Principles of management

Generalized convulsive SE should be considered a medical emergency, and the immediate goals of management are to support vital functions, to terminate seizure activity, and to prevent recurrence. The medical team must also diagnose and treat the etiology of SE, and manage morbidity relating to SE itself, as well as any underlying conditions. Since early treatment of SE is more successful than late treatment, and SE duration is a risk factor for mortality, treatment should be initiated as soon as possible. Hospitals should have a written protocol for the initial therapy of convulsive SE, to ensure that appropriate care and treatment are provided expeditiously (see Table 106.1). The initial steps of stabilization, assessment, and treatment should be undertaken almost simultaneously. Airway, breathing, and circulation should be immediately assessed and maintained. Hemodynamic and cardiac monitoring should be initiated, and intravenous access should be obtained. Blood should be sent for initial laboratory studies (toxin screen, antiepileptic drug levels, alcohol level, complete blood count, and metabolic panel). Intravenous glucose should be administered empirically, and malnourished or alcoholic individuals should also receive thiamine concurrently. Antiepileptic drug treatment with a benzodiazepine should be initiated immediately (see below, and Table 106.1).

Benzodiazepines

The initial treatment of SE should be a benzodiazepine. Several randomized blinded trials of treatments for SE have compared lorazepam and diazepam in the treatment of SE, and found a higher response rate for lorazepam (Leppik et al. 1983; Alldredge et al. 2001). The Veterans Affairs Status Epilepticus Cooperative study randomized SE patients into four treatment groups. Each patient received: either 0.1 mg/kg lorazepam, 15 mg/kg phenobarbital, 18 mg/kg phenytoin, or 0.15 mg/kg diazepam followed by 18 mg/kg phenytoin. Among 384 veterans with overt SE, lorazepam had the highest response rate (64.9%), followed by phenobarbital (58.2%), diazepam plus phenytoin (55.8%), and then phenytoin alone (43.6%). Lorazepam was the most effective treatment overall, and was significantly more effective than phenytoin alone, although other paired comparisons were not statistically significant (Treiman et al. 1998).

While both diazepam and lorazepam have demonstrated efficacy in the treatment of SE, in general lorazepam is preferred. Diazepam has high lipid solubility and enters the brain within minutes, but it rapidly redistributes to other parts of the

Table 106.1 Sample protocol for the treatment of convulsive status epilepticus in adults

0–5 min

Give oxygen. Assess airway and apply pulse oximeter.

Perform venipuncture and secure intravenous access.

Send blood for STAT basic metabolic panel, liver function tests, calcium, magnesium, phosphate, complete blood count, toxicology screens, troponin, and antiepileptic drug levels. Check finger-stick glucose.

Start a continuous IV infusion of normal saline.

6–10 min

Administer thiamine and dextrose:

  100 mg thiamine IV

50 mL of 50% dextrose IV (unless serum glucose is normal).

Give lorazepam at 0.1 mg/kg by IV at a rate less than 2 mg per min. Repeat if seizures persist. If IV access is not available, consider rectal diazepam.

11–30 min

Give fosphenytoin IV (20 PE mg/kg), no faster than 150 PE mg/min **or** IV phenytoin (20 mg/kg) by slow IV push no faster than 50 mg/min. Phenytoin is incompatible with glucose-containing solutions.

Monitor cardiac rhythm and blood pressure and be prepared to adjust dosage and rate accordingly.

For refractory SE

The patient will likely need to be intubated, and consider **ONE** of the following:

  Pentobarbital IV 5 mg/kg (at 25 mg/min), then 0.5–5 mg/kg/hr.

  Midazolam IV 0.2 mg/kg (at up to 4 mg/min). Dose may be repeated in 5 min if seizures persist. Then continuous infusion at 0.05–0.4 mg/kg/hr.

  Propofol IV 2 mg/kg bolus. Dose may be repeated in 5 min if seizures persist. Initial infusion rate is 2 mg/kg/hr, then 1–5 mg/kg/hr.

Order STAT EEG.

Titrate IV infusion dose of pentobarbital, midazolam, or propofol to desired level of EEG suppression.

body, resulting in a reduced clinical effect. The distribution half-life of lorazepam is several hours, and it binds more tightly to the GABA receptor, resulting in a longer duration of action and a lower risk for recurrent seizures. Potential complications of benzodiazepine administration include respiratory suppression, hypotension, and sedation. If resuscitation and cardiorespiratory monitoring facilities are available, a benzodiazepine should be administered intravenously. If not, or if intravenous access is not available, diazepam can be administered rectally, or midazolam can be administered intramuscularly, or rectally. In some countries midazolam is also available for intranasal and buccal administration. These alternate routes of administration facilitate out-of-hospital treatment of SE.

Both European and American groups that have published SE treatment protocols recommend an initial dose of lorazepam or diazepam, followed by a loading dose of a second agent (Dodson *et al.* 1993; Meierkord *et al.*, 2006; Shorvon *et al.* 2008). While the usual initial dose of lorazepam in North America is 0.1 mg/kg, the European report recommends a dose of 4 mg, which may be repeated once. Thus individuals weighing more than 40 kg would receive a lower initial dose of lorazepam in Europe than in North America.

Second-line treatment

Although the Veterans Affairs study found that a second medication rarely succeeded in terminating SE when the first treatment was unsuccessful (Treiman *et al.* 1998), European and American groups recommend a second non-benzodiazepine treatment for continuing seizures. Phenytoin or fosphenytoin are widely used as second-line agents. Fosphenytoin has advantages over phenytoin, because it can be administered more quickly, has lower risk for tissue damage through a peripheral intravenous line, and is compatible with other intravenous solutions. Other options include phenobarbital, which causes significant sedation and respiratory suppression, valproate, or levetiracetam. While levetiracetam and valproate lack the drawbacks of phenobarbital, there are limited data regarding their efficacy for SE. For SE in the setting of known idiopathic generalized epilepsy, valproate is an appropriate drug to use if there is an incomplete response to lorazepam.

Treatment of refractory generalized tonic–clonic status epilepticus

Status epilepticus is considered refractory if it continues despite treatment with adequate doses of two or more antiepileptic drugs. Refractory SE is generally treated with anesthetic agents (Table 106.2), requiring that the patient be mechanically ventilated, and monitored with EEG to assess response to treatment. Continuous infusions of propofol, midazolam, thiopental, or pentobarbital suppress seizures, but the doses required to do so often cause hypotension, requiring support with vasopressors. Maintenance infusion of any of these medications should be titrated to suppression of seizures and burst suppression on the EEG. Propofol may induce a potentially fatal infusion syndrome, with cardiocirculatory collapse, lactic acidosis, hypertriglyceridemia, and rhabodmyolysis. Concurrent use of a benzodiazepine may reduce this risk by reducing the dose of propofol required (Rossetti *et al.* 2004). Paraldehyde, ketamine, isoflurane, lidocaine, and topiramate have also been reported as treatments for refractory SE, but have not been extensively studied.

Table 106.2 Medications used in the treatment of generalized convulsive status epilepticus in adults

Drug	Loading dose	Maximal loading rate	Route	Maintenance
Options for initial response, 0–10 min				
Lorazepam (preferred)	0.1 mg/kg	2 mg/min	IV	
Diazepam	0.2 mg/kg	5 mg/min	IV or rectal	
Midazolam	0.1 mg/kg	Bolus	Buccal or nasal	
Clonazepam	0.025 mg/kg	2 min	IV	
Options for continued seizures, 20–60 min				
Fosphenytoin	18–20 PE mg/kg	150 mg/min	IV	5 PE mg/kg/day
Phenytoin	18–20 mg/kg	50 mg/min	IV	5 mg/kg/day
Phenobarbital	10–20 mg/kg	100 mg/min	IV	Pentobarbital preferred for ongoing continuous infusion
Valproate	25 mg/kg	5 mg/kg/min	IV	15–30 mg/kg/day
Options for refractory SE				
Propofol[a]	1–2 mg/kg	Bolus. May repeat in 5 min if needed	IV	2 mg/kg/hr initially, then 1–5 mg/kg/hr[b]
Midazolam	0.2 mg/kg	4 mg/min	IV	0.05–0.4 mg/kg/hr[b]
Pentobarbital	2–8 mg/kg	Bolus at 25 mg/min	IV	0.5–5 mg/kg/hr[b]
Thiopental	2–3 mg/kg	Bolus over 20 s, with additional 50-mg boluses every 2–3 min until seizures are controlled	IV	3–5 mg/kg/hr[b]

Notes:
[a]Concurrent use of a benzodiazepine may lower risk of propofol-associated infusion syndrome.
[b]Titrate to suppression of seizures and burst suppression.

Treatment of other forms of status epilepticus

The management of EPC involves treating the seizure activity as well as its cause. Antiepileptic drugs are used in an attempt to alleviate convulsive activity, and prevent secondary generalization. If the patient is awake, sedating medications that may lead to respiratory depression and ventilatory support should be avoided. In cases of progressive EPC, treatment with typical antiepileptic medications is rarely successful. Additional options for treatment of EPC include steroids, intravenous immunoglobulin, or plasma exchange, which likely suppress inflammation rather than exert a specific antiepileptic effect (Shorvon 2008). Surgical treatment offers the best prognosis for EPC in the setting of Rasmussen encephalitis.

There is little guidance regarding the treatment of postanoxic myoclonic SE. The EEG may show a burst-suppression pattern, generalized or lateralized periodic discharges, or sometimes evolving seizures in addition to one of these patterns. Continuous infusion with an anesthetic dose of a barbiturate, propofol, or benzodiazepine will lead to suppression of the EEG activity, and therapeutic levels of antiepileptic drugs should be maintained as anesthesia is eventually reduced. Induction of hypothermia is used at some centers following resuscitation after a cardiac arrest, and has a similar depressant effect on the EEG as anesthetic agents. Because the mortality associated with anoxic brain injuries is high, it is unclear to what degree SE treatment measures lead to a meaningful improvement in outcome. A recent study showed improved survival in patients treated with antiepileptic drugs and hypothermia after cardiac arrest (Rossetti *et al.* 2009).

Future directions

Convulsive SE remains a significant cause of patient morbidity and mortality despite more than 60 years of antiepileptic drugs, including parenteral forms and anesthetics. Differentiating the effects of the underlying causes of SE from the consequences of SE itself remains an epidemiological challenge, and studies are giving increased attention to these etiological distinctions. Genetic, immunological, and enhanced imaging techniques may all play important future roles in better understanding the nature and consequences of CSE, and in separating genetic underpinnings from acquired causes.

Future studies are needed that will take into account these etiological and methodological factors, and might incorporate newer investigations such as PET, SPECT, perfusion sequences on CT, fluid-attenuated inversion recovery (FLAIR) and T2-weighted images on MRI, and functional MRI. These elements may help in determining the respective effects of cause, underlying epilepsy syndrome, duration of CSE, comorbid conditions, effects and timing of treatment, and emerging interventions such as hypothermia and neuroprotective agents.

References

Adachi N, Kanemoto K, Muramatsu R, *et al.* (2005) Intellectual prognosis of status epilepticus in adult epilepsy patients: analysis with Wechsler Adult Intelligence Scale-revised. *Epilepsia* **46**:1502–9.

Alldredge BK, Gelb AM, Isaacs SM, *et al.* (2001) A comparison of lorazepam, diazepam, and placebo for the treatment of out-of-hospital status epilepticus. *N Engl J Med* **345**:631–7.

Aminoff MJ, Simon RP (1980) Status epilepticus: causes, clinical features and consequences in 98 patients. *Am J Med* **69**:657–66.

Bancaud J, Bonis A, Trottier S, Talairach J, Dulac O (1982) L'épilepsie partielle continue: syndrome et maladie. *Rev Neurol* **138**:803–14.

Barry E, Hauser WA (1994) Pleocytosis after status epilepticus. *Arch Neurol* **51**:190–3.

Blennow G, Brierley JB, Meldrum BS, Siesjo BK (1978) Epileptic brain damage: the role of systemic factors that modify cerebral energy metabolism. *Brain* **101**:687–700.

Coeytaux A, Jallon P, Galobardes B, Morabia A (2000) Incidence of status epilepticus in French-speaking Switzerland. *Neurology* **55**:693–7.

Cole AJ (2004) Status epilepticus and periictal imaging. *Epilepsia* **45**(Suppl 4):72–7.

Corey LA, Pellock JM, DeLorenzo RJ (2004) Status epilepticus in a population-based Virginia Twin Sample. *Epilepsia* **45**:159–65.

DeGiorgio CM, Heck CN, Rabinowicz AL, *et al.* (1999) Serum neuron-specific enolase in the major subtypes of status epilepticus. *Neurology* **52**:746–9.

DeLorenzo RJ, Pellock JM, Towne AR, Boggs JG (1995) Epidemiology of status epilepticus. *J Clin Neurophysiol* **12**:316–25.

DeLorenzo RJ, Hauser WA, Towne AR, *et al.* (1996) A prospective, population-based epidemiologic study of status epilepticus in Richmond, Virginia. *Neurology* **46**:1029–35.

DeLorenzo RJ, Waterhouse EJ, Towne AR, *et al.* (1998) Persistent nonconvulsive status epilepticus after the control of convulsive status epilepticus. *Epilepsia* **39**:833–40.

DeLorenzo RJ, Garnett LK, Towne AR, *et al.* (1999) Comparison of status epilepticus with prolonged seizure episodes lasting from 10–29 minutes. *Epilepsia* **40**:164–9.

Dodson WE, DeLorenzo RJ, Pedley TA, *et al.* (1993) The treatment of convulsive status epilepticus: recommendations of the Epilepsy Foundation of America's Working Group on Status Epilepticus. *J Am Med Ass* **270**:854–9.

Dworetsky BA, Bromfield EB (2005) Differential diagnosis of status epilepticus: pseudostatus epilepticus. In: Drislane F (ed.) *Status Epilepticus: A Clinical Perspective.* Totowa, NJ: Humana Press, pp. 33–54.

Fujikawa DG, Shinme SS, Cai B (2000) Kainic acid-induced seizures produce necrotic, not apoptotic, neurons with internucleosomal DNA cleavage: implications for programmed cell death mechanisms. *Neuroscience* **98**:41–53.

Hauser WA (1990) Status epilepticus: epidemiological considerations. *Neurology* **40**(Suppl 2):9–12.

Helmstaedter C (2007) Cognitive outcome of status epilepticus in adults. *Epilepsia* **48**(Suppl 8):85–90.

Hesdorffer DC, Logroscino G, Cascino G, Annegers JF, Hauser WA (1998) Incidence of status epilepticus in Rochester, Minnesota, 1965–1984. *Neurology* **50**:735–41.

Holtkamp M, Othman J, Buchheim K, Meierkord H (2005) Predictors and prognosis of refractory status epilepticus treated in a neurological intensive care unit. *J Neurol Neurosurg Psychiatry* **76**:534–9.

Hope O, Blumenfeld H (2005) Cellular phsyiology of status epilepticus. In: Drislane F (ed.) *Status Epilepticus: A Clinical Perspective.* Totowa, NJ: Humana Press, pp. 159–80.

Hui AC, Joynt GM, Li H, Wong KS (2003) Status epilepticus in Hong Kong Chinese: etiology, outcome and predictors of death and morbidity. *Seizure* **12**:478–82.

Jumao-as A, Brenner RP (1990) Myoclonic status epilepticus: a clinical and electroencephalographic study. *Neurology* **40**:1199–202.

Knake S, Rosenow F, Vescovi M, *et al.* (2001) Incidence of status epilepticus in adults in Germany: a prospective, population-based study. *Epilepsia* **42**:714–18.

Krumholz A, Stern BJ, Weiss HD (1998) Outcome from coma after cardiopulmonary resuscitation: relation to seizures and myoclonus. *Neurology* **38**:401–5.

Krumholz A, Sung GY, Fisher RS, *et al.* (1995) Complex partial status epilepticus accompanied by serious morbidity and mortality. *Neurology* **45**:1499–504.

Labovitz SL, Hauser WA, Sacco RL (2001) Prevalence and predictors of early seizure and status epilepticus after first stroke. *Neurology* **57**:200–6.

Leppik I, Derivan A, Homan R, *et al.* (1983) Double-blind study of lorazepam and diazepam in status epilepticus. *J Am Med Ass* **249**:1452–4.

Logroscino G, Hesdorffer DC, Cascino G, Annegers JF, Hauser WA (1997) Short-term mortality after a first epilsode of status epilepticus. *Epilepsia* **38**:1344–9.

Logroscino G, Hesdorffer DC, Cascino G (2005) Mortality after a first episode of status epilepticus in the United States and Europe. *Epilepsia* **46**(Suppl 11):46–8.

Lothman E (1990) The biochemical basis and pathophysiology of status epilepticus. *Neurology* **40**(Suppl 5):13–23.

Lowenstein DH, Alldredge BK (1993) Status epilepticus at an urban public hospital in the 1980s. *Neurology* **43**:483–98.

Lowenstein DH, Bleck T, MacDonald RL (1999) It's time to revise the definition of status epilepticus. *Epilepsia* **40**:120–2.

Mbodj I, Ndiaye M, Sene F, *et al.* (2000) Treatment of status epilepticus in a developing country. *Neurophysiol Clin* **30**:165–9.

Meldrum BS, Vigouroux RA, Brierley JB (1973) Systemic factors and epileptic brain damage: prolonged seizures in paralyzed, artificially ventilated baboons. *Arch Neurol* **28**:10–17.

Meierkord H (2007) The risk of epilepsy after status epilepticus in children and adults. *Epilepsia* **48**(Suppl 8):94–5.

Meierkord H, Boon P, Engelsen B, *et al.* (2006) EFNS guidline on the management of status epilepticus. *Eur J Neurol* **13**:445–50.

Monaghan DT, Cotman DW (1985) Distribution of *N*-methyl-D-aspartate-sensitive L-(3H)glutamate-binding sites in rat brain. *J Neurosci* **5**:2909–18.

Nair PP, Kalita J, Misra UK (2009) Role of cranial imaging in epileptic status. *Eur J Radiol* **70**:475–80.

Ozawa S, Kamiya H, Tuzuki K (1998) Glutamate receptors in the mammalian central nervous system. *Prog Neurobiol* **54**:581–618.

Pakalnis A, Drake ME, Phillips BB (1991) Neuropsychiatric aspects of psychogenic status epilepticus. *Neurology* **41**:1104–6.

Panayiotopoulos CP, Obeid T, Tahan AR (1994) Juvenile myoclonic epilepsy: a 5-year prospective study. *Epilepsia* **35**:285–96.

Rossetti AO, Logroscino G, Liaudet L, *et al.* (2007) Status epilepticus: an independent outcome predictor after cerebral anoxia. *Neurology* **69**:255–60.

Rossetti AO, Reichhart MD, Schaller MD, Despland PA, Bogousslavsky J (2004) Propofol treatment of refractory status epilepticus: a study of 31 episodes. *Epilepsia* **45**:757–63.

Rossetti AO, Oddo M, Liaudet L, Kaplan PW (2009) Predictors of awakening from postanoxic status epilepticus after therapeutic hypothermia. *Neurology* **72**:744–9.

Schomer DL (2005) Focal status epilepticus. In: Drislane F (ed.) *Status Epilepticus: A Clinical Perspective.* Totowa, NJ: Humana Press, pp. 265–88.

Shorvon S (2008) Controversial topics in epilepsy. *Epilepsia* **49**:1277–84.

Shorvon S, Walker M (2005) Status epilepticus in idiopathic generalized epilepsy. *Epilepsia* **46**(Suppl 9):73–9.

Shorvon S, Baulac M, Cross H, Trinka E, Walker M (2008) The drug treatment of status epilepticus in Europe: consensus document from a workshop at the 1st London Colloquium on Status Epilepticus. *Epilepsia* **49**: 1277–85.

Theodore WH, Porter RJ, Albert P, *et al.* (1994) The secondarily generalized tonic–clonic seizure: a videotape analysis. *Neurology* **44**:1403–7.

Towne AR, Pellock JM, Ko D, DeLorenzo RJ (1994) Determinants of mortality in status epilepticus. *Epilepsia* **35**:27–34.

Treiman DM (1995) Electroclinical features of status epilepticus. *J Clin Neurophysiol* **12**:343–62.

Treiman DM, Walton NY, Kendrick C (1990) A progressive sequence of electroencephalographic changes during generalized convulsive status epilepticus. *Epilepsy Res* **5**:49–60.

Treiman DM, Meyers PD, Walton NY, *et al.* (1998) A comparison of four treatments for generalized convulsive status epilepticus. *N Engl J Med* **339**:792–8.

Velio SK, Ozmeno M, Boz C, Alio Z (2001) Status epilepticus after stroke. *Stroke* **32**:169–72.

Vignatelli L, Tonon C, D'Alessandro R (2003) Incidence and short-term prognosis of status epilepticus in adults in Bologna, Italy. *Epilepsia* **44**:964–8.

Waterhouse E (2005) The epidemiology of status epilepticus. In: Drislane F (ed.) *Status Epilepticus: A Clinical Perspective.* Totowa, NJ: Humana Press, pp. 55–75.

Waterhouse E (2008) The epidemiology of nonconvulsive status epilepticus. In: Drislane F, Kaplan P (eds.) *Nonconvulsive Status Epilepticus.* New York: Demos Medical Publishing, pp. 23–40.

Waterhouse EJ, Vaughan JK, Barnes TY, *et al.* (1998) Synergistic effect of status epilepticus and ischemic brain injury on mortality *Epilepsy Res* **29**:175–83.

Waterhouse EJ, Garnett LK, Towne AR, *et al.* (1999) Prospective population-based study of intermittent and continuous convulsive status epilepticus in Richmond, Virginia. *Epilepsia* **40**:752–8.

Wu YW, Shak DW, Garcia PA, Zhao S, Johnston SC (2002) Incidence and mortality of generalized convulsive status epilepticus in California. *Neurology* **58**:1070–6.

Young GB, Gilber JJ, Zochodne DW (1990) The significance of myoclonic status epilepticus in postanoxic coma. *Neurology* **40**:1843–8.

Zandbergen EG, Hijdra A, Koelman JH, *et al.* (2006) PROPAC Study Group: prediction of poor outcome within the first three days of postanoxic coma. *Neurology* **66**:62–8.

Chapter

107

Uncommon causes of status epilepticus

Simon D. Shorvon, Raymond Y. L. Tan, and Aidan Neligan

Status epilepticus (SE) can be the result of many different underlying causes. The two previous chapters in this book deal with the common causes, and here the less common causes are briefly catalogued. As the frequency of SE in these conditions is largely unstudied, and therefore no exact figures are available, we have defined "uncommon cause" as "a cause of SE not reported in the major epidemiological studies of SE" (Tan *et al.* 2010).

This listing is based on a systematic search of the available English-language literature over the last 20 years (literature between 1990 and 2008) (Tan *et al.* 2010). The search identified 181 causes of SE after reviewing 513 articles. The reports of SE in almost all these conditions were confined to single cases or small case series, and there are no reliable estimates as to the frequency of SE in these conditions or of the frequency of these underlying causes in SE. These causes fell naturally into five categorical groups (see below). In this chapter, we outline the clinical features of the SE in the most important of these "uncommon causes," while listing the others.

Knowledge of the range of conditions is obviously important to clinical practice. Appropriate investigation will depend on the cause. Treatment is often directed at the underlying cause, as well as at the SE, and prognosis will usually depend to a large extent on the nature of the underlying cause (Neligan and Shorvon 2010).

The etiologies identified in this review include conditions where SE is a frequent or predominant manifestation of the epileptic disorder (e.g., *POLG1* mutations, anti-NMDA-receptor encephalitis, ring chromosome 20, and domoic acid intoxication) and these conditions are of particular interest from the point of view of understanding the mechansms of SE. These mechanisms include: derangements of neurotransmitter function, in particular γ-aminobutyric acid A (GABA$_A$) function (for instance, by agents such as tiagabine, valproic acid, vigabatrin, cephalosporins, and endosulfan) (Wasterlain and Chen 2008), inflammatory or autoimmune processes (e.g., autoimmune limbic encephalitis due to circulating antibodies, Rasmussen encephalitis) (Vezzani and Granata 2005), infectious processes

(e.g., cat-scratch encephalopathy), mitochondrial oxidative stress and dysfunction (Patel 2004; Cock 2007), and genetic alteration (e.g., in ring chromosome 20) (Steinlein *et al.* 1995; Inoue *et al.* 1997).

Uncommon underlying causes of status epilepticus

Immunologically mediated causes of status epilepticus

These are a particularly interesting group of conditions, in which SE is often a prominent clinical feature (Table 107.1). Pathological findings vary depending on the specific condition, but all share an immunological inflammatory response as the basic pathological finding. These conditions are increasingly recognized in recent years and no doubt account for a significant number of those cases of SE that previously were categorized as "of unknown cause." As more circulating antibodies are identified, it is likely that a greater number of causal conditions will be described.

The encephalitis associated with high concentrations of anti-thyroid antibodies (Hashimoto disease) was the first recognized of these conditions (Brain *et al.* 1966), and SE is a common feature (Brain *et al.* 1966; Tsai *et al.* 2007). Anti-NMDA-receptor encephalitis seems particularly common in cases of SE presenting de novo in young females (91%; median age 23 years) and may be associated with an underlying ovarian tumor (53%) (Dalmau *et al.* 2008). Paraneoplastic conditions such as paraneoplastic limbic encephalitis may present with focal motor or non-convulsive SE, and on rare occasions, may have multiple semiologies (Koide *et al.* 2007; Nahab *et al.* 2008).

Mitochondrial diseases causing status epilepticus

This is another important category which has attracted significant interest in the recent literature. Any mitochondrial

Table 107.1 Immunological disorders causing status epilepticus

Paraneoplastic encephalitis
Hashimoto encephalopathy
Anti-NMDA-receptor encephalitis
Anti-VGKC-receptor encephalitis
Rasmussen encephalitis
Cerebral lupus
Adult-onset Still disease
Anti-GAD antibody associated encephalitis
Goodpasture syndrome
Thrombotic thrombocytopenic purpura
Antibody-negative limbic encephalitis

Notes: GAD, glutamic acid decarboxylase; NMDA, *N*-methyl-D-aspartate; VGKC, voltage-gated potassium channel.

Table 107.2 Mitochondrial diseases causing status epilepticus

Alpers disease
Occipital lobe epilepsy/mitochondrial spinocerebellar ataxia and epilepsy (MSCAE)
Mitochondrial encephalopathy, lactic acidosis, and stroke-like episodes (MELAS)
Leigh syndrome
Myoclonic encephalopathy with ragged red fibers (MERRF)
Neuropathy, ataxia, and retinitis pigmentosa (NARP)

disease affecting cerebral functioning can cause SE, and the SE is often a predominant feature of these conditions (Table 107.2). It can take the form of convulsive or non-convulsive SE or typically also epilepsia partialis continua (EPC). Defects in the mitochondrial genome or in nuclear DNA regulating mitochondrial function can occur (the latter for instance in the *POLG1* mutations). Alpers disease has recently been found to be due to *POLG1* mutation (Naviaux and Nguyen 2004), and intractable SE is a characteristic feature of this condition (Narkewicz *et al.* 1991; Nguyen *et al.* 2005). There is no known curative treatment for the mitochondrial defects, and the control of SE relies on anti-epileptic drugs. Valproate however can seriously worsen the condition, due to its metabolism via mitochondrial pathways, and should be avoided (Krähenbühl *et al.* 2000; Tzoulis *et al.* 2006).

Uncommon infectious disorders causing status epilepticus

Status epilepticus is a common feature of a number of rare or geographically restricted infectious disorders causing encephalitis (Table 107.3). An example is cat-scratch disease, caused by a pleomorphic Gram-negative bacillus *Bartonella henselae*, in which generalized tonic–clonic SE is a predominant neurological feature (Armengol and Hendley 1999). Between 4% and 11% of HIV seropositive patients have new-onset seizures, and of these 8.1% to 18% develop SE (Wong *et al.* 1990; Van Paesschen *et al.* 1995; Lee *et al.* 2005; Sinha *et al.* 2005). The seizures and SE may be due to an opportunistic infection, HIV encephalitis, associated central nervous system lymphoma or other complications, metabolic disturbance, or drug treatment. Non-convulsive SE

Table 107.3 Uncommon infectious disease causing status epilepticus

Atypical bacterial infections	Viral infections	Prion disease	Other infections
Bartonella/cat-scratch disease	HIV and HIV-related infections	Creutzfeldt–Jakob disease	Paracoccidioidomycosis
Coxiella burnetti (Q fever)	West Nile encephalitis		Paragonimiasis
Neurosyphilis	JC virus (progressive multifocal leukoencephalopathy)		Mucormycosis
Scrub typhus	Parvovirus B19		
Shigellosis	Varicella encephalitis		
Mycoplasma pneumonia	Subacute sclerosing panencephalitis		
Chlamydophila psittaci	Measles encephalitis		
	Rubella encephalitis, Rous sarcoma virus (RSV) associated SE		
	Polioencephalomyelitis		
	St. Louis encephalitis		

Table 107.4 Status epilepticus due to genetic diseases

Chromosomal aberrations	Inborn errors of metabolism	Malformations of cortical development	Neurocutaneous syndromes	Others
Ring chromosome 20	Porphyria	Focal cortical dysplasias	Sturge–Weber syndrome	Rett syndrome
Angelman syndrome	Menkes disease	Hemimegalencephaly	Tuberous sclerosis	Dravet syndrome and *SCN1A* gene mutation spectrum
Wolf–Hirschhorn syndrome	Wilson disease Adrenoleukodystrophy	Polymicrogyria		Migrating partial seizures in infancy
Fragile X syndrome	Alexander disease	Heterotopias		Pyridoxine dependency
X-linked mental retandation syndrome	Cobalamin C/D deficiency	Schizencephaly		Familial hemiplegic migraine
Ring chromosome 17	Ornithine transcarbamylase (OTC) deficiency			Lafora disease
	Hyperprolinemia			Dentato-rubro-pallido-luysian atrophy
	Maple–syrup urine disease			Infantile-onset spinocerebellar ataxia
	3-Methylcrotonyl CoA carboxylase deficiency			Wrinkly-skin syndrome
	Lysinuric protein intolerance			Neurocutaneous melanomatosis
	Hydroxyglutaric aciduria			Neuroserpin mutation
	Metachromatic leukodystrophy			Wolfram syndrome
	Kuf disease			Autosomal recessive hyperekplexia
	Late infantile ceroid lipofuscinosis			Cockayne syndrome
	Beta-ureidopropionase deficiency			Cerebral autosomal dominant arteriopathy with subcortical infarcts and leukoencephalopathy (CADASIL)
	3-Hydroxyaxyl CoA dehydrogenase deficiency			Jeavon syndrome
	Carnitine palmitoyltransferase deficiency			Robinow syndrome
	Succinic semialdehyde dehydrogenase deficiency			*LYK5* mutation
				MECP2 mutation
				Malignant hyperpyrexia

Table 107.5 Some drugs/toxins that cause or precipitate status epilepticus

Antiepileptic drugs	Antimicrobials and antiviral drugs	Antidepressants	Antipsychotics	Contrast media	Toxins	Chemotherapeutic drugs	Others
Carbamazepine	Cephalosporins[a]	Amitriptyline	Olanzapine	Fluorescein	Aluminium-containing biomaterial	Cisplatin	4-Aminopyridine
Gapapentin	Quinolones	Amoxapine	Sertindole	Iohexol	Camphor	Cyclosporin A	Allopurinol
Lamotrigine	Isoniazid[a]	Bupropion[a]		Iopamidol	Carbon monoxide	Ifosfamide[a]	Baclofen
Levetiracetam	Antivirals	Citalopram		Diatriazoate	Colloidal silver	Methotrexate	Calcium carbonate
Pregabalin	Antihelminthics	Clomipramine			Cocaine	Tacrolimus	Clonidine
Tiagabine[a]	Antimalarials	Fluoxetine			Domoic acid[a]	Etoposide	Corticosteroids
Topiramate		Fluvoxamine			Ecstasy		Dramamine
Valproic acid					Endosulfan		Flumazenil
Vigabatrin					Lead		Gelatine
					Lysergic acid amide		Fligrastim/ molgramostim
					Maneb		Interferon
					Neem oil		Lithium[a]
					Nitromethane		Mexiletine
					Petrol sniffing		Morphine
					Star fruit[a]		N-Acetylcysteine
					Tetramine[a]		Propofol
							Sulfasalazine
							Theophylline[a]
							Thyroxine

Note: [a]Most frequently reported causes of SE.

and epilepsia partialis continua have been reported (Wong *et al.* 1992), particularly in association with concurrent progressive multifocal leukoencephalopathy (Ferrari *et al.* 1998). *Creutzfeldt–Jakob disease* is another infectious condition in which SE may be the presenting feature (Rees *et al.* 1999). The treatment and prognosis of SE associated with infectious diseases depends on the underlying cause.

Status epilepticus in genetic disorders

Status epilepticus may be a common feature in a number of rare genetic disorders (Table 107.4). Ring chromosome 20 typically presents with non-convulsive SE and has a characteristic electroencephalogram (EEG) pattern (Inoue *et al.* 1997). Long bursts or trains of rhythmic theta waves, with a sharply contoured or notched appearance, and generalized spike waves of probable frontotemporal origin (Canevini *et al.* 1998), as well as ictal EEG of prolonged high-voltage slow waves with occasional spikes, either unilateral or bilateral, frontal or frontopolar mostly with preponderance to generalize, with changing frequencies every few seconds, and sharp waves of 5–6 Hz, diffuse and irregular, located centroparietally, have been reported (Kobayashi *et al.* 1998). Most cases are treatment refractory. Other inherited disorders in which SE is common include *Angelman syndrome* and *Rett syndrome* (Sugimoto *et al.* 1992; Ohtsuka *et al.* 2005). Status epilepticus is also common in the neurocutaneous disorders and in other congenital cortical dysgeneses (Lago *et al.* 1994; Fauser *et al.* 2006). Amongst causes of adult cases of SE, *porphyria* should not be overlooked, as the treatment of SE by phenytoin or barbiturate can worsen the condition (Bhatia *et al.* 2008).

Drugs or toxins as a cause of status epilepticus

Status epilepticus is a characteristic feature of many toxin or drug-induced encephalopathies (Table 107.5). Amongst the drugs implicated are a number of antiepileptics. The most important is tiagabine (TGB), which not infrequently results in non-convulsive SE (Schapel and Chadwick 1996; Koepp *et al.* 2005). Other GABAergic drugs such as vigabatrin are also causes of non-convulsive SE (Rogers *et al.* 1993). The drugs most commonly implicated in the production of SE are the antibiotics, notably the cephalosporins and isoniazid (Martinez-Rodriguez *et al.* 2001; Caksen *et al.* 2003). Drug-induced SE usually resolves rapidly with conventional therapy and the removal of the causative agent.

Amongst the toxins, domoic acid produces severe generalized tonic–clonic SE which is often fatal and results from the stimulation of glutaminergic receptors by the toxin (Teitelbaum *et al.* 1990). Severe SE is also a characteristic feature of poisoning with star fruit (*Averrhoa carambola*), especially among cases of renal insufficiency (Neto *et al.* 2003; Chang and Yeh 2004).

Table 107.6 Other causes of status epilepticus

Iatrogenic	Other medical conditions
Electroconvulsive therapy	Multiple sclerosis
Temporal lobectomy and other neurosurgery	Hypertension-induced posterior reversible encephalopathy syndrome
Insertion of intracranial electrode	Panayiotopoulos syndrome
Ventriculoperitoneal shunt	Thyroid disease
Blood transfusion	Pyridoxine-dependent seizure
Carotid angioplasty and stenting	Neuroleptic malignant syndrome
	Ulcerative colitis
	Behçet syndrome
	Celiac disease
	Cobalamin deficiency
	Folinic acid responsive seizures
	Renal artery stenosis
	Pituitary apoplexy
	Renal artery dissection
	Hypomelanosis of Ito
	Cerebral palsy
	Hemophagocytic lymphohistiocytosis
	Anhidrotic ectodermal dysplasia
	Methemoglobinemia

Other rare causes of status epilepticus

Other rarer causes of SE reported in the literature include the conditions shown in Table 107.6. In most of these conditions, SE is an uncommon but serious complication.

Investigation

The choice of investigation depends on the underlying cause. A total of 181 different etiologies causing SE were identified in the literature search, and of these most can be diagnosed by magnetic resonance imaging (MRI), or by serological (infectious or inflammatory causes), biochemical (metabolic and toxic causes), genetic, biopsy, or other clinical investigations. The EEG findings may be helpful in diagnosing the underlying cause, in particular with *POLG1* mutations and Creutzfeldt–Jakob disease although generally the findings on EEG are nonspecific. In any person presenting with SE of uncertain cause, the net should be set widely and intensive investigation may be necessary. The range depends on the age of the patient, the clinical context, and on other factors such as geographic location, comorbidities, and past medical and drug histories.

Treatment

Treatment of the SE itself is often with conventional antiepileptic drug (AED) therapy. It is important to avoid valproate in mitochondrial disease and enzyme-inducing AEDs in porphyria. However, the success of the treatment strategy is largely dependent on knowing the underlying etiology, because in many of these conditions, it is not AED therapy that leads to abolition of the SE, but rather treatment of the underlying cause. In infectious disorders, the priority should be to control the infection and this will often in itself terminate the SE.

Similarly, in drug-induced or toxin-induced SE, the removal of the causative agent will control the SE. In immunological disorders, the SE often responds to high-dose steroids or the use of intravenous immunoglobulin or plasma exchange – and these should be considered as blind trials of therapy in any case of intractable SE of unknown cause.

Acknowledgment

This article and the tables are derived from the article by Tan, Neligan and Shorvon 2010.

References

Armengol CE, Hendley JO (1999) Cat-scratch disease encephalopathy: a cause of status epilepticus in school-aged children. *J Pediatr* **13**:635–8.

Bhatia R, Vibha D, Srivastava MV, *et al.* (2008) Use of propofol anesthesia and adjunctive treatment with levetiracetam and gabapentin in managing status epilepticus in a patient of acute intermittent porphyria, *Epilepsia* **49**:934–6.

Brain L, Jellinek EH, Ball K (1966) Hashimoto's disease and encephalopathy. *Lancet*, **2**:512–14.

Caksen H, Odabas D, Erol M, *et al.* (2003) Do not overlook acute isoniazid poisoning in children with status epilepticus. *J Child Neurol* **18**:142–3.

Canevini MP, Sgro V, Zuffardi O, *et al.* (1998) Chromosome 20 ring: a chromosomal disorder associated with a particular electroclinical pattern. *Epilepsia* **39**:942–51.

Chang CH, Yeh JH (2004) Non-convulsive status epilepticus and consciousness disturbance after star fruit (*Averrhoa carambola*) ingestion in a dialysis patient. *Nephrology* **9**:362–5.

Cock H (2007) The role of mitochondria in status epilepticus. *Epilepsia* **48**(Suppl 8):24–7.

Dalmau J, Gleichman AJ, Hughes EG, *et al.* (2008) Anti-NMDA-receptor encephalitis: case series and analysis of the effects of antibodies. *Lancet Neurol* **7**:1091–8.

Fauser S, Huppertz HJ, Bast T, *et al.* (2006) Clinical characteristics in focal cortical dysplasia: a retrospective evaluation in a series of 120 patients. *Brain* **129**:1907–16.

Ferrari S, Monaco S, Morbin M, *et al.* (1998) HIV-associated PML presenting as epilepsia partialis continua. *J Neurol Sci* **161**:180–4.

Inoue Y, Fujiwara T, Matsuda K, *et al.* (1997) Ring chromosome 20 and nonconvulsive status epilepticus: a new epileptic syndrome. *Brain* **120**:939–53.

Kobayashi K, Inagaki M, Sasaki M, *et al.* (1998) Characteristic EEG findings in ring 20 syndrome as a diagnostic clue. *Electroencephalogr Clin Neurophysiol* **107**:258–62.

Koepp MJ, Edwards M, Collins J, Farrel F, Smith S (2005) Status epilepticus and tiagabine therapy revisited. *Epilepsia* **46**:1625–32.

Koide R, Shimizu T, Koike K, Dalmau J (2007) EFA6A-like antibodies in paraneoplastic encephalitis associated with immature ovarian teratoma: a case report. *J Neurooncol* **81**:71–4.

Krahenbuhl S, Brandner S, Kleinle, S, Liechti S, Straumann D (2000) Mitochondrial diseases represent a risk factor for valproate-induced fulminant liver failure. *Liver* **20**:346–8.

Lago P, Boniver C, Casara GL, *et al.* (1994) Neonatal tuberous sclerosis presenting with intractable seizures. *Brain Dev* **16**:257–9.

Lee KC, Garcia PA, Alldredge BK (2005) Clinical features of status epilepticus in patients with HIV infection. *Neurology* **65**:314–16.

Martínez-Rodríguez JE, Barriga FJ, Santamaria J, *et al.* (2001). Nonconvulsive status epilepticus associated with cephalosporins in patients with renal failure. *Am J Med* **111**:115–19.

Nahab F, Heller A, Laroche SM (2008) Focal cortical resection for complex partial status epilepticus due to a paraneoplastic encephalitis. *Neurologist* **14**:56–9.

Narkewicz MR, Sokol RJ, Beckwith B, Sondheimer J, Silverman A (1991) Liver involvement in Alpers disease. *J Pediatr* **119**:260–7.

Naviaux RK, Nguyen KV (2004) *POLG* mutations associated with Alpers syndrome and mitochondrial DNA depletion. *Ann Neurol* **55**:706–12.

Neligan A, Shorvon SD (2010) The frequency and prognosis of convulsive status epilepticus of different causes: a systematic review. *Arch Neurol* **67**:931–40.

Neto MM, da Costa JA, Garcia-Cairasco N, *et al.* (2003) Intoxication by star fruit (*Averrhoa carambola*) in 32 uraemic patients: treatment and outcome. *Nephrol Dial Transplant* **18**:120–5.

Nguyen KV, Østergaard E, Ravn SH, *et al.* (2005) *POLG* mutations in Alpers syndrome. *Neurology* **65**:1493–5.

Ohtsuka Y, Kobayashi K, Yoshinaga H, *et al.* (2005). Relationship between severity of epilepsy and developmental outcome in Angelman syndrome *Brain Dev* **27**:95–100.

Patel M (2004) Mitochondrial dysfunction and oxidative stress: cause and consequence of epileptic seizures. *Free Radic Biol Med* **37**:1951–62.

Rees JH, Smith SJ, Kullmann DM, Hirsch NP, Howard RS (1999) Creutzfeldt–Jakob disease presenting as complex partial status epilepticus: a report of two cases. *J Neurol Neurosurg Psychiatry* **66**:406–7.

Rogers D, Bird J, Eames P (1993) Complex partial status after starting vigabatrin. *Seizure* **2**:155–6.

Schapel G, Chadwick D (1996) Tiagabine and non-convulsive status epilepticus. *Seizure* **5**:153–6.

Sinha S, Satishchandra P, Nalin A, *et al.* (2005) New-onset seizures among HIV-infected drug naive patients from south India. *Neurology Asia* **10**:29–33.

Steinlein OK, Mulley JC, Propping P, *et al.* (1995) A missense mutation in the neuronal nicotinic acetylcholine receptor alpha 4 subunit is associated with autosomal dominant nocturnal frontal lobe epilepsy. *Nat Genet* **11**:201–3.

Sugimoto T, Yasuhara A, Ohta T, *et al.* (1992) Angelman syndrome in three siblings: characteristic epileptic seizures and EEG abnormalities. *Epilepsia* **33**:1078–82.

Tan R, Neligan A, Shorvon SD (2010) Uncommon causes of status epilepticus: a systematic review. *Epilepsy Res* **91**:11–22.

Teitelbaum JS, Zatorre RJ, Carpenter S, *et al.* (1990) Neurologic sequelae of domoic acid intoxication due to the ingestion of contaminated mussels. *N Engl J Med* **322**:1781–7.

Tsai MH, Lee LH, Chen SD, *et al.* (2007) Complex partial status epilepticus as a manifestation of Hashimoto's encephalopathy *Seizure* **8**:713–16.

Tzoulis C, Engelsen BA, Telstad W, *et al.* (2006) The spectrum of clinical disease caused by the A467T and W748S *POLG* mutations: a study of 26 cases. *Brain* **129**:1685–92.

Van Paesschen W, Bodian C, Maker H (1995) Metabolic abnormalities and new-onset seizures in human immunodeficiency virus-seropositive patients. *Epilepsia* **36**:146–50.

Vezzani A, Granata T (2005) Brain inflammation in epilepsy: experimental and clinical evidence. *Epilepsia* **46**:1724–43.

Wasterlain CG, Chen JW (2008) Mechanistic and pharmacologic aspects of status epilepticus and its treatment with new antiepileptic drugs. *Epilepsia* **49**(Suppl 9):63–73.

Wong MC, Suite ND, Labar DR (1990). Seizures in human immunodeficiency virus infection. *Arch Neurol* **47**:640–2.

Wong MC, Suite ND, Labar DR (1992). Nonconvulsive generalized status epilepticus and AIDS. *Ann Intern Med* **116**:171–2.

Chapter

108

Causes of non-convulsive status epilepticus in adults

Pierre Thomas

Introduction

Non-convulsive status epilepticus (NCSE) is characterized by episodes of altered consciousness of variable length and intensity that are directely related to continuous or recurrent epileptic activity (Meierkord and Holtkamp 2007). Emergency electroencephalograph (EEG) recording will solve the problem of what is a sometimes difficult diagnosis. It also distinguishes between two main electroclinical varieties of NCSE, absence status (AS) and complex partial status epilepticus (CPSE).

Absence status consists of a confusional state of variable intensity, ranging from simple cognitive slowing to catatonic stupor, lasting for hours to days (Andermann and Robb 1972). The EEG shows bursts of rhythmic bilateral synchronous and symmetric paroxysmal activity, which may be continuous or recurrent. Absence status is a very heterogeneous condition that may occur in a number of clinical settings (Thomas and Carter-Snead 2007). Some AS occurs as part of a pre-existing idiopathic generalized epilepsy (IGE), most often with absence seizures ("typical AS"). Others occur as a complication of a chronic epileptogenic encephalopathy ("atypical" AS), such as the Lennox–Gastaut syndrome. A third group concerns elderly patients without pre-existing epilepsy in the context of toxic, metabolic, or drug-related factors ("de novo" AS of late onset). Finally, AS "with focal characteristics" may be considered a transitional form between CPSE, especially of frontal origin: it often involves patients with symptomatic or cryptogenic partial epilepsy, and the EEG shows bilateral synchronous abnormalities with a marked interhemispheric asymmetry in amplitude, raising the possibility of secondary bisynchrony from a focal onset.

Complex partial status epilepticus consist, of "a prolonged epileptic episode in which fluctuating or frequently recurring focal electrographic epileptic discharges, arising in temporal or extratemporal regions, result in a confusional state with variable clinical symptoms" (Shorvon 1994). Apart from confusion, miscellaneous clinical signs correlate to the diversity of the epileptogenic networks involved. Although rare, one of the most characteristic presentations is mesial temporal CPSE that is characterized by a cycle of repeated complex partial seizures

with altered awareness and stereotyped automatisms, interrupted by a more subtle disorder of awareness and reactive automatisms (Treiman and Delgado-Escueta 1983). More frequently, there is a continuous confusional state without any marked cycling which has been attributed to disorganization of extratemporal function, especially of the frontal lobe (Thomas *et al.* 1999).

Causes of absence status epilepticus
Non-specific precipitating factors

Non-specific precipitating factors for AS in IGE patients are similar to those found in other seizure types: withdrawal or impaired compliance of appropriate antiepileptic drugs (AEDs), alcohol, stress, grief, fatigue, sleep deprivation, disturbances of the sleep–wake cycle (see review in Thomas and Carter-Snead 2007). At the EEG laboratory, hyperventilation and intermittent photic stimulation can occasionally trigger AS in unstable IGE patients. Endocrine factors appear important in women of childbearing age. The catamenial period, pregnancy, the immediate postpartum period, and menopause have all been implicated (Ming and Kaplan 1998).

Other non-specific triggering factors have also been reported occasionally, but the mechanism by which they lead to AS is speculative. Cases have been reported following surgery, mild or severe head trauma, fever, paraneoplastic syndrome, and neurosyphilis (Primavera *et al.* 1994).

Antiepileptic drugs

Aggravation of IGE syndromes by inappropriate AEDs is increasingly recognized as a serious and common problem. Therapeutic concentrations of carbamazepine and/or phenytoin may exacerbate AS in IGE (Snead and Hosey 1985). In a retrospective video-EEG documented series of 14 misdiagnosed IGE patients treated by either carbamazepine alone or associated with other potentially aggravating AEDs (phenytoin, vigabatrin, gabapentin), AS was documented in 10 cases, and was atypical in half of them

The Causes of Epilepsy, eds. S. D. Shorvon, F. Andermann, and R. Guerrini. Published by Cambridge University Press. © Cambridge University Press 2011.

(Thomas *et al.* 2006a). All patients had experienced seizure aggravation or new seizure types before AS developed. Withdrawal of the aggravating agents and adjustment of medication resulted in full seizure control. Patients with absence seizures appear to have a heightened risk for this paradoxical response, underscoring the value of an adequate syndromic approach (Osorio *et al.* 2000). Replacement of valproate with lamotrigine precipitated AS in a single patient (Trinka *et al.* 2002). Levetiracetam has also been implicated in two patients with symptomatic partial epilepsy (Atefy and Tettenborn 2005).

Tiagabine deserves special mention. True syndromic aggravation related to tiagabine use in recommended doses has been associated with typical AS in IGE (Knake *et al.* 1999) and in AS with focal features as well as in CPSE in lesional focal epilepsy (Koepp *et al.* 2005; Vinton *et al.* 2005). However, in some cases, EEG data were not really convincing of the ictal nature of the disorder, and this issue remains controversial (Shinnar *et al.* 2001), because a benzodiazepine-responsive toxic encephalopathy may also be considered (de Borchgrave *et al.* 2003). It is also possible that AS can be triggered by other GABAergic agonists such as baclofen (Zak *et al.* 1994) and vigabatrin (Perucca *et al.* 1998).

Drug-related factors

Drug-related factors are clearly a major precipitant, especially in de novo AS of late onset (Fig. 108.1). Many authors (Thomas *et al.* 1992; Primavera *et al.* 1994; Kaplan 1996) suggest an etiologic role for psychotropic medication either taken in excess, alone, or in association with other drugs, or during rapid drug withdrawal (Fernandez-Torre 2001). A large number of psychotropic drugs have been implicated, in order of frequency and probable causality: benzodiazepines (especially during withdrawal), neuroleptics (especially butyrophenones), tricyclic antidepressants (especially amitriptyline), lithium, meprobamate, viloxazine, methaqualone, barbiturates, and monoamine oxidase inhibitors.

Many cases have also been reported to occur in relation to other drugs. Only some of these are known to lower the convulsive threshold: theophylline, ifosfamide, baclofen, metformin, cimetidine, cefepime, and ceftazidine (see review in Thomas and Carter-Snead 2007).

Metabolic and toxic factors

Metabolic disturbances, either isolated or associated with drugs, are frequently reported to be associated with AS, realizing an unhappy conjunction of synergistc epileptogenic factors: hyponatremia, hypocalcemia, hypoglycemia, decompensated chronic renal or hepatic failure, hyperthyroidism, psychogenic polydipsia with metabolic imbalance, electroconvulsive therapy, and cobalamin deficiency (see review in Thomas and Carter-Snead 2007).

Metrizamide and other contrast-enhancing products deserve special mention. A number of AS case reports have been documented following the use of these agents during myelography (Pritchard and O'Neal 1984; Vollmer *et al.* 1985), carotid angiography, or intrathecal fluorescein injection (Coeytaux *et al.* 1999).

Absence status and epileptic syndromes

Absence status has been described in various subgroups of the syndrome of IGE, especially in patients with the "eyelid myoclonia with absences syndrome" (Yang *et al.* 2008), and in another syndrome of "idiopathic generalized epilepsy with phantom absences" of undetermined onset (Panayiotopoulos *et al.* 2001). It is is supposed to occur in a high proportion of patients with the "perioral myoclonias with absences syndrome" (Agathonikou *et al.* 1998). A recently identified "absence status epilepsy" (Genton *et al.* 2008) may be a rare and distinctive IGE syndrome in which the main seizure type is recurrent, unprovoked AS. The onset is during adolescence or adulthood and the evolution is favorable with adequate treatment.

Absence status has also been associated with a peculiar chromosomal abnormality: Inoue *et al.* (1997) reported six cases of mosaic ring chromosome 20 (RC20) and epilepsy with prolonged confusional states resistant to AEDs associated with bilateral high-voltage ictal slow waves occasionally beginning with focal frontal EEG activity. Patients present with a marked pharmacoresistance, but have no distinctive feature on neurological examination, except mild retardation for some of them (Fig. 108.2). Positron emission tomography studies in RC20 syndrome suggest that dysfunction of dopaminergic neurotransmission in putamen and caudate regions could result in the inability of striatal structures to interrupt the epileptic discharges (Biraben *et al.* 2004).

Structural abnormalities

No focal lesions have been documented in AS on imaging studies. However, in elderly patients with de novo AS of late-onset type, frontal mild to moderate cortical–subcortical atrophy of vascular and/or degenerative origin is often present, and it has been suggested that the various causal toxic and/or metabolic factors may express themselves more easily in brains structurally damaged by such non-specific lesions (Thomas and Andermann 1994). An isolated case report of atypical AS has been reported in the context of a syndrome of increased intracranial pressure and transient magnetic resonance imaging (MRI) abnormalities (Callahan and Noetzel 1992). Another patient with new-onset AS (Thomas and Andermann 1994) had unilateral frontal hyperperfusion on ictal single photon emission computed tomography (SPECT); these images were similar to those found in patients with focal NCSE (Kutluay *et al.* 2005).

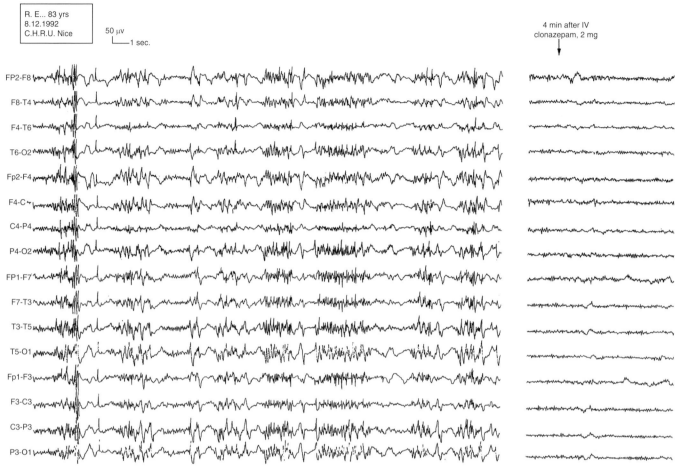

Fig. 108.1. A positive diagnostic and therapeutic trial of intravenous benzodiazepines in an 82-year-old woman with de novo absence status of late onset, related to multiple psychotropic drugs intake (tricyclic antidepressants) and withdrawal (benzodiazepines). The EEG shows continuous irregular polyspike and slow wave activity which stops 140 s after injection of 1 mg of clonazepam, while her level of consciousness returned to normal.

Causes of complex partial status epilepticus

In contrast to AS, structural abnormalities, most often documented on MRI or computed tomography (CT) scans, are usually present in the etiological investigations of CPSE, especially if this type of NCSE is the first manifestation of epilepsy.

Complex partial status epilepticus occurring in the context of pre-existing partial epilepsy

The majority of published CPSE cases with a pre-existing partial temporal or extratemporal epilepsy are more often remote symptomatic than cryptogenic (Tomson *et al.* 1992; Kaplan 1996; Scholtes *et al.* 1996). Non-specific risk factors for CPSE in patients with established epilepsy include stopping or changing AEDs, alcohol use, sleep deprivation, fever, the catamenial period, anesthesia, and surgery (Cockerell *et al.* 1994). Episodes of CPSE are rare in patients with mesial temporal lobe epilepsy, perhaps because chronic AED treatment, despite its limitations to control all seizures in this syndrome, prevents the evolution into status epilepticus.

Complex partial status epilepticus occurring as the presenting symptom of epilepsy

Complex partial status epilepticus more often appears at the onset of epilepsy in adults than in children (Shalev and Amir 1983). In a review of 70 reported cases of CPSE of frontal origin in 25 studies, no history of epilepsy was found in more than one-third of cases. A focal frontal lesion was present in 35% of cases (Fig. 108.3). Benign or malignant brain tumors and post-traumatic or postneurosurgical antecedents were the most frequent etiologies (Thomas and Zifkin 2008).

In contrast to AS, toxic and metabolic precipitating factors are relatively uncommon. Acute or chronic causes of situation-related CPSE include crack cocaine use, electroconvulsive therapy, intravenous contrast media, drugs such as cyclosporin, ciprofloxacin, lithium, or theophylline, a paradoxic response to diazepam and midazolam, and vigabatrin (see review in Thomas *et al.* 2006b). Among unusual causes, Fujiwara *et al.* (1991) reported a patient with recurrent CPSE clearly correlated with alcohol use, and Thomas *et al.* (1991) reported CPSE during pregnancy which could only be controlled after the induction of labor and delivery.

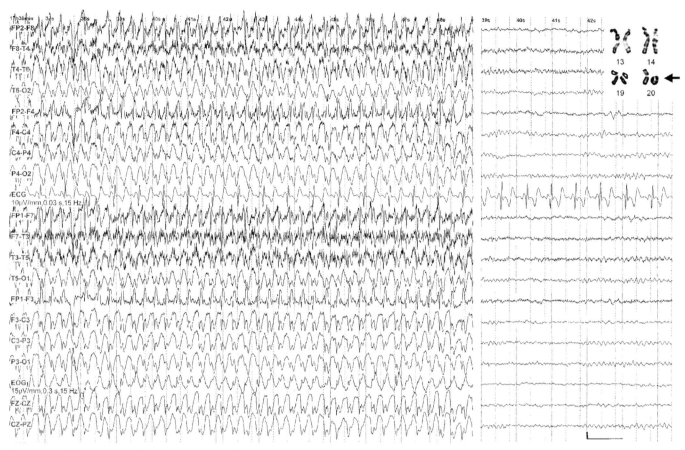

Fig. 108.2. Absence status epilepticus in a 19-year-old girl with the ring chromosome 20 syndrome (see part of the karyotype in the upper right part of the figure). This patient had several daily episodes of obtundation with staring, motor impersistency, and monosyllabic answers, which spontaneously resolved. The EEG shows the progressive build-up of rhythmic 3-Hz generalized spikes and waves (left part) that spontaneously resolve after 15 to 30 min (right part).

Complex partial status epilepticus may complicate a number of neurological conditions, including the late-onset form of mitochondrial encephalopathy, lactic acidosis, and stroke-like episodes (MELAS) (Leff *et al.* 1998), meningeal carcinomatosis (Dexter *et al.* 1990), epidural metastases (Steg *et al.* 1993), neurosyphilis (Marano *et al.* 2004), and Alzheimer disease (Armon *et al.* 2000). Mesial temporal CPSE is often the presenting symptom of newly recognized non-paraneoplastic forms of adult-onset limbic encephalitis, either related to auto-antibodies against voltage-dependent potassium channels (Bien and Elger 2007) or to autoantibodies against *N*-methyl-D-aspartate (NMDA) receptors (Dalmau *et al.* 2008). Hippo-campal swelling with an increased T2-weighted fluid attenu-ated inversion recovery (FLAIR) MRI signal are early findings, and hippocampal atrophy can subsequently develop.

The outcome of complex partial status epilepticus: the causal factors complicate assessment

Despite the fact that most documented reports of CPSE have a favorable outcome with or without prompt medical treatment (Kaplan 2002), there is no consensus regarding the risk of morbidity of CPSE (Krumholz 1999). Unfavorable outcomes in patients without underlying comorbid factors have been only very occasionally documented. Patients with cryptogenic mesial temporal CPSE of very long duration reported by Treiman *et al.* (1981) and Engel *et al.* (1978) had severe and prolonged amnesia, which was permanent in one case. Con-versely, patients with an acute brain lesion causing CPSE have a much more unfavorable prognosis. Krumholz *et al.* (1995) reported a series of 10 consecutive patients with three deaths, four patients with permanent memory disturbance (two of which were severe), and three with memory and cognitive disturbances lasting longer than 3 months. However, most of these patients had lesions that could in themselves produce permanent sequelae, such as viral encephalitis or acute stroke. Furthermore, when the episode of NCSE is related to an acute central nervous system insult, the clinical findings related to the lesions can mask those that are related to the status, making the initial EEG and clinical evaluation difficult (Hilkens and De Weed 1995; Kaplan 1996). Similarly, it can be particularly difficult to separate what is really related to NCSE from the effects of the underlying lesion, in terms of elec-troclinical presentation and of prognosis, in patients with pre-existing degenerative or vascular dementia (Bottaro *et al.* 2007), or in critically ill comatose elderly patients (Litt *et al.* 1998).

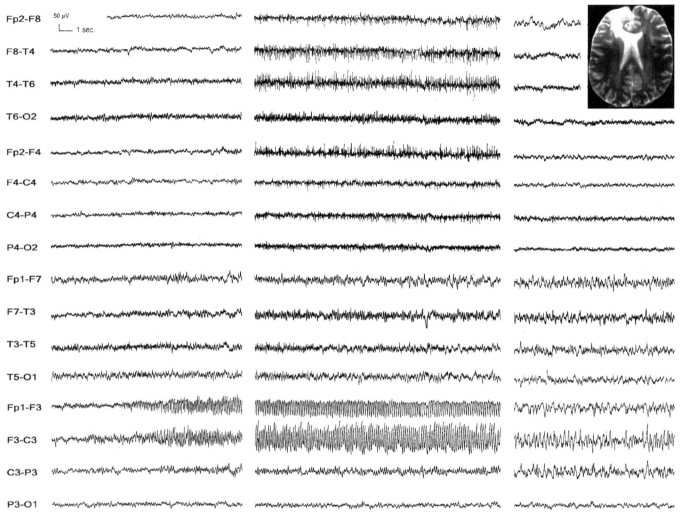

Fig. 108.3. Frontal non-convulsive status epilepticus developed in recurrent seizures in a 36-year-old patient with a remote symptomatic etiology. Onset of seizure is marked by the build up of a 12-Hz sustained rhythmic left frontal spike activity. At the end of the seizure, there is ipsilateral, unihemispheric spread of the discharge. The patient showed a continuous state of affective disinhibition with temporospatial disorientation. The MRI scan (right upper part of the figure) showed left frontal brain abscess sequelae. A 20-s delay separates each epoch.

Another problem is that CPSE occurring with an acute brain lesion may cause long-term worsening of the associated neurologic dysfunction (Hilkens and de Weerd 1995). Significant increase in neurospecific enolase, a marker of neuronal damage, has been reported in a series of eight consecutive adult patients with CPSE (De Giorgo *et al.* 1996), but this can also be the result of seizure activity itself.

If CPSE is considered to carry a risk of cerebral damage, vigorous treatment is needed, and this may be the case especially when CPSE complicates an acute brain lesion, because seizures and lesion may act synergistically to worsen brain damage. In a retrospective assessment of acute morbidity and mortality in NCSE (Shnecker and Fountain 2003), mortality rates were much higher in patients with an acute medical etiology (27%) compared to the epilepsy (3%) and the cryptogenic (18%) groups. However, usually CPSE has no propensity to cause damage, and early and aggressive treatment with intravenous anticonvulsants carries its own risks of morbidity which must be balanced, especially in ambulatory patients, with the relatively benign outcome.

References

Agathonikou A, Panayiotopoulos CP, Giannakodimos S, Koutroumanidis M (1998) Typical absence status in adults: diagnostic and syndromic considerations. *Epilepsia* **39**:1265–76.

Andermann F, Robb JP (1972) Absence status: a reappraisal following review of thirty-eight patients. *Epilepsia* **13**:177–87.

Armon C, Peterson GW, Liwnicz BH (2000) Alzheimer's disease underlies some cases of complex partial status epilepticus. *J Clin Neurophysiol* **17**:511–18.

Atefy R, Tettenborn B (2005) Nonconvulsive status epilepticus on treatment with levetiracetam. *Epilepsy Behav* **6**:613–16.

Bien CG, Elger CE (2007) Limbic encephalitis: a cause of temporal lobe epilepsy with onset in adult life. *Epilepsy Behav* 10:529–38.

Biraben A, Semah F, Ribeiro MJ, *et al.* (2004) PET evidence for a role of the basal ganglia in patients with ring chromosome 20 and epilepsy. *Neurology* 63:73–7.

de Borchgrave V, Lienard F, Willemart T, van Rijckevorsel K (2003) Clinical and EEG findings in six patients with altered mental status receiving tiagabine therapy. *Epilepsy Behav* 4:326–37.

Bottaro FJ, Martinez OA, Pardal MM, Bruetman JE, Reisin RC (2007) Nonconvulsive status epilepticus in the elderly: a case-control study. *Epilepsia* 48:966–72.

Callahan DJ, Noetzel MJ (1992) Prolonged absence status epilepticus associated with carbamazepine therapy, increased intracranial pressure, and transient MRI abnormalities. *Neurology* 42:2198–201.

Cockerell OC, Walker MC, Sander JW, Shorvon SD (1994) Complex partial status epilepticus: a recurrent problem. *J Neurol Neurosurg Psychiatry* 57:835–7.

Coeytaux A, Reverdin A, Jallon P, Nahory A (1999) Non-convulsive status epilepticus following intrathecal fluorescein injection. *Acta Neurol Scand* 100:278–80.

Dalmau J, Gleichman AJ, Hughes EG, *et al.* (2008) Anti-NMDA-receptor encephalitis: case series and analysis of the effects of antibodies. *Lancet Neurol* 7:1091–8.

De Giorgio CM, Gott PS, Rabinowicz AL, *et al.* (1996) Neuron-specific enolase, a marker of acute neuronal injury, is increased in complex partial status epilepticus. *Epilepsia* 37:606–9.

Dexter DD Jr., Westmoreland BF, Cascino TL (1990) Complex partial status epilepticus in a patient with leptomeningeal carcinomatosis. *Neurology* 40:858–9.

Engel J, Ludwig B, Fetell M (1978) Prolonged partial complex status epilepticus: EEG and behavioral observations. *Neurology* 28:863–9.

Fernandez-Torre JL (2001) De novo absence status of late onset following withdrawal of lorazepam: a case report. *Seizure* 10:433–7.

Fujiwara T, Watanabe M, Matsuda K, *et al.* (1991) Complex partial status epilepticus provoked by the ingestion of alcohol: a case report. *Epilepsia* 32:650–6.

Genton P, Ferlazzo E, Thomas P (2008) Absence status epilepsy: delineation of an adult idiopathic generalized epilepsy syndrome. *Epilepsia* 49:642–9.

Hilkens PHE, De Weerd AW (1995) Non-convulsive status epilepticus as cause for focal neurological deficit. *Acta Neurol Scand* 92:193–7.

Inoue Y, Fujiwara T, Matsuda K, *et al.* (1997) Ring chromosome 20 and nonconvulsive status epilepticus: a new epileptic syndrome. *Brain* 120:939–53.

Kaplan PW (1996) Nonconvulsive status epilepticus in the emergency room. *Epilepsia* 37:643–50.

Kaplan PW (2002) Prognosis in nonconvulsive status epilepticus. *Epileptic Disord* 2:185–93.

Knake S, Hamer HM, Schomburg U, Oertel WH, Rosenow F (1999) Tiagabine-induced absence status in idiopathic generalized epilepsy. *Seizure* 8:314–17.

Koepp MJ, Edwards M, Collins J, Farrel F, Smith S (2005) Status epilepticus and tiagabine therapy revisited. *Epilepsia* 46:1625–32.

Krumholz A (1999) Epidemiology and evidence for morbidity of nonconvulsive status epilepticus. *J Clin Neurophysiol* 16:314–22.

Krumholz A, Sung GY, Fisher RS, *et al.* (1995) Complex partial status epilepticus accompanied by serious morbidity and mortality. *Neurology* 45:1449–504.

Kutluay E, Beattie J, Passaro EA, *et al.* (2005) Diagnostic and localizing value of ictal SPECT in patients with nonconvulsive status epilepticus. *Epilepsy Behav* 6:212–17.

Leff AP, McNabb AW, Hanna MG, Clarke CR, Larner AJ (1998) Complex partial status epilepticus in late-onset MELAS. *Epilepsia* 39:438–41.

Litt B, Wityk RJ, Hertz SH, *et al.* (1998) Nonconvulsive status epilepticus in the critically ill elderly. *Epilepsia* 39:1194–202.

Marano E, Briganti F, Tortora F, *et al.* (2004) Neurosyphilis with complex partial status epilepticus and mesiotemporal MRI abnormalities mimicking herpes simplex encephalitis. *J Neurol Neurosurg Psychiatry* 75:833.

Meierkord H, Holtkamp M (2007) Non-convulsive status epilepticus in adults: clinical forms and treatment. *Lancet Neurol* 6:329–39.

Ming X, Kaplan PW (1998) Fixation-off and eyes closed catamenial generalized nonconvulsive status epilepticus with eyelid myoclonic jerks. *Epilepsia* 39:664–8.

Osorio I, Reed RC, Peltzer JN (2000) Refractory idiopathic absence status epilepticus: a probable paradoxical effect of phenytoin and carbamazepine. *Epilepsia* 41:887–94.

Panayiotopoulos CP, Ferrie CD, Koutroumanidis M, Rowlinson S, Sanders S (2001) Idiopathic generalized epilepsy with phantom absences and absence status in a child. *Epileptic Disord* 3:63–6.

Perucca E, Gram L, Avanzini G, Dulac O (1998) Antiepileptic drugs as a cause of worsening seizures. *Epilepsia* 39:5–17.

Primavera A, Giberti L, Scotto P, Cocito L (1994) Nonconvulsive status epilepticus as a cause of confusion in later life: a report of 5 cases. *Neuropsychobiology* 302:148–52.

Pritchard PB, O'Neal DB (1984) Non-convulsive status epilepticus following metrizamide myelography. *Ann Neurol* 16:252–4.

Scholtes FB, Renier WO, Meinardi HM (1996) Non-convulsive status epilepticus: causes, treatment, outcome in 65 patients. *J Neurol Neurosurg Psychiatry* 61:93–5.

Shalev RS, Amir N (1983) Complex partial status epilepticus. *Arch Neurol* 40:90–2.

Shinnar S, Berg AT, Treiman DM, *et al.* (2001) Status epilepticus and tiagabine therapy: review of safety data and epidemiologic comparisons. *Epilepsia* 42:372–9.

Shneker BF, Fountain NB (2003) Assessment of acute morbidity and mortality in nonconvulsive status epilepticus. *Neurology* 61:1066–73.

Shorvon S (1994) *Status Epilepticus: Its Clinical Features and Treatment in Children and Adults.* Cambridge, UK: Cambridge University Press.

Snead OC, Hosey LC (1985) Exacerbation of seizures in children by carbamazepine. *N Engl J Med* 313:916–21.

Steg RE, Frank AR, Lefkowitz DM (1993) Complex partial status epilepticus in a patient with dural metastases. *Neurology* 43:2389 92.

Thomas P, Andermann F (1994) Absence status in elderly patients is most often situation-related. In: Malafosse A, Genton P, Hirsch E, *et al.* (eds.) *Idiopathic Generalized Epilepsies: Clinical, Experimental and Genetic Aspects.* London: John Libbey, pp. 95–109.

Thomas P, Carter Snead O III (2007) Absence status epilepticus. In: Engel J, Pedley T (eds.) *Epilepsy: A Comprehensive Textbook* 2nd edn. Philadelphia PA: Lippincott William and Wilkins, pp. 693–703.

Thomas P, Zifkin B (2008) Frontal lobe non convulsive status epilepticus In: Kaplan PWA, Drislane F (eds.) *Non Convulsive Status Epilepticus*. New York: Demos Biomedical, pp. 91–101.

Thomas P, Barrès P, Chatel M (1991) Complex partial status epilepticus of extra-temporal origin: report of a case. *Neurology* **41**:1147–9.

Thomas P, Beaumanoir A, Genton P, Dolisi C, Chatel M (1992) De novo absence status: report of 11 cases. *Neurology* **42**:104–10.

Thomas P, Zifkin B, Migneco O, *et al.* (1999) Nonconvulsive status epilepticus of frontal origin. *Neurology* **52**:1174–83.

Thomas P, Valton L, Genton P (2006a) Absence and myoclonic status epilepticus precipitated by antiepileptic drugs in idiopathic generalized epilepsy. *Brain* **129**:1281–92.

Thomas P, Zifkin B, Andermann F (2006b) Complex partial status epilepticus. In: Wasterlain CG, Treiman DM (eds.) *Status Epilepticus: Mechanisms and Management*. Cambridge, MA: MIT Press, pp. 69–90.

Tomson T, Lindbom U, Nilsson BY (1992) Non-convulsive status epilepticus in adults: thirty-two consecutive patients from a general hospital population. *Epilepsia* **33**:829–35.

Treiman DM, Delgado-Escueta AV (1983) Complex partial status epilepticus. In: Delgado-Escueta AV, Wasterlain CG, Treiman DM, Porter RJ (eds.) *Status Epilepticus*. New York: Raven Press, pp. 69–81.

Treiman DM, Delgado-Escueta AV, Clark MA (1981) Impairement of memory following complex partial status epilepticus. *Neurology* **31**(Suppl 4):S109.

Trinka E, Dilitz E, Unterberger I, *et al.* (2002) Non-convulsive status epilepticus after replacement of valproate with lamotrigine. *J Neurol* **249**:1417–22.

Vinton A, Kornberg AJ, Cowley M, *et al.* (2005) Tiagabine-induced generalized non-convulsive status epilepticus in patients with lesional focal epilepsy. *J Clin Neurosci* **12**:128–33.

Vollmer ME, Weiss H, Beanland C, Krumholz A (1985) Prolonged confusion due to absence status following metrizamide myelography. *Arch Neurol* **42**:1005–7.

Yang T, Liu Y, Liu L, *et al.* (2008) Absence status epilepticus in monozygotic twins with Jeavons syndrome. *Epileptic Disord* **10**:227–30.

Zak R, Solomon G, Petito F, Labar D (1994) Baclofen-induced generalized nonconvulsive status epilepticus. *Ann Neurol* **36**:113–14.

Causes of epilepsia partialis continua

Hirokazu Oguni and Frederick Andermann

Definition and prevalence

Epilepsia partialis continua (EPC) is a special type of focal status epilepticus, first described by Kojewnikov in 1894. He considered it a "peculiar form of cortical epilepsy" comprising localized continuous jerks intermingled from time to time with spreading Jacksonian seizures (Kozhevnikov 1991). Kojewnikov's syndrome was later found to occur in patients with Russian spring–summer tick-borne encephalitis in which EPC develops mostly within 2–3 weeks after the end of the acute period of illness (Zemskaya et al. 1991). However, EPC has now been recognized as a complication of various neurological disorders whose onset age ranges from infancy to adulthood. Although the incidence of EPC remains unknown, Cockerell et al. (1996) estimated a prevalence of less than 1 per 1 000 000 based on EPC cases registered by the British Neurological Surveillance Unit in the United Kingdom. Thus, it is a rare seizure type. Various definitions of EPC have been proposed either on semiological, etiological, or neurophysiological grounds (Juul-Jensen and Denny-Brown 1966; Thomas et al. 1977; Obeso et al. 1985; Engel 2001). In the most recent ILAE-proposed Epilepsy Classification, EPC is classified into focal status epilepticus among continuous seizure types, and defined simply as a combination of focal seizures with continuous twitching in the same area correlated with Rasmussen syndrome, focal cerebral lesions of miscellaneous causes, or inborn errors of metabolism (Engel 2001). The definition of EPC most strongly semiology-based has been that of Obeso et al. (1985), who defined it as spontaneous regular or irregular clonic muscle twitching of cerebral cortical origin, sometimes aggravated by action or sensory stimuli, confined to one part of the body, and continuing for a period of hours, days, or weeks.

Clinical manifestations

Epilepsia partialis continua manifests with rhythmic or partially rhythmic twitching of muscle groups, mostly in distal rather than proximal muscles, preferentially involving the fingers, hands, feet, arms, or legs (Juul-Jensen and Denny-Brown 1966; Thomas et al. 1977; Obeso et al. 1985). It sometimes involves the unilateral periorbital area, cheek, perioral area of the face, or tongue (Thomas et al. 1977; Nayak et al. 2006). It rarely involves the pharyngeal area and abdominal muscles (Tezer et al. 2008). Rasmussen syndrome may manifest with writhing or choreiform movements, and may be misdiagnosed as Sydenham chorea or hemidyskinesia (Frucht 2002; Kankirawatana et al. 2004). These atypical clinical features taking the form of choreoathetosis are considered to arise from simultaneous involvement of the basal ganglia. The frequency of muscle twitching has been reported to be mostly less than 10 jerks/min, followed by 10–20 jerks/min (Cockerell et al. 1996; Pandian et al. 2002). However, these studies did not identify differences in clinical EPC manifestations among patients with different ages and etiologies. The condition has not been defined by the frequency and duration of each muscle twitch, although this may help in its differential diagnosis from other mimicking involuntary movements such as tremor, myoclonus, or choreoathetosis. Spinal segmental myoclonus preferentially manifests with continuous rhythmic jerking of the arm, legs, or trunk innervated by one or two spinal segments, at a frequency ranging from 0.2 to 8 Hz, with a median of 3.5 Hz (range 12 to 480 jerks/min; median 210 jerks/min) (Jankovic and Pardo 1986) Cortical tremor is a special type of rhythmic myoclonus, predominantly involving the distal limbs, mainly fingers, and enhanced by action. It resembles essential or myoclonic tremor, and is considered a unique form of cortical reflex myoclonus because of the presence of giant sensory evoked potential, C-reflex, and a preceding cortical spike based on a jerked-locked averaging (JLA) study (Ikeda et al. 1990). It is mostly a complication of a special type of familial generalized epilepsy (Terada et al. 1997). Thus, it is necessary to differentiate such movement disorders from EPC. In contradistinction to many movement disorders, EPC usually continues during sleep despite being milder in intensity. Other types of epileptic seizure are frequently combined or precede the occurrence of EPC, or are even interspersed during EPC.

The Causes of Epilepsy, eds. S. D. Shorvon, F. Andermann, and R. Guerrini. Published by Cambridge University Press. © Cambridge University Press 2011.

They are focal sensorimotor seizures or secondarily unilateral or generalized tonic–clonic seizures. When they are interspersed, EPC changes in rhythm and intensity, spreads to neighboring muscles, and may initiate simple or complex somatomotor seizures, sometimes with secondary generalization (Juul-Jensen and Denny-Brown 1966; Thomas *et al.* 1977; Obeso *et al.* 1985).

Etiology

The underlying pathology of EPC reported until now is diverse, including metabolic disorders (especially non-ketotic hyperglycemia and mitochondrial encephalomyopathy), cerebrovascular disorders (including stroke, intracranial bleeding, cerebral venous thrombosis, and vasculitis), inflammation (especially Creutzfeldt–Jakob disease, progressive multifocal leukoencephalopathy due to HIV infection, multiple sclerosis, Behçet disease, tuberculous meningitis, tuberculoma, or neurocysticercosis), neoplasms (astrocytoma, hemangioma, lymphoma, and metastasis), and cerebral dysplastic lesions (focal cortical dysplasia and hemimegalencephaly) (Oguni *et al.* 1991; Veggiotti *et al.* 1995; Lee *et al.* 2000; Placidi *et al.* 2001; Pandian *et al.* 2002; Huang *et al.* 2005; Wieser and Chauvel 2005; Aydin-Ozemir *et al.* 2006; Kinirons *et al.* 2006; Sinha and Satishchandra 2007; Bien and Elger 2008; Wolf *et al.* 2008; Yeh and Wu 2008) (Table 109.1). In the three largest EPC series, cerebrovascular disorders, encephalitides or other infectious disorders, neoplasms, and metabolic disorders accounted for 24–28%, 15–19%, 5–16%, and 6–14%, respectively (Fig. 109.1).

In 19–28% of cases, the causes of EPC can not be determined (Thomas *et al.* 1977; Cockerell *et al.* 1996; Sinha and Satishchandra 2007). The etiology of EPC is age-dependent. During childhood, Rasmussen syndrome is the most frequent cause of EPC, followed by cortical malformations, and mitochondrial encephalopathy including Alpers disease (Bien and Elger 2008).

These pathological lesions involve the sensorimotor cortex and the features of EPC are the same regardless of the etiology.

Pathophysiology

The ictal scalp electroencephalogram (EEG) in EPC often does not show any time-locked epileptic abnormality except for uncharacteristic, often polyphasic slow waves either in the contralateral hemisphere or both hemispheres. Because of this, there has been debate about whether EPC is of cortical or subcortical origin (Juul-Jensen and Denny-Brown 1966; Cockerell *et al.* 1996; Wieser and Chauvel 2005). The cortical origin of EPC is primarily supported by the combination of focal or generalized epileptic seizures occurring either in isolation or interspersed with EPC and by the presence of interictal epileptic EEG abnormality. Recently, the cortical origin has been confirmed by computer-based JLA EEG and magnetoencephalography (MEG) studies, demonstrating preceding spike discharges (Kuroiwa *et al.* 1985; Shigeto *et al.* 1997), and by the finding of ictal single photon emission computed tomography (SPECT) or positron emission tomography (PET) studies, showing increased perfusion or glucose uptake in the corresponding cortical area (Cowan *et al.* 1986; Katz *et al.* 1990). The

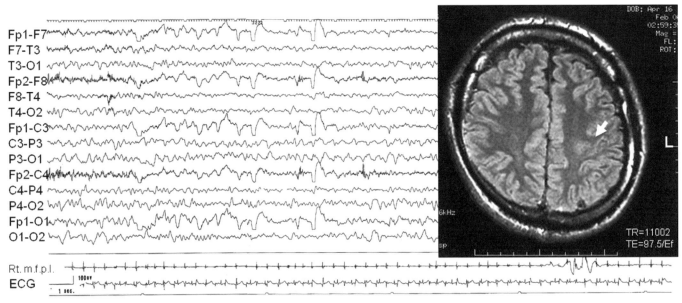

Fig. 109.1. Polygraphic recording of EPC and brain MRI in a 6-year-old boy with a history of perinatal distress. He was born at 33 weeks of gestation, weighing 210 g, and underwent intensive care for 1 month in a neonatal intensive care unit. He started to experience frequent episodes of EPC involving his right hand at a frequency of 2.5 Hz, lasting up to 1 hr. At 6 years of age, polygraphic analysis of EPC showed continuous, irregular partially rhythmic 3–5-Hz slow-wave activity in the left centroparietal area but no epileptic EEG discharges. Fluid-attenuated inversion recovery magnetic resonance imaging (FLAIR-MRI) demonstrated a high-intensity signal lesion immediately beneath the left sensorimotor cortex, suggesting gliosis. His EPC continued with occasional aggravations until he was 17 years of age, without any neurological deterioration. Rt. f. p. l., right flexor pollicis longus.

Table 109.1 Causes of epilepsia partialis continua

Age period	EPC type 1 (static cause)	Diagnostic test[a]	EPC type 2 (progressive cause)	Diagnostic test[a]
Infancy	Hemimegalencephaly		Mitochondrial disease (Alpers disease)	Serum and cerebrospinal fluid lactate, muscle biopsy, mitochondrial DNA (mutation of *POLG1*)
	Focal cortical dysplasia			
	Sturge–Weber syndrome			
Childhood	Focal cortical dysplasia		Rasmussen syndrome	Cerebrospinal fluid oligoclonal banding, immunoglobulin G index
	Tuberous sclerosis	Repeated skin examinations	Mitochondrial encephalomyopathy, lactic acidosis and stroke-like episodes (MELAS)	Serum and cerebrospinal fluid lactate, muscle biopsy, mitochondrial DNA
	Neurocysticercosis	Immunoelectrotransfer blot assay	Delayed type of measles encephalitis (complication of measles in immunocompromised children)	Immunosuppresive treatment, contact with measles
	(Tick-borne) encephalitis	Cerebrospinal fluid study, serologic test for virus		
	Gliomatosis cerebri			
	Other foreign tissue lesions			
	Non-ketotic (ketotic) hyperglycemia	Serum glucose, urinary ketones		
Adults	Cerebrovascular disorders (stroke, intracranial bleeding, cerebral venous thrombosis, vascultis)		Adult-onset Rasmussen syndrome	Cerebrospinal fluid oligoclonal banding, immunoglobulin G index
	Non-ketotic (ketotic) hyperglycemia	Serum glucose	Creutzfeldt–Jakob disease	14–3–3 proteins in cerebrospinal fluid
	Focal cortical dysplasia		Myoclonus epilepsy with ragged-red fibers (MERFF)	Serum and cerebrospinal fluid lactate, muscle biopsy, mitochondrial DNA
	Paraneoplastic limbic encephalopathy	Cerebrospinal fluid study, chest computed tomography, anti-Hu test	Kufs disease	Skin or rectal mucosal biopsy
	Neoplasms			
	Tuberculous meningitis (tuberculoma)	Cerebrospinal fluid study, chest XP, tuberculin skin test		
	(Tick-borne) encephalitis	Cerebrospinal fluid study, serologic test for virus		
	Autoimmune thyroid encephalopathy	Thyroid function tests, anti-thyroglobulin antibody, antimicrosomal antibody		

Table 109.1 (*cont.*)

Age period	EPC type 1 (static cause)	Diagnostic test[a]	EPC type 2 (progressive cause)	Diagnostic test[a]
	Behçet disease	Neuroimaging, recurrent oral and genital ulceration, skin lesions, HLA-B5 positivity		
	Sjögren syndrome	Hypergammaglobulinemia, positive antinuclear antibody, anti-SSA, SSB, rheumatoid factor		
	Multiple sclerosis	Cerebrospinal fluid oligoclonal banding, immunoglobulin G index		
	HIV encephalopathy	Serologic test for HIV		

Note:
[a]Diagnostic test includes neuroimaging study, routine EEG examination with or without long-term EEG monitoring in all cases.
Sources: Juul-Jensen and Denny-Brown (1966); Thomas *et al.* (1977); Oguni *et al.* (1991); Veggiotti *et al.* (1995); Lee *et al.* (2000); Placidi *et al.* (2001); Pandian *et al.* (2002); Huang *et al.* (2005); Wieser and Chauvel (2005); Aydin-Ozemir *et al.* (2006); Kinirons *et al.* (2006); Sinha and Satishchandra (2007); Yeh and Wu (2008); Bien and Elger (2008); Wolf *et al.* (2008).

most reliable evidence for a cortical origin is the disappearance of EPC after surgical resection of the sensorimotor cortex, although this was rarely performed (Cowan *et al.* 1986; Molyneux *et al.* 1998). As EPC and some forms of myoclonus (cortical reflex myoclonus and cortical tremor) share clinical manifestations and polygraphic findings, a similar underlying neurophysiologic mechanism has been postulated (Kuroiwa *et al.* 1985; Cockerell *et al.* 1996). Obeso *et al.* (1985) studied 11 selected patients with cortical myoclonus with or without EPC, and concluded that cortical reflex myoclonus, spontaneous cortical myoclonic jerks, EPC, and Jacksonian motor seizures, with or without secondary generalization, form a continuum of epileptic activity centered on the sensorimotor cortex. Sensorimotor neurons may discharge spontaneously and repetitively, with or without afferent triggers, to produce EPC. If such discharges spread within the sensorimotor cortex, Jacksonian motor seizures occur, with or without secondary generalization.

The scalp EEG often cannot pick up electrical sources generated by the deep layers of the sensorimotor cortex sufficiently distant from electrodes, or the cortical neurons horizontal to the scalp surface forming a horizontal dipole. Thus, a JLA study eliminating the ongoing background EEG noise and isolating the small hidden spike discharges time-locked with the EPC jerks has been employed to identify the origin of EPC or myoclonus (Kuroiwa *et al.* 1985; Ikeda *et al.* 1990; Wieser and Chauvel 2005) However, the absence of JLA spike discharges does not always exclude the cortical origin of jerks because some of them may be too small to pick up using the EEG (Obeso *et al.* 1985). Even if potentials can be measured, the latency between JLA spike discharges and the jerks may not consistently show either a cortical or subcortical origin.

Features of epilepsy in epilepsia partialis continua

Epilepsia partialis continua is most frequently encountered in chronic neurological conditions, for example Rasmussen syndrome, symptomatic focal epilepsy due to focal cortical dysplasia, and mitochondrial encephalopathy (including Alpers disease). The first two are the most common (Andermann 1992).

Rasmussen syndrome

Rasmussen syndrome (RS) is characterized by intractable partial epilepsy often associated with EPC and slowly progressive neurological deficits affecting one side of the body due to chronic localized encephalitis. Although RS is fundamentally a clinicopathological entity requiring pathological confirmation for a definite diagnosis, recent progress in clinical studies of RS allows a presumptive clinical diagnosis to be made based on characteristic clinical features and progressive tissue loss with a relatively high degree of accuracy. Although EPC has been considered to be a hallmark of RS, it occurred in 56% to 100% of the patients in combination with other seizure types at ages between 2 and 16 years (peak at 6 years of age) (Oguni *et al.* 1991; Granata *et al.* 2003) (Fig. 109.2). The initial seizures are either focal motor or secondarily generalized. The time from the onset of epilepsy to the development of EPC ranged from 0 to 10 years (most often within 3 years from the onset of epilepsy) in the Montreal series (Oguni *et al.* 1991). It involves fingers, arms, legs, or the mouth.

Epilepsia partialis continua may initially manifest with choreic or hemidyskinetic movements in association with

A

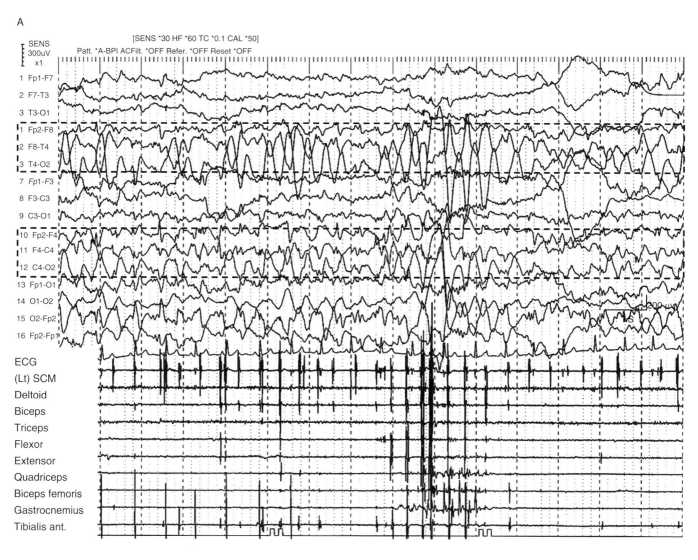

[SENS *30 HF *60 TC *0.1 CAL *50]
Patt. *A-BPI ACFilt. *OFF Refer. *OFF Reset *OFF

SENS
300uV
x1

1 Fp1-F7
2 F7-T3
3 T3-O1
1 Fp2-F8
2 F8-T4
3 T4-O2
7 Fp1-F3
8 F3-C3
9 C3-O1
10 Fp2-F4
11 F4-C4
12 C4-O2
13 Fp1-O1
14 O1-O2
15 O2-Fp2
16 Fp2-Fp1
ECG
(Lt) SCM
Deltoid
Biceps
Triceps
Flexor
Extensor
Quadriceps
Biceps femoris
Gastrocnemius
Tibialis ant.

B

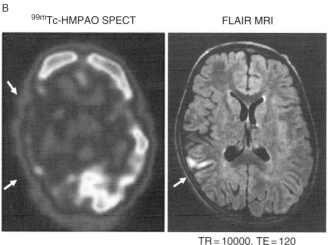

⁹⁹ᵐTc-HMPAO SPECT   FLAIR MRI

TR = 10000, TE = 120

Fig. 109.2. Polygraphic recording of EPC and brain MRI in a 10-year-old girl with Rasmussen syndrome. Polygraphic recording showed myoclonic jerks involving the left sternocleidomastoid (SCM), deltoid, and biceps muscles as well as quadriceps recurring at 2 Hz, corresponding to EPC (A). The EEG demonstrated continuous high-amplitude, irregular, slow activity at 2–3 Hz lateralized throughout the entire right hemisphere without apparent preceding spikes prior to myoclonic EMG jerks. Background EEG activity was faster and lower in amplitude in the left hemisphere. FLAIR-MRI showed right-sided mild, diffuse cortical atrophy with a high-intensity signal in the sensorimotor cortex, and ⁹⁹ᵐTc-hexamethylpropyleneamine oxime (HMPAO) demonstrated low-level cerebral perfusion in the right frontoparietal regions (B).

magnetic resonance imaging (MRI) involvement of contralateral cortical and basal ganglia regions (Frucht 2002; Kankirawatana *et al.* 2004). A diagnosis of RS is suggested when choreic or hemidyskinetic movements are strictly unilateral, and associated with MRI and EEG abnormalities in the contralateral hemisphere. The epileptic seizures progressively increase in frequency along with neurological deterioration up to the point when patients develop ipsilateral hemiparesis, cortical sensory loss, mental impairment, and visual field deficit. The treatment of EPC is extremely difficult except for functional hemispherectomy. Focal resection has not been shown to control EPC (Olivier 1991).

Symptomatic focal epilepsy due to focal cortical dysplasia

Epilepsia partialis continua also occurs in patients with focal cortical dysplasia involving the sensorimotor cortex as well as in hemimegalencephaly. They usually develop EPC in combination with other focal motor seizures, mostly during childhood. The epileptic seizures including EPC are generally resistant to antiepileptic drug (AED) therapy, but neurological deterioration is not evident except for that seizure-generated. Scanning with MRI can detect focal cortical dysplasia in the sensorimotor cortex with or without involvement of the adjacent cortex. Interestingly, those with perisylvian polymicrogyria do not show accompanying EPC despite involvement of the sensorimotor cortex (Guerrini *et al.* 2005).

Symptomatic focal epilepsy due to mitochondrial encephalopathy

Epilepsia partialis continua may be the first symptom of Alpers disease (Alpers–Huttenlocher syndrome), in which the onset of epilepsy usually occurs between the ages of 1 and 3 years, although there have been an increasing number of reports in older children and adults (Gordon 2006). Most cases are caused by recessive mutations in the *POLG1* gene encoding the catalytic subunit of polymerase γ, which is essential for the replication of mitochondrial DNA (mDNA). Epilepsia partialis continua, involving either one or both sides, is associated with focal clonic or partial seizures of predominantly occipital onset. The seizures including EPC are refractory to AEDs. Neurological deterioration and subsequent hepatic failure ensue. An initial EEG characterized by unilateral occipital rhythmic high-amplitude delta with superimposed (poly) spikes (RHADS) has been shown to be an important hallmark of this syndrome (Wolf *et al.* 2008). Diagnosis is based on rapidly progressive encephalopathy with EPC, progressive brain atrophy, the association of hepatic dysfunction, and increased cerebrospinal fluid (CSF) lactate. It is important to make an early diagnosis because of the potentially familial nature of the disorder and the possible worsening of liver dysfunction by valproic acid.

Epilepsia partialis continua can be associated with mitochondrial encephalomyopathy, lactic acidosis and stroke-like episodes (MELAS), Leigh syndrome, and myoclonus epilepsy with ragged-red fibers (MERFF) syndrome, although the incidence appears to be lower than that in Alpers disease (Veggiotti *et al.* 1995). Patients usually develop epilepsy associated with other neurological symptoms including mental deterioration, ataxia, muscle weakness, and stroke-like episodes during childhood. Other rare specific disorders associated with EPC are shown in Table 109.1.

Diagnostic tests for causal conditions

Bancaud classified EPC into two types: type 1 caused by static focal lesions of the sensorimotor cortex, and type 2 caused by progressive cerebral disorders with neurological and intellectual deterioration (Bancaud 1992). The latter largely comprises Rasmussen encephalitis. This classification is clinically useful for approaching the etiology of EPC (Wieser and Chauvel 2005). The causes of types 1 and 2 EPC in relation to onset age and their specific diagnostic tests are shown in Table 109.1. Type 1 EPC is caused by static focal or unilateral cerebral lesions including focal cortical dysplasia, hemimegalencephaly, or neoplasms in children, and cerebrovascular disorders and non-ketotic (ketotic) hyperglycemia in adults. High-resolution MRI study can facilitate a diagnosis of certain cortical lesions, although this may require sophisticated methodology to identify cortical malformations. Barkovich recommends T1-weighted volumetric three-dimensional (3D) fast spoiled gradient echo sequences using a 1.0 or 1.5 mm partition size and T2-weighted 3D fast spin echo volumetric acquisition or 2–3 mm spin-echo or fast spin-echo sequences in two planes. In addition, he also suggests the use of a proton-density-weighted or fluid-attenuated inversion recovery (FLAIR) sequence to identify subtle white matter lesions associated with focal balloon cell dysplasia (Barkovich 2005). The ^{99m}Tc-hexamethylpropyleneamine oxime (HMPAO) or ^{99m}Tc-ethylcysteine dimer single photon emission computed tomography (ECD SPECT) and ^{18}F-fluorodeoxyglucose PET study also help identify the location of the seizure focus, demonstrating a focally increased signal when these scans are performed during EPC and a focally decreased signal during the interictal period, but have little pathological specificity.

In type 2 EPC, the neurological findings and the clinical course are important in diagnosis. The neuroimaging findings may be normal or non-contributory during the early stages. A CSF study including cell count, protein, lactic acid, immunoglobulin G, and oligoclonal bands is recommended to identify acute and chronic encephalitis, as well as mitochondrial disorders. Serum studies including glucose, HIV titer, serum organic acid, and amino acid analyses may be helpful.

On neurophysiological examination, EEG and sensory evoked potentials are mandatory. Magnetoencephalography is sometimes helpful if available. A routine awake and sleep EEG study with intermittent photic stimulation should be performed. In RS, there is usually a lateralized, severe disturbance of background activity contralateral to the side of EPC, while there should be bilateral disturbances in patients who have metabolic disorders. Polygraphic recording of EPC with EEG and surface electromyograph (EMG) is recommended to confirm visually whether epileptic discharges precede each myoclonic EMG potential. In addition, a JLA study may help to distinguish more precisely a cortical from a subcortical origin of EPC (Kuroiwa *et al.* 1985; Obeso *et al.* 1985). Somatosensory evoked potential may show hyperexcitability of the sensorimotor cortex, indicating the presence of cortical reflex myoclonus. When surgery is considered, depth EEG studies may identify the responsible cortical areas. Genetic study does not help in the diagnosis except for mitochondrial encephalomyopathy.

Principles of management

The treatment strategy for EPC depends largely on the underlying disorders, and whether they are treatable or not. Patients with type 1 EPC show mild impairment of functional status with varying responses to treatment, while those with type 2 EPC due to RS or mitochondrial encephalomyopathy show cognitive decline, motor deficits, and pharmacoresistance. The long-term prognosis depends upon the underlying cause rather than on the EPC itself. Symptomatic treatment for EPC (and associated seizures) is with AEDs and, at times, antimyoclonic drugs (Wieser and Chauvel 2005). Although the evidence is based largely on uncontrolled clinical observation, valproate or clonazepam are often used as first-line AEDs for EPC. Piracetam and levetiracetam, often effective for myoclonus, are also widely used. High-dose steroid administration and high-dose γ-globulin treatment may be effective for inflammatory causes. Recently, repetitive transcranial magnetic stimulation has been applied to reduce hyperexcitability due to cortical lesions in EPC (Misawa *et al.* 2005). If these treatments fail, and in the presence of a significant reduction in the quality of life due to the EPC, surgery should be considered. The choice of multiple subpial transections, focal resection, or hemispherectomy depends on the extent of the cortical pathology and on the presence of hemiplegia.

References

Andermann F (1992) Epilepsia partialis continua and other seizures arising from the precentral gyrus: high incidence in patients with Rasmussen syndrome and neuronal migration disorders. *Brain Dev* **14**:338–9.

Aydin-Ozemir Z, Tüzün E, Baykan B, *et al.* (2006) Autoimmune thyroid encephalopathy presenting with epilepsia partialis continua. *Clin Electroencephalogr Neurosci* **37**:204–9.

Bancaud J (1992) Kojewnikov's syndrome (epilepsia partialis continua) in children. In: Roger J, Dravet C, Bureau M, Dreifuss FE, Wolf P (eds.) *Epileptic Syndromes in Infancy, Childhood and Adolescence*, 2nd edn. London: John Libbey Eurotext, pp. 363–79.

Barkovich AJ (2005) Congenital malformation of the brain and skull. In: Barkovich AJ (ed.) *Pediatric Neuroimaging*, 4th edn. Philadelphia, PA: Lippincott Williams and Willkins, pp. 291–439.

Bien CG, Elger CE (2008) Epilepsia partialis continua: semiology and differential diagnoses. *Epilept Disord* **10**:3–7.

Cockerell OC, Rothwell J, Thompson PD, Marsden CD, Shorvon SD (1996) Clinical and physiological features of epilepsia partialis continua: cases ascertained in the UK. *Brain* **119**:393–407.

Cowan JM, Rothwell JC, Wise RJ, Marsden CD (1986) Electrophysiological and positron emission studies in a patient with cortical myoclonus, epilepsia partialis continua and motor epilepsy. *J Neurol Neurosurg Psychiatry* **49**:796–807.

Engel J Jr. (2001) A proposed diagnostic schema for people with epileptic seizures and with epilepsy: report of the ILAE Task Force on Classification and Terminology. *Epilepsia* **42**:796–803.

Frucht S (2002) Dystonia, athetosis, and epilepsia partialis continua in a patient with late-onset Rasmussen's encephalitis. *Mov Disord* **17**:609–12.

Gordon N (2006) Alpers syndrome: progressive neuronal degeneration of children with liver disease. *Dev Med Child Neurol* **48**:1001–3.

Granata T, Gobbi G, Spreafico R, *et al.* (2003) Rasmussen's encephalitis: early characteristics allow diagnosis. *Neurology* **60**:422–5.

Guerrini R, Holthausen H, Parmeggiani L, Parrini E, Chiron C (2005) Epilepsy and malformation of the cerebral cortex. In: Roger J, Bureau M, Dravet C, *et al.* (eds.) *Epileptic Syndromes in Infancy, Childhood, and Adolescence*, 4th edn. Montrouge, France: John Libbey Eurotext, pp. 493–528.

Huang CW, Hsieh YJ, Pai MC, Tsai JJ, Huang CC (2005) Nonketotic hyperglycemia-related epilepsia partialis continua with ictal unilateral parietal hyperperfusion. *Epilepsia* **46**:1843–4.

Ikeda A, Kakigi R, Funai N, *et al.* (1990) Cortical tremor: a variant of cortical reflex myoclonus. *Neurology* **40**:1561–5.

Jankovic J, Pardo R (1986) Segmental myoclonus: clinical and pharmacological study. *Arch Neurol* **43**:1025–31.

Juul-Jensen P, Denny-Brown D (1966) Epilepsia partialis continua. *Arch Neurol* **15**:563–78.

Kankirawatana P, Dure LS IV, Bebin EM (2004) Chorea as manifestation of epilepsia partialis continua in a child. *Pediatr Neurol* **31**:126–9.

Katz A, Bose A, Lind SJ, Spencer SS (1990) SPECT in patients with epilepsia partialis continua. *Neurology* **40**:1848–50.

Kinirons P, O'Dwyer JP, Connolly S, Hutchinson M (2006) Paraneoplastic limbic encephalitis presenting as lingual epilepsia partialis continua. *J Neurol* **253**:256–7.

Kozhevnikov AY (1991) A particular type of cortical epilepsy. (Translated from the Russian by David M. Asher.) In: Andermann F (ed.) *Chronic Encephalitis and Epilepsy: Rasmussen's Syndrome*. Boston, MA: Butterworth-Heinemann, pp. 245–61.

Kuroiwa Y, Tohgi H, Takahashi A, Kanaya H (1985) Epilepsia partialis continua:

active cortical spike discharges and high cerebral blood flow in the motor cortex and enhanced transcortical long loop reflex. *J Neurol* 232:162–6.

Lee K, Haight E, Olejniczak P (2000) Epilepsia partialis continua in Creutzfeldt–Jakob disease. *Acta Neurol Scand* 102:398–402.

Misawa S, Kuwabara S, Shibuya K, Mamada K, Hattori T (2005) Low-frequency transcranial magnetic stimulation for epilepsia partialis continua due to cortical dysplasia. *J Neurol Sci* 234:37–9.

Molyneux PD, Barker RA, Thom M, *et al.* (1998) Successful treatment of intractable epilepsia partialis continua with multiple subpial transections. *J Neurol Neurosurg Psychiatry* 65:137–8.

Nayak D, Abraham M, Kesavadas C, Radhakrishnan K (2006) Lingual epilepsia partialis continua in Rasmussen's encephalitis. *Epilept Disord* 8:114–17.

Obeso JA, Rothwell JC, Marsden CD (1985) The spectrum of cortical myoclonus: from focal reflex jerks to spontaneous motor epilepsy. *Brain* 108:193–224.

Oguni H, Andermann F, Rasmussen T (1991) The natural history of the syndrome of chronic encephalitis and epilepsy: a study of the MNI series of forty-eight cases. In: Andermann F (ed.) *Chronic Encephalitis and Epilepsy: Rasmussen's Syndrome*. Boston, MA: Butterworth-Heinemann, pp. 7–35.

Olivier A (1991) Cortical resection for diagnosis and treatment of seizures due to chronic encephalitis. In: Andermann F (ed.) *Chronic Encephalitis and Epilepsy: Rasmussen's Syndrome*. Boston, MA: Butterworth-Heinemann, pp. 205–11.

Pandian JD, Thomas SV, Santoshkumar B, *et al.* (2002) Epilepsia partialis continua: a clinical and electroencephalography study. *Seizure* 11:437–41.

Placidi F, Floris R, Bozzao A, *et al.* (2001) Ketotic hyperglycemia and epilepsia partialis continua. *Neurology* 57:534–7.

Shigeto H, Tobimatsu S, Morioka T, *et al.* (1997) Jerk-locked back averaging and dipole source localization of magnetoencephalographic transients in a patient with epilepsia partialis continua. *Electroencephalogr Clin Neurophysiol* 103:440–4.

Sinha S, Satishchandra P (2007) Epilepsia partialis continua over last 14 years: experience from a tertiary care center from south India. *Epilepsy Res* 74:55–9.

Terada K, Ikeda A, Mima T, *et al.* (1997) Familial cortical myoclonic tremor as a unique form of cortical reflex myoclonus. *Movement Disord* 2:370–7.

Tezer FI, Celebi O, Ozgen B, Saygi S (2008) A patient with two episodes of epilepsia partialis continua of the abdominal muscles caused by cortical dysplasia. *Epilept Disord* 10:306–11.

Thomas JE, Raegan TJ, Klass DW (1977) Epilepsia partialis continua: a review of 32 cases. *Arch Neurol* 34:266–75.

Veggiotti P, Colamaria V, Dalla Bernardina B, *et al.* (1995) Epilepsia partialis continua in a case of MELAS: clinical and neurophysiological study. *Neurophysiol Clin* 25:158–66.

Wieser HG, Chauvel P (2005) Simple partial status epilepticus and epilepsia continua of Kozhevnikov. In: Engel J Jr., Pedley TA (eds.) *Epilepsy: A Comprehensive Textbook*, 2nd edn. Philadelphia, PA: Lippincott-Raven, pp. 705–24.

Wolf NI, Rahman S, Schmitt B, *et al.* (2009) Status epilepticus in children with Alpers disease caused by POLG1 mutations: EEG and MRI features. *Epilepsia* 50:1596–607.

Yeh SJ, Wu RM (2008) Neurocysticercosis presenting with epilepsia partialis continua: a clinicopathologic report and literature review. *J Formos Med Ass* 107:576–81.

Zemskaya AG, Yatsuk SL, Samoilov VI (1991) Intractable or partial epilepsy of infectious or inflammatory etiology: recent surgical experience in the USSR. In: Andermann F (ed.) *Chronic Encephalitis and Epilepsy: Rasmussen's Syndrome*. Boston, MA: Butterworth-Heinemann, pp. 271–9.

Simon D. Shorvon, Renzo Guerrini, and Frederick Andermann

When the editors set out on the planning of this book, the idea that all the causes of epilepsy could be corralled into a single book seemed outlandish. Kinnier Wilson's memorable statement, that the listing of all causes of epilepsy would be an *act of supererogation*, echoed in our heads. However, as the book proceeded, it became clear that knowledge has now reached a level that a comprehensive text could be produced. This has been largely the result of advances in the past two decades in molecular chemistry and genetics and in magnetic resonance imaging (MRI). It is now feasible to produce a comprehensive listing of all known causes, and this is what is attempted here. We hope the result will stimulate, and be a useful framework, for future studies. Knowledge though is, of course, incomplete, and in this final section, we point very briefly to six topics in which we predict that clinical and research work will advance knowledge and in which our concepts of causation may evolve in the next few years.

Etiology in clinical practice

No one doubts that the underlying etiology is a primary influence on many clinical aspects of epilepsy. However, it is remarkable how little etiology features in the broader management or the drug treatment of epilepsy. This is in spite of the obvious fact that etiology often determines prognosis and the response to therapy, and such knowledge also provides an explanatory model for patients to assist in the greater understanding of their epilepsy (the value of such self-knowledge should not be underestimated). Etiology also should be more fully addressed by regulatory agencies, researchers, and the pharmaceutical industry as a variable in the design of antiepileptic drug trials. A greater emphasis on etiology, and greater efforts to determine etiology, should in the future improve clinical practice.

Etiology or mechanism?

One most interesting aspect of Hughling Jackson's thoughts on etiology was his emphasis on etiology as "mechanism" rather than on etiology as "underlying cause." This position was taken because Jackson believed that, whatever the underlying cause, the final common pathway to the production of an epileptic fit was always similar (in his view, instability of nervous elements due to vascular congestion). Whilst the vascular theories are now no longer held, the concept of common final pathways is attractive and more emphasis could be placed on how epilepsy is caused by such a wide range of underlying causes. It does seem likely that there may well be only a limited number of ways in which a causal condition can result in epilepsy, and the elucidation of these translational mechanisms would be of potential value in the conceptualization and discovery of novel therapy.

Idiopathic epilepsy

Amongst the most exciting developments in recent years in the field of epilepsy is undoubtedly the explosion of knowledge in the field of molecular genetics. This "new genetics" has covered the whole of medicine in a tidal wave of discovery, and no area has been left unaffected. In epilepsy, the most important advances have been made in relation to the symptomatic epilepsies of metabolic or congenital origin (including the cortical dysplasias). Despite intense efforts, the genetic bases of the idiopathic epilepsies remain largely obscure. It seems likely to us that the current emphasis on finding causal single-nucleotide polymorphisms will be replaced by more sophisticated genetic investigation, including exome sequencing in small homogeneous groups of patients and studies for instance of such mechanisms as copy-number variation, genomic imprinting, chromosomal imbalance, X inactivation, trinucleotide repeats, mitochondrial mechanisms, gene–environment interactions, and polygenic mechanisms. Further, the translation of genomic to proteonomic discovery presents a formidable challenge but promises much, perhaps yielding molecular insights into the final common pathways of epileptogenesis referred to above.

Symptomatic epilepsy

Is it too much to claim that the structural deficits causing epilepsy are now all largely defined? The clinical data have

The Causes of Epilepsy, eds. S. D. Shorvon, F. Andermann, and R. Guerrini. Published by Cambridge University Press. © Cambridge University Press 2011.

been provided largely by MRI, and the rate of incrementation of useful new information in this area is now relatively slight. It seems likely that future advances in useful clinical knowledge are probably going to be marginal at best, and the emphasis is moving to molecular histological and neuropathological studies. It is hoped that ultra-high-field MRI will help to deepen knowledge in this area, in vivo and non-invasively, in a much large number of patients than can currently be done with neuropathology. Unraveling the chemistry of the rarer metabolic disorders is one area that continues to grow, and to link this molecular knowledge to structure is one way in which genetic and non-genetic factors can be integrated. Perhaps the greatest advances will be in understanding the processes of neurodevelopment, both genetic and acquired, that result in pathological lesions and epilepsy.

Provoked epilepsy

The environmental causation of epilepsy remains largely *terra incognita*, and yet is most intriguing not least because of the tantalizing possibility of fresh approaches to therapy. As Lennox noted, epilepsy is almost always (perhaps always) multifactorial, and whilst the contribution of seizure precipitants varies, a recent estimate was that in 17% of cases, these were a predominant factor. It is clear that seizure provocation can influence genetic and acquired epilepsies, focal or generalized epilepsies, and does not map easily across conventional seizure-type or syndromic classifications, but how such precipitants produce seizures is largely obscure. This is a topic in which research in the next few years could yield valuable insight.

Classification

Finally to classification. As emphasized in the historical introduction to this book, one of the most remarkable features of the widely used epilepsy classification schemes is that they do not incorporate etiology to any detailed degree. A classification scheme based on etiology would be a very different animal from the current schemes based on semiology or electroencephalography. Both surely have a place, but the absence of any etiological scheme requires urgent remediation. There are significant drawbacks to current schemes for clinical work and for research and conceptualization in epilepsy. For instance, genetic studies have been in our opinion significantly thwarted by reliance on what are artificial classification schemes of seizures and syndromes. In Chapter 2 a draft classification scheme is proposed, with causation divided into three major, and redefined, categories: idiopathic, symptomatic, and provoked epilepsy. This scheme can certainly be improved upon, but we hope that it will provide at least a framework for further work in this area. If a new classification scheme for epilepsy fully acknowledging etiology is one result of this book, then this would be the source of some considerable satisfaction to the editors and authors.

This book breaks new ground by attempting to integrate all (or almost all) the known etiologies of epilepsy into a single text. We have tried to structure this in the form of a draft "blueprint" of epilepsy etiology, reflecting the current state of knowledge in this area. We consider that the focusing of attention on etiology may facilitate the opening of new research avenues and new concepts, and look forward to including these in any future edition of this book. We hope that this is a useful contribution to epilepsy studies, and as is our overriding objective, that the book will assist in improving clinical practice.

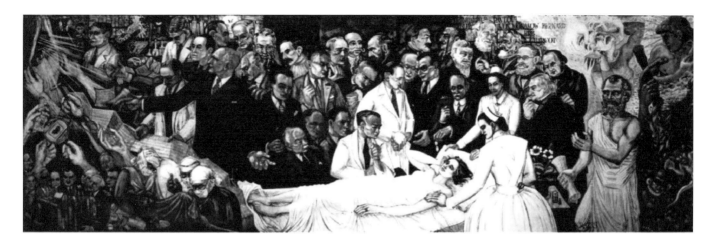

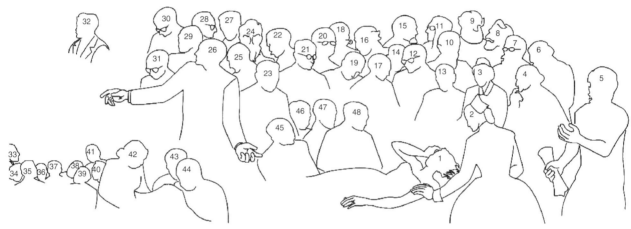

1. Patient (Filer)	13. Dr. William Osler	25. Dr. S. Edward Archibald	37. Maurice Duplessis
2. Mary Filer (artist)	14. Dr. Roma Amyot	26. Dr. Wilder Penfield	38. Camillien Houde
3. Eileen Flanagan	15. Dr. Franz Nissl	27. Dr. Harvey Cushing	39. Dr. Allan Gregg
4. Dr. Jean-Martin Charcot	16. Dr. Ramon y Cajal	28. Dr. Donald Mcrae	40. Paul Martin, Senator
5. Hippocrates	17. Dr. Francis McNaughton	29. Dr. Theodore Rasmussen	41. Dean Charles Martin
6. Dr. Claude Bernard	18. Camillo Golgi	30. K.A.C. Elliott	42. Mlle Phoebe Stanley
7. Dr. Wilhelm Heinrich Erb	19. Dr. Jean Saucier	31. Dr. Herbert Jasper	43. Stanley, préposé patient
8. Dr. Konstantin von Monakov	20. Sir Charles Sherrington	32. Dr. Jerzy Olszewski	44. Dr. Wilder Penfield
9. Dr. Ivan Pavlov	21. Dr. Arthur Elvidge	33. Dr. Cyril James	45. Dr. Colin Russel
10. Dr. Alois Alzheimer	22. Sir Victor Horsely	34. Mme McConnell	46. Dr. Arthur Young
11. Dr. S. Weir Mitchell	23. Dr. William Cone	35. J.W. McConnell	47. Dr. Preston Robb
12. Dr. John Kershman	24. Dr. John Hughlings Jackson	36. W.H. Donner	48. Dr. Donald McEachern

Key: The title of this mural is "The advance in Neurology." It is a mural in the Montreal Neurological Institute, by Mary Filer, painted in 1954. It illustrates the contribution of neurologists and physicians to advancing knowledge in neurology and particularly in epilepsy; and so seemed an appropriate illustration to include on the back cover of this book. (Reproduced with kind permission of the Montreal Neurological Institute.)

Jean Paul Acco; Neuro Media Services, Montreal Neurological Institute

Index

propensity, circadian rhythm
643
sleep deprivation 644
sleep starts 120, 386
small-cell lung cancer (SCLC) 587
smallpox vaccine 390
Sneddon syndrome 567
socioeconomic differences,
convulsive status
epilepticus in childhood
732
sodium balance, disturbances in
655–658
sodium channels see voltage-
gated Na$^+$ channels
somatosensory-evoked seizures
627, 684, 695–698, 709
sparganosis 501–503, 508
spatial-task-induced seizures 684
speech dyspraxia, familial
rolandic epilepsy
with 106
Spielmeyer–Vogt syndrome
(juvenile neuronal ceroid
lipofuscinosis) 158, 209
spinal segmental myoclonus 759
spinocerebellar degenerations 174
Spirometra 501–503, 508
Spratling, W. 6
SPRED1 gene 183
SRPX2 gene 311, 312, 313
star fruit poisoning 749
startle, non-epileptic 386
startle epilepsy 711
auditory-evoked seizures
704–706
with infantile hemiplegia
695–697, 711
startle reaction 695–696
startle seizures 695–697, 698
in epileptic syndromes 697
localization 627, 695, 697
status epilepticus (SE) 723–727
absence 752–753, 754, 755
Angelman syndrome 203,
204, 749
antiepileptic-drug-induced
670, 749
children 724, 725, 730–733
classification 723
complex partial (CPSE) 752,
754–756
convulsive (CSE) 735–743
acute bacterial meningitis
476, 731–732
children 730–732
clinical features 737–738
definition 730, 735
epidemiology 735–737
etiologies 730–732, 735–736
fever 632, 731–732
incidence 730, 735
intracerebral hemorrhage
538, 539
management 740–743

pathophysiology 737
social/geographic factors
738–739
socioeconomic/ethnic
differences 732
definition 723
diagnostic tests 739–740, 749
Dravet syndrome 78, 732
drug-induced 664, 669, 724,
748, 749
electrical, during sleep
see continuous spikes
and waves during sleep
epidemiology 723–724
etiologies 724, 736
adults 735–743
children 730–733
uncommon 745–750
febrile 633, 730–731
genetic disorders 747, 749
genetic factors 738
hypothermia treatment 634, 742
immunologically-mediated
causes 745, 746
as initial manifestation of
epilepsy 738
Lennox–Gastaut syndrome
128, 732
mechanistic causes 725–727
mitochondrial cytopathies
150, 151, 152, 154,
745–746
non-accidental brain injury
427, 430
non-convulsive (NCSE) 723,
752–756
children 732–733
etiologies 733, 752–756
intracerebral hemorrhage 538
raised body temperature 632
outcome/mortality 725, 730,
736–737, 740
Panayiotopoulos syndrome 108
in previously diagnosed
epilepsy 738
refractory 634, 725, 741
toxin-induced 748, 749
treatment 724–725, 750
tuberculosis 514
uncommon infectious causes
746–749
stereotactic radiosurgery
see radiosurgery,
stereotactic
sterilization, enforced 13
steroid hormones, reproductive
636–638, 651
steroid responsive
encephalopathy
associated with
autoimmune thyroiditis
(SREAT) 589–590
steroid therapy
see corticosteroids
stiff person syndrome 587

stimulant drugs 597, 598, 631,
632, 669
Streptococcus pneumoniae
(pneumococcal)
meningitis 475, 482
epilepsy risk 484
treatment 478, 488
vaccine 475, 478, 488
stress 593–595
in adult life (in humans) 594
evaluation 594
link with depression 595
prenatal/early postnatal
(in rats) 593–594
as seizure precipitant
593, 594
treatment 594–595
stroke
antiphospholipid syndrome 567
clinical features 545
definition 544
diagnostic tests 547
epilepsy risk factors 545–547
hemorrhagic 537–540, 565
ischemic 544, 545, 565
management of epilepsy 548
neonatal and perinatal 376
older adults 544, 547
pathophysiology 544, 545
pediatric 544, 545, 548
status epilepticus 736
vascular dementia 619
stroke-like episodes
MELAS 149–150
Sturge–Weber syndrome
189, 192
strongyloidiasis 502
structural causes of epilepsy
767–768
structural–metabolic epilepsies
44–47
Sturge–Weber syndrome (SWS)
189–193, 196
clinical features 189–191,
193, 378
CNS abnormalities 190,
191, 192
epilepsy in 190–191
etiology 191–192
subtypes 189
treatment 192–193
subacute sclerosing
panencephalitis (SSPE)
471, 472
subarachnoid hemorrhage (SAH)
541–542
de novo epilepsy after
treatment 408
fever 632
neonatal seizures 376–377
non-accidental brain injury 426
subclinical electrical activity 39
subcortical band heterotopia
(SBH) (double cortex
syndrome) 298

clinical features 300
genetic basis and diagnosis
298–299
pathogenesis 300, 350, 352
undulating band heterotopia
350
subcortical vascular
encephalopathy
(SVE) 548
subdural empyema 482
children 479, 480
diagnostic tests 487–488
epilepsy after 485–486
management 489
pathology and clinical
features 483
subdural hematoma (SDH)
540, 541
diagnostic tests 540
epilepsy and 540
neonatal seizures 376–377
non-accidental brain injury
426, 429, 430
seizures after surgery for
407–408
subependymal giant cell tumors
(SGCT) 179
subependymal nodules 178, 179
subgaleal abscess 483
substance misuse, psychoactive
596–598, 669–670
substrate reduction therapy (SRT)
Gaucher disease 167
Niemann–Pick disease
type C 208
succinic semialdehyde
dehydrogenase (SSADH)
deficiency 216, 223,
228, 259
sugar disturbances 655–661
suicide, attempted 664
sulfite oxidase deficiency 218,
225, 652
SUMF1 gene 210
supernatural theories 1
supernumerary marker
chromosomes (SMCs) 281
suppurative intracranial
infections, focal
adults 482–490
children 478–480
definition and epidemiology
482
diagnostic tests 487–488
epilepsy after 485–486
management 488–490
surgery
arteriovenous malformations
555
cavernous malformations
562–563
de novo epilepsy after 407
dysembryoplastic
neuroepithelial tumors 444
epilepsy see epilepsy surgery